W9-APR-848

Radiology Review Manual

Radiology Review Manual

Wolfgang Dähnert, M.D.

Assistant Professor
Department of Radiology
Good Samaritan Medical Center
Phoenix, Arizona

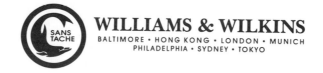

WILLIAMS & WILKINS
BALTIMORE · HONG KONG · LONDON · MUNICH
PHILADELPHIA · SYDNEY · TOKYO

Editor: Timothy H. Grayson
Associate Editor: Carol Eckhart
Copy Editor: Janis Oppelt, Susan Vaupel, Klemie Bryte
Designer: Wilma E. Rosenberger
Production Coordinator: Charles E. Zeller

Copyright © 1991
Williams & Wilkins
428 East Preston Street
Baltimore, Maryland 21202, USA

All rights reserved. This book is protected by copyright. No part of this book may be reproduced in any form or by any means, including photocopying, or utilized by any information storage and retrieval system without written permission from the copyright owner.

Accurate indications, adverse reactions, and dosage schedules for drugs are provided in this book, but it is possible that they may change. The reader is urged to review the package information data of the manufacturers of the medications mentioned.

Printed in the United States of America

Library of Congress Cataloging–in–Publication Data

Dähnert, Wolfgang.
 Radiology review manual / Wolfgang Dähnert.
  p. cm.
 Includes bibliographical references.
 ISBN 0–683–02339–X
 1. Diagnosis, Radioscopic—Outlines, syllabi, etc. 2. Radiology, Medical—Outlines, syllabi, etc. I. Title.
 (DNLM: 1. Radiology—outlines. WN 18 D131r)
RC78. D29 1989
616.07'57—dc20
DNLM / DLC
for Library of Congress

89–25040
CIP

92 93 94
4 5 6 7 8 9 10

Toward the end of an intensive 4-year training program, the resident in radiology is usually well-equipped to prove his/her diagnostic ability. Although most residency programs prepare well for the written and oral examination, the board candidate who rests comfortably on the accumulated knowledge has yet to be born. Faced with the large amount of material to be reviewed in a short period of time, residents often find themselves in a state of mental paralysis, which is soon overcome and replaced by frantic study activity.

In preparation for the exam, of course, hundreds of books can be found in the department's library and many have, hopefully, been read during the residency program. But day and night wouldn't be enough to go through just a fraction of these in the little time that remains. There are those textbooks that are especially popular to review certain topics. Naturally, they are checked out when you need them, and few residents have the resources to purchase them. The multi-volume books covering every aspect of a subspecialty rest in peace. Who has the time now to read them from cover to cover?

It has struck me as peculiar that I was unable to find a comprehensive review textbook to help me prepare for the exam, in contrast to most other subspecialties for which such material is available. Instead, I joined the ranks of previous generations of examinees going through the same routine: the typical study room is crammed with handouts, review articles, various textbooks, ACR syllabi, hand-written notes taken during lectures, etc. All this is seasoned by mountains of photocopies containing hand- or type-written reports from previous exams diligently prepared by returning board candidates, which often enough provide more questions than answers. All these resources are organized into various piles and commonly spread on the floor for lack of desk top space. It is a formidable task indeed trying to look up some minutia, probably unimportant and irrelevant for one's performance, but seemingly so vital at that particular moment. Valuable time is wasted thumbing through piles of paper in an effort to track down trivia. How frustrating an experience to come up empty-handed. More precious time is lost organizing lists of differential diagnosis or etiologies into memorable groups and categories, possibly acronyms or other mnemonics. In short, much of one's effort is directed toward the task of collecting and hunting rather than digesting. Every 3rd or 4th year resident is doing over again those things that generations of board candidates have gone through — but their collections and recollections have never been passed on in a readily available and organized fashion.

Radiology Review Manual was created in preparation for the specialty exam as the "book under the pillow." It served me as a quick review on a large number of topics. In its original concept, generated as computer printouts in file format, it represents a very personal choice and includes topics that were unfamiliar to me or with which I had struggled. However, I learned that my choices were appropriate for many examinees. I have to credit the idea to publish this material to several residents who urged me to do so. Over the years, this material has been continuously changed, upgraded and expanded — even as we speak. Our voluminous field of diagnostic radiology makes it necessary to use a short-hand style for the sake of conserving space and thus provides only an extract of information, a quintessence if you will. This may, at times, jeopardize the full meaning of statements when taken out of context. It should be kept in mind that this book is not intended for the novice and that it requires familiarity with the subject of radiology and the background information of major textbooks. In addition, it provides such a density of information that it is quite unsuitable to be read from cover to cover.

How to use this book:
The organization of this book has caused a major headache as any topic can be looked at from various points of view. I have selected just one of many possibilities to avoid redundancy. The material is presented in a manner that is in keeping with the topics of the current board exam. Unfortunately, this grouping is inconsistent, sectioning off by age (Pediatric Radiology) and image modality (Nuclear Medicine, Ultrasound). In order to avoid repetition, pediatric entities are subsumed within organ systems. Ultrasound and Nuclear Medicine are used from head to heel and consequently are mentioned in all body sections. However, Nuclear Medicine is additionally treated in a separate section when emphasis is on technique and functional aspects not covered elsewhere. A section on ear, nose, and throat topics is placed at the end of the section on CNS disorders. The skull and spine are dealt with as the first part of the CNS section.

The organization within the individual chapters follows the practical approach of reading films. The initial step of film interpretation is the description of radiologic patterns which serves to identify categories in which they belong. Therefore, radiologic patterns for differential diagnoses are found in the first portion of a chapter. Once the diagnostic possibilites have been reviewed in brief outline, one can look up detailed information about a disease entity in the last segment of a chapter. The disease entities are presented in alphabetical order. Both these segments are separated by a few pages of functional, anatomic, or embryologic aspects. Occasionally, important clinical signs and their differential diagnoses are included in the first portion of a chapter.

The backbone of the book is disease entities, radiological symptoms, as well as lists of differential diagnosis. Disease entities are headed by their most commonly used name with other designations listed below. As a radiologic diagnosis should be entertained in context with its probability to be correct, percentages in regard to frequency of signs and symptoms are included liberally, often giving the lowest and the highest number found in the literature. The truth may be somewhere in between for a non-selected patient population. Arbitrary choices have been made in situations when different or contradictory results are found in the literature — unfortunately, an occurrence not at all infrequent.

Lists of differential diagnoses can be presented in many fashions. There is no right or wrong way, but there certainly is a chaotic versus an organized approach. An orderly thought process portrays familiarity with a problem. Examinees have always felt that "nailing" the diagnosis is secondary, but including it in one's consideration is paramount to a successful exam. Accordingly, an attempt is made to categorize differential diagnostic considerations or etiologies of certain diseases in a manner digestible for recapitulation. It is common experience that this is not always possible, satisfactory, or complete.

A table of contents and abbreviations used throughout the book are found in front. A user-friendly index, which selectively refers to those pages with significant information concludes the manual. Notice that most systemic diseases will be mentioned in more than one chapter with some unavoidable redundancy. However, emphasized are those manifestations of the disease that occur within the organ under which it is listed. The index also includes so-called "buzz words" that are miraculously attached to diseases.

Radiology Review Manual is not exclusive to the near-term resident. It has continued to refresh my memory bank for years beyond the specialty exam. In fact, the stimulus to go through with this project has been the challenge found in daily practice as well as my encounters in teaching residents and fellow radiologists. Just as the cases presented in the oral exam apply to the real world of a radiologist, so do the topics in this book. Thus, I can recommend it to any practicing radiologist. I sincerely hope that *Radiology Review Manual* will serve its users in the same manner it has helped me in preparation for the board exam and beyond this scope in daily practice and teaching.

Acknowledgement:
The information contained herein has been gathered over several years and stems from various sources. Data from numerous radiological articles and textbooks are incorporated and anecdotal contributions can no longer be traced. I realize, in retrospect, that this may present a problem when certain statements appear unlikely and their verification has to be left up to the user. For my defense, I can only say that I have tried to extract all data as diligently as possible. I would like to acknowledge the input of numerous teachers, residents, fellows, past and present board candidates at the Johns Hopkins Hospital, Baltimore, and Thomas Jefferson University Hospital, Philadelphia.

The following textbooks have been particularly helpful and deserve mention: Burgener FA, Kormano M: *Differential Diagnosis in Conventional Radiology;* Chapman S, Nakielny R: *Aids to Radiological Differential Diagnosis;* Davidson AJ: *Radiology of the Kidney;* Edeiken J: *Roentgen Diagnosis of Diseases of Bone;* Fraser RG, Pare JAP: *Diagnosis of Diseases of the Chest;* Gedgaudas E, Moller JH, Castaneda-Zuniga WR, Amplatz K: *Cardiovascular Radiology;* Kadir S: *Diagnostic Angiography;* Kirks DR: *Practical Pediatric Imaging;* Reed JC: *Chest Radiology: Plain Film Patterns and Differential Diagnosis;* Reeder MM, Felson B: *Gamuts in Radiology;* Sanders RC, James AE: *Ultrasonography in Obstetrics and Gynecology;* Swischuk LE: *Plain Film Interpretation in Congenital Heart Disease;* Taveras JM, Ferrucci JT: *Radiology – Diagnosis – Imaging – Intervention.*

I am particularly indebted to the following individuals for reviewing the separate sections of this book: Christopher Canino, Thomas Chang, Adam E. Flanders, Keith Haidet, Charles Intenzo, David Karasick, Stephen Karasick, Alfred B. Kurtz, Esmond M. Mapp, Joel Raichlen, Paul Spirn, Robert M. Steiner, and C. Amy Wilson.

Phoenix, September 1990

I would appreciate any comments and suggestions which you feel would improve *Radiology Review Manual.* Your input is of value to me and will be considered in future editions.

Wolfgang Dähnert, M.D.
c/o Williams & Wilkins
428 East Preston Street
Baltimore, MD 21202

CONTENTS

ABBREVIATIONS

√	radiologic sign	BPH	benign prostatic hyperplasia	ECA	external carotid artery
•	clinical sign, symptom	Ca	calcium	ECD	endocardial cushion defect
=	equals, is	CAD	coronary artery disease	ECF	extracellular fluid space
@	at anatomic location of	CAM	cystic adenomatoid	ECG	electrocardiogram
/	or		malformation	ECHO	echocardiogram
+	and, plus, with	CBD	common bile duct	ED	end-diastole
±	with or without	CCA	common carotid artery	EDV	end-diastolic volume
<	less than	CCAM	congenital cystic adenomatoid	EEG	electroencephalogram
>	more than, over		malformation	EF	ejection fraction
		CCK	cholecystokinin	EG	eosinophilic granuloma
ABC	aneurysmal bone cyst	CECT	contrast-enhanced computed	EHDP	ethylene hydroxydiphosphonate
AC	abdominal circumference		tomography	ERC	endoscopic retrograde
ACA	anterior cerebral artery	CHD	congenital heart defect		cholangiography
ACE	angiotensin I-converting	CHF	congestive heart failure	ES	end-systole
	enzyme	CLL	chronic lymphatic leukemia	ESV	end-systolic volume
ACom	anterior communicating artery	CMC	carpometacarpal	F	female
ACTH	adrenocorticotropic hormone	CML	chronic myelogenous leukemia	FDA	Federal Drug Administration
ADH	antidiuretic hormone	CMV	cytomegalovirus	FEV	forced expiratory volume
AICA	anterior inferior cerebellar	CNS	central nervous system	FN	false negative
	artery	CO	carbon monoxide	FNH	follicular nodular hyperplasia
AIDS	acquired immune deficiency	CoA	coarctation of aorta	FP	false positive
	syndrome		computed tomography	FRC	functional residual capacity
AMA	antimitochondrial antibodies	COPD	chronic obstructive pulmonary	FS	fractional shortening
AML	acute myeloblastic leukemia		disease	FSH	follicle stimulating hormone
AML	angiomyolipoma	CPA	cerebellopontine angle	FWHM	full-width at half-maximum
aML	anterior mitral valve leaflet	CPPD	calcium pyrophosphate	GA	gestational age
ANA	antinuclear antibodies		dihydrate	GB	gallbladder
Angio	angiography	CPR	cardiopulmonary resuscitation	GBS	group B streptococcus
Ao	aorta	CRT	cathode ray tube	GE	gastroesophageal
AP	anteroposterior	CSF	cerebrospinal fluid	GFR	glomerular filtration rate
APUD	amine precursor uptake and	CST	contraction stress test	GI	gastrointestinal
	decarboxylation	CT	cardiothoracic ratio	GMRH	germinal matrix related
APVR	anomalous pulmonary venous	CT	computed tomography		hemorrhage
	return	CVA	cerebrovascular accident	GN	glomerulonephritis
ARA-C	arabinoside C	CWP	coal worker's pneumoconiosis	GU	genitourinary
ARDS	acute respiratory distress	Cx	complication	Hb	hemoglobin
	syndrome	CXR	chest X-ray	HC	head circumference
AS	aortic stenosis	DDx	differential diagnosis	hCG	human chorionic gonadotropin
ASA	acetylsalicylic acid	DES	diethylstilbestrol	HIAA	hydroxyindole acetic acid
ASD	atrial septal defect	DIC	disseminated intravascular	HIDA	hepatic 2,6-dimethyl
ASH	asymmetric septal hypertrophy		coagulation		iminodiacetic acid
aTL	anterior tricuspid valve leaflet	DIDA	diethyl iminodiacetic acid	HIP	health insurance plan
ATN	acute tubular necrosis	DIL	drug-induced lupus	Histo	histology
AV	arteriovenous		erythematosus	HIV	human immunodeficiency virus
AV	atrioventricular	DIP	desquamative interstitial	HL	Hodgkin lymphoma
AVM	arteriovenous malformation		pneumonia	HOCM	hypertrophic obstructive
AVN	avascular necrosis	DIP	distal interphalangeal		cardiomyopathy
AVNA	atrioventricular node artery	DISH	diffuse idiopathic skeletal	HPT	hyperparathyroidism
Ba	barium		hyperostosis	HSA	human serum albumin
BCDDP	breast cancer detection	DISIDA	diisopropyl iminodiacetic acid	HSE	herpes simplex encephalitis
	demonstration project	DIT	diiodotyrosine	HTLV	human T-cell lymphotropic
BCG	bacille Calmette-Guérin	DMSA	dimercaptosuccinic acid		virus
BE	barium enema	DORV	double outlet right ventricle	HU	Hounsfield units
BIDA	butyl iminodiacetic acid	DSMA	dimercaptosuccinic acid	HWP	hepatic wedge pressure
BIH	benign intracranial	DTPA	diethylenetriamine penta-	Hx	history
	hypertension		acetic acid	ICA	internal auditory canal
BKG	background	DVT	deep venous thrombosis	ICA	internal carotid artery
BP	blood pressure	Dx	diagnosis	IDA	iminodiacetic acid
BPD	biparietal diameter	EAC	external auditory canal	IDP	imidodiphosphonate

IHSS	idiopathic hypertrophic subaortic stenosis	MHF	malignant fibrous histiocytoma	PEEP	positive end expiratory pressure
IM	intramuscular	MIBG	meta-iodobenzylguanidine	PEP	preejection period
IMA	inferior mesenteric artery	MID	multi-infarct dementia	PET	positron emission tomography
In	indium	MIT	monoiodotyrosine	pHPT	primary hyperparathyroidism
IPF	idiopathic pulmonary fibrosis	ML	middle lobe	PICA	posterior inferior cerebellar artery
IPH	idiopathic pulmonary hemosiderosis	MLCN	multilocular cystic nephroma		
		MMAA	mini-microaggregated albumin colloid	PIE	pulmonary infiltration with eosinophilia
IUD	intrauterine device	MMFR	maximal midexpiratory flow rate		
IUGR	intrauterine growth retardation	MPS	mucopolysaccharidosis	PIE	pulmonary interstitial emphysema
IV	intravenous	MRI	magnetic resonance imaging		
IVC	inferior vena cava	MS-AFP	maternal serum alpha-fetoprotein	PIP	proximal interphalangeal
IVH	intraventricular hemorrhage			PIPIDA	paraisopropyl iminodiacetic acid
IVP	intravenous pyelogram	MTP	metatarsophalangeal		
KCC	Kulchitzky cell carcinoma	MUGA	multiple gated acquisition	PLES	parallel-line-equal spacing
L	left	MV	mitral valve	PM	photomultiplier
L-DOPA	3-(3,4-dihydroxyphenyl)-levo-alanin	Myelo	myelography	PMF	progressive massive fibrosis
		NBS	National Bureau of Standards	PML	progressive multifocal leukoencephalopathy
LA	left atrium	NEC	necrotizing enterocolitis		
LAD	left anterior descending	NECT	non-enhanced computed tomography	pML	posterior mitral valve leaflet
LAO	left anterior oblique			PMN	polymorphonuclear
LAT	lateral	NHL	non-Hodgkin lymphoma	PMT	photomultiplier tube
LATS	long-acting thyroid stimulating	NPH	normal pressure hydrocephalus	PNET	permeative neuroectodermal tumor
LAV	lymphadenopathy-associated virus	NPH	nucleus pulposus herniation		
		NST	non-stress test	PPLO	pleuropneumonia-like organism
LCA	left coronary artery	NTD	neural tube defect	ppm	posterior papillary muscle
LCX	left circumflex coronary artery	NUC	nuclear medicine	PS	pulmonary stenosis
LDH	lactate dehydrogenase	OB-US	obstetrical ultrasound	PSS	progressive systemic sclerosis
LE	lupus erythematosus	OCG	oral cholecystogram	PTC	percutaneous transhepatic cholangiography
LES	lower esophageal sphincter	OCVM	occult vascular malformation		
LGA	large for gestational age	OHP	orthogonal-hole test pattern	PTH	parathyroid hormone
LH	luteinizing hormone	OHSS	ovarian hyperstimulation syndrome	pTL	posterior tricuspid valve leaflet
LIP	lymphocytic interstitial pneumonitis			PTU	propylthiouracil
		OIH	orthoiodohippurate	PVC	polyvinyl chloride
LL	lower lobes	P	phosphorus	PVE	periventricular echogenicity
LLL	left lower lobe	PA	posteroanterior	PVH	pulmonary venous hypertension
LLQ	left lower quadrant	PA	pulmonary artery		
LPA	left pulmonary artery	PAC	premature atrial contractions	PVL	periventricular leukomalacia
LSD	lysergic acid diethylamide	PAH	para-aminohippurate	PVNS	pigmented villonodular synovitis
LUL	left upper lobe	PAP	primary atypical pneumonia		
LUQ	left upper quadrant	PAP	pulmonary alveolar proteinosis	PYP	pyrophosphate
LV	left ventricle	PAPVR	partial anomalous pulmonary venous return	R	right
LVET	left ventricular ejection time			RA	rheumatoid arthritis
LVFT$_2$	left ventricular slow filling time	PAS	periodic acid Schiff	RAO	right anterior oblique
LVOT	left ventricular outflow tract	PAS	pulmonary alveolar proteinosis	RBC	red blood cell
LVT$_1$	left ventricular fast filling time	Path	pathology	RCA	right coronary artery
LVW/HW	lateral ventricular width to hemispheric width	PAVM	pulmonary arteriovenous malformation	RCC	renal cell carcinoma
				RDS	respiratory distress syndrome
M	male	PBF	pulmonary blood flow	RES	reticuloendothelial system
MA	menstrual age	PCA	posterior cerebral artery	RIND	reversible ischemic neurologic deficit
MAA	macroaggregated albumin	PCAVC	persistent complete atrioventricular canal		
MCA	middle cerebral artery			RISA	radioiodine serum albumin
MCDK	multicystic dysplastic kidney	PCKD	polycystic kidney disease	RLL	right lower lobe
MCK	multicystic kidney	PCom	posterior communicating artery	RLQ	right lower quadrant
MCP	metacarpophalangeal	PCWP	pulmonary capillary wedge pressure	RML	right middle lobe
MDP	methylene diphosphonate			ROC	receiver operating characteristics
MEA	multiple endocrine adenomas	PD	posterior descending artery		
MEN	multiple endocrine neoplasms	PDA	patent ductus arteriosus	ROI	region of interest
MFH	malignant fibrous histiocytoma	PE	pulmonary embolism	RPA	right pulmonary artery

RPF	renal plasma flow	SPECT	single photon emission	TSH	thyroid stimulating hormone
RTA	renal tubular acidosis	SV	stroke volume	TV	tidal volume
RUL	right upper lobe	SVC	superior vena cava	TW1I	T1 weighted image
RV	residual volume	T2WI	T2 weighted image	UGI	upper gastrointestinal series
RV	right ventricle	TAPVR	total anomalous pulmonary	UIP	usual interstitial pneumonia
RVOT	right ventricular outflow tract		venous return	UL	upper lobe
Rx	therapy	TB	tuberculosis	UPJ	uteropelvic junction
S/P	status post	TBG	thyroxin binding globulin	US	ultrasound
SAE	subcortical arteriosclerotic	TBPA	thyroxin binding prealbumin	USP	United States Pharmacopeia
	encephalopathy	TCC	transitional cell carcinoma	UTI	urinary tract infection
SAM	systolic anterior motion of	TE	tracheo-esophageal	UVJ	urethrovesical junction
	mitral valve	TGA	transposition of great arteries	V/Q	ventilation perfusion
SANA	sinoatrial node artery	tHPT	tertiary hyperparathyroidism	VC	vital capacity
SGA	small for gestational age	TIA	transitory ischemic attack	VIP	vasoactive intestinal peptides
sHPT	secondary hyperparathyroidism	TLC	total lung capacity	VMA	vanillylmandelic acid
SIJ	sacroiliac joint	TN	true negative	VQ	ventilation perfusion
SLE	systemic lupus erythematosus	TOF	tetralogy of Fallot	VS	interventricular septum
SMA	superior mesenteric artery	TORCH	toxoplasmosis, rubella,	VSD	ventricular septal defect
SMV	superior mesenteric vein		cytomegalovirus, herpes virus	WBC	white blood cells
Sn	stannum	TP	true positive	WDHA	watery diarrhea, hypokalemia,
SONK	spontaneous osteonecrosis of	TR	repetition time		achlorhydria
	knee	TRH	thyrotropin releasing hormone	XGP	xanthogranulomatous
					pyelonephritis

ACRONYMS AND MNEMONICS

DIFFERENTIAL DIAGNOSIS OF MUSCULOSKELETAL DISORDERS

Differential-diagnostic gamut of bone disorders

Conditions to be considered = "dissect bone disease with a DIATTOM"

Dysplasia + **D**ystrophy
Infection
Anomalies of development
Tumor + tumorlike conditions
Trauma
Osteochondritis + ischemic necrosis
Metabolic disease

DYSPLASIA = disturbance of bone growth
DYSTROPHY = disturbance of nutrition

BONE SCLEROSIS

Constitutional sclerosing bone disease

1. Engelmann-Camurati disease
2. Infantile cortical hyperostosis
3. Melorheostosis
4. Osteopathia striata
5. Osteopetrosis
6. Osteopoikilosis
7. Pachydermoperiostosis
8. Pyknodysostosis
9. Van Buchem disease
10. William syndrome

Diffuse osteosclerosis

mnemonic: "FROM"

Fluorosis
Renal osteodystrophy
Osteopetrosis
Myelosclerosis, Metastases (blastic), Mastocytosis

Solitary osteosclerotic lesion

A. Developmental
    1. Bone island
B. Vascular
    1. Old bone infarct
    2. Aseptic / ischemic / avascular necrosis
C. Healing bone lesion
    (a) Trauma: Callus formation
    (b) Benign tumor: fibrous cortical defect / nonossifying fibroma, brown tumor; bone cyst
    (c) Malignant tumor: lytic metastasis after radiation, chemo-, hormone therapy
D. Infection / inflammation (low-grade chronic infection / healing infection)
    1. Osteoid osteoma
    2. Chronic / healed osteomyelitis: bacterial, tuberculous, fungal
    3. Sclerosing osteomyelitis of Garré
    4. Granuloma
    5. Brodie abscess

E. Benign tumor
    1. Osteoma
    2. Ossifying fibroma
    3. Enchondroma / osteochondroma
    4. Osteoblastoma
F. Malignant tumor
    1. Osteoblastic metastasis (prostate, breast)
    2. Lymphoma
    3. Sarcoma: osteo-, chondro-, Ewing sarcoma
G. Others
    1. Sclerotic phase of Paget disease
    2. Fibrous dysplasia

Multiple osteosclerotic lesions

A. FAMILIAL
    1. Osteopoikilosis
    2. Enchondromatosis = Ollier disease
    3. Melorheostosis
    4. Multiple osteomas: associated with Gardner syndrome
    5. Osteopetrosis
    6. Pyknodysostosis
    7. Osteopathia striata
    8. Chondrodystrophia calcificans congenita = congenital stippled epiphyses
    9. Multiple epiphyseal dysplasia = Fairbank disease

B. SYSTEMIC DISEASE
    1. Mastocytosis = urticaria pigmentosa
    2. Tuberous sclerosis

Blastic metastases

mnemonic: "5 Bees Lick Pollen"

Brain (medulloblastoma)
Bronchus
Breast
Bowel (especially carcinoid)
Bladder
Lymphoma
Prostate

Dense metaphyseal bands

mnemonic: "Heavy Cretins Sift Scurrilously through Rickety Systems"

Heavy metal poisoning (lead, bismuth, phosphorus)
Cretinism
Syphilis, congenital
Scurvy
Rickets (healed)
Systemic illness
also: normal variant; methotrexate therapy

mnemonic: "DENSE LINES"
D-vitamin intoxication
Elemental arsenic, bismuth, phosphorus
Normal variant
Systemic illness
Estrogen to mother during pregnancy
Leukemia, **L**ead poisoning
Infection (TORCH), **I**diopathic hypercalcemia
Never forget rickets
Early hypothyroidism
Scurvy, **S**ickle cell disease

Bone-within-bone appearance
= endosteal new bone formation
1. Normal
   (a) thoracic + lumbar vertebrae (in infants)
   (b) growth recovery lines (after infancy)
2. Infantile cortical hyperostosis (Caffey)
3. Sickle cell disease / thalassemia
4. Congenital syphilis
5. Osteopetrosis / oxalosis
6. Radiation
7. Acromegaly
8. Paget disease

OSTEOPENIA
= decrease in bone density
Categories: 1. Osteoporosis = decreased osteoid
                  production
              2. Osteomalacia = undermineralization of
                  osteoid
              3. Hyperparathyroidism
              4. Multiple myeloma / diffuse metastases

Osteoporosis
= reduced bone mass of normal composition secondary
to (a) osteoclastic resorption (85%) (trabecular,
endosteal, intracortical, subperiosteal) (b) osteocytic
resorption (15%)
Incidence: 7% of all women between ages 35 – 40
               years; 1 in 3 women > age 65 years
Etiology:
   A. Congenital disorders
      1. Osteogenesis imperfecta (the only
         osteoporosis with bending)
      2. Homocystinuria
   B. Idiopathic (bone loss begins earlier + proceeds
      more rapidly in women)
      1. Juvenile osteoporosis: < 20 years
      2. Adult osteoporosis: 20 – 40 years
      3. Postmenopausal osteoporosis: > 50 years
      4. Senile osteoporosis: > 60 years
         progressively decreasing bone density at a rate
         of 8% in females; 3% in males
   C. Nutritional disturbances
      Scurvy; protein deficiency (malnutrition, nephrosis,
      chronic liver disease, alcoholism, anorexia
      nervosa, kwashiorkor, starvation), calcium
      deficiency

   D. Endocrinopathy
      Cushing disease, hypogonadism (Turner
      syndrome, eunuchoidism), hyperthyroidism,
      hyperparathyroidism, acromegaly, Addison
      disease, diabetes mellitus, pregnancy
   E. Immobilization = disuse osteoporosis
   F. Collagen disease, rheumatoid arthritis
   G. Bone marrow replacement
      infiltration by lymphoma / leukemia, multiple
      myeloma, diffuse metastases, marrow hyperplasia
      secondary to hemolytic anemia
   H. Drug therapy
      Heparin (15,000 – 30,000 U for > 6 months),
      methotrexate, steroids, vitamin A
   I. Localized osteoporosis
      Sudeck dystrophy, transient osteoporosis of hip,
      regional migratory osteoporosis of lower
      extremities
• serum calcium, phosphorus, alkaline phosphatase
  frequently normal
• hydroxyproline may be elevated during acute stage
Technique:
   (1) Single photon absorptiometry
        measures primarily cortical bone
        Site: distal radius (= wrist bone density), os
                calcis
        Dose: 2 – 3 mrem; Precision: 1 – 3%
   (2) Dual photon absorptiometry
        measures vertebrae + hips; should be reserved
        for patients < 65 years of age because of
        interference from osteophytosis + vascular
        calcifications
        Site: spine, femur
        Dose: 5 – 10 mrem; Precision: 2 – 4%
   (3) Quantitative Computed Tomography
        Site: spine
        (a) single energy: 300 – 500 mrem;
                             6 – 25% precision
        (b) dual energy : 750 – 800 mrem;
                            5 – 10% precision
   (4) Dual energy radiography
        Site: spine, femur
        Dose: < 3 mrem; Precision: 0.3 – 0.4%
   Δ radiographs are insensitive prior to bone loss of 25
     – 30%
   Δ bone scans do NOT show a diffuse increase in
     activity
Location: axial skeleton (lower dorsal + lumbar spine),
            proximal humerus, neck of femur, wrist, ribs
√ decreased number + thickness of trabeculae
√ cortical thinning (endosteal + intracortical resorption)
√ juxtaarticular osteopenia with trabecular bone
  predominance
√ delayed fracture healing with poor callus formation
  (DDx: abundant callus formation in osteogenesis
  imperfecta + Cushing syndrome)
@ Spine
  √ diminished radiographic density

√ vertical striations (= marked thinning of transverse trabeculae with relative accentuation of vertical trabeculae along lines of stress)
√ prominence of endplates
√ "picture framing" (= accentuation of cortical outline with preservation of external dimensions secondary to endosteal + intracortical resorption)
√ compression deformities with protrusion of intervertebral discs
  √ biconcave vertebrae
  √ Schmorl nodes
  √ wedging
  √ decreased height of vertebrae
√ absence of osteophytes
Cx: (1) compression fractures of lower dorsal + lumbar spine
        (2) complete fractures of extremities (ribs, hips, wrists)

Osteomalacia
= accumulation of excessive amounts of uncalcified osteoid with bone softening + insufficient mineralization of osteoid due to
  (a) high remodeling rate: excessive osteoid formation + normal / little mineralization
  (b) low remodeling rate: normal osteoid production + diminished mineralization
Etiology:
  (1) dietary deficiency of vitamin D3 + lack of solar irradiation
  (2) deficiency of metabolism of vitamin D:
       — chronic renal tubular disease
       — chronic administration of phenobarbital (alternate liver pathway)
       — diphenylhydantoin (interferes with vitamin D action on bowel)
  (3) decreased absorption of vitamin D:
       — malabsorption syndromes (most common)
       — partial gastrectomy (self-restriction of fatty foods)
  (4) decreased deposition of calcium in bone
       — diphosphonates (for treatment of Paget disease)
Histo: excess of osteoid seams + decreased appositional rate
• bone pain / tenderness
• muscular weakness
• serum calcium slightly low / normal
• decreased serum phosphorus
• elevated serum alkaline phosphatase
√ uniform osteopenia
√ fuzzy indistinct trabecular detail of endosteal surface
√ thin cortices of long bone
√ coarsened frayed trabeculae decreased in number + size
√ bone deformity from softening: hourglass thorax, bowing of long bones, buckled / compressed pelvis
√ increased incidence of fractures, biconcave vertebral bodies

√ mottled skull
√ pseudofractures = Milkman syndrome = Looser zones = 2 – 3 mm wide radiolucent ribbon-like band of osteoid seams formed within stress-induced infractions (PATHOGNOMONIC) + nonunion (= incomplete healing due to mineral deficiency)
  Location: bilateral + symmetrical; at right angles to bone margin; outer border of scapula, femoral neck, pubic + ischial rami, ribs

Localized osteopenia
  1. Disuse atrophy
      Etiology: local immobilization secondary to
                    (1) fracture (more pronounced distal to fracture site)
                    (2) neural paralysis
                    (3) muscular paralysis
  2. Reflex sympathetic dystrophy = Sudeck dystrophy
  3. Shoulder-hand syndrome
      after acute illness (e.g., myocardial infarction)
      • pain + stiffness in shoulder + hand
      • swelling of upper extremity
  4. Regional migratory osteoporosis, transient osteoporosis of hip
  5. Osteolytic tumor
  6. Lytic phase of Paget disease
  7. Inflammation: rheumatoid arthritis, osteomyelitis, tuberculosis
  8. Early phase of bone infarct and hemorrhage
  9. Burns + frostbite

Transverse lucent metaphyseal lines
  mnemonic: "LINING"
  Leukemia
  Illness, systemic (rickets, scurvy)
  Normal variant
  Infection, transplacental (congenital syphilis)
  Neuroblastoma metastases
  Growth lines

OSTEOLYSIS
  1. Acroosteolysis
  2. Massive osteolysis
  3. Essential osteolysis
  4. Ainhum disease

Idiopathic acroosteolysis
  May be unilateral
  • fingernails remain intact; sensory changes + plantar ulcers rare

Acquired acroosteolysis
  Causes:
  Burns; frostbite; electric shock; PVC; syringomyelia; diabetes; congenital insensitivity to pain; leprosy; Raynaud disease; thrombangiitis obliterans; collagen disease; sarcoidosis; psoriasis; yaws; Ehlers-Danlos syndrome; HPT; Kaposi sarcoma; progeria; pyknodysostosis; pachydermoperiostosis

mnemonic: "RADISH"
  Raynaud disease
  Arteriosclerosis
  Diabetes
  Injury (burns, frostbite)
  Scleroderma, **S**arcoidosis
  Hyperparathyroidism

√ lytic destructive process involving distal + middle phalanges
√ NO periosteal reaction
√ epiphyses resist osteolysis until late

Frayed metaphyses
mnemonic: "CHARMS"
  Congenital infections (Rubella, Syphilis)
  Hypophosphatasia
  Achondroplasia
  Rickets
  Metaphyseal dysostosis
  Scurvy

PERIOSTEAL REACTION
1. Trauma, hemophilia
2. Infection
3. Inflammatory: arthritis
4. Neoplasm
5. Congenital: physiologic in newborn
6. Metabolic: hypertrophic osteoarthropathy, thyroid acropachy, hypervitaminosis A
7. Vascular: venous stasis

Solid periosteal reaction
= reaction to periosteal irritant
√ even + uniform thickness > 1 mm
√ persistent + unchanged for weeks
Patterns:
  (a) thin: eosinophilic granuloma, osteoid osteoma
  (b) dense undulating: vascular disease
  (c) thin undulating: pulmonary osteoarthropathy
  (d) dense elliptical: osteoid osteoma; longstanding malignant disease (with destruction)
  (e) cloaking: storage disease; chronic infection

Interrupted periosteal reaction
= pleomorphic, rapidly progressing process undergoing constant change
  (a) lamellated = "onion skin": acute osteomyelitis; malignant tumor (osteosarcoma, Ewing sarcoma)
  (c) perpendicular = "sunburst": osteosarcoma; Ewing sarcoma; chondrosarcoma; fibrosarcoma; leukemia; metastasis; acute osteomyelitis
  (d) amorphous: malignancy (deposits may represent extension of tumor / periosteal response); osteosarcoma
  (a) Codman triangle: hemorrhage; malignancy (osteosarcoma, Ewing sarcoma); acute osteomyelitis; fracture

Symmetric periosteal reaction in adulthood
1. Vascular insufficiency (lower extremity)
2. Hypertrophic osteoarthropathy
3. Pachydermoperiostosis
4. Thyroid acropachy
5. Fluorosis

Periosteal reaction in childhood
  (a) benign
    1. Physiologic (up to 35%): symmetric involvement of diaphyses during first 1 – 6 months of life
    2. Battered child syndrome
    3 Infantile cortical hyperostosis < 6 months of age
    4. Hypervitaminosis A
    5. Scurvy
    6. Osteogenesis imperfecta
    7. Congenital syphilis
  (b) malignant
    1. Multicentric osteosarcoma
    2. Metastases from neuroblastoma + retinoblastoma
    3. Acute leukemia

BONE TUMOR
Age incidence of malignant bone tumors
80% of bone tumors are correctly determined on the basis of age alone!

Age (years)	Tumor
0.1	Neuroblastoma
0.1 – 10	Ewing tumor in tubular bones (diaphysis)
10 – 30	Osteosarcoma (metaphysis); Ewing tumor in flat bones
30 – 40	Reticulum cell sarcoma (similar histology to Ewing tumor); fibrosarcoma; malignant giant cell tumor (similar histology to fibrosarcoma); parosteal sarcoma; lymphoma
> 40	Metastatic carcinoma; multiple myeloma; chondrosarcoma

SARCOMAS BY AGE:
mnemonic: "Every Other Runner Feels Crampy Pain On Moving"

Ewing sarcoma	0 – 10 years
Osteogenic sarcoma	10 – 30 years
Reticulum cell sarcoma	20 – 40 years
Fibrosarcoma	20 – 40 years
Chondrosarcoma	40 – 50 years
Parosteal sarcoma	40 – 50 years
Osteosarcoma	60 – 70 years
Metastases	60 – 70 years

ROUND CELL TUMORS:
  arise in midshaft; osteolytic; reactive new bone formation; no tumor new bone
  mnemonic: "LEMON"
    Leukemia, **L**ymphoma
    Ewing sarcoma, **E**osinophilic granuloma
    Multiple myeloma
    Osteomyelitis
    Neuroblastoma

Tumor matrix

Cartilage-forming tumors
(a) benign
  1. Enchondroma
  2. Parosteal chondroma
  3. Chondroblastoma
  4. Chondromyxoid fibroma
  5. Osteochondroma
(b) malignant
  1. Chondrosarcoma
√ centrally located ring-like / flocculent / fleck-like radiodensities

Bone-forming tumors
(a) benign
  1. Osteoma
  2. Osteoid osteoma
  3. Osteoblastoma
  4. Ossifying fibroma
(b) malignant
  1. Osteogenic sarcoma
√ inhomogeneous / homogeneous radiodense collections of variable size + extent

Fibrous connective tissue tumors
(a) benign
  1. Nonossifying fibroma
  2. Periosteal desmoid = avulsive cortical irregularity
  3. Desmoplastic fibroma
(b) malignant
  1. Fibrosarcoma

BENIGN FIBROUS BONE LESIONS
  (a) cortical
    1. Benign cortical defect
    2. Avulsion cortical irregularity
  (b) medullary
    1. Herniation pit
    2. Nonossifying fibroma
    3. Ossifying fibroma
    4. Congenital generalized fibromatosis
  (c) corticomedullary
    1. Nonossifying fibroma
    2. Ossifying fibroma
    3. Fibrous dysplasia
    4. Cherubism
    5. Desmoplastic fibroma
    6. Fibromyxoma

Tumors of histiocytic origin
(a) locally aggressive
  1. Giant cell tumor
  2. Benign fibrous histiocytoma
(b) malignant
  1. Malignant fibrous histiocytoma

Tumors of fatty tissue origin
(a) benign
  1. Intraosseous lipoma
  2. Parosteal lipoma
(b) malignant
  1. Intraosseous liposarcoma

Tumors of vascular origin
< 1% of all bone tumors
(a) benign
  1. Hemangioma
  2. Glomus tumor
  3. Lymphangioma
  4. Cystic angiomatosis
  5. Hemangiopericytoma
(b) malignant
  1. Malignant hemangiopericytoma
  2. Angiosarcoma = hemangioendothelioma
     Metastatic sites: lung, brain, lymph nodes, other bones

Tumors of neural origin
(a) benign
  1. Solitary neurofibroma
  2. Neurilemoma
(b) malignant
  1. Neurogenic sarcoma = malignant schwannoma

Pattern of bone destruction
A. Geographic bone destruction:
   Indicative of slow-growing usually benign tumor
   √ well-defined smooth / irregular margin
   √ short zone of transition
B. Motheaten bone destruction
   Indicative of more rapid growth as in malignant bone tumor / osteomyelitis
   √ less well-defined / demarcated lesional margin
   √ longer zone of transition
C. Permeative bone destruction
   Aggressive bone lesion with rapid growth potential (e.g., Ewing sarcoma)
   √ poorly demarcated lesion imperceptibly merging with uninvolved bone
   √ long zone of transition
D. Size of lesion
   Primary malignant tumors are larger than benign tumors
E. Elongated lesion
   √ greatest lesional diameter is > 1 1/2 times the least diameter
   Ewing sarcoma, reticulum cell sarcoma, chondrosarcoma, angiosarcoma

Tumor position in transverse plane
A. Central medullary lesion
   1. Enchondroma
   2. Solitary bone cyst
B. Eccentric medullary lesion
   1. Giant cell tumor
   2. Osteogenic sarcoma, chondrosarcoma, fibrosarcoma
   3. Chondromyxoid fibroma
C. Cortical lesion
   1. Nonossifying fibroma
   2. Osteoid osteoma
D. Parosteal / juxtacortical lesion
   1. Juxtacortical chondroma
   2. Osteochondroma
   3. Parosteal osteogenic sarcoma

Tumor position in longitudinal plane
A. Epiphyseal lesion
   1. Chondroblastoma
   2. Intraosseous ganglion
   3. Giant cell tumor (originating in metaphysis)
B. Metaphyseal lesion
   1. Nonossifying fibroma
   2. Chondromyxoid fibroma
   3. Solitary bone cyst
   4. Osteochondroma
   5. Brodie abscess
   6. Osteogenic sarcoma, chondrosarcoma
C. Diaphyseal lesion
   1. Round cell tumor (e.g., Ewing sarcoma)
   2. Nonossifying fibroma
   3. Solitary bone cyst
   4. Aneurysmal bone cyst
   5. Enchondroma
   6. Osteoblastoma
   7. Fibrous dysplasia

Tumor-like conditions
1. Solitary bone cyst
2. Juxtaarticular ("synovial") cyst
3. Aneurysmal bone cyst
4. Nonossifying fibroma; cortical defect; cortical desmoid
5. Eosinophilic granuloma
6. Reparative giant cell granuloma
7. Fibrous dysplasia (monostotic; polyostotic)
8. Myositis ossificans
9. "Brown tumor" of hyperparathyroidism
10. Massive osteolysis

INTRAOSSEOUS LESION
Bubbly bone lesion
mnemonic: "FOG MACHINES"
Fibrous dysplasia, Fibrous cortical defect
Osteoblastoma
Giant cell tumor
Myeloma (plasmacytoma), Metastases from kidney, thyroid, breast
Aneurysmal bone cyst / Angioma
Chondromyxoid fibroma, Chondroblastoma
Histiocytosis X, Hyperparathyroid brown tumor, Hemophilia
Infection (Brodie abscess, echinococcus, coccidioidomycosis)
Nonossifying fibroma
Enchondroma, Epithelial inclusion cyst
Simple unilocular bone cyst

Infectious bubbly lesion
1. Brodie abscess (Staph. aureus)
2. Coccidioidomycosis
3. Echinococcus
4. Atypical mycobacterium
5. Cystic tuberculosis

Blow out lesion
A. Metastases
   Carcinoma of thyroid, kidney, breast
B. Primary bone tumor
   1. Fibrosarcoma
   2. Multiple myeloma (sometimes)
   3. Aneurysmal bone cyst
   4. Hemophilic pseudotumor

Nonexpansile unilocular well-demarcated bone defect
1. Fibrous cortical defect
2. Nonossifying fibroma
3. Simple unicameral bone cyst
4. Giant cell tumor
5. Brown tumor of HPT
6. Eosinophilic granuloma
7. Enchondroma
8. Epidermoid inclusion cyst
9. Posttraumatic / degenerative cyst
10. Pseudotumor of hemophilia
11. Intraosseous ganglion
12. Histiocytoma
13. Arthritic lesion
14. Endosteal pigmented villonodular synovitis
15. Fibrous dysplasia
16. Infectious lesion

Nonexpansile multilocular well-demarcated bone defect
1. Aneurysmal bone cyst
2. Giant cell tumor
3. Fibrous dysplasia
4. Simple bone cyst

Expansile unilocular well-demarcated bone defect
1. Simple unicameral bone cyst
2. Enchondroma
3. Aneurysmal bone cyst
4. Juxtacortical chondroma

5. Nonossifying fibroma
6. Eosinophilic granuloma
7. Brown tumor of HPT

Poorly demarcated osteolytic lesion without periosteal reaction
A. Nonexpansile
   1. Metastases from any primary
   2. Multiple myeloma
   3. Hemangioma
B. Expansile
   1. Chondrosarcoma
   2. Giant cell tumor
   3. Metastasis from kidney / thyroid

Poorly demarcated osteolytic lesion + periosteal reaction
1. Osteomyelitis
2. Ewing sarcoma
3. Osteosarcoma

Mixed sclerotic and lytic lesion
(a) with sequestrum
   1. Osteomyelitis

(b) without sequestrum
   1. Osteomyelitis
   2. Tuberculosis
   3. Ewing sarcoma
   4. Metastasis
   5. Osteosarcoma

Marked sclerosis surrounding osteolysis
1. Osteoid osteoma
2. Benign osteoblastoma
3. Chronic osteomyelitis
4. Tuberculosis

Moth-eaten bone destruction
mnemonic: "H LEMMON"
Histiocytosis X
Lymphoma
Ewing sarcoma
Metastasis
Multiple myeloma
Osteomyelitis
Neuroblastoma

Trabeculated bone lesions
1. Giant cell tumor: delicate thin trabeculae
2. Chondromyxoid fibroma: coarse thick trabeculae
3. Nonossifying fibroma: loculated
4. Aneurysmal bone cyst: delicate, horizontally oriented trabeculae
5. Hemangioma: striated radiating trabeculae

DWARFISM
Micromelic dwarfism
= disproportionate shortening of entire leg
A. Mild micromelic dwarfism
   1. Jeune syndrome
   2. Ellis-Van Creveld syndrome
      = chondroectodermal dysplasia
   3. Diastrophic dwarfism
B. Mild bowed micromelic dwarfism
   1. Camptomelic dysplasia
   2. Osteogenesis imperfecta, type III
C. Severe micromelic dwarfism
   1. Thanatophoric dysplasia
   2. Homozygous achondroplasia
   3. Osteogenesis imperfecta, type II
   4. Achondrogenesis
   5. Hypophosphatasia
   6. Short-rib polydactyly syndrome

Acromelic dwarfism
= distal shortening (hands, feet)
1. Asphyxiating thoracic dysplasia

Mesomelic dwarfism
= shortening of intermediate segments (radius + ulna or tibia + fibula)
1. Langer syndrome: autosomal recessive
2. Nievergelt syndrome: autosomal dominant
3. Reinhardt syndrome: autosomal dominant
4. Robinow syndrome: autosomal dominant
5. Werner syndrome: autosomal dominant

Rhizomelic dwarfism
= shortening of proximal segments (humerus, femur)
1. Heterozygous achondroplasia
2. Chondrodysplasia punctata, rhizomelic type

Lethal dwarfism
1. Achondrogenesis
2. Thanatophoric dwarfism
3. Achondroplasia (homozygous)
4. Osteogenesis imperfecta (congenital)
5. Chondrodysplasia punctata (recessive)

Nonlethal dwarfism
1. Achondroplasia (heterozygous)
2. Asphyxiating thoracic dysplasia
3. Chondroectodermal dysplasia
4. Chondrodysplasia punctata
5. Spondyloepiphyseal dysplasia (congenital)
6. Diastrophic dwarfism
7. Metatrophic dwarfism
8. Hypochondroplasia

Late onset dwarfism
1. Spondyloepiphyseal dysplasia tarda
2. Multiple epiphyseal dysplasia
3. Pseudoachondroplasia

4. Metaphyseal chondrodysplasia
5. Dyschondrosteosis
6. Cleidocranial dysplasia
7. Progressive diaphyseal dysplasia

Osteochondrodysplasia
A. Failure of
  (a) articular cartilage: spondyloepiphyseal dysplasia
  (b) ossification center: multiple epiphyseal dysplasia
  (c) proliferating cartilage: achondroplasia
  (d) spongiosa formation: hypophosphatasia
  (e) spongiosa absorption: osteopetrosis
  (f) periosteal bone: osteogenesis imperfecta
  (g) endosteal bone: idiopathic osteoporosis
B. Excess of
  (a) articular cartilage: dysplasia epiphysealis hemimelica
  (b) hypertrophic cartilage: enchondromatosis
  (c) spongiosa: multiple exostosis
  (d) periosteal bone: progressive diaphyseal dysplasia
  (e) endosteal bone: hyperphosphatemia

Limb reduction anomalies
Amelia   = absence of limb
Hemimelia   = absence of distal parts
Phocomelia = proximal reduction with distal parts attached to trunk

Aplasia / hypoplasia of radius
1. Aplasia / hypoplasia of radius
2. Thrombocytopenia absent radius syndrome
3. Fanconi anemia
4. Cornelia de Lange syndrome
5. Holt-Oram syndrome

Pubic bone maldevelopment
mnemonic: "CHIEF"
  Cleidocranial dysostosis
  Hypospadia, epispadia
  Idiopathic
  Extrophy of bladder
  F for syringomyelia

Bone overdevelopment
1. Marfan syndrome
2. Klippel-Trenaunay syndrome
3. Macrodystrophia lipomatosa

Erlenmeyer flask deformity
= expansion of distal end of long bones, usually femur
1. Gaucher disease, Niemann-Pick disease
2. Rickets
3. Anemias
4. Fibrous dysplasia
5. Osteopetrosis

6. Heavy metal poisoning
7. Metaphyseal dysplasia
8. Down syndrome
9. Achondroplasia
10. Rheumatoid arthritis

JOINTS
Classification of Arthritides
A. BACTERIAL ARTHRITIS
  1. Tuberculous
  2. Pyogenic
  3. Lyme arthritis
B. ARTHRITIS OF COLLAGEN / COLLAGEN-LIKE DISEASE
  1. Rheumatoid arthritis
  2. Ankylosing spondylitis
  3. Psoriatic arthritis
  4. Rheumatic fever
  5. Sarcoidosis
C. BIOCHEMICAL ARTHRITIS
  1. Gout
  2. Chondrocalcinosis
  3. Ochronosis
  4. Hemophilic arthritis
D. DEGENERATIVE JOINT DISEASE = Osteoarthritis
E. TRAUMATIC
  1. Secondary osteoarthritis
  2. Neurotrophic arthritis
  3. Pigmented villonodular synovitis
F. ARTHRITIS OF INFLAMMATORY BOWEL DISEASE
  1. Ulcerative colitis (in 10 – 20%)
  2. Crohn disease (in 5%)
  3. Whipple disease (in 60 – 90% transient intermittent polyarthritis: sacroiliitis, spondylitis)

SPONDYLOARTHRITIS + HLA-B 27 HISTOCOMPATIBILITY COMPLEX
positive testing in:
1. Ankylosing spondylitis 95%
2. Reiter disease 80%
3. Psoriatic spondylitis...70%
4. Arthropathy of inflammatory bowel disease 70%
5. Normal population 10%

Articular disorders of the hand + wrist
1. **Osteoarthritis** = degenerative joint disease
   = abnormal stress with minor + major traumatic episodes
   target areas: DIP, PIP, 1st CMC, trapezioscaphoid
   √ sclerosis + osteophytes
2. **Erosive Osteoarthritis** = inflammatory osteoarthritis
   Age: predominantly middle-aged / postmenopausal women
   • acute inflammatory episodes
   target areas: DIP, PIP, 1st CMC, trapezioscaphoid

√ subchondral "gull wing" erosions
√ rare ankylosis

3. **Psoriatic Arthritis**
   = rheumatoid variant / seronegative spondyloarthropathy; peripheral manifestation in monarthritis / asymmetric oligoarthritis / symmetric polyarthritis
   target areas: all hand + wrist joints (commonly distal)
   √ "mouse ears" marginal erosions
   √ new bone formation

4. **Rheumatoid Arthritis**
   = synovial proliferative granulation tissue = pannus
   target areas: PIP, MCP, all wrist joints, ulnar styloid
   √ marginal poorly defined erosions
   √ joint deformities

5. **Gouty Arthritis**
   • monosodium urate crystals in synovial fluid
   • asymptomatic periods from months to years
   target areas: commonly CMC + all hand joints
   √ development of chronic tophaceous gout
   √ well-defined erosions with overhanging edge (often periarticular)
   √ joint space narrowing

6. **Calcium pyrophosphate dihydrate crystal deposition disease** = CPPD
   target areas: MCP, radiocarpal
   √ chondrocalcinosis
   √ "degenerative changes" in unusual locations
   √ no erosions

7. **SLE**
   = myositis, symmetric polyarthritis, deforming nonerosive arthropathy, osteonecrosis
   target areas: PIP, MCP
   √ reversible deformities

8. **Scleroderma** = progressive systemic sclerosis (PSS)
   target areas: DIP, PIP, 1st CMC
   √ tuft resorption
   √ soft tissue calcifications

Arthritis with periostitis
1. Juvenile rheumatoid arthritis
2. Psoriatic arthritis
3. Reiter syndrome
4. Infectious arthritis

Arthritis with demineralization
mnemonic: "HORSE"
Hemophilia
Osteomyelitis
Rheumatoid arthritis, Reiter disease
Scleroderma
Erythematosus, systemic lupus

Arthritis without demineralization
1. Gout
2. Neuropathic arthropathy
3. Psoriasis
4. Reiter disease
5. Pigmented villonodular synovitis

Premature osteoarthritis
mnemonic: "COME CHAT"
Calcium pyrophosphate dihydrate arthropathy
Ochronosis
Marfan syndrome
Epiphyseal dysplasia
Charcot joint = neuroarthropathy
Hemophilic arthropathy
Acromegaly
Trauma

Arthritis of interphalangeal joint of great toe
1. Psoriatic arthritis
2. Reiter disease
3. Gout
4. Degenerative joint disease

Ankylosis of interphalangeal joints
mnemonic: "S - Lesions"
1. Psoriatic arthritis
2. Ankylosing spondylitis
3. Erosive osteoarthritis
4. Still disease

Loose intraarticular bodies
1. Osteochondrosis dissecans
2. Synovial osteochondromatosis
3. Chip fracture from trauma
4. Degenerative joint disease
5. Neuropathic arthropathy

Sacroiliitis
A. BILATERAL SYMMETRICAL:
   1. Ankylosing spondylitis
   2. Reiter syndrome
   3. Enteropathic
B. BILATERAL ASYMMETRICAL:
   1. Psoriatic arthritis
   2. Rheumatoid arthritis
   3. Juvenile rheumatoid arthritis
C. UNILATERAL:
   1. Gout
   2. Infection
   3. Osteoarthritis

Protrusio acetabuli
= acetabular floor bulging into pelvis
√ crossing of medial + lateral components of pelvic "teardrop"
A. UNILATERAL
   1. Tuberculous arthritis

2. Trauma
3. Fibrous dysplasia
B. BILATERAL
  1. Rheumatoid arthritis
  2. Paget disease
  3. Osteomalacia

mnemonic: "PROT"
  Paget disease
  Rheumatoid arthritis
  Osteomalacia (HPT)
  Trauma

Subchondral cyst
= SYNOVIAL CYST = SUBARTICULAR PSEUDOCYST
= NECROTIC PSEUDOCYST = GEODES
Etiology: bone necrosis allows pressure-induced
    intrusion of synovial fluid into subchondral
    bone; in conditions with synovial
    inflammation
Causes: (1) Osteoarthritis (2) Rheumatoid arthritis
    (3) Osteonecrosis (4) CPPD
√ size of cyst usually 2 – 35 mm
√ may be large + expansile (especially in CPPD)
DDx: (1) Giant cell tumor
    (2) Pigmented villonodular synovitis
    (3) Metastasis
    (4) Intraosseous ganglion
    (5) Hemophilia

Chondrocalcinosis
mnemonic: "WHIP A DOG"
  Wilson disease
  Hemochromatosis, **H**emophilia, **H**ypothyroidism,
    1° **H**yperparathyroidism (15%), **H**ypophosphatasia,
    Familial **H**ypomagnesemia
  Idiopathic (aging)
  Pseudogout (CPPD)
  Arthritis (rheumatoid, postinfectious, traumatic),
    Amyloidosis
  Diabetes mellitus
  Ochronosis
  Gout

Enthesis
= bone proliferation + erosion at site of tendon +
  ligament attachment
1. Seronegative arthropathies: Ankylosing spondylitis,
  Reiter disease, psoriatric arthritis
2. Rheumatoid arthritis
3. Osteoarthritis
4. Acromegaly

EPIPHYSIS
Stippled epiphyses
  1. Normal variant
  2. Avascular necrosis
  3. Hypothyroidism

  4. Chondrodysplasia punctata
  5. Multiple epiphyseal dysplasia
  6. Spondyloepiphyseal dysplasia
  7. Hypoparathyroidism
  8. Down syndrome
  9. Trisomy 18
  10. Fetal warfarin syndrome
  11. Homocystinuria (distal radial + ulnar epiphyses =
    pathognomonic)
  12. Zellweger cerebrohepatorenal syndrome

Epiphyseal overgrowth
  1. Juvenile rheumatoid arthritis
  2. Hemophilia
  3. Healed Legg-Perthes disease
  4. Tuberculous arthritis
  5. Pyogenic arthritis (chronic)
  6. Fungal arthritis
  7. Epiphyseal dysplasia hemimelica
  8. Fibrous dysplasia of epiphysis
  9. Winchester syndrome

Ring epiphysis
  1. Severe osteoporosis
  2. Healing rickets
  3. Scurvy

Epiphyseolysis
= SLIPPED EPIPHYSIS (zone of maturing
  hypertrophic cartilage affected, not zone of
  proliferation)
1. Idiopathic / juvenile epiphyseolysis
  Age: 12 – 15 years (? puberty-related hormonal
    dysregulation)
  • adiposogenital type; tall stature
2. Renal osteodystrophy
3. Hyperparathyroidism in chronic renal disease
4. Hypothyroidism
5. Radiotherapy

Epiphyseal lesions
mnemonic: "DELCO"
  Degenerative
  Enchondroma
  Lipoma
  Cyst, **C**hondroblastoma
  Osteomyelitis

Tibiotalar slanting
= downward slanting of medial tibial plafond
1. Hemophilia
2. Still disease
3. Sickle cell disease
4. Epiphyseal dysplasia
5. Trauma

TRAUMA
Trauma in childhood
1. Greenstick fracture
   = incomplete fracture of soft growing bone with intact periosteum
2. Bowing fracture
3. Traumatic epiphyseolysis
4. Battered child syndrome
5. Epiphyseal plate injury

Pseudarthrosis in long bones
1. Nonunion of fracture
2. Fibrous dysplasia
3. Neurofibromatosis
4. Osteogenesis imperfecta
5. Congenital: clavicular pseudarthrosis

Excessive callus formation
1. Steroid therapy / Cushing syndrome
2. Neuropathic arthropathy
3. Osteogenesis imperfecta
4. Congenital insensitivity to pain
5. Paralysis
6. Renal osteodystrophy
7. Multiple myeloma

WRIST & HAND
Resorption of terminal tufts
A. Trauma
   1. Amputation
   2. Burns, electric injury
   3. Frostbite
   4. Vinyl chloride poisoning
B. Neuropathic
   1. Congenital indifference to pain
   2. Syringomyelia
   3. Myelomeningocele
   4. Diabetes mellitus
   5. Leprosy
C. Collagen-vascular disease
   1. Scleroderma
   2. Dermatomyositis
   3. Raynaud disease
D. Metabolic
   1. Hyperparathyroidism
E. Inherited
   1. Familial acroosteolysis
   2. Pyknodysostosis
   3. Progeria = Werner syndrome
   4. Pachydermoperiostosis
F. Others
   1. Sarcoidosis
   2. Psoriatic arthropathy
   3. Epidermolysis bullosa

Carpal angle
= angle of 130° formed by tangents to proximal row of carpal bones

A. DECREASED CARPAL ANGLE (< 124°)
   1. Turner syndrome
   2. Hurler syndrome
   3. Morquio syndrome
   4. Madelung deformity
B. INCREASED CARPAL ANGLE (> 139°)
   1. Down syndrome
   2. Arthrogryposis
   3. Bone dysplasia with epiphyseal involvement

Metacarpal sign
= tangent between 4th + 5th metacarpals intersects 3rd metacarpal = shortening of 4th metacarpal
1. Idiopathic
2. Gonadal dysgenesis: Turner syndrome, Klinefelter syndrome
3. Pseudo- and Pseudopseudohypoparathyroidism
4. Ectodermal dysplasia = Cornelia de Lange syndrome
5. Hereditary multiple exostoses
6. Peripheral dysostosis
7. Basal cell nevus syndrome
8. Melorheostosis

mnemonic: **"Ping Pong Is Tough To Teach"**
   Pseudohypoparathyroidism
   Pseudopseudohypoparathyroidism
   Idiopathic
   Trauma
   Turner syndrome
   Trisomy 13–18

Brachydactyly
= shortening / broadening of metacarpals ± phalanges
1. Idiopathic
2. Trauma
3. Osteomyelitis
4. Arthritis
5. Turner syndrome
6. Pseudohypoparathyroidism, Pseudopseudohypoparathyroidism
7. Osteochondrodysplasia
8. Mucopolysaccharidoses
9. Cornelia de Lange syndrome
10. Basal cell nevus syndrome
11. Hereditary multiple exostoses

Syndactyly
= osseous ± cutaneous fusion of digits
1. Apert syndrome
2. Carpenter syndrome
3. Down syndrome
4. Neurofibromatosis
5. Poland syndrome
6. Others

Polydactyly
Frequently associated with:
1. Carpenter syndrome
2. Ellis-van Creveld syndrome
3. Meckel-Gruber syndrome
4. Polysyndactyly syndrome
5. Short rib-polydactyly syndrome
6. Trisomy 13

Clinodactyly
= curvature of finger in mediolateral plane
1. Normal variant
2. Down syndrome
3. Multiple dysplasia
4. Trauma, arthritis, contractures

Lucent lesion in finger
(a) benign tumor
   1. Giant cell tumor
   2. Aneurysmal bone cyst
   3. Brown tumor
   4 Hemophilic pseudotumor
   5. Epidermoid inclusion cyst
   6 Glomus tumor
   7. Solitary bone cyst
   8. Osteoblastoma
   9. Enchondroma
(b) malignant tumor
   1. Osteosarcoma
   2. Fibrosarcoma
   3. Metastasis from lung, breast, malignant melanoma

mnemonic: **"GAMES PAGES"**
Glomus tumor
Arthritis (gout, rheumatoid)
Metastasis (lung, breast)
Enchondroma
Simple cyst (inclusion)
Pancreatitis
Aneurysmal bone cyst
Giant cell tumor
Epidermoid
Sarcoid

Finger tip calcifications
1. Scleroderma / CREST syndrome
2. Raynaud disease
3. Systemic lupus erythematosus
4. Dermatomyositis
5. Calcinosis circumscripta universalis

RIBS
Rib lesions
A. BENIGN RIB LESION
   1. Healing fracture
     (a) cough fractures: 4 – 9th rib in anterior axillary line
     (b) fatigue fracture: 1st rib (from carrying a heavy back pack)
   2. Fibrous dysplasia (most common benign lesion)
     √ predominantly posterior location
   3. Enchondroma: at costochondral / costovertebral junction
   4. Osteochondroma: at costochondral / costovertebral junction
   5. Eosinophilic granuloma
   6. Osteomyelitis
B. MALIGNANT RIB LESION
   1. Metastasis (most common malignant lesion)
   2. Multiple myeloma
   3. Chondrosarcoma
   4. Osteosarcoma
   5. Ewing sarcoma
   6. Malignant lymphoma

Rib notching on inferior margin
A. <u>Vascular</u>
   (a) Aorta: coarctation, thrombosis
   (b) Subclavian artery: Blalock-Taussig shunt
   (c) Pulmonary artery: pulmonary stenosis, tetralogy of Fallot, absent pulmonary artery
   (d) AV fistula
   (e) Superior vena cava obstruction
B. <u>Neurogenic</u>
   1. Intercostal neuroma
   2. Neurofibromatosis
   3. Poliomyelitis / quadriplegia / paraplegia
C. <u>Osseous</u>
   1. Hyperparathyroidism
   2. Thalassemia
   3. Melnick-Needles syndrome

Rib notching on superior margin
1. Rheumatoid arthritis
2. Scleroderma
3. Systemic lupus erythematosus
4. Hyperparathyroidism
5. Restrictive lung disease
6. Marfan syndrome

Ribbon ribs
1. Osteogenesis imperfecta
2. Neurofibromatosis

Bulbous enlargement of costochondral junction
1. Rickets rosary
2. Scurvy
3. Achondroplasia

Wide ribs
1. Marrow hyperplasia (anemias)
2. Fibrous dysplasia
3. Paget disease
4. Achondroplasia
5. Mucopolysaccharidoses

Expansile rib lesion
mnemonic: "THELMA"
Tuberculosis
Hematopoiesis
Eosinophilic granuloma, Ewing sarcoma, Enchondroma
Leukemia, Lymphoma
Myeloma, Metastases
Aneurysmal bone cyst

Short ribs
1. Achondroplasia
2. Achondrogenesis
3. Thanatophoric dysplasia
4. Asphyxiating thoracic dysplasia
5. Mesomelic dwarfism
6. Short rib-polydactyly syndrome
7. Spondyloepiphyseal dysplasia
8. Enchondromatosis
9. Chondroectodermal dysplasia (Ellis-Van Creveld)

Dense ribs
1. Osteopetrosis
2. Mastocytosis
3. Fluorosis

Hyperlucent ribs
1. Osteopetrosis
2. Cushing disease
3. Acromegaly
4. Scurvy

Absence of outer end of clavicle
1. Rheumatoid arthritis
2. Hyperparathyroidism
3. Posttraumatic osteolysis
4. Metastasis / multiple myeloma
5. Cleidocranial dysplasia

Penciled distal end of clavicle
mnemonic: "SHIRT Pocket"
Scleroderma
Hyperparathyroidism
Infection
Rheumatoid arthritis
Trauma
Progeria

Destruction of medial end of clavicle
mnemonic: "MILERS"
Metastases
Infection
Lymphoma
Eosinophilic granuloma
Rheumatoid arthritis
Sarcoma

FOOT
Clubfoot
= Talipes equinovarus (talipes = inversion of foot along long axis; equinus = plantar flexion of ankle; metatarsus varus = lateral deviation of metatarsals)
1. Arthrogryposis multiplex congenita
2. Chondrodysplasia punctata
3. Neurofibromatosis
4. Spina bifida
5. Myelomeningocele

Vertical talus
= "Rocker-bottom foot"
√ vertically oriented talus with increased lateral talocalcaneal angle
√ dorsal navicular displacement
√ heel equinus
√ rigid deformity
Associated with: Arthrogryposis multiplex congenita; spina bifida; trisomy 13–18

Heel pad thickening
= heel pad thickening > 25 mm (normal < 21 mm)
mnemonic: "MAD COP"
Myxedema
Acromegaly
Dilantin therapy
Callous
Obesity
Peripheral edema

SOFT TISSUE CALCIFICATION
Metastatic calcification
= deposit of calcium salts in previously normal tissue
(1) as a result of elevation of Ca x P product above 60 – 70
(2) with normal Ca x P product after renal transplant
Location: lung (alveolar septa, bronchial wall, vessel wall), kidney, gastric mucosa, heart, peripheral vessels
Causes:
(a) Skeletal deossification:
  1. 1° HPT
  2. Ectopic HPT production (lung / kidney tumor)
  3. Renal osteodystrophy + 2° HPT
  4. Hypoparathyroidism
(b) Massive bone destruction:
  1. Widespread bone metastases
  2. Plasma cell myeloma
  3. Leukemia
(c) Increased intestinal absorption:
  1. Hypervitaminosis D
  2. Milk-alkali syndrome
  3. Excess ingestion / IV administration of calcium salts
  4. Prolonged immobilization
  5. Sarcoidosis
(d) Idiopathic hypercalcemia

Dystrophic calcification
= in presence of normal serum Ca + P levels secondary to local electrolyte / enzyme alterations in areas of tissue injury
(a) Metabolic disorder without hypercalcemia
  1. Renal osteodystrophy with 2° HPT
  2. Hypoparathyroidism
  3. Pseudohypoparathyroidism
  4. Pseudopseudohypoparathyroidism
  5. Gout
  6. Pseudogout = chondrocalcinosis
  7. Ochronosis = alkaptonuria
  8. Diabetes mellitus
(b) Connective tissue disorder
  1. Scleroderma
  2. Dermatomyositis
  3. Systemic lupus erythematosus
(c) Trauma
  1. Neuropathic calcifications
  2. Frostbite
  3. Myositis ossificans progressiva
  4. Calcific tendinitis / bursitis
(d) Infestation
  1. Cysticercosis
  2. Dracuncolosis (guinea worm)
  3. Loiasis
  4. Bancroft filariasis
  5. Hydatid disease
  6. Leprosy
(e) Vascular disease
  1. Atherosclerosis
  2. Media sclerosis (Mönckeberg)
  3. Venous calcifications
  4. Tissue infarction (e.g., myocardial infarction)
(f) Miscellaneous
  1. Ehlers-Danlos syndrome
  2. Pseudoxanthoma elasticum
  3. Werner syndrome = progeria
  4. Calcinosis (circumscripta, universalis, tumoral calcinosis)
  5. Necrotic tumor

Soft tissue ossification
= formation of trabecular bone
1. Myositis ossificans progressiva / circumscripta
2. Paraplegia
3. Soft tissue osteosarcoma
4. Parosteal osteosarcoma
5. Surgical scar
7. Severely burned patient

Generalized calcinosis
(a) Collagen vascular disorders
  1. Scleroderma
  2. Dermatomyositis
(b) Idiopathic tumoral calcinosis
(c) Idiopathic calcinosis universalis

Interstitial calcinosis
Calcinosis circumscripta
1. Acrosclerosis: granular deposits around joints of fingers + toes, fingertips
2. Scleroderma: acrosclerosis + absorption of ends of distal phalanges
3. Dermatomyositis: extensive subcutaneous deposits
4. Varicosities: particularly in calf
5. 1° Hyperparathyroidism: infrequently periarticular calcinosis
6. Renal osteodystrophy with 2° hyperparathyroidism: extensive vascular deposits even in young individuals
7. Hypoparathyroidism: occasionally around joints; symmetrical in basal ganglia
8. Vitamin D intoxication: periarticular in rheumatoid arthritis (putty-like); calcium deposit in tophi

Calcinosis universalis
Progressive disease of unknown origin
Age: children + young adults
√ plaque-like calcium deposits in skin + subcutaneous tissues; sometimes in tendons + muscles
√ NO true bone formation

ANATOMY AND METABOLISM OF BONE

Calcium
A. 99% in bone
B. serum calcium
   (a) protein-bound fraction (albumin)
   (b) ionic (pH-dependent) 3% as calcium citrate / phosphate in serum
Absorption: facilitated by vitamin D
Excretion : related to dietary intake; >500 mg/24 hours = hypercalciuria

Phosphorus
Absorption: requires sodium; decreased by aluminum hydroxide gel in gut
Excretion : increased by estrogen, parathormone decreased by vitamin D, growth hormone, glucocorticoids

Parathormone
Major stimulus: low levels of serum calcium ions (action requires vitamin D presence)
Target organs:
   (a) BONE: increase in osteocytic + osteoclastic activity mobilizes calcium + phosphate = bone resorption
   (b) KIDNEY: (1) increase in tubular reabsorption of calcium
                (2) decrease in tubular reabsorption of phosphate (+ amino acids) = phosphate diuresis
   (c) GUT: increased absorption of calcium + phosphorus

Major function: • increase of serum calcium levels
              • increase in serum alkaline phosphatase (50%)

Vitamin D Metabolism
required for
   (1) adequate calcium absorption from gut
   (2) synthesis of calcium-binding protein in intestinal mucosa
   (3) parathormone effects (stimulation of osteoclastic + osteocytic resorption of bone)

Biochemistry:
inactive form of vitamin D3 present through diet / exposure to sunlight; vitamin D3 is converted into 25-OH-vitamin D3 by liver and then converted into 1,25-OH vitamin D3 (= hormone) by kidney
Stimulus for conversion: (1) hypophosphatemia
                              (2) PTH elevation
Action:
   (a) INTESTINE: (1) increased absorption of calcium from bowel
                   (2) increased absorption of phosphate from distal small bowel
   (b) BONE: (1) proper mineralization of osteoid
             (2) mobilization of calcium + phosphate (potentiates parathormone action)
   (c) KIDNEY: (1) increased absorption of calcium from renal tubule
               (2) increased absorption of phosphate from renal tubule

Calcitonin
secreted by parafollicular cells of thyroid
Major stimulus: increase in serum calcium
Target organs:
   (a) BONE: (1) inhibits parathormone-induced osteoclasis by reducing number of osteoclasts
             (2) enhances deposition of calcium phosphate; responsible for sclerosis in renal osteodystrophy
   (b) KIDNEY: inhibits phosphate reabsorption in renal tubule
   (c) GUT: increases excretion of sodium + water into gut
Major function: decreases serum calcium + phosphate

	PTH ACTION	NET EFFECT
Principal:	(1) phosphate diuresis (2) resorption of Ca + P from bone	(1) Serum: increase in Ca decrease in P
Secondary:	(3) resorption of Ca from gut (4) reabsorption of Ca from renal tubule	(2) Urine: increase in Ca increase in P

Occurrence of bone centers at elbow
mnemonic: "CRITOE"

Capitellum	1 year	(< 1 year)
Radial head	5 years	(3 – 6 years)
Internal humeral epicondyle	7 years	(5 – 7 years, last to fuse)
Trochlea	10 years	(9 – 10 years)
Olecranon	10 years	(6 – 10 years)
External humeral epicondyle	11 years	(9 – 13 years)

Rotator cuff muscles
mnemonic: "SITS"
- **S**upraspinatus
- **I**nfraspinatus
- **T**eres minor
- **S**ubscapularis

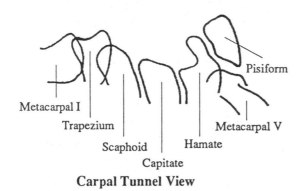

Carpal Tunnel View

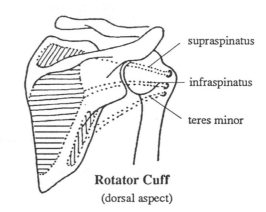

Rotator Cuff
(dorsal aspect)

Muscle Attachments of Thigh

	Origin	Insertion
Gracilis	inferior pubic ramus	pes anserinus
Semimembranosus	ischial tuberosity	medial tibial condyle
Semitendinosus	ischial tuberosity	pes anserinus
Biceps femoris		
— long head:	ischial tuberosity	fibular head
— short head:	lateral linea aspera	fibular head
Adductor		
— longus	superior pubic ramus	medial linea aspera
— magnus	inferior pubic ramus	medial linea aspera
Sartorius	anterior superior iliac spine	pes anserinus
Quadriceps		
— rectus	anterior inferior iliac spine	patellar tendon
— vastus lateralis	greater trochanter	patellar tendon
— vastus medialis	medial intertrochanteric line	patellar tendon
Iliopsoas		
— iliacus	ilium	lesser trochanter
— psoas	lumbar spine	lesser trochanter
Tensor fasciae latae	anterior superior iliac spine	anterolateral tibia

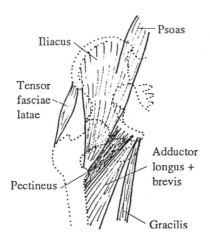

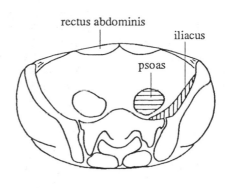

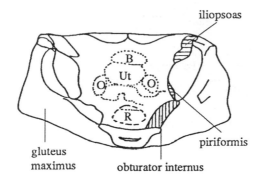

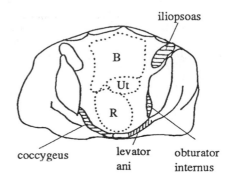

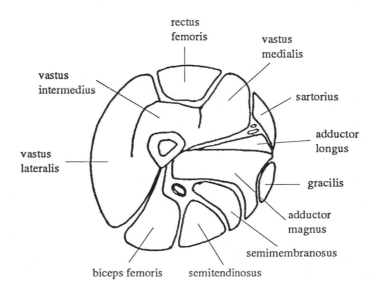

Cross section through right thigh

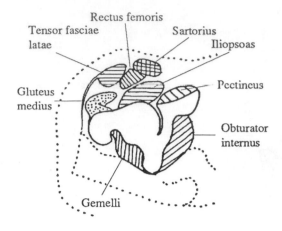

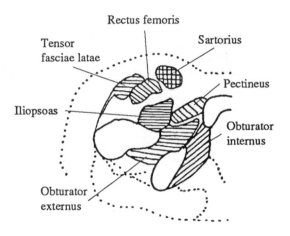

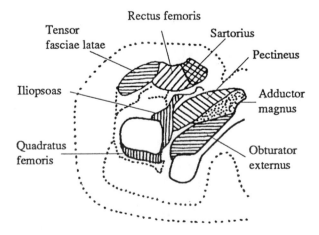

Cross section through right hip
(consecutive sections toward feet)

DISEASE ENTITIES OF BONE AND SOFT TISSUE

ACHONDROGENESIS
- = autosomal recessive lethal chondrodystrophy characterized by extreme micromelia, short trunk, large cranium
- TRIAD: (1) severe short limb dwarfism (2) lack of vertebral calcification (3) large head with normal / decreased calvarial ossification
- *Birth prevalence:* 2.3:100,000
- *Path:* disorganization of cartilage
- A. TYPE I = Parenti-Fraccaro
  - defective enchondral + membranous ossification
  - √ complete lack of ossification of calvarium + spine + pelvis
  - √ absent sacrum + pubic bone
  - √ extremely short long bones without bowing, especially femur, radius, ulna
  - √ thin ribs with multiple fractures (frequent)
- B. TYPE II = Langer-Saldino
  - defective enchondral ossification only
  - √ good ossification of skull vault
  - √ nonossification of lower lumbar vertebrae + sacrum
  - √ short + stubby ribs without fractures
- √ flared metaphyses
- √ short trunk with narrow chest + protruding abdomen
- √ redundant soft tissues
- √ polyhydramnios
- √ increase in HC:AC ratio
- *Prognosis:* uniformly lethal in utero / shortly after birth

ACHONDROPLASIA
Heterozygous Achondroplasia
- = autosomal dominant / sporadic (80%) disease with quantitatively defective endochondral bone formation; related to advanced paternal age; prototype of rhizomelic dwarfism; epiphyseal maturation + ossification unaffected
- *Incidence:* 1:26,000 – 66,000 births, most common nonlethal bone dysplasia
- • normal intelligence + motor function
- • neurologic defects
- @ Skull
  - • receding bridge of nose (hypoplastic base of skull)
  - • brachycephaly with enlarged bulging forehead (nonprogressive hydrocephalus)
  - • relative prognathism
  - √ large calvarium with frontal bossing
  - √ broad mandible
  - √ shortened base of skull + small foramen magnum
  - √ communicating hydrocephalus caused by obstruction of basal cisterns + aqueduct secondary to small foramen magnum
- @ Chest & Spine
  - • protuberant abdomen
  - • prominent buttocks

√ squaring of inferior scapular margin
√ narrow chest
√ narrowing of spinal canal (ventrodorsal + interpediculate space) in lumbar spine
√ hypoplastic bullet- / wedge-shaped vertebra = rounded anterior beaking of vertebra in upper lumbar spine (DDx: Hurler disease)
√ wide intervertebral foramina
√ posterior vertebral scalloping
√ lumbar angular kyphosis (gibbus) + sacral lordosis
@ Pelvis
- • rolling gait from backward tilt of pelvis and hip joints
- √ square-shaped flat nonflared pelvic bones with tomb-stone configuration
- √ flattened iliac wings ("champagne glass")
- √ horizontal acetabuli (decreased acetabular angle)
- √ small sacrosciatic notch
@ Extremities
- • trident hand = separation of 2nd + 3rd digit and inability to approximate 3rd + 4th finger
- √ predominantly rhizomelic shortness of long bones (femur, humerus); may not be observed until 3rd trimester
- √ limb bowing
- √ "ball-in-socket" epiphysis = broad V-shaped metaphysis in which the epiphysis is incorporated
- √ high position of fibular head (fibula less short)
- √ short ulna with thick proximal + slender distal end
- √ brachydactyly (uniform length of short bones) + divergent fingers
OB-US (> 27th week GA):
- √ shortening of proximal long bones
- √ increased BPD, HC, HC:AC ratio
- √ decreased FL:BPD ratio
- √ normal mineralization, no fractures
- √ normal cardiothoracic ratio
Cx: (1) Hydrocephalus + syringomyelia (small foramen magnum)
  (2) Recurrent ear infection (poorly developed facial bones)
  (3) Crowded dentition + malocclusion
  (4) Neurologic complications (spinal cord compression)

Homozygous Achondroplasia
- = hereditary autosomal dominant disease with severe features of achondroplasia
- • ± lethal in neonatal period
- *DDx:* thanatophoric dysplasia

ACROCEPHALOSYNDACTYLY
- = syndrome characterized by (1) increased height of skull vault due to generalized craniosynostosis (= acrocephaly, oxycephaly) (2) syndactyly of fingers / toes

Type I   : Apert syndrome = acrocephalosyndactyly
Type II   : Vogt cephalosyndactyly
Type III : Acrocephalosyndactyly with asymmetry of skull
            + mild syndactyly
Type IV   : Wardenburg type
Type V   : Pfeiffer type

ACROOSTEOLYSIS, FAMILIAL
dominant inheritance
Age: onset in 2nd decade; M:F = 3:1
• sensory changes in hands + feet
• destruction of nails
• joint hypermobility
• swelling of plantar of foot with deep wide ulcer + ejection
  of bone fragments
@ Skull
    √ Wormian bones
    √ craniosynostosis
    √ basilar impression
    √ protuberant occiput
    √ resorption of alveolar processes + loss of teeth
@ Spine
    √ spinal osteoporosis ± fracture
    √ kyphoscoliosis + progressive decrease in height

ACROMEGALY
Etiology: excess growth hormone due to eosinophilic
            adenoma / hyperplasia
• gigantism in children (DDx: **Soto syndrome** of cerebral
  gigantism = large skull, mental retardation, cerebral
  atrophy, advanced bone age)
√ osseous enlargement (phalangeal tufts, vertebrae)
√ flared ends of long bone
√ cystic changes in carpals, femoral trochanters
√ osteoporosis
@ Hand
    • spade-like hand
    √ widening of terminal tufts
@ Skull
    √ prognathism (= elongation of mandible) in few cases
    √ sellar enlargement + erosion
    √ enlargement of paranasal sinuses: large frontal
      sinuses (75%)
    √ calvarial hyperostosis (especially inner table)
    √ enlarged occipital protuberance
@ Vertebrae
    √ posterior scalloping in 30% (secondary to pressure
      of enlarged soft tissue)
    √ anterior new bone
    √ loss of disc space (weakening of cartilage)
@ Soft tissue
    √ heel pad > 25 mm
@ Joints
    √ premature osteoarthritis (commonly knees)

ACTINOMYCOSIS
Types: (1) cervicofacial (poor oral hygiene, common)
        (2) lungs (hematogenous / inhalation)
        (3) ileocecal (after rupture / surgery of appendix)

• draining cutaneous sinuses
Location: predilection for thorax + spine
@ Mandible
    √ destruction of mandible (most frequently involved)
      around tooth socket without new bone formation,
      spread to soft tissues at angle of jaw + into neck
@ Vertebra
    √ destruction of vertebra with preservation of disc +
      small paravertebral abscess without calcification
      (DDx to tuberculosis: disc destroyed, large abscess
      with calcium)
    √ thickening of cervical vertebrae around margins
@ Tubular bones of hands
    √ destructive lesion of a mottled permeating type
    √ cartilage destruction + subarticular erosive defects
      in joints (simulating TB)
    √ destruction / thickening of ribs + pleuritis
@ Abdomen
    Initially localized to cecum / appendix
    √ ulcerations with abscess (containing yellow sulphur
      granules)
    √ abscesses in liver, retroperitoneum, psoas muscles,
      chronic sinus in groin

ADAMANTINOMA
= (MALIGNANT) ANGIOBLASTOMA = locally aggressive
/ malignant lesion
Histo: pseudoepithelial cell masses with peripheral
          columnar cells in a palisade pattern with varying
          amounts of fibrous stroma; areas of squamous /
          tubular / alveolar / vessel transformation; --
          prominent vascularity; resembles ameloblastoma
          of the jaw
Age: 25 – 50 years, commonest in 3rd – 4th decade
• frequently history of trauma
• local swelling ± pain
Location: middle 1/3 of tibia (90%), fibula, ulna, carpals,
           metacarpals, humerus, shaft of femur
√ eccentric round osteolytic lesion with sclerotic margin,
  may have additional foci in continuity with major lesion
  (CHARACTERISTIC)
√ may show mottled density
√ **bone expansion frequent**
√ **often multiple**
Prognosis: tendency to recur after local excision; after
              several recurrences pulmonary metastases
              may develop
DDx: fibrous dysplasia (possibly related)

AINHUM DISEASE
= DACTYLOLYSIS SPONTANEA
ainhum = fissure, saw, sword
Etiology: unknown
Histo: hyperkeratotic epidermis with fibrotic thickening
          of collagen bundles below; chronic lymphocytic
          inflammatory reaction may be present; arterial
          walls may be thickened with narrowed vessel
          lumina
Incidence: up to 2%

Age: usually in males in 4th + 5th decades; blacks (West Africa) + American descendants; M>F
- deep soft tissue groove forming on medial aspect of plantar surface of proximal phalanx with edema distally
- painful ulceration may develop

Location: mostly 5th / 4th toe (rarely finger); near interphalangeal joint; mostly bilateral

√ sharply demarcated progressive bone resorption of distal / middle phalanx with tapering of proximal phalanx to complete autoamputation (after an average of 5 years)

√ osteoporosis

Rx: early surgical resection of groove with Z plasty

DDx: (1) Neuropathic disorders (diabetes, leprosy, syphilis)
(2) Trauma (burns, frostbite)
(3) Acroosteolysis from inflammatory arthritis, infection, polyvinylchloride exposure
(4) Congenitally constricting bands in amniotic band syndrome

AMYLOIDOSIS
= accumulation + infiltration of a protein polysaccharide in body tissues; tends to form around capillaries + endothelial cells of larger blood vessels causing ultimately vascular obliteration with infarction
- rubbery soft tissue swelling

√ periarticular soft tissue swelling (amyloid deposited in synovium, joint capsule, tendons, ligaments)

√ subluxation of proximal humerus + femoral neck

√ osteoporosis

√ coarse trabecular pattern (DDx: sarcoidosis)

√ solitary osteolytic lesion (secondary invasion + erosion of articular bone) in ribs, olecranon, coronoid process

√ pathologic fractures may occur (vertebral fracture)

PRIMARY AMYLOIDOSIS
In 10 – 15% of multiple myeloma; may precede development of multiple myeloma; sporadic, familial; predominantly connective tissue involvement
- progressive cardiac failure
- bone pain
- periarticular soft tissue swelling + stiffness (shoulders, hips, fingers)
- Bence Jones protein (without myeloma)

Location:

heart (90%)	GI tract (70%)	tongue (40%)
spleen(40%)	liver (35%)	lungs (30%)
skin + subcutis (25%)		

SECONDARY AMYLOIDOSIS
Chronic suppurative disease of lungs / skeleton; chronic inflammatory disease of GI tract (ulcerative colitis); lymphoproliferative disorders (multiple myeloma, Waldenström, heavy chain disease); rheumatoid arthritis, amyloidosis of aging

Location: spleen, liver, kidneys, GI tract

ANEURYSMAL BONE CYST
Etiology: (a) primary nonneoplastic lesion (2/3)
(b) arising in preexisting bone tumor: giant cell tumor, fibrous dysplasia, chondroblastoma, xanthoma, chondromyxoid fibroma, solitary bone cyst, nonossifying fibroma, osteosarcoma, metastatic carcinoma (1/3)

Histo: honey-combed spaces filled with blood + lined by granulation tissue / osteoid; areas of free hemorrhage; sometimes multi-nucleated giant cells

Types:
1. INTRAOSSEOUS ABC
= primary cystic / telangiectatic tumor of giant cell family, originating in bone marrow cavity, slow expansion of cortex; rarely related to history of trauma
2. EXTRAOSSEOUS ABC
= postraumatic hemorrhagic cyst; originating on surface of bones, erosion through cortex into marrow

Age: peak age 16 years (range 10 – 30 years) in 75% < 20 years; F > M
- pain of relatively acute onset with rapid increase of severity over 6 – 12 weeks
- ± history of trauma
- neurologic signs (radiculopathy to quadriplegia) if in spine

Location:
(a) spine (30%) with slight predilection for posterior elements + lumbar spine, cervical spine (22%); involvement of vertebral body (40%); may involve two contiguous vertebrae (25%)
(b) long bones: eccentric in metaphysis of femur, tibia, humerus, fibula; pelvis

√ purely lytic eccentric radiolucency

√ aggressive expansile ballooning lesion of "soap-bubble" pattern

√ rapid progression within 6 weeks to 3 months

√ sclerotic inner portion

√ almost invisible thin cortex (CT shows integrity)

√ tumor respects epiphyseal plate

√ no periosteal reaction (except when fractured)

Cx: (1) pathologic fracture (frequent)
(2) extradural block with paraplegia

DDx: (1) Giant cell tumor (particularly in spine)
(2) Hemorrhagic cyst (end of bone / epiphysis, not expansile)

ANKYLOSING SPONDYLITIS
= chronic inflammatory disease primarily affecting spine

Age: young men; M:F = 15:1; caucasians:blacks = 3:1
- HLA-B 27 positive in 96%

Location: bilateral + asymmetric; hips + shoulders (80%), small peripheral joints (50%)

Associated with: (1) ulcerative colitis, regional enteritis
(2) iritis in 25%

(3) aortic insufficiency + atrioventricular conduction defect

@ HAND (30%)
Target area:MCP, PIP, DIP
√ exuberant osseous proliferation
√ osteoporosis, joint space narrowing, osseous erosions (deformities less striking than in rheumatoid arthritis)

@ SACROILIAC / SYMPHYSIS PUBIS
√ initially sclerosis of joint margins primarily on iliac side (bilateral, symmetric)
√ later irregularities + widening of joint (cartilage destruction)

@ SPINE
√ straightening / squaring of anterior vertebral margins = osteitis of anterior corners
√ reactive sclerosis of corners of vertebral bodies
√ asymmetric erosions of laminar + spinous process at level of lumbar spine
√ ossification of annulus fibrosus (NOT anterior longitudinal ligament)
√ apophyseal + costovertebral ankylosis
√ marginal syndesmophyte formation = thin vertical radiodense spicules
√ "bamboo" spine = undulating contour of ligamentous calcifications; prone to fracture resulting in pseudarthrosis
√ periostitic "whiskering": ischial tuberosity, iliac crest, ischiopubic rami, greater femoral trochanter, external occipital protuberance, calcaneus
√ dorsal arachnoid diverticula in lumbar spine
√ atlantoaxial subluxation
√ temporomandibular joint space narrowing, erosions, osteophytosis

@ CHEST
√ bilateral upper lobe pulmonary fibrosis (uncommon)

ANTERIOR TIBIAL BOWING
= WEISMANN-NETTER SYNDROME = congenital painless nonprogressive bilateral anterior leg bowing
Age: beginning in early childhood
• may be accompanied by mental retardation, goiter, anemia
√ anterior bowing of tibia + fibula, bilaterally, symmetrically at middiaphysis
√ thickening of posterior tibial + fibular cortices
√ minor radioulnar bowing
√ kyphoscoliosis
√ extensive dural calcification
DDx: Luetic sabre shin (bowing at lower end of tibia + anterior cortical thickening)

APERT SYNDROME
Autosomal dominant; may be mentally retarded
@ Skull
√ oxycephalic skull + flat occiput
√ hypertelorism + bilateral exophthalmus
√ underdeveloped paranasal sinuses
√ underdeveloped maxilla with prognathism
√ high pointed arch of palate
√ prominent vertical crest in middle of forehead (increased intracranial pressure)
√ V-shaped anterior fossa due to elevation of lateral margins of lesser sphenoid
√ sella may be enlarged
√ cervical spine may be fused

@ Hand & feet
√ fusion of distal portions of phalanges, metacarpals / carpals (2nd, 3rd + 4th digit)
√ absence of middle phalanges
√ missing / supernumerary carpal / tarsal bones
√ pseudarthroses

ARTERIOVENOUS FISTULA OF BONE
Etiology: (a) acquired (usually gun shot wound)
(b) congenital
Location : lower extremity most frequent
√ soft tissue mass
√ presence of large vessels
√ phleboliths (DDx: long standing varicosity)
√ accelerated bone growth
√ cortical osteolytic defect (= pathway for large vessels into medulla)
√ increased bone density

ARTHROGRYPOSIS
= ARTHROGRYPOSIS MULTIPLEX CONGENITA
= nonprogressive congenital syndrome complex characterized by poorly developed + contracted muscles, deformed joints with thickened periarticular capsule and intact sensory system
Etiology:
congenital / acquired defect of motor unit (anterior horn cells, nerve roots, peripheral nerves, motor end plates, muscle) early in fetal life with immobilization of joints at various stages in their development
Cause: ? neurotropic agents, toxic chemicals, hard drugs, hyperthermia, neuromuscular blocking agents, mytotic abnormalities, mechanical immobilization
Incidence: 0.03% of newborn infants; 5% risk of recurrence in sibling
Associated with: (1) neurogenic disorders (90%)
(2) myopathic disorders
(3) skeletal dysplasias
(4) intrauterine limitation of movement (myomata, amniotic band, twin, oligohydramnios)
(5) connective tissue disorders
Distribution: all extremities (46%), lower extremities only (43%), upper extremities only (11%); - symmetrical; peripheral joints >> proximal joints
• club feet
• congenital dislocation of hip
• claw hand
• diminished muscle mass

√ osteopenia + pathologic fractures
√ carpal coalition
√ vertical talus
√ calcaneal valgus deformity

ASPHYXIATING THORACIC DYSPLASIA
= JEUNE DISEASE = autosomal recessive disorder
Incidence: 100 cases
Associated with: renal anomalies (hydroureter), PDA
• reduced thoracic mobility + frequent pulmonary
  infections
• progressive renal failure + hypertension
@ Chest
  √ narrow + elongated cylindrical chest with flared base
  √ normal sized heart leaving little room for lungs
  √ horizontal clavicles at level of 6th cervical vertebra
  √ short horizontal ribs + bulbous costochondral
    junction
@ Pelvis
  √ trident pelvis
  √ small iliac bone flared + shortened in cephalocaudal
    diameter ("wine glass" pelvis)
  √ short ischial + pubic bones
  √ prematue ossification of capital femoral epiphysis
@ Extremities
  √ rhizomelic brachymelia (humerus, femur)
  √ postaxial hexadactyly
  √ shortening of distal phalanges in hands + cone-
    shaped epiphyses in feet
@ Kidneys
  √ enlarged kidneys with linear streaking on
    nephrogram
OB-US:
  √ proportionate shortening of long bones
  √ small thorax with decreased circumference
  √ increased cardiothoracic ratio
  √ occasionally polydactyly
  √ polyhydramnios
Prognosis: neonatal death in 80% (respiratory failure +
  infections)
DDx: Ellis-van Creveld syndrome

AVASCULAR NECROSIS
= AVN = consequence of interrupted blood supply to bone
  with death of cellular elements
Histo: (a) cellular ischemia leading to death of
  osteocytes + marrow cells
  (b) necrotic debris in intertrabecular spaces +
  proliferation and infiltration of mesenchymal
  cells + capillaries
  (c) mesenchymal cells differentiate to
  osteoblasts on the surface of dead
  trabeculae synthezising new bone layers +
  resulting in trabecular thickening
Pathogenesis:
  (1) obstruction of extra- and intraosseous vessels by
  embolism, thrombosis, external compression
  (2) cumulative stress from cytotoxic factors

Causes:
  mnemonic: "PLASTIC RAGS"
  Pancreatitis, **P**regnancy
  Lupus
  Alcoholism
  Steroids
  Trauma
  Idiopathic, **I**nfection
  Caisson disease, **C**ollagen disease (SLE)
  Rheumatoid arthritis, **R**adiation
  Amyloid
  Gaucher disease
  Sickle cell disease
MRI:
  √ low-intensity band / ring (= mesenchymal + fibrous
    repair tissue, amorphous cellular debris, thickened
    trabecular bone) on T1WI
  √ central area of high signal intensity (= necrotic bone +
    marrow not invaded by capillaries + mesenchymal
    tissue) on T1WI
  √ cleft of low-signal intensity on T1WI + high signal
    intensity on T2WI (= subchondral fracture)

BASAL CELL NEVUS SYNDROME
= GORLIN SYNDROME = syndrome of autosomal
  dominant inheritance characterized by (1) multiple
  cutaneous basal cell carcinomas (2) jaw cysts
  (3) ectopic calcifications (4) skeletal anomalies
• nevoid basal cell carcinomas (nose, mouth, chest, back)
  at mean age of 19 years; after puberty aggressive,
  may metastasize
• pitlike defects in palms + soles
Associated with: high incidence of medulloblastoma in
  children
√ multiple mandibular + maxillary cysts (dentigerous cysts
  + ectopic dentition)
√ anomalies of upper 5 ribs: bifid, fused, dysplastic
√ bifid spinous processes, spina bifida
√ scoliosis (cervical + upper thoracic)
√ hemivertebrae + block vertebrae
√ Sprengel deformity (scapula elevated, hypoplastic,
  bowed)
√ brachydactyly
√ calcification of falx
√ ectopic calcifications of subcutaneous tissue, ovaries,
  sacrotuberous ligaments, mesentery
√ bony bridging of sella turcica

BATTERED CHILD SYNDROME
= CAFFEY-KEMPE SYNDROME = CHILD ABUSE =
  PARENT / INFANT TRAUMATIC STRESS SYNDROME
= NONACCIDENTAL TRAUMA
  Most common cause of serious intracranial injuries in
  children < 1 year of age
Incidence: 5 – 10% of children seen in emergency
  rooms
@ Skeletal Trauma (20%)

Site: multiple ribs, sternum, costochondral /
         costovertebral separation, clavicles, scapula,
         skull, vertebral compression, tibia, metacarpus
√ multiple asymmetric fractures in different stages of
  repair
√ separation of distal epiphysis
√ marked irregularity + fragmentation of metaphyses
  (DDx: osteochondritis stage of congenital syphilis;
  infractions of scurvy)
√ "bucket-handle" fracture = avulsion of an arcuate
  metaphyseal fragment overlying the lucent
  epiphyseal cartilage
√ corner fracture secondary to sudden twisting motion
  of extremity around knee, elbow, distal tibia, fibula,
  radius, ulna
√ isolated spiral fracture (15%) secondary to external
  rotatory force applied to femur / humerus
√ extensive periosteal reaction from subperiosteal
  hemorrhage (DDx: scurvy, copper deficiency)
√ exuberant callus formation at fracture sites
√ cortical hyperostosis extending to epiphyseal plate
  (DDx: not in infantile cortical hyperostosis)
√ avulsion fracture of ligamentous insertion; frequently
  seen without periosteal reaction
@ Head Trauma (15 – 25%)
  Major cause of death
  (1)   Impact injury with translational force: extraaxial
        hemorrhage, brain contusion, cerebral
        hemorrhage, infarction, generalized edema;
        flexible calvaria + meninges decrease likelihood
        of skull fractures
  (2)   Whiplash injury with rotational force: subdural
        hemorrhage
  • bulging fontanelles, convulsions
  Skull film (associated fracture in 1%):
        √ linear fracture > comminuted fracture > diastases
          (conspicuously absent)
  CT:
        √ subdural hemorrhage (most common):
          interhemispheric location most common
        √ epidural hemorrhage (uncommon)
        √ cerebral edema (focal, multifocal, diffuse)
        √ intracerebral hematoma
@ Viscera
  √ small bowel / gastric rupture
  √ traumatic pancreatic pseudocyst
  √ lacerations of lung / liver / spleen
Cx: (1)   Brain atrophy (up to 100%)
      (2)   Infarction (50%)
      (3)   Subdural hygroma
      (4)   Encephalomalacia
      (5)   Porencephaly

BENIGN CORTICAL DEFECT
= developmental intracortical bone defect
Age: usually 1st – 2nd decade; uncommon in boys < 2
       years of age; uncommon in girls < 4 years of age
• asymptomatic

Site: metaphysis of long bone
√ well-defined intracortical round / oval lucency
√ usually < 2 cm long
√ sclerotic margins
Cx: pathologic / avulsion fracture following minor
       trauma (infrequent)
Prognosis:
  (1)   Spontaneous healing resulting in sclerosis /
        disappearance
  (2)   Ballooning of endosteal surface of cortex = fibrous
        cortical defect
  (3)   Medullary extension resulting in nonossifying
        fibroma

BLASTOMYCOSIS
= NORTH AMERICAN BLASTOMYCOSIS
Organism: Blastomyces dermatitidis
Primary lesions usually in skin with direct extension into
  bone; occasionally hematogenous spread (resembles
  actinomycosis)
√ marked destruction ± surrounding sclerosis
√ multiple osseous lesions are frequent
√ vertebral bodies + intervertebral discs are destroyed
  (similar to tuberculosis)
√ lytic skull lesions + soft tissue abscess

BLOUNT DISEASE
= TIBIA VARA = avascular necrosis of medial tibial
  condyle
Age: > 6 years
• limping, lateral bowing of leg
√ medial tibial condyle enlarged + deformed (DDx: Turner
  syndrome)
√ irregularity of metaphysis (medially + posteriorly
  prolonged with beak)

BONE INFARCT
Etiology:
A. Occlusion of vessel:
    (a) Thrombus: thromboembolic disease, sickle cell
         anemia (SS + SC hemoglobin), polycythemia
         rubra vera
    (b) Fat: pancreatitis (intramedullary fat necrosis from
         circulating lipase), alcoholism
    (c) Gas: caisson disease, astronauts
B. Vessel wall disease:
    1. Arteritis: SLE, rheumatoid arthritis, polyarteritis
        nodosa, sarcoidosis
    2. Arteriosclerosis
C. Vascular compression by deposition of:
    (a) fat: corticosteroid therapy (e.g. renal transplant,
         Cushing disease)
    (b) blood: trauma (fractures + dislocations)
    (c) inflammatory cells: osteomyelitis, infection,
         histiocytosis X
    (d) edema: radiation therapy, hypothyroidism,
         frostbite
    (e) substances: Gaucher disease (vascular

compression by lipid-filled histiocytes), gout
D. Others: idiopathic, hypopituitarism,
pheochromocytoma (microscopic thrombotic
disease), osteochondroses

Medullary Infarction
Nutrient artery is the sole blood supply for diaphysis!
Location: distal femur, proximal tibia, iliac wings, ribs,
humeri
(a) Acute phase:
√ NO radiographic changes without cortical
involvement
√ area of rarefaction
√ bone marrow scan: diminished uptake in
medullary RES for long period of time
√ bone scan: photon-deficient lesion within 24 – 48
hours; increased uptake after collateral
circulation established
(b) Healing phase: (complete healing / fibrosis /
calcification)
√ demarcation by zone of serpiginous / linear
calcification + ossification parallel to cortex
√ dense bone indicating revascularization

Cortical Infarction
Requires compromise of
(a) nutrient artery and (b) periosteal vessels
Age: particularly in childhood where periosteum is
easily elevated by edema
√ avascular necrosis = osteonecrosis
√ osteochondrosis dissecans
Cx: (1) Growth disturbances
√ cupped / triangular / coned epiphyses
√ "H-shaped" vertebral bodies
(2) Fibrosarcoma (more common), malignant
fibrous histiocytoma, benign cysts
(3) Osteoarthritis

BONE ISLAND
= ENOSTOSIS = COMPACT ISLAND = FOCAL
SCLEROSIS = SCLEROTIC BONE ISLAND
= CALCIFIED MEDULLARY DEFECT
• asymptomatic
Age: any age; grows more rapidly in children
Location: ilium, ribs, femur, humerus, phalanges (not in
skull)
√ round solitary density of trabeculated bone < 2 cm in
size
√ "brush" border margins = sharply demarcated with
thorny radiations
√ may show activity on bone scan
√ may demonstrate slow growth
Prognosis: may increase to 8-12 cm over years (40%);
may decrease / disappear

BRUCELLAR OSTEOMYELITIS
Organism: small Gram-negative nonencapsulated
coccobacilli

Location: commonest site of involvement is
reticuloendothelial system; spine > long bones
√ sharply demarcated lesion with little sclerosis
(resembling TB)
DDx: fibrous dysplasia, benign tumor, osteoid osteoma

BURKITT LYMPHOMA
Endemic in areas with malaria (tropical Africa, New
Guinea)
Age: < 10 years of age
Path: resemblance to Hodgkin disease
Location: maxilla, mandible (first); multifocal (10%);
soft tissues: abdominal lymph nodes, ovaries,
kidneys
@ Mandible / maxilla
√ grossly destructive lesion, spicules of bone growing
at right angles
√ large soft tissue mass
@ Other skeleton
√ reminiscent of Ewing tumor / reticulum cell sarcoma
√ lamellated periosteal reaction around major long
bones
Prognosis: long-term survival in 50%

CAISSON DISEASE
= DECOMPRESSION SICKNESS = THE BENDS
Etiology: during too rapid decompression = reduction of
surrounding pressure (ascent from dive, exit
from caisson / hyperbaric chamber, ascent to
altitude) nitrogen bubbles form (nitrogen more
soluble in fat of panniculus adiposus, spinal
cord, brain, bones containing fatty marrow)
• "the bends" = local pain in knee, elbow, shoulder, hip
• neurologic symptoms (paresthesia, major cerebral /
spinal involvement)
• "chokes" = substernal discomfort + coughing
(embolization of pulmonary vessels)
Location: mostly in long tubular bones of lower extremity
(distal end of shaft + epiphyseal portion);
symmetrical lesions
√ early: area of rarefaction
√ healing phase: irregular new bone formation with
greater density
√ peripheral zone of calcification / ossification
√ ischemic necrosis of articular surface with secondary
osteoarthritis

CALCIUM PYROPHOSPHATE DIHYDRATE DEPOSITION DISEASE
= CPPD = PSEUDOGOUT = FAMILIAL
CHONDROCALCINOSIS
Types
1. Osteoarthritic form (50%)
2. Pseudogout = acute synovitis (20%)
3. Rheumatoid form (5%)
4. Neuropathic arthropathy
5. Asymptomatic with tophaceous pseudogout
(common)

M:F = 3:2
- calcium pyrophosphate crystals in synovial fluid + within leukocytes (characteristic weakly positive birefringent diffraction pattern)

Location:
- (a) knee (especially meniscus + cartilage of patellofemoral joint)
- (b) wrist (triangular fibrocartilage in distal radioulnar joint bilaterally)
- (c) pelvis (sacroiliac joint, symphysis)
- (d) spine (annulus fibrosis of lumbar intervertebral disc; NEVER in nucleus pulposus as in ochronosis)
- (e) shoulder, hip, elbow, ankle, acromioclavicular joint
- √ polyarticular chondrocalcinosis (in fibro- and hyaline cartilage)
- √ involvement of tendons, bursae, pinnae of the ear
- √ pyrophosphate arthropathy resembles osteoarthritis: joint space narrowing, subchondral eburnation, cyst formation
- √ numerous intraarticular bodies (fragmentation of subchondral bone)

CALVÉ-KÜMMEL-VERNEUIL DISEASE
= VERTEBRAL OSTEOCHONDROSIS = VERTEBRA PLANA = avascular necrosis of vertebral body
Age: 2 – 15 years
- √ uniform collapse of vertebral body into flat thin disc
- √ increased density of vertebra
- √ neural arches NOT affected
- √ discs are normal with normal intervertebral disc space
- √ intervertebral vacuum cleft sign (PATHOGNOMONIC)
DDx: Eosinophilic granuloma, Metastatic disease

CAMPOMELIC DYSPLASIA
= sporadic / autosomal recessive dwarfism
Incidence: 0.05:10,000 births
Associated with:
1. Hydrocephalus (23%)
2. Congenital heart disease (30%): VSD, ASD, Tetralogy, AS
3. Hydronephrosis (30%)
- pretibial dimple
- √ macrocephaly, cleft palate, micrognathia (90-99%)
- √ hypoplastic scapulae (92%)
- √ narrow bell-shaped chest
- √ hypoplastic vertebral bodies + nonmineralized pedicles (especially lower cervical spine)
- √ vertically narrowed iliac bones
- √ bowing (= campo) of long bones, in particular tibiae + femurs

OB-US:
- √ bowing of tibia + femur
- √ decreased thoracic circumference
- √ hypoplastic scapula
- √ ± cleft palate
Prognosis: death within first year in 97% (respiratory insufficiency)

CARPENTER SYNDROME
= ACROCEPHALOPOLYSYNDACTYLY
autosomal recessive
- retardation • hypogonadism
- √ patent ductus arteriosus
- √ acro(oxy)cephaly
- √ polysyndactyly

CHONDROBLASTOMA
= CODMAN TUMOR = CARTILAGE-CONTAINING GIANT CELL TUMOR = BENIGN CHONDROBLASTOMA; occurs before cessation of enchondral bone growth
Incidence: 1% of primary bone neoplasms (700 cases in world literature)
Age: peak in 2nd decade (range of 8 – 59 years); 5 – 25 years (88%); M:F = 2:1
Histo: polyhedral chondroblasts + multinucleated giant cells = epiphyseal chondromatous giant cell tumor (resembles chondromyxoid fibroma)
- mild joint pain, tenderness, swelling, limitation of motion
Location: proximal femur + greater trochanter (23%), distal femur (20%), proximal tibia (17%), proximal humerus (17%), tarsal bones; 2/3 lower extremity, 50% about knee; may occur in apophyses (minor + greater trochanter, patella, greater tuberosity of humerus), near triradiate cartilage of innominate bone
Site: eccentric medullary, subarticular location with open growth plate, growth may continue to involve metaphysis
- √ oval / round radiolucency usually 1 – 4 cm in diameter
- √ well-defined sclerotic margin, may be lobulated
- √ punctate / irregular calcifications in 25 – 50%
- √ no periosteal reaction / joint involvement
- √ periostitis of adjacent metaphysis / diaphysis (30%)
Rx: curettage
DDx: (1)   Ischemic necrosis of femoral head (may be indistinguishable, more irregular configuration)
        (2)   Giant cell tumor (usually larger + less well demarcated, not calcified, older age group)
        (3)   Chondromyxoid fibroma

CHONDRODYSPLASIA PUNCTATA
= CONGENITAL STIPPLED EPIPHYSES = CHONDRODYSTROPHIA CALCIFICANS CONGENITA
Etiology: peroxisomal disorder characterized by fibroblast plasmalogen deficiency
Incidence: 1:110,000 births
A.   AUTOSOMAL RECESSIVE CHONDRODYSPLASIA PUNCTATA = RHIZOMELIC TYPE
     potentially lethal variety; autosomal recessive
     - flat face
     - joint contractures
     - congenital cataracts
     - ichthiotic skin lesions
     - √ marked limb shortening (in particular arms)

√ occasional asymmetric shortening of a long bone (rarely all limbs symmetrically affected)

√ metaphyseal splaying of proximal tubular bones (in particular about knee)

√ multiple small punctate calcifications of varying size in epiphyses (knee, hip, shoulder, wrist) + in respiratory cartilage and soft tissues (neck, rib ends) before appearance of ossification centers

√ prominent vertebral + paravertebral calcifications

√ coronal clefts in vertebrae

B   CONRADI-HÜNERMANN DISEASE
= NONRHIZOMELIC TYPE
more common nonlethal variety; autosomal dominant (+ recessive)

Cx: respiratory failure (severe underdevelopment of ribs), tracheal stenosis, spinal cord compression

DDx: (1) Cretinism (may show epiphyseal fragmentation, much larger calcifications within epiphysis)
       (2) Warfarin embryopathy
       (3) Zellweger syndrome

CHONDROECTODERMAL DYSPLASIA
= ELLIS-VAN CREVELD SYNDROME = MESODERMAL DYSPLASIA
= autosomal recessive acromesomelic dwarfism

Incidence: 120 cases; in inbred Amish communities

Associated with: congenital heart disease in 50% (ASD, VSD)

• ectodermal dysplasia:
  • absent / hypoplastic brittle spoon-shaped nails
  • irregular + pointed teeth, partial anodontia, teeth may be present at birth
  • scant / fine hair
• obliteration of maxillary mucobuccal space (thick frenula between alveolar mucosa + upper lip)
• strabismus
• undescended testicles
√ hepatosplenomegaly
√ accelerated skeletal maturation
√ normal spine
@ Skull
  √ Wormian bones
  √ cleft lip
@ Chest
  √ long narrow thorax in ap + transverse dimensions
  √ horizontal ribs + elevated clavicles
@ Pelvis
  √ small falttened ilia
  √ trident shape of acetabulum with indentation in roof (almost pathognomonic)
  √ acetabular + tibial exostoses
@ Extremities
  √ shortening of all long bones, more severe in forearms + lower legs
  √ dislocation of radial head
  √ frequent fusion of two / more carpal + tarsal bones (hamate + capitate)

√ hypoplasia / absence of distal phalanges

√ postaxial polydactyly (usually finger, rarely toe) ± syndactyly of hands + feet

√ carpal fusion (after complete ossification)

OB-US:
  √ proportional shortening of long bones
  √ small thorax with decreased circumference
  √ increased cardiothoracic ratio
  √ ASD
  √ polydactyly

Prognosis: death within first month of life in 33%

DDx: Jeune disease (difficult distinction)

CHONDROMYXOID FIBROMA
Benign tumor derived from cartilage; initially arising in cortex

Incidence: < 1% of all bone tumors

Histo: chondroid + fibrous + myxoid tissue (related to chondroblastoma); may be mistaken for chondrosarcoma

Age: peak 2nd – 3rd decade (range of 5 – 79 years)
         M:F = 1:1

• slowly progressive local pain, swelling, restriction of motion

Location: proximal tibia (common), proximal + distal femur and fibula, pelvis, short tubular bones of hand + feet, ribs (classic but uncommon)

Site: eccentric meta- / diaphyseal, sparing epiphyseal plate (epiphysis rarely involved)

√ expansile ovoid lesion with radiolucent center + oval shape at each end of lesion

√ long axis parallel to long axis of host bone (1 – 10 cm in length and 4 – 7 cm in width)

√ thick scalloped sclerotic inner border (characteristic)

√ scalloped margins (common) may mimic trabeculations

√ stippled calcifications within tumor (in advanced lesions)

√ usually bulged + thinned overlying cortex

√ NO cortical destruction / periosteal reaction

Prognosis: 25% recurrence rate following currettage

Cx: malignant degeneration distinctly unusual

DDx: (1) Aneurysmal bone cyst (2) Solitary bone cyst (3) Nonossifying fibroma (4) Fibrous dysplasia (5) Enchondroma (6) Chondroblastoma (7) Eosinophilic granuloma (8) Fibrous cortical defect

CHONDROSARCOMA
A.   PRIMARY CHONDROSARCOMA
B.   SECONDARY CHONDROSARCOMA
     as a complication of a preexisting skeletal abnormality such as
     1. Osteochondroma
     2. Enchondroma
     3. Parosteal chondroma

Peripheral Chondrosarcoma
= EXOSTOTIC CHONDROSARCOMA = malignant degeneration of hereditary multiple exostoses and

rarely of a solitary exostosis (beginning in cartilaginous cap of osteochondroma)

Peak age: 5th – 6th decade; M:F = 1.5:1
- asymptomatic / pain + swelling

Location: pelvis, scapula, sternum, ribs, ends of humerus / femur, skull, facial bones

√ unusually large soft tissue mass attached to bone
√ flocculent / streaky chondroid calcification (characteristic)
√ dense radiopaque center with streaks radiating to periphery (not marginated)
√ thickening of cortex at site of attachment
√ late destruction of bone

DDx:
(1) Osteochondroma (densely calcified with multiple punctate calcifications) (2) Parosteal osteosarcoma (more homogeneous density of calcified osteoid)

Central Chondrosarcoma

= ENDOSTEAL CHONDROSARCOMA = 3rd most common primary bone tumor (1st multiple myeloma, 2nd osteosarcoma)

Histo: arises from chondroblasts (tumor osteoid is never formed)

Age: median 45 years; 50% > 40 years; 10% in children (rapidly fatal); M:F = 2:1
- hyperglycemia as paraneoplastic syndrome (85%)

Location: neck of femur, pubic rami, proximal humerus, ribs, skull (sphenoid bone, cerebellopontine angle, mandible), sternum

Site: central + meta- / diaphysis

√ expansile osteolytic lesion 1 – several cm in size
√ short transition zone ± sclerotic margin (well defined from host bone)
√ ± small irregular punctate / snowflake type of calcification; single / multiple
√ late: loss of definition + break through cortex
√ endosteal cortical thickening, sometimes at a distance from the tumor
√ presence of large soft tissue mass

DDx: Benign enchondroma, osteochondroma, osteosarcoma, fibrosarcoma

Clear Cell Chondrosarcoma

Low grade malignancy, usually mistaken for chondroblastoma (may be related)

Histo: small lobules of tissue composed of cells with centrally filled vesicular nuclei surrounded by large clear cytoplasm

Age: 19 – 68, predominantly after epiphyseal fusion

Location: proximal femur, proximal humerus, proximal ulna, lamina vertebrae (5%); pubic ramus; head of femur / humerus

Site: close to end of bone

√ single lobulated oval / round sharply marginated lesion of 1 – 2 cm in size
√ surrounding increased bone density
√ aggressive rapid growth over 3 cm

√ may contain calcifications
√ bone often enlarged
√ indistinguishable from conventional chondrosarcoma / chondroblastoma (slow growth over years)

CLEIDOCRANIAL DYSOSTOSIS

= CLEIDOCRANIAL DYSPLASIA = MUTATIONAL DYSOSTOSIS

Autosomal dominant inheritance; delayed ossification of midline structures

@ Skull
√ diminished / absent ossification of skull (in early infancy)
√ Wormian bones
√ widened fontanelles + sutures with delayed closure
√ persistent metopic suture
√ brachycephaly + prominent bossing
√ large mandible
√ high narrow palate (may be cleft)
√ hypoplastic paranasal sinuses
√ delayed / defective dentition

@ Chest & Upper extremity
√ hypoplasia / absence (10%) of clavicles (defective development, predominantly on right side) (DDx: congenital pseudarthrosis of clavicle)
√ thorax may be narrowed + bell-shaped
√ supernumerary ribs
√ incompletely ossified sternum
√ radius short / completely absent
√ pointed terminal tufts
√ hemivertebrae, spondylosis (frequent)

@ Pelvis & lower extremity
√ delayed ossification of bones at symphysis pubis (DDx: bladder extrophy)
√ hypoplastic iliac bones
√ deformed / absent femoral necks

COCCIDIOIDOMYCOSIS

Endemic in southern California + southern Arizona (San Joaquin Valley)

(1) primary / respiratory phase: usually asymptomatic; erythema nodosum in 5%
(2) secondary phase: disseminated infection from bronchial ulceration in 10 – 20%

Histo: granulomatous bone lesions

Location: most frequent site at end of bone / bony prominences of tibial tubercle, ankle, acromion, medial end of clavicle, spine, ribs, pelvis

√ focal areas of destruction, formation of cavities (early) followed by sclerosis of surrounding bone (later) = bubbly bone lesion
√ proliferation of overlying periosteum
√ joints generally not infected
√ destruction of vertebra with preservation of disc space
√ psoas abscess indistinguishable from tuberculosis, may calcify
√ soft tissue abscesses common

CONGENITAL GENERALIZED FIBROMATOSIS
= INFANTILE MULTIPLE FIBROMATOSIS
= rare disorder of fibroblastic origin
Type 1: <u>CONGENITAL GENERALIZED FIBROMATOSIS</u>
Involvement of bone + visceral organs (lungs, intestines, liver, pancreas, kidney)
Age: lesions present at birth / first 4 months with progressive growth
√ multiple focal fibrous lesions anywhere in the body
Prognosis: 80% die within 4 months
Type 2: <u>CONGENITAL DIFFUSE FIBROMATOSIS</u>
= CONGENITAL MULTIPLE FIBROMATOSIS
Predominant involvement of bone, no visceral involvement (occasionally colon)
Prognosis: good, spontaneous regression may occur
Location: bilateral, symmetric
Site: metaphyseal in long bones
√ destructive bone lesions with smooth margins 0.5 – 1.0 cm in size
√ well-defined sclerotic margin occasionally
√ any bone may be involved
DDx: (1) Letterer-Siwe (skin lesions)
(2) Neurofibromatosis (multiple masses)
(3) Osseous hemangiomas / lymphangiomatosis / lipomatosis
(4) Metastatic neuroblastoma

CONGENITAL INSENSITIVITY TO PAIN
CRITERIA: (1) defect must be present at birth
(2) general insensitivity to pain
(3) no general mental / physical retardation
Causes: (1) sensory neuropathies (e.g. diabetes)
(2) hysteria (3) syphilis (4) mental deficiency
(5) syringomyelia (6) organic brain disease
• history of painless injuries + burns
√ Charcot joints = neurotrophic joints (usually weight-bearing joints)
√ bizarre deformities + gross displacement + considerable hemorrhage (unnoticed fractures + dislocations)
√ osteomyelitis + septic arthritis may occur + progress extensively

CORNELIA DE LANGE SYNDROME
= Amsterdam dwarfism
• mental retardation (IQ < 50)
• hirsutism; hypoplastic genitalia
• feeble growling cry
• high forehead; short neck
• arched palate
• bushy eyebrows meeting in midline + long curved eyelashes
• small nose with depressed bridge; upward tilted nostrils; excessive distance between nose + upper lip
√ small + brachycephalic skull
√ hypoplasia of long bones (upper extremity more involved)

√ forearm bones may be absent
√ short radius + elbow dislocation
√ thumbs placed proximally (hypoplastic 1st metacarpal)
√ short phalanges + clinodactyly of 5th finger

CORTICAL DESMOID
= AVULSIVE CORTICAL IRREGULARITY
= PERIOSTEAL / SUBPERIOSTEAL DESMOID
= SUBPERIOSTEAL / CORTICAL ABRASION
= SUBPERIOSTEAL CORTICAL DEFECT
= rare fibrous lesion of the periosteum
Age: peak 14 – 16 years (range of 3 – 17 years);
M:F = 3:1
Histo: shallow defect filled with proliferating fibroblasts, multiple small fragments of resorbing bone (microavulsions) at tendinous insertions
• no localizing signs / symptoms
Location: posterior aspect of medial femoral condyle along medial ridge of linea aspera at adductor magnus aponeurosis; 1/3 bilateral
√ area of cortical thickening
√ 1 – 2 cm irregular, shallow, concave saucer-like crater with sharp margin
√ lamellated periosteal reaction
√ localized cortical hyperostosis proximally (healing phase)
CAVE: may be confused with a malignant tumor (osteosarcoma) / osteomyelitis

CRI-DU-CHAT SYNDROME
= deletion of short arms of 5th chromosome (5 p)
• peculiar high-pitched cat cry (hypoplastic larynx)
• low set ears
• strabismus
• marked mental + growth retardation
• microcephaly
Associated with: congenital heart disease
√ agenesis of corpus callosum
√ hypertelorism
√ small mandible
√ faulty long bone development
√ short 3rd, 4th, 5th metacarpals
√ long 2nd, 3rd, 4th, 5th proximal phalanges
√ horseshoe kidney

CROUZON DISEASE
= CRANIOFACIAL SYNOSTOSIS = Apert syndrome without syndactyly
• parrot-beaked nose
• strabismus
• deafness
• mental retardation
• dental abnormalities
√ acro(oxy)cephaly (premature craniosynostosis)
√ hypertelorism + exophthalmus
√ hypoplastic maxilla (relative prominence of mandible)

CUSHING SYNDROME
√ most often axial osteoporosis
√ stippled calvarium
√ demineralized dorsum sellae
Cx: (1) pathologic fractures of vertebrae + ribs with excessive callus formation
(2) aseptic necrosis of hips
(3) bone infarcts
(4) delayed skeletal maturation in children

CYSTIC ANGIOMATOSIS
= LYMPHANGIOMATOSIS / HEMANGIOMATOSIS
Histo: endothelial lined cysts in bone
Age: peak 10 – 15 years; range of 3 months – 55 years
Location: long bones, skull, flat bones
√ multiple osteolytic metaphyseal lesions of 1 – 2 mm to several cm with fine sclerotic margins + relative sparing of medullary cavity
√ may show overgrowth of long bone
√ endosteal thickening
√ sometimes associated with soft tissue mass ± phleboliths
√ chylous pleural effusion suggests fatal prognosis
DDx: (other polyostotic diseases): histiocytosis X, fibrous dysplasia, metastases, Gaucher disease, congenital fibromatosis, neurofibromatosis, enchondromatosis, Maffucci syndrome

DERMATOMYOSITIS
= POLYMYOSITIS = damaged chondroitin sulfate no longer inhibiting calcification
Histo: atrophy of muscle bundles followed by edema and coagulation necrosis; mucoid degeneration with round cell infiltrates concentrated around blood vessels
Age: 4th – 6th decade, F > M
@ Skeleton
√ linear + confluent calcifications in soft tissues (extremities, hands, abdominal wall, chest wall, axilla, inguinal region)
√ pointing of terminal tufts
√ rheumatoid-like arthritis (rare)
√ "floppy-thumb sign"
@ Chest
√ disseminated pulmonary infiltrates (reminiscent of scleroderma)
@ Myocardium
√ changes similar to skeletal muscle
@ GI tract
√ atony + dilatation of esophagus
√ atony of small intestines + colon
ACUTE FORM
• fever, joint pain, lymphadenopathy, splenomegaly, subcutaneous edema
Prognosis: death within a few months
CHRONIC FORM
• low-grade fever, musclular aches + pains, muscle weakness, edema, skin erythema

Cx: high incidence of malignant neoplasms in GI tract, lung, kidney, ovary, breast

DESMOPLASTIC FIBROMA
= rare locally aggressive benign neoplasm of bone with borderline malignancy resembling soft tissue desmoids / musculoaponeurotic fibromatosis
Histo: intracellular collagenous material in fibroblasts
Age: 2nd decade; in 90% < 30 years; M:F = 1:1
• slowly progressive pain + local tenderness
Location: > 50% in long bones (humerus, tibia, femur, radius, clavicle), scapula, vertebra, calcaneus, ilium, mandible
Site: central meta- / diaphyseal (if growth plate open); may extend into epiphysis with subarticular location (if growth plate closed)
√ well-defined area of bone destruction
√ residual columns of bone with trabeculated / honeycombed / bubbly appearance
√ may grow to massive size (simulating aneurysmal bone cyst / metastatic renal cell carcinoma)
√ soft tissue mass may be present
Cx: pathologic fracture (10%)
Prognosis: high rate of local recurrence

DIASTROPHIC DYSPLASIA
= DIASTROPHIC DWARFISM = EPIPHYSEAL DYSOSTOSIS
= autosomal recessive severe rhizomelic dwarfism secondary to generalized disorder of cartilage followed by fibrous scars + ossifications
• diastrophic = "twisted" habitus
• "cauliflower ear" = ear deformity from inflammation of pinna
• laryngomalacia
• lax + rigid joints with contractures
• normal intellectual development
@ Axial skeleton
√ cleft palate
√ progressive kyphoscoliosis (not present at birth)
√ cervical spina bifida occulta
√ narrowed interpedicular space in lumbar spine
√ short + broad bony pelvis
√ posterior tilt of sacrum
@ Extremities
√ severe micromelia (predominantly rhizomelic = humerus + femur shorter than distal long bones)
√ flattened epiphysis + widened metaphysis
√ multiple joint flexion contractures (notably of major joints)
√ dislocation of multiple joints, lateral dislocation of patella
√ clubfoot = severe talipes equinovarus
√ ulnar deviation of hands
√ oval + hypoplastic 1st metacarpal = "hitchhiker's thumb" (CHARACTERISTIC)
√ widely spaced fingers

OB-US:
- √ proportionately shortened long bones
- √ hitchhiker thumb
- √ clubfeet
- √ joint contractures
- √ abnormal spinal curvature

DIFFUSE IDIOPATHIC SKELETAL HYPEROSTOSIS

= DISH = FORESTIER DISEASE = ANKYLOSING HYPEROSTOSIS
= bony outgrowths at osseous sites of tendinous + ligamentous attachment
Etiology: (1) may be caused by altered vitamin A metabolism (elevated plasma levels of unbound retionol) (2) long-term ingestion of retinoid derivates for dermatologic disorders (e.g., Accutane®)
Age: > 50 years; M > F
- hyperglycemia
- positive HLA-B27 in 34%
Location: lower thoracic > lower cervical > entire lumbar spine
- √ anterior + lateral right-sided syndesmophytes of vertebral column (aorta on left)
- √ disc spaces well preserved, no apophyseal ankylosis, no sacroiliitis
- √ continuous flowing ossification along anterolateral spine of at least 4 vertebrae
- √ "whiskering" at iliac crest, ischial tuberosity, trochanters
- √ spurs of olecranon process of ulna + calcaneus (plantar + posterior surface) + anterior surface of patella
- √ broad osteophytes at lateral acetabular edge, inferior portions of sacroiliac joints, superior aspect of symphysis pubis
- √ ossification in iliolumbar + sacrotuberous ligaments (DDx: fluorosis)
- √ ossification of coracoclavicular ligament, patellar ligament, tibial tuberosity, interosseous membranes
- √ increased incidence of hyperostosis frontalis interna
DDx: (1) Fluorosis (increased skeletal density)
(2) Acromegaly (posterior scalloping, skull features)
(3) Ankylosing spondylitis (squaring of vertebral bodies, coarser syndesmophytes, sacroiliitis, apophyseal alteration)

DISLOCATION

Shoulder Dislocation
Glenohumeral joint dislocations make up > 50% of all dislocations
A. ANTERIOR / SUBCORACOID SHOULDER DISLOCATION (96%)
Mechanism: external rotation + abduction; 40% recurrent
Age: in younger individuals
May be associated with:
- √ fracture of greater tuberosity (15%)
- √ Bankart lesion = fracture of inferior glenoid rim (detachment of labrum)
- √ fracture of anterior rim of glenoid
- √ Hill-Sachs defect (50%) = depression fracture of posterolateral surface of humeral head (impaction against glenoid rim)

B. POSTERIOR SHOULDER DISLOCATION (2 – 4%)
in patients with convulsive disorders /electric shock therapy
- √ rim sign (66%) = distance between medial border of humeral head + anterior glenoid rim < 6 mm
May be associated with:
- √ trough sign (75%) = "reverse Hill-Sachs" = compression fracture of anteromedial humeral head (tangential Grashey view of glenoid!)
- √ fracture of posterior glenoid rim
- √ avulsion fracture of lesser tuberosity

C. INFERIOR SHOULDER DISLOCATION
= LUXATIO ERECTA
rare type with extremity held over head in fixed position

Wrist Dislocation
Mechanism: fall on outstretched hand
Incidence: 10% of all carpal injuries
A. LUNATE DISLOCATION
B. PERILUNATE DISLOCATION
2 – 3 times more common than lunate dislocation accompanied by fracture in 75% (= transscaphoid perilunate dislocation)
- √ most commonly dorsal dislocation
C. ROTARY SUBLUXATION OF SCAPHOID
Mechanism: acute dorsiflexion of wrist; may be associated with rheumatoid arthritis
= tearing of interosseous ligaments of lunate, scaphoid, capitate
- √ gap > 4 mm between scaphoid + lunate (PA radiograph)
- √ foreshortening of scaphoid
- √ ring sign of distal pole of scaphoid
D. MIDCARPAL DISLOCATION

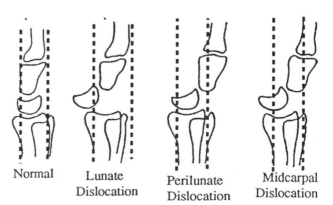

Normal   Lunate Dislocation   Perilunate Dislocation   Midcarpal Dislocation

DOWN SYNDROME
= MONGOLISM = TRISOMY 21 (95% nondisjunction,
  5% translocation)
- mental retardation   • hypotonia
- characteristic facies   • Simian crease
@ Skull
  √ hypotelorism
  √ persistence of metopic suture (40 – 79%) after age
    10
  √ hypoplasia of sinuses + facial bones
  √ microcrania (brachycephaly)
  √ delayed closure of sutures + fontanelles
  √ dental abnormalities (underdeveloped tooth No. 2)
  √ flat-bridged nose
  NO Wormian bones / intracranial calcifications /
  craniostenosis
@ Axial skeleton
  √ atlantoaxial subluxation (25%)
  √ anterior scalloping of vertebral bodies
  √ "squared vertebral bodies" = centra high and narrow
    = positive lateral lumbar index (ratio of horizontal to
    vertical diameters of L2)
@ Chest
  √ Congenital heart disease (40%): endocardial
    cushion defect
  √ hypersegmentation of manubrium = 2 – 3
    ossification centers (90%)
  √ 11 pairs of ribs (25%)
@ Pelvis
  √ flaring of iliac wings (decreased iliac angle)
    = "Mickey Mouse ears"
  √ flattening of acetabular roof (decreased acetabular
    angle)
  √ tapering of ischial rami
@ Extremities
  √ metaphyseal flaring
  √ clinodactyly (50%); widened space between first two
    digits of hands + feet
  √ hypoplastic and triangular middle + distal phalanges
    of 5th finger = acromicria (DDx: normal individuals,
    cretins, achondroplastic dwarfs)
  √ pseudoepiphyses of 1st + 2nd metacarpals
@ Gastrointestinal
  √ umbilical hernia
  √ "double bubble" sign = duodenal atresia / stenosis /
    annular pancreas
  √ tracheo-esophageal fistula
  √ anorectal anomalies
  √ Hirschsprung disease
OB-US:
  Incidence: 1:800 births
  • low alpha-fetoprotein (25%)
  • advanced maternal age (25% of fetuses with Down
    syndrome are born to mothers > 35 years of age;
    75% are born to mothers < 35 years of age)
  √ mild cerebral ventricular dilatation
  √ cystic hygroma
  √ occipital-nuchal skin thickening > 6 mm (42%) on
    transcerebellar diameter view

√ double bubble of duodenal atresia (8%)
√ omphalocele
√ hyperechogenic bowel < 20 weeks GA
√ VSD / AV canal defect (50%)
√ elevated BPD / femur ratio (secondary to short
  femur)
√ ratio of measured-to-expected femur length ≤ 0.91
  (sensitivity 40%, specificity 95%); no screening
  procedure (positive predictive value 0.33%)
√ hypoplasia of middle phalanx of 5th digit
√ IUGR
Cx: Leukemia (increased frequency 3 – 20 x)

DYSCHONDROSTEOSIS
= LÉRI-LAYANI-WEILL SYNDROME = mesomelic long
  bone shortening; autosomal dominant; M:F = 1:4
√ bilateral Madelung deformity
  √ short radius
  √ dorsal ulnar subluxation
  √ carpal wedging between radius + ulna

DYSPLASIA EPIPHYSEALIS HEMIMELICA
= TREVOR DISEASE = TARSOEPIPHYSEAL ACLASIS
= eccentric epiphyseal cartilaginous overgrowth of one /
  more epiphyses; spontaneous occurrence
Age: 2 – 4 years; M>F
May be associated with hemihypertrophy
• joint immobility
Location: localized (tarsus, carpus, knee, ankle);
            sometimes generalized
√ osteochondroma-like growth from one side of epiphysis

ECHINOCOCCUS OF BONE
Occurs occasionally in the U.S.; usually in foreign-born
  individuals; bone involvement in 1%
Histo: no connective tissue barrier; daughter cysts
         extend directly into bone
@ Pelvis, sacrum, rarely long tubular bones
  √ round / irregular regions of rarefaction
  √ multiloculated lesion (bunch of grapes)
  √ no sharp demarcation (DDx: chondroma, giant cell
    tumor) with secondary infection:
    √ thickening of trabeculae with generalized
      perifocal condensation
    √ cortical breakthrough with soft tissue mass
@ Vertebra
  √ sclerosis without pathologic fracture
  √ intervertebral discs not affected
  √ vertebral lamina often involved
  √ frequently involvement of adjacent ribs

EHLERS-DANLOS SYNDROME
= group of autosomal dominant diseases of connective
  tissue characterized by abnormal collagen synthesis
Types: 10 types have been described which differ
         clinically, biochemically and genetically
Age: present at birth
• hyperelasticity of skin

- fragile brittle skin with gaping wounds and poor healing
- molluscoid pseudotumors over pressure points
- hyperextensibility of joints
- joint contractures with advanced age
- bleeding tendency (fragility of blood vessels)
- blue sclera, microcornea, myopia, keratoconus, ectopia lentis
√ multiple ovoid calcifications (2 – 10 mm) in subcutis / in fatty cysts ("spheroids"), most frequently in periarticular areas of legs
√ ectopic bone formation
√ hemarthrosis (particularly in knee)
√ malalignment./ subluxation / dislocation on stress radiographs
√ recurrent dislocations (hip, patella, shoulder, radius, clavicle)
√ precocious osteoarthrosis (predominantly in knees)
√ ulnar synostosis
√ kyphoscoliosis
√ spondylolisthesis
√ spina bifida occulta
√ diaphragmatic hernia
√ aneurysm of great vessels, aortic dissection, tortuosity of arch, ectasia of pulmonary arteries
√ ectasia of gastrointestinal tract
AORTOGRAPHY CONTRAINDICATED!
(Cx following arteriography: aortic rupture, hematomas)

ENCHONDROMA
Benign cartilaginous growth in medullary cavity; bones preformed in cartilage are affected (NOT skull)
Age: 10 – 30 years; M:F = 1:1
Histo: lobules of hyaline cartilage
- usually asymptomatic, painless swelling
Location. (frequently multiple = enchondromatosis)
  (a) in 40% small bones of wrists + hand (most frequent tumor here), distal + mid aspects of metacarpals, proximal / middle phalanges
  (b) femur, tibia, humerus, radius, ulna, foot, rib
Site: central + diaphyseal, epiphysis only affected after closure of growth plate
√ oval / round lucency near epiphysis with fine marginal line
√ scalloped endosteum
√ ground glass appearance
√ calcification: pinhead, stippled, flocculent, "rings and arcs" pattern
√ bulbous expansion of bone with thinning of cortex
√ Madelung deformity = bowing deformities of limb, discrepant length
√ NO cortical breakthrough / periosteal reaction
Cx: (1) pathologic fracture
      (2) malignant degeneration in long bone enchondromas in 15 – 20%
DDx:
  (1) Epidermoid inclusion cyst (phalangeal tuft, Hx of trauma, more lucent)
  (2) Unicameral bone cyst (rare in hands, more radiolucent)
  (3) Giant cell tumor of tendon sheath (commonly erodes bone, soft tissue mass outside bone)
  (4) Fibrous dysplasia (rare in hand, mostly polyostotic)
  (5) Bone infarct
  (6) Chondrosarcoma

ENCHONDROMATOSIS
= OLLIER DISEASE = DYSCHONDROPLASIA
= MULTIPLE ENCHONDROMATOSIS = nonhereditary failure of cartilage ossification
Age: childhood presentation
- leg / arm shortening
- hand + feet deformity
Location: predominantly unilateral monomelic distribution
          (a) localized (b) regional (c) generalized
√ rounded masses / columnar streaks of decreased density from epiphyseal plate into diaphysis
  = cartilaginous rests
√ bony spurs pointing toward the joint (DDx: exostosis points away from it)
√ cartilaginous areas show punctate calcifications with age
√ associated with dwarfing of the involved bone due to impairment of epiphyseal fusion
√ club-like deformity of metaphyseal region
√ cartilaginous metaphyseal expansion with cortical breakthrough
√ bowing deformities of limb bones
√ discrepancy in length = Madelung deformity (radius, ulna)
√ small bones of feet + hands: deforming tumors that may break through cortex secondary to tendency to continue to proliferate
√ fan-like radiation of cartilage from center to crest of ilium
Cx: sarcomatous transformation (in 25 – 50%): osteosarcoma (young adults); chondro- / fibrosarcoma (in older patients)

<u>MAFFUCCI SYNDROME</u>
= nonhereditary enchondromatosis + multiple soft tissue hemangiomas
- multiple cavernous hemangiomas
Location: unilateral involvement / marked asymmetry; hands + feet
√ phleboliths may be present
Cx: malignant transformation even higher than in Ollier disease

ENGELMANN-CAMURATI DISEASE
= PROGRESSIVE DIAPHYSEAL DYSPLASIA
= ENGELMANN DISEASE = RIBBING DISEASE
autosomal dominant
Age: early childhood, M > F
- neuromuscular dystrophy = delayed walking (18 – 24 months) with wide-based waddling gait; often misdiagnosed as muscular dystrophy / poliomyelitis
- weakness + easy fatigability
- bone pain + tenderness
- underdevelopment of muscles secondary to malnutrition

- NORMAL laboratory values
Location: NO involvement of hands, feet, ribs, scapulae
@ Skull (initially affected)
  √ amorphous increase in density at base of skull
@ Long bones (bilateral symmetrical distribution)
  √ fusiform enlargement of diaphyses with cortical
    thickening (endosteal + periosteal accretion of
    mottled new bone) and progressive obliteration of
    medullary cavity; symmetrical involvement
  √ progression of lesions along long axis of bone
    toward either end
  √ abrupt demarcation of lesions (metaphyses +
    epiphyses spared)
  √ relative elongation of extremities
√ NORMAL epiphyses + metaphyses
√ hands + feet UNAFFECTED
DDx:
  (1) Chronic osteomyelitis (single bone)
  (2) Hyperphosphatasemia (high alkaline phosphatase
      levels)
  (3) Paget disease (age, new bone formation, increased
      alkaline phosphatase)
  (4) Infantile cortical hyperostosis (fever; mandible, rib,
      clavicles; regresses, < 1 year)
  (5) Fibrous dysplasia (predominantly unilateral,
      subperiosteal new bone)
  (6) Osteopetrosis (very little bony enlargement)
  (7) Vitamin A poisoning

EPIDERMOID INCLUSION CYST
  = INTRAOSSEOUS KERATIN CYST = IMPLANTATION
    CYST
Age: 2nd – 4th decade;   M > F
Histo: squamous epithelium, keratin, cholesterol
           crystals
- history of trauma (implantation of epithelium under skin
  with secondary bone erosion)
- asymptomatic
Location: terminal tuft of phalanx, may occur in other
            phalanges of hand, L > R hand, calvarium,
            occasionally in foot
√ usually solitary cyst in centric location
√ cortex frequently expanded
√ NO calcifications, periosteal reaction, soft tissue
  swelling
√ pathologic fracture

EPIPHYSEOLYSIS OF FEMORAL HEAD
  = SLIPPED CAPITAL FEMORAL EPIPHYSIS; Salter-
    Harris type I epiphyseal injury
Age: in overweight adolescent males
Etiology: trauma, renal osteodystrophy, rickets,
              childhood irradiation, growt hormone therapy
- knee / hip pain
Location: usually unilateral
√ widening of epiphyseal plate + slight irregularity of
  margins
√ irregularity + rarefaction of metaphysis of femoral neck
√ blurring of junction between metaphysis and epiphysis

√ posteromedial displacement (frogleg view)

ESSENTIAL OSTEOLYSIS
Progressive, slow, bone-resorptive disease
Histo: proliferation + hyperplasia of smooth muscle cells
           of synovial arterioles
√ progressive osteolysis of carpal + tarsal bones
√ thinned pointed proximal ends of metacarpals +
  metatarsals
√ elbows show same type of destruction
√ bathyrocephalic depression of base of skull
DDx:
  (1) Massive osteolysis = Gorham disease (local
      destuction of contiguous bones, usually not affecting
      hands / feet) (2) Tabes dorsalis (3) Leprosy
  (4) Syringomyelia (5) Scleroderma (6) Raynaud disease
  (7) Regional post-traumatic osteolysis (8) Ulcero-
      mutilating acropathy (9) Mutilating forms of rheumatoid
      arthritis (10) Acrodinia mutilante (nonhereditary)

EWING SARCOMA
  = EWING TUMOR = 4 – 10% of all bone tumors (less
    common than osteo- / chondrosarcoma)
Histo:
    small round cells, uniformly sized + solidly packed (DDx:
    lymphoma, osteosarcoma, myeloma, neuroblastoma,
    carcinoma, eosinophilic granuloma) invading medullary
    cavity and entering subperiosteum via Haversian canals
    producing periostitis, soft tissue mass, osteolysis;
    glycogen granules present (DDx to reticulum cell
    sarcoma); absence of alkaline phosphatase (DDx to
    osteosarcoma)
Age: peak 15 years (range 5 months – 54 years); in 30%
        < 10 years; in 39% 11 – 15 years; in 31% > 15
        years; in 50% < 20 years; in 95% 4 – 25 years;
        M:F = 3:2; caucasians in 96%
- severe localized pain
- soft tissue mass
- fever, leukocytosis, anemia (in early metastases)
  simulating infection
Location:
  (a) limb bones in 40%: humerus / femur (31%), tibia,
      fibula, clavicle, distal extremity (27%); lower
      extremity (50%)
  (b) flat bones in 50%: pelvis (21%), scapula, skull,
      vertebrae (4%, sacrum > lumbar > thoracic >
      cervical spine); ribs (14%; in 7% > age 10; in 30%
      < age 10); > 20 years of age predominantly in flat
      bones; < 20 years of age predominantly in
      cylindrical bones (tumor derived from red marrow)
Site: metaphyseal (59%); diaphyseal (35%); no
        involvement of epiphysis (originates in medullary
        cavity with invasion of Haversian system)
√ long lytic lesion in shaft of long bone (62% lytic, 23%
  minimally dense, 15% dense)
√ mottled destructive permeative lesion (72%) (late)
√ penetration into soft tissue (55%) with preservation of
  tissue planes (DDx: osteomyelitis with diffuse soft tissue
  swelling)

√ early fusiform lamellated "onion-peel" periosteal reaction (53%) / spiculated = "sunburst" / "hair-on-end" (23%), Codman triangle
√ cortical thickening (16%)
√ cortical destruction (18%)
√ cortical sequestration may occur
√ reactive sclerotic new bone (30%)
√ bone expansion (12%)
Cx: pathologic fracture (5 – 14%)
Metastases to lung + bones: in 11 – 30% at time of diagnosis, in 40 – 45% within 2 years of diagnosis
Prognosis: 60% 5-year survival
DDx:
(1) Multiple myeloma (older age group)
(2) Osteomyelitis (duration of pain < 2 weeks)
(3) Eosinophilic granuloma (solid periosteal reaction)
(4) Osteosarcoma (ossification in soft tissue, near age 20, no lamellar periosteal reaction)
(5) Reticulum cell sarcoma (clinically healthy, between 30 and 50 years, no glycogen)
(6) Neuroblastoma (< age 5)
(7) Anaplastic metastatic carcinoma (> 30 years of age)

EXTRAMEDULLARY HEMATOPOIESIS
Causes: prolonged erythrocyte deficiency due to
(1) destruction of RBC:
congenital hemolytic anemia, sickle cell anemia, idiopathic severe anemia, erythroblastosis fetalis
(2) inability of normal blood-forming organs to produce erythrocytes: myelofibrosis, polycythemia, leukemia, Hodgkin disease, carcinomatosis
• absence of pain, bone erosion, calcification
Sites: in areas of fetal erythropoiesis = liver, spleen, adrenal, heart, thymus, lung, lymphnodes, renal pelvis, gastrointestinal lymphatics, dura mater (falx cerebri and over brain convexity)
@ Chest:
√ paraspinal masses with round + lobulated margins between T8 and T12, may be bilateral
√ extramedullary hematopoiesis may compress cord

FARBER DISEASE
= DISSEMINATED LIPOGRANULOMATOSIS
Histo: foam cell granulomas; lipid storage of neuronal tissue (accumulation of ceramide + gangliosides)
• hoarse weak cry
• swelling of extremities; generalized joint swelling
• subcutaneous + periarticular granulomas
• intermittent fever, dyspnea
• lymphadenopathy
√ capsular distension of multiple joints (hand, elbow, knee)
√ juxtaarticular bone erosions from soft tissue granulomas
√ subluxation / dislocation
√ disuse / steroid deossification
Prognosis: death from respiratory failure within 2 years

FANCONI ANEMIA
= autosomal recessive disease with severe hypoplastic anemia + skin pigmentation + skeletal and urogenital anomalies
• skin pigmentation (melanin deposits) in 74% (trunk, axilla, groin, neck)
• anemia onset between 17 months and 22 years of age
• bleeding tendency (pancytopenia)
• hypogonadism (40%)
• microphthalmia (20%)

√ anomalies of radial component of upper extremity (strongly suggestive): absent / hypolastic / supernumerary thumb; hypoplastic / absent radius; absent / hypoplastic navicular / greater multangular bone
√ slight / moderate dwarfism
√ minimal microcephaly
√ renal anomalies (30%): renal aplasia, ectopia, horseshoe kidney
Prognosis: fatal within 5 years after onset of anemia; patient's family shows high incidence of leukemia

FIBROCHONDROGENESIS
= autosomal recessive lethal short limb skeletal dysplasia
Incidence: 5 cases
√ severe micromelia + broad dumbbell-shaped metaphyses
√ flat + clefted pear-shaped vertebral bodies
√ short + cupped ribs
√ frontal bossing
√ low set abnormally formed ears
Prognosis: stillbirth / death shortly after birth
DDx: (1) Thanatophoric dysplasia
(2) Metatropic dysplasia
(3) Spondyloepiphyseal dysplasia

FIBROSARCOMA
Incidence: 4% of all primary bone neoplasm
Etiology:
A. PRIMARY FIBROSARCOMA (70%)
B. SECONDARY FIBROSARCOMA (30%)
1. following radiotherapy of giant cell tumor / lymphoma / breast cancer
2. underlying benign lesion: Paget disease (common); giant cell tumor, bone infarct, osteomyelitis, desmoplastic fibroma, enchondroma, fibrous dysplasia (rare)
3. dedifferentiation of low grade chondrosarcoma
Histo: spectrum of well to poorly differentiated fibrous tissue proliferation; will not produce osteoid / chondroid / osseous matrix
Age: predominantly in 3rd – 5th decade (range of 8 – 88 years); M:F = 1:1
Metastases to: lung, lymph nodes
• localized painful mass

Location: tubular bones in young, flat bones in older
            patients; femur (40%), tibia (16%) (about knee
            in 30 – 50%), jaw, pelvis (9%); rare in small
            bones of hand + feet or spinal column
Site: eccentric at diaphyseal-metaphyseal junction into
        metaphysis; intramedullary / periosteal

A. CENTRAL FIBROSARCOMA
   = intramedullary
   √ well-defined lucent bone lesion
   √ thin expanded cortex
   √ aggressive osteolysis with geographic / ragged /
      permeative bone destruction + wide zone of
      transition
   √ occasionally large osteolytic lesion with cortical
      destruction, periosteal reaction + soft-tissue
      invasion
   √ sequestration of bone may be present (DDx:
      eosinophilic granuloma, bacterial granuloma)
   √ sparse periosteal proliferation (uncommon)
   √ intramedullary discontinuous spread
   √ no calcification
   DDx: malignant fibrous histiocytoma, myeloma,
            telangiectatic osteosarcoma, lymphoma,
            desmoplastic fibroma, osteolytic metastasis

B. PERIOSTEAL FIBROSARCOMA
   = rare tumor arising from periosteal connective tissue
   Location: long bones of lower extremity, jaw
   √ contour irregularity of cortical border
   √ periosteal reaction with perpendicular bone
      formation may be present
   √ rarely extension into medullary cavity

Cx: pathologic fracture (uncommon)
Prognosis: 20% 10-year survival
DDx: (1) Osteolytic osteosarcoma (2nd – 3rd decade)
        (2) Chondrosarcoma (usually contains
             characteristic calcifications)
        (3) Aneurysmal bone cyst (eccentric blown-out
             appearance with rapid progression)
        (4) Malignant giant cell tumor (begins in
             metaphysis extending towards joint)

FIBROUS CORTICAL DEFECT
Incidence: 30% of children; M:F = 2:1
Age: peak age of 7 – 8 years (range of 2 – 10 years);
         mostly before epiphyseal closure
Histo: fibrous tissue from periosteum invading
           underlying cortex
• asymptomatic
Location: metaphyseal cortex of long bone; posterior
            medial aspect of distal femur, proximal tibia,
            proximal femur, proximal humerus, ribs, ilium,
            fibula
√ round when small, average diameter of 1 – 2 cm
√ oval, extending parallel to long axis of host bone
√ cortical thinning + expansion may occur
√ smooth, well-defined / scalloped margins
√ larger lesions are multilocular
√ involution over 2 – 4 years

Prognosis:
(a) potential to grow and encroach on the medullary
     cavity leading to non-ossifying fibroma
(b) bone islands of the adult may be residue of
     incompletely involuted cortical defect

FIBROUS DYSPLASIA
= LICHTENSTEIN-JAFFE DISEASE
= benign fibro-osseous developmental anomaly of
  unknown origin
Age: 1st – 2nd decade (highest incidence between 3 and
         15 years), 75% before age 30; progresses until
         growth ceases; M=F
Histo: medullary cavity replaced by myxofibrous +
           woven bone trabeculae containing spindle cells
           and fluid-filled cysts
monostotic:polyostotic = 3:1
Types:
   A. <u>MONOSTOTIC FORM</u> (85%)
      • mostly asymptomatic
      Location: ribs (28%), proximal femur (23%),
                craniofacial bones (20%)
   B. <u>POLYOSTOTIC FORM</u> (15%)
      Age: mean age of 8 years
      Location: unilateral predominance (uncommon)
      • 2/3 symptomatic by age 10
      • leg pain, limp, pathologic fracture (75%)
      • abnormal vaginal bleeding (25%)
      Location: femur (91%), tibia (81%), pelvis (78%),
                foot (73%), ribs, skull, upper extremities,
                lumbar spine (14%), clavicle (10%),
                cervical spine (7%)
      √ leg length discrepancy (70%)
      √ shepherd's crook deformity (35%)
      √ facial asymmetry
      √ tibial bowing
      √ rub deformity
   C. CRANIOFACIAL FORM = LEONTIASIS OSSEA
      involved in 30% of monostotic form / in 50% of
      polyostotic form / isolated
      √ unilateral overgrowth of facial bones + calvarium
         (NO extracranial lesions)
      Cx: neurologic deficit secondary to narrowed
              cranial foramina
   D. CHERUBISM (special variant)
      = autosomal dominant disorder of variable
        penetrance
      Age: childhood; more severe in males
      √ symmetric involvement of mandible + maxilla
      Prognosis: regression after adolescence

May be associated with
(a) endocrine disorders:
    — precocious puberty in girls
    — hyperthyroidism
    — hyperparathyroidism
    — acromegaly
    — diabetes mellitus
    — Cushing syndrome

(b) soft-tissue myxoma (rare): typically multiple
intramuscular lesions

VARIANT: McCune-Albright Syndrome (10%)
(1) polyostotic unilateral fibrous dysplasia
(2) "coast of Maine" café-au-lait spots (35%)
(3) endocrine dysfunction: precocious puberty in
females (20%), hyperthyroidism

- swelling + tenderness
- limp, pain (± pathologic fracture)
- increased alkaline phosphatase
- advanced skeletal + somatic maturation (early)
- coast of Maine café-au-lait spots = yellowish / brownish
patches of cutaneous pigmentation with irregular /
serrated border, predominantly on back of trunk (30 –
50%), often ipsilateral to bone lesions (DDx: "coast of
California" spots of neurofibromatosis)

Common location:
rib cage (30%), craniofacial bones (calvarium, mandible)
(25%), femoral neck + tibia (25%), pelvis

Site: metaphysis primary site with extension into
diaphysis (rarely entire length of bone)

√ normal bone architecture altered + remodelled
√ lesions in medullary cavity: radiolucent / ground glass /
increased density
√ trabeculated appearance due to reinforced
subperiosteal bone ridges in wall of lesion
√ expansion of bones (ribs, skull, long bones)
√ well-defined sclerotic margin of reactive bone = rind
√ endosteal scalloping with thinned / lost cortex (ribs, long
bones)
√ lesion may undergo calcification + enchondral bone
formation = fibrocartilaginous dysplasia
√ increased activity on bone scan during early perfusion +
on delayed images

@ Skull
- skull deformity with cranial nerve compromise
- proptosis

Location: frontal bone > sphenoid bone; hemicranial
involvement (DDx: Paget disease is
bilateral)
√ sclerotic skull base, may narrow neural foramina
(visual + hearing loss)
√ widened diploe with displacement of outer table,
inner table spared (DDx: Paget disease, inner table
involved)
√ obliteration of sphenoid + frontal sinuses due to
encroachment by fibrous dysplastic bone
√ inferolateral displacement of orbit
√ sclerosis of orbital plate + small orbit + hypoplasia of
frontal sinuses (DDx: Paget disease, meningioma
en plaque)
√ occipital thickening
√ cystic calvarial lesions, commonly crossing sutures
√ mandibular cystic lesion (very common)
= osteocementoma, ossifying fibroma

@ Pelvis + Ribs
√ cystic lesions (extremely common)

√ protrusio acetabuli
@ Extremities
- short stature as adult (late) / dwarfism
√ premature fusion of ossification centers
√ epiphysis rarely affected before closure of growth
plate
√ bowing deformities + discrepant limb length (tibia,
femur)
√ "shepherd's crook" deformity of femoral neck = coxa
vara
√ pseudarthrosis in infancy = osteofibrous dysplasia
(DDx: neurofibromatosis)

Cx:
(1) Transformation into osteo- / chondro- /
fibrosarcoma or malignant fibrous histiocytoma
(0.5 – 1%, more often in polyostotic form)
- increasing pain
√ enlarging soft-tissue mass
√ previously mineralized lesion turns lytic
(2) Pathologic fractures

DDx:
(1) HPT (chemical changes, generalized
deossification, subperiosteal resorption)
(2) Neurofibromatosis (rarely osseous lesions, cystic
intraosseous neurofibroma rare, café-au-lait spots
smooth, familial disease)
(3) Paget disease (histological mosaic pattern,
radiographically identical to monostotic cranial
lesion)
(4) Osteofibrous dysplasia (almost exclusively in tibia
of infants, monostotic, lesion begins in cortex)
(5) Nonossifying fibroma
(6) Simple bone cyst
(7) Giant cell tumor (no sclerotic margin)
(8) Enchondromatosis
(9) Eosinophilic granuloma
(10) Osteoblastoma
(11) Hemangioma
(12) Meningioma

FIBROUS HISTIOCYTOMA
Benign Fibrous Histiocytoma
Incidence: 0.1% of all bone tumors
Histo: interlacing bundles of fibrous tissue in storiform
pattern (whorled / woven) interspersed with
mono- / multinucleated cells resembling
histiocytes, benign giant cells, and lipid-laden
macrophages; resembles nonossifying fibroma
/ fibroxanthoma
Age: 23 – 60 years
- localized intermittently painful soft-tissue swelling
Location: long bone, pelvis, vertebra (rare)
Site: typically in epiphysis / epiphyseal equivalent
√ well-defined radiolucent lesion with septae / soap-
bubble appearance / no definable matrix
√ may have reactive sclerotic rim
√ narrow transition zone (= nonaggressive lesion)
√ no periosteal reaction

Rx: curretage
DDx: nonossifying fibroma (childhood / adolescence, asymptomatic, eccentric metaphyseal location)

Atypical Benign Fibrous Histiocytoma
Histo: "atypical / aggressive" features = mitotic figures present
√ lytic defect with irregular edges
Prognosis: may metastasize

FRACTURE
NUC:

Typical time course:
1. Acute phase (3 – 4 weeks)
   abnormal in 80% < 24 hours, in 95% < 72 hours
   Δ elderly patients show delayed appearance of positive scan
   √ broad area of increased tracer uptake (wider than fracture line)
2. Subacute phase (2 – 3 months) = time of most intense tracer accumulation
   √ more focal increased tracer uptake corresponding to fracture line
3. Chronic phase (1 – 2 years)
   √ slow decline in tracer accumulation
   √ in 65% normal after 1 year; > 95% normal after 3 years
Return to normal:
Δ rib fractures return to normal most rapidly
Δ complicated fractures with orthopedic fixation devices take longest to return to normal
1. Simple fractures   : 90% normal by 2 years
2. Open reduction / fixation : < 50% normal by 3 years
3. Delayed union   : slower than normal for type of fracture
4. Nonunion   : persistent intense uptake in 80%
5. Complicated union (true pseudarthrosis, soft tissue interposition, impaired blood supply, presence of infection)
   √ intense uptake at fracture ends
   √ decreased uptake at fracture site
6. Vertebral compression fractures: 60% normal by 1 year; 90% by 2 years; 97% by 3 years

Stress fracture
A. INSUFFICIENCY FRACTURE = normal physiologic stress applied to bone with abnormal elastic resistance / deficient mineralization
    Cause: 1. Osteoporosis
               2. Rheumatoid arthritis
               3. Osteomalacia / rickets
               4. Paget disease
               5. Hyperparathyroidism
               6. Renal osteodystrophy
               7. Radiation therapy
               8. Steroid induced osteopenia
    Location: lower extremity, sacrum, ilium, pubic bone

B. FATIGUE FRACTURE = abnormal muscular stress applied to bone with normal elastic resistance
    1. **Clay shoveler's fracture**: spinous process of lower cervical / upper thoracic spine
    2. **Clavicle**: postoperative (radical neck dissection)
    3. **Coracoid process of scapula**: trap shooting
    4. **Ribs**: carrying heavy pack, golf, coughing
    5. **Distal shaft of humerus**: throwing ball
    6. **Coronoid process of ulna**: pitching ball, throwing javelin, pitchfork work, propelling wheelchairs
    7. **Hook of hamate**: swinging golf club / tennis raquet / baseball bat
    8. **Spondylolysis** = pars interarticularis of lumbar vertebrae: ballet, lifting heavy objects, scrubbing floors
    9. **Femoral neck**: ballet, long-distance running
    10. **Femoral shaft**: ballet, marching, long-distance running, gymnastics
    11. **Obturator ring of pelvis**: stooping, bowling, gymnastics
    12. **Patella**: hurdling
    13. **Tibial shaft**: ballet, joggers
    14. **Fibula**: long-distance running, jumping, parachuting
    15. **Calcaneus**: jumping, parachuting, prolonged standing, recent immobilization
    16. **Navicular**: stomping on ground, marching, prolonged standing, ballet
    17. **Metatarsal**: marching, stomping on ground, prolonged standing, ballet, postoperative bunionectomy
    18. **Sesamoids of metatarsal**:   prolonged standing
X-Ray:
   (a) compression fracture in cancellous bone (notoriously difficult to detect)
   (b) distraction fracture in compact bone
   √ sclerosis due to trabecular compression + callus formation
   √ lucency through cortex / focal area of sclerosis (early)
   √ solid thick lamellar periosteal + endosteal reaction (later)
MRI:
   Signal intensity pattern consistent with edema in soft tissue adjacent to fracture + in subperiosteal space.
   √ diminished marrow signal intensity on T1WI
   √ increased marrow signal intensity on T2WI
NUC:
   √ positive bone scan 3 – 4 weeks prior to radiographic abnormality
   √ focal fusiform area of increased tracer accumulation
DDx: (1) Shin splints
              √ long linear uptake on posterior tibial cortex where soleus muscle insertion pulls on periosteum
        (2) Osteoid osteoma (eccentric, without periosteal reaction)

(3) Chronic sclerosing osteomyelitis (dense, sclerotic, involving entire circumference)
(4) Osteomalacia (looser zones, smudged appearance of trabeculae)
(5) Osteogenic sarcoma (metaphyseal, aggressive periosteal reaction)
(6) Ewing tumor (lytic destructive appearance)

Epiphyseal Plate Injury

Mechanism: 80% shearing force; 20% compression
Resistance to trauma: ligament > bone > physis
<u>Salter-Harris classification</u> (considering probability of growth disturbance)
Type I (5 – 6%)
= slip of epiphysis due to shearing force separating epiphysis from physis
√ growth plate involvement only
(includes: apophyseal avulsion, slipped capital femoral epiphysis)
Prognosis: good
Type II (50 – 75%)
= shearing force splits growth plate, fracture line extends into metaphysis
Prognosis: good
Type III (8%)
= intra-articular fracture
√ epiphysis split vertically
Prognosis: fair (imprecise reduction leads to alteration in linearity of articular plane)
Type IV (8 – 12%)
√ fracture involves metaphysis + physis + epiphysis
Prognosis: guarded (germinal cells of physis usually injured)
Type V (1%)
= crush injury with injury to vascular supply
√ no fracture line (diagnosis difficult + often made retrospectively)
Prognosis: poor (impairment of growth)
Cx:
(1) progressive angular deformity from segmental arrest of germinal zone growth
(2) limb length discrepancy from total cessation of growth
(3) articular incongruity from disruption of articular surface

Apophyseal injury

Physis under secondary ossification center is weakest part.
Mechanism: avulsive force
Location: tibial tubercle, ischial apophysis, lesser trochanter of femur, anterior superior + anterior inferior iliac spine, iliac crest

Hand fracture

Bennett Fracture

Mechanism: forced abduction of thumb
√ intraarticular fracture / dislocation of base of 1st metacarpal
√ small fragment of metacarpal continues to articulate with trapezium
√ lateral retraction of metacarpal shaft by abductor pollicis longus
Rx: anatomic reduction important, difficult to keep in anatomic alignment
Cx: pseudarthrosis

Boxer's Fracture

Mechanism: direct blow with clenched fist
√ transverse fracture of distal metacarpal (usually 5th)

Gamekeeper's Thumb

= SKIER'S THUMB
Mechanism: hyperextension of ulnar collateral ligament in 1st MCP (faulty handling of ski pole)
√ disruption of ulnar collateral ligament of 1st MCP joint
√ stress examination necessary to document ligament damage

Navicular fracture

Mechanism: fall on outstretched hand
Location: 80% through waist of navicular
Cx: avascular necrosis of proximal fragment (blood supply derived from distal part)

Rolando fracture

√ comminuted intraarticular fracture through base of thumb

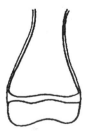 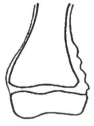 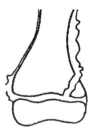 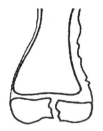 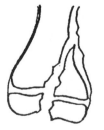 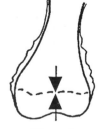

| normal | Type 1 | Type 2 | Type 3 | Type 4 | Type 5 |

Salter-Harris classification of epiphyseal plate injuries

Prognosis: worse than Bennett's fracture (difficult to reduce)

Forearm fracture

Barton Fracture
Mechanism: fall on outstretched hand
√ intraarticular oblique fracture of dorsal lip of distal radius
√ carpus dislocates with distal fragment up and back on radius

Chauffer Fracture
Mechanism: acute dorsiflexion + abduction of hand
√ triangular fracture of radial styloid process

Colles Fracture
Most common fracture in this region
Mechanism: fall on outstretched hand
√ radial fracture in distal 2 cm ± ulnar styloid fracture
√ dorsal displacement of distal fragment
√ "silver-fork" deformity
Cx: posttraumatic arthritis
Rx: anatomic reduction important

Galeazzi Fracture
Mechanism: fall on outstretched hand with elbow flexed
√ radial fracture in distal third + subluxation / dislocation of distal radioulnar joint
√ dorsal angulation
Cx: (1) high incidence of nonunion, delayed union, malunion (unstable fracture)
      (2) limitation of pronation / supination

Smith Fracture
= REVERSE COLLES FRACTURE
Mechanism: hyperflexion with fall on back of hand
√ distal radial fracture
√ ventral displacement of fragment
√ radial deviation of hand
√ "garden spade" deformity
Cx: altered function of carpus

Monteggia Fracture
Mechanism: fall on outstretched hand with elbow flexed
√ anteriorly angulated proximal ulnar fracture + anterior dislocation of radiohumeral joint
√ may have associated wrist injury
Cx: nonunion, limitation of motion at elbow, nerve abnormalities
REVERSE MONTEGGIA FRACTURE = dorsally angulated proximal ulnar fracture + posterior dislocation of radial head

Pelvic Fracture

Malgaigne Fracture
Mechanism: direct trauma

• shortening of involved extremity
√ vertical fractures through one side of pelvic ring
   (1) superior to acetabulum
   (2) inferior to acetabulum
   (3) ± sacroiliac dislocation / fracture

Bucket Handle Fracture
√ double vertical fracture through superior and inferior pubic rami + sacroiliac joint dislocation on contralateral side

Foot fracture

Ankle Fracture
Incidence: ankle injuries account for 10% of all emergency room visits; 85% of all ankle sprains involve lateral ligaments
Ligamentous connections at ankle:
   (a) binding tibia + fibula
     1. anterior inferior tibiofibular ligament (= tibiofibular syndesmosis)
     2. posterior inferior tibiofibular ligament
     3. transverse tibiofibular ligament
     4. interosseous membrane
   (b) lateral malleolus
     85% of all ankle sprains involve these ligaments:
     1. anterior talofibular ligament
     2. posterior talofibular ligament
     3. calcaneofibular ligament
   (c) medial malleolus = deltoid ligament with
     1. navicular portion
     2. sustentaculum portion
     3. talar portion

A. SUPINATION-ADDUCTION
   = INVERSION-ADDUCTION INJURY
   Mechanism: (1) avulsive forces affect lateral ankle structures
              (2) impactive forces secondary to talar shift stress medial structures
   √ sprain / rupture of lateral collateral ligament
   √ transverse avulsion of malleolus sparing tibiofibular ligaments
   √ oblique fracture of medial malleolus ± posterior lip fracture

B. SUPINATION-ABDUCTION
   = EVERSION / EXTERNAL ROTATION
   Mechanism: (1) avulsive forces on medial structures
              (2) impacting forces on lateral - structures (talar impact)
   √ lateral subluxation of talus
   √ oblique / spiral fracture of lateral malleolus
   √ partial disruption of tibiofibular ligament
   √ sprain / rupture / avulsion of deltoid ligament
   √ transverse fracture of medial malleolus

(a) **Pott Fracture**
√ fracture of fibula above an intact tibiofibular ligament
(b) **Dupuytren Fracture**
√ fracture of fibula above a disrupted tibiofibular ligament
C. PRONATION-EXTERNAL ROTATION
= EVERSION + EXTERNAL ROTATION
√ tear of tibiofibular ligament / avulsion of anterior tubercle (Tillaux-Chaput) / avulsion of posterior tubercle (Volkmann)
√ tear of interosseous membrane = lateral instability
√ fibular fracture higher than ankle joint --- (Maisonneuve fracture if around knee)

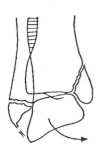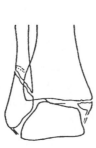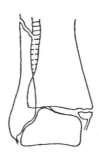

| supination-adduction | supination-abduction | pronation-external rotation |

Jones Fracture
Mechanism: plantar flexion + inversion (stepping off a curb)
√ transverse avulsion fracture of base of 5th --- metatarsal (insertion of peroneus brevis tendon)

Lisfranc Fracture
Mechanism: metatarsal heads fixed and hindfoot forced plantarwards and into rotation
√ fracture / dislocation of tarsometatarsal joints

FREIBERG DISEASE
= osteochondrosis of head of 2nd metatarsal
Age: 10 – 15 years; girls
√ compression of 2nd metatarsal head

FROSTBITE
CHILD
√ destruction of phalangeal epiphyses + DIP
√ shortening + deformity of fingers
ADULT
√ osteoporosis (4 – 10 weeks after injury)
√ acromutilation (secondary to osteomyelitis + surgical removal)
√ small round punched-out areas near edge of joint
√ periostitis
Rx: selective angiography with intraarterial reserpine

GARDNER SYNDROME
= autosomal dominant syndrome characterized by (1) osteomas (2) soft tissue tumors (3) colonic polyps
Location of osteomas: paranasal sinuses; outer table of skull (frequent); mandible (at angle)
√ endosteal cortical thickening / osteomas in any bone
√ may have solid periosteal cortical thickening
√ osteomas / exostoses may protrude from periosteal surface
√ wavy cortical thickening of superior aspect of ribs
√ polyps: colon, stomach, duodenum, ampulla of Vater, small intestine
Cx: high incidence of carcinoma of duodenum / ampulla of Vater

GAUCHER DISEASE
= rare autosomal recessive disorder / dominant (in a few), common among Ashkenazi Jews
Etiology: deficiency of lysosomal hydrolase acid ß-glycosidase leads to accumulation of glucosyl ceramide within cells of RES
Histo: bone-marrow aspirate shows Gaucher cells (kerasin-laden histiocytes)
Types: (1) rapidly fatal infantile form (2) adult form
• hepatosplenomegaly, impairment of liver function, ascites
• anemia, leukopenia, thrombocytopenia
• hemochromatosis (yellowish-brown pigmentation of conjunctiva + skin)
• dull bone pain; bone involvement in 75%
Location: distal femur, pelvis, other long bones
√ generalized osteopenia (decrease in trabecular bone density)
√ striking cortical thinning + bone widening
√ Erlenmeyer flask deformity of distal femur
√ numerous sharply circumscribed lytic lesions resembling metastases / multiple myeloma (marrow replacement)
√ periosteal reaction = cloaking
√ weakening of subchondral bone + degenerative arthritis
√ bone infarction in long bone metaphyses (common)
√ H-shaped / "step-off" / biconcave "fish mouth" vertebra
√ aseptic necrosis of femoral head, humeral head, wrist, ankle (common)
Cx: (> 90% with orthopedic complications at some time)
(1) pathologic fractures + compression fractures of vertebrae
(2) osteomyelitis (increased incidence)
(3) myelosclerosis in long-standing disease

GIANT CELL REPARATIVE GRANULOMA
= GIANT CELL REACTION
Histo: numerous giant cells in exuberant fibrous matrix, osteoid formation, areas of hemorrhage
Peak age: 2nd + 3rd decade (range from childhood to 76 years); M:F = 1:1
Location: mandible, maxilla, small bones of hand + feet

- pain + mass in affected bone
√ expansile lytic defect with thinning of overlying cortex
√ periosteal reaction may be present
√ soft tissue swelling / extension beyond cortex
√ no matrix calcification
Cx: pathologic fracture
Rx: currettage (50% recurrence rate) / local excision
DDx: (1) Enchondroma (same location, matrix
             calcification)
        (2) Aneurysmal bone cyst (rare in small bones of
             hand + feet, typically prior to epiphyseal
             closure)
        (3) Giant cell tumor (more aggressive appearance)
        (4) Infection (clinical)
        (5) Brown tumor of HPT (periosteal bone
             resorption, abnormal Ca + P levels)

GIANT CELL TUMOR
= OSTEOCLASTOMA
Incidence: 4.2% of all primary bone tumors
Histo: multinucleated giant cells within fibroid stroma
           (giant cells characteristic of all reactive bone
           disease, seen in pigmented villonodular synovitis,
           benign chondroblastoma, nonosteogenic fibroma,
           chondromyxoid fibroma)
Age: after epiphyseal plate fusion; 14% < age 20;
         65% between 20 and 40 years; M:F = 1:1
Location:
  (a) 85% in long bones: distal end of femur, proximal
       end of tibia (50 – 60% about knee), distal end of
       radius, proximal end of humerus
  (b) 15% in flat bones: pelvis, sacrum near SIJ
       (common — 2nd to chordoma), spine (5%), rib
       (anterior / posterior end), skull
Site: eccentric in metaphysis of long bones, adjacent to /
          in ossified epiphyseal line, subarticular if epiphyseal
          plate is fused (MOST TYPICAL)
√ expansile solitary radiolucent lesion ("soap bubble"),
  large at diagnosis
√ no sclerosis / periosteal reaction (aggressive rapid
  growth)
√ may break through bone cortex with cortical thinning,
  soft tissue invasion (25%), pathologic fracture (5%)
√ destruction of vertebral body with secondary invasion of
  posterior elements
√ may cross joint space (exceedingly unusual)
Cx: 15% malignant within first 5 years (M:F = 3:1);
        metastases to lung
DDx: (1) Aneurysmal bone cyst (in posterior elements of
             spine with invasion of vertebral body)
        (2) Brown tumor of HPT (lab values)
        (3) Enchondroma (not epiphyseal)
        (4) Chondroblastoma
        (5) Chondromyxoid fibroma

GLOMUS TUMOR OF BONE
= rare benign lesion composed of cells derived from
  neuromyoarterial glomus

Age: most in 4 – 5th decade
- painful
Location: distal aspect of terminal phalanx of finger
√ resembles enchondroma

GOUT
= deposition of positively birefringent monosodium urate
  monohydrate crystals in poorly vascularized tissues
  (synovial membranes, articular cartilage, ligaments,
  bursae) leading to destruction of cartilage
Age: > 40 years; males (in women gout may occur after
         menopause)
Causes:
  A. Idiopathic Gout
     (1) Overproduction of uric acid (phophoribosyl
          transferase deficiency)
     (2) Abnormality of renal urate excretion
     Incidence: 0.3%; M:F = 20:1
  B. Secondary Gout
     (1) Myeloproliferative disorders + sequelae of their
          treatment: polycythemia vera, leukemia,
          lymphoma, multiple myeloma
     (2) Blood dyscrasias
     (3) Endocrinologic:
          myxedema, hyperparathyroidism
     (4) Chronic renal failure
     (5) Enzyme defects: glycogen storage disease
     (6) Vascular: myocardial infarction, hypertension
     (7) Lead poisoning
Location:
  (a) joints: hands + feet (1st MTP joint most commonly
       affected = podagra), elbow, wrist (carpometacarpal
       compartment especially common), knee, shoulder,
       hip, sacroiliac joint (15%, unilateral)
  (b) ear, tendon, bursae
Stages:
  (1) asymptomatic hyperuricemia
  (2) acute monarticular gout
  (3) polyarticular gout
  (4) large multiple urate deposits
√ calcific deposits in gouty tophi in 50% (sodium urate
  crystals not radiopaque, only after calcium deposition)
√ juxtaarticular lobulated soft issue masses (hands +
  feet)
√ "overhanging margin" = elevated osseous spicule in
  sites of tophus formation associated with erosion of
  adjacent bone (in intra- and extraarticular locations)
  (HALLMARK)
√ erosion of joint margins (resembling rheumatoid arthritis)
  but with sclerosis
√ round / oval subarticular cysts up to 3 cm
√ preservation of joint space (important clue!)
√ absence of periarticular demineralization (DDx:
  rheumatoid arthritis)
√ cartilage destruction (late)
√ periarticular swelling
√ chondrocalcinosis (menisci, articular cartilage of knee)
√ bilateral effusion of bursae olecrani
  (PATHOGNOMONIC)

√ aural calcification
√ ischemic necrosis of femoral / humeral heads
√ bone infarction due to deposits at vascular basement
  membrane (DDx: bone island)
Coexisting disorders:
  1. Psoriasis
  2. Glycogen storage disease Type I
  3. Hypo- and hyperparathyroidism
  4. Down syndrome
  5. Lesch-Nyhan syndrome (choreaatetosis, spasticity,
     mental retardation, self-mutilation of lips + fingers tips)
     NOT associated with rheumatoid arthritis
Rx: colchicine, allopurinol

HEMANGIOENDOTHELIAL SARCOMA
= ANGIOSARCOMA = HEMANGIOENDOTHELIOMA
= HEMANGIOEPITHELIOMA
Histo: irregular anastomosing vascular channels lined
         by one / several layers of atypical anaplastic
         endothelial cells
Age: 4th − 5th decade; M:F = 2:1
• history of trauma / irradiation
Location: femur, tibia, humerus, pelvis, skull; multicentric
            lesions in 30% often with regional distribution
            (less aggressive)
√ eccentric lesion in metaphysis of long bones
√ osteolytic aggressively destructive area with indistinct
  margins (high grade)
√ well-demarcated margins with scattered bony trabeculae
  (low grade)
√ osteoblastic in vertebrae, contigious through several
  vertebrae
Metastases to: lung (early)
Prognosis: 26% 5-year survival rate
DDx: Aneurysmal bone cyst, poorly differentiated
       fibrosarcoma, highly vascular metastasis, alveolar
       rhabdomyosarcoma

HEMANGIOMA OF BONE
Incidence: 10%
Histo: mostly cavernous; capillary type is rare
Age: 4th − 5th decade; M:F = 1:2
Location: (a) vertebral body in lower thoracic / upper
                 lumbar spine
            (b) calvarium with predilection for frontal bone
@ VERTEBRA (30%)
  Incidence: 11% (autopsy)
  Age: > 40 years; female
  √ "accordion" / "corduroy" / "honeycomb" vertebra
    = exaggerated vertical trabeculae (also in multiple
    myeloma, lymphoma, metastasis)
  √ posterior bulge of cortex
  √ extraosseous extension beyond bony lesion (with
    cord compression)
  √ paravertebral soft tissue extension
  MRI:
    √ mottled pattern of increased intensity on
      T1WI + T2WI (increase in adipose tissue)

Cx: vertebral collapse (unusual), spinal cord
      compression
@ Calvarium
  √ < 4 cm round osteolytic lesion
  √ sunburst appearance without definite margin
  √ may occur in diploe, producing palpable lump
    secondary to widening of diploe
@ Flat bones & long bones (rare)
  ribs, clavicle, mandible, zygoma, nasal bones,
  metaphyseal ends of long bones (frequently capillary
  type of hemangioma)

HEMANGIOPERICYTOMA
= borderline tumor with benign / locally aggressive /
  malignant behavior (counterpart of glomus tumor)
Age: 4th − 5th decade
Location: lower extremities, vertebrae, pelvis, skull (dura
            similar to meningioma)
√ osteolytic lesions in metaphysis of long bone / flat bone
√ subperiosteal large blowout lesion (similar to
  aneurysmal bone cyst)
Angio:
  √ displacement of main artery
  √ pedicle of tumor feeder arteries
  √ spider-shaped arrangement of vessels encircling
    tumor
  √ small corkscrew arteries
  √ dense tumor stain

HEMOCHROMATOSIS
1. <u>PRIMARY HEMOCHROMATOSIS</u>
   = autosomal recessive / indeterminate inheritance
     (abnormal iron loading gene) in thalassemia,
     sideroblastic anemia
2. <u>SECONDARY HEMOCHROMATOSIS</u>
   = excessive iron absorption in anemias, myelofibrosis,
     portocaval shunt, exogenous administration of iron,
     porphyria cutanea tarda, beer brewed in iron vessels
     + deposition of excessive iron in liver, pancreas,
     spleen, GI-tract, kidney, gonads, heart, endocrine
     glands (pituitary, hypothalamus)
Age: > age 40 years; M:F = 10:1 (females protected by
       menstruation)
• cirrhosis
• "bronzed diabetes"
• congestive heart failure
• skin pigmentation
• hypogonadism
• arthritic symptoms (30%)
• increase in serum iron
Site: most commonly in hands (metacarpal heads,
        particularly 2nd + 3rd MCP joints), carpal + proximal
        interphalangeal joints, knees, hips
√ generalized osteoporosis
√ small subchondral cystlike rarefactions with fine rim of
  sclerosis (metacarpal heads)
√ arthropathy in 50% with iron deposition in synovium
√ uniform joint space narrowing

√ enlargement of metacarpal heads
√ eventually osteophyte formation
√ chondrocalcinosis in > 60%, knees most commonly affected
  (a) calcium pyrophosphate deposition (inhibition of pyrophosphatase enzyme within cartilage which hydrolyzes pyrophosphate to soluble orthophosphate)
  (b) calcification of triangular cartilage of wrist, menisci, annulus fibrosus, ligamentum flavum, symphysis pubis, Achilles tendon, plantar fascia
Cx: hepatoma (in 30%)
Prognosis: death from CHF (30%), death from hepatic failure (25%)
DDx: (1) Pseudogout (no arthropathy)
  (2) Psoriatric arthritis (skin + nail changes)
  (3) Osteoarthritis (predominantly distal joints in hands)
  (4) Rheumatoid arthritis
  (5) Gout (may also have chondrocalcinosis)

HEMOPHILIA
= X-linked deficiency / functional abnormality of coagulation factor VIII
Incidence: 1:10,000 males
@ Hemarthrosis (most common)
  Histo: hypertrophic synovial membrane with pannus formation that erodes cartilage, loss of subchondral bone plate, formation of subarticular cysts
  • tense red warm joint with decreased range of motion (muscle spasm)
  • fever, elevated WBC (DDx: septic arthritis)
  Location: in knee, ankle, elbow
  √ soft tissue swelling of joint
  √ enlargement of epiphysis (secondary to synovial hyperemia)
  √ thinning of joint cartilage (particularly patella) secondary to cartilage destruction
  √ erosions of articular surface with multiple subcondral cysts
  √ superimposed degenerative joint disease
  √ "squared" patella
  √ widening of intercondylar notch
  √ medial "slanting" of tibiotalar joint
  √ juxtaarticular osteoporosis

@ Hemophilic pseudotumor (1%)
  √ mixed cystic expansile lesion
  √ bone erosion + pathologic fracture
  (a) juvenile form = usually multiple intramedullary expansile lesions without soft tissue mass in small bones of hand / feet (before epiphyseal closure)
  (b) adult form = usually single intramedullary expansile lesion with large soft tissue mass in ilium / femur
  (c) into soft tissues of retroperitoneum (psoas muscle), bowel wall, renal collecting system

HEREDITARY HYPERPHOSPHATASIA
= "JUVENILE PAGET DISEASE" = rare autosomal recessive disease with sustained elevation of serum alkaline phosphatase, especially in individuals of Puerto Rican descent
Histo: rapid turnover of lamellar bone without formation of cortical bone; immature woven bone is rapidly laid down, but simultaneous rapid destruction prevents normal maturation
Age: 1st – 3rd year; usually stillborn
• rapid enlargement of calvarium + long bones
• dwarfism
• cranial nerve deficit (blind, deaf)
• hypertension
• frequent respiratory infections
• pseudoxanthoma elasticum
• elevated akaline phosphatase
√ metaphyseal growth deficiency
√ wide irregular epiphyseal lines (resembling rickets in childhood), persistent metaphyseal defects (40% of adults)
√ deossification = decreased density of long bones with coarse trabecular pattern
√ widened medullary canal with cortical thinning (cortex modeled from trabecular bone)
√ bowing of long bones + fractures with irregular callus
√ skull greatly thickened with wide tables, cotton wool appearance
√ vertebra plana
OB-US: √ diagnosis suspected in utero in 20%
Cx: pathologic fractures; vertebra plana universalis
DDx: (1) Osteogenesis imperfecta
  (2) Polyostotic fibrous dysplasia
  (3) Paget disease (> age 20, not generalized)
  (4) Pyle disease (spares midshaft)
  (5) van Buchem syndrome (only diaphyses > age 20, NO long bone bowing)
  (6) Engelmann syndrome (lower limbs)

HEREDITARY MULTIPLE EXOSTOSES
= DIAPHYSEAL ACLASIS
Inheritance: autosomal dominant (unaffected female may be carrier)
Age: discovered between 2 and 10 years; M:F = 2:1
Path: ectopic cartilaginous rest in metaphysis + defect in periosteum; cap of hyaline cartilage; often bursa formation over cap
• usually painless mass near joints
• tendons, blood vessels, nerves may be impaired
• sudden painful growth spurt indicates malignancy (exostosis begins in childhood + stops growing when nearest epiphyseal center fuses)
Location: metaphyses; multiple + usually bilateral; common sites are knee, elbow, scapula, pelvis, ribs
Site: metaphyses of long bones (distance to epiphyseal line increases with growth)
√ cortex + cancellous bone of exostosis contiguous to host bone

√ slope on epiphyseal side + right angle on diaphyseal side of stalk = points away from joint
√ occasionally small punctate calcifications in cartilaginous cap
√ shortening of 4th + 5th metacarpals
√ supernumerary fingers / toes
√ Madelung / reversed Madelung deformity = radius usually longer + bowed
√ occasionally results in disproportionate shortening of an extremity, radioulnar synostosis, dislocation of radial head
Cx:
  (1) Cord compression secondary to involvement of posterior spinal elements
  (2) Malignant transformation to chondrosarcoma in < 5% (growth with irregularity of outline + fuzziness)

HEREDITARY SPHEROCYTOSIS
= autosomal dominant congenital hemolytic anemia
Age: anemia begins in early infancy to late adulthood
- rarely severe anemia
- jaundice
- spherocytes in peripheral smear
√ bone changes rare (due to mild anemia); long bones rarely affected
√ widening of diploe with displacement + thinning of outer table
√ hair-on-end appearance
Rx: splenectomy corrects anemia even though spherocytemia persists
  √ improvement in skeletal alterations following splenectomy

HERNIATION PIT
= CONVERSION DEFECT
= localized bone erosion caused by herniated synovium from adjacent joint
Histo: fibroalveolar tissue
Age: usually in older individuals
- asymptomatic
- no clinical significance
Location: superolateral aspect of proximal femoral neck
Site: subcortical
√ well-circumscribed round lucency
√ usually < 1 cm in diameter
√ reactive thin sclerotic border

HISTIOCYTOSIS X
Path: influx of eosinophilic leukocytes simulating inflammation; reticulum cells accumulate cholesterol + lipids (= foam cells); sheets or nodules of histiocytes may fuse to form giant cells, cytoplasm contains Langerhans bodies

Letterer-Siwe Disease
= acute disseminated, fulminant form of histiocytosis X
Incidence: 1: 2,000,000; 10% of histiocytosis X

Age: several weeks after birth – 2 years
Path: generalized involvement of reticulum cells; may be confused with leukemia
- hemorrhage, purpura
- severe progressive anemia
- intermittent fever
- failure to grow
√ hepatosplenomegaly + lymphadenopathy
@ Bone involvement (50%):
  √ widespread multiple lytic lesions; "raindrop" pattern in calvarium
Prognosis: 70% mortality rate

Hand-Schüller-Christian Disease
= chronic disseminated form of histiocytosis X (15 – 40%) in 10% characterized by a triad of
  (1) exophthalmus
  (2) diabetes insipidus
  (3) lytic skull lesions
Path: proliferation of histiocytes, may simulate Ewing sarcoma
Age at onset: 5 – 10 years (range of birth to 40 years); M:F = 1:1
- diabetes insipidus (30 – 50%) often with large lytic lesion in sphenoid bone
- exophthalmus (33%), sometimes with orbital wall destruction
- otitis media with mastoid + inner ear invasion
- generalized eczematoid skin lesions (30%)
- ulcers of mucous membranes
@ Bone
  √ osteolytic skull lesions with overlying soft tissue nodules
  √ "geographic skull" = ovoid / serpiginous destruction of large area
  √ "floating teeth" with mandibular involvement
  √ destruction of petrous ridge + mastoids, sella turcica, orbit
@ Soft tissue
  √ hepatosplenomegaly (rare) with scattered granuloma
  √ lymphadenopathy (may be massive)
@ Lung
  √ cyst + bleb formation with spontaneous pneumothorax (25%)
  √ ill-defined diffuse nodular infiltration often progressing to fibrosis + honeycomb lung
Prognosis: spontaneous remissions + exacerbations

Eosinophilic Granuloma
= form of histiocytosis X (60 – 80%) localized to bone
Age: 5 – 10 years (highest frequency); range 2 – 30 years; M:F = 3:2
Path: bone lesions arise within medullary canal (RES)
Location: monostotic involvement in 50 – 75%; calvarium > mandible > spine > ribs > large long bones

@ Skull (50%)
  Site: diploic space of parietal bone (most
          commonly involved) + temporal bone (petrous
          ridge, mastoid)
  √ round / ovoid punched-out area with well-defined
    border
  √ sclerotic margin during healing phase (50%)
  √ "hole-within-hole" appearance = uneven
    involvement of inner + outer table with bevelled
    edge
  √ "button sequester" = bony sequester within lytic
    lesion
  √ soft tissue mass overlying the lytic process in
    calvarium (often palpable)
@ Axial skeleton (25%)
  √ "vertebra plana" = "coin on edge" = Calvé
    disease (6%) = collapse of vertebra (most
    commonly thoracic); preserved disc space; rare
    involvement of posterior elements; no kyphosis;
    most common cause of vertebra plana in children
  √ lytic lesion in supraacetabular region
@ Proximal long bones (15%)
  • painful bone lesion
  Site: mostly diaphyseal, epiphyseal lesions are
          uncommon
  √ expansile lytic lesion with ill-defined / sclerotic
    edges
  √ erosion of cortex + soft tissue mass
  √ laminated periosteal reaction (frequent), may
    show interruptions
  √ may appear rapidly within 3 weeks
  √ lesions respect joint space + growth plate
@ Lung involvement (20%)
  Incidence: 0.05 to 0.5 / 100,000 annually
  Age: peak between 20 and 40 years
  √ 3 – 10 mm nodules
  √ reticulonodular pattern with predilection for
    apices
  √ may develop into honeycomb lung
  √ recurrent pneumothoraces (25%)
  √ rib lesions with fractures (common)
  √ pleural effusion, hilar adenopathy (unusual)
NUC:
  √ negative bone scans in 35% (radiographs more
    sensitive)
  √ bone lesions generally not Ga-67 avid
  √ Ga-67 may be helpful for detecting nonosseous
    lesions

Prognosis: excellent with spontaneous resolution of
               bone lesions in 6 – 18 months

HOLT-ORAM SYNDROME
Autosomal dominant; M < F
Associated with CHD: secundum type ASD (most
                         common), VSD, persistent left
                         SVC, Tetralogy, Coarctation
• intermittent cardiac arrhythmia
• bradycardia (50 – 60/min)
Location: upper extremity only involved; symmetry of
            lesions is the rule; left side may be more
            severely affected
√ aplasia / hypoplasia of radial structures: thumb, 1st
  metacarpal, carpal bones, radius
√ "fingerized" hypoplastic thumb / triphalangeal thumb
√ slender elongated hypoplastic carpals + metacarpals
√ hypoplastic radius; absent radial styloid
√ shallow glenoid fossa (voluntary dislocation of shoulder
  common)
√ hypoplastic clavicula
√ high arched palate
√ cervical scoliosis
√ pectus excavatum

HOMOCYSTINURIA
Autosomal recessive disorder
Etiology: cystathionine B synthetase deficiency results
              in defective methionine metabolism with
              accumulation of homocystine + homocysteine
              in blood and urine; causes defect in collagen /
              elastin structure
• thromboembolic phenomena due to stickiness of
  platelets
• ligamentous laxity
• downward dislocation of lens (DDx: upward dislocation
  in Marfan syndrome)
• mild / moderate mental retardation
• crowding of maxillary teeth and protrusion of incisors
• malar flush
√ arachnodactyly in 1/3 (DDx: Marfan syndrome)
√ microcephaly
√ enlarged paranasal sinuses
√ osteoporosis of vertebrae (biconcave / flattened /
  widened vertebrae)
√ scoliosis
√ pectus excavatum / carinatum (75%)

	Marfan syndrome	**Homocystinuria**
Inheritance:	autosomal dominant	autosomal recessive
Biochemical defect:	not known	cystathionine synthetase
Osteoporosis:	no	yes
Spine:	scoliosis	biconcave vertebrae
Lens dislocation:	upward	downward
Arachnodactyly:	100 %	33 %

√ osteoporosis of long bones (75%) with bowing + fractures

√ children: metaphyseal cupping (50%); enlargement of ossification centers in 50% (knee, carpal bones); epiphyseal calcifications (esp. in wrist, resembling phenylketonuria); delayed ossification

√ Harris lines = multiple growth lines

√ genu valgum, coxa valga, coxa magna, pes cavus

√ premature vascular calcifications

Prognosis: death from occlusive vascular disease / minor vascular trauma

HYPERPARATHYROIDISM

Age: middle age; M:F = 1:3

Histo: decreased bone mass secondary to increased number of osteoclasts, increased osteoid volume (defect in mineralization), slightly increased number of osteoblasts

A. BONE RESORPTION
  (a) subperiosteal: radial margins of middle phalanges, phalangeal tufts, proximal tibial shaft medially, femoral neck medially, humeral neck, upper margins of ribs in midclavicular line, lamina dura of skull and teeth
  (b) subchondral = pseudowidening of joint space: acromioclavicular joint, sternoclavicular joint, sacroiliac joint, symphysis pubis, Schmorl nodes
  (c) intracortical: scalloped inner surface + tunneling of cortex
  (d) trabecular = granular deossification with indistinct + coarse trabecular pattern, ground glass appearance, salt and pepper skull
  (e) subligamentous: ischial + humeral tuberosity, greater + lesser trochanter, inferior surface of calcaneus, interior aspect of distal clavicle
B. BONE SOFTENING
  √ basilar impression of skull
  √ wedged vertebrae, kyphoscoliosis, biconcave vertebral deformities
  √ bowing of long bones
  √ slipped capital femoral epiphysis
C. BROWN TUMOR
  More frequent in 1° HPT
  Location: jaw, pelvis, rib, metaphyses of long bones, facial bones
  √ expansile lytic well-marginated cystlike lesion = osteoclastoma (DDx: giant cell tumor)
  √ destruction of midportions of distal phalanges with telescoping
D. OSTEOSCLEROSIS
  More frequent in 2° HPT
  √ "rugger jersey spine" = sclerosis of vertebral end plates; skull; metaphyses
E. SOFT-TISSUE CALCIFICATION
  More frequent in 2° HPT; metastatic calcification when Ca x P product > 70 mg/dl
  (a) cornea, viscera (lung, stomach, kidney)
  (b) periarticular in hip, knee, shoulder, wrist
  (c) arterial wall (resembling diabetes mellitus)

  (d) Chondrocalcinosis (15 – 18%) = calcification of hyaline / fibrous cartilage in menisci, wrist, shoulder, hip, elbow
F. EROSIVE ARTHROPATHY
  • asymptomatic
  √ simulates rheumatoid arthritis with preserved joint spaces

NUC:
  √ normal bone scan in 80%
  √ foci of abnormal uptake in periphery of calvarium, mandible, sternum, acromioclavicular joint, lateral humeral epicondyles, hands, brown tumors
  √ extraskeletal uptake in cornea, cartilage, joint capsule, tendons, lung, stomach
  √ "superscan" in 2° HPT = absent kidney, increased uptake in calvarium, mandible, acromioclavicular joint, sternum, vertebrae, distal 1/3 of long bones, ribs

Sequelae:
  1. Renal stones / nephrocalcinosis (70%)
  2. Increased osteoblastic activity (25%)
     • increased alkaline phosphatase
     (a) osteitis fibrosa cystica
        √ subperiosteal bone resorption + cortical tunneling
        √ brown tumors (primary HPT)
     (b) bone softening
        √ fractures
  3. Peptic ulcer disease (increased gastric secretion from gastrinoma)
  4. Calcific pancreatitis
  5. Soft tissue calcifications (secondary HPT)
  6. Marginal joint erosions + subarticular collapse (DIP, PIP, MCP)

Primary Hyperparathyroidism
  =pHPT = 1° HPT = intrinsic abnormality of parathyroid gland featuring
  (1) brown tumor
  (2) chondrocalcinosis (20 – 30%); requires surgical Rx
Incidence: 25 / 100,000 per year; incidence of bone lesions in HPT is 25 – 40%
Etiology:
  (a) Parathyroid adenoma (87%): single (80%); multiple (7%)
  (b) Parathyroid hyperplasia (10%): chief cell (5%); clear cell (5%)
  (c) Parathyroid carcinoma (3%)
Histo: increased number of osteoclasts, increased osteoid volume (defect in mineralization), slightly increased osteoblasts = decreased bone mass
Age: 3rd – 5th decade; M:F = 1:3
Associated with:
  (a) Wermer syndrome = MEA I (+ pituitary adenoma + pancreatic islet cell tumor)
  (b) Sipple syndrome = MEA II (+ medullary thyroid carcinoma + pheochromocytoma)

- elevation of serum calcium + decrease in serum phosphate (30%)
- increase in serum alkaline phosphatase (50%)
- increase in parathyroid hormone (100%)
- hypotonicity of muscles, weakness, constipation, difficulty in swallowing, duodenal / gastric peptic ulcer disease (secondary to hypercalcemia)
- polyuria, polydypsia (hypercalciuria + hyperphosphaturia)
- renal colic + renal insufficiency (nephrocalculosis + nephrocalcinosis)
- rheumatic bone pain + tenderness (particularly at site of brown tumor), pathologic fracture secondary to brown tumor

X-ray: (skeletal involvement in 20%)
√ thin cortices with lacy cortical pattern (subperiosteal bone resorption)
√ brown tumor (particularly in jaw + long bones)
√ osteitis cystica fibrosa (= intertrabecular fibrous connective tissue)

NUC:
√ normal bone scan in 80%
√ foci of abnormal uptake: calvarium (esp. periphery), mandible, sternum, acromioclavicular areas, lateral humeral epicondyles, hands
√ increased uptake in brown tumors
√ extraskeletal uptake: cornea, cartilage, joint capsules, tendons, periarticular areas, lungs, stomach
√ normal renal excretion [except in stone disease / calcium nephropathy (10%)]

Secondary Hyperparathyroidism
= sHPT = 2° HPT = diffuse / adenomatous hyperplasia of all four parathyroid glands as a compensatory mechanism in any state of hypocalcemia featuring (1) soft-tissue calcifications (2) osteosclerosis; requires medical Rx

Etiology:
(a) renal osteodystrophy (renal insufficiency + osteomalacia / rickets)
(b) calcium deprivation, maternal hypoparathyroidism, pregnancy, hypovitaminosis D
(c) rise in serum phosphate leading to decrease in calcium by feedback mechanism

NUC:
√ absent kidney sign
√ increased bone-to-soft tissue ratio
√ increased uptake in calvarium, mandible, acromioclavicular region, sternum, vertebrae, distal third of long bones, ribs

Tertiary Hyperparathyroidism
= tHPT = 3° HPT = development of autonomous PTH adenoma in patients with chronically overstimulated hyperplastic parathyroid glands (renal insufficiency); requires surgical Rx

Clue: (a) intractable hypercalcemia
(b) inability to control osteomalacia by vitamin D

Ectopic Parathormone-Production
= pseudohyperparathyroidism as paraneoplastic syndrome in bronchogenic carcinoma + renal cell carcinoma

HYPERTROPHIC OSTEOARTHROPATHY
= HYPERTROPHIC PULMONARY OSTEOARTHROPATHY

Etiology:
(1) release of vasodilators which are not metabolized by lung
(2) increased flow through AV shunts
(3) reflex peripheral vasodilation (vagal impulses)
(4) hormones: estrogens, growth hormone, prostaglandin

A. THORACIC CAUSES
(a) Malignant tumor (0.7 – 12%): bronchogenic carcinoma, mesothelioma, lymphoma, pulmonary metastasis from osteogenic sarcoma, melanoma, renal cell carcinoma, breast cancer
(b) Benign tumor: benign pleural fibroma, tumor of ribs, thymoma, esophageal leiomyoma, pulmonary hemangioma, pulmonary congenital cyst
(c) Chronic infection / inflammation: pulmonary abscess, bronchiectasis, blastomycosis, TB (very rare); cystic fibrosis, interstitial fibrosis
(d) congenital heart disease

B. EXTRATHORACIC CAUSES
(a) GI tract: ulcerative colitis, amebic + bacillary dysentery, intestinal TB, Whipple disease, Crohn disease, gastric ulcer, bowel lymphoma, gastric carcinoma
(b) Liver disease: biliary + alcoholic cirrhosis, posthepatic cirrhosis, chronic active hepatitis, bile duct carcinoma, benign bile duct stricture, amyloidosis, liver abscess
(c) undifferentiated nasopharyngeal carcinoma, pancreatic carcinoma, chronic myelogenous leukemia

- hypocratic fingers + toes (clubbing)
- hypertrophy of extremities (soft tissue swelling)
- burning pain, painful swelling of limbs, and stiffness of joints: ankles (88%), wrists (83%), knees (75%), elbows (17%), shoulders (10%), fingers (7%)
- peripheral neurovascular disorders: local cyanosis, areas of increased sweating, paresthesia, chronic erythema, flushing + blanching of skin

Location: tibia + fibula (75%), radius + ulna (80%), proximal phalanges (60%), femur (50%), metacarpus + metatarsus (40%), humerus + distal phalanges (25%), pelvis (5%); unilateral (rare)

Site: in diametaphyseal regions

√ periosteal proliferation of new bone, at first smooth then undulating + rough, most conspicuous on concavity of long bones (dorsal + medial aspects)
√ regression of periosteal reaction after thoracotomy
√ soft tissue swelling ("clubbing") of distal phalanges
Bone scan (reveals changes with greater clarity):
  √ symmetric diffusely increased uptake along cortical margins of diaphysis + metaphysis of tubular bones of the extremities with irregularities
  √ increased periarticular uptake (= synovitis)
  √ scapular involvement in 2/3
  √ mandible ± maxilla abnormal in 40%

HYPERVITAMINOSIS A

Age: usually infants + children
• anorexia, irritability
• loss of hair, dry skin, pruritus, fissures of lips
• jaundice, enlargement of liver
√ separation of cranial sutures secondary to hydrocephalus (coronal > lambdoid) in children < 10 years of age, may appear within a few days
√ symmetrical solid periosteal new bone formation along shafts of long + short bones (ulna, calvicle)
√ premature epiphyseal closure + thinning of epiphyseal plates
√ accelerated growth
√ tendinous, ligamentous, pericapsular calcifications
√ changes usually disappear after cessation of vitamin A ingestion
DDx: Infantile cortical hyperostosis (mandible involved)

HYPERVITAMINOSIS D

= excessive ingestion of vitamin D (large doses act like parathormone)
• loss of appetite, drowsiness, headaches
• polyuria, polydipsia, renal damage
• anemia
• diarrhea
• convulsions
• excessive phosphaturia (parathormone decreases tubular absorption)
• hypercalcemia + hypercalciuria
√ deossification

√ widening of provisional zone of calcification
√ cortical + trabecular thickening
√ alternating bands of increased + decreased density near / in epiphysis (zone of provisional calcification)
√ vertebra outlined by dense band of bone + adjacent radiolucent line within
√ dense calvarium
√ metastatic calcinosis in (a) arterial walls (between age 20 and 30) (b) kidneys = nephrocalcinosis (c) periarticular tissue (putty-like) (d) premature calcification of falx cerebri (most consistent sign!)

HYPOPARATHYROIDISM

Etiology:
  A. Idiopathic Hypoparathyroidism
    = rare condition of unknown cause
    • round face, short dwarf-like, obese
    • mental retardation
    • cataracts
    • dry scaly skin, atrophy of nails
    • dental hypoplasia (delayed tooth eruption, impaction of teeth, supernumerary teeth)
  B. Secondary Hypoparathyroidism
    = accidental removal / damage to parathyroid glands in thyroid surgery / radical neck dissection (5%); I-131 therapy (rare); external beam radiation; hemorrhage; infection; thyroid carcinoma; hemochromatosis (iron deposition)
• tetany = neuromuscular excitability (numbness, cramps, carpopedal spasm, laryngeal stridor, generalized convulsions)
• hypocalcemia + hyperphosphatemia
• normal / low serum alkaline phosphatase
√ premature closure of epiphyses
√ hypoplasia of tooth enamel + dentine; blunting of roots
√ generalized increase in bone density in 9%
  √ localized thickening of skull
  √ sacroiliac sclerosis
  √ band-like density in metaphysis of long bones (25%), iliac crest, vertebral bodies
  √ thickened lamina dura (inner table) + widened diploe
  √ deformed hips with thickening + sclerosis of femoral head + acetabulum

	HypoPT	PseudoHypoPT	PseudopseudoHypoPT
Serum-Ca	down	down	norm
Serum-P	up	up	norm
AlkaPhos	down/norm	down/norm	norm

Response to PTH-Injection	norm / HypoPT	PseudoHypoPT
Urine-AMP	up	norm
Urine-P	up	norm
Plasma-AMP	up	norm

@ Soft tissue
√ intracranial calcifications in basal ganglia, choroid plexus, occasionally in cerebellum
√ calcification of spinal and other ligaments
√ subcutaneous calcifications
√ osslfication of muscle insertions
√ ectopic bone formation

HYPOPHOSPHATASIA
= autosomal recessive congenital disease with low activity of serum-, bone-, liver-alkaline phosphatase resulting in poor mineralization (deficient generation of bone crystals)
Incidence: 1:100,000
Histo: indistinguishable from rickets
• phosphoethanolamine in urine as a precursor of alkaline phosphatase
• normal serum calcium + phosphorus
A. GROUP I = neonatal = congenital lethal form
√ marked demineralization of calvarium ("caput membranaceum" = soft skull)
√ lack of calcification of metaphyseal end of long bones
√ streaky, irregular, spotty margins of calcification
√ cupping of metaphysis
√ angulated shaft fractures with abundant callus formation
√ short poorly ossified ribs
√ poorly ossified vertebrae (especially neural arches)
√ small pelvic bones
OB-US:
√ high incidence of intrauterine fetal demise
√ increased echogenicity of falx (enhanced sound transmission secondary to poorly mineralized calvarium)
√ short bowed poorly mineralized tubular bones + multiple fractures
√ poorly mineralized spine
√ short poorly ossified ribs
√ polyhydramnios
Prognosis: death within 6 months
B. GROUP II = juvenile severe form
onset of symptoms within weeks to months
• moderate / severe dwarfism
• delayed weight bearing
√ resembles rickets
√ separated cranial sutures; craniostenosis in 2nd year
Prognosis: 50% mortality
C. GROUP III = adult mild form
recognized later in childhood / adolescence / adulthood
• dwarfism
√ clubfeet, genu valgum
√ demineralization of ossification centers (at birth / 3 – 4 months of age)
Prognosis: excellent — after 1 year no further progression
D. GROUP IV = latent form
heterozygote state
• normal / borderline levels of alkaline phosphatase

• patients are small for age
• disturbance of primary dentition
√ bone fragility + healed fractures
√ enlarged chondral ends of ribs
√ metaphyseal notching of long bones
√ Erlenmeyer flask deformity of femur

HYPOTHYROIDISM
= CRETINISM
A. Childhood:
√ delayed skeletal maturation (appearance + growth of ossification centers, epiphyseal closure)
√ fragmented, stippled epiphyses
√ wide sutures / fontanelles with delayed closure
√ delayed dentition
√ delayed / decreased pneumatization of sinuses + mastoids
√ hypertelorism
√ dense vertebral margins
√ demineralization
√ hypoplastic phalanges of 5th finger
B. Adulthood:
√ calvarial thickening / sclerosis
√ wedging of dorsolumbar vertebral bodies
√ coxa vara with flattened femoral head
√ premature atherosclerosis
No skeletal changes with adult onset!

INFANTILE CORTICAL HYPEROSTOSIS
= CAFFEY DISEASE; may be of familial origin; remission + exacerbations (common)
Age: < 5 months, reported in utero
• sudden hard, extremely tender soft tissue swellings over bone
• irritability, fever
Location: mandible > clavicle > ulna + others (except phalanges + vertebrae); hyperostosis affects diaphysis of tubular bones, epiphyses spared
√ massive periosteal new bone formation + perifocal soft tissue swelling
√ "double exposed" ribs
Prognosis: usually complete recovery after a few months
Rx: steroids

CHRONIC INFANTILE HYPEROSTOSIS
Disease may persist or recur intermittently for years
• delayed muscular development, crippling deformities
DDx: (1) Hypervitaminosis A (2) Infection (3) Hyperphosphatasia

IRON DEFICIENCY ANEMIA
Age: infants affected
Causes:
(1) inadequate iron stores at birth (2) deficient iron in diet (3) impaired gastrointestinal absorption of iron (4) excessive iron demands from blood loss (5) polycythemia vera (6) cyanotic CHD

√ widening of diploe + thinning of tables with sparing of occiput (no red marrow)
√ hair-on-end appearance of skull
√ osteoporosis in long bones (most prominent in hands)
√ absence of facial bone involvement

JACCOUD ARTHROPATHY
After subsidence of frequent severe attacks of rheumatic fever
Path: periarticular fascial + tendon fibrosis without synovitis
• rheumatic valve disease
Location: primarily involvement of hands; occasionally in great toe
√ muscular atrophy
√ periarticular swelling of small joints of hands + feet
√ ulnar deviation + flexion of MCP joints most marked in 4th + 5th finger
√ NO joint narrowing / erosion

JUVENILE APONEUROTIC FIBROMA
Rare benign fibrous tumor
Histo: cellular dense fibrous tissue with focal chondral elements infiltrating adjacent structures (= cartilaginous tumor)
Age: children + adolescents; male preponderance
Location: deep palmar fascia of hand + wrist
√ soft tissue mass overlying inflamed bursa (often mistaken for calcified bursitis)
√ stippled calcifications
√ interosseous soft tissue mass of forearm + wrist
√ bone erosion may occur
DDx: Synovial sarcoma, Chondroma, Fibrosarcoma, Osteosarcoma, Myositis ossificans

KAPOSI SARCOMA
Histo: simulates malignant angioma
Associated with: AIDS
Location: lower extremities
√ lytic cortical lesion
√ subcutaneous nodules

KIENBÖCK DISEASE
= avascular necrosis of carpal lunate bone; frequently a result of trauma

KLINEFELTER SYNDROME
47,XXY (rarely XXYY) chromosomal abnormality
Incidence: 1:750 live births
• testicular atrophy (hyalinization of seminiferous tubules), sterility (azoospermia)
• gynecomastia; paucity of hair on face + chest; female pubic escutcheon
• mild mental retardation
• high level of urinary gonadotropins + low level of 17-ketosteroids
√ may have delayed bone maturation
√ failure of frontal sinus to develop

√ ± scoliosis, kyphosis
√ ± coxa valga
√ ± metacarpal sign
√ accessory epiphyses of 2nd metacarpal bilaterally

XXX = SUPERFEMALE SYNDROME
• usually over 6 feet tall; subnormal intelligence; frequently antisocial behavior

KLIPPEL-TRENAUNAY SYNDROME
= sporadic disease of equal sex distribution characterized by a triad of:
(1) port-wine nevus = unilateral flat cutaneous capillary hemangioma often in dermatomal distribution on affected limb; may fade in 2nd – 3rd decade
(2) varicose veins on lateral aspect of affected limb; usually ipsilateral to hemangioma
(3) limb overgrowth (especially during adolescent growth spurt)
Associated with:
— polydactyly, syndactyly, clinodactyly, congenital dislocation of hip
— hemangiomas of colon / bladder (3 – 10%)
— spinal hemangiomas + AVMs
— hemangiomas in liver / spleen
— lymphangiomas of limb
Location: lower extremity (10 – 15 x more common than upper extremity); bilateral in < 5%
√ increased metatarsal / metacarpal + phalangeal size
√ cortical thickening
√ valveless lateral venous channels
√ punctate calcifications (phleboliths) in pelvis (bowel wall, urinary bladder)
DDx:
(1) **Parkes-Weber Syndrome** (similar triad + arteriovenous fistula)
(2) Neurofibromatosis (café-au-lait spots, axillary freckling, cutaneous neurofibromas, macrodactyly secondary to plexiform neurofibromas, wavy cortical reaction, early fusion of growth plate, limb hypertrophy not as extensive / bilateral)
(3) Beckwith-Wiedemann syndrome (aniridia, macroglossia, cryptorchidism, Wilms tumor, broad metaphyses, thickened long bone cortex, advanced bone age, periosteal new bone formation, entire side of body may be enlarged)
(4) Macrodystrophia lipomatosis (hyperlucency of fat, distal phalanges most commonly affected, overgrowth ceases with puberty, usually limited to digits)
(5) Maffucci syndrome (cavernous hemangiomas, soft tissue hypertrophy, phleboliths, multiple enchondromas)

KÖHLER DISEASE
= avascular necrosis of tarsal scaphoid
Age: 3 – 10 years; boys
√ irregular outline

√ fragmentation
√ disc-like compression in AP dimension
√ increased density
√ joint space maintained
√ decreased / increased uptake on radionuclide study

LAURENCE-MOON-BIEDL SYNDROME
- retardation
- obesity
- hypogonadism
√ craniosynostosis
√ polysyndactyly

LEAD POISONING
= PLUMBISM
Path: lead concentrates in metaphyses of growing
           bones (distal femur > both ends of tibia > distal
           radius) leading to failure of removal of calcified
           cartilaginous trabeculae in provisional zone
- loss of appetite, vomiting, constipation, abdominal
  cramps
- peripheral neuritis (adults), meningoencephalitis
  (children)
- anemia
- lead line at gums (adults)
√ bands of increased density at metaphyses of tubular
  bones (only in growing bone)
√ lead lines may persist
√ clubbing if poisoning severe (anemia)
√ bone-in-bone apppearance
DDx: (1)   Healed rickets
         (2)   Normal increased density in infants < 3 years
               of age

LEGG-PERTHES-CALVÉ DISEASE
= COXA PLANA = idiopathic avascular necrosis of
   femoral head in children; one of the most common sites
   of AVN; 10% bilateral
Age: (a)   4 – 7 years: more frequent in females
         (b)   adulthood: **Chandler disease**
Causes:
   Trauma 30% (subcapital fracture, epiphyseolysis, esp.
   posterior dislocation), closed reduction of congenital hip
   dislocation, prolonged interval between injury and
   reduction
Pathophysiology:
   femoral head blood supply insufficient (epiphyseal plate
   acts as a barrier in ages 4 – 10; ligamentum teres
   vessels become nonfunctional; blood supply is from
   medial circumflex artery + lateral epiphyseal artery only
Stages:
   Stage I = histologic + clinical diagnosis without
              radiographic findings
   Stage II = sclerosis ± cystic changes with preservation
              of contour + surface of femoral head
   Stage III = loss of structural integrity of femoral head
   Stage IV = in addition loss of structural integrity of
               acetabulum

- 1 week – 6 months (mean 2.7 months) duration of
  symptoms prior to initial presentation
NUC (may assist in early diagnosis):
   √ decreased uptake (early) in femoral head =
     interruption of blood supply
   √ increased uptake (late) in femoral head =
     (a) revascularization + bone repair
     (b) degenerative osteoarthritis
   √ increased acetabular activity with associated
     degenerative joint disease
X-RAY:
   Early signs:
      √ femoral epiphysis smaller than on contralateral side
        (96%)
      √ sclerosis of femoral head epiphysis (sequestration
        + compression) (82%)
      √ slight widening of joint space (thickening of
        cartilage, failure of epiphyseal growth, joint fluid,
        joint laxity) (60%)
      √ ipsilateral bone demineralization (46%)
      √ alteration of pericapsular soft tissue outline due to
        atrophy of ipsilateral periarticular soft tissues (73%)
      √ rarefaction of lateral + medial metaphyseal areas of
        neck
      √ NEVER destruction of articular cortex as in bacterial
        arthritis
   Late signs:
      √ delayed osseous maturation of a mild degree
      √ "radiolucent crescent line" of subchondral fracture
        = small archlike subcortical lucency (32%)
      √ subcortical fracture on anterior articular surface
        (better seen on frogleg view)
      √ femoral head fragmentation
      √ femoral neck cysts (intramedullary hemorrhage in
        response to stress fractures)
      √ loose bodies (only found in males)
      √ coxa plana = flattened collection of sclerotic
        fragments (over 18 months)
      √ coxa magna = remodeling of femoral head to
        become wider + flatter in mushroom configuration
        to match widened metaphysis + epiphyseal plate
CT:
   √ "asterisk" sign = remodeled compact trabecular bone
MRI:
   √ "double-line" sign (80%) = sclerotic non-signal rim
     producing line between necrotic + viable bone edged
     by a hyperintense rim of granulation tissue
   √ fluid within fracture plane
   √ central low-signal intensity region = "asterisk" sign
Cx: severe degenerative joint disease in early
       adulthood

LEPROSY
= HANSEN DISEASE
Organism: Mycobacterium leprae
Types:
   (1)   lepromatous: in cutis, mucous membranes, viscera

(2) neural: enlarged indurated nodular nerve trunks; anesthesia, muscular atrophy, neurotrophic changes
(3) mixed form
Osseous changes in 15 – 54% of patients:
SPECIFIC SIGNS
  Location: center of distal end of phalanges / eccentric
  √ ill-defined areas of decalcification, reticulated trabecular pattern, small rounded osteolytic lesions, cortical erosions
  √ joint spaces preserved
  √ healing phase: complete resolution / bone defect with sclerotic rim + endosteal thickening
  √ nasal spine absorption + destruction of maxilla, nasal bone, alveolar ridge
  √ enlarged nutrient foramina in hands, claw-like hand
  √ erosive changes of ungual tufts
NONSPECIFIC SIGNS
  √ soft tissue swelling; calcification of nerves
  √ contractures / deep ulcerations
  √ neurotrophic joints (distal phalanges in hands, MTP in feet, Charcot joints in tarsus)

LEUKEMIA OF BONE
A. CHILDHOOD
  Histo: almost always acute + lymphoblastic leukemia
  • arthritic symptoms (confused with acute rheumatic fever / rheumatoid arthritis)
  • fever, elevated sedimentation rate
  • splenomegaly, occasionally lymphadenopathy
  Skeletal manifestations in 50%:
  √ multiple small clearly defined ovoid / spheroid osteolytic lesions (destruction of spongiosa, later cortex) in 30 – 60%
  √ diffuse demineralization of long bones + spine (leukemic infiltrates + katabolic protein / mineral metabolism) in 30%
  √ coarse trabeculation of spongiosa (due to destruction of finer trabeculae)
  √ periosteal reaction: smooth / lamellated / sunburst pattern (cortical penetration by sheets of leukemic cells into subperiosteum) in 12 – 25%
  √ transverse radiolucent metaphyseal bands around large joints (tibia, femur, proximal humerus, distal radius + ulna) in 10 – 20% in vertebral bodies; become dense after treatment
  √ horizontal / curvilinear bands in vertebral bodies + edges of iliac crest
  √ multiple biconcave / partially collapsed vertebrae (14%)
  √ osteosclerotic lesions (late in disease due to reactive osteoblastic proliferation)
  √ mixed lesions (lytic + bone-forming) in 18%
  Dx: sternal marrow / peripheral blood smear
  Cx: proliferation of leukemic cells in marrow leads to extraskeletal hematopoiesis
  DDx: metastatic neuroblastoma

B. ADULTHOOD
  Death usually occurs before skeletal abnormalities manifest
  √ osteoporosis
  √ solitary radiolucent foci (vertebral collapse)
  √ permeating radiolucent mottling (proximal humerus)

LIPOMA OF BONE
Age: any; M:F = 1:1
May be associated with: hyperlipoproteinemia
Location: calcaneus, skull, ribs, extremities (tibia, fibula, humerus, femur)
Site: metaphysis
√ expansile radiolucent lesion + thinned cortex
√ may contain small central calcification (= fat necrosis)
√ loculated / septated appearance (trabeculae)

LYME ARTHRITIS
Agent: spirochete Borrelia burgdorferi; transmitted by tick Ixodes dammini
Histo: inflammatory synovial fluid, hypertrophic synovia with vascular proliferation + cellular infiltration
• history of erythema chronicum migrans
• endemic areas (Lyme,Connecticut first recognized location; now throughout United States, Europe, Australia)
• recurrent attacks of arthralgias within days to 2 years after disease onset (80%)
Location: mono- / oligoarthritis of large joints (especially knee)
√ erosion of cartilage / bone (4%)
Rx: antibiotics
DDx: (1) Rheumatic fever (2) Rheumtoid arthritis (3) Gonococcal arthritis (4) Reiter syndrome

LYMPHOMA OF BONE
= RETICULUM CELL SARCOMA = HISTIOCYTIC LYMPHOMA = PRIMARY LYMPHOMA OF BONE (generalized form of reticulum cell sarcoma = lymphoma)
Incidence of bone marrow involvement:
  5 – 15% in Hodgkin disease;
  25 – 40% in Non-Hodgkin lymphoma
  Δ bone marrow involvement indicates progression of disease
  NUC: 40% sensitivity; 88% specificity
  MRI: 65% sensitivity; 90% specificity
Histo: sheets of reticulum cells, larger than those in Ewing sarcoma (DDx: myeloma, inflammation, osteosarcoma, eosinophilic granuloma)
Age: any age; peak age in 3rd – 5th decade; 50% < 40 years; 35% < 30 years; M:F = 2:1
• striking contrast between size of lesion + patient's well-being
Location: lower femur, upper tibia (40% about knee), humerus, pelvis, scapula, ribs, vertebra
Site: dia- / metaphysis
√ cancellous bone erosion (earliest sign)

√ mottled permeative pattern of separate coalescent areas

√ late cortical destruction

√ lamellated / sunburst periosteal response (less than in Ewing sarcoma)

√ lytic / reactive new bone formation

√ associated soft tissue mass without calcification

√ synovitis of knee joint common

Cx: pathologic fracture (most common among malignant bone tumors)

Prognosis: 50% 5-year survival

DDx: (1) Osteosarcoma (less medullary extension, younger patients)
(2) Ewing tumor (systemic symptoms, debility, younger patients)
(3) Metastatic malignancy (multiple bones involved, more destructive)

MACRODYSTROPHIA LIPOMATOSA

= increase in size of all elements + structures of a digit

√ overgrowth of distal end of digit; stops at puberty

√ dorsal deviation

√ clinodactyly

√ overgrowth of fat

√ long, broad, splayed phalanges

DDx: Neurofibromatosis

MALIGNANT FIBROUS HISTIOCYTOMA

= MFH = MALIGNANT FIBROUS XANTHOMA
= XANTHOSARCOMA = MALIGNANT HISTIOCYTOMA
= FIBROSARCOMA VARIANT

Incidence: most common primary malignant soft tissue tumor of extremities / retroperitoneum after age 45

Histo: spindle-cell neoplasm with a mixture of fibroblasts + cells resembling histiocytes with nuclear atypia and pleomorphism in pinwheel arrangement; closely resembles high-grade fibrosarcoma

Age: 1st – 8th decade; average age of 50 years; M:F = 3:2

• painless soft tissue mass present for a few months

Location: potential to arise in any organ (ubiquitous mesenchymal tissue); meta-diaphyseal in long bones (75%): femur (45%), tibia (20%), 50% about knee; humerus (10%); ilium (10%); spine; sternum; clavicle; rarely small bones of hand + feet

@ Soft tissue

Location: lower extremity (1/3) > upper extremity > retroperitoneum

√ mass usually > 5 cm in size

√ poorly defined calcifications (7 – 20%)

√ occasional secondary involvement of adjacent bone with periosteal reaction, cortical erosion, pathologic fracture

DDx: (1) Liposarcoma (younger patient, presence of fat, calcifications rare)
(2) Rhabdomyosarcoma

(3) Synovial sarcoma

@ Bone (130 cases only)

associated with prior radiation therapy / bone infarcts./ Paget disease / fibrous dysplasia

• painful, tender, rapidly enlarging mass

Site: metaphysis of long bones (most common)

√ radiolucent defect with ill-defined margins (2.5 – 10 cm in diameter)

√ extensive mineralization / small areas of focal calcification

√ permeation + cortical destruction

√ expansion in smaller bones (ribs, sternum, fibula, clavicle)

√ occasionally lamellated periosteal reaction (especially in presence of pathologic fracture)

√ soft tissue extension

Cx: pathologic fracture (30 – 50%)

DDx: (1) metastasis (2) fibrosarcoma (often with sequestrum) (3) reticulum cell sarcoma (4) osteosarcoma

@ Lung (extremely rare)

√ solitary pulmonary nodule without calcification

√ diffuse infiltrate

NUC: √ increased uptake of Tc-99m MDP (mechanism not understood)

√ increased uptake of Ga-67 citrate

US: √ well-defined mass with hyperechoic + hypoechoic (necrotic) areas

CT: √ mass of muscle density with hypodense areas (necrosis)

√ invasion of abdominal musculature, but not IVC / renal veins (DDx to renal cell carcinoma)

Angio: √ hypervascularity + early venous return

Prognosis: 2-year survival rate of 60%; 5-year survival rate of 50%; local recurrence rate of 44%; metastatic rate of 42% (lung, lymph nodes, liver, bone)

MARFAN SYNDROME

= ARACHNODACTYLY = autosomal dominant familial disorder of connective tissue (abnormal cross-linking of collagen fibers) with high penetrance but extremely variable expression, new mutations in 15%

Prevalence: 5:100,000; M:F = 1:1

A. MUSCULOSKELETAL MANIFESTATIONS

• tall thin stature with long limbs, arm span greater than height

• muscular hypoplasia + hypotonicity

• scarcity of subcutaneous fat (emaciated look)

@ Skull

• elongated face

√ dolichocephaly

√ prominent jaw

√ high-arched palate

@ Hand

• Steinberg sign = protrusion of thumb beyond the confines of the clenched fist (found in 1.1% of normal population)

- metacarpal index (averaging the 4 ratios of length of 2nd through 5th metacarpals divided by their respective middiaphyseal width) > 8.8. (male) or 9.4 (female)
- √ arachnodactyly = elongation of phalanges + metacarpals
- √ flexion deformity of 5th finger
@ Foot
- √ pes planus
- √ club feet
- √ hallux valgus
- √ hammer toes
- √ disproportionate elongation of 1st digit of foot
@ Spine
- ratio of measurement between symphysis and floor + crown and floor > 0.45
- √ pectus carinatum / excavatum (common)
- √ scoliosis / kyphoscoliosis (45 – 60%)
- √ increased incidence of Scheuermann disease and spondylosis
- √ increased interpeduncular distance
- √ posterior scalloping
- √ presacral + lateral sacral meningoceles
- √ expansion of sacral spinal canal
- √ enlargement of sacral foramina
- √ winged scapulae
@ Joints
- ligamentous laxity + hypermobility + instability
- √ premature osteoarthritis
- √ patella alta
- √ genu recurvatum
- √ recurrent dislocations of patella, hip, clavicle, mandible
- √ slipped capital femoral epiphysis
- √ progressive protrusio acetabuli (50%), bilateral > unilateral, F > M

B. OCULAR MANIFESTATIONS
- bilateral ectopia lentis, usually upwards
- contracted pupils (absence of dilator muscle)
- myopia
- strabismus
- retinal detachment

C. CARDIOVASCULAR MANIFESTATIONS (60%)
Cause of death in 93%
- chest pain, palpitations, shortness of breath, fatigue
- mid-to-late systolic murmur + one/more clicks
Associated with congenital heart defect (33%): incomplete coarctation, ASD
@ AORTA (cause of death in 55%)
- √ aneurysm of ascending aorta (cystic medial necrosis) without calcifications
- √ "tulip bulb" = symmetrical dilatation of aortic sinuses of Valsalva (58%)
- √ myxomatous degeneration of aortic annulus
@ MITRAL VALVE
- √ "floppy valve syndrome" (95%) = redundant chordae tendineae

Cx: (1) aortic dissection (2) aortic regurgitation (in 81% if root diameter > 5 cm; in 100% if root diameter > 6 cm) (3) mitral regurgitation (4) cor pulmonale (secondary to chest deformity)
D. PULMONARY MANIFESTATIONS
- √ cystic lung disease
- √ recurrent spontaneous pneumothoraces
DDx: (1) Homocystinuria (osteoporosis)
(2) Ehlers-Danlos syndrome
(3) Congenital contractural arachnodactyly (ear deformities, NO ocular / cardiac abnormalities)
(4) Type III MEN (medullary thyroid carcinoma, mucosal neuromas, pheochromocytoma, marfanoid habitus)

MASSIVE OSTEOLYSIS
= GORHAM DISEASE = "VANISHING BONE" SYNDROME = PHANTOM BONE = HEMANGIOMA OF BONE
Infrequent disorder of unknown etiology with unpredictabe course + progression
Histo: massive proliferation of hemangiomatous / lymphangiomatous tissue with large sinusoid spaces + fibrosis
Age: children + adults < 40 years
Associated with: soft tissue hemangiomas without calcifications
- frequently history of severe trauma
- little / no pain
Location : any bone; most commonly major long bones, innominate bones, spine, thorax, short tubular bones of hand + feet (unusual)
- √ progressive relentless destruction of bone
- √ lack of reaction (no periosteal reaction, no repair)
- √ advancing edge of destruction not sharply delineated
- √ tapering margins of bone ends at sites of osteolysis with conelike spicule of bone (early changes)
- √ no respect for joints
- √ may destroy all bones in a particular area

MASTOCYTOSIS
= URTICARIA PIGMENTOSA = mast cell accumulation in multiple organs
Age: < 6 months (50%)
Associated with leukemia
- skin lesions
- hepatomegaly
- lymphadenopathy
- pancytopenia

@ Skeletal involvement (70%)
- √ osteoporosis
- √ coarsened trabeculae
- √ scattered well-defined sclerotic foci with focal / diffuse involvement; often alternating with areas of bone rarefaction;
Predilected sites: skull, spine, ribs, pelvis, humerus, femur

MELORHEOSTOSIS

Nonhereditary disease of unknown etiology

Age: slow chronic course in adults; rapid progression in children

Associated with osteopoikilosis, osteopathia striata

- severe pain + limited joint motion (bone may encroach on nerves, blood vessels, or joints)
- thickening + fibrosis of overlying skin
- tumors / malformations of blood vessels (hemangioma, vascular nevi, glomus tumor, AVM, aneurysm, lymphedema, lymphangiectasia)

Location:

diaphysis, usually limited to single extremity with at least two bones involved in dermatomal distribution (follows spinal sensory nerve sclerotomes); entire cortex / limited to one side of cortex; skull, spine, ribs rarely involved

√ "candle wax dripping" = continuous / interrupted streaks / blotches of sclerosis along tubular bone beginning at proximal end extending distally with slow progression

√ may cross joint with joint fusion

√ small opacities in scapula + hemipelvis (similar to osteopoikilosis)

DDx: (1) Osteopoikilosis (generalized)
(2) Fibrous dysplasia (normal bone structure not lost, not as dense)
(3) Engelmann disease
(4) Hyperostosis of neurofibromatosis, tuberous sclerosis, hemangiomas
(5) Osteoarthropathy

MESOMELIC DWARFISM

Heritable bone dysplasia

√ shortening of all long bones

√ hypoplasia of fibula with absent lateral malleolus

√ short + thick ulna with hypoplastic distal end

√ hypoplasia of mandible with short condyles

√ radius + tibia proportionally shorter than humerus + femur

√ hypoplasia of a vertebral body may be present

METAPHYSEAL CHONDRODYSPLASIA

A. Jansen type
B. Schmid type
C. Spahr type
D. **Pyle disease** = Metaphyseal dysplasia
- may be tall
- often asymptomatic
√ craniofacial hyperostosis
√ genu valgum

√ short-limbed dwarfism

√ decreased bone density

√ metaphyseal flaring (Erlenmeyer flask deformity) extending into diaphysis, irregularity, calcification

METASTATIC MALIGNANCY

15 – 100 times more common than primary skletal neoplasms

SOLITARY BONE LESION

Δ of all causes only 7% due to metastasis

Δ in patients with known malignancy due to metastasis (55%), trauma (25%), infection (10%)

Location: axial skeleton (64 – 68%), ribs (45%), extremities (24%), skull (12%)

METASTASES IN PRIMARY BONE TUMORS

1. Osteosarcoma: 2% with distant metastases, adjuvant therapy has changed the natural history of the disease in that bone metastases occur in 10% of osteosarcomas without mets to the lung
2. Ewing sarcoma: 13% with distant metastases

FREQUENCY

in known primary		in unknown primary	
breast	35%	prostate	25%
prostate	30%	lymphoma	15%
lung	10%	breast	10%
kidney	5%	lung	10%
uterus	2%		
thyroid	2%		
stomach	2%		
colon	1%		
others	13%		

Breast cancer: extensive osteolytic lesions; involvement of entire skeleton; pathologic fractures common

Thyroid + kidney: often solitary; rapid progression with bone expansion (bubbly); frequently associated with soft tissue mass (distinctive)

Rectum + colon: may resemble osteosarcoma with sunburst pattern + osteoblastic reaction

Neuroblastoma: extensive destruction, resembles leukemia (metaphyseal band of rarefaction), mottled skull destruction + increased intracranial pressure, perpendicular spicules of bone

Hodgkin tumor: upper lumbar + lower thoracic spine, pelvis, ribs; osteolytic / occasionally osteoblastic lesions

Ewing tumor: extensive osteolytic / osteoblastic reaction

Mode of spread: through blood stream / lymphatics / direct extension

Location: predilection for marrow-containing skeleton (skull, spine, ribs, pelvis, humeri, femora)

√ single / multiple lesions of variable size

√ usually nonexpansile

√ joint spaces + intervertebral spaces preserved (cartilage resistant to invasion)

(a) OSTEOLYTIC

Most common cause: neuroblastoma (in childhood); lung cancer (in adult male); breast cancer (in adult female), thyroid cancer; kidney; colon

√ may begin in spongy bone (associated with soft tissue mass in ribs)

√ vertebral pedicles often involved (not in multiple myeloma)

(b) <u>OSTEOBLASTIC</u>

= evidence of slow-growing neoplasm

Primary:

prostate, breast, lymphoma, malignant carcinoid, medulloblastoma, mucinous adenocarcionma of GI-tract, TCC of bladder, pancreas, neuroblastoma

Most common cause: prostate cancer (in adult male); breast cancer (in adult female)

√ frequent in vertebrae + pelvis

√ may be indistinguishable from Paget disease

(c) <u>MIXED</u>: breast, prostate, lymphoma

(d) <u>EXPANSILE / BUBBLY</u>: kidney, thyroid

(e) <u>PERMEATIVE</u>: Burkitt lymphoma, Mycosis fungoides

(f) "Sunburst" periosteal reaction (infrequent): prostatic carcinoma, retinoblastoma, neuroblastoma (skull), GI tract

(g) Soft tissue mass: thyroid, kidney

(h) Calcifying metastases

mnemonic: " BOTTOM"

Breast

Osteosarcoma

Testicular

Thyroid

Ovary

Mucinous adenocarcinoma of GI tract

NUC:

Pathophysiology: accumulation of tracer at sites of reactive bone formation

<u>Baseline scan:</u>

(a) high sensitivity for many metastatic tumors to bone (particularly carcinoma of breast, lung, prostate); 5% of metastases have normal scan; 5 – 40% occur in appendicular skeleton

(b) substantially less sensitive than radiographs in infiltrative marrow lesions (multiple myeloma, neuroblastoma, histiocytosis)

(c) screening of asymptomatic patients

— useful in: prostate cancer, breast cancer

— not useful in: non-small cell bronchogenic carcinoma, gynecologic malignancy, head and neck cancer

√ multiple asymmetric areas of increased uptake

√ axial > appendicular skeleton (dependent on distribution of bone marrow); vertebrae, ribs, pelvis involved in 80%

√ superscan with diffuse bony metastases

<u>Follow-up scan:</u>

√ stable scan = suggestive of relative good prognosis

√ increased activity:

(a) enlargement of bone lesions / appearance of new lesions indicate progression of the disease

(b) "flare phenomenon" (in 20 – 61%) = transient increase in lesion activity secondary to healing under antineoplastic treatment, maximum

between 1 and 3 months, unrelated to eventual therapeutic response

(c) steroid therapy may cause avascular necrosis particularly in hips, knees, shoulders

(d) increased activity in osteoradionecrosis / radiation-induced osteosarcoma

√ decreased activity:

(a) lytic destruction predominates

(b) photopenic areas under radiotherapy; as early as 2 – 4 months with minimum of 2000 rads

ROLE OF BONE SCAN IN BREAST CANCER

<u>Routine preoperative bone scan</u> not justified:

Stage I : unsuspected mets in 2%, mostly single lesion

Stage II : unsuspected mets in 6%

Stage III: unsuspected mets in 14%

<u>Follow-up bone scan:</u>

At 12 months no new cases; at 28 months in 5% new metastases; at 30 months in 29% new metastases

Conversion from normal: Stage I : in 7%

Stage II : in 25%

Stage III: in 58%

With axillary lymph node involvement conversion rate 2.5 x of those without

ROLE OF BONE SCAN IN PROSTATE CANCER

Stage B : 5% with skeletal metastases

Stage C : 10% with skeletal metastases

Stage D : 20% with skeletal metastases

Test sensitivities for detection of osseous metastases:

(a) Scintigraphy 1.0

(b) Radiographic survey 0.68

(c) Alkaline phosphatase 0.5

(d) Acid phosphatase 0.5

Serial follow-ups are important to assess therapeutic efficacy + prognosis

Skeletal metastases in children

1. Neuroblastoma (most often)
2. Retinoblastoma
3. Embryonal rhabdomyosarcoma
4. Hepatoma
5. Ewing tumor

Skeletal metastases in adult

mnemonic: " Common Bone Lesions Can Kill The Patient"

Colon

Breast

Lung

Carcinoid

Kidney

Thyroid

Prostate

Osteoblastic metastases
mnemonic: "5 Bees Lick Pollen"
Brain (medulloblastoma)
Bronchus
Breast
Bowel (especially carcinoid)
Bladder
Lymphoma
Prostate

METATROPHIC DYSPLASIA
= HYPERPLASTIC ACHONDROPLASIA
= METATROPHIC DWARFISM
metatrophic = "changeable" (change in proportions of trunk to limbs over time secondary to developing kyphoscoliosis in childhood)
√ dumbbell-like / trumpet-shaped configuration of long bones with shortening
√ "hour-glass" phalanges
√ narrow thorax of normal length
√ progressive kyphoscoliosis
√ platyspondyly
√ coccygeal appendage similar to a tail (rare but CHARACTERISTIC)
Prognosis: compatible with life, increased disability from kyphoscoliosis

MUCOPOLYSACCHARIDOSES
= defect in mucopolysaccharide degradation
Type   I = Hurler   Type   IV= Morquio
Type   II = Hunter   Type   V = Scheie
Type   III= Sanfilippo   Type   VI= Maroteaux-Lamy
— all autosomal recessive except for Hunter (x-linked)
• corneal clouding
• retardation
Associated with: valvular heart disease
√ scaphocephaly, hydrocephaly; thick calvarium; hypertelorism
√ platyspondyly with kyphosis + dwarfism
√ irregularity at anterior aspect of vertebral bodies
√ hypoplastic ondotoid
√ limb contractures
√ broad hands
√ hepatosplenomegaly

Hurler Syndrome
= GARGOYLISM = PFAUNDLER-HURLER DISEASE
= MPS I; autosomal recessive disease with excess chondroitin sulfate B
Incidence: 1:10,000 births
Age: usually appears > 1st year
• dwarfism
• progressive mental + physical deterioration
• large head; sunken bridge of nose; hypertelorism
• corneal opacities progressing to blindness
• "gargoyle" features = everted lips + protruding tongue
• teeth widely separated + poorly formed
• protuberant abdomen (dorsolumbar kyphosis + hepatosplenomegaly)

• urinary excretion of chondroitin sulfate B + heparin sulfate
• Reilly bodies (metachromic granules) in white blood cells or bone marrow cells
√ thick periosteal cloaking of long bone diaphyses (early changes)
√ swelling of diaphyses + tapering of either end: distal humerus, radius, ulna, proximal ends of metacarpals, ribs
√ enlargement of shaft due to dilatation of medullary canal
√ deossification
√ flexion deformitites of knees + hips
√ trident hands; clawing
√ enlarged J-shaped sella
√ dorsolumbar kyphosis with lumbar gibbus
√ oval centra with normal / increased height; anterior beak at T12/L1/L2

Morquio Syndrome
= KERATOSULFATURIA = MPS IV;
autosomal recessive; excess keratosulfate
Incidence: 1:40,000 births
Etiology: N-acetylgalactosamine-6-sulfatase deficiency resulting in defective degradation of keratin sulfate (mainly in cartilage, nucleus pulposus, cornea)
Age: manifest at end of first year
• excretion of keratin sulfate in urine
• dwarfism with short trunk (< 4 feet tall)
• head thrust forward + sunken between high shoulders
• normal intelligence
• corneal opacification evident around age 10
• progressive deafness
• broad-mouthed face, spacing between teeth
• semicrouching stance + knock knees from flexion deformities of knees + hips
@ Skull
    √ mild dolichocephaly
    √ hypertelorism
    √ poor mastoid air cell development
    √ short nose + depression of bridge of nose
    √ prominent maxilla
@ Chest
    √ increased A-P diameter + marked pectus carinatum
    √ slight lordosis with wide short ribs
    √ bulbous costochondral junctions
@ Spine
    √ hypoplasia / absence of odontoid process of C2
    √ C1-C2 instability with anterior subluxation
    √ thick C2-body with narrowing of vertebral canal
    √ atlas close to occiput / posterior arch of C1 within foramen magnum
    √ platyspondyly = universal vertebra plana esp. affecting lumbar spine (DDx: normal height in Hurler syndrome)
    √ ovoid thoracic vertebral bodies with central beak / tongue

√ mild gibbus at thoracolumbar transition = low dorsal kyphosis

√ wide disc spaces

@ Pelvis

√ "goblet-shaped" / wine glass" pelvis = constricted iliac bodies + elongated pelvic inlet + flared iliac wings

√ oblique hypoplastic acetabular roofs

@ Femur

√ initially well-formed capital epiphysis, involution by age 3 – 6 years

√ fragmentation of femoral head epiphysis; later hip dislocation

√ lateral subluxation of femoral heads

√ wide femoral neck + coxa valga deformity

@ Tibia

√ delayed ossification of lateral proximal tibial epiphysis

√ sloping of superior margin of tibia plateau laterally + severe genu valgum

@ Hand

√ small irregular carpal bones

√ proximal pointing of metacarpals 2 – 5

√ enlarged joints; hands + feet deformities (flat feet)

Cx: cervical myelopathy (traumatic quadriplegia / leg pains / subtle neurologic abnormality); most common cause of death secondary to C2 abnormality

Rx: early fusion of C1 – C2

DDx:

(1) Spondyloepiphyseal dysplasia (autosomal dominant, present at birth, absent flared ilia / deficient acetabular ossification, small acetabular angle, deficient ossification of pubic bones, varus deformity of femoral neck, minimal involvement of hand + feet, myopia)

(2) Hurler syndrome (normal / increased vertebral height; vertebral beak inferior)

MULTIPLE EPIPHYSEAL DYSPLASIA

= FAIRBANK DISEASE = ? tarda form of chondrodystrophia calcificans congenita

√ mild limb shortening

√ irregular mottled calcifications of epiphyses (in childhood + adolescence)

√ epiphyseal irregularities + premature degenerative joint disease, esp. of hips (in adulthood)

√ short phalanges

DDx: Legg-Perthes disease, Hypothyroidism

MULTIPLE MYELOMA

Most common primary malignant neoplasm in adults

Histo: normal / pleomorphic plasma cells (not pathognomonic), may be mistaken for lymphocytes (lymphosarcoma, reticulum cell sarcoma, Ewing tumor, neuroblastoma)

Age: usually 5th – 8th decade; 98% > 40 years; rare < age 30; M:F = 2:1

(a) DISSEMINATED FORM: > 40 years of age (98%); M:F = 3:2

(b) SOLITARY FORM: mean age 50 years

• bone pain (68%)

• normochromic normocytic anemia (62%)

• RBC rouleau formation

• renal insufficiency (55%)

• hypercalcemia (30 – 50%)

• proteinuria (88%)

• Bence-Jones proteinuria (50%)

• increased globulin production (monoclonal gammopathy)

Location:

A. DISSEMINATED FORM:
scattered; axial skeleton predominant site; vertebrae (50%) > ribs > skull > pelvis > long bones (distribution correlates with normal sites of red marrow)

B. SOLITARY FORM:
vertebrae > pelvis > skull > sternum > ribs

C. SPINAL PLASMA CELL MYELOMA

√ sparing of posterior elements

√ paraspinal soft tissue mass with extradural extension

√ scalloping of anterior margin of vertebral bodies (osseous pressure from adjacent enlarged lymph nodes)

√ generalized osteoporosis with accentuation of trabecular pattern, esp. in spine (early)

√ punched out appearance of widespread osteolytic areas (skull, long bones) with endosteal scalloping and uniform size

√ diffuse osteolysis (pelvis, sacrum)

√ expansile osteolytic lesions (ballooning) in ribs, pelvis, long bones

√ soft tissue mass adjacent to bone destruction (= extrapleural + paraspional mass adjacent to ribs / vertebral column)

√ periosteal new-bone formation exceedingly rare

√ involvement of mandible (rarely affected by metastatic disease)

√ vertebral pedicles usually spared (no red marrow) (DDx: metastatic disease)

√ sclerosis may occur after chemotherapy, radiotherapy, fluoride administration

√ sclerotic form of multiple myeloma (1 – 3%)
(a) solitary sclerotic lesion: frequently in spine
(b) diffuse sclerosis
associated with POEMS syndrome:
Polyneuropathy
Organomegaly
Endocrine abnormalities
M-protein
Skin changes

<u>SENSITIVITY OF BONE SCANS VS. RADIOGRAPHS</u>
Radiographs: in 90% of patients and 80% of sites

Bone scan :   in 75% of patients and 24 – 54% of
               sites
Gallium scan : in 55% of patients and 40% of sites
Δ 30% of lesions only detected on radiographs
Δ 10% of lesions only detected on bone scans
Cx: (1) renal involvement frequent
       (2) predilection for recurrent pneumonias
            (leukopenia)
       (3) secondary amyloidosis in 6 – 15%
       (4) pathologic fractures occur often
Prognosis: 20% 5-year survival; death from renal
               insufficiency, bacterial infection,
               thromboembolism
DDx:
— with osteopenia: (1) Postmenopausal osteoporosis
                      (2) Hyperparathyroidism
— with lytic lesion: (1) Metastatic disease
                      (2) Amyloidosis
                      (3) Myeloid metaplasia
— with sclerotic lesion: (1) Osteopoikilosis
                      (2) Lymphoma
                      (3) Osteoblastic metastasis
                      (4) Mastocytosis
                      (5) Myelosclerosis
                      (6) Fluorosis
                      (7) Lymphoma
                      (8) Renal osteodystrophy

MYELOMATOSIS
√ generalized deossification without discrete tumors
√ vertebral flattening

MYELOPROLIFERATIVE DISORDERS
= autonomous clonal disorder initiated by an acquired
  pluripotential hematopoietic stem stell
Types:
  1. Polycythemia vera
  2. Chronic granulomatous leukemia = chronic
     myelogenous leukemia
  3. Essential idiopathic thrombocytopenia
  4. Agnogenic myeloid metaplasia (= primary
     myelofibrosis + extramedullary hematopoiesis in
     liver + spleen)
Pathophysiology:
  — self-perpetuating intra- and extramedullary
     hematopoietic cell proliferation without stimulus
  — trilinear panmyelosis (RBCs, WBCs, platelets)
  — myelofibrosis with progression to myelosclerosis
  — myeloid metaplasia = extramedullary hematopoiesis
     (normocytic anemia, leukoerythroblastic anemia,
     reticulocytosis, low platelet count, normal / reduced
     WBC count)

MYELOSCLEROSIS
= AGNOGENIC MYELOID METAPLASIA
= MYELOPROLIFERATIVE SYNDROME
= PSEUDOLEUKEMIA
= hematologic disorder of unknown etiology with gradual
  replacement of bone marrow elements by fibrosis

Characterized by
  (1) extramedullary hematopoiesis
  (2) progressive splenomegaly
  (3) anemia
  (4) variable changes in number of granulocytes ı
       platelets; often predated by polycythemia vera
Age: usually > 50 years
Path: fibrous / bony replacement of bone marrow;
           extramedullary hematopoiesis
Associated with:
    metastatic carcinoma, chemical poisoning, chronic
    infection (TB), acute myelogenous leukemia,
    polycythemia vera, McCune-Albright syndrome,
    histiocytosis
• dyspnea, weakness, fatigue, weight loss, hemorrhage
• normochromic normocytic anemia; polycythemia may
   precede myelosclerosis in 59%
• dry marrow aspirate
√ splenomegaly
Location: red marrow containing bones in 40% (thoracic
            cage, pelvis, femora, humeral shafts, lumbar
            spine, skull, peripheral bones)
√ widespread diffuse increase in density (ground glass)
√ "jail bar" ribs
√ sandwich / rugger jersey spine
√ generalized increase in bone density in skull +
   obliteration of diploic space; scattered small rounded
   radiolucent lesions; or combination of both
NUC:
   √ diffuse increased uptake of bone tracer in affected
      skeleton, possibly "superscan"
   √ increased uptake at ends of long bones
DDx:
   (a) with splenomegaly: chronic leukemia, lymphoma,
        mastocytosis
   (b) without splenomegaly: osteoblastic metastases,
        fluorine poisoning, osteopetrosis, chronic renal
        disease

MYOSITIS OSSIFICANS
(1) Myositis ossificans progressiva
(2) Localized myositis ossificans secondary to TRAUMA
     (60%)
     Site: periosteal at tendon insertion; **"rider's bone"**
             (adductor longus); **"fencer's bone"**
             (brachialis); **"dancer's bone"** (soleus);
             Pellegrini-Stieda disease (adductor magnus
             tendon)
     √ radiolucent zone towards bone (DDx: periosteal
        sarcoma on stalk)
     √ irregular ossified mass (5 – 6 weeks)
     √ resorption in 1 year
(3) Myositis ossificans associated with NEUROLOGIC
     DISORDERS = Paraosteoarthropathy
(4) Localized myositis ossificans of UNKNOWN ORIGIN
     ? trauma; ? healed phase of dermatomyositis

MYOSITIS OSSIFICANS PROGRESSIVA

= congenital / idiopathic disease
Age: onset within 1st decade; exacerbation
- initially subcutaneous swelling on neck, back,
  ± extremities
- lesions may ulcerate and bleed
- muscles of back + proximal extremities become rigid
- inanition secondary to jaw trismus (masseter, temporal muscle)
- "wry neck"
- respiratory failure (thoracic muscles affected)
√ microdactyly of big toes (90%) and thumbs (50%)
  = usually only one large phalanx present / synostosis of metacarpal + proximal phalanx (first sign)
√ hallux valgus
√ progressive fusion of vertebral bodies
√ rounded / linear calcification in neck / shoulders, hips, proximal extremity, trunk, palmar + plantar fascia
√ ossification of voluntary muscles, complete by 20 – 25 years (sparing of sphincters + head)

NAIL-PATELLA SYNDROME

= FONG DISEASE = ILIAC HORNS = FAMILIAL ONYCHO-OSTEODYSPLASIA = OSTEO-ONYCHODYSOSTOSIS
- aplasia / hypoplasia of thumb + index finger nails
- renal failure in later life
√ hypoplasia / absence of patella
√ bilateral posterior iliac horns in 80% (independent ossification center) DIAGNOSTIC
√ flared iliac crest with prominent anterior spines
√ radial head / capitellum hypoplasia (DDx: congenital dislocation of radial head)
√ clinodactyly
√ short 5th metacarpals

NEUROBLASTOMA

Age at presentation: < 2 years (50%); < 4 years (75%);
 < 8 years (90%); peak age < 3 years
- abdominal mass (45%)
- neurologic signs (20%)
- bone pain / limp (20%)
- orbital ecchymosis / proptosis (12%)
- catecholamine production (95%) with paroxysmal episodes of flushing, tachycardia, hypertension, headaches, sweating, intractable diarrhea, acute cerebellar encephalopathy
- positive bone marrow aspiration (70%)
Location: adrenal gland (67%), chest (13%), neck (5 %), intracranial (2%); commonly involvement of multiple skeletal sites
NUC: (overall sensitivity of detection better than radiography)
  CAVE: symmetric lytic neuroblastoma metastases occur frequently in metaphyseal areas where normal epiphyseal activity obscures lesions
√ purely lytic lesions may present as photopenic areas
√ soft tissue uptake of Tc-99m phosphate in 60%

√ frequently GA-67 uptake in primary site of neuroblastoma
Prognosis: 2-year survival (a) in 60% for age < 1 year (b) in 20% for ages 1 – 2 years (c) 10% for ages > 2 years

NEUROPATHIC ARTHROPATHY

= CHARCOT JOINT = change in sensory nerves associated with trauma
Pathogenesis: (1) decreased pain sensation produces repetitive trauma
 (2) sympathetic dysfunction results in local hyperemia + bone resorption
Causes:
  A. Congenital
    1. Myelomeningocele
    2. Congenital indifference to pain = asymbolia
  B. Acquired
    (a) Central neuropathy
      1. Injury to brain / spinal cord
      2. Syringomyelia (in 1/3 of patients): shoulder joint affected
      3. Neurosyphilis = tabes dorsalis (in 15 – 20% of patients): knees, hips, tarsals, ankles affected
      4. Spinal cord tumors / infection
    (b) Peripheral neuropathy
      1. Diabetes mellitus (most common cause, although incidence low): hands + feet affected
      2. Leprosy
      3. Peripheral nerve injury
    (c) Others
      1. Scleroderma, Raynaud disease, Ehlers-Danlos syndrome
      2. Rheumatoid arthritis, psoriasis
      3. Amyloid infiltration of nerves, adrenal hypercorticism
  C. Iatrogenic
    prolonged use of pain-relieving drugs
mnemonic: "DS6"
  Diabetes
  Syphilis
  Steroids
  Spinal cord injury
  Spina bifida
  Syringomyelia
  Scleroderma
√ persistent joint effusion (first sign)
√ narrowing of joint space
√ hypertrophic spurs
√ increased density of subchondral bone
√ calcification of synovial membrane
√ fragmentation of eburnated subchondral bone
√ joint subluxation (laxity of periarticular soft tissues) + dislocations
√ progressive rapid resorption of head + neck of humerus or femur

√ "pencilpoint" deformity of metatarsal heads
√ NO juxtaarticular osteoporosis
√ "bags-of-bones" effect in late stage (= marked deformities around joint)
mnemonic: "5 Ds"
√ **D**ense subchondral bone
√ **D**estruction of articular cortex
√ **D**eformity (pencil point)
√ **D**ebris (loose bodies)
√ **D**islocation

NONOSSIFYING FIBROMA

= NONOSTEOGENIC FIBROMA = XANTHOMA
= XANTHOGRANULOMA OF BONE = FIBROUS METAPHYSEAL-DIAPHYSEAL DEFECT = FIBROUS MEDULLARY DEFECT
Incidence: up to 40% of all children > 2 years of age
Etiology: lesion resulting from proliferative activity of a fibrous cortical defect which has expanded into medullary cavity
Histo: whorled bundles of connective tissue cells + multinucleated giant cells + foamy xanthomatous cells
Age: 8 – 20 years; 75% in 2nd decade of life
• usually asymptomatic
Location: shaft of long bone; mostly in bones of lower extremity, especially about knee (distal femur + proximal tibia); distal tibia; fibula
Site: eccentric metaphyseal, several cm shaftwards from epiphysis, mostly intramedullary, rarely purely diaphyseal
√ multilocular ovoid bubbly osteolytic area
√ alignment along long axis of bone, about 2 cm in length
√ dense sclerotic border toward medulla; V- or U-shaped at one end
√ endosteal scalloping +thinning ± overlying bulge
√ migrates toward center of diaphysis
√ resolves with age
√ minimal / mild uptake on bone scan
Prognosis: spontaneous healing in most cases
Cx: (1) Pathologic fracture (not uncommon)
(2) Hypophosphatemic vitamin D-resistant rickets + osteomalacia (tumor may secrete substance that increases renal tubular resorption of phosphorus)
DDx: (1) Adamantinoma (midshaft of tibia)
(2) Chondromyxoid fibroma (more bulging of cortex)

JAFFE-CAMPANACCI SYNDROME

= nonossifying fibroma with extraskeletal manifestations in children
• mental retardation
• hypogonadism
• ocular defect
• cardiovascular congenital defect
• café-au-lait spots

NOONAN SYNDROME

= PSEUDO-TURNER = MALE TURNER SYNDROME
= somatic abnormalities similar to Turner syndrome but with normal karyotype
• short / may have normal height
• webbed neck
• agonadism / normal gonads
• mental retardation
√ osteoporosis
√ retarded bone age
√ cubitus valgus
@ Skull
√ mandibular hypoplasia with dental malocclusion
√ hypertelorism
√ biparietal foramina
√ dolichocephaly, microcephaly / cranial enlargement
√ webbed neck
@ Chest
√ sternal deformity: pectus cavus / carinatum
√ right-sided congenital heart disease (pulmonary stenosis, PDA, VSD)
√ coronal clefts of spine
@ Gastrointestinal tract
√ intestinal lymphangiectasia
√ eventration of diaphragm
√ renal duplication, renal malrotation, hydronephrosis, large redundant extrarenal pelvis

OCHRONOSIS

= ALKAPTONURIA = inherited absence of homogentisic acid oxidase with excessive homogentisic acid production + deposition in connective tissue;
M:F = 2:1
• black pigment in soft tissues (in 2nd decade): yellowish skin; gray pigmentation of sclera; bluish tinge of ears + nose cartilage
• alkaptonuria with black staining of diapers
• heart failure, renal failure (pigment deposition)
√ laminated calcification of multiple intervertebral discs
√ disc space drastically narrowed
√ multiple "vacuum" phenomena (common)
√ osteoporosis in adjoining vertebrae
√ massive osteophytosis + ankylosis of spine (in older patient)
√ hypertrophic changes in humeral head
√ severe premature progressive osteoarthritic changes in shoulder, knee, hip, spine of young patients
√ spotty calcifications in tissue anterior to vertebral bodies
√ small calcifications in paraarticular soft tissues + tendons

OSGOOD-SCHLATTER DISEASE

= avascular necrosis of tibial tuberosity
• local pain + tenderness on pressure, swelling of overlying soft tissue
Age: 10 – 15 years; boys
√ fragmentation of tibial tubercle displaced away from the shaft

√ sometimes increased density
√ comparison with other side (irregular development normal)

OSSIFYING FIBROMA
Closely related to fibrous dysplasia + adamantinoma
Age: 2nd – 4th decade; M < F
Histo: maturing cellular fibrous spindle cells with osteoblastic activity producing many calcific cartilaginous + bone densities
Location: frequently in face
@ Mandible, maxilla
  • painless expansion of tooth-bearing portion of jaw
  √ 1 – 5 cm well-circumscribed round / oval tumor
  √ moderate expansion of intact cortex
  √ homogeneous tumor matrix
  √ dislodgement of teeth
@ Tibia
  √ eccentric ground-glass lesion (resembling fibrous dysplasia)
Cx: frequent recurrences

OSTEITIS CONDENSANS ILII
Age: in women during childbearing age
  • may be associated with low back pain
  √ increased triangular sclerosis of inferior aspect of ileum (joint space uninvolved)
  √ usually bilateral + symmetric; occasionally unilateral
  √ sclerosis may dissolve in 3 – 20 years
DDx:
  (1) Ankylosing spondylitis (affects ilium + sacrum, joint space narrowing, involvement of other bones)
  (2) Rheumatoid arthritis (asymmetric, joint destruction)

OSTEOARTHRITIS
= DEGENERATIVE JOINT DISEASE = decreased chondroitin sulfate with age creates unsupported collagen fibrils followed by cartilage degeneration
Radiologic signs:
  √ joint space narrowing
  √ sclerosis / eburnation of subchondral bone in areas of stress
  √ subchondral cyst formation (geodes)
  √ osteophytosis at articular margin / non-stressed area

@ Hand + foot
  Target area: 1st MCP; trapezioscaphoid; DIP > PIP; 1st MTP
  √ radial subluxation of 1st metacarpal base
  √ Bouchard nodes = osteophytosis at PIP joint
  √ Heberden nodes = osteophytosis at DIP joint: M:F = 1:10
@ Hip
  √ superior migration of femoral head (less frequently medial / axial)
  √ femoral + acetabular osteophytes, sclerosis, cyst formation
  √ thickening / buttressing of medial femoral cortex

@ Knee
  √ medial femorotibial compartment usually first to be involved
  √ varus deformity
@ Spine
  √ sclerosis + narrowing of intervertebral apophyseal joints
  √ osteophytosis usually associated with discogenic disease

EROSIVE OSTEOARTHRITIS
= inflammatory form of osteoarthrosis
Predisposed: postmenopausal females
Site: DIP + PIP joints of hands; bilateral + symmetric
√ "bird-wing" / "sea-gull" joint configuration = central erosions
√ may lead to bony ankylosis
DDx: Rheumatoid arthritis, Wilson disease, chronic liver disease, hemochromatosis

EARLY OSTEOARTHRITIS
mnemonic: "**E**arly **O**steo**A**rthritis"
  E piphyseal dysplasia, multiple
  O chronosis
  A cromegaly

OSTEOBLASTOMA
= GIANT OSTEOID OSTEOMA = OSTEOGENIC FIBROMA OF BONE = OSSIFYING FIBROMA; rare benign tumor with unlimited growth potential + capability of malignant transformation
Incidence: < 1% of all primary bone tumors; 3% of all benign bone tumors
Age: 16 – 19 years mean age; 6 – 30 years (90%); 2nd decade (55%); 3rd decade (20%); M:F = 2:1
Path: lesion > 1.5 cm; smaller lesions are classified as osteoid osteoma
Histo: numerous multinucleated giant cells (osteoclasts), irregularly arranged osteoid + bone; very vascular connective tissue stroma; trabeculae broader + longer than in osteoid osteoma
Location: (rarely multifocal)
  (a) spine (33 – 37%): 62 – 94% in dorsal elements, secondary extension into vertebral body (28%); cervical spine (31%), dorsal spine (34%), lumbar spine (31%), sacrum (3%)
  (b) long bones (26 – 32%): femur (50%), tibia (19%), humerus (19%), radius (8%), fibula (4%); unusual in neck of femur
  (c) small bones of hand + feet (15 – 26%): dorsal talus neck (62%), calcaneus (4%), scaphoid (8%), metacarpals (8%), metatarsals (8%)
  (d) calvarium + mandible (= cementoblastoma)
Site: diaphyseal (58%), metaphyseal (42%); eccentric (46%), intracortical (42%), centric (12%), may be periosteal
  • asymptomatic in < 2%

- dull pain of insidious onset (84%), worse at night in 7 – 13%
- response to salicylates in 7%
- localized swelling, tenderness, decreased range of motion (29%)
- painful scoliosis in 50% (with spinal / rib location) secondary to muscle spasm
- mild muscle weakness to paraplegia due to cord compression
- occasional systemic toxicity (high WBC, fever)
√ radiolucent nidus > 2 cm (range of 2 – 12 cm) in size
√ well demarcated (83%)
√ ± stippled / ringlike small flecks of matrix calcification
√ tumor matrix radiolucent (25 – 64%) / ossified (36 – 72%)
√ no reactive sclerosis (9 – 56%)
√ reactive sclerosis (22 – 91%)
√ cortical expansion (75 – 94%)
√ cortical destruction (20 – 22%)
√ progressive expansile lesion that may rapidly increase in size (25%)
√ sharply defined soft tissue component
√ thin shell of periosteal new bone (58 – 77%) / no periosteal reaction
√ scoliosis (35%)
√ osteoporosis due to disuse + hyperemia in talar location
√ rapid calcification after radiotherapy
NUC:
    √ intense focal accumulation of bone agent (100%)
Angio:
    √ tumor blush in capillary phase (50%)
MRI:
    √ low to intermediate intensity on T1WI
    √ mixed to high intensity on T2WI
    √ surrounding edema
Prognosis: 10% recurrence after excision; incomplete currettage can effect cure due to cartilage production + trapping of host lamellar bone
DDx:
    (1) Osteo- / chondrosarcoma (periosteal new bone)
    (2) Osteoid osteoma (dense calcification + halo of bone sclerosis, < 2 cm due to limited growth potential)
    (3) Cartlagineous tumors (lumpy matrix calcification)
    (4) Giant cell tumor (no calcification, epiphyseal involvement)
    (5) Aneurysmal bone cyst
    (6) Osteomyelitis
    (7) Hemangioma
    (8) Lipoma
    (9) Epidermoid
    (10) Fibrous dysplasia
    (11) Metastasis
    (12) Ewing sarcoma

OSTEOCHONDROSIS DISSECANS
= OSTEOCHONDRAL FRACTURE
Etiology: subchondral fatigue fracture

Age: adolescence; M > F
- asymptomatic / vague complaints
Location:
    (a) capitellum of elbow
    (b) knee (medial femoral condyle close to fossa intercondylaris (90%); rarely lateral; bilateral in 20 – 30%
    (c) talus
√ mouse = osteochondrotic fragment
√ mouse bed = sclerosed pit in articular surface

OSTEOGENESIS IMPERFECTA
= PSATHYROSIS = FRAGILITAS OSSIUM = LOBSTEIN DISEASE
= heterogeneous group of a generalized connective tissue disorder leading to micromelic dwarfism characterized by bone fragility, blue sclerae, and dentinogenesis imperfecta
Incidence: overall in 1:28,500 (20,000 – 60,000) live births; M:F = 1:1
Histo: immature collagen matrix
Clinical types:
    1. OSTEOGENESIS IMPERFECTA CONGENITA
        = disease manifest at birth (occurring in utero); autosomal dominant; corresponds to Type II
    2. OSTEOGENESIS IMPERFECTA TARDA
        = usually not manifest at birth; recessive / sporadic corresponds to Type I + IV
- soft skull (caput membranaceum)
- hyperlaxity of joints
- blue sclerae
- poor dentition
- otosclerosis
- thin loose skin
√ diffuse demineralization, deficient trabecular structure, cortical thinning
√ defective cortical bone: increase in diameter of proximal ends of humeri + femora; slender fragile bone; multiple cyst-like areas
√ multiple fractures + pseudarthrosis with bowing (vertebral bodies, long bones)
√ normal / exuberant callus formation
√ rib thinning / notching
√ thin calvarium
√ sinus + mastoid cell enlargement
√ Wormian bones persisting into adulthood
√ basilar impression (= platybasia)
√ biconcave vertebral bodies + Schmorl nodes, increased height of intervertebral disc space
√ bowing deformities after child begins to walk
Cx: (1) impaired hearing / deafness from otosclerosis (20 – 60%)
        (2) death from intracranial hemorrhage (abnormal platelet function)

Osteogenesis Imperfecta Type I
Autosomal dominant; compatible with life
Age at presentation: 2 – 6 years

- blue sclerae
- presenile deafness
- normal / abnormal dentinogenesis
- √ infants of normal weight + length
- √ osteoporosis
- √ fractures in neonate (occurring during delivery)
- OB-US: √ marked bowing of long bones
  - √ NO IUGR

Osteogenesis Imperfecta Type II
Autosomal recessive / sporadic; perinatal lethal form
Incidence: 1:54,000 births; most frequent variety
- blue sclerae
- ligamentous laxity + loose skin
- √ shortened broad crumpled long bones
- √ bone angulations, bowing, demineralization
- √ localized bone thickening from callus formation
- √ thin beaded ribs ± fractures resulting in bell-shaped / narrow chest
- √ thin poorly ossified skull
- √ spinal osteopenia
- √ platyspondyly
- √ infants small for gestational age (frequent)
- OB-US:
  - √ abnormal compressibility of skull vault with transducer
  - √ increased through-transmission (extremely poor mineralization)
    - √ unusually good visualization of orbits
    - √ increased visualization of intracranial arterial pulsations
  - √ decreased visualization of skeleton
  - √ multiple fetal fractures + deformities of long bones + ribs
  - √ abnormally short limbs
  - √ small thorax (collapse of thoracic cage)
  - √ decreased fetal movement
- *Prognosis:* stillborn / death shortly after birth due to pulmonary hypoplasia

Osteogenesis Imperfecta Type III
Autosomal recessive / dominant; progressively deforming disorder compatible with life
- bluish sclerae during infancy which turn pale with time
- joint hyperlaxity (50%)
- √ decreased ossification of skull
- √ progressive deformities of limbs + spine into adulthood
- √ normal vertebrae + pelvis
- √ shortened + bowed long bones
- √ ± rib fractures
- √ multiple fractures present at birth in 2/3 of cases
- √ fractures heal well
- OB-US:
  - √ short + bowed long bones
  - √ fractures
  - √ humerus almost normal in shape
  - √ normal thoracic circumference

Prognosis: progressive limb + spine deformities during childhood / adolescence

Osteogenesis Imperfecta Type IV
Autosomal dominant; mildest form with best prognosis
- normal scleral color
- little tendency to develop hearing loss
- √ tubular bones of normal length; mild femoral bowing may occur
- √ osteoporosis
- OB-US: √ bowing of long bones

OSTEOID OSTEOMA
No growth progression, infrequent regression
Etiology: ? (inflammatory response)
Histo: small highly vascularized nidus of osteoid-laden trabeculae surrounded by zone of reactive bone sclerosis; indistinguishable from osteoblastoma
Age: peak age 2nd decade (51%); 2nd + 3rd decade (73%); 5 – 25 years (90%); range of 2 – 50 years; M:F = 2:1
- tender to touch + pressure
- local pain, worse at night, decreased by activity
- salicylates give relief in 20 – 30 minutes in 90%
- prostaglandin E2 elevated 100 x normal
- Location:
  - (a) metaphysis of long bones (73%): upper end of femur (43%), hands (8%), feet (4%); frequent in proximal tibia + femoral neck, fibula, humerus; no bone exempt
  - (b) spine (14%): predominantly in posterior elements (pedicle, lamina, spinous process) of lower thoracic + upper lumbar spine
- Site:
  - (a) CORTICAL: nidus within cortex; solid / laminated periosteal reaction
  - (b) CANCELLOUS = intramedullary: femoral neck, vertebral centra, small bones of hands + feet; little osteosclerosis / sclerotic cortex distant to nidus
  - (c) PAROSTEAL: round soft tissue mass adjacent to bone; bony pressure atrophy affecting neighboring joints; posterior elements of spine, femoral neck, hands, feet
- √ small nidus of < 1.0 cm in size surrounded by dense bone
- √ radiolucent nidus (75%) ± central calcifications
- √ scoliosis concave toward lesion
- √ intensely increased radiotracer uptake (increased blood flow + new bone formation)
- √ radiographically difficult areas: vertebral column, femoral neck, small bones of hand + feet
- *DDx:* Brodie abscess, bone island, stress fracture, osteosarcoma, Ewing sarcoma, metastasis, subperiosteal aneurysmal bone cyst

OSTEOFIBROUS DYSPLASIA
= entity previously mistaken for fibrous dysplasia
Age: newborn up to 5 years

Histo: fibrous tissue surrounding trabeculae in a whirled
            storiform pattern
Location: normally confined to tibia (mid-diaphysis in
            50%), lesion begins in anterior cortex;
            ipisilateral fibula affected in 20%
√ enlargement of tibia with anterior bowing
√ cortex thin / invisible
√ periosteal expansion
√ sclerotic margin (DDx: nonosteogenic fibroma,
  chondromyxoid fibroma)
√ spontaneous regression in 1/3
Cx: pathologic fracture in 25%, fractures will heal with
        immobilization; infrequently complicated by
        pseudarthrosis
DDx: Fibrous dysplasia, Paget disease

OSTEOMA
= benign tumor of membranous bone (hamartoma)
Age: adult life
Associated with: Gardner syndrome (multiple osteomas +
                    colonic polyposis)
Location: inner / outer table of calvarium (usually from
            external table), paranasal sinuses (frontal /
            ethmoid sinuses), mandible, nasal bones
√ well-circumscribed round extremely dense +
  structureless lesion usually < 2 cm in size

FIBROUS OSTEOMA
Probably a form of fibrous dysplasia
Age: childhood
√ less dense than osteoma / radiolucent
√ expanding external table without affecting internal
  table
DDx: enostoma, bone island, bone infarct (located in
        medulla)

OSTEOMYELITIS
Acute Osteomyelitis
Age: most commonly affects children
Organisms:
   (a) newborns: St. aureus, group B streptococcus,
                    Escherichia coli
   (b) children: St. aureus (blood cultures in 50%
                    positive)
   (c) adults: St. aureus (60%), Enteric species
                    (29%), Streptococcus (8%)
   (d) drug addicts: Pseudomonas (86%), Klebsiella,
                        Enterobacteriae; (57 days
                        average delay in diagnosis)
   (e) sickle cell disease: Salmonella
Cause:
   (a) genitourinary tract infection (72%) (b) lung
   infection (14%) (c) dermal infection (14%)
Sites:
   @ Lower extremity (75%)
   @ Vertebrae (53%):   lumbar (75%) > thoracic >
                         cervical
   @ Radial styloid (24%)
   @ Sacroiliac joint (18%)

• leukocytosis + fever (66%)

A. ACUTE NEONATAL OSTEOMYELITIS
    Age: onset < 30 days of age
    • little / no systemic disturbance
    √ multicentric involvement more common; often
      joint involvement
    √ bone scan falsely negative / equivocal in 70%
B. ACUTE OSTEOMYELITIS IN INFANCY
    (< 18 months of age)
    Pathomechanism:
        spread to epiphysis because transphyseal
        vessels cross growth plate into epiphysis
    √ striking soft tissue component
    √ subperiosteal abscess with extensive periosteal
      new bone
    Cx: frequent joint involvement
    Prognosis: rapid healing
C. ACUTE OSTEOMYELITIS IN CHILDHOOD
    (2 – 16 years of age)
    Pathomechanism:
        transphyseal vessels closed; metaphyseal
        vessels adjacent to growth plate loop back
        toward metaphysis locating the primary focus of
        infection into metaphysis; abscess formation in
        medulla with cortical spread
    √ sequestration frequent
    √ periosteal elevation
    √ small single / multiple osteolytic areas in
      metaphysis
    √ extensive periosteal reaction parallel to shaft (3 –
      6 weeks); may be "lamellar nodular"
      (DDx: osteoblastoma, eosinophilic granuloma)
    √ shortening of bone with destruction of epiphyseal
      cartilage
    √ growth stimulation by hyperemia + premature
      maturation of adjacent   epiphysis
    √ midshaft osteomyelitis less frequent site
    √ serpiginous tract with small sclerotic rim
      (PATHOGNOMONIC)
D. ACUTE OSTEOMYELITIS IN ADULTHOOD
    √ delicate periosteal new bone
    √ joint involvement common

Radiographs:
√ initial radiographs often normal (in early phase
  notoriously poor)
√ localized soft tissue swelling adjacent to
  metaphysis with obliteration of usual fat planes (3 –
  10 days)
√ area of bone destruction (lags 7 – 14 days behind
  pathologic changes)
√ involucrum = cloak of laminated / spiculated
  periosteal reaction (develops after 20 days)
√ sequestrum = detached necrotic cortical bone
  (develops after 30 days)
√ cloaca formation = space in which dead bone
  resides

NUC (accuracy approx. 90%):
  (1) Ga-67 scans: 100% sensitivity; increased
      uptake 1 day earlier than for Tc-99m MDP
  (2) Static Tc-99m diphosphonate: 83% sensitivity
      5 – 60% false-negative rate in neonates +
      children because of (a) masking effect of
      epiphyseal plates (b) early diminished blood flow
      with infection (c) spectrum of uptake pattern from
      hot to cold
  (3) Three-phase skeletal scintigraphy:
      92% sensitivity, 87% specificity
      Phase 1 : Radionuclide angiography = perfusion
                 phase of regional blood flow
      Phase 2: "blood pool" images
      Phase 3: "bone uptake"
      DDx: Cellulitis (decrease in activity over time)
  (4) In-111-labeled leukocytes: best agent for acute
      infections
  √ local increase in radiopharmaceutical uptake
    (positive within 24 – 72 hours)
  √ "cold" area in early osteomyelitis subsequently
    becoming "hot " if localized to long bones / pelvis
    (not seen in vertebral bodies)
Cx:
  (1) Soft tissue abscess (2) Fistula formation
  (3) Pathologic fracture (4) Extension into joint
  (5) Growth disturbance due to epiphyseal involvement
  (6) Neoplasm (7) Amyloidosis (8) Severe deformity
  with delayed treatment

Chronic Osteomyelitis
  √ thick irregular sclerotic bone with radiolucencies,
    elevated periosteum, chronic draining sinus

Sclerosing Osteomyelitis of Garré
    = low grade infection, no purulent exudate
    Location: mandible (most commonly)
    √ focal bulge of thickened cortex (sclerosing
      periosteal reaction)
    DDx: Osteoid osteoma, stress fracture

Chronic Recurrent Multifocal Osteomyelitis
    = benign self-limited disease of unknown etiology
    Age: children + adolescents; M:F = 1:2
    Histo: nonspecific subacute / chronic osteomyelitis
    • pain, soft tissue swelling, limited motion
    Location: tibia > femur > clavicle > fibula
    Site: metaphyses of long bones; often symmetric
    √ small areas of bone lysis, often confluent

Brodie Abscess
    = subacute pyogenic osteomyelitis (smoldering -
      indolent infection)
    Organism: S. aureus (most common)
    Histo: granulation tissue + eburnation
    Age: more common in children; M > F
    Location: tibial metaphysis (most common)
    √ central area of lucency surrounded by dense
      reactive sclerosis

√ channel-like configuration toward growth plate
√ may persisit for many months
DDx: Osteoid osteoma

Epidermoid Carcinoma
    Etiology: Complication of chronic osteomyelitis (0.5 –
                1.6%)
    Histo: squamous cell carcinoma (90%);
             occasionally: basal cell carcinoma,
             adenocarcinoma, fibrosarcoma,
             angiosarcoma, reticulum cell sarcoma,
             spindle cell sarcoma, rhabdomyosarcoma,
             parosteal osteosarcoma, plasmacytoma
    Age: 30 – 80 (mean 55) years; M >> F; after 20
           years of osteomyelitis
    • exacerbation of symptoms with increasing pain,
      enlarging mass
    • change in character / amount of sinus drainage
    Location: at site of chronically / intermittently draining
                sinus; tibia (50%), femur (20%)
    √ lytic lesion superimposed on changes of chronic
      osteomyelitis
    √ soft tissue mass
    √ pathologic fracture
    Prognosis: (1) early metastases in 20% (within 18
                      months)
                 (2) no recurrence in 80%

OSTEOPATHIA STRIATA
    = VOORHOEVE DISEASE
    • usually asymptomatic (similar to osteopoikilosis)
    Location: all long bones affected; the only bone sclerosis
                primarily involving metaphysis (with extension
                into epi- and diaphysis)
    √ longitudinal striations of dense bone in metaphysis
    √ radiating densities of "sunburst" appearance from
      acetabulum into ileum

OSTEOPETROSIS
    = ALBERS-SCHÖNBERG DISEASE = MARBLE BONE
      DISEASE = rare hereditary disorder
    • anemia
    • cranial nerve compression (optic atrophy, deafness)
    • hepatosplenomegaly
    • lymphadenopathy
    • subarachnoid hemorrhage
    Path: failure of resorptive mechanisms of calcified
            cartilage which interferes with its normal
            replacement by mature bone
    √ osteosclerosis = generalized dense amorphous
      structureless bones
    √ cortical thickening with medullary encroachment
    √ Erlenmeyer flask deformity = lack of modeling of tubular
      bones + flaring of ends
    √ bone-within-bone appearance
    √ alternating dense + radiolucent transverse metaphyseal
      lines (phalanges, iliac bones)
    √ longitudinal metaphyseal striations

√ obliteration of mastoid cells, paranasal sinuses, basal foramina by osteosclerosis

√ calvaria often spared

Cx: (1) usually transverse fractures (common) with abundant callus
      (2) crowding of marrow (myelophthisic anemia + extramedullary hematopoiesis)
      (3) frequently terminates in acute leukemia

Rx: bone marrow transplant

DDx: (1) Heavy metal poisoning
      (2) Melorheostosis (limited to one extremity)
      (3) Hypervitaminosis D
      (4) Pyknodysostosis
      (5) Fibrous dysplasia of skull / face

OSTEOPOIKILOSIS

= OSTEOPATHIA CONDENSANS DISSEMINATA

Autosomal dominant; M > F

• asymptomatic

Histo: compact bone islands

Location: in most metaphyses + epiphyses (rarely extending into midshaft); concentrated at glenoid + acetabulum; rare in skull, ribs, vertebral centra, mandible

√ small foci of ovoid / lenticular opacification (2 – 20 mm)

√ long axis of lesions parallel to long axis of bone

Prognosis: not progressive, no change after cessation of growth

DDx: (1) Epiphyseal dysplasia (metaphyses normal)
      (2) Melorheostosis (diaphyseal involvement)

OSTEOSARCOMA

TYPES & FREQUENCY

A. Conventional osteosarcoma   72%
    osteoblastic / chondroblastic / fibroblastic
B. Variants
    (a) Clinical variants
         1. Osteosarcoma of jaw   6%
         2. Postradiation osteosarcoma   4%
         3. Osteosarcoma in Paget disease   3%
         4. Multifocal osteosarcoma   < 1%
         5. Osteosarcoma in benign condition   < 1%
             (fibrous dysplasia, osteoblastoma)
    (b) Surface variants
         1. Parosteal osteosarcoma   4%
         2. Dedifferentiated parosteal osteosa.
         3. Periosteal osteosarcoma   < 1%
         4. High-grade surface osteosarcoma   < 1%
    (c) Morphological variants
         1. Telangiectatic osteosarcoma   3%
         2. Dedifferentiated chondrosarcoma   3%

Osteosarcomatosis

= SCLEROSING OSTEOGENIC SARCOMA
= OSTEOBLASTIC OSTEOGENIC SARCOMA
= SCLEROSING OSTEOGENIC SARCOMATOSIS

Etiology: (a) multicentric type of osteosarcoma
            (b) multiple metastastic lesions

Age: 6 – 9 years

Site: metaphysis of long bones; may extend into epiphyseal plate / begin in epiphysis

√ multicentric simultaneously appearing lesions

√ densely opaque (osteoblastic)

√ lesions bilateral + symmetrical

√ early: bone islands

√ late: entire metaphysis fills with sclerotic lesions breaking through cortex

√ lesions are of same size

√ lung metastases common

Prognosis: uniformly poor with early death

DDx: heavy metal poisoning, sclerosing osteitis, progressive diaphyseal dysplasia, melorheostosis, osteopoikilosis, bone infarction, osteopetrosis

Central Osteosarcoma

Most common malignant primary bone tumor in young adults + children; 2nd most common primary malignant bone tumor after multiple myeloma

Histo: arising from undifferentiated mesenchymal tissue; forming fibrous / cartilaginous / osseous matrix (mostly mixed) that produces osteoid / immature bone

Age: bimodal distribution 10 – 25 years and > 60 years; 21% < 10 years; 68% < 15 years; 70% between 10 and 30 years; M:F = 3:2;
        > 35 years: related to preexisting conditions (Paget disease, previously irradiated bone)

• painful swelling (1 – 2 months duration)

• fever (frequent)

• slight elevation of alkaline phosphatase

• diabetes mellitus (paraneoplastic syndrome) in 25%

Location: long bones, femur (40%), tibia (16%);
            50 – 75% at knee; proximal humerus (15%);
            cylindrical bone < 30 years; flat bone (ilium) > 50 years

Site: meta- / diaphysis

√ usually large bone lesion > 5 cm when first detected

√ osteolytic / almost normal / extremely dense (50%) lesion

√ sunburst / onion-peel periosteal reaction + Codman triangle

√ motheaten bone destruction + cortical disruption

√ soft tissue mass with tumor new bone (osseous / cartilaginous type)

√ transepiphyseal spread after plate closure only

√ intensely increased activity on bone scan (vascularity, new bone formation)

√ bone scan establishes local extent, skip lesions, metastases to bone + soft tissues

Cx:
    (1) pathologic fracture (significant number)
    (2) radiation-induced osteosarcoma (30 years delay)

Metastases (in 2% at presentation):
    (a) hematogeneous lung metastases (15%):

calcifying; spontaneous pneumothorax secondary to subpleural cavitating nodules rupturing into pleural space
(b) lymph nodes, liver, brain (may be calcified)
(c) skeletal metastases uncommon (unlike Ewing sarcoma)
Prognosis:
(1) amputation: 20% 5-year survival; 15% develop skeletal metastases; 75% dead within < 2 years
(2) multidrug chemotherapy: 55% 4-year survival more proximal lesions carry higher mortality (0% 2-year survival for axial primary)
DDx: Osteoid osteoma, sclerosing osteomyelitis, Charcot joint

Periosteal Osteosarcoma
1% of all osteosarcomas
Histo: centrally malignant osteoid with peripheral lobules of cartilage extending perpendicular from cortical surface
Age: peak 10 – 20 years (range of 13 – 70 years)
Location: proximal tibia, distal femur at the medial / anterior aspects, humerus, fibula, ilium
Site: metaphysis / diaphysis of long bone; limited to periphery of cortex with normal endosteal margin + medullary canal (resembles parosteal sarcoma)
√ sessile elliptical growth at periosteum
√ short spicules of bone at right angles to shaft
√ tumor 7 – 12 cm in length, 2 – 4 cm in width
√ small uncalcified soft tissue component beyond calcified margins
√ tumor base closely attached to cortex over entire extent of tumor
√ NO cortical destruction / medullary cavity invasion
√ may lie in apparent depression on bone surface
Prognosis: 80 – 90% cure rate (better prognosis than central osteosarcoma with 50% 5-year survival)
DDx: juxtacortical chondrosarcoma

Parosteal Osteosarcoma
= JUXTACORTICAL OSTEOSARCOMA;
4% of osteosarcomas; slowly growing lesion with fulminating course if tumor reaches medullary canal
Histo: often cartilaginous cap (as in benign osteo- / chondrosarcoma)
Age: peak age 38 years (range of 12 – 58 years); 50% > age 30 (for central osteosarcoma 75% < age 30); M:F = 2:3
Location: posterior aspect of distal femur (50%), either end of tibia, proximal humerus, rare in other long bones
Site: adjacent to metaphyseal cortex in close relationship to periosteum
√ dense masses of homogeneous new bone extending away from cortex
√ lobulated round tumor periphery
√ small trabeculae may be present

√ initially fine radiolucent line separating tumor mass from cortex (30 – 40%)
√ tumor stalk grows with tumor obliterating radiolucent line
√ occasionally periphery more dense than center (DDx: myositis ossificans)
√ large soft tissue component with osseous + cartilaginous elements
Prognosis: 80 – 90% treated successfully (best prognosis of all osteosarcomas)
DDx: osteochondroma, myositis ossificans, juxtacortical hematoma, extraosseous osteosarcoma

Extraosseous Osteosarcoma
Infrequent
Histo: same as in osseous osteosarcoma
Mean age: 45 years
Location: thigh, retroperitoneum, buttock, back, orbit, submental, upper + lower extremities, axilla, abdomen, neck, kidney, breast
√ large soft tissue tumor
√ > 50% calcified

OXALOSIS
Rare inborn error of metabolism
Etiology: excessive amounts of oxalic acid combine with calcium and deposit throughout body (kidneys, soft tissue, bone)
• hyperoxaluria = urinary excretion of oxalic acid > 50 mg/ day
• progressive renal failure
√ osteoporosis = cystic rarefaction + sclerotic margins in tubular bones on metaphyseal side, may extend throughout diaphysis
√ erosions on concave side of metaphysis near epiphysis (DDx: hyperparathyroidism)
√ bone-within-bone appearance of spine
√ nephrocalcinosis (2° HPT: subperiosteal resorption, rugger jersey spine, sclerotic metaphyseal bands)
Cx: pathologic fractures

PACHYDERMOPERIOSTOSIS
= OSTEODERMOPATHIA HYPERTROPHICANS (TOURAINE-SOLENTÉ-GOLÉ)= PRIMARY HYPERTROPHIC OSTEOARTHROPATHY
Autosomal dominant
Age: 3 – 38 years with progression into late 20s / 30s; M >> F
• large skin folds of face + scalp
Location: epiphyses + diametaphyseal region of tubular bones; distal third of bones of legs + forearms (early); distal phalanges rarely involved
√ enlargement of paranasal sinuses
√ irregular periosteal proliferation of phalanges + distal long bones (hand + feet) beginning in epiphyseal region at tendon / ligament insertions
√ thick cortex, BUT NO narrowing of medulla

√ clubbing
√ may have acro-osteolysis
Prognosis: progression ceases after several years
DDx: pulmonary osteoarthropathy, thyroid acropachy

PAGET DISEASE
= OSTEITIS DEFORMANS = chronic skeletal disease of probable viral etiology
Incidence: 3% of individuals > 40 years; higher incidence in northern latitudes
Age: > 55 years (in 3%); > 80 years (in 10%); unusual < 40 years; M:F = 2:1
Histo: increased resorption + increased bone formation; newly formed bone is abnormally soft with disorganized trabecular pattern ("mosaic pattern") causing deformity
(a) ACTIVE PHASE = OSTEOLYTIC PHASE = aggressive bone resorption with lytic lesions, replacement of hematopoietic bone marrow by fibrous connective tissue with numerous large vascular channels
(b) INACTIVE PHASE = QUIESCENT PHASE = decreased bone turnover with skeletal sclerosis + cortical accretion
(c) MIXED PATTERN (common) = lytic + sclerotic phases usually coexist
• asymptomatic (1/5)
• fatigue
• enlarged hat size
• peripheral nerve compression
• neurologic disorders from compression of brain stem (basilar invagination)
• hearing loss, blindness, facial palsy (narrowing of neural foramina) — rare
• pain (a) from primary disease process — rare (b) pathologic fracture (c) malignant transformation (d) degenerative joint disease / rheumatic disorder aggravated by skeletal deformity
• local hyperthermia of overlying skin
• high-output congestive heart failure from markedly increased perfusion (rare)
• increased alkaline phosphatase (increased bone formation)
• hydroxyproline increased (increased bone resorption)
• normal serum calcium + phosphorus
Sites: usually polyostotic + asymmetric; pelvis (75%) > lumbar spine > thoracic spine > proximal femur > calvarium > scapula > distal femur > proximal tibia > proximal humerus
Sensitivity: scintigraphy + radiography (60%) scintigraphy only (27%) radiography only (13%)
√ thick coarse trabeculae, cortical thickening, cyst-like areas
@ Skull (inner + outer table involved)
√ osteoporosis circumscripta = well-defined lysis, most commonly in calvarium anteriorly, occasionally in long bones (destructive active stage)

√ "cotton wool" appearance = mixed lytic + blastic pattern of thickened calvarium (late stage)
√ diploic widening
√ basilar invagination with encroachment on foramen magnum
√ deossification + sclerosis in maxilla
@ Long bones (almost invariable at end of bone; rarely in diaphysis)
√ "candle flame" / "blade of grass" lysis = advancing tip of V-shaped lytic defect in diaphysis of long bone originating in subarticular site (CHARACTERISTIC)
√ lateral curvature of femur, anterior curvature of tibia (commonly resulting in fracture)
@ Small / flat bones
√ bubbly destruction + periosteal successive layering
@ Pelvis
√ thickened trabeculae in sacrum, ilium; rarefaction in central portion of ilium
√ thickening of ileopectineal line
√ acetabular protrusion (DDx: metastatic disease not deforming) + secondary degenerative joint disease
@ Spine (upper cervical, low dorsal, midlumbar)
√ lytic / coarse trabeculations at periphery of bone
√ "picture frame vertebra" = bone-within-bone appearance = enlarged square vertebral body with reinforced peripheral trabeculae + radiolucent inner aspect, typically in lumbar spine
√ "ivory vertebra = blastic vertebra with increased density
√ ossification of spinal ligaments, paravertebral soft tissue, disc spaces
Bone scan:
√ usually markedly increased uptake (symptomatic lesions strikingly positive)
√ normal scan in some sclerotic burned-out lesions
√ marginal uptake in lytic lesions
√ enlargement + deformity of bones
Bone marrow scan:
√ sulfur colloid bone marrow uptake is decreased (marrow replacement by cellular fibrovascular tissue)
Cx:
(1) Sarcomatous transformation into chondro- / osteo- / fibrosarcoma in < 5%
(2) Fracture: "banana fracture" = tiny horizontal cortical infractions on convex surfaces of lower extremity long bones (lateral bowing of femur, anterior bowing of tibia); compression fractures of vertebrae (soft bone despite increased density)
(3) Extradural spinal block (bone-forming phase / compression fractures) with neurologic deficits
(4) Giant cell tumor, especially in skull + facial bones
Rx: calcitonin, diphosphonate, mithramycin
Detection of recurrence:
(a) in 1/3 detected by bone scan
(b) in 1/3 detected by biomarkers (alkaline phosphatase, urine hydroxyproline)
(c) in 1/3 by scan + biomarkers simultaneously

√ diffuse (most common) / focal increase in tracer uptake

√ extension of uptake beyond boundaries of initial lesion

DDx: Osteosclerotic metastases, Hodgkin disease, Vertebral hemangioma

PANNER DISEASE

= osteonecrosis of capitellum

PARAOSTEOARTHROPATHY

= HETEROTOPIC BONE FORMATION = ECTOPIC OSSIFICATION = MYOSITIS OSSIFICANS

common complication following surgical manipulation, total hip replacement (62%) and chronic immobilization (spinal cord injury / neuromuscular disorders)

Etiology: pluripotent mesenchymal cell lays down matrix for formation of heterotopic bone similar to endosteal bone

Causes: Para- / quadriplegia (40 – 50%), myelomeningocele, poliomyelitis, severe head injury, cerebrovascular disease, CNS infections (tetanus, rabies), surgery (commonly following total hip replacement)

Evolution: calcifications seen 4 – 10 weeks following insult; progression for 6 – 14 months; trabeculations by 2 – 3 months; stable lamellar bone ankylosis in 5% by 12 – 18 months

√ largest quantity of calcifications around joints, especially hip, along fascial planes

√ disuse osteoporosis of lower extremities

√ renal calculi (elevation of serum calcium levels)

Radiographic grading system (Brooker):

0   no soft-tissue ossification

I   separate small foci of ossification

II > 1 cm gap between opposing bone surfaces of heterotopic ossifications

III < 1 cm gap between opposing bone surfaces

IV bridging ossification

Bone scan:

√ tracer accumulation in ectopic bone

√ assessment of maturity for optimal time of surgical resection (indicated by same amount of uptake as normal bone)

Cx: Ankylosis in 5%

Rx: 1000 – 2000 rad within 4 days following surgical removal

PHENYLKETONURIA

High incidence of X-ray changes in phenylalanine-restricted infants:

√ metaphyseal cupping of long bones (30 – 50%), especially wrist

√ calcific spicules extending vertically from metaphysis into epiphyseal cartilage (DDx to rickets)

√ sclerotic metaphyseal margins

√ osteoporosis

√ delayed skeletal maturation

DDx: Homocystinuria

PHOSPHORUS POISONING

Etiology: (1) ingestion of metallic phosphorus (yellow phosphorus)

(2) treatment of rachitis or TB with phosphorized cod liver oil

Location: long tubular bones, ilium

√ multiple transverse lines (intermittent treatment with phosphorus)

√ disappear after some years

PIERRE ROBIN SYNDROME

May be associated with: CHD, defects of eye and ear, hydrocephalus, microcephaly

• glossoptosis

√ micrognathia = hypoplastic receding mandible

√ arched ± cleft palate

√ rib pseudarthrosis

Cx: airway obstruction (relatively large tongue), aspiration

PIGMENTED VILLONODULAR SYNOVITIS

= PVNS

Histo: (1) hyperplasia of undifferentiated connective tissue with large cells ingesting hemosiderin / lipoid (foam / giant cells)

(2) villonodular appearance of synovial membrane ± fibrosis

(3) pressure erosion / invasion of adjoining bone

Age: mainly 2nd – 4th decade (range 12 – 68 years); 50% < 40 years

• hemorrhagic "chocolate" effusion without trauma

• pain of long duration, decreased range of motion, joint locking

Location: knee, ankle, hip, elbow, shoulder, tarsal + carpal joints; predominantly monarticular (DDx: degenerative arthritis)

√ soft tissue swelling around joint (effusion + synovial proliferation)

√ dense soft tissues (hemosiderin deposits)

√ subchondral pressure erosion at margins of joint

√ multiple sites of deossification appearing as cysts

√ NO calcifications, osteoporosis, joint space narrowing (until late)

DDx: Synovial sarcoma (solitary calcified mass outside joint)

INTRA-ARTICULAR LOCALIZED NODULAR SYNOVITIS
= synovial lining without hemosiderin

POLAND SYNDROME

May be associated with aplasia of mamilla / breast;

Autosomal recessive

√ unilateral absence of the sternocostal head of the pectoralis major muscle

√ ipsilateral syndactyly + brachydactyly

√ rib anomalies

POLIOMYELITIS
√ osteoporosis
√ soft tissue calcification / ossification
√ intervertebral disc calcification
√ rib erosion commonly on superior margin of 3rd + 4th rib (secondary to pressure from scapula)
√ "bamboo" spine (resembling ankylosing spondylitis)
√ sacroiliac joint narrowing

POPLITEAL CYST
= BAKER CYST = herniation of synovium through posterior joint capsule of knee
Etiology: (1) rheumatoid arthritis (most)
              (2) medial meniscal tear
• pseudophlebitis syndrome
√ cyst may dissect down calf between gastrocnemius + soleus
√ communicates with bursa

PROGERIA
= WERNER SYNDROME
Age: shortly after adolesence; M:F = 1:1
• premature aging
• shallow orbits + beaking of nose
• graying of hair + premature baldness
• diabetes + hypogonadism
• dwarf with short stature and spindly extremities
• scleroderma-like skin with hyperkeratosis + atrophy
√ generalized osteoporosis
√ slender long bones, short thin clavicles
√ hypoplastic facial bones, delayed sutural closure
√ coxa valga
√ acro-osteolysis of terminal phalanges

@ Soft tissue
  √ soft-tissue atrophy of extremities
  √ soft tissue calcifications around bony prominences (ankles, wrists, elbows)
  √ peripheral vascular calcifications = premature atherosclerosis
  √ coronary artery + heart valve calcifications with cardiac enlargement
@ Joints
  √ flexion + extension deformities of toes (hallux valgus, pes planus)
  √ excessive degenerative joint disease of major + peripheral joints
  √ neurotrophic joint lesions (feet)
  √ widespread osteomyelitic + suppurative arthritic foci (hands, feet, limbs)
Prognosis: rare survival beyond age 20

PSEUDOACHONDROPLASIA
• normal face + head
√ limb shortening
√ irregular epiphyses
√ scoliosis
√ coxa vara
√ marked shortening of bones in hand + feet

PSEUDOFRACTURES
= LOOSER LINES = LOOSER ZONES = OSTEOID SEAMS = MILKMAN SYNDROME = insufficiency stress fractures + nonunion (incomplete healing due to mineral deficiency)
Associated with:
  (1) Osteomalacia / rickets (2) Paget disease ("banana fracture") (3) Osteogenesis imperfecta tarda (4) Fibrous dysplasia (5) Organic renal disease (6) Renal tubular dysfunction (7) Congenital hypophosphatasia (8) Congenital hyperphosphatasia ("juvenile Paget disease") (9) Vitamin D malabsorption / deficiency (10) Neurofibromatosis
  mnemonic: "POOF"
    Paget disease
    Osteomalacia
    Osteogenesis imperfecta
    Fibrous dysplasia
Common sites:
  scapulae (axillary margin, lateral + superior margin), femoral neck + shaft, pubic + ischial rami, ribs, proximal 1/3 of ulna, distal 1/3 of radius, phalanges, metatarsals, metacarpals, clavicle
√ typically bilateral + symmetric at right angles to bone margin
√ 2 – 3 mm stripe of lucency perpendicular to cortex
√ paralleled by marginal sclerosis in later stage

PSEUDOHYPOPARATHYROIDISM
= PHypoPT = congenital X-linked dominant abnormality with renal + skeletal resistance to PTH due to (1) end organ resistance (2) presence of antienzymes (3) defective hormone
May be associated with hyperparathyroidism due to hypocalcemia; F > M
• short obese stature
• mental retardation
• corneal + lenticular opacity
• abnormal dentition (hypoplasia, delayed eruption, excessive caries)
• hypocalcemia + hyperphosphatemia (resistant to PTH injection)
• normal levels of PTH
√ brachydactyly in bones in which epiphysis appears latest (metacarpal, metatarsal bones I, IV, V) (75%)
√ accelerated epiphyseal maturation resulting in dwarfism + coxa vara / valga
√ multiple diaphyseal exostoses (occasionally)
√ calcification of basal ganglia + dentate nucleus
√ calcification / ossification of skin + subcutaneous tissue

PSEUDOPSEUDOHYPOPARATHYROIDISM
= PPHypoPT = different expression of same familial disturbance with identical clinical + radiographic features as Pseudohypoparathyroidism
• short stature, round facies
• NO blood chemical changes (normal calcium + phosphorus)

	PHypoPT	PPHypoPT
√ calcification of basal ganglia	44 %	8 %
√ soft tissue calcifications	55 %	40 %
√ metacarpal shortening (4 + 5 always involved)	75 %	90 %
√ metatarsal shortening (3 + 4 involved)	70 %	99 %

- normal response to injection of PTH
- √ brachydactyly

PSORIATIC ARTHRITIS
Types:
  (1) true psoriatic arthritis (31%)
  (2) psoriatic arthritis resembling rheumatoid arthritis (38%)
  (3) concomitant rheumatoid + psoriatic arthritis (31%)
- pitting, discoloration, hyperkeratosis, subungual separation, ridging of nails (in 80%)
- positive HLA-B27 in 80%; negative rheumatoid factor
Location: widely variable distribution + asymmetry
- √ NO juxta-articular osteoporosis (DDx: rheumatoid arthritis)
- √ periosteal reaction frequent

@ Hands + feet
  Target area: DIP, PIP, MCP
- √ asymmetrical destruction of distal interphalangeal joints + ankylosis
- √ resorption of terminal tufts with "pencil-in-cup" deformity (hands + feet)
- √ ivory phalanx
- √ destruction of interphalangeal joint of 1st toe with exuberant periosteal reaction + bony proliferation at distal phalangeal base (PATHOGNOMONIC)
@ Axial skeleton
- √ asymmetrical + incomplete nonmarginal syndesmophyte formation (thoracic area, lower cervical and upper lumbar regions)
- √ squaring of vertebrae in lumbar region
- √ paravertebral soft tissue calcifications, separate from edges of vertebrae
- √ bilateral sacroiliac joint widening, increased density, fusion

PYKNODYSOSTOSIS
= autosomal recessive disease
Age: children; M:F = 2:1;
- dwarfism (resembling osteopetrosis)
- mental retardation (10%)
- widened hands + feet
- dystrophic nails
- yellowish discoloration of teeth
- characteristic facies (beak nose, receding jaw)
- √ brachycephaly + platybasia

- √ wide cranial sutures, Wormian bones
- √ thick skull base
- √ hypoplasia of mandible + loss of mandibular angle
- √ hypoplasia + nonpneumatization of paranasal sinuses
- √ nonsegmentation of C1/2 and L5/S1
- √ generalized increased density of long bones with thickened cortices
- √ clavicular dysplasia
- √ hypoplastic tapered terminal tufts
- √ multiple spontaneous fractures
DDx:
  (1) Osteopetrosis (no mandibular / skull abnormality, no phalangeal hypoplasia, no transverse metaphyseal bands, anemia, Erlenmeyer flask deformity; "bone-within-bone" appearance)
  (2) Cleidocranial dysostosis (no dense bones / terminal phalangeal hypoplasia, short stature)

RADIATION INJURY TO BONE
Pathogenesis: vascular compromise with obliterative endarteritis + periarteritis followed by damage to osteoblasts with decreased matrix production (growing bone + periosteal new bone most sensitive)
A. RADIATION OSTEITIS
  Dose: (a) 600 – 1200 rad: histological recovery retained
       (b) > 1200 rad : pronounced cellular damage
- √ temporary growth cessation with recovery
- √ periostitis
- √ increased fragility with sclerosis
- √ aseptic necrosis
- √ osteoradionecrosis
MRI:
- √ increased intensity of spinal bone marrow on T1WI + T2WI corresponding to radiation port (fatty infiltration)
B. BENIGN NEOPLASM
  Most likely in patients < 2 years of age at treatment; with doses of 1600 – 6425 rads; latent period of 9 – 14 years
  1. Exostosis = Osteochondroma
  2. Osteoblastoma
C. MALIGNANT NEOPLASM
  1. Sarcoma (5.5% of all osteogenic sarcomas)

Criteria: (a) microscopic evidence of altered
histology of the original lesion
(b) malignancy occuring within radiated
field
(c) latency period of > 5 years
(d) histologic proof of sarcoma
- pain, soft tissue mass, rapid progression of lesion

REGIONAL MIGRATORY OSTEOPOROSIS
Age: middle-aged males
- gradual pain + swelling
√ rapid osteoporosis around knee, ankle, foot migrating
from one joint to another

REITER SYNDROME
= triad of (1) arthritis (2) uveitis (3) urethritis; 98% male
Types:
(1) endemic type (venereal)
(2) epidemic (postdysenteric)
- Hx of sexual exposure / diarrhea 3 – 11 days before
onset of urethritis
- mucocutaneous lesions (keratosis blennorrhagia,
balanitis circinata sicca)
- uveitis, conjunctivitis
- positive HLA-B27 in 76%
Location: asymmetric mono- / pauciarticular
√ polyarthritis
√ articular soft tissue swelling + joint space narrowing in
50% (particularly knees, ankles, feet)
√ widening + inflammation of achilles + patella tendons
√ "fluffy" periosteal reaction (DISTINCTIVE) at metatarsal
necks, proximal phalanges, calcaneal spur, tibia + fibula
at ankle and knee
√ juxtaarticular osteoporosis (rare in acute stage)
CHRONIC CHANGES
- recurrent joint attacks in a few cases
√ calcaneal spur at insertion of plantar fascia + achilles
tendon
√ periarticular deossification
√ marginal erosions, loss of joint space
√ bilateral sacroiliac changes indistinguishable from
ankylosing / psoriatic spondylitis
√ isolated osteophyte usually in thoracolumbar area,
separated from vertebral body
Cx: gastric ulcer + hemorrhage; aortic incompetence;
heart block; amyloidosis

RELAPSING POLYCHONDRITIS
= generalized recurring inflammation of cartilage in joints,
ears, nose, airways probably related to abnormality in
mucopolysaccharide metabolism
Etiology: acquired metabolic disorder / hypersensitivity /
altered immunity
- saddle-nose deformity
- cauliflower ear
@ Chest
√ ectasia + collapsibility of trachea
√ generalized + localized emphysema
√ dissecting aortic aneurysm + cystic medial necrosis

@ Bone
√ erosive changes in carpal bones resembling
rheumatoid arthritis
√ soft tissue swelling around joints + styloid process
of ulna
√ erosive irregularities in sacroiliac joints
√ disc space erosion + increased density of articular
plates

RENAL OSTEODYSTROPHY
= combination of (1) Osteomalacia (adults) / rickets
(children) (2) 2° HPT with osteitis cystica fibrosa + soft
tissue calcifications (3) Osteosclerosis
Classification:
(1) Glomerular form = acquired renal disease: chronic
glomerulonephritis (common)
(2) Tubular form = congenital renal osteodystrophy:
1. Vitamin D-resistent rickets = Hypophosphatemic
rickets
2. Fanconi syndrome = impaired resorption of
glucose, phosphate, amino acids, bicarbonate,
uric acid, sodium, water
3. Renal tubular acidosis
Pathogenesis:
(A) Renal insufficiency causes a decrease in vitamin D
conversion + vitamin D deficiency which slows
intestinal calcium absorption; *vitamin D resistance
predominates* and calcium levels stay low (Ca x P
product remains almost normal secondary to
hyperphosphatemia); low calcium levels lead to
OSTEOMALACIA
(B) Renal insufficiency with diminished filtration results
in phosphate retention; maintenance of Ca x P -
product lowers serum calcium directly which in turn
increases PTH production (2° HPT); *2° HPT
predominates* associated with mild vitamin D
resistance and leads to an increase in Ca x P -
product with SOFT TISSUE CALCIFICATION in
kidney, lung, joints, bursae, blood vessels, heart as
well as OSTEITIS FIBROSA
(b) Mixture of (A) and (B): increased serum phosphate
inhibits vitamin D activation via feedback regulation
- phosphate retention
- hypocalcemia
A. OSTEOMALACIA (adult)
Due to acquired insensitivity to vitamin D / antivitamin
D factor
(a) diffuse form:
√ osteopenia = diminution in number of trabeculae
+ thickening of stressed trabeculae = increased
trabecular pattern
(b) focal form:
√ Milkman fracture / Looser zones = incomplete
compression fractures with little or no callus
response; bilateral symmetric
B. RICKETS (children)
Most apparent in areas of rapid growth such as knee
joints

√ diffuse bone demineralization
√ widened growth plate
√ irregular zone of provisional calcification
√ metaphyseal cupping + fraying
√ bowing of long bones
√ slipped capital femoral epiphysis

C. OSTEITIS FIBROSA
Secondary to hypocalcemia + hyperphosphatemia
followed by increased parathormone production
√ subperiosteal bone resorption (most constant +
specific): radial aspect of phalanges, distal end of
clavicles, medial tibia plateau, medial humerus
neck, distal ulna, phalangeal tufts, lamina dura of
teeth
√ subchondral + subligamentous bone resorption
= widening of symphysis, sacroiliac joints,
resorption of ischial tuberosity
√ spotty deossification of skull (wooly / granular salt
and pepper skull)
√ metaphyseal fractures, slipped epiphyses
√ brown tumor + chondrocalcinosis (more common in
1° HPT)

D. OSTEOSCLEROSIS
One of the most common radiologic manifestations;
most commonly with chronic glomerulonephritis
√ diffuse chalky density: thoracolumbar spine in 60%
(rugger-jersey spine); also in pelvis, ribs, long
bones, facial bones, base of skull (children)

E. SOFT TISSUE CALCIFICATIONS
(a) metastatic secondary to hyperphosphatemia
(elevated Ca x P product)
(b) dystrophic secondary to tissue injury
Location: arteries, periarticular, cutaneous +
subcutaneous, viscera
√ fluffy amorphous "tumoral" calcification
Rx:
1. Decrease of phosphorus absorption in bowel (in
hyperphosphatemia)
2. Vitamin D3 administration (if vitamin D resistance
predominates)
3. Parathyroidectomy for 3° HPT (= autonomous
HPT)

Congenital Renal Osteodystrophy
Vitamin D-resistant Rickets
= PHOSPHATE DIABETES = X-linked dominant
renal tubular abnormality characterized by
(1) impaired resorption of phosphate in proximal
renal tubule (2) decreased intestinal resorption of
calcium + phosphate
Age: < 1 year
• hypophosphatemia + hyperphosphaturia
• increased alkaline phosphatase
• hypocalcemia (secondary to intestinal
malabsorption)
√ classic rachitic changes, occasionally dwarfism
Rx: phosphate infusion + large doses of vitamin D

Fanconi Syndrome
Triad of
(1) hyperphosphaturia
(2) amino aciduria
(3) renal glucosuria (normal blood glucose)
Etiology: renal tubular defect
√ rickets, osteomalacia, osteitis fibrosa,
osteosclerosis
Prognosis: functional renal impairment likely when
bone changes occur
Rx: large doses of vitamin D + alkalinization

Renal Tubular Acidosis
• systemic acidosis, bone lesions
√ rickets, osteomalacia, pseudofractures,
nephrocalcinosis, osteitis fibrosa (rare)
(a) Lightwood syndrome = salt-losing nephritis (self-
limited form)
• NO nephrocalcinosis
(b) Butler-Albright syndrome (severe form)
• nephrocalcinosis

RHEUMATOID ARTHRITIS
= generalized connective tissue disease
Age: highest incidence 40 – 50 years;
M:F = 1:3 if < 40 years; M:F = 1:1 if > 40 years
Pathogenesis: synovitis with synovial hypertrophy leads
to impaired nutrition with chondronecrosis,
joint narrowing, subluxation, and ankylosis
• morning stiffness
• fatigue, weight loss
• carpal tunnel syndrome
• positive rheumatoid factor (94%)
• positive latex flocculation test
Location: symmetric involvement of diarthrodial joints
Target areas:
all five MCP, PIP, interphalangeal joint of thumb, all
wrist compartments (especially radiocarpal, inferior
radioulnar, pisiform-triquetral joints); medial aspect of
MTP + interphalangeal joints of foot (esp. great toe);
earliest changes seen in 2nd + 3rd MCP, 3rd PIP
EARLY SIGNS:
√ fusiform periarticular soft tissue swelling (result of
effusion)
√ regional osteoporosis (disuse + local hyperemia)
√ widened joint space
√ marginal + central bone erosions (less common in
large joints); site of first erosion is classically base of
proximal phalanx of 4th finger
√ changes in the ulnar styloid + distal radioulnar joint
√ atlantoaxial dislocation > 2.5 mm
√ giant synovial cysts

LATE SIGNS:
√ diffuse loss of interosseous space
√ flexion + extension contractures with ulnar subluxation
+ dislocation
√ marked destruction + fractures of joint space

√ extensive destruction of bone ends
√ bony fusion
√ elevation of humeral heads (tear / atrophy of rotator cuff)
√ resorption of distal clavicle
√ erosion of superior margins of posterior portions of ribs 3 – 5
√ destruction + narrowing of disc spaces
√ destruction of zygapophyseal joints without osteophyte formation
√ resorption of spinous processes
√ protrusio acetabuli (from osteoporosis)
√ calcaneal plantar spur

EXTRAARTICULAR MANIFESTATIONS (76%)
  A. **Felty Syndrome** (< 1%)
     = rheumatoid arthritis (present for > 10 years) + splenomegaly + neutropenia
     Age: 40 – 70 years; F > M; rare in blacks
     • rapid weight loss
     • therapy refractory leg ulcers
     • brown pigmentation over exposed surfaces of extremities
  B. SJÖGREN SYNDROME (15%)
     = keratoconjunctivitis + xerostomia + rheumatoid arthritis
  C. PULMONARY MANIFESTATIONS
     √ pleural effusion, mostly unilateral, without change for months, usually not associated with parenchymal disease
     √ interstitial fibrosis with lower lobe predominance
     √ rheumatoid nodules (30%): well-circumscribed, peripheral, with frequent cavitation
     √ Caplan syndrome (= hyperimmune reactivity to silica inhalation with rapidly developing multiple pulmonary nodules)
     √ pulmonary hypertension secondary to arteritis
  D. SUBCUTANEOUS NODULES
     (in 5 – 35% with active arthritis) over extensor surfaces of forearm + other pressure points (e.g. olecranon) without calcifications (DDx to gout)
  E. CARDIOVASCULAR INVOLVEMENT
     1. Pericarditis (20 – 50%)
     2. Myocarditis (arrhythmia, heartblock)
  F. RHEUMATOID VASCULITIS
     Mimicks periarteritis nodosa;
     • polyneuropathy, cutaneous ulceration, gangrene, polymyopathy, myocardial / visceral infarction
  G. NEUROLOGIC SEQUELAE
     1. Distal neuropathy (related to vasculitis)
     2. Nerve entrapment (atlantoaxial subluxation, carpal tunnel syndrome, Baker cyst)
  H. LYMPHADENOPATHY (up to 25%)
     √ splenomegaly (1 – 5%)

Juvenile Rheumatoid Arthritis

= rheumatoid arthritis in patients < 16 years of age; M < F

Classification:
  (1) Juvenile-onset adult type (10%)
      • IgM RA factor positive; age 8 – 9; poor prognosis
      √ erosive changes; perfuse periosteal reaction; hip disease with protrusio
  (2) Polyarthritis of the ankylosing spondylitic type
      • iridocyclitis; boys age 9 – 11 years
      √ peripheral arthritis; fusion of greater trochanter; complete fusion of both hips; heel spur
  (3) **Still disease**
      (a) systemic (b) polyarticular (c) pauciarticular + iridocyclitis (30%)
      • fever, rash, lymphadenopathy, hepatosplenomegaly; pericarditis, dwarfism
      • fatal kidney disease in 20%
      Age: 2 – 4 and 8 – 11 years of age; M < F
      Location: involvement of carpometacarpal joints ("squashed carpi" in adulthood), hind foot, hip (40 – 50%)
      √ periosteal reaction of phalanges; broadening of bones; accelerated bone maturation + early fusion (stunting of growth)

• morning stiffness, arthralgia
• subcutaneous nodules (10%)
• skin rash (50%)
• fever, lymphadenopathy
Location: early involvement of large joints (hips, knees, ankles, wrists, elbows); later of hands + feet
√ radiologic signs similar to rheumatoid arthritis (except for involvement of large joints first, late onset of bony changes, more ankylosis, wide metaphyses)
√ periarticular soft tissue swelling
√ thinning of joint cartilage
√ large cyst-like lesions removed from articular surface (invasion of bone by inflammatory pannus); rare in children
√ articular erosions at ligamentous + tendinous insertion sites
√ joint destruction may resemble neuropathic joints
√ juxtaarticular osteoporosis
√ "balloon epiphyses" + "gracile bones" (epiphyseal overgrowth + early fusion with bone shortening secondary to hyperemia)
@ Hand / foot
  √ "rectangular" phalanges (periostitis + cortical thickening)
  √ ankylosis in carpal joints
@ Axial skeleton
  √ ankylosis of cervical spine (apophyseal joints), sacroiliac joints
  √ subluxation of atlantoaxial joint (66%)
  √ thoracic spinal compression fractures
@ Chest
  √ ribbon ribs
  √ pleural + pericardial effusions
  √ interstitial pulmonary lesions (simulating scleroderma, dermatomyositis)
  √ solitary pulmonary nodules, may cavitate

Prognosis: complete recovery (30%); secondary amyloidosis

RICKETS
= osteomalacia during enchondral bone growth
Age: 4 – 18 months
Histo: zone of preparatory calcification does not form, heap up of maturing cartilage cells; failure of osteoid mineralization also in shafts so that osteoid production elevates periosteum

- irritability, bone pain, tenderness
- craniotabes
- rachitic rosary
- bowed legs
- delayed dentition
- swelling of wrists + ankles

Location: metaphyses of long bones subjected to stress are particularly involved (wrists, ankles, knees)
√ poorly mineralized epiphyseal centers with delayed appearance
√ irregular widened epiphyseal plates (increased osteoid)
√ increase in distance between end of shaft and epiphyseal center
√ cupping + fraying of metaphysis with thread-like shadows into epiphyseal cartilage (weight-bearing bones)
√ cortical spurs projecting at right angles to metaphysis
√ coarse trabeculation (NO ground glass pattern as in scurvy)
√ periosteal reaction may be present
√ deformities common (bowing of soft diaphysis, molding of epiphysis, fractures)
√ bowing of long bones
√ frontal bossing

Causes & Classification of Rickets
I. *ABNORMALITY IN VITAMIN D METABOLISM*
Associated with reactive hyperparathyroidism
A. Vitamin D deficiency
(a) Dietary lack of vitamin D
= famine osteomalacia
(b) Lack of sunshine exposure
(c) Malabsorption of vitamin D
= gastroenterogenous rickets
1. pancreatitis + biliary tract disease
2. steatorrhea, celiac disease, postgastrectomy
3. inflammatory bowel disease
B. Defective conversion of vitamin D to 25-OH-cholecalciferol in liver
1. Liver disease
2. Anticonvulsant drug therapy (= induction of hepatic enzymes which accelerate degradation of biologically active vitamin D metabolites)
C. Defective conversion of 25-OH-D3 to 1,25-OH-D3 in kidney
1. Chronic renal failure = renal osteodystrophy

2. Vitamin D-dependent rickets = autosomal recessive enzyme defect of 1-OHase

II. *ABNORMALITY IN PHOSPHATE METABOLISM*
not associated with hyperparathyroidism secondary to normal serum calcium
A. Phosphate deficiency
1. Intestinal malabsorption of phosphates
2. Ingestion of aluminum salts [$Al(OH)_2$] forming insoluble complexes with phosphate
3. Low phosphate feeding in prematurely born infants
4. Severe malabsorption state
5. Parenteral hyperalimentation
B. Disorders of renal tubular reabsorption of phosphate
1. Renal tubular acidosis (renal loss of alkali)
2. deToni-Debré-Fanconi syndrome
= hypophosphatemia, glucosuria, aminoaciduria
3. Primary hypophosphatemia = vitamin D resistant rickets = familial hypophosphatemic rickets (X-linked dominant)
4. Cystinosis
5. Tyrosinosis
6. Lowe syndrome
C. Hypophosphatemia with nonendocrine tumors
= Oncogenic rickets = elaboration of humeral substance which inhibits tubular reabsorption of phosphates
1. Sclerosing hemangioma
2. Hemangiopericytoma
3. Ossifying mesenchymal tumor
4. Nonossifying fibroma
D. Hypophosphatasia

III. *CALCIUM DEFICIENCY*
1. Dietary rickets = milk-free diet (extremely rare)
2. Malabsorption
3. Consumption of substances forming chelates with calcium

CLASSIFICATION OF RICKETS
I. Primary vitamin D deficiency rickets
II. Gastrointestinal malabsorption
A. Partial gastrectomy
B. Small intestinal disease: gluten-sensitive enteropathy / regional enteritis
C. Hepatobiliary disease: chronic biliary obstruction / biliary cirrhosis
D. Pancreatic disease: chronic pancreatitis
III. Primary hypophosphatemia; vitamin D deficiency rickets
IV. Renal disease
A. Chronic renal failure
B. Renal tubular disorders: renal tubular acidosis
C. Multiple renal defects
V. Hypophosphatasia + pseudohypophosphatasia

VI.   Fibrogenesis imperfecta osseum
VII.   Axial osteomalacia
VIII.   Miscellaneous
Hypoparathyroidism, hyperparathyroidism, thyrotoxicosis, osteoporosis, Paget disease, fluoride ingestion, ureterosigmoidostomy, neurofibromatosis, osteopetrosis, macroglobulinemia, malignancy

RUBELLA

Age: infants
- neonatal dwarfism (growth retardation)
- failure to thrive
- cataracts, deafness
- mental deficiency
- thrombocytopenic purpura
- √ "celery-stalk" sign (50%) = metaphyseal irregular margins + coarsened trabeculae extending longitudinally from epiphysis; distal end of femur > proximal end of tibia, humerus
- √ no periosteal reaction
- √ congenital heart disease (PDA)
- √ peripheral pulmonary artery stenosis
- √ hepatosplenomegaly
- √ pneumonia
- √ necrosis of myocardium

Prognosis: osseous manifestations disappear in 1 – 3 months

DDx: (1)   CMV (brain calcifications, not seen in rubella)
(2)   Congenital syphilis (diaphysitis + epiphysitis)
(3)   Toxoplasmosis

SARCOIDOSIS

Osseous involvement in 15 – 20%
Location: small bones of hands + feet (middle + distal phalanges)
- unimpaired joint function, joints are rarely involved
- √ reticulated "lace-like" trabecular pattern in metaphyseal ends of middle + distal phalanges, metacarpals, metatarsals
- √ well-defined cystlike lesions of varying size
- √ neuropathic-like destruction of terminal phalanges (DDx: scleroderma)
- √ endosteal sclerosis + periosteal new bone (infrequent)
- √ vertebral involvement unusual: destructive lesions with sclerotic margin
- √ diffuse sclerosis of multiple vertebral bodies
- √ paravertebral soft tissue mass (DDx: indistinguishable from tuberculosis)
- √ osteolytic changes in skull

SCHEUERMANN DISEASE

= SPINAL OSTEOCHONDROSIS = KYPHOSIS DORSALIS JUVENILIS = VERTEBRAL EPIPHYSITIS
Age: onset at puberty
Location: lower thoracic / upper lumbar vertebrae; in mild cases limited to 3 – 4 vertebral bodies

- √ anterior wedging of vertebral body with increased anteroposterior diameter
- √ irregular-shaped + narrowed disc spaces
- √ kyphosis / loss of lordosis; scoliosis
- √ Schmorl nodes (herniation of nucleus pulposus into vertebral body)
- √ flattened area in superior surface of epiphyseal ring anteriorly
- √ detached epiphyseal ring anteriorly

DDx: (1)   Developmental notching of anterior vertebrae (NO wedging or Schmorl nodes)
(2)   Osteochondrodystrophy (earlier in life, extremities show same changes)

SCLERODERMA

= PROGRESSIVE SYSTEMIC SCLEROSIS = initial hypertrophy and finally atrophy of collagen fibers; sclerotic process affecting small arteries (e.g., nephrosclerosis)
Age: 4th – 5th decade; F > M
- atrophy + thickening of skin and musculature
- difficulty in swallowing
- weakness, generalized debility
- cough, dyspnea

@   Hands
- √ punctate soft tissue calcifications (finger tips, shoulders, hips)
- √ "tapered fingers" = atrophy of soft tissues of finger tips
- √ "penciling" / "autoamputation" of terminal tufts
- √ NO significant osteoporosis
- √ intercarpal joint space narrowing (late)

@   Chest
- √ pulmonary fibrosis with diffuse reticulate infiltrate predominantly in lower lungs

@   GI tract
- √ atony of esophagus, duodenum
- √ segmentation, dilatation, delay in transit of small bowel
- √ sacculations + pseudosacculations in colon; wide-mouthed small bowel diverticula / pseudodiverticula on mesenteric side

SCURVY

= BARLOW DISEASE = vitamin C deficiency with defective osteogenesis from abnormal osteoblast function
Age: 6 – 19 months (maternal vitamin C protects for first 6 months)
- irritability
- tenderness + weakness of lower limbs
- scorbutic rosary of ribs
- bleeding of gums (teething)
- legs drawn up + widely spread = pseudoparalysis

Location: distal femur (esp. medial side), proximal and distal tibia + fibula, distal radius + ulna, proximal humerus, sternal end of ribs
- √ Wimberger ring = sclerotic ring around epiphysis

√ white line of Fränkel = metaphyseal zone of preparatory calcification (DDx: lead / phosphorus poisoning, bismuth treatment, healing rickets)

√ Trümmerfeld zone = radiolucent zone on shaft side of Fränkel's white line (site of subepiphyseal infraction)

√ Parke corner sign = subepiphyseal infraction / comminution resulting in mushrooming / cupping of epiphysis (DDx: syphilis, rickets)

√ Pelkan spurs = metaphyseal spurs projecting at right angles to shaft axis

√ "ground glass" osteoporosis (CHARACTERISTIC)

√ cortical thinning

√ subperiosteal hematoma with calcification of elevated periosteum (sure radiographic sign of healing)

√ soft tissue edema (rare)

SEPTIC ARTHRITIS

Organism:

most often due to S. aureus; Gonorrhea (indistinguishable from tuberculous arthritis, but more rapid); Brucellar arthritis (indistinguishable from tuberculosis, slow infection); Salmonella (commonly associated with sickle cell disease / Gaucher disease)

(a) < 4 years of age: Streptococcus pyogenes, S. aureus, Hemophilus influenzae

(b) > 4 years of age: S. aureus

(c) > 10 years of age: S. aureus, Neisseria gonorrhea

Location: lower extremity (75%) with hip + knee in 90%

• pain, limp, pseudoparalysis
• warmth, swelling
• septic clinical picture
• bacteremia, leukocytosis

ACUTE SIGNS:

√ initial radiographs frequently normal

√ soft tissue swelling (first sign secondary to local hyperemia + edema)

√ joint distension (effusion)

√ subluxation may occur (in hip + humerus of children)

√ joint space narrowing ▪ rapid development of destruction of articular cartilage (not in tuberculous arthritis)

SUBACUTE SIGNS after 8 – 10 days:

√ small erosions in articular cortex / loss of entire cortical outline (marginal erosions in tuberculosis)

√ reactive bone sclerosis in underlying bone

√ subchondral bone destruction (by synovial proliferation)

√ defective reparation / ankylosis (if entire cartilage is destroyed)

√ local bone atrophy (immobility)

√ metaphyseal bone destruction (osteomyelitis as source of septic joint)

Dx: prompt arthrocentesis + blood culture

Cx: (1) bone growth disturbance (lengthening, shortening, angulation)

     (2) chronic degenerative arthritis

     (3) ankylosis

     (4) osteonecrosis

SHORT RIB-POLYDACTYLY SYNDROME

= group of autosomal recessive disorders characterized by short limb dysplasia, constricted thorax, postaxial polydactyly (on ulnar / fibular side)

TYPE I   = SALDINO-NOONAN SYNDROME

TYPE II = MAJEWSKI TYPE

TYPE III = NAUMOFF TYPE

√ severe micromelia

√ pointed femurs at both ends (Type I); widened metaphyses (Type III)

√ narrow thorax

√ extremely short horizontally oriented ribs

√ distorted underossified vertebral bodies + incomplete coronal clefts

√ polydactyly

√ cleft lip / palate

Prognosis: uniformly lethal

SICKLE CELL ANEMIA

Abnormal Hemoglobins:

Hb S = DNA mutation substituting glutamic acid in position 6 on beta-chain with valine

Hb C = DNA mutation substituting glutamic acid in position 6 on beta-chain with lysine

(a) homozygous   = Hb SS with sickle cell anemia

(b) heterozygous = Hb SA with sickling trait but no anemia

                   = Hb SC with sickle cell S-C disease (less severe form)

                   = Hb S-thalassemia, seen occasionally

Incidence: 8 – 13% of American negroes carry sickling factor (Hb S); 1:40 with sickle cell trait will manifest sickle cell anemia (Hb SS); 1:120 with sickle cell trait will manifest Hb SC disease

Pathogenesis:

altered shape + plasticity of RBCs under lowered oxygen tension lead to increased blood viscosity, stasis, "log jam" occlusion of small blood vessels, infarction, necrosis, superinfection; sickling occurs in areas of

(a) slow flow (spleen, liver, renal medulla)

(b) rapid metabolism (brain, muscle, fetal placenta)

• hemolytic anemia (altered RBCs rapidly destroyed by RES), jaundice

• chronic leg ulcers, priapism

• abdominal crisis

• rheumatic-like joint pain

• skeletal pain (osteomyelitis, cellulitis, bone marrow infarction)

• splenomegaly (in children + infants), later organ atrophy

Cx: high incidence of infections (lung, bone, brain)

Prognosis: death < 40 years

(1) DEOSSIFICATION DUE TO MARROW HYPERPLASIA

√ porous decrease in bone density of skull (25%)

√ widening of diploe with decrease in width of outer table (22%)

√ vertical hair-on-end striations (5%)
√ osteoporosis with thinning of trabeculae
√ biconcave "fish" vertebrae (bone softening) in 70%
√ widening of medullary space + thinning of cortices
√ coarsening of trabecular pattern in long + flat bones
√ rib notching
√ pathologic fractures

(2) THROMBOSIS AND INFARCTION
Location: in diaphysis of small tubular bones
(children); in metaphysis + subchondrium
of long bones (adults)
√ osteolysis (in ACUTE infarction)
√ dystrophic medullary calcification
√ periosteal reaction (bone-within-bone appearance)
√ juxtacortical sclerosis
√ Lincoln log = Reynold sign = H-vertebrae = step-like
endplate depression
√ articular disintegration
√ collapse of femoral head (DDx: Perthes with
involvement of metaphysis)
MRI:
√ diffusely decreased signal of marrow on short +
long TR/TE images (= hematopoietic marrow
replacing fatty marrow)
√ focal areas of decreased signal intensity on short
TR/TE + increased intensity on long TR/TE
(= acute marrow infarction)
√ focal areas of decreased signal intensity on short
TR/TE + long TR/TE images (= old infarction /
fibrosis)

(3) SECONDARY OSTEOMYELITIS
Organism: salmonella in unusual frequency, also
staphylococcus
√ periostitis (DDx: indistinguishable from bone
infarction)
√ dactylitis = hand-foot syndrome

(4) GROWTH EFFECTS (secondary to diminished blood
supply)
Location: particularly in metacarpal / phalanx
√ bone shortening = premature epiphyseal fusion
√ epiphyseal deformity with cupped metaphysis
√ cup / peg-in-hole defect of distal femur
√ diminution in vertebral height (shortening of stature
+ kyphoscoliosis)

@ Abdomen
√ splenomegaly < age 10
√ episodes of splenic sequestration (= functional
drainage obstruction)
√ small fibrotic spleen
√ autoinfarction of spleen (function lost by age 5)
√ cholelithiasis

@ Kidney
• hematuria
• hyposthenuria
• nephrotic syndrome
• renal tubular acidosis (distal)
• hyperuricemia
• progressive renal insufficiency

√ normal urogram (70%)
√ papillary necrosis (20%)
√ focal renal scarring (20%)
√ smooth large kidney (4%)
MRI:
√ decreased cortical signal on T2-weighted
images
@ Chest
√ cardiomegaly + congestive heart failure

Bone marrow scintigraphy:
√ usually symmetric marked expansion of hematopoietic
marrow beyond age 20 involving entire femur,
calvarium, small bones of hand + feet (normally only
in axial skeleton + proximal femur and humerus)
√ bone marrow defects indicative of acute / old
infarction
Tc-99m diphosphonate scan:
√ increased overall skeletal uptake (high bone-to-soft
tissue ratio)
√ prominent activities at knees, ankles, proximal
humerus (delayed epiphyseal closure / increased
blood flow to bone marrow)
√ bone marrow expansion (calvarial thickening with
relative decrease in activity along falx insertion)
√ decreased / normal uptake on bone scan within 24
hours in acute infarction / posthealing phase
following infarction (cyst formation)
√ increased uptake on bone scan after 2 – 10 days
persistent for several weeks in healing infarction
√ increased uptake on bone scan within 24 – 48 hours
in osteomyelitis
√ increased blood-pool activity + normal delayed image
on bone scan in cellulitis
√ renal enlargement with marked retention of tracer in
renal parenchyma (medullary ischemia + failure of
countercurrent system) in 50%
√ persistent splenic uptake (secondary to
degeneration, atrophy, fibrosis, calcifications)
Tc-99m sulfur colloid scan:
√ functional asplenia

SICKLE CELL TRAIT
Hb SA carrier; mild disease with few episodes of crisis +
infection; sickling provoked only under extreme stress
(unpressurized aircraft, anoxia with CHD, prolonged
anesthesia, marathon running)
Incidence: in 8 – 10% of American blacks
• may have normal blood count
• recurrent gross hematuria
√ splenic infarction

SC DISEASE
Hb SC carrier
Incidence: 3% of American blacks
• retinal hemorrhages
• hematuria due to multiple infarctions
√ aseptic necrosis of hip

SICKLE-THAL DISEASE
Resembling clinically Hb SS patients
• anemia (no normal adult hemoglobin)
√ persistent splenomegaly

SJÖGREN SYNDROME
= multisystem disorder associated with collagen-vascular
disease affecting (1) salivary + lacrimal glands
(2) mucosa + submucosa of pharynx
(3) tracheobronchial tree (4) reticuloendothelial system
(5) joints
TRIAD: keratoconjunctivitis sicca, xerostomia, rheumatoid
arthritis
Age: 35 – 70; female predominance
• dry eyes
• dry mouth
• decreased sweating
• decreased vaginal secretions
√ sialectasis
√ rheumatoid arthritis
√ interstitial lymphocytic pneumonitis + fibrosis
√ pseudolymphoma (disorder between lymph node
hyperplasia and neoplasm)
√ bilateral lower lobe bronchiectasis
√ acute focal / lipoid pneumonia (oils taken to combat dry
mouth)
Cx: Lymphoma (occurs in significant number of
patients)

SMALLPOX
5% of infants
Location: elbow bilateral; metaphysis of long bones
√ rapid bone destruction spreading along shaft
√ periosteal reaction
√ endosteal + cortical sclerosis frequent
√ premature epiphyseal fusion with severe deformity
√ ankylosis is frequent

SOFT TISSUE CHONDROMA
Age: 3rd – 4th decade; M > F
Histo: adult-type hyaline cartilage
Location: hand + feet
√ slow-growing lobular well-demarcated mass
√ may contain calcifications / ossifications
√ scalloping of adjacent bone with sclerotic reaction

SOLITARY OSTEOCHONDROMA
= OSTEOCARTILAGINOUS EXOSTOSIS = hyperplastic /
dysplastic bone disturbance originating from displaced
or aberrant cartilage of the growth plate; growth ends
when nearest epipyseal plate fuses; most common
benign growth of the skeleton
Age: 1st – 3rd decade; M:F = 1:1
Histo: cartilage cap containing a basal surface with
enchondral ossification
• usually painless mass; painful with impingement of
nerves / blood vessels

Location: long bone metaphysis of femur, humerus,
proximal radius, tibia (50% about knee);
scapula; rib; pelvis; spine (1 – 5%, commonly
thoracic); in any bone that develops by
enchondromal calcification
Type: (a) pedunculated form (b) broad-based form
(c) calcific form
√ cortical bone with cartilaginous cap
√ grows at right angles + towards diaphysis (tendon pull)
√ continuity of bone cortex to host bone
√ continuity of medullary marrow space to host bone
√ metaphyseal widening
Cx: (1) Impingement on nerves / blood vessels
(2) Malignant transformation into chondro- /
osteosarcoma (< 1%)
√ enlargement after epiphyseal fusion (usually
starts in cartilaginous cap)

SOLITARY BONE CYST
= UNICAMERAL / SIMPLE BONE CYST
Etiology: ? trauma (synovial entrapment at capsular
reflection), ? vascular anomaly (blockage of
interstitial drainage)
Histo: fluid-filled cyst, wall lined with fibrous tissue +
hemosiderin, giant cells may be present
Age: 3 – 19 years (80%); occurs during active phase
of bone growth; M:F = 2:1
• asymptomatic, unless fractured
Location: proximal femur + proximal humerus (60 -
75%), fibula, at base of calcaneal neck (> 12
years of age), talus; rare in ribs, ilium, small
bones of hand + feet (rare), (NOT in spine /
calvarium)
Sites: centric metaphyseal, adjacent to epiphyseal
cartilage (during active phase) / migrating into
diaphysis with growth (during latent phase), does
not cross epiphyseal plate
√ 2 – 3 cm oval radiolucency with long axis parallel to long
axis of host bone
√ fine sclerotic boundary
√ scalloping + erosion of internal aspect of underlying
cortex
√ photopenic area on bone scan (if not fractured)
√ "fallen fragment" sign if fractured
Prognosis: mostly spontaneous regression
DDx: (1) Enchondroma (calcific stipplings) (2) Fibrous
dysplasia (more irregular lucency) (3) Eosinophilic
granuloma (4) Chondroblastoma (epiphyseal)
(5) Chondromyxoid fibroma (more eccentric +
expansile) (6) Giant cell tumor (7) Aneurysmal bone
cyst (eccentric) (8) Hemorrhagic cyst (9) Brown
tumor

SOLITARY PLASMACYTOMA
= represents early stage of multiple myeloma, precedes
multiple myeloma by 1 – 20 years
Age: 5th – 7th decade
• negative marrow aspiration; no IgG spike in serum /
urine

A. <u>SOLITARY MYELOMA OF BONE</u>
Sites: thoracic / lumbar spine (most common) > pelvis > ribs > sternum, femora, humeri (common)
√ solitary "bubbly" osteolytic grossly expansile lesion
√ poorly defined margins, swiss-cheese pattern
√ frequently pathologic fracture (collapse of vertebra)
DDx: Giant cell tumor, Aneurysmal bone cyst, Osteoblastoma, Solitary metastasis from renal cell / thyroid carcinoma

B. <u>EXTRAMEDULLARY PLASMACYTOMA</u>
Location: majority in head + neck; 80% in nasal cavity, paranasal sinuses, upper airways of trachea, lung parenchyma

SPONDYLOEPIPHYSEAL DYSPLASIA

Spondyloepiphyseal Dysplasia Congenita
Autosomal dominant
• retinal detachment
√ hypoplasia of odontoid process (Cx: cervical myelopathy)
√ cleft palate
√ ovoid vertebral bodies + severe platyspondyly (flattened vertebral bodies)
√ progressive kyphoscoliosis (short trunk)
√ bell-shaped thorax
√ normal / slightly shortened limbs
√ coxa vara + genu valgum
√ talipes equinovarus
Cx: (1) Retinal detachment, myopia (50%)
        (2) Secondary arthritis in weightbearing joints

Spondyloepiphyseal Dysplasia Tarda
Sex-linked recessive; exclusive to males
Age: 10 years
√ hyperostotic new bone along posterior aspect of vertebral end-plate
√ premature osteoarthritis
√ platyspondyly
√ short trunk
√ flattened femoral heads
DDx: Ochronosis

SPONTANEOUS OSTEONECROSIS OF KNEE
= SONK
Causes: ? degenerative joint disease, gout, rheumatoid arthritis, meniscal tear (78%), trauma, joint bodies, intraarticular steroid injection (45 – 85%)
Age: 7th decade (range 13 – 83 years)
• acute onset of pain
Location: weight-bearing medial condyle more toward epicondylus (95%), lateral condyle (5%), may involve tibial plateau
√ radiographs usually normal (within 3 months after onset)
√ positive bone scan within 5 weeks (most sensitive)
√ flattening of weight-bearing segment of medial femoral epicondyle
√ radiolucent focus in subchondral bone + peripheral zone of osteosclerosis

√ horizontal subchondral fracture (within 6 – 9 months) + osteochondral fragment
√ periosteal reaction along medial side of femoral shaft (30 – 50%)
Cx: osteoarthritis

SPRENGEL DEFORMITY
= failure of descent of scapula secondary to fibrous / osseous omovertebral connection
Associated with: Klippel-Feil syndrome, renal anomalies
• webbed neck
• shoulder immobility
√ elevation of scapula

SUDECK DYSTROPHY
= REFLEX SYMPATHETIC DYSTROPHY = CAUSALGIA
= SHOULDER-HAND SYNDROME = POST-TRAUMATIC OSTEOPOROSIS
Etiology: (1) Injury (fracture, frost bite; may be trivial)
             (2) Immobilization (3) Infection (4) Myocardial infarction
• pain, tenderness, soft tissue swelling out of proportion to degree of injury
• atrophic skin changes
• vasomotor instability (Raynaud phenomenon, local vasoconstriction /-dilatation, hyperhydrosis)
• end-stage (after 6 – 12 months): contractures, atrophy of skin + soft tissues
Location: hands and feet distal to injury
√ periarticular soft tissue swelling
√ patchy demineralization = ground glass appearance (endosteal + intracortical excavation; subperiosteal bone resorption; lysis of juxtaarticular + subchondral bone)
Bone scan:
    √ increased uptake particularly in periarticular bone (radiocarpal, intercarpal, carpometacarpal, metacarpophalangeal, interphalangeal joints) on delayed images
    √ perfusion + blood pool phase not sensitive

SYNOVIAL CHONDROMATOSIS
= OSTEOCHONDROMATOSIS = JOINT CHONDROMA
Histo: cartilage / osteochondroma formed by synovial membrane / joint capsule; hyperplastic synovia with cartilage metaplasia (foci < 2 – 3 cm)
Age: presents in 4th decade; M > F
• progressive joint pain
Sites: knee (most often involved), hip, elbow, ankle, shoulder, wrist; usually monarticular, occasionally bilateral
√ multiple calcified / ossified loose bodies in a single joint
√ varying degrees of bone mineralization (1/3 of chondromas show no radiopacity)
√ pressure erosion of adjacent bone
√ widening of joint space
√ long-standing disease may lead to degenerative joint disease

DDx:
(1) Synovial sarcoma
(2) Osteochondral fracture (Hx of trauma)
(3) Joint surface disintegration (rheumatoid arthritis, neurotrophic arthropathy, tuberculous arthritis, degenerative joint disease)

SYNOVIOMA
= SYNOVIAL SARCOMA
originating in the synovial lining / bursa / tendon sheath; uncommonly intraarticular
Incidence: 10% of soft-tissue sarcomas
Histo: fibrosarcomatous + synovial component
Age: young adults to middle age
• painful soft tissue mass
Location: knee (most common), hip, ankle, elbow, wrist, hands, feet
√ about 1 cm removed from joint cartilage
√ bone erosion (1/3) with wide zone of transition
√ amorphous calcifications (1/3)
√ juxtaarticular osteoporosis
√ large spheroid well-defined soft tissue mass
MRI:
    √ low signal intensity on T1WI
    √ inhomogeneously increased signal intensity on T2WI

SYPHILIS OF BONE
Congenital Syphilis
Transplacental transmission cannot occur < 16 weeks gestational age
√ pneumonia alba
√ hepatomegaly
Location: symmetrical bilateral osteomyelitis involving multiple bones (HALLMARK)
A. Early phase
    1. Metaphysitis
        √ lucent band on diaphyseal side = widened zone of provisional calcification = wide epiphyseal plate
        √ frayed edge of metaphyseal-physeal junction (osteochondritis)
    2. Diaphyseal periostitis = "luetic diaphysitis"
        √ solid / lamellated periosteal new bone growth = bone-within-bone appearance
    3. Spontaneous epiphyseal fractures causing Parrot pseudopalsy (DDx: battered child syndrome)
    4. Bone destruction
        √ marginal destruction of spongiosa + cortex along side of shaft with widening of medullary canal (in short tubular bones)
        √ patchy rarefaction in diaphysis
    5. Wimberger sign
        √ symmetrical focal bone destruction of medial portion of proximal tibial metaphysis (ALMOST PATHOGNOMONIC)
B. Late phase
    • Hutchinson triad = dental abnormality, interstitial keratitis, 8th nerve deafness

√ frontal bossing of Parrot = diffuse thickening of outer table
√ saddle nose + high palate (syphilitic chondritis + rhinitis)
√ short maxilla (maxillary osteitis)
√ thickening at sternal end of clavicle
√ "saber-shin" deformity = anteriorly convex bowing in upper 2/3 of tibia with bone thickening

Acquired Syphilis
= TERTIARY SYPHILIS resembling chronic osteomyelitis
√ dense bone sclerosis of long bones
√ irregular periosteal proliferation + endosteal thickening with narrow medulla
√ extensive calvarial bone proliferation with mottled pattern (anterior half + lateral skull) in outer table (DDx: fibrous dysplasia, Paget disease)
√ ill-defined lytic destruction in skull, spine, long bones (gumma formation)
√ enlargement of clavicle (cortical + endosteal new bone)
√ Charcot arthropathy = neuropathic joints (lower extremities + spine)

THALASSEMIA SYNDROMES
PHYSIOLOGIC HEMOGLOBINS
(a) in adulthood:
    Hb A (98% = 2 alpha- and 2 beta-chains); Hb A_2 (2% = 2 alpha- and 2 delta-chains)
(b) in fetal life, rapidly decreasing up to 3 months of newborn period:
    Hb F (= 2 alpha- and 2 gamma-chains)
A. ALPHA-THALASSEMIA
= decreased synthesis of alpha chains leading to excess of beta-chains + gamma-chains (Hb H = 4 beta-chains; Hb Bart = 4 gamma-chains)
• disease begins in intrauterine life as no fetal hemoglobin is produced
• homozygosity is lethal (lack of oxygen transport)
B. BETA-THALASSEMIA
= decreased synthesis of beta-chains leading to excess of alpha-chains + gamma-chains (= fetal hemoglobin)
• disease manifest in early infancy
(a) homozygous defect = thalassemia major = Cooley anemia
(b) heterozygous defect = thalassemia minor

Thalassemia major
= COOLEY ANEMIA = MEDITERRANIAN ANEMIA
= HEREDITARY LEPTOCYTOSIS = beta-thalassemia trait inherited from both parents (= homozygous)
Incidence: 1% for American Blacks; 7.4% for Greek population; 10% for certain Italian populations
Age: develops after newborn period
• retarded growth
• elevated serum bilirubin

- hyperpigmentation of skin
- hyperuricemia
- secondary sexual characteristics retarded, normal menstruation rare
- hypochromic microcytic anemia (Hb 2 – 3 g/dl), nucleated RBC, target cells, reticulocytosis, decrease in RBC survival, leukocytosis
- susceptible to infection (leukopenia secondary to splenomegaly)
- bleeding diathesis (secondary to thrombocytopenia)
@ Skull:
  √ widening of diploic space with displacement + thinning of outer table
  √ severe hair-on-end appearance (frontal bone, NOT inferior to internal occipital protuberance)
  √ impediment of pneumatization of maxillary antra + mastoid sinuses
  √ lateral displacement of orbits
  √ rodent facies = ventral displacement of incisors (marrow overgrowth in maxillary bone) with dental malocclusion
@ Peripheral skeleton:
  √ earliest changes in small bones of hands + feet (> 6 months of age)
  √ widened medullary spaces with thinning of cortices
  √ osteoporosis = atrophy + coarsening of trabeculae (marrow hyperplasia)
  √ Erlenmeyer flask deformity = bulging of normally concave outline of metaphyses
  √ premature fusion of epiphyses (10%), usually at proximal humerus + distal femur
  √ arthropathy (secondary to hemochromatosis + CPPD + acute gouty arthritis)
  √ regression of peripheral skeletal changes (as red marrow becomes yellow)
@ Chest:
  √ cardiac enlargement + congestive heart failure (secondary to anemia)
  √ paravertebral masses (= extramedullary hematopoiesis)
  √ costal osteomas = expanded posterior aspect of ribs with thinned cortices
@ Abdomen:
  √ hepatosplenomegaly
  √ gallstones
Cx:
  (1) Pathologic fractures
  (2) Sequelae of iron overload from transfusion therapy (absent puberty, diabetes mellitus, adrenal insufficiency, myocardial insufficiency)
Prognosis: usually death within 1st decade

Thalassemia minor

= beta-thalassemia trait inherited from one parent (= heterozygous)
- usually asymptomatic except for periods of stress (pregnancy, infection)

- microcytic hypochromic anemia (Hb 9 – 11 g/dl)
- occasionally jaundice + splenomegaly

THANATOPHORIC DYSPLASIA

= sporadic lethal skeletal dysplasia characterized by severe rhizomelia (micromelic dwarfism)
Incidence: 6.9:100,000 births; 1:6,400 – 16,700 births; most common bone dysplasia
√ large head with short base of skull + prominent frontal bone
√ occasionally trilobed clover leaf skull = "Kleeblattschädel" (huge coronal + lambdoid sutures)
√ narrow chest + short ribs (pulmonary hypoplasia)
√ normal length of trunk
√ iliac wings small + square
√ narrow sacrosciatic notch
√ reduction of interpediculate space of last few lumbar vertebrae
√ platyspondyly = severe H-shaped universal vertebra plana
√ excessive intervertebral space height
√ severe micromelia + bowing of extremities
√ metaphyseal flaring = "telephone handle" appearance of long bones
OB-US: (findings may not be present before last trimester)
  √ polyhydramnios (71%)
  √ short-limbed dwarfism with extremely short + bowed femurs
  √ hypoplastic thorax narrowed in anteroposterior dimension
  √ protuberant abdomen
  √ short ribs
  √ macrocrania with frontal bossing ± hydrocephalus (increased HC:AC ratio)
  √ "cloverleaf skull" (in 14%) (DDx: encephalocele)
  √ redundant soft tissues
Prognosis: uniformly fatal shortly after birth (cardiorespiratory failure)
DDx:
  (1) Ellis-van-Creveld syndrome (extra digit, acromesomelic short limbs)
  (2) Asphyxiating thoracic dysplasia (less marked bone shortening, vertebrae spared)
  (3) Short rib-polydactyly syndrome
  (4) Homozygous achondroplasia (both parents affected)

THROMBOCYTOPENIA-ABSENT RADIUS SYNDROME

= TAR SYNDROME = rare autosomal recessive disorder
Age: presentation at birth
May be associated with CHD (33%): ASD, tetralogy
- platelet count < 100,000 / mm³ (decreased production by bone marrow)
√ usually bilateral radial aplasia / hypoplasia
√ uni- / bilaterally hypoplastic / absent ulna / humerus
√ defects of hands, feet, legs
Prognosis: death in 50% in early infancy (hemorrhage)

THYROID ACROPACHY

Onset: occurs 18 months following thyroidectomy for hyperthyroidism (no occurrence with antithyroid medication)

Incidence: 1 – 10%

- clubbing, soft tissue swelling
- eu- / hypo- / hyperthyroid state

Location: diaphyses of phalanges + metacarpals of hand; less commonly feet, lower legs, forearms

√ thick spiculated lacy periosteal reaction

DDx: (1) Pulmonary osteoarthropathy (painful)
(2) Pachydermoperiostosis
(3) Fluorosis (ligamentous calcifications)

TRANSIENT OSTEOPOROSIS OF HIP

= self-limiting disease of unknown etiology

Age: typically in middle-aged males, related to pregnancy in females

- spontaneous onset of hip and groin pain
- painful swelling of joint followed by progressive demineralization
- rapid development of disability, limp, decreased range of motion

Site: hip most commonly affected; generally only one joint at a time

√ progressive marked osteoporosis of femoral head, neck, acetabulum (3 – 6 weeks after onset of illness)

√ NO joint space narrowing / subchondral bone collapse

√ diffuse increased uptake on bone scan without cold spots / inhomogeneities

Cx: pathologic fracture common

Prognosis: spontaneous recovery within 2 – 6 months; recurrence in another joint within 2 years possible

DDx:
(1) AVN (cystic + sclerotic changes, early subchondral undermining
(2) Septic / tuberculous arthritis (joint aspiration)
(3) Monoarticular rheumatoid arthritis
(4) Metastasis
(5) Reflex sympathetic dystrophy
(6) Disuse atrophy
(7) Synovial chondromatosis
(8) Villonodular synovitis

TRANSIENT SYNOVITIS OF HIP

= OBSERVATION HIP = TRANSITORY SYNOVITIS
= TOXIC SYNOVITIS = COXITIS FUGAX
= nonspecific inflammatory reaction; most common nontraumatic cause of acute limp in a child

Etiology: unknown

Age: 5 – 10 (average 6) years; M:F = 2:1

- developing limp over 1 – 2 days
- pain in hip, thigh, knee
- Hx of recent viral illness (65%)
- mild fever (25%)

√ radiographs usually normal

√ joint effusion

√ displacement of femur from acetabulum

√ displacement of psoas line

√ lateral displacement of gluteal line (least sensitive + least reliable)

√ regional osteoporosis (? hyperemia, disuse)

Prognosis: complete recovery within a few weeks

Dx: per exclusion

Rx: non-weight-bearing treatment

DDx: trauma, Legg-Perthes disease, acute rheumatoid arthritis, acute rheumatic fever, septic arthritis, tuberculosis, malignancy

TREACHER COLLINS SYNDROME

= MANDIBULOFACIAL DYSOSTOSIS
autosomal dominant

- antimongoloid eye slant, deficient lashes in lower eye lids, coloboma
- dysplastic ears; deafness

√ craniosynostosis

√ egg-shaped orbits

√ marked hypoplasia of zygomatic arches, maxilla, paranasal sinuses

√ mandibular hypoplasia with broad concave curve on lower border of body

TRISOMY 18

trisomy 16 – 18 group syndrome

- low-set deformed ears
- small buccal cavity

Associated with: congenital heart disease in 100% (PDA, VSD); hernias; renal anomalies; eventration of diaphragm

√ persistent metopic suture

√ prominent occiput

√ hypoplastic mandible (most constant feature)

√ increase in a.p.-diameter of thorax

√ hypoplastic sternum

√ hypoplastic clavicles (DDx: cleidocranial dysostosis)

√ slender + tapered ribs

√ small pelvis + forward rotation of iliac wings

√ stippled epiphyses

√ overlapping of fingers

√ ulnar deviation of 3rd + 4th + 5th fingers (wide gap between 2nd + 3rd)

√ varus deformities of forefoot + dorsiflexion of toes

√ rocker bottom / club foot deformity

OB-US:
√ hydrocephalus
√ cystic hygroma
√ diaphragmatic hernia
√ club feet
√ overlapping index finger
√ choroid plexus cyst (30%)

Prognosis: child rarely survives infancy

TUBERCULOSIS

Age: Tuberculosis of bone in first 3 decades (prepubertal child)

- history of active pulmonary disease (in 50%)
Location: joints in 84%; bone in 16% (epiphyseal, occasionally diaphyseal)
√ epiphysis + diaphysis affected secondary to joint disease
√ initially destructive lesion with minimal / no surrounding sclerosis
√ spina ventosa = tuberculous dactylitis = digit with exuberant periosteal new bone formation of fusiform appearance secondary to erosion of endosteal cortex with lamellated / solid periosteal thickening in hands + feet
√ cystic tuberculosis = symmetric disseminated destructive osseous lesions
√ Pott disease = tuberculous spondylitis = destructive lesions in spine ± sclerosis, vertebral disc space maintained longer than in pyogenic arthritis, involvement of contiguous vertebra frequent
√ kyphosis (gibbus)
√ large cold paravertebral abscess with subligamentous spread anteriorly (common)
ADULT TUBERCULOSIS
   predilection for greater trochanter associated with soft tissue disease; not necessarily accompanied by hip joint involvement

TUBERCULOUS ARTHRITIS
Pathophysiology: synovitis with pannus formation leads to chondronecrosis
Location: hip, knee, tarsal joints (spine no longer commonest site)
√ Phemister triad:
   1. slow cartilage destruction
   2. peripheral articular defects
   3. osteoporosis
√ early: extensive deossification adjacent to joint, soft tissues normal
√ late: small cyst-like erosions along joint margins in non-weightbearing line opposing one another (DDx: pyogenic arthritis erodes articular cartilage)
√ no joint space narrowing for months
√ articular cortical bone destruction earlier in joints with little unopposed surfaces (hip, shoulder)
√ infection of subchondral bone forming "kissing sequestra"
√ increased density with extensive soft tissue calcifications in healing phase
@ SPINE
   √ narrowed vertebral interspaces (first change)
   √ cold abscess in paravertebral gutters
   √ "gouge defect" = erosion of anterior third of vertebral body
   √ erosion of vertebral plates, destruction of centra; gibbus deformity

TUMORAL CALCINOSIS
= LIPOCALCINOGRANULOMATOSIS = progressive large nodular juxtaarticular calcified soft tissue masses in

patients with normal serum calcium + phosphorus and no evidence of renal, metabolic, or collagen-vascular disease
Etiology: unknown; familial
Path: multilocular cystic lesions with creamy white fluid (calcium phosphate / carbonate) + many giant cells reminiscent of foreign body reaction surrounded by fibrous capsule
Age: 6 – 25 years; M > F; predominantly in blacks
- progressive painful / painless soft-tissue mass with overlying skin ulceration
- swelling
- limitation of motion
- normal serum calcium + phosphorus
Location: periarticular in hips, shoulders, elbows, toes, wrists, ankles, ribs, ischial spines, (single / multiple joints); ALMOST NEVER knees
√ dense loculated homogeneously calcified mass of 1 – 20 cm in size
√ radiolucent septa (= connective tissue)
√ may have fluid levels
√ bones NORMAL
√ increased tracer uptake of soft tissue masses on bone scan
Prognosis: tendency for recurrence after incomplete excision
DDx: Hyperparathyroidism, paraosteoarthropathy, CPPD

TURNER SYNDROME
= due to (1) complete monosomy (45,XO) (2) partial monosomy (structurally altered second X-chromosome (3) mosaicism (XO + another sex karyotype)
Incidence: 1:3,000 live births
Associated with: coarctation, aortic stenosis, horseshoe kidney
- primary amenorrhea; absent secondary sex characteristics
- short stature; absence of prepubertal growth spurt
- webbed neck; low irregular nuchal hair line
- shield-shaped chest + widely spaced nipples
- mental deficiency
- high palate; thyromegaly
- multiple pigmented nevi; keloid formation
- idiopathic hypertension; elevated urinary gonadotropins
@ General
   √ normal skeletal maturation with growth arrest at skeletal age of 15 years
   √ delayed fusion of epiphyses > age 20 years
   √ osteoporosis during / after 2nd decade (gonadal hormone deficiency)
   √ coarctation of aorta (10%); aortic stenosis
   √ renal ectopia / horseshoe kidney
   √ lymphedema
@ Skull
   √ basilar impression; basal angle > 140°
   √ small bridged sella
   √ hypertelorism

@ Axial skeleton + chest
  √ hypoplasia of odontoid process + C1
  √ osteochondritic changes; squared lumbar vertebrae; kyphoscoliosis
  √ small iliac wings; android pelvic inlet; late fusion of iliac crests
  √ thinning of lateral aspects of clavicles
  √ thinned + narrowed ribs with pseudonotching
@ Hand + arm
  √ positive metacarpal sign = relative shortening of 4th metacarpal
  √ positive carpal sign = proximal row of carpal bones forms angle < 117°
  √ shortening of 2nd + 5th middle phalanx (also in Down syndrome)
  √ "drumstick" phalanges = slender shaft + large distal head
  √ "insetting" of epiphyses into bases of adjacent metaphyses (phalanges + metacarpals)
  √ Madelung deformity = shortening of ulna / absence of ulnar styloid process
  √ radial tilt of articular surface of trochlea (cubitus valgus deformity)
@ Knee
  √ tibia vara = enlarged medial femoral condyle + depression of medial tibial plateau
  √ exostosis-like projections from medial border of proximal tibiae

BONNEVIE-ULLRICH SYNDROME
– infantile form of Turner syndrome
  (1) congenital webbed neck
  (2) widely separated nipples
  (3) lymphedema of hands + feet

VAN BUCHEM DISEASE
= GENERALIZED CORTICAL HYPEROSTOSIS may be related to hyperphosphatasemia
• paralysis of facial nerve
• auditory + ocular disturbances (in late teens secondary to foraminal encroachment)
• increased alkaline phosphatase
Location: skull, mandible, clavicles, ribs, long bone diaphyses
√ symmetrical generalized sclerosis + thickening of endosteal cortex
√ obliteration of diploe
√ spinous processes thickened + sclerotic
DDx:
  (1) Osteopetrosis (sclerosis of all bones, not confined to diaphyses)
  (2) Generalized hyperostosis with pachydermia - (involves entire long bones, considerable pain, skin changes)
  (3) Hyperphosphatasia (infancy, widened bones but decreased cortical density)
  (4) Engelmann disease (rarely generalized, involves lower limbs)

  (5) Pyle disease (does not involve middiaphyses)
  (6) Polyostotic fibrous dysplasia (rarely symmetrically generalized, paranasal sinuses abnormal, skull involvement)

WILLIAMS SYNDROME
= IDIOPATHIC HYPERCALCEMIA OF INFANCY
• elfin facies, dysplastic dentition
• neonatal hypercalcemia
• mental retardation
@ Skeletal manifestations
  √ osteosclerosis (secondary to trabecular thickening)
  √ dense broad zone of provisional calcification
  √ radiolucent metaphyseal bands
  √ dense vertebral endplates + acetabular roofs
  √ bone islands in spongiosa
  √ metastatic calcification
  √ craniostenosis
@ Cardiovascular manifestations
  √ supravalvular aortic stenosis, aortic hypoplasia
  √ pulmonic stenosis
  √ stenoses of major vessels (innominate, carotids, renal arteries)
@ GI and GU tract:
  √ colonic diverticula
  √ bladder diverticula
Prognosis: spontaneous resolution after 1 year in most
Rx: withhold vitamin D + calcium
DDx: Hypervitaminosis D

WILSON DISEASE
= HEPATOLENTICULAR DEGENERATION = autosomal recessive disease with excessive copper retention due to decreased ceruloplasmin in liver
Incidence: 1:200,000
Age of onset: 7 – 50 years
• tremor, rigidity, dysarthria (excessive copper deposition in lenticular region of brain)
• Kayser-Fleischer ring surrounding limbus corneae
• liver cirrhosis
Skeletal manifestations (in 2/3):
  √ generalized deossification may produce pathologic fractures
@ Joints: shoulder (frequent), knee, hip, wrist, 2nd – 4th MCP joints
  • articular symptoms in 75%: pain, stiffness, gelling of joints
  √ subarticular cysts
  √ premature osteoarthritis (narrowing of joint space + osteophyte formation)
  √ osteochondritis dissecans
  √ chondrocalcinosis
  √ premature osteoarthrosis of spine, prominent Schmorl nodes, wedging of vertebrae, irregularities of vertebral plates
Cx: rickets + osteomalacia (secondary to renal tubular dysfunction) in minority of patients

DIFFERENTIAL DIAGNOSIS OF SKULL AND SPINE DISORDERS

Basilar invagination
= bulging of C-spine and foramen magnum into cranial cavity
A. Primary form: associated with narrow foramen magnum + occipitalization of atlas
B. Secondary form: osteogenesis imperfecta, Paget disease
mnemonic: "COOP"
Congenital
Osteogenesis imperfecta
Osteomalacia
Paget disease
√ C-spine + foramen magnum bulge into cranial cavity
√ distance from Chamberlain line (= line between roof of hard palate to posterior lip of foramen magnum) to dens < 5 mm
√ elevation of posterior arch of C1

Platybasia
= flattened skull base
Cause: osteomalacia, rickets, hyperparathyroidism, fibrous dysplasia, Paget disease, Arnold-Chiari malformation
• cord symptoms
√ sphenoid angle (= angle between roof of sphenoid and clivus) > 150 °

Sutural abnormalities
Wide sutures
= > 10 mm at birth, > 3 mm at 2 years, > 2 mm at 3 years of age; (sutures are splittable up to age 12 – 15; complete closure by age 30)
A. NORMAL VARIANT
in neonate + prematurity; growth spurt occurs at 2 – 3 years and 5 – 7 years
B. CONGENITAL UNDEROSSIFICATION
Osteogenesis imperfecta, Hypophosphatasia, Rickets, Hypothyroidism, Pyknodysostosis, Cleidocranial dysplasia
C. METABOLIC DISEASE
Hypoparathyroidism; Lead intoxication; Hypo- / hypervitaminosis A
D. RAISED INTRACRANIAL PRESSURE
Cause: (1) intracerebral tumor (2) subdural hematoma (3) hydrocephalus
Age: seen only if < 10 years of age
Location: coronal > sagittal > lambdoid > squamosal suture
E. INFILTRATION OF SUTURES
Cause: metastases to meninges from (1) neuroblastoma (2) leukemia (3) lymphoma
√ poorly defined margins
F. RECOVERY

from (1) deprivational dwarfism (2) chronic illness (3) prematurity (4) hypothyroidism

Craniosynostosis
= CRANIOSTENOSIS = premature closure of sutures (normally at about 30 years of age)
Age: often present at birth; M:F = 4:1
√ sharply defined thickened sclerotic suture margins
Etiology:
A. Primary Craniosynostosis
B. Secondary Craniosynostosis
  (a) Hematologic: Sickle cell anemia, thalassemia
  (b) Metabolic: Rickets, hypercalcemia, hyperthyroidism, hypervitaminosis D
  (c) Bone dysplasia: Hypophosphatasia, achondroplasia, metaphyseal dysplasia, Mongolism, Hurler disease, skull hyperostosis, Rubinstein-Taybi syndrome
  (d) Syndromes: Crouzon, Apert, Carpenter, Treacher-Collins, cloverleaf skull, craniotelencephalic dysplasia, arhinencephaly
  (e) Microcephaly: brain atrophy / dysgenesis
  (f) after shunting procedures
TYPES:
Sagittal suture most commonly affected followed by coronal suture
  1. Scaphocephaly= Dolichocephaly (55%)
     premature closure of sagittal suture (long skull)
  2. Brachycephaly = Turricephaly (10%)
     premature closure of coronal / lambdoid sutures (short tall skull)
  3. Plagiocephaly (7%)
     unilateral early fusion of coronal + lambdoidal suture (lopsided skull)
  4. Trigonocephaly: premature closure of metopic suture (forward pointing skull)
  5. Oxycephaly: premature closure of coronal, sagittal, lambdoid sutures
  6. Cloverleaf skull = Kleeblattschädel:
     intrauterine premature closure of sagittal, coronal, lambdoid sutures
√ delayed growth of BPD in early pregnancy

Wormian bones
= intrasutural ossicles in lambdoid, posterior sagittal, temperosquamosal sutures; normal up to 6 months of age (most frequently)
mnemonic: "PORKCHOPS"
Pyknodysostosis
Osteogenesis imperfecta
Rickets in healing phase
Kinky hair syndrome
Cleidocranial dysplasia

Hypothyroidism / Hypophosphatasia
Otopalatodigital syndrome
Primary acro-osteolysis (Hajdu-Cheney) /
   Pachydermoperiostosis
Syndrome of Down

Increase in skull thickness

A. Generalized
  1. Chronic severe anemia (e.g. thalassemia, sickle cell disease)
  2. Cerebral atrophy following shunting of hydrocephalus
  3. Engelmann disease: mainly skull base
  4. Hyperparathyroidism
  5. Acromegaly
  6. Osteopetrosis
B. Focal
  1. Meningioma
  2. Fibrous dysplasia
  3. Paget disease
  4. Dyke-Davidoff syndrome = unilateral cerebral atrophy + ipsilateral small skull
  5. Hyperostosis frontalis interna
    = dense hyperostosis of inner table of frontal bone;
     M < F
mnemonic: "HIPFAM"
Hyperostosis frontalis interna
Idiopathic
Paget disease
Fibrous dysplasia
Anemia (sickle cell, iron deficiency, thalassemia, spherocytosis)
Metastases

Leontiasis ossea

= overgrowth of facial bones causing leonine (lion-like) facies
1. Fibrous dysplasia
2. Paget disease
3. Craniometaphyseal dysplasia
4. Hyperphosphatasia

Abnormally thin skull

A. Generalized
  1. Obstructive hydrocephalus
  2. Cleidocranial dysostosis
  3. Progeria
  4. Rickets
  5. Osteogenesis imperfecta
  6. Craniolacuna
B. Focal
  1. Neurofibromatosis
  2. Chronic subdural hematoma
  3. Arachnoid cyst

Inadequate cranial calcification

1. Achondroplasia
2. Osteogenesis imperfecta
3. Hypophosphatasia

Osteolytic lesion of skull

A. Normal variant
  1. Venous lake, Pacchionian granulations
    = usually multiple lesions with irregular contour in parasagittal location (within 3 cm of superior sagittal sinus) primarily involving the inner table; associated with impressions by arachnoid granulations
  2. Parietal foraminae
    nonossification of embryonal rests in parietal fissure; bilateral at superior posterior angles of parietal bone; hereditary transmission
B. Trauma
  1. Surgical burr hole
  2. Leptomeningeal cyst
C. Infection
  1. Osteomyelitis
  2. Hydatid disease
  3. Syphilis
  4. Tuberculosis
D. Congenital
  1. Epidermoid / Dermoid
  2. Neurofibromatosis (asterion defect)
  3. Meningoencephalocele
  4. Fibrous dysplasia
  5. Osteoporosis circumscripta of Paget disease
E. Benign tumor
  1. Hemangioma
  2. Brown tumor
  3. Eosinophilic granuloma
F. Malignant tumor
  1. Solitary / multiple metastases
  2. Multiple myeloma
  3. Leukemia
  4. Neuroblastoma

Absent greater sphenoid wing

mnemonic: "M FOR MARINE"
Meningioma
Fibrous dysplasia
Optic glioma
Relapsing hematoma
Metastasis
Aneurysm
Retinoblastoma
Idiopathic
Neurofibromatosis
Eosinophilic granuloma

Button sequestrum

mnemonic: "TORE ME"
Tuberculosis
Osteomyelitis
Radiation
Eosinophilic granuloma
Metastasis
Epidermoid

Mandibular hypoplasia
1. Pierre-Robin syndrome
2. Treacher-Collins syndrome
3. Chromosomal abnormalities
4. Pyknodysostosis

Destruction of temporomandibular joint
mnemonic: "HIRT"
Hyperparathyroidism
Infection
Rheumatoid arthritis
Trauma

Radiolucent lesion of mandible
A. SHARPLY MARGINATED LESION
  (a) around apex of tooth
    1. Radicular cyst
    2. Cementinoma
  (b) around unerupted tooth
    3. Dentigerous cyst
    4. Ameloblastoma
  (c) unrelated to tooth
    5. Simple bone cyst
    6. Fong disease (symmetrical meso- and ectodermal anomalies): iliac horns, absence of fingernails, mandibular cysts (occasionally)
    7. Basal cell nevus syndrome: multiple basal cell epitheliomas, mandibular cysts, extensive calcification of falx + tentorium, brachydactyly, bifid ribs, scoliosis
B. POORLY MARGINATED LESIONS
  √ "floating tooth": suggestive of primary / secondary malignancy
  √ resorption of tooth root: hallmark of benign process
  (a) Infection
    1. Osteomyelitis: actinomycosis
  (b) Radiotherapy
    1. Osteoradionecrosis
  (c) Malignant neoplasm
    1. Osteosarcoma (1/3 lytic, 1/3 sclerotic, 1/3 mixed)
    2. Local invasion from gingival / buccal neoplasms (more common)
    3. Metastasis from breast, lung, kidney in 1 % (in 70 % adenocarcinoma)
  (d) Other
    1. Eosinophilic granuloma: "floating tooth"
    2. Fibrous dysplasia
    3. Osteocementoma
    4. Ossifying fibroma (very common)

Tooth Mass
A. CYSTIC LESION
  1. Radicular cyst (commonest)
    Cause: deep carious lesion / deep filling / trauma
    Site: intimately associated with apex of nonvital tooth
    √ apical lucency

2. Ameloblastoma = adamantinoma of jaw
    locally aggressive lesion from enamel-type epithelial tissue elements around tooth; 1/3 arise from dentigerous cyst
    Age: 4 – 5th decade; M:F = 1:1
    Location: mandible (75 %), maxilla (25 %), in region of bicuspids + molars (angle of mandible commonly affected)
    √ uni- / multilocular lytic lesion with scalloped margin + cortical expansion
    √ may be associated with impacted tooth / resorption of the root of a tooth
    Prognosis: frequently local recurrence even more aggressive after excision
3. Primordial cyst
    arising from follicle of tooth that never developed
    √ absent tooth
4. Giant cell reparative granuloma
    unrelated to tooth (nonodontogenic)
    √ lucent smooth multiloculated lesion
5. Traumatic bone cyst
    in association with vital tooth
    √ sharply marginated lucent lesion with finger-like projections between roots
6. Dentigerous cyst
    = epithelial-lined cyst from odontogenic epithelium developing around unerupted tooth
    Location: maxilla (may expand into maxillary sinus), posterior mandible
    √ cystic expansile lesion containing tooth
    Cx: may degenerate into ameloblastoma (rare)
B. SCLEROTIC LESION
  1. Cementinoma = fibro-osteoma = periapical cemental dysplasia
    Histo: spindle-cell fibroblastic proliferation + cementum
    Age: 30 – 40 years of age; most common in women
    Location: in anterior portion of mandible, at apex of vital tooth
    √ often multicentric
    √ mixed lucent + sclerotic lesion with little expansion, calcifies with time
    DDx: ossifying fibroma, fibrous dysplasia, Paget disease
  2. True cementoma = benign cementoblastoma
  3. Gigantiform cementoma
  4. Hypercementosis
    = bulbous enlargement of a root
    (a) idiopathic (b) associated with Paget disease
  5. Benign fibro-osseous lesions
    (a) ossifying fibroma: young adults; mandible > maxilla
    (b) monostotic fibrous dysplasia: M < F, younger patients
    (c) condensing osteitis = focal chronic sclerosing osteitis
    √ near apex of nonvital tooth

6. Paget Disease
   involvement of jaw in 20 %; maxilla > mandible
   Location: bilateral, symmetric involvement
   √ widened alveolar ridges
   √ flat palate
   √ loosening of teeth
   √ hypercementosis
   √ may cause destruction of lamina dura
7. **Torus mandibularis** = exostosis
   Site: midline of hard palate; lingual surface of
          mandible in region of bicuspids

Small vertebral body

1. Radiation therapy
   during early childhood in excess of 1000 rads
2. Juvenile rheumatoid arthritis
   Location: cervical spine
   √ atlantoaxial subluxation may be present
   √ vertebral fusion may occur
3. Eosinophilic granuloma
   Location: lumbar / lower thoracic spine
   √ compression deformity / vertebra plana
4. Gaucher disease
   = deposits of glucocerebrosides within RES
   √ compression deformity
5. Platyspondyly generalisata
   = flattened vertebral bodies associated with many
     hereditary systemic disorders (achondroplasia,
     spondyloepiphyseal dysplasia tarda,
     mucopolysaccharidosis, osteopetrosis,
     neurofibromatosis, osteogenesis imperfecta,
     thanatophoric dwarfism)
   √ disc spaces of normal height

VERTEBRA PLANA
   mnemonic: "FETISH"
   Fracture
   Eosinophilic granuloma
   Tumor (metastasis, myeloma)
   Infection
   Steroids
   Hemangioma

Enlarged vertebral body

1. Paget disease
   √ "picture framing"; bone sclerosis
2. Gigantism
   √ increase in height of body + disc
3. Myositis ossificans progressiva
   √ bodies greater in height than width
   √ osteoporosis
   √ ossification of ligamentum nuchae

Enlarged vertebral foramen

1. Neurofibroma
2. Congenital absence / hypoplasia of pedicle
3. Dural ectasia (Marfan syndrome, Ehlers-Danlos
   syndrome)

3. Intraspinal neoplasm
4. Metastatic destruction of pedicle

Vertebral border abnormality
Straightening of anterior border

1. Ankylosing spondylitis
2. Paget disease
3. Psoriatric arthritis
4. Reiter disease
5. Rheumatoid arthritis
6. Normal variant

Anterior scalloping of vertebrae

1. Aortic aneurysm
2. Lymphadenopathy
3. Tuberculosis
4. Multiple myeloma (paravertebral soft tissue mass)

Posterior scalloping of vertebrae

in conditions associated with dural ectasia
A. Increased intraspinal pressure
    1. Communicating hydrocephalus
    2. Ependymoma
B. Mesenchymal tissue laxity
    1. Neurofibromatosis (secondary to dural ectasia /
       spinal tumor)
    2. Marfan syndrome
    3. Ehlers-Danlos syndrome
    4. Posterior meningocele
C. Bone softening
    1. Mucopolysaccharidoses: Hurler, Morquio,
       Sanfillipo
    2. Acromegaly (lumbar vertebrae)
    3. Ankylosing spondylitis (lax dura acting on
       osteoporotic vertebrae)
    4. Achondroplasia

   mnemonic: "HAMENTS"
   Hurler disease, **H**ydrocephalus
   Achondroplasia, **A**cromegaly
   Marfan syndrome
   Ehlers-Danlos syndrome
   Neurofibromatosis
   Tumor (meningioma, ependymoma)
   Syringohydromyelia

Bony projections from vertebra

1. Hurler syndrome = gargoylism
   √ rounded appearance of vertebral bodies
   √ mild kyphotic curve with smaller vertebral body at
     apex of kyphosis displaying tongue-like beak at
     anterior half (usually at T12 / L1)
   √ "step-off" deformities along anterior margins
2. Hunter syndrome
   less severe changes than in Hurler syndrome
3. Morquio disease
   √ flattened + widened vertebral bodies

√ anterior "tongue-like" elongation of central portion of vertebral bodies

4. Hypothyroidism = cretinism
   √ small flat vertebral bodies
   √ anterior "tongue-like" deformity (in children only)
   √ widened disc spaces + irregular endplates

5. Spondylosis deformans
   √ osteophytosis along anterior + lateral aspects of endplates with horizontal + vertical course as a result of shearing of the outer annular fibers (Sharpey fibers connecting the annulus fibrosus to adjacent vertebral body)

6. Diffuse idiopathic skeletal hyperostosis (DISH) = Forrestier disease
   √ flowing calcifications + ossifications along anterolateral aspect of > 4 contiguous thoracic vertebral bodies ± osteophytosis

7. Ankylosing spondylitis
   √ bilateral symmetric syndesmophytes (ossification of annulus fibrosus)
   √ "bamboo spine"
   √ "discal ballooning" = biconvex intervertebral discs secondary to osteoporotic deformity of endplates
   √ straightening of anterior margins of vertebral bodies (erosion)
   √ ossification of paraspinal ligaments

8. Fluorosis
   √ vertebral osteophytosis + hyperostosis
   √ sclerotic vertebral bodies + kyphoscoliosis
   √ calcification of paraspinal ligaments

Spine ossification

A. Syndesmophyte = ossification of annulus fibrosus
   associated with: ankylosing spondylitis, ochronosis

B. Osteophyte
   = ossification of anterior longitudinal ligament
   associated with: osteoarthritis

C. Flowing anterior ossification
   = ossification of disc, anterior longitudinal ligament, paravertebral soft tissues
   associated with: diffuse idiopathic skeletal hyperostosis

D. Paravertebral ossification
   associated with: psoriatric arthritis, Reiter syndrome

Vertebral endplate abnormality

1. Osteoporosis (senile / steroid-induced)
   √ "fish vertebrae" (DDx: osteomalacia, Paget disease, Hyperparathyroidism)
   √ bone sclerosis along endplates

2. Sickle cell disease
   √ "H vertebrae" = compression of central portions from subchondral infarcts (DDx: other anemias, Gaucher disease)

3. Schmorl node
   = intraosseous herniation of nucleus pulposus at center

of weakened endplate in disc herniation / Scheuermann disease

4. Limbus vertebrae
   = intraosseous herniation of disc material at junction of vertebral bony rim of centra + endplate (anterosuperior corner)

5. "Ring" epiphysis
   = normal aspect of developing vertebra (between 6 and 12 years of age)
   √ small step-like recess at corner of anterior edge of vertebral body

6. Renal osteodystrophy
   √ "rugger-jersey spine" = horizontal bands of increased opacity subjacent to vertebral endplates

7. Myelofibrosis
   √ "rugger-jersey spine"

8. Osteopetrosis
   √ "sandwich" / "hamburger" vertebrae = sclerotic endplates alternate with radiolucent midportions of vertebral bodies

Schmorl node

= chondrification defects where periosteal vessels penetrate cartilage plates of disc
√ concave defects at upper and lower vertebral endplates with sharp margins produced by superior / inferior herniation of disc material

MRI: √ node of similar signal intensity as disc
   √ low signal intensity of rim
   √ associated with narrowed disc space

DDx: mnemonic: "SHOOT"
   Scheuermann disease
   Hyperparathyroidism
   Osteoporosis
   Osteomalacia
   Trauma

Vacuum phenomenon in intervertebral disc space

= liberation of nitrogen gas from surrounding tissues into clefts with an abnormal nucleus or annulus attachment

Incidence: in up to 20% of plain radiographs / in up to 50% of spinal CT in patients > age 40

Cause:
1. Primary / secondary degeneration of nucleus pulposus
2. Intraosseous herniation of disc (= Schmorl node)
3. Spondylosis deformans
4. Adjacent vertebral metastatic disease with vertebral collapse
5. Infection (extremely rare)

Bone-within-bone vertebra

= "ghost vertebra" following stressful event during vertebral growth phase in childhood
1. Stress line of unknown cause
2. Leukemia
3. Heavy metal poisoning
4. Thorotrast injection

5. Rickets
6. Scurvy
7. Hypothyroidism
8. Hypoparathyroidism

Ivory vertebra
mnemonic: "**M**y **O**nly **S**ister **L**eft **H**ome **O**n **F**riday **P**ast"
Myelosclerosis
Osteoblastic metastasis
Sickle-cell disease
Lymphoma
Hemangioma
Osteopetrosis
Fluorosis
Paget disease

Expansile lesion of vertebrae
A. INVOLVEMENT OF MULTIPLE VERTEBRAE
Metastases, multiple myeloma / plasmacytoma, lymphoma, hemangioma, Paget disease, angiosarcoma, eosinophilic granuloma
B. INVOLVEMENT OF TWO / MORE CONTIGUOUS VERTEBRAE
Osteochondroma, chordoma, aneurysmal bone cyst, myeloma
C. BENIGN LESION
1. Osteochondroma (1 – 5 % in spine)
commonly thoracic, posterior elements, large dense calcified mass with ill-defined borders
2. Osteoblastoma (40 % in spine)
M:F = 2:1; commonly cervical, posterior elements, may involve body if large, well-defined borders, calcified tumor matrix in 50 %, rarely malignant degeneration
3. Giant cell tumor (5 % in spine)
commonly sacrum, expansile lytic lesion of vertebral body with well-defined borders; secondary invasion of posterior elements; malignant degeneration in 15 – 20 %
4. Osteoid osteoma (25 % in spine)
commonly lower thoracic / upper lumbar spine, posterior elements (pedicle, lamina, spinous process), painful scoliosis with concavity toward lesion
5. Aneurysmal bone cyst (30 % in spine)
commonly lower thoracic / upper lumbar spine, posterior elements, well-defined margins, arising from primary bone lesion (giant cell tumor, fibrous dysplasia) in 50 %, may involve two contiguous vertebrae
6. Hemangioma (30 % in spine)
10 % incidence in general population; commonly lower thoracic / upper lumbar spine, vertebral body, "accordion" / "corduroy" appearance
7. Hydatid cyst (1 % in spine)
slow-growing destructive lesion, well-defined sclerotic borders, endemic areas

8. Paget disease
vertebral body ± posterior elements, enlargement of bone, "picture framing"; bone sclerosis
9. Eosinophilic granuloma (6 % in spine)
most often cervical / lumbar spine, vertebral body, "vertebra plana"; multiple involvement common
10. Fibrous dysplasia (1 % in spine)
vertebral body, nonhomogeneous trabecular "ground glass" appearance
D. MALIGNANT
1. Chordoma
particularly 2nd cervical vertebra, within vertebral body
√ total destruction + collapse + anterior soft tissue mass
√ violates disc space
2. Metastases (especially from lung, breast)
Age: > 50 years of age;
Clue: pedicles often destroyed
3. Multiple myeloma / plasmacytoma
Clue: vertebral pedicles usually spared
4. Angiosarcoma
10 % involve spine, most commonly lumbar
5. Osteosarcoma, chondrosarcoma, lymphoma

Blow out lesion of posterior elements
mnemonic: "**GO APE**"
Giant cell tumor
Osteoblastoma
Aneurysmal bone cyst
Plasmacytoma
Eosinophilic granuloma

Bone tumors favoring vertebral bodies
mnemonic: "**CALL HOME**"
Chordoma
Aneurysmal bone cyst
Leukemia
Lymphoma
Hemangioma
Osteoid osteoma, **O**steoblastoma
Myeloma, **M**etastasis
Eosinophilic granuloma

Segmentation anomalies of vertebral bodies
during 9 – 12th week of gestation two ossification centers form for the ventral + dorsal half of vertebral body
1. **Asomia** = agenesis of vertebral body
√ complete absence of vertebral body
√ hypoplastic posterior elements may be present
2. **Hemivertebra**
(a) Unilateral wedge vertebra
√ right / left hemivertebra
√ scoliosis at birth
(b) Dorsal hemivertebra
√ rapidly progressive kyphoscoliosis
(c) Ventral hemivertebra (extremely rare)

3. **Coronal cleft**
   = failure of fusion of anterior + posterior ossification centers
   may be associated with: premature male infant, chondrodystrophia calcificans congenita
   Location: usually in lower thoracic + lumbar spine
   √ vertical radiolucent band just behind midportion of vertebral body; disappears mostly by 6 months of life
4. **Butterfly vertebra**
   = failure of fusion of lateral halves secondary to persistence of notochordal tissue
   may be associated with: anterior spina bifida ± anterior meningocele
   √ widened vertebral body with butterfly configuration (AP view)
   √ adaptation of vertebral endplates of adjacent vertebral bodies
5. **Block vertebra**
   = congenital vertebral fusion
   Location: lumbar / cervical
   √ height of fused vertebral bodies equals the sum of heights of involved bodies + intervertebral diisc
   √ "waist" at level of intervertebral disc space
6. **Hypoplastic vertebra**
7. **Klippel-Feil Syndrome**

Cervical spine fusion
mnemonic: "SPAR BIT"
Senile hypertrophic ankylosis (DISH)
Psoriasis
Ankylosing spondylitis
Reiter disease
Block vertebra (Klippel-Feil)
Infection
Trauma

Spinal dysraphism
= abnormal / incomplete fusion of midline embryologic mesenchymal, neurologic, bony structures
External signs (in 50 %)
- subcutaneous lipoma
- hypertrichosis
- pigmented nevi
- skin dimple
- bladder + bowel dysfunction
- pathologic plantar response
- spastic gait disturbance
- foot deformities
- absent tendon reflexes
- sinus tract

Spina bifida occulta
= skin covered defect; 15 % of spinal dysraphism
- rarely leads to neurologic deficit in itself
associated with: 1. Diastematomyelia
2. Lipomeningocele
3. Tethered cord syndrome
4. Filum terminale lipoma
5. Intraspinal dermoid
6. Epidermoid cyst

Spina bifida aperta
= incomplete fusion of posterior elements of vertebrae + overlying soft tissue; 85 % of spinal dysraphism
- associated with neurologic deficit in > 90 %
1. Meningocele
   = herniation of CSF-filled sac without neural elements
2. Meningomyelocele
   = herniation of neural elements covered by a meningeal sac
3. Myeloschisis
   = surface presentation of neural elements completely uncovered by meninges
4. Myelocystocele
   = herniation of meninges + spinal cord with grossly dilated central canal

Atlantoaxial subluxation
= distance between dens + anterior arch of C1 (measurement along midplane of atlas on lateral view):
  (a) predental space: > 2.5 mm; > 5 mm (in children)
  (b) retrodental space: < 18 mm
Causes of subluxation:
  (a) Congenital:
    1. Occipitalization of atlas
       0.75 % of population; fusion of basion + anterior arch of atlas
    2. Congenital insufficiency of transverse ligament
    3. Os odontoideum / aplasia of dens
    4. Down syndrome (20 %)
    5. Morquio syndrome
    6. Bone dysplasia
  (b) Arthritis: due to laxity of transverse ligament or erosion of dens
    1. Rheumatoid arthritis
    2. Psoriatric arthritis
    3. Reiter syndrome
    4. Ankylosing spondylitis
    5. SLE
    rare: in gout + CPPD
  (c) Inflammatory process:
    Pharyngeal infection in childhood, Retropharyngeal abscess, Coryza, Otitis media, Mastoiditis, Cervical adenitis, Parotitis, Alveolar abscess
    √ dislocation 8 – 10 days after onset of symptoms
  (d) Trauma (very rare)
  (e) Marfan disease

Intramedullary lesion
15% of spinal canal tumors in adults
A. Tumor
  (a) primary: low grade astrocytoma I and II (25%), high grade astrocytoma III and IV (8%), ependymoma (63%), oligodendroglioma (3%), lipoma
     Location: (a) cervical region: astrocytoma
              (b) thoracic region: teratoma-dermoid
              (c) lumbar region: ependymoma, astrocytoma, dermoid
  (b) metastatic: e.g. malignant melanoma, breast, lung

B. Cystic lesion
   may show delayed filling of cystic space on CT-
   myelography
   1. Syringomyelia
   2. Hydromyelia
   3. Reactive cyst
   4. Hemangioblastoma
C. Vascular
   1. Cord concussion = reversible local edema
   2. Hemorrhagic contusion
   3. Cord transection
   4. AVM
D. Chronic infection
   1. Sarcoid
   2. Transverse myelitis
   3. Multiple sclerosis

mnemonic: "HAM LEGS"
   Hematoma, Hydromyelia
   Astrocytoma, Abscess
   Metastasis
   Lipoma
   Ependymoma
   Glioma
   Syrinx

Intradural extramedullary mass
1. Neurofibroma (25 – 35%)
   may be associated with neurofibromatosis; M:F = 1:1
   Location: any level, but particularly cervical
   √ bone erosion + scalloping of vertebral bodies
   √ widening of intervertebral foramen + erosion of
     pedicles
   √ dumbbell configuration of mass = extension through
     neural foramen
   MRI:
     √ isointense to cord on T1W images
     √ hyperintense tumor on T2W images compared
       with surrounding fat
2. Meningioma (25 – 45% of all spinal tumors)
3. Lipoma
4. Dermoid
   commonly conus / cauda equina; associated with
   spinal dysraphism (1/3)
5. Ependymoma
   commonly filum terminale; NO spinal dysraphism
6. "Drop" metastases from CNS tumors
   Common: medulloblastoma, ependymoblastoma,
     pineal germinoma
   Less common: high grade astrocytoma, mature
     ependymoma, malignant choroid plexus
     papilloma, angioblastic meningioma
7. Metastases from outside CNS
   with subarachnoid hemorrhage: malignant melanoma,
     choriocarcinoma, hypernephroma, bronchogenic
     carcinoma
   others: breast, lymphoma,
   √ predominantly dorsal location

√ single / multiple nodules
√ thickening of meninges
√ matted nerve roots
8. Arachnoid Cyst
   Etiology: ? congenital, traumatic, inflammatory
   Location: thoracic spine, posterior to cord, over
     several vertebral segments
9. Neurenteric Cyst
10. Hemangioblastoma

Epidural extramedullary lesion
Epidural space = space between dura mater + bone
   containing epidural venous plexus, lymphatic channels,
   connective tissue, fat
Incidence: 30 % of all spinal tumors
A. Tumor
   (a) benign
     1. Dermoid, Epidermoid
     2. Lipoma: over several segments
     3. Fibroma
     4. Neurinoma (with intradural component)
     5. Meningioma (with intradural component)
   (b) malignant
     1. Hodgkin disease
     2. Lymphoma: most commonly in dorsal space
     3. Metastasis: breast, lung — most commonly from
       involved vertebrae without extension through
       dura
     4. Paravertebral neuroblastoma
B. Disc disease
     1. Bulging disc
     2. Herniated nucleus pulposus
     3. Sequestered nucleus pulposus
C. Osseous spinal stenosis, Spondylosis
D. Inflammation: epidural abscess
E. Hematoma

Cord atrophy
1. Multiple sclerosis
2. Amyotrophic lateral sclerosis
3. Cervical spondylosis
4. Sequelae of trauma
5. Ischemia
6. Radiation therapy
7. AVM of cord

Delayed uptake of water-soluble contrast in cord lesion
1. Syringohydromyelia
2. Cystic tumor of cord
3. Osteomalacia
exceedingly rare: 4. Demyelinating disease
                  5. Infection
                  6. Infarction

Extraarachnoid myelography
A. SUBDURAL INJECTION
   √ spinal cord, nerve roots, blood vessels not outlined

√ irregular filling defects
√ slow flow of contrast material
√ CSF pulsations diminished
√ contrast material pools at injection site within anterior / posterior compartments

B. EPIDURAL INJECTION
   √ contrast extravasation along nerve roots
   √ contrast material lies near periphery of spinal canal
   √ intraspinal structures are not well outlined

ANATOMY OF SKULL AND SPINE

FORAMINA OF BASE OF SKULL
on inner aspect of middle cranial fossa 3 foramina are oriented along an oblique line in the greater sphenoidal wing from anteromedial behind the superior orbital fissure to posteromedial
> mnemonic: "rotos"
> foramen **ro**tundum
> foramen **o**vale
> foramen **s**pinosum

Foramen rotundum
> = canal within greater sphenoid wing connecting middle cranial fossa + pterygopalatine fossa
> Location: inferior and lateral to superior orbital fissure
> Course: extends obliquely forward + slightly inferiorly in a sagittal direction parallel to superior orbital fissure
> Contents:
> (a) nerves: V_2 (maxillary nerve)
> (b) vessels: 1. artery of foramen rotundum
> 2. emissary vv.

Foramen ovale
> = canal connecting middle cranial fossa + infratemporal fossa
> Location: medial aspect of sphenoid body, situated posterolateral to foramen rotundum (endocranial aspect) + at base of lateral pterygoid plate (exocranial aspect)
> Contents:
> (a) nerves: 1. V_3 (mandibular nerve)
> 2. lesser petrosal nerve (occasionally)
> (b) vessels: 1. accessory meningeal artery
> 2. emissary vv.

Foramen spinosum
> Location: on greater sphenoid wing posterolateral to foramen ovale (endocranial aspect) + lateral to eustacian tube (exocranial aspect)
> Contents:
> (a) nerves: 1. recurrent meningeal branch of mandibular nerve
> 2. lesser superficial petrosal nerve
> (b) vessels: 1. middle meningeal a.
> 2. middle meningeal v.

Foramen lacerum
> Fibrocartilage cover (occasionally), carotid artery rests on endocranial aspect of fibrocartilage
> Location: at base of medial pterygoid plate
> Contents: (inconstant)
> (a) nerve: nerve of pterygoid canal (actually pierces cartilage)
> (b) vessel: meningeal branch of ascending pharyngeal a.

Superior orbital fissure
> Boundaries: — medial: body of sphenoid
> — above: lesser wing of sphenoid
> — below: greater wing of sphenoid
> — lateral: frontal bone
> Contents:
> (a) nerves: 1. oculomotor n.
> 2. trochlear n.
> 3. abducens n.
> 4. V_1
> 5. sympathetic filaments of internal carotid plexus
> (b) vessels: 1. orbital branch of middle meningeal a.
> 2. recurrent meningeal branches of lacrimal a.
> 3. ophthalmic vv.

Foramen magnum
> Contents:
> (a) nerves: 1. medulla oblongata
> 2. spinal accessory n.
> (b) vessels: 1. vertebral a.
> 2. anterior spinal a.
> 3. posterior spinal a.

Pterygoid canal
> = VIDIAN CANAL
> = within sphenoid body connecting pterygopalatine fossa anteriorly to foramen lacerum posteriorly
> Location: at base of pterygoid plate below foramen rotundum
> Contents:
> (a) nerves: Vidian nerve = nerve of pterygoid canal = continuation of greater superficial petrosal nerve (from cranial nerve VII) after its union with deep petrosal nerve
> (b) vessel: Vidian artery = artery of pterygoid canal = branch of terminal portion of internal maxillary a. arises in pterygopalatine fossa + passes through foramen lacerum posterior to Vidian n.

Hypoglossal canal
> = ANTERIOR CONDYLAR CANAL
> Location: in posterior cranial fossa anteriorly above condyle starting above anterolateral part of foramen magnum, continuing in an anterolateral direction + exiting medial to jugular foramen
> Contents:
> (a) nerves: cranial nerve 12 (hypoglossal nerve)
> (b) vessels: 1. pharyngeal artery
> 2. branches of meningeal artery

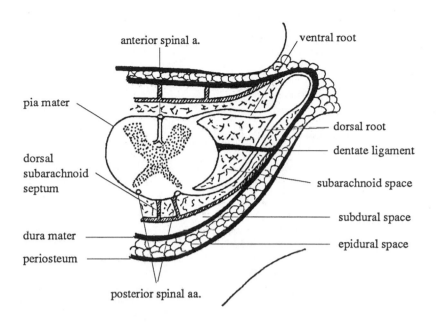

anterior spinal a.

ventral root

pia mater

dorsal root

dentate ligament

dorsal
subarachnoid
septum

subarachnoid space

subdural space

dura mater

epidural space

periosteum

posterior spinal aa.

Meninges of Spinal Cord

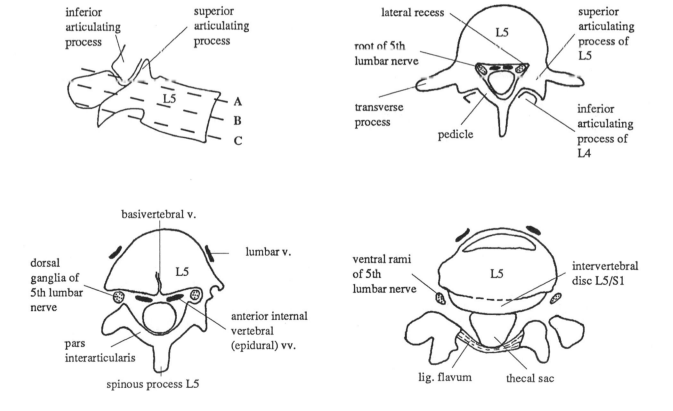

inferior
articulating
process

superior
articulating
process

L5

A
B
C

lateral recess

L5

superior
articulating
process of
L5

root of 5th
lumbar nerve

transverse
process

pedicle

inferior
articulating
process of
L4

basivertebral v.

lumbar v.

dorsal
ganglia of
5th lumbar
nerve

L5

ventral rami
of 5th
lumbar nerve

L5

intervertebral
disc L5/S1

anterior internal
vertebral
(epidural) vv.

pars
interarticularis

spinous process L5

lig. flavum

thecal sac

Cross-sections through 5th lumbar vertebra

Jugular foramen
Location: at the posterior end of petro-occipital suture
            directly posterior to carotid orifice
A.   anterior part:
     (1)   inferior petrosal sinus
     (2)   meningeal branches of pharyngeal artery +
           occipital artery
B.   intermediate part:
     (1)   cranial nerve 9 (glossopharyngeal nerve)
     (2)   cranial nerve 10 (vagus nerve)
     (3)   cranial nerve 11 (accessory nerve)
C.   posterior part: internal jugular vein

MENINGES OF SPINAL CORD
A.   Periosteum
     = continuation of outer layer of cerebral dura mater
B.   Epidural space
     consists of loose areolar tissue + rich plexus of veins
     —   cervical + thoracic spine: spacious posteriorly,
         potential space anteriorly
     —   lower lumbar + sacral spine: may occupy more
         than half of cross-sectional area

C.   Dura
     = continuation of meningeal / inner layer of cerebral
       dura mater; ends at 2nd sacral vertebra + forms
       coccygeal ligament around filum terminale; sends
       tubular extensions around spinal nerves; is
       continuous with epineurium of peripheral nerves
     Attachment: at circumference of foramen magnum,
                  bodies of 2nd + 3rd cervical vertebrae,
                  posterior longitudinal ligament (by
                  connective tissue strands)
D.   Subarachnoid space
     = space between arachnoid and pia mater containing
       CSF, reaching as far lateral as spinal ganglia
     dentate ligament partially divides CSF space into an
       anterior + posterior compartment extending from
       foramen magnum to 1st lumbar vertebra, is
       continuous with pia mater of cord medially + dura
       mater laterally (between exiting nerves)
     dorsal subarachnoid septum connects the arachnoid
       to the pia mater (cribriform septum)
E.   Pia mater
     = firm vascular membrane intimately adherent to
       spinal cord, blends with dura mater in intervertebral
       foramina around spinal ganglia, forms filum
       terminale, fuses with periosteum of 1st coccygeal
       segment

DISEASE ENTITIES OF SKULL AND SPINE DISORDERS

ARACHNOIDITIS
Etiology: Pantopaque (inflammatory effect potentiated by blood), back surgery, hemorrhage, trauma, idiopathic
associated with syrinx
Myelo: √ blunting of nerve root sleeves
√ blocked nerve roots without cord displacement (2/3)
√ streaking + clumping of contrast
CT: √ fusion / clumping of nerve roots
√ featureless empty-looking sac with roots adherent to wall (final stage)

BRACHIAL PLEXUS INJURY
1. Erb-Duchenne: adduction injury affecting C5/6 (downward displacement of shoulder)
2. Klumpke: abduction injury at C7, C8, T1 (arm stretched over head)
√ pouch-like root sleeve at site of avulsion
√ asymmetrical nerve roots
√ contrast extravasation collecting in axilla
√ metrizamide in neural foraminae (CT-myelography)

CHORDOMA
1 – 4% of all primary malignant neoplasms of bone
Incidence: 1:2,000,000
Etiology: originates from embryonic notocordal remnants / ectopic cordal foci (notocord appears between 4 – 7th week of embryonic development and forms nucleus pulposus)
Age: 30 – 70 years (peak age in 5th – 7th decade); M:F = 2:1; highly malignant in children
Histo: large vacuolated (physaliferous) cells containing intracytoplasmic mucous droplets; areas of hemorrhage + abundant extracellular mucus deposition
Location: (a) 50% in sacrum (b) 35% in skull base (c) 15% spinal axis (d) other sites (5%) in mandible, maxilla, scapula
Metastases (in 10 – 30%) to: lung, lymph nodes, bone, liver, skin (late)

SACROCOCCYGEAL CHORDOMA (50 – 70%)
Age: older patient; M:F = 2:1
• low back pain
• constipation
• fecal incontinence
• sciatica
• frequency, urgency, straining on micturition
√ large presacral mass extending superiorly + inferiorly; rarely posterior location
√ displacement of rectum + bladder
√ solid tumor with cystic areas (in 50%)

√ may contain amorphous calcifications (15 – 89%)
√ osteolytic midline mass in sacrum + coccyx
√ secondary bone sclerosis in tumor periphery (50%)
Prognosis: 66% 5-year survival rate (adulthood)
DDx: Giant cell tumor, Plasmacytoma, Metastatic adenocarcinoma, Aneurysmal bone cyst, Chondrosarcoma, Osteomyelitis, Ependymoma

SPHENO-OCCIPITAL CHORDOMA (15 – 25%)
Age: younger patient (peak 3rd – 4 th decade); M:F - 1:1
• localized pain
• 6th nerve palsy / paraplegia
Location: clivus, sphenoid sinus
√ bone destruction (in 90%): clivus > sella > petrous bone > orbit > floor of middle cranial fossa > jugular fossa > atlas > foramen magnum
√ reactive bone sclerosis (rare)
√ calcifications (20 – 70%)
√ soft tissue extension into nasopharynx (common), into sphenoid + ethmoid sinuses possible
√ variable degree of enhancement
DDx: meningioma, metastasis, plasmacytoma, giant cell tumor, sphenoid sinus cyst, nasopharyngeal carcinoma

VERTEBRAL CHORDOMA (15 – 20%)
more aggressive than sacral / cranial chordomas
Age: younger patient; M:F = 2:1
• low back pain + radiculopathy
Location: cervical (particularly axis) > lumbar > thoracic spine
√ total destruction of vertebra, initially unaccompanied by collapse
√ variable extension into spinal canal
√ violates disc space to involve adjacent bodies (common)
√ anterior soft tissue mass
Cx: complete spinal block
DDx: Metastasis, Primary bone tumor, Primary soft tissue tumor, Neuroma, Meningioma

DEGENERATIVE DISC DISEASE
Pathophysiology:
loss of disc height leads to malalignment (= rostrocaudal subluxation) of facet joints causing spine instability with arthritis, capsular hypertrophy, hypertrophy of posterior ligaments, facet fracture
Plain film:
√ narrowing of disc space
√ disc calcification
√ vacuum disc phenomenon = radiolucent interspace accumulation of nitrogen gas at sites of negative pressure

√ intervertebral osteochondrosis = loss of disc space height + bone sclerosis of adjacent vertebral bodies
√ cartilaginous nodes = intraosseous disc herniation
√ spondylosis deformans = endplate osteophytosis secondary to anterolateral disc displacement resulting in traction osteophytes at site of osseous attachment of annulus fibrosus fibers of Sharpey

Myelography:
√ delineation of thecal sac, spinal cord, exiting nerve roots

CT (accuracy > 90%):
√ facet joint disease (marginal sclerosis, joint narrowing, cyst formation, bony overgrowth)

MRI:
√ endplate changes (Modic & DeRoos):
(a) Type I   (4%) with decreased signal on T1WI + increased signal on T2WI (= vascularized fibrous tissue)
(b) Type II   (16%) with increased signal on T1WI + isointensity on T2WI (= local fatty replacement of marrow)
(c) Type III with decreased signal on T1WI + T2WI (= advanced sclerosis)

NUC:
√ eccentrically placed increased uptake on either side of an intervertebral space (osteophytes, discogenic sclerosis)

Sequelae: (1) disc bulging (2) disc herniation (3) spinal stenosis (4) facet joint disease

Bulging Disc
= broad-based disc extension outward in all directions with intact but weakened annulus fibrosus + posterior longitudinal ligament
Age: common finding in individuals > 40 years of age
Location: lumbar, cervical spine
√ rounded symmetric defect localized to disc space level
√ concave anterior margin of thecal sac
MRI: √ nucleus pulposus hypointense on T1WI + hyperintense on T2WI (water loss through degeneration)

Herniation of Nucleus Pulposus
= HNP = focal protrusion of disc material beyond margins of adjacent vertebral end plates secondary to rupture of annulus fibrosus confined within posterior longitudinal ligament
• local somatic spinal pain = sharp / aching, deep, localized
• centrifugal radiating pain = sharp, well-circumscribed, superficial, "electric", confined to dermatome
• centrifugal referred pain = dull, ill-defined, deep or superficial, aching or boring, confined to somatome (= dermatome + myotome + sclerotome)
Location: L4/5 (35%) > L5/S1 (27%) > L3/4 (19%) > L2/3 (14%) > L1/2 (5%); thoracic spine affected in 3:1,000 disc operations

(a) posterolateral (49%) = weakest point along posterolateral margin of disc at lateral recess of spinal canal (posterior longitudinal ligament tightly adherent to posterior margins of disc)
(b) posterocentral (8%)
(c) bilateral (on both sides of posterior ligament)
(d) lateral / foraminal (< 10 %)
(e) intraosseous / vertical = Schmorl node (14%)
(f) extraforaminal = anterior (commonly overlooked) (29%)

Myelography:
√ sharply angular indentation on lateral aspect of thecal sac with extension above or below level of disc space (ipsilateral oblique projection best view)
√ asymmetry of posterior disc margin
√ double contour secondary to superimposed normal + abnormal side (horizontal beam lateral view)
√ narrowing of intervertebral disc space (most commonly a sign of disc degéneration)
√ deviation of nerve root / root sleeve
√ enlargement of nerve root secondary to edema ("trumpet sign")
√ amputated / truncated nerve root (nonfilling of root sleeve)

MRI: √ herniated disc material of low-signal intensity displaces the posterior longitudinal ligament and epidural fat of relative high signal intensity on T1WI

Cx: spinal stenosis

Free Fragment Herniation
= DISC SEQUESTRATION
= complete separation of disc material with rupture through posterior longitudinal ligament into epidural space
√ migration superiorly / inferiorly away from disc space with compression of nerve root above / below level of disc herniation
√ disc material noted > 9 mm away from intervertebral disc space

DDx: (1) Postoperative scarring (retraction of thecal sac to side of surgery)
(2) Epidural abscess
(3) Epidural tumor
(4) Conjoined nerve root (2 nerve roots arising from thecal sac simultaneously representing mass in ventrolateral aspect of spinal canal; normal variant in 1 – 3% of population)

Cervical Disc Herniation
• neck stiffness, muscle splinting
• dermatomic sensory loss
• weakness + muscle atrophy
• reflex loss
Sites: C6-7 (69%); C5-6 (19%); C7-T1 (10%); C4-5 (2%)
Sequelae:
(1) compression of exiting nerve roots

(2) cord compression (spinal stenosis + massive disc rupture)

DIASTEMATOMYELIA

= SPLIT CORD = MYELOSCHISIS = congenital malformation secondary to continued infolding of neural tube leading to division of spinal cord / filum terminale by fibrous (25%), cartilaginous / bony spurs (75%) in a sagittal plane

M:F = 1:3

associated with: myelomeningocele
- hair patch / lumbar nevus (26 – 81 %)
- muscle wasting + ankle weakness in one leg

Location: lower thoracic / upper lumbar spine
√ congenital scoliosis (75%);
   Δ 5% of patients with congenital scoliosis have diastematomyelia
√ spina bifida over multiple levels
√ anteroposterior narrowing of vertebral bodies
√ widening of interpediculate distance
√ narrowed disc spaces with fusion of adjacent laminae / hemivertebrae
√ abnormalities of posterior neural arch (90%)
√ bony spur through center of spinal canal arising from posterior aspect of centra
√ tethered cord with low conus medullaris (60%)
√ defect in thecal sac on myelogram
Cx: progressive spinal cord dysfunction

DISCITIS

most common pediatric spine problem

Etiology: blood borne bacterial invasion of vertebrae infecting disc via communicating vessels through end plate

Age peak: 6 months – 4 years and 10 – 14 years
- fever, irritability, malaise
- back / referred hip pain, limp
- failure to bear weight

Location: L3/4, L4/5, unusual above T9
Plain film: (positive 2 – 4 weeks after onset of symptoms)
√ disc space narrowing (earliest sign) = intraosseous herniation of nucleus pulposus into vertebral body through weakened end plate
√ indistinctness of both end plates with destruction
√ end-plate sclerosis (during healing)
CT:
√ paravertebral inflammatory mass
√ epidural soft tissue extension with deformity of thecal sac
MRI:
√ decreased intensity on T1WI + increased intensity on T2WI
NUC: (90% sensitivity on Tc-99m phosphate / Ga-67 scans)
√ positive before radiographs
√ bone scan usually positive in adjacent vertebrae (until age 20) secondary to vascular supply via endplates; may be negative after age 20
Cx: kyphosis

EOSINOPHILIC GRANULOMA

= most benign variety of Histiocytosis X with skull as most frequent site of involvement of skeletal system

Age: < 20 years (in 75%)
- intractable otitis media with chronically draining ear (temporal bone involvement)
- eosinophilia in blood + CSF

Sites: frontal bone > temporal bone
√ purely lytic lesion with serrated + beveled edge
√ sharply marginated without sclerotic rim (DDx: epidermoid with bone sclerosis)
√ central bone density = "button" sequestrum
√ destructive lesion near mastoid antrum (resembling cholesteatoma)
√ infiltration of orbital bones / mandible
√ isodense homogeneously enhancing mass in hypothalamus / pituitary gland

EPIDURAL HEMATOMA OF SPINE

Etiology: (1) vertebral fracture / dislocation (2) traumatic lumbar puncture (3) hypertension (4) AVM (5) vertebral hemangioma (6) bleeding diathesis / anticoagulation / hemophilia (7) idiopathic (45%)

Peak age: 40 – 50 years
- acute radicular pain
- paraplegia

Location: thoracic spine (most common)
√ compression of posterior aspect of cord
√ high attenuation lesion on CT
√ iso- / slightly hypointense lesion on T1WI with marked increase in intensity on T2WI

FRACTURES OF SKULL

1. Linear fracture (most common type)
   (DDx: vascular groove, suture)
2. Depressed fracture
   surgery indicated if depression > 5 mm
3. Basal fracture
   - CSF rhinorrhea
   - 7th / 8th nerve palsy
   √ air-fluid level in sinuses + mastoid

LeFort Fracture

= all LeFort fractures involve pterygoid process
A. LeFort I = Transverse maxillary fracture caused by blow to premaxilla
   Fracture line: (a) alveolar ridge (b) lateral aperture of nose (c) inferior wall of maxillary sinus
   √ detachment of alveolar process of maxilla
B. LeFort II = "Pyramidal fracture"
   Fracture line: arch through (a) posterior alveolar ridge (b) medial orbital rim (c) across nasal bones
   √ separation of midportion of face
C. LeFort III = "cranio-facial dysjunction"

Fracture line: horizontal course through (a) naso-frontal suture (b) maxillo-frontal suture (c) orbital wall (d) zygomatic arch
√ separation of entire face from base of skull

Zygomaticomaxillary Fracture
= "TRIPOD" FRACTURE = MALAR / ZYGOMATIC COMPLEX FRACTURE
Cause: direct blow to malar eminence
- loss of sensibility of face below orbit
- deficient mastication
- double vision / ophthalmoplegia
- facial deformity
Fracture line:

(a) lateral wall of maxillary sinus (b) orbital rim close to infraorbital foramen (c) floor of orbit (d) zygomatico-frontal suture / zygomatic arch

Blow-out Fracture
= isolated fracture of orbital floor
Cause: sudden direct blow to globe with increase in intraorbital pressure transmitted to the weak orbital floor, often associated with fracture of the thin lamina papyracea
- diplopia on upward gaze (entrapment of inferior rectus + inferior oblique muscles)
- enophthalmus
- facial anesthesia

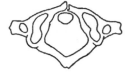 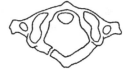 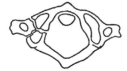 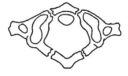

Anterior arch fracture   Posterior arch fracture   Lateral mass fracture   Jefferson fracture
Atlas Fracture

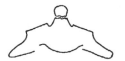 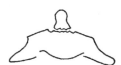 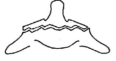

Type I   Type II   Type III
Axis Fracture

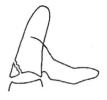

Tear drop fracture   Hangman's fracture
Dens Fractures

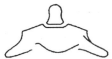 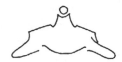 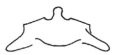 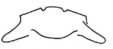

Os odontoideum   Ossiculum terminale   Hypoplasia of dens   Aplasia of dens

√ soft tissue mass extending into maxillary sinus
√ complete opacification of maxillary sinus (edema + hemorrhage)
√ depression of orbital floor
√ posttraumatic atrophy of orbital fat leads to enophthalmus

FRACTURES OF CERVICAL SPINE

Frequency: C2, C6 > C 5, C 7 > C3, C4 > C1
Location:
  (a)   upper cervical spine = C1/2 (19 – 25%): atlas (4%), odontoid (6%)
  (b)   lower cervical spine = C3 – 7 (75 – 81%)
Site: vertebral arch (50%), vertebral body (30%), intervertebral disc (25%), posterior ligaments (16%), dens (14%), locked facets (12%), anterior ligament (2%)
associated with
    thoracic / lumbar spine fracture in 5 – 15%

A. HYPERFLEXION INJURY (46 – 79%)
  1. Odontoid fracture
  2. Simple wedge fracture (stable)
  3. Tear drop fracture: most severe + unstable injury of C-spine
  4. Anterior subluxation
  5. Bilateral locked facets (unstable)
  6. Anterior disc space narrowing
  7. Widened interspinous distance
  8. spinous process fracture = clay shoveler's fracture = sudden load on flexed spine with avulsion fracture of C6 / C7 / T1 (stable)

B. HYPEREXTENSION INJURY (20 – 38%)
  1. Anteriorly widened disc space
  2. Prevertebral swelling
  3. **Tear drop fracture** = avulsion of anteroinferior corner by anterior ligament (unstable) typically at C2
  4. Neural arch fracture of C1 (stable: anterior ring + transverse ligament intact)
  5. Subluxation (anterior / posterior)
  6. **Hangman's fracture** = bilateral neural arch fracture of C2 (unstable)
    √ prevertebral soft tissue swelling
    √ anterior subluxation of C2 on C3
    √ avulsion of anteroinferior corner of C2 (rupture of anterior longitudinal ligament)

C. FLEXION-ROTATION INJURY (12%)
  1. Unilateral locked facets (oblique views !, stable)

D. VERTICAL COMPRESSION (4%)
  1. **Jefferson fracture** = comminuted fracture of ring of C1 (unstable)
    √ lateral displacement of lateral massa (self-decompressing)
  2. Burst fracture = intervertebral disc driven into vertebral body below (stable)

√ several fragments, fragment from posterior superior margin often in spinal canal

E. LATERAL FLEXION / SHEARING (4 – 6%)
  1. Uncinate fracture
  2. Isolated pillar fracture
  3. Transverse process fracture
  4. Lateral vertebral compression

Atlas fracture
Incidence: 4% of cervical spine injuries
Site: posterior arch, anterior arch, massa lateralis, Jefferson fracture
associated with:
    fractures of C7 (25%), C2 pedicle (15%), extraspinal fractures (58%)

Axis fracture
Incidence: 6% of cervical spine injuries
associated with   fractures of C1 in 8%
  Type I   = avulsion of tip of ondontoid (5 – 8%)
      √ difficult to detect
  Type II   = fracture through base of dens (54 – 67%)
      Cx: nonunion
  Type III   = subdental fracture (30 – 33%)
      Prognosis: good
  DDx: os ondontoideum, ossiculum terminale, hypoplasia of dens, aplasia of dens

Chance Fracture
  = SEATBELT FRACTURE
  Mechanism: shearing flexion injury (lap-type seatbelt injury)
  √ oblique horizontal splitting of spinous process, neural arch + superior portion of vertebral body
  Cx: often associated with visceral injury

FRACTURES OF THORACOLUMBAR SPINE
40% of all vertebral fractures that cause neurologic deficit, mostly complex (body + posterior elements involved)
√ diastasis of apophyseal joints
√ disruption of interspinal ligament
√ retropulsion of body fragments into spinal canal
√ "burst" fragments at superior surface of body

GLIOMA OF SPINE
often associated with syrinx
  1. Ependymoma (60 – 70%)
    Location: lower spinal cord, conus medullaris, filum terminale; extends over several vertebral segments
    √ focal mass with areas of extensive cystic degeneration, hemorrhage, and calcification
    √ erosion of vertebral body (uncommon)
  2. Astrocytoma (30%)
    Histo: low grade astrocytoma (I + II) in 75%
    Location: thoracic + cervical spine; often extending into lower brainstem

√ usually homogeneous extensive cord tumor with widening of spinal cord

√ dilated veins on surface of cord

√ mass may be cystic with water-soluble myelographic contrast entering cystic space on delayed CT images

HEMANGIOBLASTOMA OF SPINE

= ANGIOBLASTOMA = ANGIORETICULOMA

Incidence: 2% of all spinal cord tumors; mostly sporadic

associated with: von Hippel-Lindau disease (in 1/3)

Age: middle age; M:F = 1:1

Location: intramedullary (75%), radicular (20%), intradural extramedullary (5%); solitary in > 90%; mostly in cervicothoracic spine

√ increased interpediculate distance (mass effect)

√ expanded cord

√ intratumoral cystic component (50 – 60%)

√ large draining veins form sinuous mass along posterior aspect of cord

√ densely staining tumor nodule

Cx: intramedullary hemorrhage

KLIPPEL-FEIL SYNDROME

= BREVICOLLIS = synostosis of two / more cervical segments

may be associated with:

platybasia, syringomyelia, encephalocele, facial + cranial asymmetry, Sprengel deformity (25 – 40%), syndactyly, clubbed foot, hypoplastic lumbar vertebrae, Renal anomalies in 50% (agenesis, malrotation, duplication)

• clinical triad of

(1)   short neck

(2)   restriction of cervical motion

(3)   low posterior hairline

Location: cervical spine

√ fusion of vertebral bodies and posterior elements

√ ± hemivertebrae

√ may have cervico-occipital fusion

√ Sprengel deformity (25 – 40%) = elevation + medial rotation of scapula (may be related to presence of anomalous omovertebral bone)

KÜMMEL DISEASE

= intravertebral vacuum phenomenon

Cause: 1. Osteonecrosis

2. weeks to months following acute fracture

Pathophysiology: likely to represent gaseous release into bony clefts within a nonhealed fracture underneath endplate

Age: > 50 years

Location: most commonly at thoracolumbar junction

√ gas collection increasing with extension + traction, decreasing with flexion

LEPTOMENINGEAL CYST

Incidence: 1% of all pediatric skull fractures

Pathogenesis:

skull fracture with dural tear leads to arachnoid herniation into dural defect; CSF pulsations produce fracture diastasis + erosion of bone margins (apparent 2 – 3 months after injury)

Age: usually < 3 years

√ skull defect with scalloped margins

√ CSF-density cyst adjacent to / in skull, may contain cerebral tissue

MRI: √ cyst isointense with CSF + communicating with subarachnoid space

LIPOMA OF SPINE

Age peak: infancy, puberty, 3rd – 5th decade; NO sex predilection

may be associated with: spinal dysraphism + low position of conus medullaris

• normal skin / cutaneous abnormality (nevus, abnormal hair, dimple)

• gait disturbance, loss of sphincter control

• elevation of protein in CSF (30%)

Location: usually lumbosacral (conus medullaris + filum terminale); lower cervical / upper thoracic spine; may extend over several vertebral segments; longitudinal extension over entire length of spinal canal (in 7%)

Site: extradural (most common) / intradural extramedullary / intramedullary / combination; mostly posterior extending from subcutaneous tissue

√ congenital vertebral anomalies: spina bifida occulta, abnormal vertebral segmentation, tethered cord

√ erosion of vertebral body + pedicles

√ posterior scalloping (50%)

√ large filling defect within capacious spinal canal

LÜCKENSCHÄDEL

= CRANIOLACUNIA = LACUNAR SKULL = mesenchymal dysplasia of calvarial ossification (developmental disturbance)

Age: present at birth

associated with: (1) meningocele / myelomeningocele (2) encephalocele (3) spina bifida (4) cleft palate (5) Arnold-Chiari II malformation

• normal intracranial pressure

Location: particularly upper parietal area

√ honeycombed appearance about 2 cm in diameter (thinning of diploic space)

√ premature closure of sutures (turricephaly / scaphocephaly)

Prognosis: spontaneous regression within first 6 months of life

DDx:

(1)   Convolutional impressions = "digital" markings (visible at 2 years, maximally apparent at 4 years, disappear by 8 years of age)

(2) "beaten brass" = "hammered silver" appearance of increased intracranial pressure

MENINGIOMA OF SPINE
Incidence: 25 – 45% of all spine tumors
Age: > 40 years + female (80%)
Location: thoracic region (82%); cervical spine on anterior cord surface near foramen magnum (2nd most common location); 90% on lateral aspect
Site: intradural extramedullary (50%); entirely epidural; intradural + epidural
√ bone erosion in < 10%
√ scalloping of posterior aspect of vertebral body
√ widening of interpedicular distance
√ enlargement of intervertebral foramen
√ solid hyperdense mass with marked enhancement
√ may calcify (not as readily as intracranial meningioma)
MRI:
√ isointense to grey matter on T1WI + T2WI
√ rapid + dense enhancement after Gd-DTPA

MYELOMENINGOCELE
= sac covered by leptomeninges containing CSF + variable amount of neural tissue; herniated through a defect in the posterior / anterior elements of spine
Incidence: 1:1,000 – 2,000 births (in Great Britain 1:200 births); twice as common in infants of mothers > 35 years of age; Caucasians > Blacks > Orientals; most common congenital anomaly of CNS
Etiology: failure of closure of caudal neuropore (usually closed by 28 days)
• positive family Hx in 10%
• normal skin / cutaneous abnormality: pigmented nevus, abnormal distribution of hair, skin dimple, angioma, lipoma
• MS-AFP (≥ 2.5 S.D. over mean) permits detection in 80% (positive predictive value of 2 – 5%) if defect not covered by full skin thickness
Recurrence rate: 3 – 7% chance of NTD with previously affected sibling / in fetus of affected parent
associated with:
(1) Hydrocephalus (70 – 90%): requiring ventriculo-peritoneal shunt (90%) [25% of patients with hydrocephalus have spina bifida], most commonly in Arnold-Chiari malformation
(2) Congenital / acquired kyphoscoliosis (90%)
(3) Vertebral anomalies (vertebral body fusion, hemivertebrae, cleft vertebrae, butterfly vertebrae)
(4) Chromosomal anomalies
Location:
(a) dorsal meningocele: lumbosacral, suboccipital
(b) anterior sacral meningocele = prolapse through anterior sacral bony defect; occasionally associated with GU tract / colonic anomalies; M:F = 1:4

(c) lateral thoracic meningocele through enlarged intervertebral foramen; right > left side; often associated with neurofibromatosis + hemivertebrae
(d) traumatic meningocele = in avulsion of spinal nerve roots secondary to tear in meningeal root sheath; in C-spine after brachial plexus injury (most commonly)
√ small irregular arachnoid diverticulum with extension outside the spinal canal
(e) cranial meningocele = encephalocele
√ bony defect in neural arch
√ deformity + failure of fusion of lamina
√ absent spinous process
√ widened interpedicular distance
√ widened spinal canal

OB-US: detection rate of 85 – 90%; sensitivity dependent on GA (fetal spine may be adequately visualized after 16 – 20 weeks GA); false-negative rate of 24%
√ may have clubfoot / rockerbottom foot
√ polyhydramnios
@ Spine:
√ soft tissue mass protruding posteriorly + visualization of sac
√ splaying / widening of lumbar spine
√ divergent position of ossification centers of laminae with cup- / wedge shaped pattern (in transverse plane = most important section for diagnosis)
√ absence of posterior line = posterior vertebral elements (in sagittal plane)
√ gross irregularity in parallelism of lines representing laminae of vertebrae (in coronal plane)
@ Head (prior to 24 weeks):
√ "lemon sign" = concave / linear frontal contour abnormality located at coronal suture (positive predictive value 81 – 84%, false-positive rate of 1%); resolves with advancing gestation
√ "banana sign" = obliteration of cisterna magna with cerebellum wrapped around posterior brain stem secondary to downward traction of spinal cord in Arnold-Chiari malformation type II
√ absence of normal cisterna magna
√ ventricular dilatation (40 – 90%), choroid incompletely filling the ventricles
Rx: possibly elective cesarian section at 36 – 38 weeks GA (may decrease risk of contaminating / rupturing the meningomyelocele sac)
Prognosis:
(1) Mortality 15% by age 10 years
(2) Intelligence: IQ < 80 (27%); IQ > 100 (27%); learning disability (50%)
(3) Urinary incontinence: 85% achieve social continence (scheduled intermittent catheterization)
(4) Motor function: some deficit (100%); improvement after repair (37%)
(5) Hindbrain dysfunction associated with Chiari II malformation (32%)

(6) Ventriculitis: 7% in initial repair within 48 hours, 7% in delayed repair > 48 hours.

NEURENTERIC CYST

= persistence of canal of Kovalevski between yolk sac + notochord

associated with:

neurofibromatosis; meningocele; spinal malformation (stalk connects cyst and neural canal; usually no stalk between cyst and esophagus)

Location: anterior to spinal canal on mesenteric side of gut

√ midline cleft in centra (accommodates stalk)

√ anterior / posterior spina bifida

√ incomplete vertebral elements

√ diastematomyelia

√ posterior mediastinal mass

OSSIFYING FIBROMA

Peak incidence: first 2 decades of life

Histo: areas of osseous tissue intermixed with a highly cellular fibrous tissue

Sites: maxilla > frontal > ethmoid bone > mandible (rarely seen elsewhere)

√ areas of increased + decreased attenuation

√ intact inner + outer table

√ slow-growing expansile lesion

√ usually unilateral + monostotic

DDx: may be impossible to differentiate from fibrous dysplasia

OSTEOMYELITIS OF VERTEBRA

Incidence: 2 – 10% of all cases of osteomyelitis

Causes:

(1) direct penetrating trauma (most common); following surgical removal of nucleus pulposus

(2) hematogenous: associated with urinary tract infections / following GU surgery / instrumentation; diabetes mellitus; drug abuse

Pathophysiology: infection begins in low-flow end-vascular arcades adjacent to subchondral plate region

Organism: Staphylococcus aureus, Streptococcus

Peak age: 5 – 7 th decade

• back pain, neurologic deficit

• fever, leukocytosis

• increased erythrocyte sedimentation rate

• positive blood / urine culture

√ disc space narrowing (earliest radiographic sign)

√ tracer uptake in adjacent portions of two vertebral bodies

Cx: secondary infection of intervertebral disc is frequent

PERINEURAL SACRAL CYST

= TARLOV CYST = cyst arising from posterior rootlets (S2 + S3 most common)

√ sacral erosion

√ may communicate with thecal sac

SACRAL AGENESIS

= CAUDAL REGRESSION SYNDROME = midline closure defect of neural tube

Incidence: 0.005 – 0.01%

predisposed: infants of diabetic mothers (16%)

associated with:

1. musculoskeletal anomalies: hip dislocation, foot deformities, hypoplasia of extremities

2. lack of bladder / bowel control

3. spina bifida (myleomeningocele often not in combination with hydrocephalus)

not associated with VATER syndrome

√ sacral agenesis

√ ± dural sac stenosis with high termination

√ ± tethered cord with associated lipoma, teratoma, cauda equina cyst

Cx: neurogenic bladder (if > 2 segments are missing)

SACROCOCCYGEAL TERATOMA

= tumor arising from pluripotential cells that are initially derived from the primitive knot (Henson node) with its final resting place in the sacrococcygeal area

Incidence: 1:40,000 live births; Type I + II (80%); most common congenital solid tumor in the newborn; M:F = 1:4

Histo:

(1) mature benign teratoma (55 – 75%) with elements from glia, bowel, pancreas, bronchial mucosa, skin appendages, striated + smooth muscle, bowel loops, bone components (metacarpal bones + digits), well-formed teeth, choroid plexus structures (production of CSF)

(2) immature teratoma (11 – 28%): neuroepithelial / renal origin

(3) malignant teratoma (7 – 17%): yolk sac / endodermal sinus tumor / embryonal carcinoma; more common in males; metastases to lung, spine, lymph nodes, liver

Age: 50 – 70% during first few days; 80% by 6 months of age; < 10% > 2 years of age; M:F = 1:4

CLASSIFICATION

Type Ia   predominantly external lesion covered by skin with a minimal presacral component (80%)

Type IIa   predominantly external tumor with significant presacral component

Type III   predominantly sacral component + external extension

Type IV   presacral tumor with no external component

associated with other congenital anomalies (in 18%):

(1) vertebral (5 – 16%) (2) musculoskeletal (3) renal anomalies (4) placentomegaly (5) nonimmune hydrops (6) curvilinear sacrococcygeal defect (+ anorectal stenosis / atresia, vesicoureteral reflux) with frequent familial occurrence, equal sex incidence, low malignant potential, absence of calcifications

• AFP only elevated with malignant degeneration

• premature labor

• uterus large for dates

Plain film:
√ amorphous, punctate, spiculated calcifications,
possibly resembling bone (36 – 50%); suggestive of
benign tumor
√ soft tissue mass in pelvis protruding anteriorly +
inferiorly
BE:
√ anterosuperior displacement of rectum
√ luminal constriction
IVP:
√ displacement of bladder anterosuperiorly
√ development of bladder neck obstruction
Myelography:
√ intraspinal component may be present
Angio:
√ neovascularity (arterial supply by middle sacral,
internal iliac, gluteal arteries)
√ enlargement of feeding vessels
√ arterial encasement
√ arteriovenous shunting
√ early venous filling with serpiginous dilated tumor
veins
US / CT:
√ solid (25%) / mixed (60%) / cystic (15%) sacral mass
√ average size of 8 cm in diameter
√ polyhydramnios (2/3)
√ oligohydramnios, hydronephrosis, urinary ascites,
hydrops are poor prognostic factors
Prognosis: prevalence of malignant germ cell tumors
increases with patient's age
√ predominantly fatty tissue tumors are usually benign
√ hemorrhage / necrosis is suggestive of malignancy
√ cystic lesions are less likely malignant
Cx: (1) dystocia in 6 – 13%
(2) massive intratumoral hemorrhage
(3) fetal death in utero / stillbirth
DDx: myelomeningocele, lipomeningocele, lipoma,
hemangioma, epidermal cyst, rectal duplication,
lymphangioma, chordoma, sarcoma, ependymoma

SPINAL STENOSIS
= abnormal narrowing of spinal canal, lateral recess, or
neuroforamen
Causes:
A. congenitally short pedicles (idiopathic /
achondroplasia)
B. acquired:
1. hypertrophy of ligamentum flavum (most
common)
2. superior facet joint hypertrophy
3. degenerative bulging disc
4. spondylosis, spondylolisthesis
5. surgical fusion
6. fracture
7. calcification of posterior longitudinal ligament
8. Paget disease
√ narrowing of cervical canal < 13 mm, of lumbar canal
< 16 mm (AP dimension)

√ distorted shape of thecal sac
√ obliteration of epidural fat

Lumbar Spinal Stenosis
Causes:
1. Achondroplasia:
√ narrowed interpediculate distance with
progression toward lumbar spine
2. Paget disease: bony overgrowth
3. Spondylolisthesis
4. Operative posterior spinal fusion
5. Herniated disc
6. Metastasis to vertebrae
7. Developmental / congenital
Age: presentation between 30 – 50 years of age
• low back pain
• cauda equina syndrome: paraparesis, incontinence,
sensory findings in saddle-like pattern, areflexia
√ unusual small quantity of contrast material to fill thecal
sac
√ anteroposterior + interpediculate diameter constricted
√ may appear as spinal block in hyperextended neck on
AP views
√ thickened articular process, pedicles, laminae,
ligaments
√ trefoil / cloverleaf configuration of spinal canal
√ bulging discs

SPONDYLOLISTHESIS
Cause: (a) usually spondylolysis
(b) pseudospondylolisthesis = degenerative /
inflammatory joint disease (e.g. rheumatoid
arthritis)
Grades I – IV (Meyerding method):
each grade equals 1/4 anterior subluxation of superior
on inferior vertebral body
• symptoms not related to grade

SPONDYLOLYSIS
= pars interarticularis defect between superior + inferior
articulating processes
Incidence: 4 – 7% of population
Cause: (a) congenital hereditary weakness / hypoplasia
of pars
(b) pseudarthrosis following stress fracture of
pars (in most)
(c) secondary spondylolysis: neoplasm,
osteomyelitis, Paget disease, osteomalacia,
osteogenesis imperfecta
• mostly asymptomatic
Location: L5; L4; C6 (rare); usually bilateral
√ fracture line resembles collar of "scotty dog"

SPONDYLOSIS OF CERVICAL SPINE
= progressive degeneration of intervertebral discs leading
to proliferative changes of bone + meninges
Incidence: 5 – 10% at age 20 – 30; > 50% at age 45;
> 90% by age 60

- spastic gait disorder
- neck pain

Sequelae: (a) direct compression of spinal cord
(b) ischemia due to vascular compromise
(c) repeated trauma from normal flexion /
extension

DDx of myelopathy:
rheumatoid arthritis, congenital anomalies of
craniocervical junction, intradural extramedullary
tumor, spine metastases, cervical spinal cord tumor,
arteriovenous malformation, amyotrophic lateral
sclerosis, multiple sclerosis, neurosyphilis

SYRINGOHYDROMYELIA

Causes:

A. Primary / Congenital syringohydromyelia
associated with:
(1) Chiari malformation in 20 – 70%
(2) Spinal dysraphism
(3) Myelocele
(4) Dandy-Walker syndrome
(5) Diastematomyelia
(6) Scoliosis in 48 – 87%
(7) Klippel-Feil syndrome
(8) Spinal segmentation defects

B. Acquired / Secondary syringohydromyelia (rare)
1. Posttraumatic syringohydromyelia:
Incidence: in 3.2% after spinal cord injury
√ 0.5 – 40 cm (average 6 cm) in length
2. Postinflammatory syringohydromyelia:
Infection, Subarachnoid hemorrhage, Arachnoid
adhesions, S/P surgery
3. Spinal cord tumors
(secondary to circulatory disturbance + thoracic
spinal cord atrophy)
4. Vascular insufficiency

Age: primarily childhood / early adult life

- loss of sensation to pain + temperature (interruption of
spinothalamic tracts)
- trophic changes [skin lesions; Charcot joints in 25%
(shoulder, elbow, wrist)]
- muscle weakness (anterior horn cell involvement)
- spasticity, hyperreflexia (upper motor neuron
involvement)
- abnormal plantar reflexes (pyramidal tract involvement)

Location: predominantly lower end of cervical cord

CT:
√ distinct area of decreased attenuation within spinal
cord (100%)
√ swollen / normal-sized / atrophic cord
√ no contrast enhancement
√ flattened vertebral border (rare) with increased
transverse diameter of cord
√ change in shape + size of cord with change in position
(rare)
√ filling of syringohydromyelia with intrathecal contrast
(a) early filling via direct communication with
subarachnoid space

(b) late filling after 4 – 8 hours (80 – 90%) secondary
to permeation of contrast material

Myelography:
√ enlarged cord (DDx: intramedullary tumor)
√ "collapsing cord sign" = collapsing of cord with gas
myelography as fluid content moves caudad in the
erect position (rare)

MRI:
√ cystic area of low signal intensity on T1WI, increased
intensity on T2WI
√ presence of CSF flow-void within cavity
√ eccentric / beaded cavity
√ cord enlargement

Syringomyelia
= any cavity within substance of spinal cord which may
communicate with the central canal, usually
extending over several vertebral segments
Histo: not lined by ependymal tissue

Hydromyelia
= dilatation of persistent central canal of spinal cord (in
70 – 80% obliterated) which communicates with 4th
ventricle
Histo: lined by ependymal tissue

Reactive Cyst
= POSTTRAUMATIC SPINAL CORD CYST
= CSF-filled cyst adjacent to level of trauma; usually
single (75%)
- late deterioration in patients with spinal cord injury
(not related to severity of original injury)
Rx: shunting leads to clinical improvement

TETHERED CORD
= LOW CONUS MEDULLARIS
= abnormally short + thickened filum terminale
Etiology: failure of ascent of conus (normal location of tip
of conus medullaris: L 4/5 at 16 weeks of
gestation, L 2/3 at birth, L1/2 > 3 months of
age)
Age at presentation: 5 – 15 years (in years of growth
spurt); M:F = 2:3
associated with: lipoma in 29 – 78%
- dorsal nevus, dermal sinus, hair patch (50%)
- paraplegia, paraparesis
- bowel, bladder, limb dysfunction in childhood
- gait abnormalities
- anal / perineal pain (in adults)
√ lumbar spina bifida with interpedicular widening
√ posteriorly located tethered conus medullaris + filum
terminale (supine views)
√ conus medullaris below level of L2 by age 12 (86%)
√ filum terminale thickened > 2mm (by definition)
√ abnormal lateral course of nerve roots (> 15° angle
relative to spinal cord)
√ triangular thecal sac pointing posteriorly (thecal sac
pulled posteriorly)

√ dorsally located cyst / lipoma may be present
Sequelae: chronic repetitive cord ischemia with
stretching of cord

Rx: decompressive laminectomy / partial removal of
lipoma ± freeing of cord

DIFFERENTIAL DIAGNOSIS OF BRAIN DISORDERS

Prolactin elevation
Causes:
1. Interference with hypothalamic-pituitary axis:
   (a) hypothalamic tumor
   (b) parasellar tumor
   (c) sarcoidosis
   (d) histiocytosis
   (e) traumatic infundibular transection
2. Pharmacologic agents
   alpha-methyldopa, reserpine, phenothiazine,
   butyrophenone, tricyclic antidepressants, oral
   contraceptives
3. Hypothyroidism
4. Renal failure
5. Cirrhosis
6. Stress / recent surgery
7. Breast examination
8. Pregnancy
9. Lactation

Stroke
Incidence: 3rd leading cause of death in United States
   (after heart disease + cancer); 2nd leading
   cause of death in patients > 75 years of age;
   leading cause of death in Orient
Age: > 55 years
Risk factors:
   heredity, hypertension, smoking, diabetes, obesity,
   familial hypercholesterolemia, myocardial infarction,
   atrial fibrillation, congestive heart failure, alcoholic
   excess, oral contraceptives, high anxiety + stress

Etiology:
A. NONVASCULAR (5%): e.g. tumor
B. VASCULAR (95%)
   1. Hemorrhage (14%)
   2. Ischemia (81%)
      (a) cerebrovascular disease (65%)
          inadequate blood flow / embolus = progressive
          atherosclerosis with intimal plaques, central
          necrosis of atheroma, release of plaque
          contents into blood stream, thrombus formation
          on intimal ulcers
      (b) cardiogenic emboli (12%)
      (c) others (4%): e.g. systemic disease

Prognosis:
(1) death during hospitalization (25%): alteration in
    consciousness, gaze preference, dense hemiplegia
    have a 40% mortality rate
(2) survival with varying degrees of neurologic deficit
    (75%)
(3) good functional recovery (40%)

Indications for cerebrovascular testing:
1. TIA = transient ischemic attack
2. Progression of carotid disease to 95 – 98% stenosis
3. Cardiogenic cerebral emboli
   Incidence: 6 – 23% of all ischemic strokes
   Etiology:
      (1) nonvalvular atrial fibrillation (6% risk/year)
      (2) acute myocardial infarction (3% risk/year)
      (3) mitral stenosis (20% risk/year)
      (4) prosthetic valves (1 – 4% risk/year)
      (5) mitral valve prolapse (low risk)
      (6) nonbacterial thrombotic endocarditis (30% risk/
          year)
      (7) infective endocarditis (20% risk/year)
      (8) left atrial myxoma (27 – 55% risk/year)

Temporal classification:
1. TIA = transient ischemic attack
2. RIND = reversible ischemic neurologic deficit
3. Progressive stroke = stroke in evolution with change
   in neurologic symptomatology
4. Completed stroke = stable neurologic
   symptomatology: 6 – 11% recurrent stroke rate

TRANSIENT ISCHEMIC ATTACK
• symptomatology < 24 hours (carotid attacks < 6 hrs.
  in 90%, vertebrobasilar events < 2 hrs. in 90%)
Prognosis: per year 12% increase of stroke /
   myocardial infarction / death; complete
   stroke in 33% within 5 years; complete
   stroke in 5% in 1 month
A. CAROTID TIA
   — motor dysfunction = weakness, paralysis,
     clumsiness of one / both limbs on same side
   — sensory alteration = numbness, loss of sensation,
     paresthesia of one / both limbs on same side
   — speech / language disturbance = difficulty in
     speaking / writing, in comprehension of language
     / reading / performing calculations
   — visual disturbance = loss of vision in one eye,
     homonymous hemianopia, transient monocular
     blindness
   • paresis (mono- , hemiparesis) in 61%
   • paresthesia (mono-, hemiparesthesia) in 57%
   • monocular visual disturbance in 32%
   • facial paresthesia in 30%
B. VERTEBROBASILAR TIA
   — motor dysfunction = as with carotid TIA but
     sometimes changing from side to side including
     quadriplegia
   — sensory alteration = as with carotid TIA usually
     involving one / both sides of face / mouth /
     tongue

— visual loss = as with carotid TIA including bilateral homonymous hemianopia
— disequilibrium of gait / postural disturbance, ataxia, imbalance / unsteadiness
— drop attack = sudden fall to the ground without loss of consciousness
- binocular visual disturbance in 57%
- vertigo in 50%
- paresthesia in 40%
- diplopia in 38%
- ataxia in 33%
- paresis in 33%
- headaches in 25%
- seizures in 1.5%

Rx: 1. Carotid endarterectomy (1% mortality, 5% stroke)
  2. Anticoagulation
  3. Aspirin

Intracranial pneumocephalus
Causes:
 A. Trauma (74%):
  in 3% of all skull fractures; in 8% of fractures involving paranasal sinuses (frontal > ethmoid > sphenoid > mastoid)
 B . Neoplasm invading sinus (13%):
  1. osteoma of frontal / ethmoid sinus
  2. pituitary adenoma
  3. mucocele, epidermoid, malignancy of paranasal sinuses
 C. Infection with gas-forming organism (9%): mastoiditis, sinusitis
 D. Surgery (4%): of paranasal sinuses, hypophysectomy
Mechanism (dural laceration):
 (1) ball-valve mechanism during straining, coughing, sneezing
 (2) vacuum phenomenon secondary to loss of CSF
Time of onset: on initial presentation (25%), usually seen within 4 – 5 days, delay up to 6 months (33%)
Mortality: 15%
Cx:
 1. CSF rhinorrhea (50%)
 2. Meningitis / epidural / brain abscess (25%)
 3. Extracranial pneumocephalus = air collection in subaponeurotic space

Cerebral atrophy
= irreversible loss of brain substance + subsequent enlargement of intra- and extracerebral CSF-containing spaces (hydrocephalus ex vacuo)
 A. DIFFUSE BRAIN ATROPHY
  Cause:
  (a) Trauma, Radiation
  (b) Drugs (dilantin, steroids, methotrexate, marijuana, hard drugs, chemotherapy), Alcoholism, Hypoxia
  (c) Demyelinating disease (multiple sclerosis, encephalitis)
  (d) Degenerative disease
   e.g. Alzheimer disease, Pick disease, Jakob-Creutzfeldt disease
  (e) Cerebrovascular disease + multiple infarcts
  (f) Advancing age, Anorexia, Renal failure
  √ enlarged ventricles + sulci
 B. FOCAL BRAIN ATROPHY
  Cause: Vascular / chemical / metabolic / traumatic / idiopathic (Dyke-Davidoff-Mason syndrome)
 C. REVERSIBLE PROCESS SIMULATING ATROPHY (in younger people)
  Cause: Anorexia nervosa, Alcoholism, Catabolic steroid treatment, Pediatric malignancy

Cerebellar atrophy
 A. Cerebellar atrophy with cerebral atrophy
  = Generalized senile brain atrophy
 B. Cerebellar atrophy without cerebral atrophy
  1. Olivopontocerebellar degeneration / Marie ataxia / Friedreich ataxia
  - onset of ataxia in young adulthood
  2. Ethanol- / phenytoin-toxicity
  3. Idiopathic degeneration secondary to carcinoma (= paraneoplastic), usually oat cell carcinoma of lung
  4. Radiotherapy
  5. Focal cerebellar atrophy: (a) infarction (b) traumatic injury

HYPERDENSE LESIONS
Increased density of falx
 1. Subarachnoid hemorrhage
 2. Interhemispheric subdural hematoma
 3. Diffuse cerebral edema (= increased density relative to low density brain)
 4. Dural calcifications (hypercalcemia from chronic renal failure, basal cell nevus syndrome, hyperparathyroidism)
 5. Normal falx (can be normal in pediatric population)

Intracranial calcifications
mnemonic: "PINEEAL"
 Physiologic
 Infection
 Neoplasm
 Endocrine
 Embryologic
 Arteriovenous
 Leftover Ls

 A. Physiologic intracranial calcifications:
  Pineal gland (> 10 years of age), choroid plexus (> 3 years of age), habenular commissure (> 10 years of age), petroclinoid ligament (> 5 years of age), falx / tentorium (> 3 years of age)
 B. Infection:
  TORCH (toxoplasmosis, rubella, CMV, herpes), healed abscess, hydatid cyst, tuberculoma, cysticercosis

mnemonic:
    CM**V** calcifications are **c**ircum**v**entricular
    Toxoplasma calcifications are in**t**raparenchymal
C. Neoplasm:
    Craniopharyngioma (40 – 80%), oligodendroglioma
    (50 – 70%), chordoma (25 – 40%), choroid plexus
    papilloma (10%), meningioma (20%), pituitary
    adenoma (3 – 5%), pinealoma (10 – 20%), dermoid
    (20%), lipoma of corpus callosum, ependymoma
    (50%), astrocytoma (15%), radiotherapy
D. Endocrine:
    Hyperparathyroidism, hypervitaminosis D,
    hypoparathyroidism, pseudohypoparathyroidism,
    CO poisoning, lead poisoning
E. Embryologic:
    Neurocutaneous syndromes (Tuberous sclerosis,
    Sturge-Weber, Neurofibromatosis), Fahr disease,
    Cockayne syndrome, basal cell nevus syndrome
F. Arteriovenous:
    Atherosclerosis, aneurysm, AVM, hemangioma,
    subdural hematoma
G. Leftover Ls:
    Lipoma, lipoid proteinosis, lissencephaly

Basal ganglia calcification
A. Physiologic with aging
B. Metabolic
    1. Hypoparathyroidism + Pseudohypoparathyroidism
       (60%)
    2. Wilson disease
    3. Fahr disease
    4. Cockayne syndrome
    5. Down syndrome
C. Trauma
    1. Childhood leukemia following methotrexate therapy
    2. Post radiation
    3. Birth anoxia
D. Drugs
    1. Carbon monoxide poisoning
    2. Lead intoxication
E. Infection
    1. Toxoplasmosis
    2. AIDS

Periventricular calcifications in a child
1. Tuberous sclerosis
2. Congenital infection: CMV, toxoplasmosis

Dense cerebral mass
Substrate: calcification / hemorrhage / dense protein
A. VESSEL
    1. Aneurysm
    2. Arteriovenous malformation
    3. Hematoma (acute / subacute)
B. TUMOR
    1. Lymphoma
    2. Medulloblastoma
    3. Meningioma

4. Metastasis
    (a) from mucinous-producing adenocarcinoma
    (b) hemorrhagic metastases: melanoma,
         choriocarcinoma, hypernephroma,
         bronchogenic carcinoma, breast carcinoma
         (rarely)

Dense lesion near foramen of Monro
A. Intraventricular lesion
    1. Colloid cyst
    2. Meningioma
    3. Choroid plexus tumor / granuloma
    4. AVM of septal, thalamostriate, internal cerebral
       veins
B. Periventricular mass
    1. Primary CNS lymphoma
    2. Tuberous sclerosis
       (a) subependymal tuber
       (b) giant cell astrocytoma
    3. Metastasis from mucin-producing adenocarcinoma
       / hemorrhagic metastasis (melanoma,
       choriocarcinoma, hypernephroma, bronchogenic
       carcinoma, breast carcinoma)
    4. Glioblastoma of septum pellucidum
C. Masses projecting superiorly from base of skull
    1. Pituitary adenoma
    2. Craniopharyngioma
    3. Aneurysm
    4. Dolichoectatic basilar artery

ENHANCING LESIONS
Sulcal enhancement
A. Meningeal tumor
    (a) Meningeal carcinomatosis from systemic tumor:
         e.g. breast carcinoma, small cell carcinoma of
         lung, malignant melanoma, lymphoma / leukemia
    (b) Seeding primary CNS tumor:
         1. Medulloblastoma
         2. Pineoblastoma
         3. Ependymoma
B. Meningitis
    pyogenic, tuberculous, fungal, cysticercosis,
    sarcoidosis
C. Sequelae of subarachnoid hemorrhage (fibroblastic
    proliferation)

Enhancing ventricular margins
A. Subependymal spread of metastatic tumor
    1. Bronchogenic carcinoma (especially small cell
       carcinoma)
    2. Melanoma
    3. Breast carcinoma
B. Subependymal seeding of CNS primary
    1. Glioma
    2. Ependymoma
C. Ependymal seeding of CNS primary
    1. Medulloblastoma
    2. Germinoma

D. Primary CNS lymphoma / systemic lymphoma
E. Inflammatory ventriculitis

Dense and enhancing lesions
1. Aneurysm
2. Meningioma
3. CNS lymphoma
4. Medulloblastoma
5. Metastasis

Multifocal enhancing lesions
1. multiple infarctions
2. arteriovenous malformations
3. multifocal primary / secondary neoplasms
4. multifocal infectious processes
5. demyelinating diseases: e.g. multiple sclerosis

Innumerable small enhancing cerebral nodules
A. METASTASES
B. PRIMARY CNS LYMPHOMA
C. DISSEMINATED INFECTION
   1. Cysticercosis
   2. Histoplasmosis
   3. Tuberculosis
D. INFLAMMATION
   1. Sarcoidosis
   2. Multiple sclerosis
E. SUBACUTE MULTIFOCAL INFARCTION
   from hypoperfusion, multiple emboli, cerebral
   vasculitis (SLE), meningitis, cortical vein thrombosis

HYPERINTENSE LESIONS
Periventricular T2W-hyperintense lesions
1. Virchow-Robin space
   = small subarachnoid space following pia mater along
     perforating nutrient end vessels into brain
     substance
   √ 1 – 2 mm round lesions (seen on high axial
     sections through hemispheres + on low sections at
     level of anterior commissure)
2. État criblé (sieve-like)
   = perivascular fluid spaces predominantly at arteriolar
     level secondary to chronic ischemia
     (arteriosclerosis + lipohyaline deposits within vessel
     walls) followed by partial demyelination, gliosis,
     interstitial edema
   Incidence: in 10% without risk factors, in 84% with
              risk factors and symptoms
   Age: > 60 years
   Location: periventricular white matter > optic
            radiation > basal ganglia > centrum
            semiovale > brainstem (usually spares
            corpus callosum + subcortical U-fibers)
3. Multiple sclerosis
4. Progressive multifocal leukoencephalopathy (PML)
5. Leukodystrophy: in children, symmetric diffuse
   confluent involvement

6. White matter encephalitis:
   acute clinical course, Hx of viral infection / vaccination
   / AIDS
7. Vasculitic disorder: SLE, Behçet disease, Sickle cell
   disease
8. Migraine: in 41% with classic migraine, in 57% with
   complicated migraine; periventricular location
9. Transependymal CSF flow secondary to
   hydrocephalus
   √ smooth halo of even thickness
10. Radiation necrosis
    √ confluent pattern with scalloped margins within
      periventricular white matter extending out to
      subcortical U-fibers

HYPODENSE LESIONS
Diffusely swollen hemispheres
A. Metabolic
   1. Metabolic encephalopathy: e.g. uremia, Reye
      syndrome, ketoacidosis
   2. Anoxia: cardiopulmonary arrest, near-drowning,
      smoke inhalation, ARDS
B. Neuro-vascular
   1. Hypertensive encephalopathy
   2. Superior sagittal sinus thrombosis
   3. Head trauma
   4. Pseudotumor cerebri
C. Inflammation
   e.g. Herpes encephalitis, CMV, Toxoplasmosis

Edema of Brain
Etiology:
   1. Vasogenic edema (most common form):
      secondary to breakdown of blood-brain barrier with
      plasma extravasation;
      associated with primary brain neoplasm, metastases,
      hemorrhage, infarction, inflammation
   2. Cytotoxic edema:
      reversible increase in intracellular water content
      secondary to ischemia / anoxia
   3. Interstitial edema:
      increase in periventricular interstitial spaces
      secondary to transependymal flow of CSF with
      elevated intraventricular pressure
   CT: √ areas of hypodensity ± mass effect
        √ nonvisualization of 4th ventricle, basal cisterns,
          cortical sulci
        √ small / absent lateral ventricles ± midline shift
   MRI: √ decreased intensity on T1WI, increased intensity
          on T2WI

Midline cystic structures
1. **Cavum septi pellucidi** = "5th ventricle"
   = thin triangular membrane consisting of two glial layers
     covered laterally with ependyma separating the
     frontal horns of lateral ventricles
   Incidence: in 80% of term infants; in 15% of adults
   √ extends to foramen of Monro
   √ may dilate + cause obstructive hydrocephalus (rare)

2. **Cavum vergae** = "6th ventricle"
= cavity posterior to columns of fornix; contracts after about 6th gestational month
Incidence: in 30% of term infants; in 15% of adults
√ posterior midline continuation of cavum septi pellucidi beyond foramen of Monro
3. **Cavum veli interpositi**
= extension of quadrigeminal plate cistern above 3rd ventricle to foramen of Monro, laterally bounded by columns of fornix + thalamus
4. Colloid cyst: anterior + superior to cavum septi pellucidi
5. Arachnoid cyst: in region of quadrigeminal plate cistern
√ curvilinear margins

Periventricular hypodensity
1. Encephalomalacia
√ slightly denser than CSF
2. Porencephaly
= cavity communicating with ventricle / cistern from intracerebral hemorrhage
associated with: dilated ventricle, sulci, and fissures
√ CSF density
3. Resolving hematoma
• Hx of previously demonstrated hematoma
√ may show ring enhancement + compression of adjacent structures
4. Cystic tumor
√ mass effect + contrast enhancement

Suprasellar low-density lesion with hydrocephalus
A. CYST
1. Arachnoid cyst
2. Ependymal cyst of 3rd vertricle
3. Parasitic cyst of 3rd ventricle (cysticercosis)
4. Dilated 3rd ventricle (in aqueductal stenosis)
B. CYSTIC MASS
1. Epidermoid
2. Hypothalamic pilocytic astrocytoma
3. Cystic craniopharyngeoma
Nota bene: Cystic lesion may be inapparent within surrounding CSF; metrizamide cisternography is helpful in detection + to exclude aqueduct stenosis

Low-attenuation lesion in basal ganglia
1. Poisoning: carbon monoxide, barbiturate intoxication, hydrogen sulfide poisoning, cyanide poisoning, methanol intoxication
2. Hypoxia
3. Hypoglycemia
4. Hypotension (lacunar infarcts)
5. Wilson disease

Mesencephalic low-density lesion
1. Normal: decussation of superior cerebellar peduncles at level of inferior colliculi
2. Syringobulbia
found in conjunction with syringomyelia, Arnold-Chiari malformation, trauma

√ CSF density centrally
√ intrathecal contrast enters central cavity
3. Brainstem Infarction
√ abnormal contrast enhancement after 1 week
√ well-defined low attenuation region without enhancement after 2 – 4 weeks
4. Central Pontine Myelinolysis
comatose patient receiving rapid correction / overcorrection of severe hyponatremia (following prolonged IV fluid administration / alcoholism)
√ central region of diminished attenuation
5. Brainstem Glioma
√ mass with indistinct margins and vague enhancement
6. Metastasis
√ well-defined contrast enhancement
7. Granuloma in TB / sarcoidosis (rare)

MASSES
Ring lesion
= ring of enhancement on CECT / MRI
Cause:
1. Primary neoplasm: high grade glioma, meningioma, lymphoma, leukemia, pituitary macroadenoma, acoustic neuroma, craniopharyngioma
2. Metastatic carcinoma + sarcoma
3. Abscess: bacterial, fungal, parasitic
4. Empyema of epidural / subdural / intraventricular spaces
5. Resolving infarction, aging hematoma
6. Thrombosed aneurysm
7. Radiation necrosis, necrotizing leukoencephalopathy after methotrexate, operative bed following resection
Pathogenesis:
(1) hypervascular margin of lesion = granulation tissue / peripheral vascular channels / hypervascular tumor capsule
(2) breakdown of blood-brain barrier = leakage of contrast out of abnormally permeable vessels into extracellular fluid space
(3) hypodense center = avascular / hypovascular (requires time to fill) / cystic degeneration
√ ring-blush
Incidence of ring blush:
abscess (in 73%); glioblastoma (in 48%); metastases (in 33%); grade II astrocytoma (in 26%); [NOT in grade I astrocytoma]
√ "garland" blush: glioblastoma (19%); RARE in others
√ perilesional edema involving entire hemisphere: metastases (19%); glioblastoma (18%); meningioma (13%) [NOT in malignant lymphoma]

Classification of primary CNS tumors
A. TUMORS OF BRAIN AND MENINGES
(a) GLIOMAS
Astrocytoma
1. Astrocytoma (astrocytoma grades I – II)
2. Glioblastoma (astrocytoma grades III – IV)
Oligodendroglioma

Intra- versus extra-axial mass		
	intraaxial	**extraaxial**
Relationship to dura / bone	no attachment until advanced	contiguous
Local bony changes	uncommon	common
Displacement of cortex	toward dura / bone	away from bone
Subarachnoid cistern	effaced	widened
Feeding arteries	pial feeding arteries	dural feeding arteries

Paraglioma
  1. Ependymoma
  2. Choroid plexus papilloma
Ganglioglioma
Medulloblastoma
(b) PINEAL TUMOR
  1. Germinoma
  2. Teratoma
  3. Pineocytoma
  4. Pineoblastoma
(c) PITUITARY TUMOR
  1. Pituitary adenoma
  2. Pituitary carcinoma
(d) MENINGIOMA
(e) NERVE SHEATH TUMOR
  1. Schwannoma
  2. Neurofibroma
(f) MISCELLANEOUS
  1. Sarcoma
  2. Lipoma
  3. Hemangioblastoma

B. TUMORS OF EMBRYONAL REMNANTS
  (a) Craniopharyngioma
  (b) Colloid cyst
  (c) Teratoid tumor
    1. Epidermoid
    2. Dermoid
    3. Teratoma

Incidence of Brain Tumors
= 9% of all primary neoplasms; account for 1.2% of
  autopsied deaths

IN ALL AGE GROUPS:		IN PEDIATRIC AGE GROUP:	
Glioma	34%	Astrocytoma	50%
Meningioma	17%	Medulloblastoma	15%
Metastasis	12%	Ependymoma	10%
Pituitary adenoma	6%	Craniopharyngioma	6%
Neurinoma	4%	Choroid plexus papilloma	2%
Sarcoma	3%		
Granuloma	3%		
Craniopharyngioma	2%		
Hemangioblastoma	2%		

Tumors possibly presenting at birth
  1. Teratoma
  2. Choroid plexus papilloma
  3. Ependymoma
  4. Craniopharyngioma
  5. Astrocytoma
  6. Medulloblastoma

Intracranial tumors in pediatric age group
Incidence: 2.4:100,000 (< 15 years of age); 15% of all
          pediatric neoplasms; M>F
• increased intracranial pressure
• increasing head size
A. SUPRATENTORIAL (50%)

Covering of brain	: dural sarcoma, schwannoma, meningioma (3%)
Cerebral hemisphere	: astrocytoma (37%), oligodendroglioma
Corpus callosum	: astrocytoma
3rd ventricle	: colloid cyst, ependymoma
Lateral ventricle	: ependymoma (5%), choroid plexus papilloma (12%)
Optic chiasm	: craniopharyngioma (12%), optic nerve glioma (13%), teratoma, pituitary adenoma
Hypothalamus	: glioma (8%), hamartoma
Pineal region	: germinoma, pinealoma, teratoma (8%)

B. INFRATENTORIAL (50%)

Cerebellum	: astrocytoma (31 – 33%), medulloblastoma (26 – 31%)
Brainstem	: glioma (16 – 21%)
4th ventricle	: ependymoma (6 – 14%), choroid plexus papilloma

SUPRATENTORIAL MIDLINE TUMORS
  1. Optic + hypothalamic glioma (39%)
  2. Craniopharyngeoma (20%)
  3. Astrocytoma (9%)
  4. Pineoblastoma (9%)
  5. Germinoma (6%)
  6. Lipoma (6%)
  7. Teratoma (3.5%)
  8. Pituitary adenoma (3.5%)
  9. Meningioma (2%)
  10. Choroid plexus papilloma (2%)

SUPRATENTORIAL INTRAVENTRICULAR TUMORS
  (a) Lateral ventricle (3/4)
    1. Choroid plexus tumor (44%)
    2. Giant cell astrocytoma in tuberous sclerosis
       (19%)
    3. Hemangioma in Sturge-Weber syndrome (12%)
  (b) Third ventricle (1/4)
    1. Astrocytoma (13%)
    2. Choroid plexus tumor (6%)
    3. Meningioma (6%)

CLASSIFICATION BY HISTOLOGY
  1. Astrocytic tumors (33.5%)
  2. "Primitive" neuroectodermal tumor = PNET (21%)
      — Medulloblastoma (16%)
      — Pineoblastoma (2.5%)
      — PNET of cerebral hemisphere (2.5%)
  3. Mixed gliomas (16%)
  4. Malformative tumors (11.5%)
      — Craniopharyngeoma (5.5%)
      — Lipoma (4.5%)
      — Dermoid cyst (1%)
      — Epidermal cyst (0.5%)
  5. Choroid plexus tumors (4%)
  6. Ependymal tumors (4%)
  7. Tumors of meningeal tissues (3.5%)
      — Meningioma (3%)
      — Meningeal sarcoma (0.5%)
  8. Germ cell tumors (2.5%)
      — Germinoma (1.5%)
      — Teratomatous tumor (1%)
  9. Neuronal tumors
      — Gangliocytoma (1.5%)
  10. Tumors of neuroendocrine origin
      — Pituitary adenoma (1%)
  11. Oligodendroglial tumors (0.5%)
  12. Tumors of blood vessels
      — Hemangioma (1%)

Multifocal CNS tumors
  A. METASTASES FROM PRIMARY CNS TUMOR
      (a) via commissural pathways: corpus callosum,
           internal capsule, massa intermedia
      (b) via CSF: ventricles / subarachnoid cisterns
      (c) satellite metastases
  B. MULTICENTRIC CNS TUMOR
      (a) true multicentric gliomas (4%)
      (b) concurrent tumors of different histology
           (coincidental)
  C. MULTICENTRIC MENINGIOMAS (3%) without
      neurofibromatosis
  D. MULTICENTRIC PRIMARY CNS LYMPHOMA
  E. PHAKOMATOSES
      1. Generalized neurofibromatosis: meningiomatosis,
         bilateral acoustic neuromas, bilateral optic nerve
         gliomas, cerebral gliomas, choroid plexus
         papillomas, multiple spine tumors, AVMs

      2. Tuberous sclerosis: subependymal tubers,
         intraventricular gliomas (giant cell astrocytoma),
         ependymomas
      3. von Hippel-Lindau disease: retinal angiomatosis,
         hemangioblastomas, congenital cysts of pancreas +
         liver, benign renal tumors, cardiac rhabdomyomas

Phakomatoses
  = NEUROCUTANEOUS SYNDROMES
  = NEUROECTODERMAL DYSPLASIAS = development of
    benign tumors / malformations especially in organs of
    ectodermal origin
  1. Neurofibromatosis
  2. Tuberous sclerosis
  3. von Hippel-Lindau disease
  4. Sturge-Weber-Dimitri syndrome

Intraventricular tumor
  1. Ependymoma   20%
  2. Astrocytoma   18%
  3. Colloid cyst   12%
  4. Meningioma   11%
  5. Choroid plexus papilloma 7%
  6. Epidermoid / dermoid   6%
  7. Craniopharyngioma   6%
  8. Medulloblastoma   5%
  9. Cysticercosis   5%
  10. Arachnoid cyst   4%
  11. Subependymoma   2%
  12. AVM   2%
  13. Teratoma   1%
  14. Metastasis

IN 4TH VENTRICLE
  1. Choroid plexus papilloma
  2. Ependymoma / glioma
  3. Hemangioblastoma
  4. Vermian metastasis
  5. AVM
  6. Epidermoid tumor (rare)
  7. Inflammatory mass
  8. Cyst

IN 3RD VENTRICLE
  1. Colloid cyst
  2. Glioma
  3. Aneurysm
  4. Craniopharyngioma
  5. Ependymoma
  6. Meningioma
  7. Choroid plexus papilloma

Jugular foramen mass
  1. Glomus tumor
  2. Meningioma
  3. Neuroma
  4. Metastasis

Dumbbell mass spanning petrous apex

1. Large trigeminal schwannoma
2. Meningioma
3. Epidermoid cyst

Posterior fossa tumor in adult

A. Extraaxial:
1. Acoustic neuroma
2. Meningioma
3. Chordoma
4. Choroid plexus papilloma
5. Epidermoid

B. Intraaxial:
1. Metastasis (lung, breast)
2. Hemangioblastoma
3. Lymphoma
4. Lipoma

CYSTIC MASS IN CEREBELLAR HEMISPHERE
IN ADULT
1. Hemangioblastoma
2. Cerebellar astrocytoma
3. Metastasis
4. Lateral medulloblastoma (="cerebellar sarcoma")
5. Choroid plexus papilloma with lateral extension

Cerebellopontine angle tumor

= extraaxial tumor arising between bone / dura and brain
√ may widen CSF space (cistern) in 25%
√ bone erosion / hyperostosis
√ sharp margination with brain
Types:
1. Acoustic neuroma (80%): from intracanalicular portion of 8th cranial nerve
2. Meningioma (13%)
   2nd most common extraaxial mass in posterior fossa; 10% of intracranial meningiomas arise there; larger than acoustic neuroma
3. Epidermoid tumor (5%): cholesterol contents
4. Trigeminal neuroma
   from Gasserian ganglion within Meckel cave in the most anteromedial portion of petrous pyramid / trigeminal nerve root
5. Glomus jugulare tumor
   within adventitia of bulb of jugular vein at base of petrous bone with invasion of posterior fossa
6. Chordoma
7. Arachnoid cyst
8. Aneurysm of basilar / vertebral artery
9. Exophytic glioma

LOW-ATTENUATION EXTRAAXIAL LESION:
1. Acoustic schwannoma (occasionally low density mass)
2. Epidermoid tumor
3. Arachnoid cyst

Lesion expanding cavernous sinus

A. TUMOR
1. Trigeminal schwannoma
2. Pituitary adenoma
3. Parasellar meningioma
4. Parasellar metastasis
5. Invasion by tumor of skull base
B. VESSEL
1. Internal carotid artery aneurysm
2. Carotid-cavernous fistula
3. Cavernous sinus thrombosis
C. Tolosa-Hunt syndrome = granulomatous invasion of cavernous sinus

CLASSIFICATION OF CNS ANOMALIES

A. DORSAL INDUCTION ANOMALY
   = defects of neural tube closure
   1. Chiari malformation: at 4 weeks
   2. Encephalocele: at 4 weeks
   3. Anencephaly
   4. Spinal dysraphism
   5. Hydromyelia
B. VENTRAL INDUCTION ANOMALY
   1. Holoprosencephaly: 5 – 6 weeks
   2. Septo-optic dysplasia: 6 – 7 weeks
   3. Dandy-Walker malformation: 7 – 10 weeks
   4. Agenesis of septum pellucidum
C. NEURONAL PROLIFERATION & HISTOGENESIS
   1. Neurofibromatosis: 5 weeks – 6 months
   2. Tuberous sclerosis: 5 weeks – 6 months
   3. Primary hydranencephaly: > 3 months
   4. Neoplasia
   5. Vascular malformation (vein of Galen, AVM, hemangioma)
D. MIGRATION ANOMALY
   1. Schizencephaly: 2 months
   2. Agyria + pachygyria: 3 months
   3. Gray matter heteropia: 5 months
   4. Dysgenesis of corpus callosum: 2 - 5 months
   5. Lissencephaly
   6. Polymicrogyria
      = excessive thickness + excessive convolutions of histologically normal cerebral cortex with paradoxic impression of smooth cortex secondary to fusion of gyri
E. DESTRUCTIVE LESIONS
   1. Hydranencephaly
   2. Porencephaly
   3. Hypoxia
   4. Toxicoses
   5. Inflammatory disease (TORCH)
      (a) Toxoplasmosis
      (b) Rubella
          √ punctate / nodular calcifications
          √ porencephalic cysts
          √ occasionally microcephaly
      (c) Cytomegalic inclusion disease
          √ typically punctate / stippled / curvilinear periventricular calcifications
          √ often hydrocephalus
      (d) Herpes simplex

SELLA
Destruction of sella
1. Pituitary adenoma
2. Suprasellar tumor
3. Carcinoma of sphenoid + posterior ethmoid sinus
   √ opacification of sinus + destruction of walls
   √ associated with nasopharyngeal mass (common)
4. Nasopharyngeal carcinoma
   (a) squamous cell carcinoma
   (b) lymphoepithelioma = Schmincke tumor = non-keratinizing form of squamous cell carcinoma
   √ sclerosis of adjacent bone
5. Metastasis to sphenoid
   from breast, kidney, thyroid, colon, prostate, lung, esophagus
6. Primary tumor of sphenoid bone (rare)
   osteogenic sarcoma, giant cell tumor, plasmacytoma
7. Chordoma
8. Mucocele of spenoid sinus (uncommon)
9. Enlarged 3rd ventricle
   aqueductal stenosis from infratentorial mass, maldevelopment

Enlarged sella
A. TUMOR
   1. Pituitary adenoma
   2. Craniopharyngioma
   3. Meningioma: hyperostosis
   4. Optic glioma: J-shaped sella
B. PITUITARY HYPERPLASIA
   1. Hypothyroidism
   2. Hypogonadism
   3. Nelson syndrome (occurring in 7% of patients subsequent to adrenalectomy)
C. CSF-SPACE
   1. Enlarged 3rd ventricle
   2. Hydrocephalus
   3. Empty sella
D. VESSEL
   1. Arterial aneurysm
   2. Ectatic internal carotid artery

Parasellar mass
1. Meningioma: tentorium cerebelli
2. Neurinoma (III, IV, V 1 + 2, VI)
3. Metastasis: lung, breast, kidney, GI tract, spread from nasopharynx
4. Epidermoid
5. Aneurysm
6. Carotid-cavernous fistula

mnemonic: "SATCHMO"
Sella neoplasm with superior extension, **S**arcoidosis
Aneurysm, **E**ctatic carotid, **C**arotid-cavernous sinus fistula, **A**rachnoid cyst
Teratoma: Dysgerminoma (usually), Dermoid, Epidermoid
Craniopharyngioma, **C**hordoma

Hypothalamic glioma, **H**istiocytoma, **H**amartoma
Metastatic disease, **M**eningioma, **M**ucocele
Optic nerve glioma, Neuroma

Intrasellar mass
1. Pituitary adenoma / carcinoma (most common cause)
2. Craniopharyngioma (2nd most common cause)
3. Meningioma: from surface of diaphragm / tuberculum sellae
4. Chordoma
5. Metastasis: lung, breast, prostate, kidney, GI tract, spread from nasopharynx
6. Intracavernous ICA aneurysm: bilateral in 25%
7. Pituitary abscess: rapidly expanding mass associated with meningitis
8. Empty sella
9. Rathke cleft cyst: commonly at junction of anterior + posterior pituitary gland
10. Granular cell tumor = Myeloblastoma: benign neoplasm of posterior pituitary gland
11. Granuloma: sarcoidosis, giant cell granuloma, TB, syphilis, eosinophilic granuloma
12. Lymphoid hypophysitis
13. Pituitary hyperplasia, e.g. in Nelson syndrome

Suprasellar mass
1. Meningioma
2. Craniopharyngioma: in 80% suprasellar
3. Chiasmal + optic nerve glioma
   in 38% of neurofibromatosis; adolescent girls;
   DDx: chiasmal neuritis
4. Hypothalamic glioma
5. Hamartoma of tuber cinereum
   • precocious puberty, seizures, mental changes
   √ isodense nonenhancing pedunculated mass between tuber cinereum + pons
6. Infundibular tumor
   metastasis (esp. breast); glioma; lymphoma; histiocytosis X; sarcoid
   √ diameter of infundibulum > 4.5 mm immediately above level of dorsum; cone-shaped (on coronal scan)
7. Germinoma
   malignant tumor similar to seminoma (= "ectopic pinealoma")
   √ frequently calcified (teratoma)
   √ CSF spread (germinoma + teratocarcinoma)
   √ enhancement on CECT (common)
8. Epidermoid / Dermoid
   √ cystic lesion containing calcifications + fat
   √ minimal / no contrast enhancement
9. Arachnoid cyst
   • hydrocephalus (common), visual impairment,
   • endocrine dysfunction
   Age: most common in infancy
10. Enlarged 3rd ventricle extending into pituitary fossa
11. Suprasellar aneurysm
    √ rim calcification + eccentric position

Suprasellar mass with low attenuation
1. Craniopharyngioma
2. Dermoid / Epidermoid
3. Arachnoid cyst
4. Lipoma
5. Simple pituitary cyst
6. Glioma of hypothalamus

Suprasellar mass with mixed attenuation
A. IN CHILDREN
   1. Hypothalamic-chiasmatic glioma
   2. Craniopharyngioma
   3. Hamartoma of tuber cinereum
   4. Histiocytosis
B. IN ADULTS
   1. Suprasellar extension of pituitary adenoma
   2. Craniopharyngioma
   3. Epidermoid cyst
   4. Thrombosed aneurysm
   5. Low-grade hypothalamic / optic glioma
   6. Inflammatory lesion: sarcoidosis, TB, sphenoid mucocele

Suprasellar mass with calcification
A. Curvilinear:
   1. Giant carotid aneurysm
   2. Craniopharyngioma
B. Granular:
   1. Craniopharyngioma
   2. Meningioma
   3. Granuloma
   4. Dermoid cyst / teratoma
   5. Optic / hypothalamic glioma (rare)

Enhancing mass with supra- and intrasellar component
1. Pituitary adenoma
2. Meningioma
3. Germinoma
4. Hypothalamic glioma
5. Craniopharyngioma

Perisellar vascular lesion
1. ICA aneurysm
   Giant aneurysms are > 2.5 cm in diameter
   √ destruction of bony sella / superior orbital fissure
   √ calcified wall / thrombus
   √ CECT enhancement, nonuniform with thrombosis
2. Ectatic carotid artery
   √ curvilinear calcifications
   √ encroachment upon sella turcica
3. Carotid-cavernous sinus fistula

PINEAL GLAND
Classification of pineal gland tumors
Incidence of pineal mass: 2% of all CNS tumors
A. PRIMARY TUMOR
   (a) Germ cell origin (most common)

1. Germinoma (seminoma)
2. Benign teratoma
3. Teratocarcinoma: embryonal cell carcinoma, yolk sac carcinoma, choriocarcinoma
   (b) Pineal parenchymal cell origin
      1. Pineocytoma
      2. Pineoblastoma
   (c) Other cell origin
      1. Retinoblastoma (Trilateral retinoblastoma = left eye + right eye + pineal gland
      2. Glioma
      3. Meningioma
      4. Hemangiopericytoma
   (d) Cysts
      1. Malignant teratoma
      2. AVM, vein of Galen aneurysm
      3. Arachnoid cyst
B. SECONDARY TUMOR
   Metastasis: e.g. lung carcinoma

- Parinaud syndrome = paralysis of upward gaze (compression / infiltration of superior colliculi)
- headache
- somnolence (related to hydrocephalus)

DDx considerations:

Δ female:	likely NOT germ cell tumor
Δ hypodense matrix:	likely NOT pineal cell tumor
Δ distinct tumor margins:	probably pineocytoma / teratoma
Δ calcification:	likely NOT teratocarcinoma, metastasis, germinoma
Δ CSF seeding:	NOT teratoma
Δ intense enhancement:	likely NOT teratoma

Intensely enhancing mass in pineal region
1. Germinoma
2. Pineocytoma
3. Glioma of brain stem / thalamus
4. Subsplenial meningioma
5. Vein of Galen aneurysm

DEGENERATIVE DISEASES OF CEREBRAL HEMISPHERES
= progressive fatal disease characterized by destruction / alteration of gray and white matter
Etiology: (a) genetic (b) viral infection (c) nutritional disorders (e.g. anorexia nervosa, Cushing syndrome) (d) immune system disorders (e.g. AIDS) (e) exposure to toxins (e.g. CO) / drugs (e.g. alcohol, methotrexate + radiation)

Leukodystrophy
= degenerative diffuse sclerosis with symmetrical bilateral white matter lesions

Leukoencephalopathy
= disease of white matter

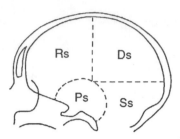

Rs = round shift   Ds = distal shift   Ps = Proximal shift   Ss = square shift

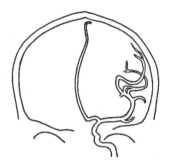

Round shift

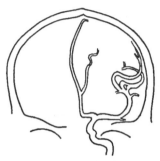

Distal shift

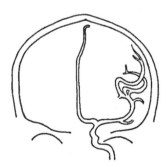

Square shift

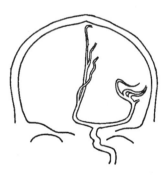

Proximal shift

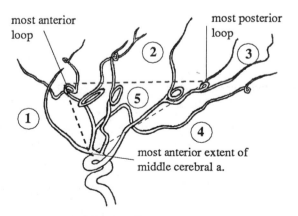

Sylvian Triangle
reference to numbers in text

A. DEMYELINATING DISEASE
= normal myelin destroyed by disease process
1. Multiple sclerosis (most frequent primary demyelinating disease)
2. Alzheimer disease (most common of diffuse gray matter degenerative diseases)
3. Parkinson disease (most common subcortical degenerative disease)
4. Creutzfeldt-Jakob disease
5. Menkes disease (sex-linked recessive disorder of copper metabolism)
6. Progressive multifocal leukoencephalopathy
7. Disseminated necrotizing leukoencephalopathy
8. Globoid cell leukodystrophy
9. Spongiform degeneration
10. Cockayne syndrome
11. Spongiform leukoencephalopathy

B. DYSMYELINATING
= metabolic abnormality resulting in formation of abnormal myelin
1. Metachromatic leukodystrophy (most common hereditary leukodystrophy)
2. Binswanger disease (SAE)
3. Multi-infarct dementia (MID)
4. Pick disease
5. Huntington disease
6. Wilson disease
7. Reye syndrome
8. Mineralizing microangiopathy
9. Diffuse sclerosis
10. Alexander disease (rare)

C. DE- AND DYSMYELINATING DISEASE
1. Adrenoleukodystrophy

Infection in immunocompromised patients

Cause: underlying malignancy, collagen disease, cancer therapy, AIDS, immunosuppressive therapy in organ transplants
Organism: Toxoplasma, Nocardia, Aspergillus, Candida, Cryptococcus
√ ring / nodular enhancement (sufficient immune defenses): Toxoplasma, Nocardia
√ enhancement may be blunted by steroid Rx
√ poorly defined hypodense zones with rapid enlargement in size + number, particularly affecting basal ganglia + centrum semiovale (poorly localized + encapsulated infection with poor prognosis)
AIDS may be associated with:
thrombocytopenia, lymphoma, plasmacytoma, Kaposi sarcoma, progressive multifocal leukoencephalopathy

Displacement of vessels

A. Arterial shift
(a) Pericallosal arteries
1. Round shift   = frontal lesion anterior to coronal suture

2. Square shift   = lesion behind foramen of Monro in lower half of hemisphere
3. Distal shift   = posterior to coronal suture in upper half of hemisphere
4. Proximal shift = basifrontal lesion / anterior middle cranial fossa including anterior temporal lobe
(b) Sylvian triangle
= branches of MCA within Sylvian fissure on outer surface of insula form a loop upon reaching the upper margin of the insula; serves as angiographic landmark for localizing supratentorial masses
Location of lesion:
1. anterior sylvian ... frontal region
2. suprasylvian   ... posterior frontal + parietal
3. retrosylvian   ... occipital, parieto-occipital
4. infrasylvian   ... temporal lobe + extracerebral region
5. intrasylvian   ... usually due to meningioma
6. lateral sylvian ... frontal, frontotemporal, parietotemporal
7. central sylvian ... deep posterior frontal, basal ganglia

B. Cerebral veins
= indicate the midline of the posterior part of the forebrain showing the exact location of the roof of the 3rd ventricle

Occlusive vascular disease

(a) Embolic state: √ single vascular territory
(b) Hypoperfusive state: √ multiple vascular territories
Causes:
1. Vasospasm from subarachnoid hemorrhage
2. Embolic infarction (50%)
(a) thrombus (atrial fibrillation, valvular disease, atheromatous plaques of extracerebral arteries, fibromuscular dysplasia, intracranial aneurysm, surgery, paradoxic emboli, sickle cell disease, atherosclerosis, thrombotic thrombocytopenic purpura)
• fluctuating blood pressures
• hypercoagulability
√ "supernormal artery" on NECT = high-density material lodged in cerebral vessel near major bifurcations
√ cerebral petechial hemorrhage within cortical / basal gray matter during 2nd week (from fragments of embolus) in up to 40%; initial ischemia is followed by reperfusion (= HALLMARK of embolic infarction)
√ atheromatous narrowing of vessels
(b) fat
(c) nitrogen
3. Watershed infarct
involving deep white matter between two adjacent vascular beds in global hypoperfusion secondary to poor cardiac output / cervical carotid artery occlusion

Δ 6% of cerebral infarcts have hemorrhage (red infarct)
- stroke (3rd most common cause of death in USA) (5% of stroke syndromes are caused by underlying tumor)
- TIA = transitory ischemic attack: clears within 24 hours
- RIND = reversible ischemic neurologic deficit: still evident > 24 hours with eventual total recovery
- amaurosis fugax = transient monocular blindness
- weakness / numbness in an extremity
- aphasia
- dizziness, diplopia, dysarthria (vertebrobasilar ischemia)

4. Hypertension
   (a) Hypertensive encephalopathy
       √ diffuse white matter hypodensity (edema secondary to arterial spasm)
   (b) Hypertensive hemorrhage
       Location: basal ganglia (putamen, external capsule), thalamus, pons, cerebellum
   (c) Lacunar infarct
       secondary to occlusion of small penetrating endarteries at base of brain
       Location: basal ganglia, thalamus, pons (territory of lenticulostriate, thalamoperforating, pontine perforating arteries)
       √ small discrete foci of hypodensity < 1 cm in diameter
   (d) Subcortical arteriosclerotic encephalopathy (SAE)

5. Amyloidosis
   involvement of small + medium-sized arteries of meninges + cortex
   - normotensive patient > 65 years of age
   √ multiple simultaneous / recurrent cortical hemorrhages

6. Vasculitis
   (a) Bacterial meningitis, TB, Syphilis, fungus, virus, Rickettsia
   (b) Collagen-vascular disease: Wegener granulomatosis, Polyarteritis nodosa, SLE, Scleroderma, Dermatomyositis
   (c) Granulomatous angitis: Giant cell arteritis, Sarcoidosis, Takayasu disease, Temporal arteritis
   (d) Inflammatory arteritis: Rheumatoid arteritis, Hypersensitivity arteritis, Behçet disease, Lymphomatoid granulomatosis

   (e) Drug-induced: IV amphetamine, ergot preparations, oral contraceptives
   (f) Radiation arteritis = mineralizing microangiopathy
   (g) Moya-Moya disease

7. Anoxic encephalopathy
   cardiorespiratory arrest, near-drowning, drug overdose, CO poisoning

8. Venous thrombosis

MULTIPLE INFARCTIONS
typical in extracranial occlusive disease, cardiac output problems, small vessel disease; in 6% from a shower of emboli
Location: usually bilateral + supratentorial (3/4); supra- and infratentorial (1/4)

Cerebrovascular malformations
1. Arteriovenous malformation
2. Vein of Galen aneurysm
3. Sinus pericranii
4. Venous angioma

Occult vascular malformation
   1. Cavernous angioma
   2. Capillary teleangiectasia

Birth Trauma
1. **Caput succedaneum**
   = localized edema in presenting portion of scalp, frequently associated with microscopic hemorrhage + subcutaneous hyperemia
2. **Cephalohematoma**
   = subperiosteal hematoma, may result from incorrect application of obstetric forceps or skull fracture during birth
   Incidence: 2% of all deliveries
   Location: most commonly parietal
   √ confined within suture lines
   √ may calcify / ossify causing thickening of diploe
3. Skull fracture
   Incidence: 1% of all deliveries
   √ CT shows associated intracranial hemorrhage
4. Subdural hematoma
   (a) convexity hematoma (b) interhemispheric hematoma
   (c) posterior fossa hematoma
5. Benign subdural effusion
   = benign condition that resolves spontaneously
   - clear / xanthochromic fluid with elevated protein level
   √ extracerebral fluid collection accompanied by ventricular dilatation (= communicating hydrocephalus caused by impaired CSF absorption of these subdural fluid collections)

ANATOMY OF BRAIN

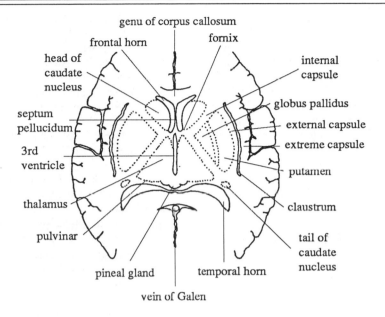

Axial section through level of 3rd ventricle

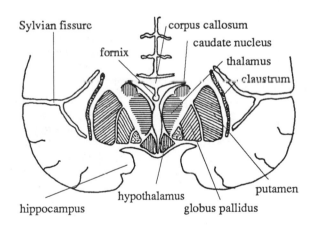

Coronal section through level of basal ganglia

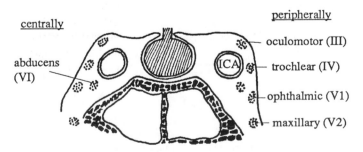

Cavernous Sinus
(coronal view)

Classification of brain anatomy
A. **Prosencephalon** = forebrain
   1. **Telencephalon** = cerebrum
      mainly comprising the two cerebral hemispheres
   2. **Diencephalon**
      = most of 3rd ventricle and adjacent dorsal
      thalamus, hypothalamus, epithalamus (= pineal
      gland + habenula), subthalamus (= ventral
      thalamus)
B. **Mesencephalon** = midbrain
   = short segment of brainstem above pons; traverses
   the hiatus in tentorium cerebelli; contains cerebral
   peduncles, tectum, colliculi (corpora quadrigemina)
C. **Rhombencephalon** = hindbrain
   1. **Cerebellum**
   2. **Metencephalon** = pons
   3. **Myelencephalon** = medulla oblongata

Basal nuclei
= BASAL GANGLIA (earlier incorrect designation)
A. Amygdaloid body
B. Claustrum
C. Corpus striatum
   (1) Caudate
   (2) Lentiform nucleus
       (a) pallidum = globus pallidus
       (b) putamen

Contents of superior orbital fissure
A. NERVES
   III oculomotor nerve
   IV   trochlear nerve
   V1   ophthalmic branch of trigeminal nerve:
        (a) lacrimal nerve
        (b) frontal nerve
   VI   abducens nerve

B. VESSELS
   1. veins: superior + inferior ophthalmic vein
   2. arteries: (a) meningeal branch of lacrimal artery
               (b) orbital branch of middle meningeal
                   artery

External carotid artery
mnemonic for branches: "All Summer Long Emily Ogled
Peter's Sporty Isuzu"
   Ascending pharyngeal artery
   Superior thyroid artery
   Lingual artery
   External maxillary = facial artery
   Occipital artery
   Posterior auricular artery
   Superficial temporal artery
   Internal maxillary artery

Internal carotid artery
A. CERVICAL SEGMENT
   ascends posterior and medial to ECA; enters carotid
   canal of petrous bone; NO branches

B. PETROUS SEGMENT
   ascends briefly, in carotid canal bends anteromedially
   in a horizontal course (anterior to tympanic cavity +
   cochlea); exits near petrous apex through posterior
   portion of foramen lacerum; ascends to juxtasellar
   location where it pierces dural layer of cavernous
   sinus
   Branches:
   1. **Caroticotympanic a.:** to tympanic cavity,
      anastomoses with anterior tympanic branch of
      maxillary a.+ stylomastoid a.
   2. **Pterygoid (vidian) a.:** through pterygoid canal;
      anastomoses with recurrent branch of greater
      palatine a.

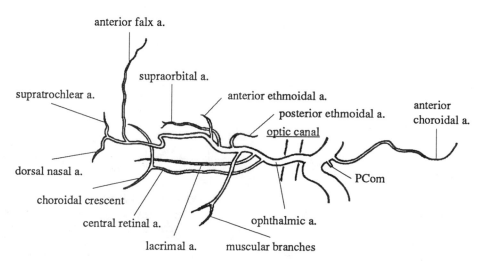

Ophthalmic artery

C. CAVERNOUS SEGMENT
ascends to posterior clinoid process, then turns anteriorly + superomedially through cavernous sinus; exits medial to anterior clinoid process piercing dura
Branches:
1. **Meningohypophyseal trunk**
   (a) tentorial branch
   (b) dorsal meningeal branch
   (c) inferior hypophyseal branch
2. **Anterior meningeal a.**: supplies dura of anterior fossa; anastomoses with meningeal branch of posterior ethmoidal a.
3. Cavernous rami supply trigeminal ganglion, walls of cavernous + inferior petrosal sinuses

D. SUPRACLINOID SEGMENT
ascends posterior + lateral between oculomotor + optic nerve
Branches:
   mnemonic   "OPA"
   Ophthalmic a.
   Posterior communicating a.
   Anterior choroidal a.
1. **Ophthalmic a.** exits from ICA medial to anterior clinoid process, travels through optic canal inferolateral to optic nerve
   (a) recurrent meningeal branch: dura of anterior middle cranial fossa
   (b) posterior ethmoidal a.: supplies dura of planum sphenoidale
   (c) anterior ethmoidal a.
2. **Superior hypophyseal a.**: optic chiasm, anterior lobe of pituitary
3. **Posterior communicating a.** (PCom)
4. **Anterior choroidal a.**
5. **Middle + anterior cerebral arteries** (MCA, ACA)

Vertebral artery
originates from subclavian a. proximal to thyrocervical trunk; left vertebral a. usually greater than right cerebral a.; left vertebral a. may originate directly from aorta (5 %)

A. PREVERTEBRAL SEGMENT
ascends posterosuperiorly between longus colli + anterior scalene muscle; enters transverse foramina at C6
Branches: muscular branches

B. CERVICAL SEGMENT
ascends through transverse foramina in close proximity to uncinate processes
Branches:
1. **Anterior meningeal a.**

C. ATLANTIC SEGMENT
exits transverse foramen of atlas; passes posteriorly in a groove on superior surface of posterior arch of atlas; pierces atlanto-occipital membrane + dura mater to enter cranial cavity
Branches:
1. **Posterior meningeal branch** to posterior falx + tentorium

D. INTRACRANIAL SEGMENT
ascends anteriorly + laterally around medulla to reach midline at pontomedullary junction; anastomoses with contralateral side to form basilar artery at clivus
Branches:
1. **Anterior + Posterior spinal a.**
2. **Posterior inferior cerebellar a.** (PICA)
3. **Anterior inferior cerebellar a.** (AICA)
4. **Internal auditory a.**
5. **Superior cerebellar a.**
6. **Posterior cerebral a.** (PCA)
7. medullary + pontine perforating branches

Anterior cerebral artery (ACA)
A. HORIZONTAL PORTION = A 1 SEGMENT = segment between origin and anterior communicating a. (ACom)
   (a) Inferior branches
      supply superior surface of optic nerve + chiasm
   (b) superior branches
      penetrate brain to supply anterior hypothalamus, septum pellucidum, anterior commissure, fornix columns, anterior inferior portion of corpus striatum (largest striatal artery = recurrent artery of Heubner for anteroinferior portion of head of caudate, putamen, anterior limb of internal capsule)

B. INTERHEMISPHERIC PORTION = A 2 SEGMENT = segment after origin of anterior communicating a. (ACom); ascends in cistern of lamina terminalis
Branches:
1. **Medial orbitofrontal a.**: along gyrus rectus
2. **Frontopolar a.**
3. **Callosomarginal a.**: within cingulus gyrus
4. **Pericallosal a.**: over corpus callosum within callosal cistern
   (a) Superior internal parietal a.: anterior portion of precuneus + convexity of superior parietal lobule
   (b) Inferior internal parietal a.
   (c) Posterior pericallosal a.
      from callosomarginal / pericallosal artery:
      — Anterior + middle + posterior internal frontal aa.
      — Paracentral a.: supplies precentral + postcentral gyri

Middle cerebral artery
= largest branch of ICA arising lateral to optic chiasm; passes horizontal in lateral direction just ventral to anterior perforated substance to enter sylvian fissure where it divides into 2 / 3 / 4 branches
Branches: 1. **Anterior temporal a.**

2. **Ascending frontal a.** (Candelabra) / Prefrontal a.
3. **Precentral a.** = Pre Rolandic a.
4. **Central a.** = Rolandic a.
5. **Anterior parietal a.** = Post Rolandic a.
6. **Posterior parietal a.**
7. **Angular a.**
8. **Middle temporal a.**
9. **Posterior temporal a.**
10. **Temporooccipital a.**

Posterior cerebral artery

originates from bifurcation of basilar artery within interpeduncular cistern (in 15% as a direct continuation of posterior communicating artery); lies above oculomotor nerve and circles midbrain above the tentorium cerebelli
Branches:
1. Mesencephalic perforating branches: tectum + cerebral peduncles

2. Posterior thalamoperforating aa.: midline of thalamus + hypothalamus
3. Thalamogeniculate aa.: geniculate bodies + pulvinar
4. Posterior medial choroidal a.: circles midbrain parallel to PCA; enters lateral aspect of quadrigeminal cistern; passes lateral and above pineal gland and enters roof of 3rd ventricle; supplies quadrigeminal plate + pineal gland
5. Posterior lateral choroidal a.: courses lateral and enters choroidal fissure; anterior branch to temporal horn + posterior branch to choroid plexus of trigone and lateral ventricle + lateral geniculate body
6. Cortical branches: (a) Anterior inferior temporal a.
　　　　　　　　　　(b) Posterior inferior temporal a.
　　　　　　　　　　(c) Parietooccipital a.
　　　　　　　　　　(d) Calcarine a.
　　　　　　　　　　(e) Posterior pericallosal a.

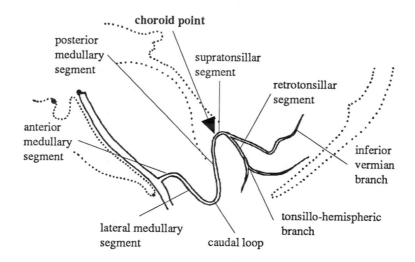

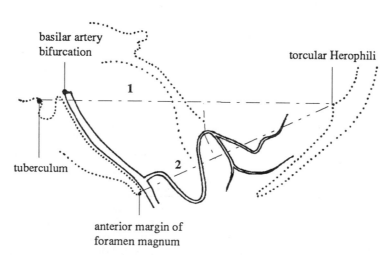

Posterior inferior cerebellar artery

Posterior inferior cerebellar artery

= PICA = last and largest branch of vertebral artery
Parts:
1. Premedullar segment = caudal loop around medulla, may descend below level of foramen magnum
2. retromedullar segment = ascending portion up to the level of 4th ventricle and tonsils
3. supratonsillar segment = the most cranial point is the choroidal point

Variations: commonly asymmetric; hypoplastic / absent in 20% [vascular supply then provided by anterior inferior cerebellar artery (AICA)]

Orthotopic **choroid point** established by:
1. perpendicular line from choroid point onto Twining's line = TTT-line (Twining's Tuberculum Torcula line) bisects TTT-line (length of anterior portion 52 – 60%)
2. perpendicular line from choroid point cuts CT-line (Clivus Torcular line) < 1 mm anterior / < 3 mm posterior to junction of anterior and middle thirds of CT-line

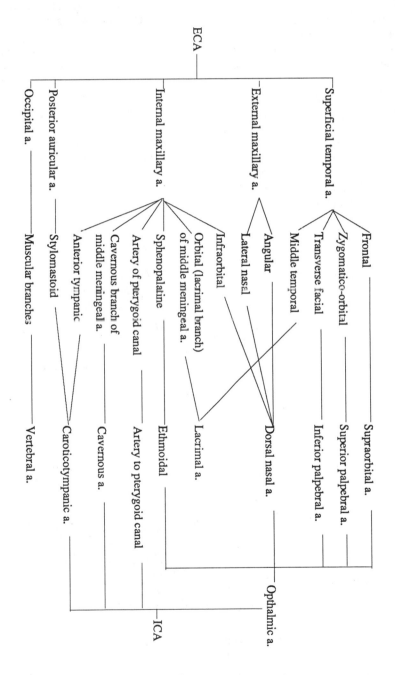

Anastomoses between ICA and ECA and Vertebral Artery

Arterial anastomoses of the brain
Anastomoses via the arteries at the base of the brain
A. <u>Circle of Willis</u>
1. right ICA — right anterior cerebral a. — anterior communicating a. — left anterior cerebral a. — left ICA
2. ICA — posterior communicating a. — basilar a.
3. ICA — anterior choroidal a. — posterior choroidal a. — posterior cerebral a. — basilar a.
B. <u>Developmental anomaly</u>
three transient embryonal carotid-basilar anastomoses appearing consecutively in fetal life:
1. **Primitive hypoglossal artery**
= arterial connection between the intrapetrosal portion of ICA and proximal portion of basilar artery
2. **Primitive acoustic (otic) artery**
= arterial connection between cervical portion of ICA + vertebral artery in region of 12th nerve
3. **Persistent primitive trigeminal artery**
Incidence: 1 – 2 / 1000 angiograms
√ short wide connection between the cavernous portion of ICA and upper third of basilar artery (beneath posterior communicating artery)

Anastomoses via surface vessels
A. Leptomeningeal anastomoses of the cerebrum: ACA — MCA — PCA
B. Leptomeningeal anastomoses of the cerebellum: Superior cerebellar a. — anterior inferior cerebellar a. — posterior inferior cerebellar a.

Rete mirabile
ECA — middle meningeal a. / superficial temporal a. — leptomeningeal aa. — ACA / MCA

Cerebral veins
Important vascular markers:
1. Pontomesencephalic v. = anterior border of brain stem
2. Precentral cerebellar v. = position of tectum
Δ colliculocentral point = midpoint of Twining's line at knee of precentral cerebellar vein
3. Venous angle = acute angle at junction of thalamostriate with internal cerebral v. = posterior aspect of foramen of Monro
4. Internal cerebral v. = caudad border of splenium of corpus callosum
5. Copular point = junction of inferior + superior retrotonsillar tributaries draining cerebellar tonsils in region of copular pyramids of vermis

Carotid duplex ultrasound
Doppler equation: fD = 2 f v cos ø / c
fD = Doppler shift frequency (in Hz)
f = frequency of the ultrasound transducer (in Hz)
v = velocity of moving blood (in m/s)
ø = angle between the direction of blood flow + axis of ultrasound beam
c = velocity of sound in the medium (in m/s)

A. LAMINAR FLOW
= narrow range of Doppler shift frequencies, esp. during systole, due to blunt velocity profile

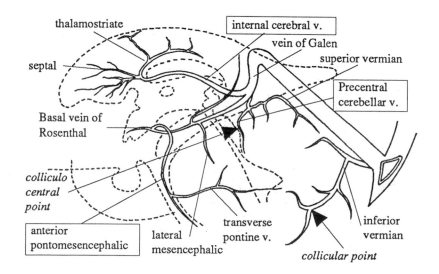

Cerebral Veins

√ window below spectral trace in systole (small sample volume located in center of vessel)

B. DISTURBED FLOW
= breakdown of laminar flow with a wide range of Doppler shifts secondary to velocity vectors whose direction varies
  (a) vortex formation = rotating flow elements forming secondary to increase in velocity during upstroke of systole
  (b) turbulence = shed vortices traveling downstream
    Cause: stenosis / tortuosity of vessel
√ increase in velocity
√ spectral broadening = reduction of size of window
√ simultaneous forward + reversed flow
√ fluctuations of flow velocity with time

DECREASE IN LUMEN DIAMETER VS. CROSS-SECTIONAL AREA

decrease in lumen diameter	decrease in cross-sectional area
20%	36%
40%	64%
60%	84%
80%	96%

INDEXED FLOW
= assessment of increased vascular resistance which reduces diastolic flow
1. Stuart index
   = S/D ratio = A/B ratio
   maximal systolic shift (S) divided by enddiastolic frequency shift (D)
2. Pourcelot index = resistive index
   (S - D)/S or 1 - (D/S)
3. Pulsatility index
   (S - D)/ mean velocity

DISEASE ENTITIES OF BRAIN

ABSCESS OF BRAIN

Pyogenic Abscess

= focal area of necrosis with formation of surrounding membrane beginning in area of cerebritis

Cause:
1. Extension from paranasal sinus infection (41%) / mastoiditis / otitis media (5%) / facial soft tissue infection / dental abscess
2. Generalized septicemia (32%):
   (a) Lung (most common): bronchiectasis, empyema, lung abscess, bronchopleural fistula, pneumonia
   (b) Heart (less common): CHD with R-L shunt, AVM, bacterial endocarditis
   (c) Osteomyelitis
3. Penetrating trauma or surgery
4. Cryptogenic (25%)

predisposed: patients on steroids / immunosuppressive drugs, congenital / acquired immunologic deficiency

Organism: anaerobic streptococcus (most common), bacteroides, staphylococcus; in 25% sterile contents

Location: typically at corticomedullary junction; frontal + temporal lobes;
supratentorial : infratentorial = 2:1

NCCT:
√ zone of low density with mass effect (92%)
√ slightly increased rim density (4%), development of collagen layer takes 10 – 14 days
√ gas within lesion (4%) is diagnostic of gas-forming organism

CECT:
√ ring-blush (90%) with peripheral zone of edema
√ edema + contrast enhancement suppressed by steroids
√ regular 1 – 3 mm thick wall with relative thinning of medial wall (secondary to poorer blood supply of white matter)
√ multiloculation + subjacent daughter abscess in white matter

MRI: (most sensitive modality)
√ centrally increased / variable intensity with hypointense rim on T2WI
√ outside border of increased signal intensity on T2WI (edema)

Cx: ependymitis from rupture into adjacent ventricle (thin medial wall predisposes)

DDx: primary / metastatic neoplasm, subacute infarction, resolving hematoma

Granulomatous Abscess

1. Tuberculoma

2. Sarcoid abscess
3. Fungal abscess
commonly in immunocompromised patients

ACRANIA

= very rare developmental anomaly characterized by partial / complete absence of calvarium + complete but abnormal development of brain tissue
√ absence of calvarium
√ hemispheres surrounded by thin membrane
Prognosis: uniformly lethal

ADRENOLEUKODYSTROPHY

Etiology: defective peroxisomal fatty acid oxidation with accumulation of very long chain fatty acids (cholesterol esters) in gray and white matter + adrenal cortex

Mode of inheritance: (a) X-linked recessive in boys (common)
(b) autosomal recessive in neonates (uncommon)

Histo: PAS cytoplasmic inclusions in brain, adrenals, other tissues

Age: 1 – 2nd decade (X-linked recessive)
• deteriorating vision (27%), loss of hearing (50%)
• ataxia
• optic disk pallor
• adrenal gland insufficiency (abnormal increased pigmentation, elevated ACTH levels)
• altered behavior, mental deterioration, death

CT:
√ large symmetric low-density lesions in occipitoparietotemporal white matter (80%) advancing toward frontal lobes + cerebellum
√ thin curvilinear / serrated enhancing rims near edges of lesion
√ initial frontal lobe involvement (12%)
√ calcifications within hypodense areas (7%)

MRI:
√ hyperintense signals on long TR sequences in subcortical white matter, auditory tract, visual pathway, pyramidal fibers

AGENESIS OF CORPUS CALLOSUM

= failure of formation of corpus callosum originating from the lamina terminalis at 7 – 13 weeks from where a phalanx of callosal tissue extends backwards arching over the diencephalon; usually developed by 20 weeks

Incidence: 0.7 – 5.3%

Histo: axons from cerebral hemispheres continue along medial walls of lateral ventricles as bundles of Probst that terminate randomly in occipital + temporal lobes

associated with:
  (a) CNS anomalies (85%):
    1. Interhemispheric cyst may be continuous with 3rd and lateral ventricles
    2. Hydrocephalus (30%)
    3. Midline intracerebral lipoma of corpus callosum often surrounded with ring of calcium (10%)
    4. Dandy-Walker cyst (11%)
    5. Arnold-Chiari II malformation (7%)
    6. Midline encephalocele
    7. Porencephaly
    8. Holoprosencephaly
    9. Hypertelorism median cleft syndrome
  (b) cardiovascular, gastrointestinal, genitourinary anomalies (62%)
- normal brain function unusual but possible; neurologic abnormalities
- intellectual impairment; seizures
√ wide separation of lateral ventricles with parallel parasagittal orientation ("bat-wing" appearance on CT)
√ dilatation of occipital horns + atria (= colpocephaly)
√ anterior pointing with concave medial wall of frontal horns
√ "high-riding third ventricle" = upward displacement of 3rd ventricle often to level of bodies of lateral ventricles
√ elongated interventricular foramina
√ radial arrangement of medial gyri + sulci fanning out to cerebral cortex and terminating superficially at the roof of the 3rd ventricle (on sagittal images)
√ failure of normal convergence of calcarine + parietooccipital sulci
√ absence of cingulate gyrus on midsagittal images (rotated inferiorly + laterally)
√ anterior interhemispheric fissure adjoins elevated 3rd ventricle (PATHOGNOMONIC)
√ absence of septum pellucidum + corpus callosum
Angio:
  √ wandering straight posterior course of pericallosal arteries (lateral view)
  √ wide separation of pericallosal arteries secondary to intervening 3rd ventricle (anterior view)
  √ separation of internal cerebral veins
  √ loss of U-shape in vein of Galen
DDx: (1) Prominent cavum septi pellucidi + cavum vergae (should not be mistaken for 3rd ventricle)
       (2) Arachnoid cyst in midline (suprasellar, collicular plate) raising and deforming the 3rd ventricle and causing hydrocephalus

ALZHEIMER DISEASE
most common of diffuse gray matter diseases with large loss of cells from cerebral cortex + other areas
- slowly progressing memory loss, dementia
√ "cracked walnut" appearance = symmetrically enlarged sulci in high convexity area

ANENCEPHALY
= failure of closure of the rostral end of the neural tube between 4 – 5th week MA
Incidence: 1:1,000 births (3.5:1,000 in South Wales); M:F = 1:4; most common congenital defect involving CNS
Etiology: multifactorial (genetic + environmental)
Path: absence of cerebral hemispheres + cranial vault; partial / complete absence of diencephalic + mesencephalic structures; hypophysis + rhombencephalic structures usually preserved
Risk factors: family Hx of neural tube defect; twin pregnancy; 4% risk of recurrence
associated anomalies:
  spinal dysraphism (17 – 50%), cleft lip / palate (2%), clubfoot (2%), umbilical hernia
√ absence of cranium cephalad to orbits
√ bulging eyes (frog-like appearance)
√ short neck
√ polyhydramnios (40 – 50%) after 26 weeks GA (due to failure of normal fetal swallowing) / oligohydramnios
Prognosis: uniformly fatal within hours to days of life; in 53% premature birth; in 68% stillbirth
DDx: microcephaly, acrania, encephalocele, amniotic band syndrome

ANEURYSM OF CNS
Etiology:
  (a) congenital (97%) = "berry aneurysm" in 2% of population (in 20% multiple); associated with aortic coarctation + adult polycystic kidney disease
  (c) infectious (3%) = mycotic aneurysm
  (b) arteriosclerotic: fusiform shape
  (d) traumatic
  (e) neoplastic
Location of aneurysm:
  A. by autopsy:
    (a) Circle of Willis (80%):
        MCA bifurcation > ICA at origin of PCom > ACom > ICA at bifurcation into ACA + MCA
    (b) Posterior fossa (20%)
  B. by angiography (= symptomatic aneurysms):
     PCom (38%) > ACom (36%) > MCA bifurcation (21%) > ICA bifurcation > tip of basilar artery (2.8%)
  C. by risk of bleeding: 1 – 2% per year
     ACom (70% bleed), PCom (2nd highest risk)

LOCATION OF BLOOD SUGGESTING SITE OF ANEURYSM:
  A. according to location of SUBARACHNOID HEMORRHAGE:
    1. Anterior chiasmatic cistern   : ACom
    2. Septum pellucidum   : ACom
    3. Intraventricular   : ACom, ICA, MCA
    4. Sylvian fissure   : MCA, ICA, PCom
    5. Anterior pericallosal cistern : ACA, ACom
    6. Symmetric distribution in subarachnoid space: ACA + basilar artery

B. according to location of <u>CEREBRAL HEMATOMA</u>:
    1. inferomedial frontal lobe   : ACom
    2. temporal lobe   : MCA
    3. corpus callosum   : pericallosal artery
C. <u>INTRAVENTRICULAR HEMORRHAGE</u>
    from aneurysms at ACom, MCA, pericallosal artery
    (CAVE: blood may have entered in retrograde
    manner from subarachnoid location)

Rupture size: 5 – 15 mm
Clues for bleeding aneurysm:
    (a) the largest aneurysm (87%)
    (b) anterior communicating artery (70%)
    (c) contralateral side of all visualized aneurysms
         (60%), non-visualization due to spasm

MULTIPLE ANEURYSMS
    Cause: congenital aneurysms in 20%, mycotic
              aneurysms in 22%
    mirror image aneurysms = 35% of patients with one
      MCA aneurysm have one on the contralateral side
    CECT: detection rate of aneurysms at PCom (40%),
            ACom / MCA, basilar artery (80%)
Prognosis:
    (1) death in 10% within 24 hours from concomitant
         intracerebral hemorrhage, extensive brain
         herniation, massive infarcts + hemorrhage within
         brain stem
    (2) survivors frequently recover completely within a few
         days
    (3) cerebral ischemia + infarction
    (4) recurrence within 2 weeks (increased mortality)
Cx: subdural hematoma

Giant Aneurysm
    = aneurysm larger than 2.5 cm in diameter, usually
      presenting with intracranial mass effect
    Incidence: 25% of all aneurysms
    Age: no age predilection; M : F = 2 : 1
    Location: (arise from arteries at the base of the brain)
        (a) Middle fossa: cavernous segement of ICA
             (43%), supraclinoid segment of ICA, terminal
             bifurcation of ICA, middle cerebral artery
        (b) Posterior fossa: at tip of basilar artery, AICA,
             vertebral artery
    Skull film:
        √ predominantly peripheral curvilinear calcification
          (22%)
        √ bone erosion (44%)
        √ pressure changes on sella turcica (18%)
    CECT:
        √ "target sign" = centrally opacified vessel lumen +
          ring of thrombus + enhanced fibrous outer wall
        √ simple ring-blush (75%) of fibrous outer wall with
          total thrombosis
        √ little / no surrounding edema
    MRI:
        √ mixed signal intensity (combination of subacute +
          chronic hemorrhage, calcification)
    Cx: subarachnoid hemorrhage in < 30%

Mycotic Aneurysm
    = 3% of all intracranial aneurysms, multiple in 20%
    Source: subacute bacterial endocarditis (65%),
                acute bacterial endocarditis (9%), meningitis
                (9%), septic thrombophlebitis (9%), myxoma
    Location: peripheral to first bifurcation of major vessel
                (64%); often located near surface of brain
                especially over convexities
        (a) suprasellar cistern = circle of Willis
        (b) inferolateral sylvian fissure = middle
             cerebral artery trifurcation
        (c) genu of corpus callosum = origin of
             callosomarginal artery
        (d) bottom of 3rd ventricle = pericallosal
             artery
    NCCT:
        √ aneurysm rarely visualized except, indirect
          evidence from focal hematoma secondary to
          rupture
        √ zone of increased density / calcification
        √ increased density in subarachnoid, intraventricular,
          intracerebral spaces (extravasated blood)
        √ focal / diffuse lucency of brain (edema / infarction /
          vasospasm)
    CECT:
        √ intense homogeneous enhancement within round /
          oval mass contiguous to vessels
        √ incomplete opacification with mural thrombus
    Cx: develop recurrent bleeding more frequently than
            congenital aneurysms

Supraclinoid Carotid Aneurysm
    = 38% of intracranial aneurysms
    Sites: (a) at origin of posterior communicating artery
                (65%)
           (b) at bifurcation of internal carotid artery (23%)
           (c) at origin of ophthalmic artery (12%) medial
                to anterior clinoid process; most likely to
                become giant aneurysm
    Presentation: • bitemporal hemianopsia (extrinsic
                       compression on chiasm)
        √ calcification is rare (frequent in atherosclerotic
          cavernous sinus aneurysm)

Cavernous Sinus Aneurysm
    Age: 20 – 70 years, peak 5 – 6th decade; F > M
    Cause: sinus thrombophlebitis
        • cavernous sinus syndrome: trigeminal nerve pain,
          oculomotor nerve paralysis
        • progressive visual failure
        √ undercutting of anterior clinoid process
        √ erosion of lateral half of sella
        √ erosion of posterior clinoid process
        √ erosion into middle cranial fossa
        √ enlargement of superior orbital fissure
        √ erosion of tip of petrous pyramid
        √ rim-like calcification (33 %)
        √ displacement of thin bony margins without sclerosis

AQUEDUCTAL STENOSIS
aqueduct develops about the 6th week of gestation
Incidence: most frequent cause of congenital
hydrocephalus (43%); M:F = 2:1
Etiology: (a) infectious (50%): toxoplasmosis, CMV,
syphilis, mumps, influenza virus
(b) developmental: forking / narrowing /
transverse septum (X-linked recessive
inheritance in 25% of males)
(c) neoplastic (extremely rare): glioma,
pinealoma, meningioma
may be associated with other congenital anomalies
(16%): thumb deformities
√ enlargement of lateral + 3rd ventricles (nonspecific)
Prognosis: 11 – 30% mortality

ARACHNOID CYST
= CSF-containing cyst without ventricular communication /
brain maldevelopment
Incidence: 1% of all intracranial masses
Origin: (1) congenital: arising from clefts / duplication
of arachnoid membrane
(2) acquired: following hemorrhage / infection in
neonatal period
Pathogenesis: growth secondary to
(1) ball-valve communication with subarachnoid space
(2) CSF-producing choroid plexus-like tissue
Age: presentation at any time during life
• often asymptomatic
• symptomatic due to mass effect
Location: (between brain + dura)
(a) floor of middle fossa near tip of temporal lobe
(sylvian fissure)
(b) cerebral convexity (interhemispheric fissure)
(c) suprasellar / chiasmatic cistern (may produce
endocrinopathy)
(d) posterior fossa (1/3): cerebellopontine angle
(11%), quadrigeminal plate cistern (10%), in
relationship to vermis (9%), prepontine /
interpeduncular cistern (3%)
√ forward bowing of anterior wall of cranial fossa +
elevation of sphenoid ridge
√ extraaxial thin-walled CSF-density cyst with well-defined
smooth angular margins
√ compression of subarachnoid space + subjacent brain
(minimal mass effect)
√ may erode inner table of calvarium
√ NO enhancement (intrathecal contrast penetrates into
cyst on delayed scans)
Cx: Hydrocephalus
CT-DDx: epidermoid, dermoid, subdural hygroma,
infarction, porencephaly
US-DDx: choroid plexus cyst, porencephalic cyst
(communicates with ventricle), cystic tumor
(solid components), midline cyst associated
with agenesis of corpus callosum, dorsal cyst
associated with holoprosencephaly, vein of
Galen aneurysm

Prognosis: favorable if removed before onset of
irreversible brain damage

ARNOLD-CHIARI MALFORMATION
A. CHIARI I MALFORMATION (adulthood)
HALLMARK: herniation of cerebellar tonsils below
foramen magnum
frequent, often isolated abnormality of little
consequence
associated with:
(1) hydromyelia (30 – 75%)
(2) hydrocephalus (25 – 44%)
(3) basilar impression (25%)
(4) occipitalization of C1 (10%)
(5) Klippel-Feil anomaly (10%)
(6) incomplete ossification of C1-ring (5%)
NOT associated with myelomeningocele !
√ slight downward displacement of cerebellar tonsils
+ medial part of the inferior lobes of the cerebellum
3 – 5 mm below the level of the foramen magnum
√ obliteration of cisterna magna
√ elongation of 4th ventricle which remains in normal
position
√ slight anterior angulation of lower brainstem

B. CHIARI II MALFORMATION (childhood)
= most common and serious complex of anomalies
secondary to a too small posterior fossa involving
many parts of neural axis
HALLMARK: dysgenesis of hindbrain with
(1) caudally displaced 4th ventricle
(2) caudally displaced brainstem
(3) tonsillar + vermian herniation through foramen
magnum
associated with:
(1) lumbar myelomeningocele (80%)
(2) dysgenesis of corpus callosum (75%)
(3) obstructive hydrocephalus (50 – 98%)
(4) absence of septum pellucidum (40%)
(5) syringohydromyelia
(6) excessive cortical gyration (stenogyria
= histologically normal cortex; polymicrogyria
= histologically abnormal cortex)
NOT associated with basilar impression / C1-
assimilation / Klippel-Feil deformity!
Skull film:
√ Lückenschadel (most prominent near torcular
Herophili / vertex)
√ scalloping of posterior aspect of petrous
pyramids + scalloped clivus (from pressure of
cerebellum) in 70 – 90%
√ small posterior fossa
√ enlarged foramen magnum + enlarged upper
spinal canal secondary to molding in 75%
@ Supratentorial
√ hydrocephalus (duct of Sylvius dysfunctional but
probe patent); may not become evident until after
repair of myelomeningocele

√ colpocephaly (= enlargement of occipital horns + atria)

√ "batwing" configuration of frontal horns on coronal views = frontal horns pointing inferiorly with blunt superolateral angle secondary to prominent impressions by caudate nucleus

√ "hour-glass ventricle" = small biconcave 3rd ventricle secondary to large massa intermedia

√ interdigitation of cerebral gyri (hypoplasia + fenestration of falx)

√ wide prepontine + supracerebellar cisterns

√ nonvisualization of aqueduct (up to 70%)

@ Cerebellum

√ "cerebellar peg" = protrusion of vermis + hemispheres through foramen magnum (90%) resulting in craniocaudal elongation of cerebellum

√ hypoplastic poorly differentiated cerebellum (poor visualization of folia on sagittal images)

√ elongated / obliterated thin-tubed 4th ventricle exiting below foramen magnum

√ obliteration of CPA cistern + cisterna magna by cerebellum growing around brain stem

√ dysplastic tentorium with wide U-shaped free edge and insertion close to foramen magnum

√ "tectal beaking" = deformed quadrigeminal plate (fusion of midbrain colliculi into a single beak) pointing posteriorly and invaginating into cerebellum

√ V-shape of quadrigeminal plate cistern

√ "towering cerebellum" = "pseudomass" = cerebellar extension above incisura of tentorium

√ triple peak configuration = corners of cerebellum pointing anteriorly + laterally (on axial images)

√ flattened superior portion of cerebellum secondary to temporoparietal herniation

√ vertical orientation of shortened straight sinus

@ Spinal cord

√ medulla + pons displaced into cervical canal

√ "cervicomedullary kink" = herniation of medulla posterior to spinal cord (up to 70%)

√ upper cervical nerve roots ascend toward their exit foramina

√ small arch of C1

√ syringohydromyelia

C. CHIARI III MALFORMATION
rare abnormality associated with occipitocervical / high cervical meningomyeloencephalocele; survival usually not beyond infancy

D. CHIARI IV MALFORMATION = severe cerebellar hypoplasia]

ARTERIOVENOUS MALFORMATION
= congenital abnormality consisting of dilated tortuous arteries + veins with racemose tangle of closely packed pathologic vessels resulting in shunting of blood from arterial to venous side without intermediary capillary network; most common vascular lesion

Age: 80% by end of 4th decade; 20% < 20 years of age
• headaches, seizures (nonfocal in 40%), mental deterioration
• progressive hemispheric neurologic deficit (50%)
• ictus from acute intracranial hemorrhage (50%)

Location:
(a) supratentorial (90%): parietal > frontal > temporal lobe > paraventricular > intraventricular region > occipital lobe
(b) infratentorial (10%)

Vascular supply:
(a) pial branches of ICA in 73% of supratentorial location, in 50% of posterior fossa location
(b) dural branches of ECA in 27% with infratentorial lesions

Skull film:
√ speckled / ring-like calcifications (15 – 30%)
√ thinning / thickening of skull at contact area with AVM
√ prominent vascular grooves on inner table of skull (dilated feeding arteries + draining veins) in 27%

NCCT:
√ irregular mass with large feeding arteries + draining veins
√ mixed density (60%): dense large vessels + hemorrhage + calcifications
√ isodense lesion (15%): may be recognizable by mass effect
√ low density (15%): brain atrophy due to ischemia
√ not visualized (10%)

CECT:
√ serpiginous dense enhancement in 80% (tortuous dilated vessels)
√ No enhancement in thrombosed AVM
√ No avascular spaces within AVM
√ lack of mass effect / edema (unless thrombosed / bleeding)
√ rapid shunting
√ thickened arachnoid covering
√ adjacent atrophic brain

MRI:
√ flow void (imaging with GRASS gradient echo + long TR sequences)

Angio:
√ grossly dilated efferent + afferent vessels with a racemose tangle ("bag of worms"), arteriovenous shunting
√ negative angiogram (compression by hematoma / thrombosis)

Prognosis: 10% mortality; 30% morbidity; 2% risk per year of recurrent bleeding

WYBURN-MASON SYNDROME
= telangiectasias of skin + retinal cirsoid aneurysm + AVM involving entire optic tract (optic nerve, thalamus, geniculate bodies, calcarine cortex);
may be associated with AVMs of posterior fossa, neck, mandible / maxilla presenting in childhood

BASAL GANGLIA HEMATOMA

= rupture of small distal microaneurysms in the lenticulostriate arteries in patients with poorly controlled systemic arterial hypertension

Cx: (1) dissection into adjacent ventricles (2/3)
(2) porencephaly
(3) atrophy with ipsilateral ventricular dilatation

BASAL GANGLIA INFARCT

= occlusion of small penetrating arteries at base of brain (lenticulostriate / thalamoperforating arteries) = lacunar infarct (infarcts < 1 cm in size)

Cause:
(1) Embolism (2) Hypoperfusion (3) Carbon monoxide poisoning (4) Drowning (5) Vasculopathy (hypertension, microvasculopathy, aging)
√ dense homogeneous enhancement outlining caudate nucleus, putamen, globus pallidus, thalamus
√ dense round nodular enhancement / peripheral ring enhancement

BINSWANGER DISEASE

= ENCEPHALOPATHIA SUBCORTICALIS PROGRESSIVA = SUBCORTICAL ARTERIOSCLEROTIC ENCEPHALOPAHTY (SAE)

Path: atherosclerosis in small arteries of subcortical white matter
Age: middle age
• psychiatric changes, intellectual impairment, slowly progressive dementia, transient neurologic deficits, seizures, spasticity, syncope
√ multifocal hypodense lesions (periventricular, centrum semiovale, spares U fibers)
√ lacunar infarcts in basal ganglia
√ sulcal enlargement + dilated lateral ventricles (brain atrophy)
DDx: Leukodystrophy, Progressive multifocal leukoencephalopathy, Multiple sclerosis

CAPILLARY TELANGIECTASIA

= abnormal dilated capillaries separated by normal neural tissue; commonly "cryptic"
may be associated with: hereditary Rendu-Osler-Weber syndrome, ataxia-telangiectasis syndrome
• usually asymptomatic (incidental finding at necropsy)
Location: mostly in pons; usually multiple / may be solitary
√ poorly defined areas of dilated vessels (resemble petechiae)
Prognosis: bleeding uncommon; bleeding in pons usually fatal

CAROTID ARTERY STENOSIS

High-grade ICA stenosis is associated with increased risk for TIA, stroke, carotid occlusion, embolism arising from thrombi forming at site of narrowing
Increased risk for stroke: (a) ICA stenosis
(b) intraplaque hemorrhage

Accuracy of Duplex scans in comparison to arteriography for ICA lesions:
91 – 94% sensitivity, 85 – 99% specificity for ICA stenosis > 50 % in diameter

DUPLEX CATEGORIES OF INTERNAL CAROTID ARTERY LESIONS

A. No lesion
√ peak systole < 125 cm/s
√ clear window under systole
√ no evidence of plaque
√ no spectral broadening
B. Minimal Disease
= 0 – 15% diameter reduction
√ peak systole < 125 cm/s
√ clear window under systole
√ minimal plaque
√ minimal spectral broadening in deceleration phase of systole
C. Moderate Disease
= 16 – 49% diameter reduction
√ peak systole < 125 cm/s
√ no window under systole
√ moderate plaque
√ spectral broadening throughout systole
D. Severe Disease = Hemodynamically Significant Lesion
(a) 50 – 79% diameter reduction
√ peak systole > 125 cm/s
√ increased diastolic flow
√ marked spectral broadening throughout cardiac cycle
√ velocity ratio of ICA/CCA > 1.5
(b) 80 – 99% diameter reduction
√ peak systole > 125 cm/s
√ end diastole > 135 cm/s
√ no window under systole
√ spectral broadening throughout systole
E. Occluded Vessel
√ no signal in ICA
√ unilateral flow to zero / flow reversal in CCA
√ increased diastolic flow in ECA (if ECA assumes the role of primary supplier of blood to brain)
√ increase in peak systolic velocities in contralateral ICA (due to collateral flow)

PLAQUE CHARACTERIZATION

A. Homogeneous plaque = stable plaque
Histo: deposition of fatty streaks + fibrous tissue; rarely shows intraplaque hemorrhage / ulcerations
Prognosis:
Δ neurologic deficits develop in 4%
Δ ipsilateral infarction on CT in 12%
Δ ipsilateral symptoms develop in 22%
Δ progressive stenosis develops in 18%
√ homogenous uniform echo pattern with smooth surface

B. Heterogeneous plaque
    = unstable plaque = mixture of high, medium and
    low level echoes with smooth / irregular surface;
    may fissure / tear resulting in intraplaque
    hemorrhage / ulceration + thrombus formation
    (embolus / increasing stenosis)
    B-mode ultrasound has 94% sensitivity, 88%
    specificity, 90% accuracy for intraplaque
    hemorrhage
    Histo: lipid-laden macrophages, monocytes,
    leukocytes, necrotic debris, cholesterol
    crystals, calcifications
    Prognosis:
    Δ neurologic deficits develop in 27%
    Δ ipsilateral infarction on CT in 24%
    Δ ipsilateral symptoms develop in 50%
    Δ progressive stenosis develops in 77%
    √ heterogeneous complex echo pattern

COURSE OF CAROTID ARTERY STENOSIS
    1. Stable stenosis (68%)
    2. Progressive stenosis to > 50% diameter reduction
       (25%)

INDIRECT METHODS OF EVALUATION
    1. Oculoplethysmography (OPG)
       = measurement of ophthalmic artery pressure by air
       calibrated system
       Contraindications: glaucoma, retinal detachment,
       recent eye surgery / trauma, lens
       implants
    2. Periorbital Doppler
       = insonation of frontal + supraorbital arteries to
       assess flow direction around orbit and to detect
       crossover flow through the circle of Willis (through
       contra- and ipsilateral compression)
    3. Transcranial Doppler
       = insonation to establish flow direction in basal
       cerebral arteries through temporal bone (MCA,
       ACA, PCA, terminal portion of ICA), foramen
       magnum (both vertebral arteries, basilar artery),
       orbit (carotid syphon)

Errors in Duplex Ultrasound
    1. Error in localization (6 %)
       Cause: ECA stenosis placed into ICA / carotid
       bifurcation or vice versa
    2. Mistaking patent ECA branches for carotid
       bifurcation (4 %)
       Cause: complete occlusion of ICA not recognized
       √ disparity in position of bifurcation
       √ no difference in pulsatility waveform
       √ high resistance waveform in CCA
    3. Interpreter error in estimating severity of stenosis
       (2.5 %)
       usually overestimation, rarely underestimation
       √ absence of one / more components for diagnosis
       which are

    (a) significant elevation of peak velocity
    (b) poststenotic turbulence
    (c) extension of high velocity into diastole
    4. Superimposition of ECA + ICA (2 %)
       Cause: strict coronal orientation of ECA + ICA
       √ superimposition can be avoided by rotation of
       head to opposite side
    5. Severe stenosis mistaken for occlusion
       minimal flow not detectable; angiogram necessary
       with delayed images
    6. Weak signals misinterpreted as occlusion
    7. Normal / weak signals in severe stenosis
       Cause: severe stenosis causes a decrease in
       blood flow + peak velocity with return to
       normal levels
       √ high resistivity in CCA
    8. Point of maximum frequency shift not identified
       Cause: extremely small lumen / short segment of
       stenosis
       √ unexplained (poststenotic) coarse turbulence
       √ ipsilateral ECA collateral flow
       √ abnormal CCA resistivity
    9. Stenosis obscured by plaque / strong Doppler shift
       in overlying vessel
    10. Inaccessible stenosis
       √ abnormal CCA resistivity
       √ abnormal oculoplethysmography

CAROTID-CAVERNOUS SINUS FISTULA
Etiology: (a)   laceration of ICA within cavernous sinus;
                    usually secondary to basal skull fracture /
                    penetrating trauma
             (b)   rupture of an intracavernous ICA
                    aneurysm
    • chemosis, pulsating exophthalmus, conjunctival edema,
    persistent bruit
    √ focal / diffuse enlargement of cavernous sinus
    √ edematous extraocular muscles
    √ arterial enlargement (pulsating exophthalmus)
    √ dilatation of superior ophthalmic vein / facial veins /
    internal jugular vein
    √ enlarged cavernous sinus
    √ occasionally sellar erosion / enlargement
    √ enlargement of superior orbital fissure (in chronic phase)

CAVERNOUS HEMANGIOMA OF BRAIN
    = CAVERNOUS ANGIOMA = CAVERNOMA = well-
    circumscribed nodule of honeycomb of large sinusoidal
    vascular spaces separated by fibrous collagenous
    bands without intervening neural tissue
Age: 3rd – 6th decade; M > F
    • seizures
Location: cerebrum (mainly subcortical) > pons >
            cerebellum; solitary > multiple
NCCT: √ extensive calcifications = hemangioma
            calcificans (20%)
            √ small round hyperdense region (CLUE)
            √ minimal surrounding edema

CECT: √ minimal / intense enhancement
    √ low attenuation areas due to thrombosed portions
Angio: √ negative ("cryptic / occult vascular malformation" = OCVM)

CEREBELLAR ASTROCYTOMA
2nd most frequent tumor of posterior fossa in children
Incidence: 10 – 20% of pediatric brain tumors
Histo: mostly grade I
Age: children > adults; no specific age peak; M:F = 1:1
Location: cerebellar hemisphere > vermis > tonsils > brainstem
√ uniformly slightly hypodense mass
√ cystic changes: within solid mass / completely cystic process (cyst fluid density > CSF); midline astrocytomas cystic in 50%, hemispheric astrocytomas cystic in 80%
√ enhancement of solid tumor portions ("mural nodule") ± cyst wall
√ calcifications (20%): dense / faint / reticular / punctate / globular
√ may develop extreme hydrocephalus (quite large when finally symptomatic)
Angio: √ avascular
DDx of solid astrocytoma:
(1) medulloblastoma (hyperdense mass, noncalcified)
(2) ependymoma (fourth ventricle, 50% calcify)
DDx of cystic astrocytoma:
(1) hemangioblastoma (lesion < 5 cm)
(2) arachnoid cyst
(3) trapped 4th ventricle
(4) megacisterna magna
(5) Dandy-Walker cyst

CEREBRITIS
= focal area of inflammation within brain substance
CT: √ area of decreased density ± mass effect
    √ no contrast enhancement (initially) / central or patchy enhancement (later)
MRI: √ focal area of increased intensity on T2WI
Cx: brain abscess

CHOROID PLEXUS CYST
= cyst arising from neuroepithelial folds within choroid plexus
Incidence: 0.9 – 3.6% in sonographic population; 50% of autopsied brains; 71% of autopsied fetuses with trisomy 18 have choroid plexus cysts bilaterally > 10 mm in diameter
Histo: no epithelial lining, filled with clear fluid
may be associated with trisomy 18
• usually asymptomatic
√ round anechoic cyst, frequently at level of atrium
√ usually 2 – 8 mm in size
Cx: hydrocephalus (if large)
Prognosis: usually disappear by 28th week; may persist; in 95% of no significance; risk of trisomy 18 is lower than risk of fetal loss with amniocentesis

CHOROID PLEXUS PAPILLOMA
Incidence: < 1% of all primary CNS tumors; 3 – 5% of brain tumors in childhood; 0.6 % of brain tumors in adults
Age: 20 – 40% < 1 year of age; 86% < 5 years of age; middle age; in 75% < 2 years of age
Location: (a) trigone of lateral ventricles, most common on L side (children)
    (b) 4th ventricle + cerebellopontine angle (adults)
    (c) multiple in 7%
√ asymmetric diffuse ventricular dilatation (CSF overproduction)
√ large mass with smooth lobulated border
√ intrinsically hyperdense with intense homogeneous enhancement on CECT
√ small foci of calcifications (common)
√ engulfment of glomus of choroid plexus (distinctive feature)
√ echogenic mass adjacent to normal choroid plexus
√ supplied by anterior + posterior choroidal arteries
Cx: (1) transformation into malignant choroid plexus papilloma
    (2) hydrocephalus (in children) secondary to increased intracranial pressure from CSF-overproduction
Rx: surgical removal (24% operative mortality)
DDx: intraventricular meningioma, ependymoma, metastasis, cavernous angioma, xanthogranuloma, astrocytoma

COCKAYNE SYNDROME
= autosomal recessive diffuse demyelinating disease
Age: beginning at age 1
• dwarfism
• progressive physical + mental deterioration
√ brain atrophy / microcephaly
√ calcifications in basal ganglia + cerebellum

COLLOID CYST
= 2% of glial tumors of ependymal origin; < 1% of CNS tumors
Histo: ciliated + columnar epithelium; mucin-secreting; squamous cells of ependymal origin; tough fibrous capsule
Age: young adults;   M > F
Location: exclusively arising from inferior aspect of septum pellucidum protruding into anterior portion of 3rd ventricle between columns of fornix
• positional headaches (transient obstruction secondary to ball valve mechanism at foramen of Monro)
• gait apraxia
• change in mental status ± dementia (related to increased intracranial pressure)
• papilledema (may become medical emergency with acute herniation)
√ ± sellar erosion

√ spherical iso- / hyperdense lesion on NCCT with smooth surface

√ fluid contents:
(a) in 20% similar to CSF (= isodense)
(b) in 80% mucinous fluid, proteinaceous debris, hemosiderin, desquamated cells (= hyperdense)

√ may show enhancement of border (draped choroid plexus / capsule)

√ 3rd ventricular enlargement (to accommodate cyst anteriorly)

√ asymmetric lateral ventricular enlargement (invariable)

√ occasionally widens septum pellucidum

MRI: √ hyperintense lesion on short TR sequences

DDx: meningioma, ependymoma of 3rd ventricle (rare) with enhancement

CONTUSION OF BRAIN

Incidence: in 21% of head trauma patients; children:adults = 2:1

Path: tissue necrosis, capillary disruption, petechial hemorrhage followed by liquefaction + edema after 4 – 7 days

Mechanism: acceleration-deceleration forces
1. **Coup** = impact on stationary brain
2. **Contrecoup** = impact of moving brain on stationary calvarium
   Location: common in frontal, particularly supraorbital, temporal, occipital region at apices of cerebral gyri with variable extension into white matter
3. **White matter shearing injury** = Diffuse impact injury with rotational forces = cortex and deep structures move at different speed resulting in shearing stress along the course of white matter tracts especially at gray-white matter junction with axonal tears followed by wallerian degeneration
   Location: corpus callosum, internal capsule, basal ganglia, thalamus, upper brain stem, cerebellar peduncles, corticomedullary junction

• confusion
• focal cerebral dysfunction
• seizures, personality changes
• focal neurologic deficits (late changes)

CT: (often not visualized by CT)
√ focal / multiple (29%) poorly defined areas of irregular contour + inhomogeneous increased density (hemorrhage) + surrounding edema
√ isodense after 2 – 3 weeks
√ some degree of contrast enhancement (leaking new capillaries)

MRI: (best modality to demonstrate exact extent of hemorrhagic contusional involvement even relatively late after trauma)
√ initially decreased intensity (deoxyhemoglobin of acute hemorrhage) surrounded by hyperintense edema on T2WI
√ later high intensity on T2WI secondary to Met-Hb

Cx: (1) encephalomalacia (= scarred brain)
(2) porencephaly (= formation of cystic cavity lined with gliotic brain and communicating with ventricles / subarachnoid space)

Prognosis: poor

CRANIOPHARYNGIOMA

Incidence: 4% of all intracranial neoplasms; 7% of all intracranial childhood tumors; most common suprasellar mass

Origin: from remnants of Rathke pouch

Path: benign tumor originating from neuroepithelium from craniopharyngeal duct + primitive buccal epithelium

Age: from birth – 7th decade; age peak in childhood + adolescence (75%); in adulthood (25%)

• diabetes insipidus (compression of pituitary gland)
• growth retardation (compresssion of hypothalamus)
• bitemporal hemianopsia (compression of optic nerve chiasm)
• headaches from hydrocephalus (compression of foramen of Monro / aqueduct of Sylvius)

Location:
(a) pituitary stalk / tuber cinereum
(b) suprasellar (20%)
(c) intrasellar (10%)
(d) intra- and suprasellar (70%)

ECTOPIC CRANIOPHARYNGIOMA
(e) floor of anterior 3rd ventricle (more common in adults)
(f) sphenoid bone

Skull films:
√ normal sella (25%)
√ enlarged J-shaped sella with truncated dorsum
√ thickening + increased density of lamina dura in floor of sella (10%)
√ extensive sellar destruction (75%)
√ curvilinear / flocculent / stippled calcifications / lamellar ossification; calcifications seen in youth in 70 – 80%, in adults in 30 – 40%

CT:
√ frequently marginal hyperdense lesion (calcification / ossification) in 100%
√ solid (15%) / mixed (30%) / cystic lesion (54 – 75%) (cystic appearance secondary to cholesterol, keratin, necrotic debris with higher density than CSF)
√ enhancement of solid lesion, peripheral enhancement of cystic lesion
√ ± obstructive hydrocephalus

MRI: (relatively ineffective in demonstrating calcifications)
√ hyper- / iso- / hypointense on T1WI (variable secondary to hemorrhage / cholesterol-containing proteinaceous fluid)
√ markedly hyperintense on T2WI
√ marginal enhancement of solid components with gadopentetate dimeglumine

Angio:
√ usually avascular
√ lateral displacement, elevation, narrowing of supraclinoid segment of ICA

√ posterior displacement of basilar artery

CYSTICERCOSIS OF BRAIN

larva of pork tape worm (taenia solium) frequently involving CNS, muscles, heart, fat tissue
Incidence: CNS involvement in up to 90%
Location: meninges (39%) esp. in basal cisterns, parenchyma (20%), intraventricular (17%), mixed (23%), intraspinal (1%)
A. Acute phase (= focal meningoencephalitis)
   • focal seizures
   √ single / multiple small focal enhancing lesions; transitory with resolution in a few months
   √ diffusely edematous white matter
   √ homogeneously enhancing small nodules often with extensive edema (DDx: metastases without edema)
B. Chronic phase (= involution with subsequent calcification + cyst formation)
   √ small focal calcifications (= probably dead larvae); may appear within 8 months – 10 years after acute infection along gray-white matter junction
   √ well-defined cystic areas of CSF density (= racemose cysts) without associated edema (= living larvae)
   √ "rice-like" muscle calcifications rarely visible
Cx: hydrocephalus (secondary to dense ependymal + arachnoid adhesions / intraventricular cysts)

DANDY-WALKER SYNDROME

= congenital atresia of foramina of **L**uschka (**l**ateral) + **M**agendie (**me**dian) characterized by (1) hydrocephalus (2) posterior fossa cyst (3) cystic dilatation of 4th ventricle (4) variable dysplasia of cerebellar vermis
Incidence: 12% of all congenital hydrocephaly
Path: defect in vermis connecting an ependyma-lined retrocerebellar cyst with 4th ventricle (PATHOGNOMONIC)
associated midline abnormalities: (> 60%)
   (1) agenesis of corpus callosum (7 – 25%), lipoma of corpus callosum
   (2) holoprosencephaly (25%)
   (3) malformation of cerebral gyri (dysplasia of cingulate gyrus) (25%)
   (4) cerebellar heterotopia + malformation of cerebellar folia (25%)
   (5) malformation of inferior olivary nucleus
   (6) hamartoma of tuber cinereum
   (7) syringomyelia
   (8) cleft palate
   (9) polydactyly
Skull film:
   √ large skull secondary to hydrocephalus + dolichocephaly
   √ diastatic lambdoid suture
   √ disproportionately large expanded posterior fossa
   √ torcular Herophili and lateral sinuses high above lambdoid angle = torcular-lambdoid inversion
CT / US / MRI:
   √ hypoplasia / absence of cerebellar vermis: total (25%), partial (75%)

√ superiorly displaced superior vermis cerebelli
√ small + widely separated cerebellar hemispheres
√ anterior + lateral displacement of ± hypoplastic cerebellar hemispheres
√ large posterior fossa cyst with extension through foramen magnum = diverticulum of roofless 4th ventricle
√ elevated insertion of tentorium cerebelli
√ absence of falx cerebelli
√ scalloping of petrous pyramids
√ hydrocephalus (in 72% open communication with 3rd ventricle; in 39% patent 4th ventricle; in 28% aqueductal stenosis; in 11 % incisural obstruction); usually develops over time but may be present at birth
√ anterior displacement of pons
Angio:
   √ high position of transverse sinus
   √ elevated great vein of Galen
   √ elevated posterior cerebral vessels
   √ anterosuperiorly displaced superior cerebellar arteries above the posterior cerebral arteries
   √ small / absent PICA with high tonsillar loop
Cx: trapping of cyst above tentorium = "keyhole configuration"
Prognosis: 22 – 50% mortality
DDx: posterior fossa extraaxial cyst, arachnoid cyst, isolated 4th ventricle, giant cisterna magna, porencephaly

DANDY-WALKER VARIANT

= large posterior fossa cyst + partially formed 4th ventricle; more common than Dandy-Walker malformation
√ 4th ventricle smaller + better formed
√ retrocerebellar cyst smaller
√ communication between retrocerebellar cyst and subarachnoid space through a patent foramen of Magendie may be present
√ posterior fossa smaller than in usual Dandy-Walker syndrome

DERMOID OF BRAIN

= pilosebaceous mass lined with skin appendages
Incidence: 0.1% of all CNS tumors
Path: ectodermal + mesodermal lesion = squamous epithelium, mesodermal cells (hair follicles, sweat + sebaceous glands)
Age: < 30 years (appears in adulthood secondary to slow growth); M < F
Location: predilection for midline
   (a) posterior fossa (most common)
   (b) base of brain (inferior frontal, parasellar, vermian)
• bouts of chemical / bacterial meningitis possible
√ thick-walled inhomogeneous mass with focal areas of fat
√ mural / central calcifications / bone (possible)

√ may have sinus tract to skin surface (dermal sinus)
√ fat-fluid level if cyst ruptures into ventricles
√ NO contrast enhancement

DIFFUSE SCLEROSIS
sporadic, young adults, fulminant course
• dementia, deafness
√ low attenuation regions in both hemispheres without symmetry

DYKE-DAVIDOFF-MASON SYNDROME
= atrophy of one hemisphere + skull
• seizures
• hemiparesis
• mental retardation
Age: presents in adolescence
√ unilateral thickening of skull
√ unilateral decrease in size of cranial fossa
√ unilateral overdevelopment of sinuses
√ contraction of a hemisphere / lobe
√ compensatory enlargement of adjacent ventricle + sulci with midline shift

EMPTY SELLA SYNDROME
= extension of subarachnoid space into sella turcica which becomes exposed to CSF pulsations secondary to defect in diaphragma sellae; characterized by normal / molded pituitary gland + normal or enlarged sella configuration (empty sella = misnomer)
Incidence: 24% in autopsy study
A.   PRIMARY EMPTY SELLA (anatomic spectrum)
     Incidence: 10% of adult population; M:F = 1:4
     Probable causes:
        (1) pituitary enlargement followed by regression during pregnancy
        (2) involution of a pituitary tumor
        (3) congenital weakness of diaphragma sellae occurs more frequently in patients with increased intracranial pressure
     • usually asymptomatic
     • increased risk for CSF rhinorrhea
     • NO endocrine abnormalities
B.   SECONDARY EMPTY SELLA
     = postsurgical when diaphragma sellae has been disrupted
     • visual disturbance
     • headaches

√ slowly progressive symmetrical / asymmetrical (double floor) enlargement of sella
√ remodeled lamina dura remains mineralized
√ small rim of pituitary tissue displaced posteriorly + inferiorly
√ infundibulum sign = infundibulum extends to floor of sella
DDx: cystic tumor, large herniated 3rd ventricle (displaced infundibulum)

EMPYEMA OF CNS
A. SUBDURAL EMPYEMA
   20% of all intracranial bacterial infections
   Cause: paranasal sinusitis, otitis media, calvarial osteomyelitis, infection after craniotomy or ventricular shunt placement, penetrating wound, contamination of meningitis-induced subdural effusion
   Location: frontal + inferior cranial space in close proximity to paranasal sinuses; 80 % over convexity extending into interhemispheric fissure or posterior fossa
   √ hypo- / isodense crescentic / lentiform zone adjacent to inner table
   √ may show mass effect (sulcal effacement, ventricular compression, shift)
   √ thin curvilinear rim of enhancement (7 – 10 days later) adjacent to brain
   √ severe sinusitis / mastoiditis (may be most significant indicator)
   Mortality: 30% (neurosurgical emergency)
   Cx: venous thrombosis, infarction, seizures, hemiparesis, hemianopsia, aphasia, brain abscess
   DDx: subacute / chronic subdural hematoma

B. EPIDURAL EMPYEMA
   same causes as above
   No neurologic deficits (dura minimizes pressure exerted on brain)
   √ thick enhancing rim

ENCEPHALITIS
= term generally reserved for diffuse inflammatory process of viral etiology
√ diffuse mild cerebral edema
√ small infarctions / hemorrhage (less frequent)

Herpes Simplex Encephalitis (HSE)
= most common cause of nonepidemic necrotizing meningoencephalitis in USA
Organism: HSV type I (in adults); HSV type II (in neonates from transplacental infection)
• confusion, disorientation
• preceding viral syndrome, fever, headache, seizures
Location: temporal > frontal > parietal lobes
CT: (principal role is to identify biopsy site)
   √ may be negative in first 3 days
   √ poorly defined bilateral areas of decreased attenuation
   √ spared putamen forms sharply defined concave / straight border (DDx: infarction, glioma)
   √ compression of lateral ventricles, sylvian fissure (brain edema)
   √ patchy peripheral / gyral / cisternal enhancement (50%), may persist for several months
   √ tendeny for hemorrhage + rapid dissemination in brain

MRI:
√ increased signal intensity on T2WI
NUC:
√ characteristic increased activity in temporal lobes on brain scan
Dx: fluorescin antibody staining / viral culture from brain biopsy
Mortality: 70%
Rx: adenine arabinoside
DDx: low-grade glioma, infarct, abscess

ENCEPHALOCELE

= failure of surface ectoderm to separate from neuroectoderm early in embryonic development characterized by herniation of cerebral tissue + meninges through a cranial bone defect
Incidence: 1 – 4 per 10,000 live births
associated with:
(1) Spina bifida (7 – 30%)
(2) Corpus callosum dysgenesis
(3) Chiari malformation
(4) Meckel-Gruber syndrome (= encephalocele + microcephaly + polycystic kidneys + polydactyly)
(5) Amniotic band syndrome: multiple irregular asymmetric encephaloceles
• alpha-fetoprotein in amniotic fluid usually elevated
Location:
(1) occipital (75%): external mass
(2) sincipital (15%): external mass near dorsum of nose, orbits, forehead (more frequent in Asian population)
(3) basal (10%): internal mass in upper nasal cavity, epipharynx, sphenomaxillary fossa
(4) occasionally eccentric frontal / parietal encephaloceles (mostly parasagittal)
√ cranium bifidum = cranioschisis = "split cranium" (= skull defect)
√ hydrocephalus in 15 – 80% (from associated aqueductal stenosis, Arnold-Chiari malformation, Dandy Walker cyst)
√ nonenhancing expansile homogeneous paracranial mass
√ mantle of cerebral tissue often difficult to image in encephalocele
√ intracranial communication often not visualized
√ metrizamide / radionuclide ventriculography diagnostic
√ microcephaly (20%)
√ polyhydramnios
DDx: may be impossible to differentiate from mucocele

EPENDYMOMA

= in majority benign slow-growing neoplasm of mature well-differentiated ependymal cells lining the ventricles
Incidence: 6% of all intracranial gliomas; 8 – 10% of childhood brain tumors; 63% of spinal intramedullary gliomas
Histo: perivascular pseudorosettes of tumor cells; may have papillary pattern (difficult DDx from choroid plexus papilloma)

Age: (a) supratentorial: at any age (atrium / foramen of Monro)
(b) posterior fossa: < 10 years; age peaks at 5 and 34 years; M:F = 0.8:1
associated with: neurofibromatosis
Location:
(a) 4th ventricle (70% of all intracranial ependymomas), lateral, 3rd ventricle
(b) conus (40% of all spinal intramedullary gliomas)
√ sharply marginated multilobulated iso- / slightly hyperdense mass
√ small cystic areas in 50% (central necrosis)
√ thin well-defined low-attenuation halo (distended effaced 4th ventricle)
√ fine punctate calcifications (50%)
√ heterogeneous / moderately uniform enhancement of solid portions (80%) + edema
√ frequently grows into brain parenchyma extending to cortical surface (particularly in frontal + parietal lobes)
√ direct invasion of brain stem / cerebellum (35%)
√ expansion frequently through foramen of Luschka into cerebellopontine angle or caudad into cisterna magna (CHARACTERISTIC)
√ communicating hydrocephalus (100%) secondary to protein exudate elaborated by tumor clogging resorption pathways
MRI:
√ low to intermediate signal intensity on T1WI
√ high signal intensity on T2WI
√ signal voids with calcifications
Cx: dissemination via CSF (10 – 33%)
Rx: surgery + radiation (partially radiosensitive) + chemotherapy
DDx of cerebellar ependymoma:
(1) astrocytoma (hypodense, displaces 4th ventricle from midline, cystic lucency)
(2) medulloblastoma (hyperdense, calcifications in only 10%)
(3) trapped 4th ventricle (no contrast enhancement)

EPIDERMOID OF CNS

Incidence: < 1% of all intracranial neoplasms; most common congenital intracranial tumor
Etiology: ectodermal lesion = inclusion of epithelial elements within neural groove
Path: lined by stratified squamous epithelium becoming cystic by progressive desquamation of keratinized debris + cholesterol crystals = PRIMARY / CONGENITAL CHOLESTEATOMA
Age: 10 – 60 years; M:F = 1:1
Location: (may be intra- / extradural)
(a) cerebellopontine angle (most common)
(b) suprasellar region (common)
(c) medial aspect of middle fossa
(d) petrous apex
(e) skull vault
√ soft infiltrating lesion surrounding vessels + cranial nerves

√ little mass effect, no edema / hydrocephalus
√ typically round low density mass without enhancement
√ bony erosion with sharply defined well-corticated margins
√ calcification (1%)
√ angiographically avascular
√ papillary / frondlike surface on cisternography

EPIDURAL HEMATOMA OF BRAIN

= EXTRADURAL HEMATOMA = within potential space between naked inner table + calvarial periosteum (dura layer) which is bound down at suture margins

Incidence: 2% of all serious head injuries; in < 1% of all children with cranial trauma; uncommon in infants

associated with: skull fracture in 40 – 85% (best demonstrated on radiograph)

Mechanism of injury:
   (a) laceration of dural vessels adjacent to inner table from fracture of calvarium (91%)
   (b) avulsion of venous vessels from points of calvarial perforations
   (c) disruption of dural venous sinuses (major cause in younger children)
• transient loss of consciousness
• lucent interval
• 3rd nerve palsy (sign of cerebral herniation)
• somnolence (24 – 96 hours after accident): medical emergency !

Types:
I   acute epidural hematoma   (58%) from arterial bleeding
II   subacute hematoma   (31%)
III   chronic hematoma   (11%) from venous bleeding

Location:
   (a) in 66% temporoparietal (most often from laceration of middle meningeal artery)
   (b) in 29% at frontal pole, parieto-occipital region, between occipital lobes, posterior fossa (most often from laceration of venous sinuses)

CT:
   √ fracture line in area of epidural hematoma
   √ biconvex elliptical extraaxial fluid collection (most frequent) = under high pressure
   √ high density in acute stage (60 – 90 HU)
   √ mass effect ("compression cone effect") with effacement of gyri + sulci from:
      √ epidural hematoma (57%)
      √ hemorrhagic contusion (29%)
      √ cerebral edematous swelling (14%)
   √ venous sinuses displaced away from inner table of skull
   √ marked stretching of vessels
   √ signs of arterial injury (rare): contrast extravasation, arteriovenous fistula, middle meningeal artery occlusion, formation of false aneurysm

Angio:
   √ meningeal arteries displaced away from inner table of skull
Rx: after surgical evacuation return of ventricular system to midline
DDx: Chronic subdural hematoma (may have similar shape as acute epidural hematoma)

GLIOMA

growth along white matter tracts, tendency to increase in grade with time; may be multifocal

CELL OF ORIGIN
   1. Astrocyte   ...Astrocytoma
   2. Oligodendrocyte ...Oligodendroglioma
   3. Ependym   ...Ependymoma
   4. Medulloblast   ...Medulloblastoma
                        (PNET = permeative neuroectodermal tumor)
   5. Choroid plexus   ...Choroid plexus papilloma

FREQUENCY OF INTRACRANIAL GLIOMAS
   Glioblastoma multiforme   51%
   Astrocytoma   25%
   Ependymoma   6%
   Oligodendroglioma   6%
   Spongioblastoma polare   3%
   Mixed gliomas   3%
   Astroblastoma   2%

Location: (a) central white matter of cerebrum (adults); 15 – 30% of all gliomas
            (b) cerebellar hemisphere + brainstem (children)
Contrast enhancement:
   Δ increases in proportion to degree of anaplasia
   Δ diminished intensity of enhancement with steroid therapy

A.   LOW-GRADE GLIOMAS (Grade I / II) = ASTROCYTOMA
     Age: 25 – 45 years; M > F
     Histo: histologically benign, nonmetastasizing; blood-brain barrier may remain intact; no significant tumor vascularity
        Location: cerebral hemisphere, thalamus, pons, midbrain
     CT:
        √ usually hypodense lesion with minimal mass effect + NO peritumeral edema
        √ well-defined tumor margins
        √ central calcifications (frequent)
        √ minimal / no contrast enhancement (normal capillary endothelial cells)
     Angio: √ majority avascular

B.   HIGH-GRADE GLIOMAS (Grade III / IV) = GLIOBLASTOMA MULTIFORME

Age: 35 – 55 years; M > F
Histo: histologically malignant; neovascularity, frequently hemorrhagic + necrotic
Dissemination: along CSF pathways / hematogenous
Location: hemisphere
CT:
√ contrast enhancement (breakdown of blood-brain barrier / neovascularity / areas of necrosis)
   (a) diffuse homogeneous enhancement
   (b) nonhomogeneous enhancement
   (c) ring pattern (occasionally enhancing mass within the ring)
   (d) low-density lesion with contrast fluid level (leakage of contrast)
Angio:
√ avascular / vascular lesion

Glioblastoma Multiforme

= most common primary brain tumor; 50% of all intracranial gliomas; most malignant form of astrocytoma (Grade IV); results from severe anaplasia of preexisting Grade I / II astrocytoma
Age: all ages; peak incidence at 45 – 55 years; M:F = 3:2
Location: frontal > temporal lobes, basal ganglia, corpus callosum ("butterfly"), thalamus, quadrigeminal region, pons, rarely in cerebellum
Spread:
follows white matter tracts into corpus callosum (36%); readily crosses midline = "butterfly" glioma (clue: invasion of septum pellucidum); frontal + temporal gliomas tend to invade basal ganglia; may invade pia, arachnoid and dura (mimicking meningioma); may reach subependymal surface of ventricles (subependymal carpet)
NECT:
√ inhomogeneous low-density mass with irregular shape + poorly defined margins (hypodense solid tumor / cavitary necrosis / tumor cyst / peritumoral edema)
√ compression + displacement of ventricles, cisterns, brain parenchyma
√ iso- / hyperdense portions (hemorrhage) in 5%
√ rarely calcifies (if coexistent with lower grade glioma / after radio- or chemotherapy)
CECT:
√ almost always ring blush of variable thickness: multiscalloped ("garland"), round / ovoid; may be seen surrounding ventricles (subependymal spread)
√ sedimentation level secondary to cellular debris / hemorrhage / accumulated contrast material in tumoral cyst
Angio:
√ neovascularity + early draining veins

Oligodendroglioma

= uncommon form of slowly growing glioma; presenting with large size at time of diagnosis
Incidence: 2 – 10% of intracranial gliomas
Histo: mixed glial cells (50%), astrocytic components (30%)
Age: 30 – 55 years
Location: most commonly in cerebral hemispheres (propensity for periphery of frontal lobes) involving cortex + white matter, thalamus, corpus callosum; rare in cerebellum + spinal cord
√ round / oval hypodense lesion with mass effect (75%)
√ large nodular clumps of calcifications (in 45% on plain film; in 90% on CT)
√ commonly no / minimal tumor enhancement (75%), pronounced in high grade tumors
√ may be adherent to dura (mimicking meningiomas)
√ cystic changes (very common)
√ edema (in 50% of low-grade, in 80% of high-grade tumors)
Cx: malignant metaplasia
DDx:
   (1) Astrocytoma (no large calcifications)
   (2) Ganglioglioma (in temporal lobes + deep cerebral tissues)
   (3) Ependymoma (enhancing tumor, often with internal bleeding producing fluid levels)
   (4) Glioblastoma (infiltrating, enhancing, edema, no calcifications)

Hypothalamic Glioma

= astrocytoma in infants
• obese child
• sexual precocity
• marked emaciation
• euphoria, unusual alertness
• diabetes insipidus
• hyperactivity
√ suprasellar mass with dense enhancement; thalamus usually involved
√ obstructive hydrocephalus

Pontine Glioma

Incidence: 1%; 12 – 15% of all pediatric brain tumors
Histo: usually anaplastic astrocytoma / glioblastoma multiforme
Age: in children + young adults; peak age 3 – 13 years; M:F = 1:1
• become clinically apparent early before ventricular obstruction occurs
• ipsilateral progressive cranial nerve palsies
• contralateral hemiparesis
• eventually respiratory insufficiency
Location: pons > midbrain > medulla; often unilateral at medullopontine junction
   Δ medullary + mesencephalic are more benign than pontine gliomas

Growth pattern:
(a) diffuse infiltration of brain stem with symmetric expansion + rostrocaudal spread into medulla / thalamus + spread to cerebellum
(b) focally exophytic growth into adjacent cisterns
CT:
√ asymmetrically expanded brainstem
√ isodense / hypodense mass with indistinct margins
√ ± hyperdense foci (hemorrhage)
√ flattening + posterior displacement of 4th ventricle + aqueduct of Sylvius
√ compression of prepontine + interpeduncular cistern (in upward transtentorial herniation)
√ absent / minimal / patchy contrast enhancement (50%)
√ ring enhancement in necrotic / cystic tumors (most aggressive)
√ prominent enhancement in exophytic lesion
√ hydrocephalus uncommon (because of early symptomatology)
Angio:
√ anterior displacement of basilar artery + anterior pontomesencephalic vein
√ posterior displacement of precentral cerebellar vein
√ posterior displacement of posterior medullary + supratonsillar segments of PICA
√ lateral displacement of lateral medullary segment of PICA
MRI: (better evaluation in subtle cases) isointense on T1WI, hyperintense on T2WI
Rx: radiation therapy
DDx: focal encephalitis, hematoma, metastasis, lymphoma, granuloma, infarct, vascular malformation, multiple sclerosis

GLOBOID CELL LEUKODYSTROPHY
= KRABBE DISEASE = deficiency of beta-galactocerebrosidase leading to cerebroside accumulation
√ low-density white matter lesions
√ brain atrophy with enlargement of ventricles
Prognosis: fatal by age 2

GLOMUS TUMOR
= CHEMODECTOMA = NON-CHROMAFFIN PARAGANGLIOMA
Origin: tumor arising from nonchromaffin paraganglion cells of neuroectodermal origin; differs from adrenal medulla only in its nonchromaffin feature
Path: histologically similar to pheochromocytoma, storage of catecholamines (usually nonfunctioning)
associated with: pheochromocytoma
Age: range of 6 months – 80 years; peak age in 5 – 6th decade; F : M = 4 : 1
Location:
anywhere in paraganglionic tissue between glomus jugulotympanicum and base of bladder: carotid body,

skull base, temporal region, trachea, periaortic region, mandible, ciliary ganglion of the eye, retroperitoneal region, cervical vagus nerve, laryngeal branches of vagus nerve
multiple in 10%: (a) autosomal dominant in 25 – 35%
(b) non-hereditary in < 5%

Glomus Tympanicum
most common tumor in middle ear
• hearing loss, bruit, reddish purple mass behind tympanic membrane
Location: on cochlear promontory
CT: √ high attenuation with high uptake of iodine
√ erosion + displacement of ossicles
√ usually small at presentation (early involvement of ossicles)
Angio: √ difficult to visualize because of small size

Glomus Jugulare
most common tumor in jugular fossa with intracranial extension
Origin: adventitia of jugular bulb
• tinnitus, hearing loss
Location: at dome of jugular bulb
√ destruction of posteroinferior petrous pyramid + corticojugular spine
√ soft tissue mass in jugular bulb region / hypotympanicum / middle ear space
√ destruction of ossicles (usually incus), otic capsule, posteromedial surface of petrous bone
MRI:
√ "salt and pepper" appearance due to multiple small tumor vessels
Angio: (filming of entire neck for concurrent glomus tumors)
√ hypervascular mass with persistent homogeneous reticular stain
√ invasion / occlusion of jugular bulb by thrombus / tumor
√ supplied by tympanic branch of ascending pharyngeal artery, meningeal branch of occipital artery, posterior auricular artery via stylomastoid branch, internal carotid artery, internal maxillary artery
√ arteriovenous shunting
Cx: malignant transformation with metastases to regional lymph nodes (in 2 – 4%)

Glomus Vagale
Origin: near ganglion nodosum of vagus nerve at base of skull close to jugular foramen
Extension (a) downward into parapharyngeal space (2/3)
(b) intracranially (dumbbell-shape)
• slow-growing + asymptomatic
√ spherical / ovoid mass with sharp interfacing margins and homogeneous enhancement
√ highly vascular mass + neovascularity + intense tumor blush

Cx: malignant transformation with metastases in 15% to regional lymph nodes + lung (other paragangliomas in 10%)

Carotid Body Tumor
Location: carotid bifurcation; bilateral in 3%
- painless pulsatile firm neck mass
√ splaying of ICA + ECA
Cx: malignant transformation in 6%

HAMARTOMA OF CNS
Age: 0 – 30 years
Location: temporal lobe
√ cyst with little mass effect, possibly with focal calcifications
√ usually no enhancement

HEMANGIOBLASTOMA OF CNS
benign autosomal dominant tumor; 2% of all intracranial neoplasms; multiple lesions in 10%
Age: (a) adulthood (common): average age of 33 years; M > F
(b) childhood: in von Hippel-Lindau disease (10%); girls
associated with:
(a) von Hippel-Lindau disease, may have multiple hemangioblastomas (only 20% of patients show other stigmata)
(b) pheochromocytoma (often familial)
(c) syringomyelia
(d) spinal cord hemangioblastomas
- erythrocytemia in 20% (stimulant elaborated by tumor)
Location: cerebellar hemisphere > spinal cord > cerebral hemisphere
√ cystic sharply marginated mass of CSF-density (2/3)
√ peripheral mural nodule with homogeneous enhancement (50%)
√ occasionally enhancement of cyst wall
√ solid tumor (1/3)
√ almost never calcifies
Angio: √ densely stained tumor nidus within cyst ("contrast loading")
√ staining of entire rim of cyst
DDx: (1) astrocytoma (> 5 cm, calcifications, no angiographic contrast blush of mural nodule, no erythrocytemia)
(2) Metastasis

HEMATOMA OF BRAIN
Etiology:
1. Aneurysm (36%)
2. Hypertension (36%):
Age: > 60 years; often large hemorrhage located in basal ganglia (putamen in 50%) / thalamus (25%), pons + brainstem (10%), cerebellum (10%), cerebral hemisphere (5%)
3. AVM (11%)

4. Trauma
(a) blunt / penetrating trauma (bullet, icepick, skull fragment)
(b) brain contusion — coup and contrecoup lesions — white matter shearing injury
5. Bleeding into tumor (e.g. metastasis, glioma)
6. Hypocoagulable state
7. Hemorrhagic infarction
Sequelae of trauma:
1. Posttraumatic hydrocephalus (1/3)
= obstruction of CSF pathways secondary to intracranial hemorrhage; develops within 3 months
2. Generalized cerebral atrophy (1/3)
= result of ischemia + hypoxia
3. Encephalomalacia
√ focal areas of decreased density, but usually higher density than CSF
4. Pseudoporencephaly
= CSF-filled space communicating with ventricle / subarachnoid space from cystic degeneration
5. Subdural hygroma
= localized collection of CSF in subdural space secondary to (a) result of chronic subdural hematoma (b) arachnoidal tear acting as a ball valve
Age: most often in elderly + young children
√ may resolve spontaneously
6. Leptomeningeal cyst
= progressive protrusion of leptomeninges through traumatic calvarial defect
7. Cerebrospinal fluid leak
- rhinorrhea, otorrhea (indicating basilar fracture with meningeal tear)
8. Carotid-cavernous fistula
9. Traumatic pseudoaneurysm
= excavated encapsulated hematoma communicating with arterial lumen
Location: branches of ACA + MCA, intracavernous portion of ICA, PCom
10. Posttraumatic abscess
secondary to (a) penetrating injury (b) basilar skull fracture (c) infection of traumatic hematoma
11. Vascular compression
compression of PCA against tentorial margin secondary to uncal herniation leads to infarction of PCA territory

Stages of cerebral hematomas
Resolution: resorption from outside toward the center; rate depends on size of hematoma (usually 1 – 6 weeks)
FALSE-NEGATIVE CT:
1. impaired clotting
2. anemia
√ iso- / hypodense stage

Acute hemorrhage
Time period: < 24 hrs.

MRI APPEARANCE OF HEMORRHAGE

	T1	T2	
Oxyhemoglobin	high	high	hyperacute bleed in < 1 hr.
Deoxyhemoglobin			deoxygenation
intracellular	iso	low	within intact hypoxic RBCs
extracellular	iso	iso	after lysis of RBCs
Methemoglobin			oxidation
intracellular	high	low	after 3 - 4 days in intact RBCs
extracellular	high	high	may be present for months to years
Hemosiderin	low	low	within macrophages present for years
Fibrous tissue	low	low	
Serous fluid	iso	high	
Edema	iso	high	

NCCT:
√ homogeneous consolidated high-density lesion with irregular well-defined margins increasing in density during day 1 – 3 (hematoma attenuation dependent on hemoglobin concentration + rate of clot retraction)
√ usually surrounded by low attenuation (edema, contusion) appearing within 24 – 48 hours
(a) irregular shape in trauma
(b) spherical + solitary in spontaneous hemorrhage
√ less mass effect compared with neoplasms
MRI:
√ center of hematoma isointense on T1WI + markedly hypointense on T2WI (= deoxygenation of blood clot forms paramagnetic deoxy-hemoglobin in intact hypoxic RBCs, dependent on degree of surrounding oxygen tension)
√ surrounding tissue isointense on T1WI / hyperintense on T2WI (edema)

Subacute hemorrhage
Time period: days – 1 month
NCCT:
√ increase in size of hemorrhagic area over days / weeks
√ high density lesion within 1st week; often with layering
√ gradual decrease in density from periphery inwards (1 – 2 HU per day) during 2nd + 3rd week
√ isodense hematoma from 3rd – 10th week with perilesional ring of lucency
CECT:
√ peripheral rim enhancement at inner border of perilesional lucency (1 – 6 weeks after injury) in 80% (secondary to blood-brain barrier breakdown / luxury perfusion / formation of hypervascular granulation tissue)
√ ring blush may be diminished by administration of corticosteroids

MRI:
√ center of hematoma isointense on T1WI , moderately hypointense onT2WI
√ periphery hyperintense on T1WI, hyperintense on T2WI (= progressive conversion of deoxy-hemoglobin to methemoglobin after 3 – 4 days)
√ rim isointense on T1WI, markedly hypointense on T2WI (= paramagnetic hemosiderin phagocytized by macrophages appearing during 2nd week; present for years)
√ surrounding edema isointense on T1WI + hyperintense on T2WI

Chronic hemorrhage
Time period: 1 month – years
CT:
√ hypodense phase (4 – 6 weeks) secondary to fluid uptake by osmosis
√ decreased density (3 – 6 months) / invisible
√ after 10 weeks lucent hematoma with ring blush (DDx: tumor)
MRI:
√ center hyperintense on T1WI + T2WI (= extracellular methemoglobin of lysed RBCs, present for months to 1 year)
√ periphery hyperintense on T1WI + T2WI
√ rim isointense on T1WI + hypointense on T2WI; rim gradually increases over weeks in thickness, eventually fills in entire hematoma (= hemosiderin laden macrophages) = HALLMARK

HETEROTOPIC GRAY MATTER
= presence of cortical neurons in an abnormal location secondary to arrest of migrating neuroblasts from ventricular walls to brain surface between 7 – 24 weeks of GA
Frequency: 3% of healthy population
may be associated with: agenesis of corpus callosum, aqueductal stenosis, microcephaly, schizencephaly
• seizures

Location: (a) nodular form: usually symmetric bilateral periventricular with predilection for posterior + anterior horns
(b) laminar form: deep / subcortical regions within white matter (less common)
√ single / multiple bilateral subependymal nodules along lateral ventricles
DDx: subependymal spread of neoplasm, subependymal hemorrhage, vascular malformation, tuberous sclerosis, intraventricular meningioma, neurofibromatosis

HOLOPROSENCEPHALY
= lack of cleavage / diverticulation of the forebrain (= prosencephalon) laterally (cerebral hemispheres), transversely (telencephalon, diencephalon), horizontally (optic + olfactory structures) as a consequence of arrested lateral ventricular growth in a 6-week embryo; cortical brain tissue develops to cover the monoventricle and fuses in the midline; posterior part of the monoventricle becomes enlarged and saclike
Incidence: 1:16,000
A. ALOBAR = no hemispheric development
B. SEMILOBAR = some hemispheric development
C. LOBAR = frontal and temporal lobation + small monoventricle
associated with: polyhydramnios (60%), renal + cardiac anomalies; chromosomal anomalies (predominantly trisomy 13)
Associated borderline syndromes secondary to diencephalic malformation:
1. Anophthalmia
2. Microphthalmia
3. Aplasia of pituitary gland
4. Olfactogenital dysplasia
5. Septo-optic dysplasia
DDx:
1. Severe hydrocephalus (roughly symmetrically thinned cortex)
2. Dandy-Walker cyst (normal supratentorial ventricular system)
3. Hydranencephaly (frontal + parietal cortex most severely affected)
4. Agenesis of corpus callosum with midline cyst (lateral ventricles widely separated with pointed superolateral margins)

Alobar Holoprosencephaly
= extreme form in which the prosencephalon does not divide
• minimal motor activity, little sensory response (ineffective brain function); seizures
• Facial features ("the face predicts the brain"):
1. Normal face in 17%
2. Cyclopia (= midline single orbit); may have proboscis (= fleshy supraorbital prominence) + absent nose
3. Ethmocephaly = 2 hypoteloric orbits + proboscis between eyes and absence of nasal structures

4. Cebocephaly = 2 hypoteloric orbits + single nostril with small flattened nose + absent nasal septum
5. Median cleft lip + cleft palate + hypotelorism
6. Others: micrognathia, trigonocephaly (early closure of metopic suture), microphthalmia, microcephaly
√ monoventricle = single large ventricle without occipital or temporal horns
√ dorsal cyst widely communicating with single ventricle; posterior fossa contents may be hypoplastic
√ "horseshoe" / "boomerang" configuration of brain = peripheral rim of cerebral cortex displaced rostrally (coronal plane)
(a) pancake configuration = cortex covers monoventricle to edge of dorsal cyst
(b) cup configuration = more cortex visible posteriorly
(c) ball configuration = complete covering of monoventricle without dorsal cyst
√ protrusion of anteriorly placed fused thalami + basal ganglia into monoventricle
√ midbrain, brainstem, cerebellum structurally normal
√ cerebral mantle pachygyric
√ absence of septum pellucidum, falx cerebri, interhemispheric fissure, corpus callosum, fornix, optic tracts, olfactory bulb (= arhinencephaly), internal cerebral veins, superior + inferior straight sagittal sinus, vein of Galen, 3rd ventricle, tentorium, Sylvian fissure, opercular cortex
√ midline clefts in maxilla + palate
Prognosis: death within 1st year of life / stillborn
DDx: massive hydrocephalus, hydranencephaly

Semilobar Holoprosencephaly
= intermediate form with incomplete cleavage of prosencephalon (more midline differentiation + beginning of sagittal separation)
• facial anomalies less severe: midline cleft lip + palate
• hypotelorism
• mental retardation
√ single ventricular chamber with partially formed occipital horns
√ peripheral rim of brain tissue is several cm thick
√ thalami anteriorly situated, abnormally rotated and fused
√ absence of septum pellucidum + corpus callosum + olfactory bulb
√ rudimentary falx cerebri + interhemispheric fissure form caudally with partial separation of occipital lobes
Prognosis: infants survive frequently into adulthood

Lobar Holoprosencephaly
= mildest form with two cerebral hemispheres + two distinct lateral ventricles
• usually not associated with facial anomalies except for hypotelorism
• mild to severe mental retardation, spasticity, athetoid movements
√ closely apposed bodies of lateral ventricles with occipital + frontal horns

√ unseparated frontal horns of angular squared shape +
  flat roof (on coronal images)
√ mild dilatation of lateral ventricles
√ falx cerebri + corpus callosum usually present
√ anterior hemispheric fissure shallow
√ septum pellucidum + sylvian fissures are usually
  absent
√ basal ganglia + thalami may be fused / separated
√ pachygyria (= abnormally wide + plump gyri),
  lissencephaly (= no gyri)
Prognosis: survival into adulthood

HYDATID DISEASE OF BRAIN
canine tapeworm (Echinococcus granulosus) in sheep-
and cattle-grazing areas
Location: liver (60%), lung (25%), CNS (2%)
                    subcortical
√ usually single, large round, sharply marginated smooth-
  walled hypodense cyst
√ no significant surrounding edema; no rim enhancement
√ development of daughter cysts (after rupture / following
  diagnostic puncture)

HYDRANENCEPHALY
= replacement of cerebral hemispheres by a thin
  membranous sac of leptomeninges + atrophic glial
  cells filled with CSF + necrotic debris
Incidence: 0.2% of infant autopsies
Etiology: absence of supraclinoid ICA system
                    (? vascular occlusion / infection) = ultimate
                    form of porencephaly
• seizures; respiratory failure; generalized flaccidity
• decerebrate state with vegetative existence
√ normal skull size / macrocrania
√ complete filling of hemicranium with membranous sac
  lined by leptomeninges
√ absence of cortical mantle (remnants of temporal,
  occipital, subfrontal cortex may be identified in some
  patients)
√ posterior fossa structures (brainstem, cerebellum)
  remain intact
√ thalamic, hypothalamic, mesencephalic structures
  project into cystic cavity
√ central brain tissue can be asymmetric
√ choroid plexus present
√ falx cerebri + tentorium cerebelli usually intact, may be
  deviated in asymmetric involvement, may be incomplete
  / absent
Prognosis: not compatible with prolonged extrauterine
                    life
DDx: (1) Severe hydrocephalus (some identifiable
                    cortex present)
          (2) Alobar holoprosencephaly (facial midline
                    anomalies)
          (3) Schizencephaly (some spared cortical mantle)

HYDROCEPHALUS
= increased intraventricular pressure

Obstructive Hydrocephalus
= obstructed CSF flow
Skull film: Signs of raised intracranial pressure
A.   YOUNG INFANT / NEWBORN:
        √ bulging of anterior fontanelle
        √ sutural diastasis
        √ macrocrania
        √ prominent digital impressions (wide range of
          normals in 4 – 10 years of age)
B.   ADOLESCENT / ADULT (changes in sella turcica)
        √ atrophy of anterior wall of dorsum sellae
        √ shortening of the dorsum sellae producing
          pointed appearance
        √ erosion / thinning / discontinuity of floor of sella
        √ depression of floor of sella with bulging into
          sphenoid sinus
        √ enlargement of sella turcica
        DDx: osteoporotic sella (aging, excessive steroid
                    hormone)

Communicating Hydrocephalus
= EXTRAVENTRICULAR HYDROCEPHALUS =
  elevated intraventricular pressure secondary to
  blockade beyond the outlet of 4th ventricle within the
  subarachnoid pathways
Incidence: 38% of congenital hydrocephaly
Pathophysiology:
  unimpeded CSF flow through ventricles, impeded
  CSF flow over convexities, impeded reabsorption by
  arachnoid villi
Cause:
  Subarachnoid hemorrhage (most common cause),
  Meningeal carcinomatosis, Purulent / tuberculous
  meningitis, Subdural hematoma, Craniosynostosis,
  Achondroplasia, Hurler syndrome, Obliteration of
  superior sagittal sinus, Absence of Pacchioni
  granulations
√ symmetric enlargement of lateral, 3rd, and often 4th
  ventricles
√ dilatation of subarachnoid cisterns
√ normal / effaced cerebral sulci
√ symmetric low attenuation of periventricular white
  matter (transependymal migration of CSF)
√ delayed ascent of radionuclide tracer over
  convexities
√ persistence of radionuclide tracer in lateral ventricles
  for up to 48 hours

Changes after successful shunting:
        √ diminished size of ventricles + increased
          prominence of sulci
        √ cranial vault may thicken
        Cx: subdural hematoma (result from precipitous
                    decompression)

Noncommunicating Hydrocephalus
= INTRAVENTRICULAR HYDROCEPHALUS =
  blockade of CNS flow within the ventricular system
  with dilatation of ventricles proximal to obstruction

Pathogenesis:
increased CSF pressure causes ependymal flattening with breakdown of CSF-brain barrier leading to myelin destruction + compression of cerebral mantle (brain damage)

Location:
(a) Lateral ventricular obstruction
Cause: choroid plexus papilloma, intraventricular glioma, meningioma
(b) Foramen of Monro obstruction
Cause: 3rd ventricular colloid cyst, tuber, papilloma, meningioma, septum pellucidum cyst / glioma, fibrous membrane (post infection)
(c) Third ventricular obstruction
Cause: large pituitary adenoma, craniopharyngloma, glioma of 3rd ventricle, hypothalamic glioma
(d) Aqueductal obstruction
Cause: Congenital web / atresia (often associated with Chiari malformation), fenestrated aqueduct, tumor of mesencephalon / pineal gland, S/P intraventricular hemorrhage or infection
(e) Fourth ventricular obstruction
Cause: Congenital obstruction, Dandy-Walker syndrome, Inflammation (TB), Tumor within 4th ventricle (glioma, ependymoma), extrinsic compression of 4th ventricle (astrocytoma, medulloblastoma, large CPA tumors, posterior fossa mass)
√ enlarged lateral ventricles (enlargement of occipital horns precedes enlargement of frontal horns)
√ effaced cerebral sulci
√ periventricular edema with indistinct margins (especially frontal horns)
√ radioisotope cisternography: no obstruction if tracer reaches ventricle

Nonobstructive Hydrocephalus
= secondary to rapid CSF production
Cause: Choroid plexus papilloma
√ ventricle near papilloma enlarges
√ intense radionuclide uptake in papilloma
√ enlarged anterior / posterior choroidal artery and blush

Congenital Hydrocephalus
= multifactorial CNS malformation during the 3rd / 4th week after conception
Incidence: 0.3 – 1.8 : 1,000 pregnancies
Etiology:
(1) aqueductal stenosis (43%)
(2) communicating hydrocephalus (38%)
(3) Dandy-Walker syndrome (13%)
(4) other anatomic lesions (6%)

(a) Genetic factors: Spina bifida, Aqueductal stenosis (X-linked recessive trait with a 50% recurrence rate for male fetuses), Congenital atresia of foramina of Luschka and Magendie (Dandy-Walker syndrome; autosomal recessive trait with 25% recurrence rate), Cerebellar agenesis, Cloverleaf skull, Trisomy 13 – 18
(b) Nongenetic etiology: Tumor compressing 3rd / 4th ventricle, Obliteration of subarachnoid pathway due to infection (syphilis, CMV, rubella, toxoplasmosis), proliferation of fibrous tissue (Hurler syndrome), Arnold-Chiari syndrome, Vein of Galen aneurysm, Choroid plexus papilloma, Vitamin A intoxication

associated with:
(a) Intracranial anomalies (37%): hypoplasia of corpus callosum, encephalocele, arachnoid cyst, arteriovenous malformation
(b) extracranial anomalies (63%): spina bifida in 25 – 30% (with spina bifida hydrocephalus is present in 80%), renal agenesis, multicystic dysplastic kidney, VSD, tetralogy of Fallot, anal agenesis, malrotation of bowel, cleft lip / palate, Meckel syndrome, gonadal dysgenesis, arthrogryposis, sirenomelia
(c) chromosomal anomalies (11%): trisomy 18 + 21, mosaicism, balanced translocation
• elevated amniotic alpha-fetoprotein level

OB-US: (assessment difficult prior to 20 weeks GA as ventricles constitute a large portion of cranial vault)
√ polyhydramnios (in 30%)
√ lateral ventricular width to hemispheric width (LVW:HW) > 50% by 17 – 20 weeks GA, > 33% after 20 weeks GA
√ BPD > 95th percentile (usually not before third trimester)
Recurrence rate: < 4%
Mortality: (1) fetal death in 24%
(2) neonatal death in 17%
Prognosis: poor with
(1) associated anomalies
(2) shift of midline (porencephaly)
(3) head circumference > 50 cm
(4) absence of cortex (hydranencephaly)
(5) cortical thickness < 10 mm

Infantile hydrocephalus
1. Communicating hydrocephalus
2. Aqueductal stenosis
3. Chiari II malformation
4. Dandy-Walker malformation

mnemonic: "**A** **V**P-Shunt **C**an **D**ecompress **T**he **H**ydrocephalic **C**hild"
Aqueductal stenosis
Vein of Galen aneurysm
Postinfectious

Superior vena cava obstruction
Chiari malformation
Dandy-Walker syndrome
Tumor
Hemorrhage
Choroid plexus papilloma

Normal Pressure Hydrocephalus
= NPH = ADAM SYNDROME
• dementia, unsteady gait, incontinence
  mnemonic: wacky, wobbly and wet
Age: 50 – 70 years
√ ventricular enlargement with prominent temporal horns
√ NO commensurate enlargement of sulci (out of proportion to atrophy)

HYGROMA
= CSF-fluid collection within subdural space following tear of leptomeninges after 6 – 30 days following trauma; common in children
Cause: (1) previous subdural hematoma
          (2) tear in arachnoid with secondary ball valve mechanism
√ radiolucent crescentic-shaped collection (as in acute subdural hematoma)
MRI: √ isointense to CSF / hyperintense to CSF on T1WI (increased protein content)
Prognosis: often spontaneous resorption

IDIOPATHIC INTRACRANIAL HYPERTENSION
= PSEUDOTUMOR CEREBRI = BENIGN INTRACRANIAL HYPERTENSION (BIH) secondary to (a) elevation in blood volume (85%) (b) decrease in regional cerebral blood flow with delayed CSF absorption (10%)
Etiology:
1. Sinovenous occlusive disease, SVC occlusion, obstruction of dural sinus, obstruction of both internal jugular veins
2. Dural AVM
3. S/P brain biopsy with edema
4. Endocrinopathies
5. Hypervitaminosis A
6. Hypocalcemia
7. Menstrual dysfunction, pregnancy, menarche, birth control pills
8. Drug therapy
predilection for   obese young to middle-aged women
• headache
• papilledema
• elevated opening pressures on lumbar puncture
√ normal ventricular size / pinched ventricles
√ increased volume of subarachnoid space

INFARCTION OF BRAIN
Acute Ischemic Infarction
  (a) Substage I (ictus – 24 hours)

NCCT:
  √ initially normal finding within first 24 – 48 hours (secondary to delayed onset of cerebral edema)
  √ focal decrease in attenuation with effacement of sulci (8%)
MRI: (positive as early as 1 – 6 hours)
  √ subtle low signal intensity on T1WI, high signal intensity on T2WI (masking of gyral infarcts on heavily T2WI due to sulcal CSF intensity)
(b) Substage II (24 hours – 7 days)
NCCT:
  √ hypodense wedge-shaped lesion with base at cortex in a vascular distribution (in 70%) due to vasogenic + cytotoxic edema
  √ mass effect (in 75%): sulcal effacement, transtentorial herniation, displaced subarachnoid cisterns + ventricles
CECT:
  √ gyral enhancement along cortex
Angio:
  √ narrowed / occluded vessels supplying the area of infarction
  √ delayed filling + emptying of involved vessels
  √ early draining vein
  √ luxury perfusion of infarcted area (rare) = loss of small vessel autoregulation due to local increase in pH
NUC:
  √ hemispheric hypoperfusion throughout all phases
  √ "flip-flop sign" in radionuclide angiogram (15%) = decreased uptake during arterial + capillary phase followed by increased uptake during venous phase
  √ "luxury perfusion syndrome" (14%) = increased perfusion

OVERALL CT-SENSITIVITY
—   on day of ictus: 48%
—   1 – 2 days later: 59%
—   7 – 10 days later: 66%
—   10 – 11 days later: 74%

Subacute Ischemic Infarction
Time period: 7 – 21 days = paradoxical phase with resolution of edema + onset of coagulation necrosis
NCCT: √ "fogging phenomenon" = low density area less apparent
       √ decrease of mass effect + ex vacuo dilatation of ventricles (in 57%)
CECT: √ gyral blush + ring enhancement (breakdown of blood brain barrier + luxury perfusion) for 2 – 8 weeks (in 65% within first 4 weeks)
       √ No enhancement in 1/5 of patients

Chronic Ischemic Infarction
= demyelination + gliosis complete (focal brain atrophy after 8 weeks)

NCCT: √ loss of volume + enlargement of subarachnoid space
√ ipsilateral dilatation of basal cisterns + ventricles
√ prominent sulci + thinning of gyri in vicinity of infarction
√ cyst development in vascular distribution

MRI: √ patchy region with increased intensity on T2WI

INIENCEPHALY
= complex developmental anomaly characterized by (1) exaggerated lordosis (2) rachischisis (3) imperfect formation of skull base at foramen magnum

M:F = 1:4

associated with other anomalies (in 84%):
anencephaly, encephalocele, hydrocephalus, cyclopia, absence of mandible, cleft lip / palate, diaphragmatic hernia, omphalocele, gastroschisis, single umbilical artery, CHD, polycystic kidney disease, arthrogryposis, club foot
√ dorsal flexion of head
√ abnormally short + deformed spine

Prognosis: almost uniformly fatal
DDx: (1) Anencephaly (2) Klippel-Feil syndrome (3) Cervical myelomeningocele

JAKOB-CREUTZFELDT DISEASE
= transmissible slow virus infection developing over weeks
• rapidly progressive dementia in middle age

LIPOMA
Incidence: < 1% of brain tumors
Age: presentation in childhood / adulthood
associated with agenesis of corpus callosum (in 50%)
• asymptomatic in 50%

Location:
midline lesion at genu of corpus callosum (25 – 50%), tuber cinereum, quadrigeminal region, chiasmatic / interpeduncular / sylvian / CP angle / cerebellomedullary cistern
√ well-circumscribed mass with CT-density of -100 HU
√ occasionally calcified rim (esp. in corpus callosum)
√ no enhancement
√ hyperintense mass on T1WI (CHARACTERISTIC)

Lipoma of Corpus Callosum
associated with:
(1) frontal bone defect (frequent)
(2) absence of corpus callosum (50%)
• in 50% symptomatic:
  • seizure disorders, mental retardation, dementia
  • emotional lability, headaches
  • hemiplegia

√ sharply marginated midline low-density mass in region of callosal genu, may involve entire corpus callosum
√ curvilinear mural calcification (common)
√ hyperintense mass on T1WI
√ encasement of ACA
DDx: Dermoid (denser, extraaxial)

LISSENCEPHALY
= AGYRIA = autosomal recessive disease with abnormal stratification (only four cortex layers are formed resulting in thick gray + thin white matter)

often associated with
(1) CNS anomalies: microcephaly, hydrocephalus, agenesis of corpus callosum, hypoplastic thalami
(2) micromelia, club foot, polydactyly, camptodactyly, syndactyly, duodenal atresia, micrognathia, omphalocele, hepatosplenomegaly, cardiac + renal anomalies
• mental retardation
√ absent sulci and gyri (brain looks similar to that in fetuses < 20 weeks GA)
√ ventriculomegaly (atrium + occipital horns)
√ widened sylvian fissures
√ midline round calcification in area of septum pellucidum (CHARACTERISTIC)
√ polyhydramnios (50%)
Prognosis: death by age 2

LYMPHOID HYPOPHYSITIS
autoimmune disorder with lymphocytic infiltration of pituitary gland;
associated with: thyrotoxicosis + hypopituitarism
Age: predilection for postpartum women
√ enlarged homogeneously enhancing pituitary gland; spontaneous regression

LYMPHOMA
Primary lymphoma more common than secondary !

A. PRIMARY LYMPHOMA = RETICULUM CELL SARCOMA = MICROGLIOMA = HISTIOCYTIC LYMPHOMA
= 1% of all CNS tumors; increased incidence in immunosuppressed (transplant, AIDS)
Sites: basal ganglia (50%), leptomeninges (30%), posterior fossa / brainstem (10 – 20%), corpus callosum, periventricular white mattter, vermis cerebelli, thalamus

B. SECONDARY = SYSTEMIC LYMPHOMA
1% of all CNS tumors
Sites: diffuse leptomeningeal spread, parenchymal mass (< 5%)

Clues: (1) multicentric involvement of deep hemispheres
(2) association with immunosuppression
(3) steroid response
√ commonly large discrete solitary lesion (57%)
√ small + symmetric multiple nodular lesions with blurred margins (43%)
√ diffusely infiltrating lesion

√ usually mildly hyperdense / occasionally isodense / low-density area (least common)

√ little mass effect with significant peritumoral edema

√ homogeneously dense + well-defined / irregular + patchy periventricular contrast enhancement

√ spontaneous regression (unique feature)

Angio: √ avascular

DDx: (1) Glioma (may be bilateral with involvement of basal ganglia + corpus callosum, may show dense homogeneous enhancement with vascularity)
(2) Meningioma
(3) Metastases (known primary, at gray-white matter junction)
(4) Abscess
(5) Progressive multifocal leukencephalopathy

SPINAL EPIDURAL LYMPHOMA
(a) invasion of epidural space through intervertebral foramen from paravertebral lymph nodes
(b) destruction of bone with vertebral collapse (less common)
(c) direct involvement of CNS (rare)

LEUKEMIA
CNS affected in 10% of patients with acute leukemia

√ sulcal / fissural / cisternal enhancement (meningeal infiltration)

MEDULLOBLASTOMA
2 – 6% of all intracranial gliomas, most malignant infratentorial neoplasm; most common neoplasm of posterior fossa in childhood

Incidence: 15 – 20% of all pediatric intracranial tumors

Origin: from external granular layer of inferior medullary velum (= roof of 4th ventricle)

Age: between ages 5 – 14 (2/3); between ages 15 – 35 (1/3); M:F = 2:1

Site: (a)   vermis cerebelli + roof of 4th ventricle (younger age group) in 91%
(b)   cerebellar hemisphere (older age group)

Size: usually > 2 cm in diameter

CT:
(a)   Classic features in 53%:
√ slightly hyperdense (70%) / isodense (20%) / mixed (10%) lesion
√ usually rapid intense homogeneous enhancement (97%)
√ rapid growth with extension into cerebellar hemisphere / brain stem
√ encroachment on 4th ventricle / aqueduct with hydrocephalus (85%)
√ shift / invagination of 4th ventricle
(b)   Atypical features
√ cystic / necrotic areas (16%) with lack of enhancement
√ calcifications in 13%
√ hemorrhage in 3%

√ supratentorial extension

MRI: √ mixed / hypointense on T1WI
√ intermediate / hyperintense on T2WI
√ usually homogeneous Gd-DTPA enhancement with hypointense rim

Cx: (1)   Subarachnoid metastatic spread (30%) to spinal cord, cerebral convexities, suprasellar cistern
(2)   Metastases outside CNS (axial skeleton, lymph nodes) after surgery

Rx: surgery + radiation therapy (extremely radiosensitive)

DDx of midline medulloblastoma:
ependymoma, astrocytoma

DDx of eccentric medulloblastoma:
astrocytoma, meningioma, acoustic neuroma

MENINGIOMA
Incidence: 15 – 18% of all intracranial tumors; most common extraaxial tumor

Origin: derived from meningothelial cells concentrated in arachnoid villi which penetrate the dura (sagittal sinus, exit of cranial nerves, choroid plexus)

Age: peak incidence 45 years (range 35 – 70 years); rare < 20 years; M:F = 1:2

associated with: Neurofibromatosis (multiple, occurrence in childhood)

TYPES:
(a)   Globular meningioma (most common): compact rounded mass with invagination of brain; flat at base; contact to falx / tentorium / basal dura / convexity dura
(b)   Meningioma-en-plaque: difficult to detect; pronounced hyperostosis of adjacent bone particularly along base of skull
(c)   Multicentric meningioma (2%) tendency to localize to a single hemicranium; present clinically at earlier age; global / mixed; CSF seeding is exceptional; in 50% associated with neurofibromatosis

Location:
(a)   common: parasagittal (anterior + middle third) > cerebral convexity > sphenoid ridge > posterior fossa (petrous bone, clivus, foramen magnum)
(b)   uncommon: tuberculum sellae, olfactory groove, tentorium, temporal fossa, falx, spinal cord
(c)   rare: pineal region, along intracranial nerve sheath (optic nerve), atrium of lateral ventricle (2 %) from infolding of meningeal tissue during formation of choroid plexus

Plain film:
√ hyperostosis at site close to / within bone (exostosis, enostosis, sclerosis)
√ blistering at paranasal sinuses (ethmoid, sphenoid) ± sclerosis (= pneumosinus dilatans)
√ enlarged meningeal grooves (if location in vault), enlarged foramen spinosum
√ calcification (= psammoma bodies)

CT:
- √ well-defined mass with smooth sharp margins
- √ abutting meningeal surface
- √ isodense / hyperdense lesion (psammomatous calcifications) on NECT
- √ calcifications in circular / radial pattern (20%) (DDx: osteoma)
- √ "intraosseous meningioma" = permeation of bone with intra- and extracerebral soft tissue component (DDx: fibrous dysplasia)
- √ hyperostosis of adjacent bone (18%)
- √ intense uniform enhancement on CECT (absence of blood-brain barrier)
- √ minimal peritumoral edema (2/3)
- √ cystic component: major in 2%, minor in 15%

MRI: (100% detection rate with gadolinium DTPA)
- √ most often isointense on T1WI + T2WI
- √ heterogeneous texture (tumor vascularity, cystic changes, calcifications)
- √ arcuate bowing of white matter + cortical effacement
- √ tumor-brain interface of low intensity vessels + high intensity cerebrospinal cleft on T2WI
- √ contrast enhancement for 3 – 60 minutes on T1WI
- √ linear "tail" extending from tumor mass along dural surface on Gd-DTPA enhanced scans in 60% (= meningothelial tumor nodules)

Angio:
- √ "mother-in-law" phenomenon (shows up early and stays late) = "sunburst" tumor vascularity with hypervascular cloudlike stain demonstrated early and persisting into venous phase
- √ early draining vein (rare: perhaps in angioblastic meningioma)
- √ en plaque-meningioma is poorly vascularized

Vascular supply:
1. vault: middle meningeal artery
2. sphenoid plane + tuberculum: recurrent meningeal branch of ophthalmic a.
3. tentorium: meningeal branch of meningohypophyseal trunk of ICA
4. intraventricular: choroidal vessels
5. clivus + posterior fossa: vertebral artery / ascending pharyngeal artery
6. falx: partly middle meningeal artery + others

ATYPICAL MENINGIOMA
1. low attenuation area of necrosis, old hemorrhage, cyst formation, fat (DDx: malignant glioma, metastasis)
2. "en plaque" morphology
3. "comma-shape" = combination of semilunar component bounded by dural interface + spherical component growing beyond dural margin
4. sarcomatous transformation with spread over hemisphere + invasion of cerebral parenchyma (leptomeningeal supply)

Suprasellar Meningioma
Origin: from arachnoid + dura along tuberculum sellae / diaphragma sellae; NOT from within pituitary fossa
- • hypothalamic / pituitary dysfunction (rare)
- √ irregular hyperostosis = blistering adjacent to sinus (HALLMARK of meningiomas at planum sphenoidale / tuberculum sellae)
- √ pneumatosis sphenoidale = increased pneumatization of sphenoid in area of anterior clinoids + dorsum sellae (DDx: normal variant)
- √ broad base of attachment
- √ intense homogeneous enhancement (may be impossible to differentiate from supraclinoid carotid aneurysm on CT)
- √ blood supply: posterior ethmoidal branches of ophthalmic artery, branches of meningohypophyseal trunk

DDx: metastasis, glioma, lymphoma

MENINGITIS
1. Pachymeningitis: affecting dura mater
2. Leptomeningitis: affecting pia matter / arachnoid (most common)
- • headaches, stiff neck
- • confusion, disorientation
- • positive CSF lab analysis

ROLE of CT and MRI:
(1) to exclude parenchymal abscess, ventriculitis, localized empyema
(2) to evaluate paranasal sinuses / temporal bone as source of infection
(3) to monitor complications: hydrocephalus, subdural effusion, infarction

Purulent Meningitis
Cause: otitis media / sinusitis
Organism:
(a) adults: Meningococcus, Streptococcus pneumoniae, Staphylococcus aureus, beta-hemolytic streptococcus
(b) children: Haemophilus influenzae, Escherichia coli, Neisseria meningitidis

NECT:
- √ often normal
- √ increased density in subarachnoid space (increased vascularity), esp. in children
- √ small ventricles secondary to diffuse cerebral edema

CECT:
- √ marked curvilinear meningeal enhancement over cerebrum (frontal + parietal lobes) and interhemispheric + sylvian fissures
- √ obliteration of basal cisterns with enhancement (common)

MRI: (most sensitive modality)
- √ hyperintense plaques on T2WI
- √ enhancement with Gd-DTPA

Cx:
- (1) Cerebritis
- (2) Ventriculitis = Ependymitis (secondary to retrograde spread)
- (3) Brain atrophy
- (4) Brain infarction (arteritis, venous thrombosis)
- (5) Subdural effusion [sterile subdural effusion secondary to H. influenzae meningitis (in children) may turn into empyema]
- (6) Hydrocephalus (cellular debris blocking foramen of Monro, aqueduct, 4th ventricular outlet / intraventricular septa / arachnoid adhesions)
- (7) Cranial nerve involvement

Prognosis:
Δ cerebral infarction + edema are predictive of poor outcome
Δ enlargement of ventricles + subarachnoid spaces + subdural effusions have no predictive value

Mortality: 10% (5th common cause of death in children between 1 and 4 years)

DDx: meningeal carcinomatosis

Granulomatous Meningitis
Histo: thick exudate, perivascular inflammation, granulation tissue + reactive fibrosis
- (1) Tuberculous meningitis = Basilar meningitis
- (2) Sarcoidosis
  may be associated with single / multiple intracerebral masses
- (3) Fungal meningitis: cryptococcosis, coccidioidomycosis, blastomycosis
- • acute life-threatening process / chronic indolent disease

may be associated with cerebritis, abscess formation
√ obliteration of basal cisterns, sylvian fissure, suprasellar cistern (isodense cisterns secondary to filling with debris)
√ intense contrast enhancement of involved subarachnoid spaces
√ calcification of meninges

Cx: (1) hydrocephalus (obliteration of basal cisterns; blocking of CSF flow + CSF absorption)
       (2) infarction (due to arteritis)

METACHROMATIC LEUKODYSTROPHY
= MLD = most common hereditary (autosomal recessive) leukodystrophy secondary to deficiency of aryl-sulfatase-A causing dysmyelinating disease

Age of presentation: before age 3 (2/3), in adolescence (1/3)
- • hypo-/ hypertonia, diminished reflexes, abnormal gait, mental regression
- • nystagmus
√ symmetric low density areas in white matter adjacent to ventricles (esp. centrum ovale and frontal horns)

Prognosis: death within several years

METASTASES TO BRAIN
40% of all intracranial tumors
Six tumors account for 95% of all brain metastases:
1. Bronchial carcinoma (47%): RARELY squamous cell carcinoma
2. Breast carcinoma (17%)
3. GI-tract tumors (15%): colon, rectum
4. Hypernephroma (10%)
5. Melanoma (8%)
6. Choriocarcinoma
Δ brain metastases from sarcomas are exceptionally rare !

Location: (a) corticomedullary junction of brain (most characteristic)
       (b) subarachnoid space = carcinomatous meningitis (15%)
       (c) subependymal spread (frequent in breast carcinoma)
       (d) skull (5%)

Presentation:
- — multiple lesions (2/3), single lesion (1/3)
- — cerebral hemispheres (57%), cerebellum (29%), brain stem (32%)
- — nodular deposits to dura are common
√ cyst formation: squamous cell / adenocarcinoma of lung
√ gross hemorrhage (in 3 – 4%): melanoma, choriocarcinoma, hypernephroma, thyroid carcinoma
√ calcification: mucin-producing neoplasm, cartilage- / bone-forming metastatic sarcoma, effective radiochemotherapy
√ multiple lesions of different sizes + locations
√ solid enhancement in small tumors / ring-like enhancement in large tumors
√ surrounding edema usually exceeds tumor volume
MRI: combination of T2WI + contrast-enhanced T1WI offer greatest sensitivity
√ asymmetric enhancement of dura with dural spread
√ leptomeningeal enhancement (e.g., in metastatic ependymoma)

MICROCEPHALY
= clinical syndrome characterized by a head circumference below the normal range
Incidence: 1.6:1,000 or 1:6,200 – 1:8,500 births
Etiology:
- (1) undiagnosed intrauterine infection (toxoplasmosis, rubella, CMV, herpes, syphilis), toxic agents, hypoxia, radiation
- (2) premature craniosynostosis
- (3) chromosomal abnormalities (trisomies)
- (4) Meckel-Gruber syndrome

often associated with:
microencephaly, macrogyria, pachygyria, atrophy of basal ganglia, decrease in dendritic arborization
√ AC:HC discrepancy
√ head circumference < 3 S.D. below the mean
√ ape-like sloping of forehead
√ dilatation of lateral ventricles

√ poor growth of fetal cranium
√ intracranial contents may not be visible (rare)
Prognosis: normal to severe mental retardation
(depending on degree of microcephaly)

MINERALIZING MICROANGIOPATHY
= RADIATION INDUCED LEUKOENCEPHALOPATHY
= sequelae of radiotherapy combined with methotrexate
therapy for leukemia
• 85% without neurologic deficits
CT:
√ thin reticular / serrated linear calcifications near
corticomedullary junction, especially in frontal +
posterior parietal lobes and in basal ganglia
√ symmetric low attenuation process in white matter
near corticomedullary area
MR:
√ confluent diffuse periventricular distribution spreading
peripherally with an irregular scalloped edge

MOYAMOYA DISEASE
= progressive obstructive / occlusive cerebral arteritis
affecting distal ICA at bifurcation into its branches
(anterior 2/3 of circle of Willis), usually involving both
hemispheres
Etiology: unknown
Age: predominantly in children + young adults
• headaches
• behavorial disturbances
• recurrent hemiparetic attacks
√ stenosis of distal internal carotid + proximal middle +
anterior cerebral arteries
√ large network of vessels in basal ganglia ("puff of
smoke") + upper brainstem fed by basilar artery, anterior
+ middle cerebral arteries (dilatation of lenticulostriate +
anterior choroidal arteries)
√ anastomoses between dural meningeal +
leptomeningeal arteries
Cx: subarachnoid hemorrhage (occasionally)

MULTIPLE SCLEROSIS
= most frequent form of chronic inflammatory
demyelinating disease of unknown etiology which
reduces the lipid content and brain volume;
characterized by a relapsing + remitting course
Histo: myelin degeneration at junctions of pial veins
resulting in scar (= plaque)
Age: young adults;   M:F = 1:1
• headaches, dizziness, nausea, recurrent sensory
changes
• Schumacher criteria:
(1) CNS dysfunction (2) involvement of two / more parts
of CNS (3) predominant white matter involvement
(4) two / more episodes lasting > 24 hours less than 1
month apart (5) slow stepwise progression of signs +
symptoms (6) at onset 10 – 50 years of age
• Rudick red flags (suggests diagnosis other than MS):
(1) no eye findings (2) no clinical remission (3) totally

local disease (4) no sensory findings (5) no bladder
involvement (6) no CSF abnormality
Location:
subependymal periventricular location (along lateral
aspects of atria + occipital horns), corpus callosum,
internal capsule, centrum semiovale, corona radiata,
optic nerves, chiasm, optic tract, brain stem
(ventrolateral aspect of pons at 5th nerve root entry),
cerebellar peduncles, cerebellum, spinal cord (most
common demyelinating process of spinal cord); rather
symmetric involvement of cerebral hemispheres
CT:
√ normal CT scan (18%)
√ nonspecific atrophy of brain (45%): enlarged
ventricles, prominent sulci
√ periventricular (near atria) multifocal nonconfluent
lesions with distinct margins + without mass effect on
ventricles (location not always correlating well with
symptoms)
(a) NECT: isodense / lucent
(b) CECT: transient enhancement during acute
stage (active demyelination) for about 2
weeks; may require double dose
contrast; ultimately disappearance /
permanent scar
MRI (modality of choice):
(a) for optic nerve lesions: short T1 inversion
recovery pulse sequence
(b) for cortical lesions: long TR pulse sequences
(c) for spinal cord lesions: dorsal + lateral elements
generally involved
√ well-marginated discrete foci of varying size with high
signal intensity on T2WI + proton density images
(= loss of hydrophobic myelin produces increase in
water content); hypointense on T1WI
√ Gd-DTPA enhancement of lesions on T1WI (up to 8
weeks following acute demyelination)

NEONATAL INTRACRANIAL HEMORRHAGE
Germinal Matrix Bleed
= GERMINAL MATRIX RELATED HEMORRHAGE
Germinal matrix = highly vascular subependymal
collection of tissue adjacent to lateral ventricles in
region of the caudate nucleus and caudothalamic
notch / groove composed of many veins; decreases in
size with increasing fetal maturity and usually
involutes by 32 – 34 weeks of gestation
Cause: (1) prematurity (2) hypoxia (3) birth trauma
(4) coagulopathy
Pathogenesis: friable vascular bed ruptures under
hypertension, hypoxia, acidosis
Incidence: in premature neonates < 32 weeks of age;
in 43% of infants < 1,500 gms
GRADES
I : subependymal hemorrhage confined to germinal
matrix
II : subependymal / choroid plexus hemorrhage
ruptured into nondilated ventricle

III : intraventricular hemorrhage with ventricular enlargement

IV : massive intraventricular + intraparenchymal hemorrhage with ventricular dilatation

Time of onset: within first 3 days of life (86%); within first week of life (91%)

Optimum for screening: 7 – 14 days of life

√ echogenic clot in ventricles (acute phase) becoming sonolucent with time

√ highly echogenic mass, commonly lateral to frontal horns / in parietal lobe, rare in occipital lobe + thalamus

√ irregular bulky choroid plexus

√ echogenic ventricular surfaces

√ ventricular dilatation (progressive / arrested hydrocephalus)

Cx:

(1) Cavitation of hemorrhage
(2) Unilocular subependymal cyst
(3) Unilocular porencephalic cyst
(4) Ventriculomegaly (scarring of pacchionian granulations, septation of ventricles)
(5) Mental retardation, cerebral palsy
(6) Death in 25% (IVH most common cause of neonatal death)

Prognosis:

(1) Grade I + II: good with normal developmental scores (12 – 18% risk of handicap)
(2) Grade III + IV: 54% mortality; motor disabilities, cognitive defects

Intraventricular Hemorrhage

Etiology: (a) germinal matrix hemorrhage (b) bleeding from choroid plexus

• seizures, dystonia, obtundation, intractable acidosis

• bulging anterior fontanelle, drop in hematocrit, bloody / proteinaceous CSF, IVH usually cleared within 7 – 14 days

Periventricular Leukoencephalopathy
Periventricular Leukomalacia

= PVL = focal necrosis of deep white matter as a result of ischemic infarction involving the watershed zones between central and peripheral vascularity; nonhemorrhagic (more often) / hemorrhagic

Incidence: 5% of premature infants; 7 – 22% at autopsy; in 34% of infants < 1500 g; in 59% of infants surviving longer than 1 week on assisted ventilation; only 28% detected by cranial sonography

Histo: edema, white matter necrosis, evolution of cysts / diminished myelin

Pathogenesis:
immature autoregulation of periventricular vessels secondary to deficient muscularis of arterioles limits vasodilation in response to hypoxemia + hypercapnia + hypotension of perinatal asphyxia

• spastic diplegia / quadriparesis (affecting descending fibers from motor cortex)

• mental retardation
• severe hearing / visual impairments
• convulsive disorders

Location: bilateral paralleling both lateral ventricles, dorsal + lateral to external angle of lateral ventricular trigones, frontal cerebral white matter near foramen of Monro

√ increased periventricular echogenicity (PVE) (appearing 2 days – 2 weeks after insult)

√ bilateral often asymmetric zones, occasionally extending to cortex

√ infrequently accompanied by IVH

Late changes:

√ periventricular cystic PVL = cystic degeneration of ischemic areas (= multiple, small, never septated periventricular cysts in relationship to lateral ventricles appearing 2 – 3 weeks after development of echodensities + disappearing after 1 – 3 months)

√ brain atrophy secondary to thinning of periventricular white matter

√ ventriculomegaly (after disappearance of cysts)

√ enlarged interhemispheric fissure

Prognosis: very poor

Periventricular Hemorrhagic Infarction

= hemorrhagic necrosis of periventricular white matter, usually large + asymmetric

associated with IVH in 80%

Incidence: 15% of infants with IVH have periventricular hemorrhagic infarction

Pathogenesis:
intraventricular / germinal matrix blood clot leads to obstruction of terminal veins

Histo: perivascular hemorrhage of medullary veins near ventricular angle

Age: peak occurrence at 4th postnatal day

• spastic hemiparesis (affects lower + upper extremities equally)

Location: dorsal + lateral to external angle of lateral ventricle; 67% unilateral; 33% bilateral but asymmetric

√ unilateral / asymmetric bilateral triangular "fan-shaped" echodensities

√ extension from frontal to parietooccipital regions / localized

Late changes:

√ single large cyst = porencephaly

√ bumpy ventricle / false accessory ventricle

Prognosis:
59% overall mortality with echodensities > 1 cm

Encephalomalacia

= more extensive brain damage than PVL; may include all of white matter in subcortex + cortex

associated with: (1) Neonatal asphyxia (2) Vasospasm (3) Inflammation of CNS

√ cysts often not communicating

NEUROBLASTOMA

A. PRIMARY CEREBRAL NEUROBLASTOMA (rare)
   Age: childhood / early adolescence
   √ large hypodense / mixed-density mass with well-defined margins
   √ intratumoral coarse dense calcifications
   √ central cystic / necrotic zones with hemorrhage
   Cx: metastasizes via subarachnoid space to dura + calvarium

B. SECONDARY NEUROBLASTOMA (common)
   metastatic to: (usually not to brain)
   @ liver
   @ skeleton
      √ osteolytic with periosteal new bone formation
      √ sutural diastasis
      √ hair-on-end appearance of skull
   @ orbit: √ unilateral proptosis

Olfactory Neuroblastoma

= very malignant tumor arising from olfactory mucosa
Types:
   1. Esthesioneuroepithelioma
   2. Esthesioneurocytoma
   3. Esthesioneuroblastoma
√ mass in superior nasal cavity with extension into ethmoid + maxillary sinuses
Cx: distant metastases in 20%

NEUROFIBROMATOSIS

= VON RECKLINGHAUSEN DISEASE = dysplasia of mesodermal + neuroectodermal tissue with potential for diffuse systemic involvement; autosomal dominant, 50% spontaneous mutants; variable expressivity
Incidence: 1:3,000; M:F = 1:1; most common of phakomatoses
Path: pure neurofibromas (nerve fibers run through mass) + neurilemmomas (nerve fibers diverge and course over the surface of the tumor mass) frequently combined
   (1) discrete round mass
   (2) plexiform = tortuous tangles / fusiform enlargement of peripheral nerves (PATHOGNOMONIC)
may be associated with:
   (1) MEA IIb (pheochromocytoma + medullary carcinoma of thyroid + multiple neuromas)
   (2) CHD (10 fold increase): pulmonary valve stenosis, ASD, VSD, IHSS
Types:
   1. CENTRAL: central CNS involvement without significant cutaneous manifestations
   2. PERIPHERAL: peripheral CNS involvement with cutaneous lesions
   3. VISCERAL: involvement of visceral nervous system
   — Neurofibromatosis 1 = von Recklinghausen disease
   — Neurofibromatosis 2 = bilateral acoustic neuromas

A. CNS MANIFESTATIONS
   1. Bilateral optic nerve gliomas = optic nerve pilocytic astrocytoma with perineural / subarachnoid spread
      Δ in up to 30% of all neurofibromatosis patients
      Δ 10% of all optic nerve gliomas are associated with neurofibromatosis
   2. Schwannomas of cranial nerves 3 – 12 (most commonly 5 + 8)
   3. Bilateral acoustic neuromas (7% of all acoustic neuromas + almost all of bilateral tumors are associated with neurofibromatosis)
   4. Multiple meningiomas: intraventricular in choroid plexus of trigone, parasagittal, sphenoid ridge, olfactory groove, spinal cord, along intracranial nerves
   5. Meningiomatosis = dura studded with innumerable small meningiomas
   6. Cerebral gliomas (most types):
      (a) brainstem glioma
      (b) astrocytoma of hypothalamus
      (c) gliomatosis cerebri (= unusual confluence of astrocytomas)
   7. Choroid plexus papilloma
   8. Spinal cord ependymoma
   9. AVM's / Angiomatosis
   10. Arachnoid cyst

B. SKELETAL MANIFESTATIONS
   (involved in 50 – 80%)
   • dwarfism caused by scoliosis
   @ Skull:
      • pulsating exopthalmus / unilateral proptosis (herniation of subarachnoid space + temporal lobe into orbit)
      √ Harlequin appearance to orbit = partial absence of greater and lesser wing of sphenoid bone + orbital plate of frontal bone (failure of development of membranous bone)
      √ enlargement of middle cranial fossa with extension into orbit
      √ concentric enlargement of optic foramen (optic glioma)
      √ enlargement of orbit + superior orbital fissure (plexiform neurofibroma of peripheral and sympathetic nerves within orbit / optic nerve glioma)
      √ sclerosis in the vicinity of optic foramen (optic nerve sheath meningioma)
      √ deformity + decreased size of ipsilateral ethmoid + maxillary sinus
      √ macrocranium + macroencephaly
      √ calvarial defect adjacent to left lambdoid suture (parietal mastoid)
   @ Spine:
      √ sharply angled kyphoscoliosis (50%) in lower thoracic + lumbar spine; kyphosis predominates over scoliosis

√ posterior scalloping of vertebral bodies with dural ectasia secondary to weakened meninges allowing transmission of normal CSF pulsations

√ enlarged intervertebral foramina
  (a) intrathoracic / lateral meningocele (protrusion of spinal meninges through intervertebral foramina)
  (b) "dumbbell" neurofibroma of spinal nerves

CT: √ fusiform / spherical low-attenuation mass (20 – 30 HU)

US: √ hypoechoic well-circumscribed cylindrical lesion

@ Chest:
  √ twisted "ribbon-like" ribs in upper thoracic segments accompanying kyphoscoliosis
  √ localized cortical notches / depression of inferior margins of ribs (DDx: aortic coarctation)
  √ intrathoracic meningoceles
  √ lung + mediastinal neurofibromas
  √ progressive pulmonary interstitial fibrosis

@ Appendicular skeleton:
  √ anterolateral bowing of lower half of tibia (most common) / fibula (frequent) / upper extremity (uncommon) ± pseudarthrosis secondary to deossification with bowing-fracture in 1st year of life
  √ atrophic thinned / absent fibulas
  √ periosteal dysplasia = traumatic subperiosteal hemorrhage with abnormally easy detachment of periosteum from bone
  √ subendosteal sclerosis
  √ bone erosion from periosteal / soft tissue neurofibromas
  √ intramedullary longitudinal streaks of increased density
  √ single / multiple cystic lesions within bone (? deossification / non-ossifying fibroma)
  √ focal gigantism = unilateral overgrowth of a limb bone; marked enlargement of a digit in a hand / foot (overgrowth of ossification center)

C. NEURAL CREST TUMORS
  1. Pheochromocytoma: • hypertension in adults
  2. Parathyroid adenomas: • hyperparathyroidism

D. VASCULAR LESIONS
  Schwann cell proliferation within vessel wall
  1. Cranial artery stenosis
  2. Renal artery stenosis: very proximal, funnel-shaped (one of the most common causes of hypertension in childhood)
  3. Renal artery aneurysm
  4. Thoracic / abdominal aortic coarctation

E. GI TRACT MANIFESTATIONS
  √ ulcerating submucosal neurofibromas (most commonly in small bowel)

F. OCULAR MANIFESTATIONS (6%)
  • buphthalmos = congenital glaucoma
  1. Pigmented iris hamartomas < 2 mm (Lisch nodules) in > 90%, mostly bilateral

  2. Plexiform neurofibroma (most common)
  3. Optic glioma: in 12% of patients, in 4% bilateral; 75% in 1st decade
    √ extension into optic chiasm (up to 25%), optic tracts + optic radiation
    √ increased intensity on T2WI if chiasm + visual pathways involved
  4. Perioptic meningioma
  5. Choroidal hamartoma: in 50% of patients

G. SKIN MANIFESTATIONS
  1. Café-au-lait spots of "coast of California" type (= smooth outline): > 6 in number + > 15 mm in size
  2. Axillary freckling
  3. Cutaneous neurofibroma
    (a) localized = fibroma molluscum = string of pearls along peripheral nerve
    (b) plexiform neurofibroma = elephantiasis neuromatosa

Cx: malignant transformation to neurofibrosarcoma (< 5%)

NEUROMA
= 8% of all intracranial tumors
• slow growth
• not painful

Acoustic Neuroma
= 5 – 7% of all intracranial tumors; 85% of all intracranial neuromas; 80% of cerebellopontine angle tumors

Age: usually 35 – 60 years; M:F = 1:2

associated with
  1. central neurofibromatosis (95%)
  2. contralateral acoustic neuroma (25%)
  3. peripheral neurofibromatosis (5%)

• unilateral sensorineural hearing loss (acoustic neuromas account for 10%)
• tinnitus
• diminished corneal reflex
• unsteadiness, vertigo, ataxia, dizziness
• pain

Doubling time: 2 years

Location:
  (a) arises from within internal auditory canal (IAC) at the glial-Schwann cell junction of the vestibular division of 8th nerve (95%)
  (b) may arise in cerebellopontine angle cistern outside IAC with intracanalicular extension (5%)

Plain film:
  √ erosion of IAC: a difference in canal height of > 2 mm is abnormal

CT:
  √ round mass based at the IAC with adjacent IAC canal widening (rarely within cerebellopontine angle cistern without bone widening)
  √ usually solid tumor with uniformly dense tumor enhancement
  √ hypodense / isodense (50% may be missed without CECT)

√ may have cyst formation in / adjacent to tumor (15%)
√ ring enhancement may be seen
√ NO calcification
√ widening / obliteration of ipsilateral cerebellopontine angle cistern
√ shift / asymmetry of 4th ventricle with hydrocephalus
√ intrathecal contrast / carbon dioxide insufflation (for tumors < 5 mm)
MRI: (most sensitive test with Gd-DTPA enhancement)
  √ intensely enhancing mass on T1W images
Angio:
  √ elevation + posterior displacement of anterior inferior cerebellar artery (AICA) on basal view
  √ elevation of the superior cerebellar artery (large tumors)
  √ displacement of basilar artery anteriorly / posteriorly + contralateral side
  √ compression / posterior + lateral displacement of petrosal vein
  √ posterior displacement of choroid point of PICA
  √ vascular supply frequently from external carotid artery branches
  √ rarely hypervascular tumor with tumor blush

Trigeminal Neuroma
3 – 5% of intracranial neuromas, 0.26% of all brain tumors
Origin: arising from Gasserian ganglion within Meckel cave at the most anteromedial portion of the petrous pyramid / trigeminal nerve root
Age. 35 – 60 years; M:F = 1:2
Symptoms of location in middle cranial fossa:
  • facial paresthesia / hypesthesia
  • exophthalmus, ophthalmoplegia
Symptoms of location in posterior cranial fossa:
  • facial nerve palsy
  • hearing impairment, tinnitus
  • ataxia, nystagmus
Location: (a) middle cranial fossa (46%) (b) posterior cranial fossa (29%) (c) in both fossae (25%)
√ erosion of petrous tip
√ enlargement of contiguous fissures, foramina, canals
√ dumbbell / saddle-shaped mass (extension into middle cranial fossa + through tentorial incisura into posterior fossa)
√ isodense mass with dense inhomogeneous enhancement (tumor necrosis + cyst formation)
√ distortion of ipsilateral quadrigeminal cistern
√ displacement + cutoff of posterior 3rd ventricle
√ anterior displacement of temporal horn
√ angiographically avascular / hypervascular mass

PARAGONIOMIASIS OF BRAIN
oriental lung fluke (paragonimus westermani) producing arachnoiditis, parenchymal granulomas, encapsulated abscesses

√ isodense / inhomogeneous masses surrounded by edema
√ ring enhancement

PICK DISEASE
= rare form of presenile dementia similar to Alzheimer disease; may be inherited with autosomal dominant mode; M < F
√ focal cortical atrophy of anterior frontal + temporal lobes
√ dilatation of frontal + temporal horns of lateral ventricle

PINEAL DYSGERMINOMA
= most common pineal tumor (50% of all pineal tumors)
= malignant primitive germ cell neoplasm
Histo: similar to seminoma
Age: 20 – 30 years; almost exclusively in males
√ infiltrating variodense mass (rarely calcified)
√ moderate / marked homogeneous contrast enhancement
√ frequently cause of aqueduct stenosis with hydrocephalus

PINEAL TERATOMA
= benign tumor containing all three germ cell layers (pineal region most common site of teratomas)
Sex: marked male predilection
√ inhomogeneous areas of fat + linear / nodular calcifications + cysts
√ minimal / no contrast enhancement

PINEAL TERATOCARCINOMA
= arising from primitive germ cells
√ intratumoral hemorrhage
√ invasion of adjacent structures
√ intense homogeneous contrast enhancement
Cx: seeding via CSF

PINEOBLASTOMA
= highly malignant tumor derived from primitive pineal parenchymal cells
Histo: similar to medulloblastoma
Age: children + adults; M < F
CT:
  √ poorly marginated iso- / slightly hyperdense mass with dense calcifications
  √ intense homogeneous contrast enhancement
MRI:
  √ intermediate intensity on T1WI + T2WI
  √ homogeneous Gd-DTPA enhancement
Cx: frequently spread through CSF

PINEOCYTOMA
= slow-growing tumor composed of mature pineal parenchymal cells
Age: any age
√ slightly hyperdense / isodense mass with dense focal calcification

√ well-defined homogeneous enhancement
Cx: some metastasize via CSF

PITUITARY ADENOMA

= benign slow-growing neoplasms arising from adenohypophysis (= anterior lobe); account for 5 – 18% of all intracranial neoplasms

FORMER CLASSIFICATION:
- A. <u>Chromophobe adenoma</u> (80%)
  associated with hypopituitarism, prolactin, TSH, GH
  √ greatest sella enlargement; calcified in 5%
  however: functioning microadenomas are part of chromophobe adenomas
- B. <u>Acidophilic / eosinophilic adenoma</u> (15%)
  increased GH secretion (acromegaly), prolactin, TSH
  √ tumor of intermediate size
- C. <u>Basophilic adenoma</u> (5%)
  associated with ACTH secretion (Cushing syndrome), LH, FSH
  √ small tumor

Plain film: (UNRELIABLE !)
  √ enlargement of sella + sloping of sella floor
  √ erosion of anterior + posterior clinoid processes
  √ erosion of dorsum sellae
  √ calcification in < 10%
  √ may present with mass in nasopharynx

Functioning Pituitary Microadenoma

= very small adenomas < 10 mm; usually become clinically apparent by hormone production (20 – 30% of all pituitary adenomas)

1. <u>PROLACTINOMA</u>
   - prolactin levels do not closely correlate with tumor size

   Female:
   - women during childbearing age
   - amenorrhea
   - galactorrhea
   - elevated prolactin levels (usually > 100 ng/ml)

   Male:
   - headache
   - impotence
   - visual disturbance
   √ characteristic lateral location, anteriorly / inferiorly; variable in size
   Rx: bromocriptine

2. <u>CORTICOTROPHIC ADENOMA</u>
   ACTH-secreting tumor
   √ central location; posterior lobe; usually < 5 mm in size
   - Cushing disease (truncal obesity, abdominal striae, glycosuria, osteoporosis, proximal muscle weakness, hirsutism, amenorrhea, hypertension, elevated cortisol levels in plasma and urine, suppression by high doses of dexamethasone of 8 mg/day)

3. <u>SOMATOTROPHIC ADENOMA</u>
   - gigantism, acromegaly, elevated GH > 10 ng/ml, no rise in GH after administration of glucose / TRH
   √ hypodense region, may be less well-defined, variable size

   CECT (dynamic bolus injection):
   √ upward convexity of gland
   √ increased height > 10 mm
   √ deviation of pituitary stalk
   √ floor erosion
   √ gland asymmetry
   √ focal hypodensity (most specific for adenoma)
   √ shift of pituitary tuft / density change in region of adenoma

   MRI :
   Highest sensitivity on coronal non-enhanced T1WI (70%) + 3 D FLASHsequence (69%) + combination of both (90%)
   Δ 1/3 of lesions are missed with enhancement
   Δ 1/3 of lesions are missed without enhancement
   √ focus of low / high signal intensity
   DDx: simple pituitary cyst

Nonfunctioning Pituitary Macroadenoma

= tumor usually > 10 mm in size, usually nonfunctioning (70 – 80% of pituitary adenomas)
Incidence: 10 %; M:F = 1:1
Age: 25 – 60 years
- hypopituitarism, bitemporal hemianopia (with superior extension), pituitary apoplexy, hydrocephalus, cranial nerve involvement (III, IV, VI)

CT: √ tumor isodense to brain tissue
       √ roughly homogeneous enhancement
       √ calcifications infrequent
MRI: allows differentiation from aneurysm
Cx: (1) Obstructive hydrocephalus (at foramen of Monro)
         (2) Encasement of carotid artery
         (3) Pituitary apoplexy (rare)

PITUITARY APOPLEXY

= massive hemorrhage into pituitary adenoma / dramatic necrosis / sudden infarction of pituitary gland; area of destruction must be > 70% to produce pituitary insufficiency

Sheehan Syndrome =   postpartum infarction of anterior pituitary gland
- severe headache, nausea, vomiting
- stiff neck
- sudden visual loss / diplopia
- obtundation (frequent)
NCCT: √ increased density

PROGRESSIVE MULTIFOCAL LEUKOENCEPHALOPATHY

= PML = progressive fatal demyelinating disease in

patients with impaired immune system (leukemia, lymphoma, AIDS, tuberculosis, sarcoidosis, organ transplant)

Etiology: ? Papovavirus infection
- visual disturbances, ataxia, spasticity

CT:
√ scalloped confluent regions in parieto-occipital white matter of low attenuation ± enhancement
√ brain atrophy without mass effect

MRI:
√ patchy high-intensity lesions of white matter away from ependyma in asymmetric distribution on T2WI

REYE SYNDROME

= hepatitis + encephalitis following viral upper respiratory tract infection with Hx of large doses of aspirin ingestion

Age: in children + young adults
- obtundation rapidly progressing to coma

√ initially (within 2 – 3 days) small ventricles
√ later progressive enlargement of lateral ventricles + sulci
√ markedly diminshed attenuation of white matter

Mortality: 15 – 85% (from white matter edema + demyelination)

Dx: liver biopsy

SARCOIDOSIS OF CNS

Incidence: CNS involvement in 3 – 8%
- cranial neuropathy (facial > acoustic > optic nerves) secondary to granulomatous infiltration + leptomeningeal fibrosis
- peripheral neuropathy + myopathy
- aseptic meningitis
- diffuse encephalopathy
- hypothalamic dysfunction
- seizures
- improvement following therapy with steroids

Location: affects meninges more often than brain
√ diffuse meningeal enhancement (most common) / meningeal nodules (less common) from leptomeningeal invasion
  Site: particularly in basal cisterns in suprasellar, sellar, subfrontal regions with extension to optic chiasm, hypothalamus, pituitary gland
√ dense enhancement of falx + tentorium (granulomatous invasion of dura)
√ isodense / hyperdense homogeneously enhancing small single / multiple nodules (invasion of brain parenchyma via perivascular spaces of Virchow-Robin)
  Site: periphery of parenchyma, intraspinal
√ hydrocephalus most common finding (from arachnoiditis / adhesions)

SCHIZENCEPHALY

= TRUE PORENCEPHALY = segmental developmental failure of cell migration to form cerebral cortex; parenchymal clefts extending from subarachnoid space to subependyma of ventricles filled by CSF + frequently communicating with subarachnoid space

often associated with micropolygyria, microcephaly
√ bilateral often symmetric intracranial cysts, usually around Sylvian fissure
√ asymmetrical dilatation of lateral ventricles with midline shift
√ wide separation of lateral ventricles + squaring of frontal lobes
√ absence of cavum septum pellucidum + corpus callosum

Prognosis: severe intellectual impairment, spastic tetraplegia, blindness

DDx:
(1) Pseudoporencephaly = Acquired porencephaly
    = local parenchymal destruction secondary to vascular / infectious / traumatic insult (almost always unilateral)
(2) Arachnoid cyst
(3) Cystic tumor

SEPTO-OPTIC DYSPLASIA

= DeMORSIER SYNDROME = rare anterior midline anomaly often considered a mild form of lobar holoprosencephaly

M:F = 1:3
- seizures, hypotonia, diabetes insipidus (in 50%), hypopituitarism
- hypotelorism, blindness (hypoplasia of optic discs), nystagmus

√ small optic canals
√ fused dilated frontal horns squared off dorsally + pointing inferiorly
√ absent septum pellucidum
√ thin corpus callosum
√ enlarged anterior recess of 3rd ventricle
√ hypoplasia of optic nerves + chiasm + infundibulum
√ large infundibular recess
√ dilatation of chiasmatic + suprasellar cisterns

SINUS PERICRANII

= subperiosteal venous angiomas adherent to skull and connected by anomalous diploic veins to a sinus / cortical vein
- soft painless scalp mass that reduces under compression

Location: frontal bone
√ calvarial thinning + defect

CT:
√ sessile sharply marginated homogeneous densely enhancing mass adjacent to outer table of skull, perforating it and connecting it with another similar structure beneath the inner table

Angio:
√ extracalvarial sinus may not opacify secondary to slow flow

SPONGIFORM DEGENERATION

= CANAVAN DISEASE = spongy degeneration of brain in infancy

Cause: unknown
• enlargement of head
√ diffuse subtly diminished white matter density

SPONGIFORM LEUKOENCEPHALOPATHY
rare, hereditary, > age 40
• deteriorating mental function
√ confluent areas of diminished attenuation

STURGE-WEBER-DIMITRI SYNDROME
= ENCEPHALO-TRIGEMINAL ANGIOMATOSIS
= vascular malformation with capillary venous angiomas due to persistence of usually transitory plexus stage of vessel development
• seizures (90%)
• facial port wine stain (nevus flammeus)
= telangiectasia of trigeminal region; usually 1st ± 2nd division of 5th nerve; usually unilateral
• mental deficiency (> 50%)
• ipsilateral glaucoma (often)
• crossed hemiparesis (35 – 65%)
• hemiatrophy of body contralateral to facial nevus (secondary to hemiparesis)
√ leptomeningeal venous angiomas
Location: parietal > occipital > frontal lobes
Angio: √ capillary blush
        √ abnormal deep medullary veins draining into internal cerebral vein
        √ failure to opacify superficial cortical veins in calcified region
√ cortical hemiatrophy beneath meningeal angioma due to anoxia (steal)
√ "tram track" cortical calcifications > 2 years of age; in layers 3-4-5 of opposing gyri
√ ipsilateral thickening of skull + orbit (bone apposition as reaction to brain atrophy)
    √ elevation of sphenoid wing + petrous ridge
    √ enlarged ipsilateral sinuses
    √ thickened calvarium

SUBARACHNOID HEMORRHAGE
Cause:
A. Spontaneous
    (1) ruptured aneurysm (72%) (2) AV malformation (10%) (3) hypertensive hemorrhage (4) hemorrhage from tumor (5) embolic hemorrhagic infarction (6) blood dyscrasia, anticoagulation therapy (7) eclampsia (8) intracranial infection (9) spinal vascular malformation (10) cryptogenic in 6% (negative 4-vessel angiography; seldom recurrent)
B. Trauma
    concomitant to cerebral contusion
    (a) injury to leptomeningeal vessels at vertex
    (b) rupture of major intracerebral vessels (less common)
    Location: (a) focal, overlying site of contusion
            (b) interhemispheric fissure, paralleling falx cerebri

(c) spread diffusely throughout subarachnoid space (rare in trauma)
NCCT: (accuracy of detection 60 – 90% depending on time of scan; high within 4 – 5 days of onset)
√ increased density in basal cisterns, superior cerebellar cistern, sylvian fissure, cortical sulci, intraventricular, intracerebral
√ along interhemispheric fissure = on lateral aspect irregular dentate pattern due to extension into paramedian sulci with rapid clearing after several days
MRI: (relative insensitive)
√ deoxyhemoglobin effects not appreciable in acute phase (secondary to higher oxygen tension in CSF, counterbalancing effects of very long T2 of CSF, pulsatile flow effects of CSF)
√ low signal intensity on brain surfaces in recurrent subarachnoid hemorrhages (hemosiderin deposition)
Prognosis: clinical course depends on amount of subarachnoid blood
Cx:
    (1) Acute obstructive hydrocephalus (in < 1 week) secondary to intraventricular hemorrhage / ependymitis obstructing aqueduct of Sylvius or outlet of 4th ventricle
    (2) Delayed communicating hydrocephalus (after 1 week) secondary to fibroblastic proliferation in subarachnoid space and arachnoid villi
    (3) Cerebral vasospasm + infarction (develops after 72 hours, at maximum between 5 – 17 days, amount of blood is prognostic parameter)
    (4) Transtentorial herniation (cerebral hematoma, hydrocephalus, infarction, brain edema)

SUBDURAL HEMATOMA OF BRAIN
Incidence: in 5% of head trauma patients
Age: predominantly in infants + elderly (large subarachnoid space with freedom to move)
Pathogenesis:
    most often due to venous bleeding from "bridging veins" (= subdural veins) which connect cerebral cortex to dural sinuses and travel through the subarachnoid space and potential space between dura and arachnoid membranes, veins tear at portion attached to sinus
Location: potential space between dura + leptomeninges
DDx: (1) Arachnoid cyst (extension into Sylvian fissure)
        (2) Subarachnoid hemorrhage (extension into sulci)

Acute Subdural Hematoma
usually follows severe trauma, manifest within hours after injury
associated with: underlying brain injury (50%) with worse long-term prognosis than epidural hematoma, skull fracture (1%)
Location: along cerebral convexity, frequent extension into interhemispheric fissure, along tentorial margins,

beneath temporal + occipital lobes; bilateral in 15 –
25% (common in elderly)
√ extraaxial peripheral crescentic fluid collection
between skull and cerebral hemisphere usually with
  √ concave inner margin (hematoma minimally
  pressing into brain substance)
  √ convex outer margin following normal contour of
  cranial vault
√ hyperdense (< 1 week) / isodense (1 – 3 weeks) /
hypodense (3 – 4 weeks)
√ occasionally with blood-fluid level
√ isodense hematoma may be recognizable by mass
effect with effacement of cortical sulci, deviation of
lateral ventricle, midline shift
  <u>False-negative CT scan:</u>
    high-convexity location, beam-hardening artifact,
    volume averaging with high density of calvarium
    obscuring flat "en plaque" hematoma, isodense
    hematoma during 10 – 20 days post injury
    Δ 38% of small subdural hematomas are missed
√ after surgical evacuation: underlying parenchymal
injury becomes more obvious
√ after healing: ventricular + sulcal enlargement
MRI:
  √ modality of choice in subacute stage because of
  high sensitivity for Met-Hb on T1WI (esp. superior
  to CT during isodense phase)
  √ allows differentiation of subdural from epidural
  blood secondary to low signal of dura
Cx: Arteriovenous fistula (meningeal artery + vein
    caught in fracture line)

<u>INTERHEMISPHERIC SUBDURAL HEMATOMA</u>
  most common acute finding in child abuse (whiplash
  forces on large head with weak neck muscles)
  √ predominance for posterior portion of
  interhemispheric fissure
  √ crescentic shape with flat medial border
  √ unilateral increased attenuation with extension
  along course of tentorium
  √ anterior extension to level of genu of corpus
  callosum

Chronic Subdural Hematoma
following minor injury some time ago; rarely associated
with parenchymal injury
Histo: hematoma enclosed by thick + vascular
    membrane which forms after 3 – 6 weeks
Pathogenesis: vessel fragility accounts for repeated
    episodes of rebleeding following minor
    injuries which tear fragile capillary bed
    within neomembrane surrounding
    subdural hematoma
√ crescentic-shaped hematoma conforming to
configuration of brain (early)
√ usually biconvex configuration (late), esp. after
compartmentalization secondary to formation of
fibrous septa

√ low density + high density components of collection
(after rebleeding)
√ fluid-fluid level
√ displacement / absence of sulci, displacement of
ventricles + parenchyma
√ No midline shift if bilateral (25%)
√ CECT demonstrates medially displaced cortical vein
or membrane around hematoma (1 – 4 weeks after
injury)
DDx: Acute epidural hematoma (similar biconvex
    shape)

TOXOPLASMOSIS OF BRAIN
= intrauterine infection with Toxoplasma gondii (found in
ventricular fluid)
Histo: inflammatory granuloma
• chorioretinitis
• mental retardation
√ multiple irregular, nodular / cyst-like / curvilinear
calcifications in periventricular area + choroid plexus
(= necrotic foci); bilateral; 1 – 20 mm in size; increasing
in number + size (usually not developed at time of birth)
√ microcephaly with little postnatal growth
√ hydrocephalus with return to normal / persistence of
large head size
√ thickened vault, sutures apposed / overlapping

TUBERCULOMA OF BRAIN
= result of granuloma formation within cerebral substance
Incidence: 0.15% of intracranial masses in Western
    countries, 30% in underdeveloped countries
Age: infant, small child, young adult
associated with: tuberculous meningitis in 50%
• Hx of previous extracranial TB (in 60%)
Location: more common in posterior fossa (62%),
    cerebellar hemispheres; may be associated
    with tuberculous meningitis
√ solitary (70%) / multiple (30 – 60%) lesions; may be
multiloculated
NCCT:
  √ isodense (72%) / hyperdense lesion of 0.5 – 4 cm in
  diameter with mass effect (93%)
  √ surrounding edema (72%) less marked than in
  pyogenic abscess
  √ central calcification (29%)
CECT:
  √ homogeneous enhancement
  √ ring blush (nearly all) with smooth / slightly shaggy
  margins + thick wall around an isodense center
  (DDx: in pyogenic abscess less thick + more regular)
  √ "target sign" = central calcification in isodense lesion
  + ring-blush (DDx: giant aneurysm)
  √ homogeneous blush in tuberculoma-en-plaque along
  dural plane (6%) (DDx : meningioma en-plaque)

TUBEROUS SCLEROSIS
= BOURNEVILLE DISEASE = EPIPLOIA = autosomal
dominant neuroectodermal disorder with frequent skips

in generations; sporadic in 50 – 80%; characterized by TRIAD consisting of
  (1) Adenoma sebaceum
  (2) Seizures
  (3) Mental retardation
  mnemonic: zits, fits, nitwits
= GENERALIZED HAMARTOMATOUS DISEASE
  1. CNS: periventricular + cortical (tubers)
  2. kidney: angiomyolipoma
  3. skin: adenoma sebaceum
  4. retina: retinal astrocytic hamartoma
Frequency: 1:150,000 live births; lower incidence in Blacks
Prognosis: 30% dead by age 5; 75% dead by age 20

@ CNS INVOLVEMENT
- Seizures (80 – 90%): often first + most common sign of tuberous sclerosis with onset at 1st – 2nd year
- Mental retardation (< 40%): progressive; observed in adulthood

1. Tubers (in 56%):
  Histo: clusters of atypical glial cells surrounded by giant cells with frequent calcifications (if > 2 years of age) = hamartomas
  Location of tubers:
    (a) Supratentorial: lateral walls of frontal horn + anterior 3rd ventricle, commonly at foramen of Monro, cortical surface, subcortical gray matter, white matter, basal ganglia
    (b) Infratentorial (less common + always associated with supratentorial lesions): cerebellum, medulla, spinal cord
  Frequency: solitary parenchymal (6%); subependymal + parenchymal (12%); subependymal (37%); multiple (75 %); bilateral (30%)
√ noncalcified hypodense brain lesions of abnormal myelination (superficial cortical, white matter, rarely subependymal)
√ subependymal tubers with "candle drippings" appearance at lining of lateral ventricles, calcified in 88 %
√ cortical tubers calcified in 54%
√ intracranial calcifications in up to 90% (15% < 1 year of age, 60% in teenagers)
√ small round dense nodules without contrast enhancement (unless malignant)
  MRI:
  √ relaxation time similar to white matter (if uncalcified)
  √ multiple nodules + confluent areas of high signal intensity on T2WI, iso- / hypointense on T1WI (fibrillary gliosis / demyelination)
  Cx: malignant degeneration into giant cell astrocytoma (10 – 12%)
  DDx:
    (1) Intrauterine CMV / toxoplasma infection (smaller lesions, brain atrophy, microcephaly)

    (2) Basal ganglia calcification in hypoparathyroidism / Fahr disease (location)
    (3) Sturge-Weber, calcified AVM (diffuse atrophy, not focal)
    (4) Heterotopic grey matter (along medial ventricular wall, isodense, associated with agenesis of corpus callosum, Chiari malformation)

2. Intraventricular glioma (in 37%)
  Histo: (a) giant cell astrocytoma
          (b) spongioblastoma (c) ependymoma
  Location: frontal horns / bodies of lateral ventricles (83%), septum pellucidum
  √ dense lesion with contrast enhancement
  √ hydrocephalus (brain atrophy / obstruction at foramen of Monro)

@ RENAL INVOLVEMENT
- renal failure in severe cases (in 5%)
- hypertension

1. Angiomyolipoma (40 – 80%): usually multiple + bilateral; risk of spontaneous hemorrhage (subcapsular / perinephric)
2. Multiple cysts of varying size in cortex + medulla mimicking adult polycystic kidney disease
  Path: cysts lined by columnar epithelium with foci of hyperplasia projecting into cyst lumen

@ BONE INVOLVEMENT
√ sclerotic calvarial patches (45%) = "bone islands" involving diploe + internal table; frontal + parietal location
√ thickening of diploe (long-term phenytoin therapy)
√ bone islands in pelvic brim, vertebrae, long bones
√ periosteal thickening of long bones
√ bone cysts with undulating periosteal reaction in distal phalanges (most common), metacarpals, metatarsals (DDx: sarcoid, neurofibromatosis)

@ LUNG INVOLVEMENT (1%)
√ interstitial fibrosis in lower lung fields + miliary nodular pattern may progress to honeycomb lung (smooth muscle proliferation around blood vessels)
√ cor pulmonale
√ spontaneous pneumothorax (50%)
√ chylothorax

@ HEART INVOLVEMENT
√ rhabdomyoma (in 5%)

@ SKIN INVOLVEMENT
- Adenoma sebaceum (80 – 90%) = wart-like nodules averaging 4 mm in size with bimalar distribution ("butterfly rash")
  Age: first discovered at age 3 – 6 years; family history in 30%
  Path: small hamartomas from neural elements with blood vessel hyperplasia = angiofibromas
- Shagreen rough skin patches (80%) = "pigskin" = "peau d'orange" = patches of fibrous hyperplasia; intertriginous + lumbar location
- Ash leaf patches = hypopigmented macules shaped like ash / spearmint leaf (earliest manifestation in infancy)

- Ungual fibromas (15 – 50%): sub-/ periungual with erosion of distal tuft
- Cafe-au-lait spots

@ RETINAL INVOLVEMENT
- Phakoma (< 50%) = whitish disc-shaped hamartoma / astrocytoma
  Path: glia cells, ganglion cells, fibroblasts
√ Optic nerve glioma

@ VASCULAR INVOLVEMENT (rare)
√ thoracic + abdominal arterial aneurysms
Path: vascular dysplasia with intimal + medial abnormalities of large muscular + musculoelastic arteries

VEIN OF GALEN ANEURYSM
= central AVM directly draining into secondarily enlarged vein of Galen (aneurysm is misnomer), fed by anterior cerebral artery, anterior + posterior choroidal arteries, lenticulostriate + thalamic perforating arteries
Age at presentation: neonatal period; detectable in utero; M:F = 2:1
- cardiac failure (36%)
- cranial bruit
- headaches
- seizures, focal neurologic signs (5%)
- macrocrania from obstructive hydrocephalus
may be associated with porencephaly, nonimmune hydrops
√ homogeneous slightly hyperdense smoothly marginated midline mass often indenting the posterior 3rd ventricle
√ dilated straight sinus + torcular Herophili
√ marked homogeneous enhancement on CECT of vein of Galen + straight sinus
√ prominent serpiginous thalamic network
√ focal hypodense zones (ischemic changes)
√ dilatation of lateral + 3rd ventricle (37%)
√ median tubular cystic space with flow demonstrated by Doppler signals
Cx: subarachnoid hemorrhage
DDx: pineal tumor (no dilated straight sinus + torcular Herophili)

VENOUS ANGIOMA
= cluster of dilated medullary veins which drain into an enlarged vein; bleed rarely
Histo: venous channels without internal elastic lamina, separated by gliotic neural tissue which may calcify; probably representing persistent fetal venous system
√ no arterial vessels
√ radially oriented veins at periphery of lesion converging to one vein
DDx: Sturge-Weber disease (diffuse pial angiomatosis with venous-type capillaries)

VENOUS SINUS THROMBOSIS
A. *Septic causes* (esp. in childhood):
   Mastoiditis, Sub- / epidural empyema, Meningitis, Encephalitis, Brain abscess, Face + scalp cellulitis, Septicemia
B. *Aseptic causes*
   (a) Tumor compressing sinuses: meningioma, leukemia
   (b) Trauma: fracture through sinus wall, cranial surgery
   (c) Low-flow state: CHF, CHD, dehydration, shock
   (d) Hypercoagulability: Polycythemia vera, Idiopathic thrombocytosis, Thrombocytopenia, Cryofibrinogenemia, Sickle cell disease, Pregnancy, Contraceptive steroids, Disseminated intravascular coagulopathy
   (e) Chemotherapy: e.g. ARA-C
- headaches, seizures
- stroke symptomatology
NCCT:
√ high attenuation material (clotted blood) in sagittal sinus / straight sinus / cerebral cortical vein = "cord sign" (rare)
√ compression of lateral ventricles in 32% (infarction / edema)
√ unilateral (2/3) / bilateral (1/3) parenchymal hemorrhage involving gray + white matter (20%)
CECT:
√ "delta sign" / "empty triangle" = filling defect in straight sinus / superior sagittal sinus (in 70%)
√ gyral enhancement in periphery of infarction (30 – 40%)
√ intense tentorial enhancement secondary to collaterals (rare)
√ dense transcortical medullary vein
Angio:
√ nonfilling of thrombosed sinus
√ filling of cortical veins, deep venous system, cavernous sinus
√ parasagittal hemorrhages (highly specific for superior sagittal sinus thrombosis) secondary to cortical venous infarction
MRI: √ high signal within sinus on T1WI + T2WI
Prognosis: high mortality

VENTRICULITIS
= EPENDYMITIS = inflammation of ependymal lining of one / more ventricles
Cause: (1) rupture of periventricular abscess (thinner capsule wall medially)
        (2) retrograde spread of infection from basal cisterns
CECT (necessary for diagnosis):
√ thin uniform enhancement of involved ependymal lining
√ often associated with intraventricular inflammatory exudate + septations
Cx: Obstructive hydrocephalus (occlusion at foramen of Monro / aqueduct)
DDx: ependymal metastases, lymphoma, infiltrating glioma

VISCERAL LARVA MIGRANS OF BRAIN
roundworm nematode (Toxocara canis)
√ small calcific nodules, especially in basal ganglia +
  periventricular
DDx: tuberous sclerosis

VON HIPPEL-LINDAU DISEASE
= vHL= RETINOCEREBELLAR ANGIOMATOSIS
  = uncommon autosomal dominant disease with variable
    penetrance; 20% familial
@ CNS MANIFESTATION
  • cerebellar symptoms
  • signs of increased intracranial pressure
  • vision changes
  1. Retinal angiomatosis (von Hippel tumor)
     √ thick calcified retinal density (calcified angioma-
       induced hematoma)
  2. Hemangioblastomas of CNS (Lindau tumor)
     = most commonly recognized manifestation of vHL
       disease; multifocal in 10%
     Δ 4 – 20% of single hemangioblastomas occur in von
       Hippel-Lindau disease
     Age: 15 – 40 years
     Site: posterior fossa (88%) mostly in cerebellar
            hemisphere (90%), some in vermis, a few
            close to 4th ventricle, medulla, spinal cord
     CT: √ cystic mass in 75%, solid (iso- / hyperdense /
           mixed) in 25%

√ intense tumor blush / blushing mural nodule
√ NO calcifications (DDx: cystic astrocytoma
  calcified in 25%)
@ ADRENAL pheochromocytoma
@ RENAL
  • elevated erythropoeitin with polycythemia (10 – 20%)
  1. multiple cortical cysts (75%)
  2. angiomas
  3. renal cell carcinoma: age of 20 – 50 years, in 10%
     bilateral

MULTIPLE ORGAN NEOPLASMS
  @   Kidney   : renal cell carcinoma (up to 35%)
                      renal angioma (up to 45%)
  @   Liver   : adenoma, angioma
  @   Pancreas   : cystadenoma / adenocarcinoma
  @   Epididymis   : adenoma
  @   Adrenal gland: pheochromocytoma

MULTIPLE ORGAN CYSTS
  (1) Kidney (usually multiple cortical cysts in 75 – 100%
       at early age, most common abdominal
       manifestation)
  (2) Pancreas (in 9 – 72% often numerous cysts;
       second most common affected abdominal organ)
  (3) Others: liver, spleen, omentum / mesentery,
       epididymis, adrenals, lung, bone

DIFFERENTIAL DIAGNOSIS OF ORBITAL DISEASES

Intraconal lesion

CONUS = incomplete fenestrated musculofascial system extending from bony orbit to anterior third of globe, consists of extraocular muscles + interconnecting fascia

Intraconal structures: optic nerve, ophthalmic artery, orbital fat

Extraconal structures: lacrimal gland, lacrimal sac, portion of superior ophthalmic vein, fat

mnemonic: "Mel Met Rita Mending Hems On Poor Charlie's Grave"

Melanoma	Optic glioma
Metastasis	Pseudotumor
Retinoblastoma	Cellulitis
Meningioma	Grave disease
Hemangioma	

Intraconal lesion with optic nerve involvement
1. Optic nerve glioma
2. Optic nerve sheath meningioma
3. Optic neuritis
4. Inflammatory pseudotumor (may surround optic nerve)
5. Intraorbital lymphoma (may surround optic nerve, older patient)

Intraconal lesion without optic nerve involvement
1. Orbital hemangioma
2. Orbital varix
3. Carotid-cavernous fistula
4. Arteriovenous malformation
   least common of orbital vascular malformations (congenital, idiopathic, traumatic)
   √ irregularly shaped intensely enhancing mass of enlarged vessels
   √ associated with dilated superior / inferior ophthalmic vein
5. Hematoma
6. Lymphangioma
7. Neurilemoma
   √ commonly adjacent to superior orbital fissure, inferior to optic nerve
   √ local bone erosion

Extraconal lesion
Extraconal-intraorbital lesion
1. Lymphoma / Leukemia
   Location: anterior extraconal space / retrobulbar
   √ slight to moderate enhancing mass on CECT
2. Dermoid cyst

3. Metastasis
   Origin: Carcinoma of breast + lung (adults); Neuroblastoma, Ewing sarcoma, Leukemia, Wilms tumor (children)
   Location: 12% intraorbital , 86% intraocular (choroid)
4. Inflammatory orbital pseudotumor

Extraconal-extraorbital lesion
A. FROM SINUS
   maxillary / sphenoid sinuses are rare locations of origin
   1. Tumor: squamous cell carcinoma (80%), adenocarcinoma, adenoid cystic carcinoma, lymphoma
   2. Paranasal sinusitis:
      most common cause of orbital infection; originating from ethmoid sinuses (in children), from frontal sinus (in adolescence)
      Organism: Staphylococcus, Streptococcus, Pneumococcus
      √ preseptal / orbital edema / cellulitis
      √ subperiosteal / orbital abscess
      √ mucormycosis (in diabetics) destroys bone + extends into cavernous sinus
      Cx: (1) epidural abscess (2) subdural empyema (3) cavernous sinus thrombosis (4) meningitis (5) cerebritis (6) brain abscess
   3. Mucocele
B. FROM SKIN
   1. Orbital cellulitis
C. FROM LACRIMAL GLAND
   √ mass arising from superolateral aspect of orbit
   1. Tumors
      (a) benign: granuloma, cyst
      (b) malignant: adenocarcinoma, adenoid cystic carcinoma, mixed tumor
   2. Dacryoadenitis
   3. **Mikulicz syndrome**
      = enlargement of gland secondary to systemic disease (sarcoidosis, TB)

mnemonic: "MOLD"
Metastasis
Others (rhabdomyosarcoma, lymphangioma, sinus lesion)
Lymphoma, **L**acrimal gland tumor
Dermoid

Intraocular lesion
Intraocular calcifications
1. Retinoblastoma

2. **Astrocytic hamartoma**
   associated with tuberous sclerosis
   + neurofibromatosis
   Location: retina / near optic disc
   √ typically unilateral (DDx to drusen)
3. **Choroidal osteoma**
   young woman; mature bone
   √ very dense curvilinear mass aligned with choroidal
   margin of globe
4. **Optic drusen**
   = accretions of hyaline material on / near surface of
   optic disc; often familial
   √ small round calcification at junction of retina + optic
   nerve
   √ usually bilateral
5. Scleral calcifications
   (a) in systemic hypercalcemic states (HPT,
   Hypervitaminosis D, Sarcoidosis, secondary to
   chronic renal disease)
   (b) in elderly: at insertion of extraocular muscles
6. Retrolental fibroplasia
7. **Phthisis bulbi**
   secondary to trauma or infection
   √ small contracted calcified disorganized
   nonfunctioning globe

Noncalcified ocular process

1. Uveal melanoma
2. Metastasis
   86% of ocular lesions within globe; usually to
   vascular choroid
   Origin: breast, lung, GI tract, GU tract, cutaneous
   melanoma, neuroblastoma
   √ bilateral in 30%
3. **Choroidal hemangioma**
   most common benign tumor in adults
   may be associated with: Sturge-Weber syndrome
   √ focal thickening of posterior wall of globe
   √ enhancement similar to choroid
4. **Vitreous lymphoma**
   √ diffuse ill-defined soft tissue density
5. Developmental anomalies
   (a) **Primary glaucoma** = enlargement of eye
   secondary to narrowing of Schlemm canal
   (b) **Coloboma** = congenital defective closure of
   embryonic choroid fissure affecting eyelid / iris /
   retina / macula
   (c) **Staphyloma** = berry-like protrusion of cornea /
   pear-shaped sacculation of posterior pole
   secondary to high myopia, glaucoma, trauma

Optic nerve enlargement

A. TUMOR:
   1. Optic nerve glioma
   2. Optic nerve sheath meningioma
   3. Infiltration by leukemia / lymphoma
B. FLUID:
   4. Perineural hematoma

5. Papilledema of intracranial hypertension
6. Patulous subarachnoid space
C.   INFLAMMATION:
   7. Optic neuritis
   8. Sarcoidosis
√ Fusiform / excrescentic lesion
   (a) with central lucency: meningioma
   (b) without central lucency: optic nerve glioma
√ Tubular enlargement
   (a) with central lucency: subarachnoid process
   (metastases, perineuritis, meningioma, perineural
   hemorrhage)
   (b) without central lucency: papilledema, leukemia,
   lymphoma, sarcoid, optic nerve glioma

Orbital tumor in childhood

1.	Dermoid cyst	46%
2.	Inflammatory lesion	16%
3.	Dermolipoma	7%
4.	Capillary hemangioma	4%
5.	Rhabdomyosarcoma	4%
6.	Leukemia / Lymphoma	2%
7.	Optic nerve glioma	2%
8.	Lymphangioma	2%
9.	Cavernous hemangioma	1%
10.	Retinoblastoma	

Mass in superolateral quadrant of orbit

1. Lacrimal gland tumor
   — Benign mixed tumor = pleomorphic adenoma
   — Malignant mixed tumor = pleomorphic
   adenocarcinoma, Adenoid cystic carcinoma)
2. Dermoid cyst
3. Metastasis (breast, prostate, lung)
4. Lymphoma
5. Sarcoidosis
6. Wegener granulomatosis
7. Pseudotumor
8. Frontal sinus mucocele

Extraocular muscle enlargement

A . Endocrine
   1. Grave disease (50%)
   2. Acromegaly
B.   Inflammation
   1. **Myositis**
   • rapid onset of proptosis, erythema of lids,
   conjunctival injection
   Location: single muscle (in adults);
              multiple muscles (in children)
   √ enlarged extraocular muscle
   √ positive response to steroids
   2. Orbital cellulitis
   3. Sjögren disease, Wegener granulomatosis, Lethal
   midline granuloma, SLE
   4. Sarcoidosis
   5. Foreign body reaction

C. Tumor
   1. Pseudotumor
   2. Rhabdomyosarcoma
   3. Metastasis, Lymphoma, Leukemia
D. Vascular
   1. Spontaneous / traumatic hematoma
   2. Arteriovenous malformation
   3. Carotid-cavernous sinus fistula

Dense vitreous in pediatric age group
1. Retinoblastoma
2. Persistent hyperplastic primary vitreous
3. Coats disease
4. Norrie disease
5. Retrolental fibroplasia
6. Sclerosing endophthalmitis

Anopia
A. Monocular defects
   1 = monocular blindness (optic nerve lesion)
B. Bilateral heteronymous defects
   2 = bitemporal hemianopia (chiasmatic lesion: pituitary tumor)
   3 = homonymous hemianopia
C. Bilateral homonymous defects
   4   = homonymous hemianopia
   5   = central hemianoptic scotoma
   6   = upper right-sided quadranopia
   3,4,5 = most common type of hemianopia (CVA, brain tumor)

Ophthalmoplegia
lesions of
1. Oculomotor nerve (III)
   innervates medial rectus, superior rectus, inferior rectus, inferior oblique muscle, pupilloconstrictor, levator palpebrae
2. Trochlear nerve (IV)
   innervates superior oblique muscle
3. Abducens nerve (VI)
   innervates lateral rectus muscle

Leukokoria
= abnormal white / pinkish / yellowish pupillary light reflex
1. Retinoblastoma
2. Persistent hyperplastic primary vitreous
3. Retrolental fibroplasia
4. Posterior cataract
5. Coloboma of choroid / optic disk
6. Uveitis
7. Larval granulomatosis
8. Coats disease

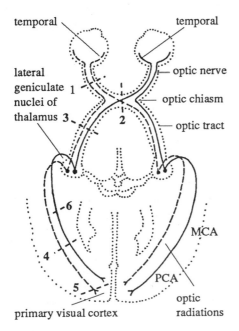

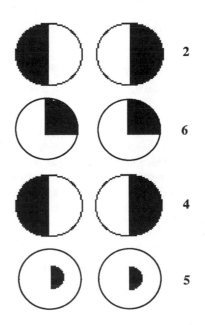

Types of Anopia
(numbers refer to bold numbers in text)

DISEASE ENTITIES OF ORBIT

ABSCESS OF ORBIT
Location: most commonly in subperiosteal space on medial wall
√ subperiosteal fluid collection
√ displacement of thickened periosteal membrane + increased enhancement
√ displacement of adjacent fat + extraocular muscles

CELLULITIS OF ORBIT
Cause: bacterial infection extending from paranasal sinuses, face, eyelid, nose, teeth, lacrimal sac through thin lamina papyracea + valveless facial veins into orbit
cannot be differentiated from edema, chloroma, leukemic infiltrate
√ thickening of eyelids + septum
√ proptosis
√ scleral thickening
√ enlargement + displacement of extraocular muscles (frequently medial rectus muscle)
√ increased attenuation of orbital fat + obliteration of fat planes
√ opacification of ethmoid + maxillary sinus

COATS DISEASE
= Pseudoglioma = primary retinal vascular anomaly with telangiectasia + detachment of retina secondary to accumulation of lipoproteinaceous exudate in retina + subretinal space
Age: 6 – 8 years
• may present with leukokoria (if retina massively detached)
√ unilateral dense vitreous without focal mass / calcification

DERMOID CYST OF ORBIT
most common orbital tumor in childhood (45% of all masses)
Age: 1st decade
Histo: contains keratin, hair, stratified epithelium + dermal appendages within thick capsule; usually arises in fetal cleavage planes (sutures)
Location: in anterior orbit superolaterally near brow (60%), upper nasal quadrant (25%)
√ well-circumscribed cystic mass ± negative HU numbers
√ ± expansion / erosion of bony orbit

EDEMA OF ORBIT
Cause: infection of skin, paranasal sinus, oral cavity, lacrimal apparatus
Location: usually confined to preseptal structures (eyelid, face); involvement of orbital structures (rare)
√ swelling of eyelids / face
√ increase in fat attenuation
√ displacement of extraocular muscles

ENDOPHTHALMITIS
A.   INFECTIOUS ENDOPHTHALMITIS
most commonly related to eye injury / surgery
√ increased attenuation of vitreous
B.   TOXOCARA CANIS ENDOPHTHALMITIS
= granulomatous uveitis resulting in subretinal exudate, retinal detachment, organized vitreous
√ obliteration of vitreous cavity with increase in density
√ contrast enhancement of sclera
C.   SCLEROSING ENDOPHTHALMITIS
= granulomatous uveitis secondary to Toxocara canis infestation
√ dense vitreous

GRAVES DISEASE OF ORBIT
= THYROID OPHTHALMOPATHY
= ENDOCRINE EXOPHTHALMUS
most common cause of bilateral proptosis, increase in orbital pressure produces ischemia, edema, fibrosis of muscles
Etiology: produced by long-acting thyroid stimulating factor (LATS)
Histo: deposition of mucopolysaccharides + collagen + glycoprotein; infiltration by mast cells and lymphocytes, edema, muscle fiber necrosis
Age: adulthood; 5% younger than 15 years; M:F = 1:4
• proptosis (> 1/3 of globe anterior to interorbital line)
• decrease in visual acuity
• hyperthyroidism; euthyroidism (in 15%)
Location: medial + inferior rectus muscle (most common) > superior + levator palpebrae > lateral rectus muscle; bilateral in 70 – 85%; asymmetrical involvement in 10 – 30%
√ swelling of muscles maximally in midportion (relative sparing of tendinous insertion of globe) = "coke-bottle" sign
√ orbital apex involved late (pressure on optic nerve)
√ increased density of orbital fat (late)

HEMANGIOMA OF ORBIT
most common benign tumor
(a) Capillary hemangioma:
most common vascular tumor of orbit in children; 5 – 15% of all pediatric orbital masses; poorly encapsulated
Age: first 2 weeks of life; 95% in < 6 months of age; M < F
• proptosis exaggerated by crying
• associated with skin angioma (90%)
√ mass with enhancement equal to / greater than orbital muscle
Prognosis: spontaneous involution within 1 – 2 years

(b) Cavernous hemangioma:
     1 – 2% of childhood orbital masses
     Age: middle-aged adult; F > M
     Histo: large dilated venous channels with flattened
              endothelial cells surrounded by fibrous
              capsule
     • slowly progressive

Location: 94% retrobulbar
√ sharply demarcated oval mass in superior-temporal
  portion of conus (2/3)
√ expansion of bony orbit
√ inhomogeneous enhancement; small calcifications
√ puddling of contrast material on angiography

LYMPHANGIOMA OF ORBIT
Incidence: 3.5:100,000; 1 – 2% of orbital childhood
              masses; 8% of expanding orbital lesions
Histo: dilated lymphatics, dysplastic venous vessels,
         smooth muscle, areas of hemorrhage
Age: 1st decade (progression slows with termination of
        body growth), may present later
• associated with lesions on lid, conjunctiva, cheek
• coincident lymphangiomatous cysts in oral mucosa
• proptosis (exacerbated during upper respiratory
   infections; sudden proptosis from spontaneous
   intratumoral hemorrhage)
√ mild to moderate enlargement of orbit
√ poorly defined multilobulated inhomogeneous lesion
  with intra- and extraconal component usually medial to
  optic nerve
√ single / multiple cystlike areas with rim enhancement
  (after hemorrhage)
√ some enhancement (venous channels)
√ rarely contains phleboliths (DDx: hemangioma, orbital
  varix)
DDx: orbital varix

NORRIE DISEASE
= X-linked recessive disease; ? inherited form of
  persistent hyperplastic primary vitreous
• seizures, mental deficiency (50%)
• hearing loss, deafness by age 4 (30%)
• leukokoria, cataract, blindness
√ microphthalmia
√ dense vitreous with blood-fluid level
√ cone-shaped central retinal detachment
√ calcifications

OPTIC NERVE GLIOMA
= JUVENILE PILOCYTIC ASTROCYTOMA
= most common cause of optic nerve enlargement
Incidence: 1% of all intracranial tumors, 2% of childhood
              orbital masses
Histo: proliferation of well-differentiated astrocytes
         = low-grade glial neoplasm
Age: 1st decade (80%); peak age around 5 years;
        M < F

associated with neurofibromatosis in 10 – 50%
                   (± bilateral optic gliomas)
• decreased visual acuity, proptosis
√ fusiform / lobulated well-circumscribed enlargement of
  optic nerve
√ ± posterior extension along optic tracts (indicates
  nonresectability)
√ globular mass; may calcify
√ same attenuation as normal optic nerve; slight contrast
  enhancement
√ ipsilateral optic canal enlargement (90%) > 3 mm /
  1 mm difference compared with contralateral side
MRI: more sensitive than CT in detecting intracanalicular
      + intracranial extent
      √ isointense to muscle on T1WI
      √ hypointense on T2WI

OPTIC NERVE SHEATH MENINGIOMA
= PERIOPTIC MENINGIOMA
Age: middle-aged + elderly females; slightly more
        aggressive in children
occasionally associated with
   neurofibromatosis (usually in teenagers)
Primary origin: arising from arachnoid rests in the
                   meningeal investiture of optic nerves
                   (a) in orbit (b) in middle fossa
• progressive loss of visual acuity (optic atrophy),
   proptosis
√ smooth fusiform tumor surrounding optic nerve
√ sphenoid bone hyperostosis
√ frequently calcified
CECT: enhancement is the rule
      √ dense linear bands (axial view) as "tram tracks" / ring-
        like (coronal view)
      √ extension into optic canal (not uncommon)
MRI:
      √ extrinsic soft tissue mass surrounding optic nerve
      √ hypointense to fat on T1WI

OPTIC NEURITIS
= nerve involvement by inflammation, degeneration,
demyelination
Etiology: (1) multiple sclerosis (involves optic nerve
             in 1/3) (2) inflammation secondary to ocular
             infection (3) degeneration (toxic, metabolic,
             nutritional) (4) ischemia (5) meningitis /
             encephalitis
√ normal / mildly enlarged optic nerve + chiasm
√ may show enhancement

PERSISTENT HYPERPLASTIC PRIMARY VITREOUS
= rare condition with persistence + hyperplasia of
  embryonic hyaloid vascular system of primary vitreous
  (= hyaloid canal of Cloquet); friable vessels may lead to
  intravitreal hemorrhage
May be associated with any severe ocular malformation /
optic dysplasia (e.g., Norrie disease)

— Primary vitreous
  = fibrillar ectodermal + mesodermal tissue consisting primarily of embryonic hyaloid vascular system
  Occupies space between lens + retina during first several months of gestation
— Hyaloid artery
  = important source of intraocular nutrition until 8th month of gestation
  Arises from dorsal opthalmic artery at 3rd week of gestation; grows anteriorly with branches supplying vitreous + posterior aspect of lens
— Secondary / adult vitreous
  Begins to form during 3rd gestational month; gradually replaces primary vitreous which is reduced to a small S-shaped remnant (hyaloid canal = Cloquet canal) and serves as lymph channel
• unilateral leukokoria
CT:
  √ microphthalmia = small hypoplastic globe
  √ small optic nerve
  √ deformity of globe + lens
  √ dense vitreous
  √ vitreous fluid-fluid levels (from breakdown of recurrent hemorrhage in subhyaloid / subretinal space)
  √ enhancing cone-shaped central retrolental density extending from lens through vitreous body to back of orbit, just lateral to optic nerve
  √ NO calcifications
MRI:
  √ hyperintense vitreous body on T1WI + T2WI from vitreous hemorrhage / proteinaceous fluid
  √ hypointense thin triangular band with base near optic disk and apex at posterior surface of lens
Cx:
  (1) Glaucoma, cataract from recurrent spontaneous intraocular hemorrhage
  (2) Proliferation of embryonic tissue
  (3) Retinal detachment from organizing hemorrhage / traction
  (4) Hydrops / atrophy of globe + resorption of lens

PSEUDOTUMOR OF ORBIT
  = nongranulomatous inflammatory process affecting all intraorbital soft tissues; may be confused with lymphoma clinically, radiographically, pathologically
Histo: nonspecific round cell infiltration of fat, muscle, sclera, (occasionally) lacrimal gland
Etiology:
  (a) cause not apparent at time of study: bacterial, viral, foreign body
  (b) systemic disease presently not apparent: sarcoidosis, collagen, endocrine
  (c) idiopathic: probably abnormal immune response
Incidence: 25% of all cases of unilateral exophthalmos
may be associated with:
  Wegener granulomatosis, Sarcoidosis, Retroperitoneal fibrosis, Thyroiditis, Cholangitis
Types: (a) local (b) diffuse (c) subconjunctival

• painful proptosis in young female
• chemosis, lid injection
• limitation of ocular movement
  √ increased density of retro-orbital fat (may involve anterior compartment)
  √ discrete / poorly defined intra- / extraconal mass = "pseudotumor" close to surface margin of globe
  √ typically involves muscles and tendon insertions (DDx to Graves disease with muscle involvement only)
  √ thickening and enhancement of sclera near Tenon capsule
  √ enlargement of one / more extraocular muscles close to insertion in globe with ill-defined margins (unusual)
  √ enlarged lacrimal gland
  √ proptosis (25% of cases presenting with unilateral proptosis)
Prognosis: (1) remitting / chronic + progressive course
            (2) dramatic response to steroids
DDx: lymphoma, thyroid ophthalmopathy, radiation therapy

RETINOBLASTOMA
  = primary intraocular malignant tumor of childhood arising from photoreceptor cells (neuroectoderm) of retina; autosomal dominant in 10%
Incidence: 1:17,000 live births
Age: 18 months at presentation; most common malignant tumor of the eye in infants < 3 years
Histo: Flexner-Wintersteiner rosettes
may be associated with:
  (1) Pinealoblastoma = **Trilateral Retinoblastoma** (rare variant) = bilateral retinoblastomas + neuroectodermal pineal tumor
  (2) Osteosarcoma + other CNS neoplasms
• "cat's eye" = leukokoria (whitish mass behind lens)
Location: posterolateral wall of globe (most commonly); multicentric within same eye (25%); hereditary form may involve both eyes in 25%
CT:
  √ solid smoothly marginated lobulated retrolental hyperdense mass in endophytic type (rarer exophytic type grows subretinally causing retinal detachment)
  √ partial / complete calcification (50 – 90%)
  √ dense vitreous (common)
  √ extraocular extension (in 25%): optic nerve enlargement, abnormal soft tissue in orbit, intracranial extension
Cx:
  (1) Metastases to: meninges (via subarachnoid space), bone marrow, liver, lymph nodes
  (2) radiation-induced sarcomas develop in 15 – 20%
Prognosis: spontaneous regression in 1%; calcifications = favorable prognostic sign; contrast enhancement = poor prognostic sign
DDx:
  (1) Retinoma = Retinocytoma (benign variant)
  (2) Toxocara canis infection

(3) Retrolental fibroplasia
(4) Coats disease (subretinal exudation)
(5) Norrie disease (retinal dysplasia)
(6) Persistent hyperplastic primary vitreous

RETROLENTAL FIBROPLASIA
= RETINOPATHY OF PREMATURITY
Predisposed: premature infants with respiratory distress
syndrome requiring prolonged oxygen
therapy
Severity directly related to:
(1) degree of prematurity
(2) birth weight
(3) amount of oxygen used in therapy
• leukokoria in severe cases (traction retinal detachment,
usually bilateral + temporal)
√ dense vitreous
√ calcifications in choroid + lens

RHABDOMYOSARCOMA
most common primary malignant orbital tumor in
childhood; arising from orbital soft tissues (not muscle)
Incidence: 3 − 4% of all pediatric orbital masses
Histo:
(1) embryonal type (75%)
(2) alveolar type (15%)
(3) pleomorphic type (10%);
arise from undifferentiated mesenchyma (not from
striated muscle)
rarely associated with neurofibromatosis
Age at presentation: average 7 years; 90% by 16 years;
M > F
• rapidly progressive proptosis
Location: orbit / retrobulbar (71%), lid (22%), conjunctiva
(7%)

√ large soft tissue density mass with ill-defined margins
(extraocular muscles not involved)
√ ± extension into preseptal space, adjacent sinus, nasal
cavity, intracranial cavity with bony erosion
√ may show significant enhancement
Metastases: lung, bone marrow, cervical lymph nodes
(rare)
Prognosis:
(1)   40% survival after exenteration
(2)   80 − 90% survival after radiation therapy
(4,000 − 5,000 rad) + chemotherapy (Vincristine,
Cyclophosphamide, Adriamycin)

UVEAL MELANOMA
most common primary intraocular neoplasm in adult
Caucasians
Age peak: 50 years
Location: choroid (93%) > ciliary body (4%) > iris (3%);
almost always unilateral
• retinal detachment, vitreous hemorrhage, astigmatism,
glaucoma
√ ill-defined hyperdense thickening of wall of globe
Metastases to: globe, optic nerve; liver, lung, subcutis

VARIX OF ORBIT
• intermittent exophthalmus associated with straining
• frequent blindness
√ involvement of superior / inferior orbital vein; phleboliths
rare
√ may produce bony erosion without sclerotic reaction
√ enlargement of mass during Valsalva maneuver /
jugular vein compression
√ well-defined markedly enhancing mass

DIFFERENTIAL DIAGNOSIS OF EAR, NOSE AND THROAT DISORDERS

Sclerosed temporal bone

1. Otosclerosis
2. Paget disease
   - hearing loss (stapes fixation in oval window / cochlear involvement)
   - √ usually lytic changes beginning in petrous pyramid + progressing laterally; otic capsule last to be affected
   - √ calvarial changes ± basilar impression
3. Fibrous dysplasia
   - painless mastoid swelling
   - conductive hearing loss (from narrowing of EAC / middle ear)
   - √ homogeneously dense thickened bone (density less than calvarial bone)
   - √ expanded bone with preserved cortex
   - √ lytic lesions (less frequent)
4. Meningioma
5. Metastasis
6. Ossifying fibroma
7. Osteosarcoma
8. Osteopetrosis

Atresia of inner ear

Incidence: 1:10,000
Etiology: (a) isolated (b) Trisomy (c) Turner syndrome (d) Maternal rubella (e) Craniofacial dysostosis (f) Mandibulofacial dysostosis
SPECTRUM
1. fibrous atresia of EAC
2. bony atresia (in position of tympanic membrane)
3. degree of pneumatization of mastoid (begins in 7th fetal month)
4. absence of tympanic cavity
5. anteriorly displaced vertical (mastoid) portion of facial nerve canal
6. decrease in number of cochlear turns (Mondini malformation) / absence of cochlea
7. dilatation of lateral semicircular canal

External ear neoplasm

1. Exostosis
   √ projecting into EAC; often multiple + bilateral
2. Osteoma
   √ may invade adjacent bone; single in EAC / mastoid
3. Ceruminoma
   from apocrine + sebaceous glands; bone erosion mimics malignancy
4. Squamous cell carcinoma
   - often long history of chronic suppurative otitis media = "malignant otitis"
5. Adenocarcinoma, Adenoid cystic carcinoma, Melanoma
6. Metastases

   (a) hematogeneous: breast, prostate, lung, kidney, thyroid
   (b) direct spread: skin, parotid, nasopharynx, brain, meninges
   (c) systemic: leukemia, lymphoma, myeloma
7. Histiocytosis X: in 15% of patients

Middle ear neoplasm

1. Glomus tumor (multiple in 10%; 8% malignant)
   (a) Glomus tympanicum: from cochlear promontory
       √ seldom erodes bone
   (b) Glomus jugulare:
       invasion of middle ear from below
       √ destruction of bony roof of jugular fossa + bony spur separating vein from carotid artery
2. Aberrant carotid artery
   √ protrusion into middle ear without bony margin
3. Enlarged jugular bulb
   √ protrusion into middle ear with dehiscent bony covering
4. Cholesteatoma
5. Rhabdomyosarcoma
   Location: orbit > nasopharynx > ear
6. Adenocarcinoma (rare)

Inner ear neoplasm

1. Acoustic neuroma
2. Meningioma = 2nd most common CPA tumor
3. Epidermoid tumor
   = Congenital / primary cholesteatoma
   3rd most common CPA tumor
   √ low attenuation (keratin content) + scalloped bone destruction
4. Glomus jugulare tumor
5. 5th nerve neurinoma
   √ may amputate petrous apex
6. Facial nerve neurinoma
   - persistent Bell palsy (in 5% caused by neurinoma)
   Location: intracanalicular > IAC
   √ expansion of bone in facial canal
7. Cholesterol granuloma
   √ isodense with brain
8. Petrous apex mucocele
9. Hemangioma, fibro-osseous lesion, metastases

Opacification of maxillary sinus

A. WITHOUT BONE DESTRUCTION
   1. Sinus aplasia / hypoplasia
      uni- / bilateral
      Age: NOT routinely visualized at birth, by age 6 antral floor at level of middle turbinate, by age 15 of adult size
      √ depression of orbital floor with enlargement of orbit

√ lateral displacement of lateral wall of nasal fossa with large turbinate
2. Maxillary dentigerous cyst
usually containing a tooth / crown; without tooth
= primordial dentigerous cyst
3. Ameloblastoma
4. Acute sinusitis
√ air-fluid level
B. WITH BONE DESTRUCTION
1. Maxillary sinus tumor
2. Infection: aspergillosis, mucormycosis, TB, syphilis
3. Wegener granulomatosis; lethal midline granuloma
4. Blow-out fracture

Paranasal sinus masses
1. Mucocele
2. Mucus retention cyst
= blockage of secretion in ducts secondary to allergy / inflammation
3. Polyp
secondary to atopic hypersensitivity (adult) / cystic fibrosis (child)
4. Antrochoanal polyp
5. Inverting papilloma
6. Sinusitis
7. Carcinoma

Granulomatous lesions of sinuses
A. Chronic irritants
1. beryllium
2. chromate salts
B. Infection
1. Tuberculosis
2. Actinomycosis
3. Rhinosclerma
4. Yaws
5. Blastomycosis
6. Leprosy
7. Rhinosporidiosis
8. Syphilis
9. Leishmaniosis
10. Glanders
C. Autoimmune disease
1. Wegener granulomatosis
D. Lymphoma-like lesions
1. Midline granuloma
E. Unclassified
1. Sarcoidosis

Parotid gland enlargement
A. Localized inflammatory disease
1. Chronic recurrent sialadenitis
2. Sialosis
3. Sarcoidosis
• diffuse bilateral painless enlargement (10 – 30%)
• xerostomia
CT: √ diffusely dense multinodular gland / enlargement of lymph nodes within gland

4. Tuberculosis
5. Cat-scratch fever
6. Syphilis
B. Systemic autoimmune related disease
1. Sjögren disease
2. Mikulicz disease
C. Neoplasm
D. Lymphoproliferative disorders

Airway obstruction in children
Nasopharyngeal narrowing
(a) Congenital: Choanal atresia, choanal stenosis, encephalocele
(b) Inflammatory: Adenoidal enlargement, polyps
(c) Neoplastic: Juvenile angiofibroma, rhabdomyosarcoma, teratoma, neuroblastoma, lymphoepithelioma
(d) Traumatic: Foreign body, hematoma, rhinolith

Oropharyngeal narrowing
(a) Congenital: Glossoptosis + micrognathia (Pierre-Robin, Goldenhar, Treacher-Collins syndrome), macroglossia (cretinism, Beckwith-Wiedemann syndrome)
(b) Inflammatory: Abscess, tonsillar hypertrophy
(c) Neoplastic: Lingular tumor / cyst
(d) Traumatic: Hematoma, foreign body

Retropharyngeal narrowing
= potential space (normally < 3/4 of AP diameter of adjacent cervical spine in infants / < 3 mm in older children)
(a) Congenital: Branchial cleft cyst, ectopic thyroid
(b) Inflammatory: Retropharyngeal abscess
(c) Neoplastic: Cystic hygroma (originating in posterior cervical triangle with extension toward midline + into mediastinum), neuroblastoma, neurofibromatosis, hemangioma
(d) Traumatic: Hematoma, foreign body
(e) Metabolic: Hypothyroidism

Vallecular narrowing
= valleys on each side of glossoepiglottic folds between base of tongue + epiglottis
(a) Congenital: Congenital cyst, ectopic thyroid, thyroglossal cyst
(b) Inflammatory: Abscess
(c) Neoplastic: Teratoma
(d) Traumatic: Foreign body, hematoma

Supraglottic narrowing
= area between epiglottis and true vocal cords
(a) Congenital: Aryepiglottic fold cyst
(b) Inflammatory: Acute bacterial epiglottitis, angioneurotic edema

(c) Neoplastic: Retention cyst, cystic hygroma, neurofibroma

(d) Traumatic: Foreign body, hematoma, radiation, caustic ingestion

(e) Idiopathic: Laryngomalacia

Glottic narrowing
= area of true vocal cords

(a) Congenital: Laryngeal atresia, laryngeal stenosis, laryngeal web (anterior commissure)

(b) Neoplastic: Laryngeal papillomatosis

(c) Neurogenic: Vocal cord paralysis (most common)

(d) Traumatic: Foreign body, hematoma

Subglottic narrowing
= short segment between undersurface of true vocal cords + inferior margin of cricoid cartilage is the narrowest portion of child's airway

(a) Congenital: Congenital subglottic stenosis

(b) Inflammatory: Croup

(c) Neoplastic: Hemangioma, papillomatosis

(d) Traumatic: Acquired stenosis (result of prolonged endotracheal intubation in 5%), granuloma

(e) Idiopathic: Mucocele = mucous retention cyst (rare complication of prolonged endotracheal intubation)

Tracheal narrowing
A. ANTERIOR COMPRESSION
  (a) Congenital
    1. Congenital goiter
    2. Innominate artery syndrome
      √ pulsatile indentation
      Rx: surgical attachment of innominate artery to manubrium
  (b) Inflammatory
    1. Cervical / mediastinal abscess
  (c) Neoplastic
    1. Cervical / intrathoracic teratoma:
      √ amorphous calcifications + ossifications
    2. Thymoma
    3. Thyroid tumors
    4. Lymphoma
  (d) Traumatic: Hematoma
B. POSTERIOR TRACHEAL COMPRESSION
  (a) Congenital
    1. Vascular ring
      —complete: double aortic arch, right aortic arch
      —incomplete: anomalous right subclavian artery
      √ posterior indentation of esophagus + trachea
    2. Pulmonary sling
      = anomalous left pulmonary artery arising

from right pulmonary artery, passing between trachea + esophagus enroute to left lung
    3. Bronchogenic cyst
      most common between esophagus + trachea at level of carina
  (b) Inflammatory: Abscess
  (c) Neoplastic: Neurofibroma
  (d) Traumatic: Esophageal foreign body, Esophageal stricture, Hematoma
C. INTRINSIC TRACHEAL CAUSES
  (a) Congenital:
    1. Congenital tracheal stenosis: generalized /segmental
      = complete cartilaginous ring (instead of horseshoe shape)
    2. Congenital tracheomalacia = immaturity of tracheal cartilage
      • expiratory stridor
      √ tracheal collapse on expiration
  (b) Neoplastic: Papilloma, Fibroma, Hemangioma
  (c) Traumatic: Acquired stenosis (endotracheal + tracheostomy tubes), Granuloma, Acquired tracheomalacia (cartilage degeneration after inflammation, extrinsic pressure, bronchial neoplasia, TE fistula, Foreign body

Inspiratory stridor in children
  1. Croup
  2. Congenital subglottic stenosis
  3. Subglottic hemangioma
  4. Airway foreign body
  5. Esophageal foreign body
  6. Epiglottitis

Epiglottic enlargement
A. Normal variant
    1. Prominent normal epiglottis
    2. Omega epiglottis
B. Inflammation
    1. Acute / chronic epiglottitis
    2. Angioneurotic edema
    3. Stevens-Johnson syndrome
    4. Caustic ingestion
    5. Radiation therapy
C. Masses
    1. Epiglottic cyst
    2. Aryepiglottic cyst
    3. Foreign body

THYROID
Congenital Dyshormonogenesis
  1. TRAPPING DEFECT
    = defective cellular uptake of iodine into thyroid, salivary glands, gastric mucosa;
    Δ high doses of inorganic iodine facilitate diffusion into thyroid permitting a normal rate of thyroid hormone synthesis

Δ   normal ratio of iodine concentrations for gastric
    juice:plasma = 20:1
√   nearly entire dose of administered radioiodine is
    excreted within 24 hours
2. ORGANIFICATION DEFECT
   =   deficient peroxidase activity which catalyzes the
       oxidation of iodide by H_2O_2 to form
       monoiodotyrosine (MIT) / diiodotyrosine (DIT)
   •   high serum TSH
   •   low serum T4
   •   diffuse symmetric thyromegaly
   √   high thyroidal uptake of radioiodine / pertechnetate
   √   rapid I-131 turnover
   √   positive perchlorate washout test
   Pendred syndrome = autosomal recessive trait of
       deficient peroxidase regeneration characterized by
       hypothyroidism + goiter + nerve deafness
3. DEIODINASE (DEHALOGENASE) DEFECT
   =   deficient deiodination of MIT / DIT to release iodide
       which is reutilized to synthesize thyroid hormone
       production
   •   hypothyroidism
   •   identification of MIT + DIT in serum + urine
       following administration of I-131
   •   "intrinsic" iodine deficiency goiter
   √   high thyroidal I-131 uptake
   √   rapid intrathyroidal turnover of I-131
4. THYROXIN-BINDING GLOBULIN (TBG) DEFICIENCY
   •   abnormal T4 transport
   •   low bound serum T4 concentration
   •   euthyroid
5. END-ORGAN RESISTANCE TO THYROID
   HORMONE
   •   high serum T4
   •   euthyroid / hypothyroid
   •   growth retardation
   √   goiter
   √   stippled epiphyses

Hyperthyroidism

1. Graves disease (most common)
2. Toxic nodular goiter
3. Iodine-induced hyperthyroidism = **Jod-Basedow**
   Most common in individuals with long standing
       multinodular goiter
   Age: > 50 years
   √   multinodular goiter with in- / decreased uptake
       (depending on iodine pool)
4. Thyroiditis
   (a) Hashimoto thyroiditis = chronic lymphocytic
       thyroiditis
   (b) Subacute thyroiditis = De Quervain thyroiditis
   (c) Painless thyroiditis
   US: √   decrease in overall echogenicity
         √   discrete nodules (50%)
5. Thyrotoxicosis medicamentosa / factitia
   surreptitious self-administration of thyroid hormones
6. Struma ovarii
   = ovarian teratoma containing thyroid tissue

7. Hydatiform mole / choriocarcinoma / testicular
   trophoblastic carcinoma
   = stimulation of thyroid by HCG
8. Pituitary hyperthyroidism = pituitary neoplasm
   •   ± acromegaly
   •   ± hyperprolactinemia
9. Thyroid carcinoma / hyperfunctioning metastases
   very rare (25 cases)

Hypothyroidism

A. PRIMARY HYPOTHYROIDISM (most common)
   =   thyroid's inability to produce sufficient thyroid
       hormone
   1. Agenesis of thyroid
   2. Congenital dyshormonogenesis
   3. Chronic thyroiditis
   4. Previous radioiodine therapy
   5. Ectopic thyroid (1:4,000)
B. SECONDARY HYPOTHYROIDISM
   =   failure of anterior pituitary to release sufficient
       quantities of TSH
   1. Sheehan disease = postpartum hemorrhage of
      anterior pituitary
   2. Head trauma
   3. Pituitary tumor (primary / secondary)
   4. Aneurysm
   5. Surgery
C. TERTIARY / HYPOTHALAMIC HYPOTHYROIDISM
   =   failure of hypothalamus to produce sufficient
       amounts of TRH

Decreased / no uptake of radiotracer

A. BLOCKED TRAPPING FUNCTION
   1. Iodine load (most common)
      =   dilution of tracer within flooded iodine pool (from
          administration of radiographic contrast / iodine-
          containing medication)
          — suppression usually lasts for 4 weeks
   2. Exogenous thyroid hormone (replacement therapy)
      suppresses TSH release
B. BLOCKED ORGANIFICATION
   1. Antithyroid medication (propylthiouracil (PTU) /
      methimazole) / goitrogenic substances
   √   Tc-99m uptake not inhibited
C. DIFFUSE PARENCHYMAL DESTRUCTION
   1. Subacute / chronic thyroiditis
D. HYPOTHYROIDISM
   1. Congenital hypothyroidism
   2. Surgical / radioiodine ablation
   3. Thyroid ectopia (struma ovarii, intrathoracic goiter)

Prominent pyramidal lobe

=   distal remnant of thyroid descent tract
1. Normal variant: present in 10%
2. Hyperthyroidism
3. Thyroiditis
4. S/P thyroid surgery
DDx: Esophageal activity from salivary excretion
         (disappears after glass of water)

Thyroid calcifications
= benign calcifications = stromal calcifications in adenoma
√ coarse calcifications with rough outline
√ alignment along periphery of lesion
√ irregular distribution

Psammoma bodies
= microcalcifications (< 1 mm) occur in 54% of thyroid neoplasms
√ seen on xeroradiography in 94%
1. Papillary carcinoma   61%
2. Follicular carcinoma   26%
3. Undifferentiated carcinoma   13%

Cystic areas in thyroid
A. Anechoic fluid + smooth regular wall:
   1. Simple cyst
   2. Colloid accumulation in goiter
B. Solid particles + irregular outline:
   1. Intranodular hemorrhage in goiter
   2. Liquefaction necrosis in adenoma / goiter
   3. Abscess

Thyroid nodule
Incidence: (increasing with age)
  (a) 4 – 8% by palpation (> 2 cm in 2%, 1 – 2 cm in 5%, < 1 cm in 1%); M:F = 1:4
  (b) 50% by autopsy / thyroid US (occult small cancers found in 4%)
A. BENIGN
   1. Adenomatous hyperplasia (50%)
   2. Follicular adenoma (20%)
   3. Ectopic parathyroid adenoma
   4. Inflammatory lymph node in subacute + chronic thyroiditis
   5. Hemorrhage / hematoma: frequently associated with adenomas
   6. Abscess
B. MALIGNANT
   1. Thyroid carcinoma
   2. Nonthyroidal neoplasm
     metastasis from breast, lung, kidney, malignant melanoma, Hodgkin disease
C. Hürtle cell carcinoma
   √ very thin hypoechoic halo
D. Carcinoma in situ
   √ echogenic area inside a goiter nodule

PROBABILITY OF A COLD NODULE FOR THYROID CANCER:
  Δ solitary cold nodules by scintigraphy are multinodular by US in 20 – 25%
  (a) 15 – 25% for solitary cold nodule
  (b) 1 – 6% for multiple nodules (DDx: multinodular goiter)

  (c) with Hx of neck irradiation in childhood
    — solitary nodule found in 70% (cancerous in 31%)
    — multiple nodules found in 25% (cancerous in 37%)
    — normal thyroid scan found in 5% (cancer detected in 20%)

Discordant thyroid nodule
= nodule hyperfunctioning on Tc-99m pertechnetate scan + hypofunctioning on I-131 scan which indicates reduced organification capacity
Causes:
  1. Malignancy : follicular / papillary carcinoma
  2. Benign lesion: follicular adenoma / adenomatous hyperplasia
   (autonomous nontoxic nodules have accelerated iodine turnover and discharge radioiodine as hormone within 24 hours)

Hot thyroid nodule
Incidence: 8% of Tc-99m pertechnetate scans
1. Adenoma
  (a) Autonomous adenoma = TSH-independent
   • hyper- / euthyroid
   √ partial / total suppression of remainder of gland
  (b) Adenomatous hyperplasia = TSH-dependent secondary to defective thyroid hormone production
2. Thyroid carcinoma (extremely rare)
  √ discordant uptake
N.B.:   any hot nodule on Tc-99m scan must be imaged with I-123 to differentiate between autonomous or cancerous lesion

Cold nodule
A. Benign tumor
   1. Nonfunctioning adenoma
   2. Cyst (11 – 20%)
   3. Involutional nodule
   4. Parathyroid tumor
B. Inflammatory mass
   1. Focal thyroiditis
   2. Granuloma
   3. Abscess
C. Malignant tumor
   1. Carcinoma
   2. Lymphoma
   3. Metastasis
US features of cold nodule:
  (1) cystic (rarely malignant)
  (2) mixed echogenicity (4%)
  (3) hyperechoic (3%)
  (4) isoechoic (22%)
  (5) hypoechoic (71%)

ANATOMY AND FUNCTION OF NECK ORGANS

Thyroid hormones

free hormone	: T4 (0.03%)
	T3 (0.4%)
Thyroxin binding globulin (TBG)	: binds T4 (70%)
	and T3 (38%)
Thyroxin binding prealbumin (TBPA)	: binds T4 (10%)
	and T3 (27%)
Albumin	: binds T4 (20%)
	and T3 (35%)

ELEVATION OF TBG
(1) Pregnancy (2) Estrogen administration (3) Genetic trait
REDUCTION IN TBG
(1) Androgens (2) Anabolic steroids (3) Glucocorticoids
(4) Nephrotic syndrome
(5) Chronic hepatic disease
INHIBITION OF T4 BINDING TO TBG: salicylates

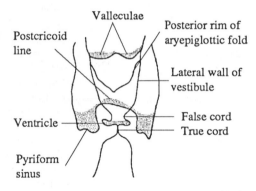

Frontal Laryngopharygogram during Phonation

Lateral Laryngogram
during phonation　　　　　　　**during quiet breathing**

DISEASE ENTITIES OF EAR, NOSE AND THROAT DISORDERS

ADENOMATOUS HYPERPLASIA OF THYROID
(1) cystic form = colloid cyst
  US: √ anechoic areas in nodule (hemorrhage / colloid degeneration)
     √ calcific deposits
(2) solid form = degenerative nodule

ANTROCHOANAL POLYP
= benign antral polyp which widens the sinus ostium and extends into nasal cavity; 5% of all nasal polyps
Age: teenagers + young adults
√ antral clouding
√ ipsilateral nasal mass
√ NO sinus expansion

APICAL PETROSITIS
Etiology: spread from middle ear + mastoid infection requires presence of air cells in petrous apices (30% of population)
• **Gradenigo syndrome:** otitis media + trigeminal pain + 6th nerve palsy
√ air cell opacification, middle ear disease, bone destruction

ARYEPIGLOTTIC CYST
= retention, lymphangioma, cystic hygroma, thyroglossal cyst
• may be symptomatic at birth
√ well-defined mass in aryepiglottic fold

CHOLESTEATOMA
= KERATOMA = epithelium-lined sac filled with keratin debris leading to bone destruction by pressure + demineralizing enzymes

Primary Cholesteatoma
= EPIDERMOID CYST (2%) = derived from embryonic ectodermal rests in temporal bone (commonly petrous apex) / epidural space / meninges
• NO history of middle ear inflammatory disease
Location:
  (a) petrous pyramid: internal auditory canal first involved
  (b) meninges: scooped out appearance of petrous ridge
  (c) cerebellopontine angle: erosion of porus, shortening of posterior canal wall
  (d) jugular fossa: erosion of posteroinferior aspect of petrous pyramid

Secondary Cholesteatoma
= INFLAMMATORY CHOLESTEATOMA (98%)
Cause: chronic inflammation of the ear + perforated ear drum with squamous cell epithelium of EAC growing through the perforation

• whitish-pearly mass behind intact tympanic membrane (invasion of middle ear cavity and mastoid) diagnosed otoscopically in 95%
• facial paralysis (compression of nerve VII at geniculate ganglion)
• sensorineural hearing loss (compromise of nerve VIII in internal auditory canal / involvement of cochlea or labyrinth)
• severe vertigo (labyrinthine fistula)
√ poorly pneumatized mastoid (frequent association)
√ perforation of tympanic membrane posterosuperiorly (pars flaccida = Shrapnell membrane)
√ initially destruction of lateral wall of attic, particularly the drum spur (scutum) with invasion of Prussak space + extension posteriorly into mastoid antrum (containing head of malleus + body of incus)
√ increasing width of attic
√ displacement of auditory ossicles
√ erosion of ossicular chain: first affecting long process of incus
√ destruction of Körner septum (= small bony projection extending inferiorly from roof of mastoid antrum)
√ erosion of tegmen tympani (with more extensive cholesteatoma)
√ destruction of labyrinthine capsule (less common) involving the lateral semicircular canal first
MRI:
  √ iso- / hypointense relative to cortex on T1WI
  √ no enhancement with Gd-DTPA (enhancement is related to granulation tissue)
DDx: chronic otitis media, granulation tissue = cholesterol granuloma, brain herniation through tegmen defect, neoplasm (rhabdomyosarcoma, squamous cell carcinoma)

CHOLESTEROL GRANULOMA
Histo: cholesterol crystals surrounded by foreign-body giant cells; embedded in fibrous connective tissue with varying proportions of hemosiderin-laden macrophages, chronic inflammatory cells and blood vessels
MRI: √ hyperintense signal on T1WI + T2WI

CHRONIC RECURRENT SIALADENITIS
• painful periodic unilateral enlargement of parotid gland
• milky discharge may be expressed
Sialography:
  √ Stenson duct irregularly enlarged / sausage-shaped
  √ pruning of distal parotid ducts
  √ ± calculi
CT: √ diffusely enlarged dense gland
    √ dilated Stenson duct ± calculi
Cx: Mucocele

CROUP
= ACUTE LARYNGOTRACHEOBRONCHITIS
= ACUTE VIRAL SPASMODIC LARYNGITIS
= lower respiratory tract infection
Organism: Parainfluenza, Respiratory Syncitial Virus
Age: > 6 months of age, peak incidence 2 – 3 years
- history of viral lower respiratory infection
- hoarse cry + "brassy" cough
- inspiratory difficulty with stridor
- fever
√ thickening of vocal cords
√ NORMAL epiglottis + aryepiglottic folds
√ "steeple sign" = subglottic "inverted V" = symmetrical funnel-shaped narrowing 1 – 1.5 cm below lower margins of pyriform sinuses on AP radiograph (loss of normal "shouldering" of air column caused by mucosal edema + external restriction by cricoid), accentuated on expiration, paradoxical inspiratory collapse, less pronounced during expiration
√ narrow + indistinct subglottic trachea on lateral radiograph
√ inspiratory ballooning of hypopharynx (nonspecific sign of any acute upper airway obstruction)
√ distension of cervical trachea on expiration
Prognosis: usually self-limiting

EPIGLOTTITIS
= ACUTE BACTERIAL EPIGLOTTITIS = life-threatening infection with edema of epiglottis + aryepiglottic folds (purely supraglottic lesion)
Organism: Hemophilus influenzae type B, Pneumococcus, Streptococcus group A
Age: > 3 years, peak incidence 6 years
- abrupt onset of respiratory distress with inspiratory stridor
- severe dysphagia
Location: purely supraglottic lesion; associated subglottic edema in 25%
Lateral radiograph should be taken in erect position only ! (frontal view irrelevant)
√ enlargement of epiglottis + thickening of aryepiglottic folds
√ circumferential narrowing of subglottic portion of trachea during inspiration
√ ballooning of hypopharynx + pyriform sinuses
√ cervical kyphosis
Cx: Mortal danger of suffocation through hazard of complete airway closure; patient needs to be accompanied by physician experienced in endotracheal intubation

FOLLICULAR ADENOMA OF THYROID
(a) Toxic adenoma
(b) Hyperfunctioning adenoma within multinodular goiter
= Toxic multinodular goiter; usually occurs in nodule > 2.5 cm in size
(c) Nonfunctioning adenoma
√ mass with increased / decreased echogenicity

√ "halo sign" = complete hypoechoic ring with regular border surrounding isoechoic solid mass

FRACTURE OF TEMPORAL BONE
A. LONGITUDINAL FRACTURE (75%)
= fracture parallel to the axis of petrous pyramid arising in squamosa of temporal bone through tegmen tympani, EAC (external auditory canal), middle ear, terminating in foramen lacerum
- bleeding from EAC (disruption of tympanic membrane)
- NO neurosensory hearing loss
- conductive hearing loss (dislocation of auditory ossicles — most commonly incus which is the least anchored ossicle)
- facial nerve palsy (10 – 20%) due to edema / fracture of facial canal near geniculate ganglion; frequent spontaneous recovery
- otorrhea (rare)
√ pneumocephalus
√ herniation of temporal lobe
√ dislocated incus (head of malleus separated from body of incus)
   √ disrupted ice cream cone relationship on direct coronal CT scan
   √ fracture of "molar tooth" on direct sagittal CT scan
√ mastoid air cells opaque / with air-fluid level
Plain film views: Stenver / Owens projection

B. TRANSVERSE FRACTURE (25%)
= fracture perpendicular to axis of petrous pyramid originating in occipital bone extending anteriorly across the base of skull + across the petrous pyramid
- neurosensory hearing loss (fracture across IAC / labyrinthine capsule)
- persistent vertigo
- facial nerve palsy in 50% (injury in IAC); less frequent spontaneous recovery because of disruption of nerve fibers
- rhinorrhea (tympanic membrane intact)
- bleeding into middle ear
Plain film views: posteroanterior (transorbital) + Towne projection

GOITER
Adenomatous Goiter
= MULTINODULAR GOITER
US: (89% sensitivity, 84% specificity, 73% positive predictive value, 94% negative predictive value)
   √ increased size + asymmetry of gland
   √ multiple 1 – 4 cm solid nodules
   √ areas of hemorrhage + necrosis
   √ coarse calcifications may occur within adenoma (hemorrhage + necrosis)

Diffuse Goiter
US: √ increase in glandular size, R lobe > L lobe
   √ NO focal textural changes
   √ calcifications not associated with nodules

Iodine-Deficiency Goiter

Not a significant problem in United States because of
supplemental iodine in food

Etiology: chronic TSH stimulation
- low serum T4
- √ high I-131 uptake

JOD-BASEDOW PHENOMENON (2%)
= development of thyrotoxicosis (= excessive amounts
of T4 synthesized + released) if normal dietary intake
is resumed / iodinated contrast medium administered

Toxic Nodular Goiter

= PLUMMER DISEASE
= autonomous function of one / more thyroid adenomas

Peak age: 4 – 5th decade; M:F = 1:3
- elevated T4
- suppressed TSH
- √ nodular thyroid with hot nodule + suppression of
remainder of gland
- √ stimulation scan will disclose normal uptake in
remainder of gland
- √ increased radioiodine uptake by 24 hours of
approx. 80%

Rx: I-131 treatment with empirical dose of 25–29 mCi

GRAVES DISEASE

= DIFFUSE TOXIC GOITER = autoimmune disorder with
thyroid stimulating antibodies (LATS) producing
hyperplasia + hypertrophy of thyroid gland

Peak age: 3rd – 4th decade; M:F = 1:7
- elevated T3 + T4
- depressed TSH production
- dermopathy = pretibial myxedema (5%)
- ophthalmopathy = periorbital edema, lid retraction,
ophthalmoplegia, proptosis, malignant exophthalmus
- √ diffuse thyroid enlargement
- √ uniform increased uptake
- √ incidental nodules superimposed on preexisting
adenomatous goiter (5%)

US: (identical to diffuse goiter)
- √ global enlargement of 2 – 3 x the normal size
- √ normal / diffusely hypoechoic pattern

Rx: I-131 treatment (for adults):
- *Dose:* 80 μCi / g of gland with 100% uptake
(taking into account estimated weight of
gland + measured uptake for 24 hours)
- *Cx:* 10 – 20% develop hypothyroidism within 1st
year + 1% added to each subsequent year

INVERTING PAPILLOMA

= most common of epithelial papillomas; commonly
occurring after nasal surgery

M > F

Path: hyperplastic epithelium inverts into underlying
stroma

Location: most often arising from the lateral nasal wall
extending into ethmoid / maxillary sinuses, at
junction of antrum + ethmoid sinuses, uniquely
unilateral
- unilateral nasal obstruction, epistaxis, postnasal drip,
sinus headache
- distinctive absence of allergic history
- √ commonly involves antrum + ethmoid sinus
- √ widening of infundibulum / outflow tract of antrum
- √ destruction of medial antral wall / lamina papyracea of
orbit (pressure necrosis)
- √ septum may be bowed to opposite side (NO invasion)

Cx: (1) cellular atypia / squamous cell carcinoma (10%)
       (2) recurrence (25 – 50%)

JUVENILE ANGIOFIBROMA

= most common benign nasopharyngeal tumor, can grow
to enormous size and invade vital structures

Age: teenagers; exclusively in males
- recurrent epistaxis
- nasal speech
- √ widening of pterygopalatine fossa (90%)
- √ anterior bowing of posterior antral wall
- √ invasion of sphenoid sinus (2/3) from tumor erosion
through floor of sinus
- √ widening of inferior + superior orbital fissures (spread
into orbit via inferior orbital fissure + into middle cranial
fossa via superior orbital fissure)
- √ highly vascular nasopharyngeal mass (only enhances
on CT scans immediately after bolus injection); supplied
primarily by internal maxillary artery

NOTE: Biopsy contraindicated !

LABYRINTHITIS

Causes: toxins, viral illness (mumps, measles), bacterial
infection
- √ no abnormalities with viral causes
- √ labyrinthitis ossificans = inner ear structures filled with
bone (suppurative infection, trauma, surgery, tumor,
severe otosclerosis)

LARYNGEAL PAPILLOMATOSIS

Squamous papilloma is the most common benign tumor of
the larynx

Etiology: human papilloma virus type 6 (papova virus)

Histo: core of vascular connective tissue covered by
stratified squamous epithelium

Age of onset: 1 – 54 years; M:F = 1:1;
bimodal distribution:
  (a) < 10 years (diffuse involvement)
  (b) 21 – 50 years (usually single papilloma)
- progressive hoarseness / aphonia
- repeated episodes of respiratory distress
- inspiratory stridor, asthma-like symptoms
- cough
- recurrent pneumonia
- hemoptysis

Location: (a) uvula, palate (b) vocal cord (c) subglottic
extension (50 – 70%) (d) pulmonary
involvement (1 – 6%)

√ thickened lumpy cords
√ bronchiectasis
Rx: CO_2 laser resection
Cx: (1) Tracheobronchial papillomatosis (2 – 5%)
        √ solid pulmonary nodules in mid + posterior lung fields
        √ 2 – 3 cm large thin-walled cavity with 2 – 4 mm thick nodular wall
        √ peripheral atelectasis + obstructive pneumonitis
    (2) Pulmonary papillomatosis from aerial metastases (bronchoscopy, laryngoscopy, tracheal intubation) 10 years after initial diagnosis
        √ irregularities of tracheal / bronchial walls
    (3) Malignant transformation into invasive squamous cell carcinoma

LARYNGOMALACIA
= immaturity of cartilage; most common cause of stridor in neonate + young infant
• only cause of stridor to get worse at rest
√ hypercollapsible larynx during inspiration (supraglottic portion only)
√ backward bent of epiglottis + anterior kink of aryepiglottic folds during inspiration
√ transient (disappears by age 1 year)

MUCOCELE
Most common lesion to cause expansion of paranasal sinus; increased incidence in cystic fibrosis
Etiology: accumulation of mucoid secretions behind an obstructed paranasal sinus ostium with expansion of sinus cavity + thinning of sinus walls
Age: usually adulthood
• history of chronic nasal polyposis + pansinusitis
• commonly present with unilateral proptosis
• palpable mass in superomedial aspect of orbit (frontal mucocele)
• pain
Sites: frontal (60%) > ethmoid (30%) > maxillary (10%) > sphenoid (rare)
√ soft tissue density mass
√ sinus cavity expansion (DDx: never in sinusitis)
√ bone erosion / remodeling at late stage (impossible DDx from neoplasm)
√ surrounding zone of bone sclerosis (from chronic infection)
√ macroscopic calcification in 5% (esp. with superimposed fungal infection)
√ pyocele = superimposed infection (rare)
√ uniform lack of enhancement
Cx: may protrude into orbit displacing medial rectus muscle laterally
DDx: Paranasal sinus carcinoma, Aspergillus infection (enlargement of medial rectus muscle + optic nerve, focal / diffuse areas of increased attenuation), Chronic infection, Inverting papilloma

OTOSCLEROSIS
= replacement of dense otic capsule by more vascular bone in active phase (misnomer) with restoration of density during reparative phase; frequently bilateral
Etiology: unknown; frequently hereditary
Age: young adult Caucasian; M:F = 1:2
(a) Stapedial otosclerosis anterior to oval window (more common)
(b) Cochlear otosclerosis
• Conductive hearing loss (stapes fixation in oval window = fenestral)
• Sensorineural hearing loss (involvement of otic capsule = retrofenestral)
• Tinnitus
√ lucent halo around cochlea
√ later bony proliferation (reparative sclerotic phase) with obliteration of oval window niche

PARANASAL SINUS CARCINOMA
Location: maxillary sinus (80%), nasal cavity (10%), ethmoid sinus (5 – 6%), frontal + sphenoid sinus (rare)

Maxillary Sinus Carcinoma
Incidence: 80% of all paranasal sinus carcinomas
Histo: squamous cell carcinoma (80%)
Age: > 40 years in 95%; M:F = 2:1
• asymmetry of face, tumor in oral / nasal cavity
√ bone destruction (in 90%) predominates over expansion
√ nodal metastases in 10 – 18%

Nasal Cavity Carcinoma
Incidence: 10% of paranasal sinus carcinomas
Histo: squamous cell carcinoma > 85%
• history of chronic sinusitis / nasal polyps (15%)
• unilateral nasal obstruction
Location: turbinates (50%) > septum > vestibule > posterior choanae > floor
√ polypoid or papillary (2/3)
√ bone invasion (1/3)

Ethmoid Sinus Carcinoma
Incidence: 5 – 6% of paranasal sinus carcinomas
Histo: squamous cell carcinoma (> 90%), sarcoma, adenocarcinoma, adenoid cystic carcinoma frequently involved secondarily from maxillary sinus carcinoma
• nasal obstruction, bloody discharge
• anosmia, broadening of nose

PHARYNGEAL ABSCESS
Etiology: spread of infection from tonsils / pharynx
Age: children > adults
• trismus (most common presenting symptom) from involvement of pterygoid muscle
• sore throat
• low-grade fever

√ isodense / low density mass with unsharp margins
√ rim enhancement
Cx: Mycotic aneurysm of carotid artery (within 10 days)

RETROPHARYNGEAL ABSCESS / HEMORRHAGE
Etiology: upper respiratory tract infection, perforating
             injury of pharynx / esophagus, suppuration of
             infected lymph node
Organism: Staphylococcus, mixed flora
Age: usually < 1 year
• fever, neck stiffness, dysphagia
√ thickness of retropharyngeal space > 3/4 of AP diameter
  of vertebral body
√ reversal of cervical lordosis
√ anterior displacement of airway
√ may contain gas and gas-fluid level

RHINOCEREBRAL MUCORMYCOSIS
= paranasal sinus infection caused by nonseptated fungi
  Rhizopus arrhizus and Rhizopus oryzae
Spread: fungus first involves nasal cavity, then extends
           into maxillary sinuses / ethmoid sinuses / orbits
           / intracranially along ophthalmic artery (frontal
           sinuses are spared)
Predisposed: (1) poorly controlled diabetes mellitus
                (2) chronic renal failure (3) cirrhosis
                (4) malnutrition (5) cancer (6) prolonged
                antibiotics (7) steroids (8) cytotoxic drug
                therapy
• black crusting of nasal mucosa (in diabetics)
• small ischemic areas (invasion of arterioles + small
  arteries)
√ nodular thickening involving nasal septum + turbinates
√ mucoperiosteal thickening + clouding of ethmoids
√ focal areas of bone destruction
Cx: (1) blindness (2) cranial nerve palsy (3) hemiparesis
Prognosis: high mortality rate

SARCOIDOSIS
Blacks:Whites = 10:1
Location: eye, lacrimal glands, salivary glands (40%),
             larynx (5%), involvement of intra- and
             extraparotid lymph nodes (rare)
√ granulomas may enhance
√ enlargement of optic canal (optic neuritis)
√ thickening of larynx with enhancement of granulomas
√ multiple small granulomas of septum + turbinates
• **Heerfordt syndrome:**
  (1) parotid enlargement
  (2) uveitis
  (3) facial nerve paralysis

SIALOSIS
= nontender noninflammatory recurrent enlargement of
  parotid gland
Cause: cirrhosis, alcoholism, diabetes, malnutrition,
          hormonal insufficiency (ovarian / pancreatic /
          thyroid), drugs (sulfisoxasole, phenylbutisone),
          radiation therapy

Histo: serous acinar hypertrophy + fatty replacement of
          gland
Sialography:
  √ sparse peripheral ducts
CT:
  √ enlarged / normal sized gland
  √ diffusely dense gland in end-stage

SINUSITIS
Most common paranasal sinus problem
A.   BACTERIAL SINUSITIS
      Cause:
      (1)   obstruction of major ostia
             (a)   middle meatus draining frontal, maxillary,
                    anterior ethmoid sinus
             (b)   sphenoethmoid recess draining posterior
                    ethmoid + sphenoid sinus
      (2)   ineffective mucociliary clearing secondary to
             contact of two mucosal surfaces
      Primary focus:
         anterior ethmoid-middle meatal complex = area
         responsible for drainage of frontal + maxillary sinuses
      Anatomic variations predisposing to osteomeatal
      narrowing:
         1. Concha bullosa = aerated middle turbinate
         2. Oversized ethmoid bulla
         3. Haller cells = inferiorly extending ethmoid cells
            below ethmoid bulla adhering to roof of maxillary
            sinus
         4. Uncinate process bulla
         5. Bowed nasal septum
         6. Paradoxical middle turbinate = convexity of
            turbinate directed toward lateral nasal wall
         7. Deviation of uncinate process
      √ solitary antral disease (obstruction of sinus ostium)
      √ air-fluid level
      √ uniform enhancement
B.   ALLERGIC SINUSITIS
      √ involves multiple sinuses
      √ bilaterally symmetric
      √ uniform enhancement
Cx: Retention cyst (10%) = smoothly marginated soft
       tissue mass from obstruction of mucous gland
       (commonly in floor of maxilla)

SUBGLOTTIC HEMANGIOMA
Most common subglottic soft tissue mass causing upper
respiratory tract obstruction in neonates
• croup-like symptoms in neonatal period
• hemangiomas elsewhere (skin, mucosal membranes) in
  50%
√ eccentric thickening of subglottic portion of trachea (AP
  view)
√ arises from posterior wall below true cords (lateral view)

SUBGLOTTIC STENOSIS
A.   Congenital subglottic stenosis
      • croup-like symptoms, often self-limiting disease

Location: 1 – 2 cm below vocal cords
√ circumferential symmetrical narrowing of subglottic
   portion of trachea during inspiration
√ NO change of degree of narrowing with expiration
B. Acquired subglottic stenosis
    following prolonged endotracheal intubation (in 5%)

THORNWALDT CYST
= persistent focal adhesion between notochord +
   ectoderm extending to the pharyngeal tubercle of the
   occipital bone which develops into a pouch / cyst lined
   by ectoderm (DDx: Rathke pouch occurs in
   craniopharyngeal canal located anterior + cephalad to
   Thornwaldt cyst)
Peak age: 15 – 30 years
• persistent nasopharyngeal drainage
• halitosis
• foul taste in mouth
Location: posterior roof of nasopharynx in midline
√ smoothly marginated cystic mass of 2 – 3 cm size
√ low density, not enhancing
√ NO bone erosion

THYROID CARCINOMA
Age: age < 30 years, M > F
• history of neck irradiation
• rapid growth
• stone-hard nodule
√ hypoechoic mass
√ irregular ill-defined border without halo
√ NO hemorrhage / liquefaction necrosis

RADIATION-INDUCED THYROID CANCER
Incidence increases with doses of thyroidal irradiation from
   6.5 – 1500 rad (higher doses are associated with
   hypothyroidism)
Peak occurrence: 5 – 30 years (up to 50 years) post
                       irradiation
Thyroid abnormalities in 20%:
   (a) in 70% adenomatous hyperplasia, follicular
        adenoma, colloid nodules, thyroiditis
   (b) in 30% thyroid cancer
   Δ nondetectable microscopic foci of cancer in 25% of
      patients operated on for benign disease
   Δ in patients with multiple cold nodules frequency of
      cancer is 40%

TREATMENT
   (1) Surgery: thyroidectomy + modified radical neck
        dissection
   (2) Postoperative radioiodine treatment with I-131
        (multiple treatments are usually necessary)
        (a) ablative dose to destroy remaining thyroid
             tissue 6 weeks following surgery; no thyroid
             hormone replacement 3 – 4 weeks prior to
             therapy
             Dose = [(weight (g) x 80-120 µCi/g) + % uptake
                of I-123 by 24 hours] x 100
                approx. 100 mCi I-131 orally

   (b) treatment of metastases
        Dose: 100 – 200 mCi
        (after administration of 150 mCi of I-131 an
        uptake of 0.5% per gram of tumor tissue with a
        biologic half-life of 4 days will produce 25,000
        rads to tumor)
        Δ rapid turnover rates may exist in some
           metastases (lower dose advisable)
        Δ treatment of large tumors incomplete (range of
           beta radiation is a few mm)
        Cx: radiation thyroiditis, radiation parotitis, GI-
                symptoms (nausea, diarrhea), minimal bone
                marrow depression, leukemia (2%),
                anaplastic transformation (uncommon)
   (3) Thyroid replacement therapy
        exogenous thyroid hormone to suppress TSH
        stimulation of metastases
   (4) External radiation therapy for anaplastic carcinoma
        + metastases without iodine uptake
FOLLOW-UP: Thyroglobulin > 50 ng/ml indicates
            functioning metastases

WHOLE-BODY SCAN in metastatic thyroid carcinoma
   Indication: to detect metastases of thyroid carcinoma
                   after total thyroidectomy; preferred over
                   bone scan (only detects 40%) for skeletal
                   metastases
   Δ metastases not detectable in presence of normal
      functioning thyroid tissue because uptake is much
      less in metastases
   Δ Tc-99m pertechnetate is useless because of high
      background activity + lack of organification
   Technique:
   (1) T4 replacement therapy is discontinued
   (2) short-acting T3 is administered for 4 – 6 weeks
   (3) T3 replacement therapy discontinued 10 – 14
        days prior to whole-body scan
   (4) measurement of TSH level to confirm adequate
        elevation (administration of exogenous TSH not
        desirable because of uneven stimulation)
   (5) oral administration of 5 – 10 mCi I-131
   (6) whole-body scan after 24, 48, 72 hours (low
        background activity)
   N.B.:   posttherapy scan (2 – 3 days after therapeutic
           dose) identifies more lesions than diagnostic
           scan
Normal sites of accumulation: nasopharynx, salivary
   glands, stomach, colon, bladder, liver (I-131-labeled
   thyroxine produced by carcinoma is metabolized in
   liver), breasts (in lactating women)

Papillary Carcinoma of Thyroid
60% of all thyroid carcinomas
Peak age: 5th decade; F > M
Histo: unencapsulated well-differentiated tumor
           (a) purely papillary
           (b) mixed with follicular elements (more
                common, esp. under age 40)

Metastases:
  (1) Lymphogenic spread to regional lymph nodes (40%, in children almost 90%)
  (2) Hematogenous spread to lung (4%), bone (rare)
NUC: √ usually concentrates radioiodine (even some purely papillary tumors)
US: √ decreased echogenicity
    √ purely solid / complex mass with areas of necrosis, hemorrhage, cystic degeneration
X-ray: √ punctate / linear psammomatous calcifications at tumor periphery
Prognosis:
  90% 10-year survival for occult + intrathyroidal cancer; 60% 10-year survival for extrathyroidal cancer; worse prognosis with increasing age

Follicular Carcinoma of Thyroid
  20% of all thyroid cancers; slow growing
  Peak age: 5th decade; F > M
  Histo: encapsulated well-differentiated tumor without papillary elements; in 25% multifocal; cytologically impossible to distinguish between well-differentiated follicular carcinoma + follicular adenoma (vascular invasion is only criteria)
  Early hematogenous spread to:
    (a) lung
    (b) bone (30%): almost always osteolytic (more frequent than in papillary carcinoma)
  √ psammoma bodies + stromal calcium deposits
  NUC:
    √ usually concentrates pertechnetate, but fails to accumulate I-131
  US:
    √ indistinguishable from benign follicular adenoma
  Prognosis:
    90% 10-year survival with slight / equivocal angioinvasion; 35% 10-year survival with moderate / marked angioinvasion

Anaplastic Carcinoma of Thyroid
  15% of all thyroid cancers
  Age: 6 – 7th decade; M:F = 1:1
  NUC: √ NO radioiodine uptake
  Prognosis: 5% 5-year survival; average survival time of 6 – 12 months

Medullary Carcinoma of Thyroid
  1 – 5% of all thyroid cancers; sporadic / familial
  Histo: arises from parafollicular C-cells, associated with amyloid deposition in primary + metastatic sites
  Mean age: 60 years
  May be associated with:
    (1) MEN IIa = pheochromocytoma + parathyroid hyperplasia
    (2) MEN IIb = without parathyroid component

Metastases: early spread to lymph nodes (50%), lung, liver, bone
• elevated calcitonin (tumor production) stimulated by pentagastrin + calcium infusion
NUC: √ NO uptake by radioiodine / pertechnetate
  √ granular calcifications within fibrous stroma / amyloid masses (50%)
Prognosis:
  90% 10-year survival without nodal metastases
  42% 10-year survival with nodal metastases
Rx: total thyroidectomy + modified radical neck dissection

THYROIDITIS
Hashimoto Thyroiditis
  = CHRONIC LYMPHOCYTIC THYROIDITIS
  Most frequent cause of goitrous hypothyroidism in adults
  Etiology: autoimmune process with marked familial predisposition; antibodies are typically present; functional organification defect
  Peak age: 4 – 5th decade; M > F
  • firm rubbery lobular goiter
  • gradual painless enlargement
  • thyrotoxicosis in early stage (4%)
  • decreased thyroid reserve
  • hypothyroidism at presentation (20%)
  √ moderate enlargement of both lobes (18%)
  NUC:
    √ low tracer uptake (occasionally increased) with poor visualization (4%)
    √ prominent pyramidal lobe
    √ positive perchlorate washout test
    √ patchy tracer distribution
    √ multiple (40%) / single cold defects (28%) / normal thyroid (8%)
  US:
    √ initially diffusely decreased echogenicity + slight lobulation of contour
    √ later dense echogenicity (fibrosis) + acoustical shadows
  Cx: Hypothyroidism

De Quervain Thyroiditis
  = SUBACUTE THYROIDITIS
  Etiology: probably viral
  Histo: lymphocytic infiltration + granulomas + foreign body giant cells
  Peak age: 2 – 5th decade; M:F = 1:5
  • upper respiratory tract infection precedes onset of symptoms by 2 – 3 weeks
  • painful tender gland + fever; only mild enlargement
  • hyperthyroidism (50%) secondary to severe destruction
  • short-lived hypothyroidism (25%) secondary to hormone-depleted gland
  √ poor visualization of thyroid (initially)
  √ single / multiple hypofunctional areas (occasionally)

√ increased uptake during phase of hypothyroidism (late event)
Cx: Permanent hypothyroidism (rare)
Prognosis: usually full recovery

Painless Thyroiditis
Histo: resembles chronic lymphocytic thyroiditis
- clinical presentation similar to subacute thyroiditis
- NOT painful / tender

Acute Suppurative Thyroiditis
US:
√ focal / diffuse enlargement; possibly abscess
√ decreased echogenicity

VOCAL CORD PARALYSIS
Causes: birth injury, Arnold-Chiari malformation, intracranial tumors, mediastinal mass, cyst, vascular ring, thyroidectomy, malignancy
√ fixed vocal cords (fluoroscopy)

WEGENER GRANULOMATOSIS
= necrotizing granulomatous vasculitis
Mean age of onset: 40 years; M:F = 2:1

Triad:
(1) Upper respiratory tract
   (a) nasal cavity:
      - erosion of nasal septum
      - saddle nose deformity
      √ progressive destruction of nasal cartilage + bone (DDx Relapsing polychondritis)
      √ granulomatous masses filling nasal cavities
   (b) sinuses (maxillary antra most frequently):
      √ thickening of mucosa
(2) Lungs
   - hemoptysis
   √ multiple pulmonary nodules
(3) Glomerulonephritis
Rx: cyclophosphamide

DIFFERENTIAL DIAGNOSIS OF CHEST DISEASES

ALVEOLAR DISEASE
Classic appearance of air space consolidation:
- √ **A**cinar rosettes: rounded poorly defined nodules in size of acini (6 – 10 mm), best seen at periphery of densities
- √ **A**ir alveologram / bronchogram
- √ **B**utterfly / batwing distribution: perihilar
- √ **C**oalescent diffuse infiltrates with ill-defined borders
- √ **C**onsolidation in segmental / lobar distribution
- √ **C**hanges occur rapidly

CT:
- √ poorly marginated densities within primary lobule (up to 1 cm in size)
- √ rapid coalescence with neighboring lesions in segmental distribution
- √ predominantly central location with sparing of subpleural zones
- √ air bronchograms

Diffuse air space disease
A. INFLAMMATORY EXUDATE = "PUS"
   1. Lobar pneumonia
   2. Bronchopneumonia: especially Gram-negative organisms
   3. Unusual pneumonias
      (a) viral: extensive hemorrhagic edema especially in immuno-compromised patients with hematologic malignancies + transplants
      (b) pneumocystis
      (c) fungal: aspergillus, candida, cryptococcus, phycomycetes
      (d) tuberculosis
   4. Aspiration
B. HEMORRHAGE = "BLOOD"
   1. Trauma: Contusion
   2. Pulmonary embolism, thromboembolism
   3. Bleeding diathesis: leukemia, hemophilia, anticoagulants, DIC
   4. Vasculitis: Wegener granulomatosis, Goodpasture syndrome, SLE, mucormycosis, aspergillosis, Rocky Mountain spotted fever, infectious mononucleosis
   5. Idiopathic pulmonary hemosiderosis
   6. Bleeding metastases: choriocarcinoma
C. TRANSUDATE / EXUDATE = "WATER"
   1. Cardiac edema
   2. Neurogenic edema
   3. Hypoproteinemia
   4. Fluid overload
   5. Renal failure
   6. Radiotherapy
   7. Shock

8. Toxic inhalation
9. Drug reaction
D. SECRETIONS = "PROTEIN"
   1. Alveolar proteinosis
   2. Adult respiratory distress syndrome
E. MALIGNANCY = "CELLS"
   1. Bronchioloalveolar cell carcinoma
   2. Lymphoma
F. INTERSTITIAL DISEASE simulating air space disease, e.g. "alveolar sarcoid"

mnemonic: "AIRSPACED"
Aspiration
Inhalation
Renal
Swimming (drowning)
Pneumonia
Alveolar proteinosis
Cardiovascular
Edema
Drug reaction

Chronic alveolar infiltrate
mnemonic: "I DALLAS"
Inflammation (TB + fungus)
DIP (not consolidative)
Alveolar proteinosis
Lymphoma
Lipoid pneumonia
Alveolar cell carcinoma
Sarcoidosis

"STALLAG"
Sarcoidosis
Tuberculosis
Alveolar cell ca.
Lymphoma
Lipoid pneumonia
Alveolar proteinosis
Goodpasture syndr.

INTERSTITIAL LUNG DISEASE
= thickening of interlobular septa:
   (a) <u>Major lymphatic trunks</u>
      1. Lymphangitic carcinomatosis
      2. Congenital pulmonary lymphangiectasia
   (b) <u>Pulmonary veins</u> (increased pulmonary venous pressure)
      1. Left ventricular failure
      2. Venous obstructive disease
   (c) <u>Supporting connective tissue network</u>
      1. Interstitial edema
      2. Chronic interstitial pneumonia
      3. Pneumoconioses
      4. Collagen-vascular disease
      5. Interstitial fibrosis
      6. Amyloid
      7. Tumor infiltration within connective tissue
      8. Desmoplastic reaction to tumor

SIGNS OF ACUTE INTERSTITIAL DISEASE
√ thickening of interlobular fissures
√ **Kerley-lines** (= thickened connective septa)
√ Kerley A lines = relatively long fine linear shadows in upper lungs, deep within lung parenchyma
√ Kerley B lines = short horizontally oriented lines extending to pleura, perpendicular to pleura in costophrenic angles + retrosternal clear space
√ Kerley C lines = "spider web" appearance covering entire lung
√ peribronchial cuffing = thickened bronchial wall + peribronchial sheath (when viewed end on)
√ perihilar haze = blurring of hilar shadows
√ blurring of pulmonary vascular markings
√ increased density at lung bases
√ small pleural effusions

SIGNS OF CHRONIC INTERSTITIAL DISEASE
√ irregular visceral pleural surface
√ **reticulations** = network of interlacing lines
  (a) fine reticulations = early potentially reversible / minimal irreversible alveolar septal abnormality
  (b) coarse reticulations
      in 75% related to environmental disease, sarcoidosis, collagen-vascular disorders, chronic interstitial pneumonia
√ **nodularity**
  in 90% related to infectious / noninfectious granulomatous process, metastatic malignancy, pneumoconioses, amyloidosis
√ **linearity**
  cardiogenic / noncardiogenic interstitial pulmonary edema, lymphangitic malignancy, diffuse bronchial wall disorders (cystic fibrosis, bronchiectasis, hypersensitivity asthma)
√ **honeycombing** = rounded radiolucencies < 1 cm in diameter set off against a background of increased lung density (end stage lung)

High resolution-CT of interstitial disease:
√ thick irregular saw-toothed appearance of interlobar fissures, vascular borders, bronchial walls
√ sharply marginated noncoalescing interstitial nodules
√ interstitial reticulation:
√ large network of polyhedral reticular elements of 15 – 25 mm in diameter with central pulmonary artery (secondary lobular architecture);
  associated with interstitial pulmonary edema, lymphangitic carcinomatosis
√ predominantly subpleural small reticular elements of 6 – 10 mm in diameter with small cystic changes ("honeycombing")
  associated with interstitial fibrosis, lymphangioleiomyomatosis, diffuse amyloidosis
√ fine diffusely distributed network of 2 – 3 mm basic elements
  associated with miliary TB, reactions to methotrexate
√ ground glass opacities (diffuse interstitial thickening + obliteration of air space)

mnemonic: "HIDE FACTS"
  Hamman-Rich, **H**emosiderosis
  Infection, **I**rradiation, **I**diopathic
  Dust, **D**rugs
  Eosinophilic granuloma, **E**dema
  Fungal, **F**armer's lung
  Aspiration (oil), **A**rthritis (rheumatoid, ankylosing spondylitis)
  Collagen disease
  Tumor, **T**BC, **T**uberous sclerosis
  Sarcoidosis, **S**cleroderma

Acute diffuse fine reticulations
A. ACUTE INTERSTITIAL EDEMA
    1. Congestive heart failure
    2. Fluid overload
    3. Uremia
    4. Hypersensitivity
B. ACUTE INTERSTITIAL PNEUMONIA
    1. Viral pneumonia
    2. Mycoplasma pneumonia
    3. Infectious mononucleosis

mnemonic: "HELP"
  Hypersensitivity
  Edema
  Lymphoproliferative
  Pneumonitis (viral)

Chronic diffuse fine reticulations
A. VENOUS OBSTRUCTION
    1. Atherosclerotic heart disease
    2. Mitral stenosis
    3. Left atrial myxoma
    4. Pulmonary veno-occlusive disease
    5. Sclerosing mediastinitis
B. LYMPHATIC OBSTRUCTION
    1. Lymphangiectasia (pediatric patient)
    2. Mediastinal mass   (lymphoma)
    3. Lymphoma / Leukemia
    4. Lymphangitic carcinomatosis: predominantly basilar distribution
       (a) bilateral (breast, stomach, colon, pancreas)
       (b) unilateral (lung tumor)
    5. Lymphocytic interstitial pneumonitis
C. INHALATIONAL DISEASE
    1. Silicosis: small nodules + reticulations
    2. Asbestosis: basilar distribution, pleural thickening + calcifications
    3. Hard metals
    4. Allergic alveolitis
D. GRANULOMATOUS DISEASE
    from a nodular to a reticular pattern if
      (a) nodules line up along bronchovascular bundles
      (b) interlobular septa show fibrotic changes
    1. Sarcoidosis: hilar + mediastinal adenopathy (may have disappeared)

2. Eosinophilic granuloma: upper lobe distribution
E. COLLAGEN-VASCULAR DISEASE
reticulations in late stages
1. Rheumatoid lung
2. Scleroderma
F. DRUG REACTIONS
G. IDIOPATHIC
1. Usual interstitial pneumonitis (UIP)
2. Desquamative interstitial pneumonitis (DIP)
3. Tuberous sclerosis: smooth muscle proliferation
4. Lymphangiomyomatosis
5. Idiopathic pulmonary hemosiderosis
6. Alveolar proteinosis (late complication)
7. Amyloidosis
8. Interstitial calcification (chronic renal failure)

mnemonic: "LIFE lines"
Lymphangitic spread
Inflammation / infection
Fibrosis
Edema

Coarse reticulations
= coarse reticular interstitial densities with intervening cystic spaces
= end-stage scarring of the lung = HONEYCOMB LUNG
√ rounded radiolucencies < 1 cm in areas of increased lung density
√ small lung volume (decreased compliance)
Cx: (1) intercurrent pneumothoraces
(2) bronchogenic carcinoma = scar carcinoma
Cause:
A. INHALATIONAL DISEASE
(a) Pneumoconioses
1. Asbestosis: basilar distribution, shaggy heart, pleural thickening + calcifications
2. Silicosis: upper lobe predominance, ± pleural thickening, ± hilar and mediastinal lymph adenopathy
3. Berylliosis
(b) Chemical inhalation (late)
1. Silo-filler's disease (nitrogen dioxide)
2. Sulfur dioxide, chlorine, phosgene, cadmium
(c) Extrinsic allergic alveolitis (hypersensitivity to organic dusts)
(d) Oxygen toxicity: sequelae of RDS therapy with oxygen
(e) Chronic aspiration
e.g. mineral oil: localized process in medial basal segments / middle lobe
B. GRANULOMATOUS DISEASE
1. Sarcoidosis
2. Eosinophilic granuloma
C. COLLAGEN-VASCULAR DISEASE
1. Rheumatoid lung
2. Scleroderma
3. Ankylosing spondylitis: upper lobes
4. SLE: rarely produces honeycombing

D. IATROGENIC
1. Drug hypersensitivity
2. Radiotherapy
E. IDIOPATHIC
1. Usual interstitial pneumonitis (UIP)
honeycombing in 50%, severe volume loss in 45%
2. Desquamative interstitial pneumonitis (DIP)
honeycombing in 12.5%, severe volume loss in 23%
√ basilar patchy air consolidations
3. Lymphangiomyomatosis
4. Tuberous sclerosis (rare)
5. Neurofibromatosis (rare)

Distribution of Interstitial Disease
mnemonics:

basilar distribution	apical distribution
"BAD LASS"	"CASSET"
Bronchiectasis	**C**ystic fibrosis
Aspiration	**A**nkylosing spondylitis
DIP + UIP, **D**rugs	**S**ilicosis
Lymphangitic spread	**S**arcoidosis
Asbestosis	**E**osinophilic granuloma
Sarcoidosis	**T**uberculosis, fungus
Scleroderma	
+ other collagen vascular diseases	

Honeycomb lung
mnemonic: "HIPS RDS"   "B CHIPS"

Histiocytosis X	**B**ronchiectasis
Interstitial pneumonia	
Pneumoconiosis	**C**ollagen-vascular disease
Sarcoidosis	**H**istiocytosis X
	Interstitial pneumonia
Rheumatoid lung	**P**neumoconiosis
Dermatomyositis	**S**arcoidosis
Scleroderma	

Reticulations + pleural effusion
A. ACUTE
1. Edema
2. Infection: viral, mycoplasma (very rare)
B. CHRONIC
1. Congestive heart failure
2. Lymphangitic carcinomatosis
3. Lymphoma + leukemia
4. SLE
5. Rheumatoid disease
6. Lymphangiectasia
7. Lymphangiomyomatosis
8. Asbestosis

Reticulations + hilar adenopathy
1. Sarcoidosis
2. Silicosis
3. Lymphoma + leukemia
4. Lung primary: particularly oat cell carcinoma
5. Metastases: lymphatic obstruction / spread

6. Fungal disease
7. Tuberculosis
8. Viral pneumonia (rare combination)

Diffuse fine nodular disease + miliary nodules
√ very small (1 – 4 mm) sharply defined nodules of interstitial disease

A. INHALATIONAL DISEASE
   1. Silicosis + coal-worker's pneumoconiosis
   2. Berylliosis
   3. Siderosis
   4. Extrinsic allergic alveolitis (chronic phase)
B. GRANULOMATOUS DISEASE
   1. Eosinophilic granuloma
   2. Sarcoidosis (with current / previous adenopathy)
C. INFECTIOUS DISEASE
   1. Tuberculosis
   2. Fungus: Histoplasmosis, Coccidioidomycosis, Blastomycosis, Aspergillosis (rare), Cryptococcosis (rare)
   3. Bacteria: Salmonella, Nocardiosis
   4. Virus: Varicella (more common in adults)
D. METASTASES
   Thyroid carcinoma, Melanoma, Adenocarcinomas of breast, stomach, colon, pancreas
E. ALVEOLAR MICROLITHIASIS (rare)
F. BRONCHIOLITIS OBLITERANS
G. GAUCHER DISEASE

mnemonic: "I SHRIMP"
   Infection (TB, fungus)
   Sarcoidosis
   Histiocytosis
   Rheumatoid lung
   Idiopathic
   Metastases (thyroid, kidney)
   Pneumoconiosis

Micronodular disease
   1. Granulomatous disease (Miliary tuberculosis, Histoplasmosis)
   2. Hypersensitivity (organic dust)
   3. Pneumoconiosis (inorganic dust, thesaurosis = prolonged hairspray exposure)
   4. Sarcoidosis
   5. Metastases (thyroid, melanoma)
   6. Histiocytosis X
   7. Chickenpox

Fine nodular disease in afebrile patient
   1. Inhalational disease
   2. Eosinophilic granuloma
   3. Sarcoidosis
   4. Metastases
   5. Fungal infection (late stage)
   6. Miliary tuberculosis (rare)

Fine nodular disease in febrile patient
   1. Tuberculosis
   2. Fungal infection (early stage)
   3. Pneumocystis
   4. Viral pneumonia

Macronodular disease
   1. Granulomatous disease (EG, fungus)
   2. Metastases
   3. Vasculitis (Wegener granulomatosis)

Chronic interstitial disease simulating air space disease
A. Replacement of lung architecture by an interstitial process
   (a) Neoplastic
        Hodgkin disease, Histiocytic lymphoma
   (b) Benign cellular infiltrate
        Lymphocytic interstitial pneumonia, Pseudolymphoma
   (c) Granulomatous disease
        Alveolar sarcoidosis
   (d) Fibrosis
B. Exudative phase of interstitial pneumonia
   1. UIP
   2. Adult respiratory distress syndrome
   3. Radiation pneumonitis
   4. Drug reaction
   5. Reaction to noxious gases
C. Cellular filling of air space
   1. Desquamative interstitial pneumonia
   2. Pneumocystis carinii pneumonia

DENSE LUNG LESION
Atelectasis
A. TUMOR
   1. Bronchogenic carcinoma (2/3 of squamous cell carcinoma occur as endobronchial mass with persistent / recurrent atelectasis or recurrent pneumonia)
   2. Bronchial carcinoid
   3. Metastases: renal cell carcinoma, breast carcinoma, melanoma
   4. Lymphoma (usually as a late presentation)
   5. Lipoma, Granular cell myoblastoma, Amyloid tumor, Fibroepithelial polyp
B. INFLAMMATION
   1. Tuberculosis (endobronchial granuloma, broncholith, bronchial stenosis)
   2. Right middle lobe syndrome (chronic right middle lobe atelectasis)
   3. Sarcoidosis (endobronchial granuloma — rare)
D. MUCUS PLUG
   1. Severe chest / abdominal pain (postoperative patient)
   2. Respiratory depressant drug (morphine; CNS illness)
   3. Chronic bronchitis / Bronchiolitis obliterans

4. Asthma
5. Cystic fibrosis
6. Bronchopneumonia (peribronchial inflammation)
D. OTHER
   1. Large left atrium (mitral stenosis + left lower lobe atelectasis)
   2. Foreign body (aspiration of food, endotracheal intubation)
   3. Amyloidosis
   4. Wegener granulomatosis
   5. Bronchial transection

√ local increase in lung density
√ crowding of pulmonary vessels
√ bronchial rearrangement
√ displacement of fissures
√ displacement of hilus
√ mediastinal shift
√ elevation of hemidiaphragm
√ cardiac rotation
√ approximation of ribs
√ compensatory overinflation of normal lung

Resorptive Atelectasis = bronchiolar obstruction by
1. Tumor
2. Stricture
3. Foreign body
4. Mucous plug
5. Bronchial rupture

Passive Atelectasis = pleural space-occupying process
1. Pneumothorax
2. Hydrothorax / Hemothorax
3. Diaphragmatic hernia
4. Pleural masses: metastases, mesothelioma

Adhesive Atelectasis = decrease in surfactant production
1. Respiratory distress syndrome of the newborn (hyaline membrane disease)
2. Pulmonary embolism: edema, hemorrhage, atelectasis
3. Intravenous injection of hydrocarbon

Cicatrizing Atelectasis = parenchymal fibrosis causing decreased lung volume
1. Tuberculosis / Histoplasmosis (upper lobes)
2. Silicosis (upper lobes)
3. Scleroderma (lower lobes)
4. Radiation pneumonitis (nonanatomical distribution)
5. Idiopathic pulmonary fibrosis

Rounded Atelectasis
√ comet-tail sign (= converging lung markings)
√ pleural thickening
√ subpleural mass lateral / posterior chest wall
√ "swiss cheese" air bronchogram (AP tomogram)

Discoid atelectasis
mnemonic: "EPIC"
Embolus
Pneumonia
Inadequate inspiration
Carcinoma, obstructing

Segmental + lobar densities
A. PNEUMONIA
   1. Lobar pneumonia
   2. Lobular pneumonia
   3. Acute interstitial pneumonia
   4. Aspiration pneumonia
   5. Primary tuberculosis
B. PULMONARY EMBOLISM
   (rarely multiple / larger than subsegmental)
C. NEOPLASM
   1. Obstructive pneumonia
   2. Bronchioloalveolar cell carcinoma
D. ATELECTASIS

Multifocal ill-defined densities
= densities 5 – 30 mm resulting in air-space filling
A. INFECTION
   1. Bacterial bronchopneumonia
     = combination of interstitial + alveolar disease (injury starts in airways involves bronchovascular bundle, spills into alveoli, which may contain edema fluid, blood, leukocytes, hyaline membranes, organisms)
     (a) Staphylococcus aureus, Pseudomonas: thrombosis of lobular artery branches with necrosis + cavitation
     (b) Streptococcus, Klebsiella, E. coli, Nocardia
     (c) Mycoplasma
   2. Fungal pneumonia
     Histoplasmosis, Blastomycosis, Actinomycosis, Coccidioidomycosis, Aspergillosis, Cryptococcosis, Mucormycosis, Sporotrichosis
   3. Viral pneumonia
     initially may have interstitial appearance
     = tracheitis, bronchitis, bronchiolitis, peribronchial infiltrate, interstitial septa infiltrates, injury to alveolar cells, hyaline membranes, necrosis of alveolar walls with blood, edema, fibrin, macrophages in alveoli
     (a) Influenza: cavitary lesion confirms superimposed infection
     (b) Varicella / herpes zoster: 10% of adults; 2 – 5 days after rash
     (c) Rubeola (measles) = before / with onset of rash; following overt measles = giant cell pneumonia
     (d) Cytomegalic inclusion virus: features suggestive of bronchopneumonia
     (e) Coxsackie, Parainfluenza, Adenovirus, Respiratory syncytial virus
   4. Tuberculosis (primary infection)

5. Rocky mountain spotted fever
6. Pneumocystis carinii
B. GRANULOMATOUS DISEASE
 1. Sarcoidosis (alveolar form secondary to
    peribronchial granulomas)
 2. Eosinophilic granuloma
C. VASCULAR
 1. Thromboembolic disease
 2. Septic emboli
 3. Vasculitis
  (a) Wegener granulomatosis
  (b) Wegener variants: Limited Wegener,
      Lymphomatoid granulomatosis
  (c) Infectious vasculitis = invasion of pulmonary
      arteries: Mucormycosis, Invasive form of
      aspergillosis, Rocky Mountain spotted fever
  (d) Goodpasture syndrome
  (e) Scleroderma
D. NEOPLASTIC
 1. Bronchioloalveolar cell carcinoma
    = only primary lung tumor to produce multifocal ill-
      defined densities with air bronchograms
 2. Alveolar type of lymphoma
    = massive accumulation of tumor cells in
      interstitium with compression atelectasis +
      obstructive pneumonia
 3. Metastases
  (a) Choriocarcinoma: hemorrhage (however rare)
  (b) Vascular tumors: malignant hemangiomas
 4. Waldenström macroglobulinemia
 5. Angioblastic lymphadenopathy
 6. Mycosis fungoides
 7. Amyloid tumor
E. IDIOPATHIC INTERSTITIAL DISEASE
 1. Lymphocytic Interstitial Pneumonitis (LIP)
 2. Desquamative Interstitial Pneumonitis (DIP)
 3. Pseudolymphoma = localized form of LIP
 4. Usual Interstitial Pneumonitis (UIP)
F. INHALATIONAL DISEASE
 1. Allergic alveolitis: acute stage (e.g. farmer's lung)
 2. Silicosis
 3. Eosinophilic pneumonia
G. DRUG REACTIONS

Ill-defined densities with holes

A. INFECTION
 1. Necrotizing pneumonias
    Staphylococcus aureus, ß-hemolytic streptococcus,
    Klebsiella pneumoniae, E. coli, Proteus,
    Pseudomonas, Anaerobes
 2. Aspiration pneumonia
    mixed Gram-negative organisms
 3. Septic emboli
 4. Fungus
    Histoplasmosis, Blastomycosis,
    Coccidioidomycosis, Cryptococcosis
 5. Tuberculosis

B. NEOPLASM
 1. Primary lung carcinoma
 2. Lymphoma (cavitates very rarely)
C. VASCULAR + COLLAGEN-VASCULAR DISEASE
 1. Emboli with infarction
 2. Wegener granulomatosis
 3. Necrobiotic rheumatoid nodules
D. TRAUMA
 1. contusion with pneumatoceles

Recurrent fleeting infiltrates

1. Löffler disease
2. Bronchopulmonary aspergillosis / Bronchocentric
   granulomatosis
3. Asthma
4. Subacute bacterial endocarditis with pulmonary emboli

Tubular density

A. Mucoid impaction
B. Vascular malformation
 1. Arteriovenous malformation
 2 Pulmonary varix

Mucoid impaction

1. Asthma (most frequent cause): esp. during acute
   attack or convalescent phase
2. Cystic fibrosis
3. Chronic bronchitis
4. Bronchial obstruction by neoplasm:
   bronchogenic carcinoma / adenoma
5. Bronchopulmonary aspergillosis: central perihilar
   bronchiectasis
6. Fluid-filled bronchiectasis: history of childhood
   pneumonia; peripheral distribution
7. Bronchial atresia

Multiple pulmonary calcifications

A. Infection
 1. Histoplasmosis
 2. Tuberculosis
 3. Chickenpox pneumonia
B. Inhalational disease
 1. Silicosis
C. Miscellaneous
 1. Hypercalcemia
 2. Mitral stenosis
 3. Alveolar microlithiasis

PULMONARY MASS
Solitary nodule / mass

Incidence:
 (a) roentgenographic survey of low risk population:
     < 5% of masses are cancerous
 (b) on surgical resection: 40% malignant tumors,
     40% granulomas
A. INFLAMMATION / INFECTION
 1. Granuloma (most common lung mass):
    Sarcoidosis (1/3), Tuberculosis, Histoplasmosis,

Coccidioidomycosis, Nocardiosis, Cryptococcosis, Talc, Dirofilaria immitis (dog heartworm), Gumma, Atypical measles infection
  CT: √ gross calcification / positive phantom study (usually > 164 HU)
  2. Fluid-filled cavity: Abscess, Hydatid cyst, Bronchiectatic cyst, Bronchocele
  3. Mass in preformed cavity: Fungus ball, Mucoid impaction
  4. Rounded atelectasis
  5. Inflammatory pseudotumor: fibroxanthoma, histiocytoma, plasma cell granuloma, sclerosing hemangioma
  6. Paraffinoma = lipoid granuloma
B. MALIGNANT TUMORS
  (a) Malignant primaries of lung
    1. Bronchogenic carcinoma (66%, 2nd most common mass)
    2. Lymphoma
    3. Primary sarcoma of lung
    4. Plasmocytoma (primary / secondary)
    5. Clear cell carcinoma, carcinoid, giant cell carcinoma
  (b) Metastases (4th most common cause)
    from kidney, colon, ovary, testes, Wilms tumor, sarcoma
C. BENIGN TUMORS
  (a) lung tissue: Hamartoma (6%, 3rd most common lung mass)
  (b) fat tissue: Lipoma (usually pleural lesion)
  (c) fibrous tissue: Fibroma
  (d) muscle tissue: Leiomyoma
  (e) neural tissue: Schwannoma, Neurofibroma, Paraganglioma
  (f) lymph tissue: Intrapulmonary lymph node
  (g) deposits: Amyloid, Splenosis, Endometrioma, Extramedullary hematopoiesis
D. VASCULAR
  1. Arteriovenous malformation
  2. Hemangioma
  3. Hematoma
  4. Organizing infarct
  5. Pulmonary vein varix
  6. Rheumatoid / vasculitic nodule
E. DEVELOPMENTAL
  1. Bronchogenic cyst (fluid-filled)
  2. Pulmonary sequestration
F. INHALATIONAL
  1. Silicosis (conglomerate mass)
  2. Mucoid impaction (allergic aspergillosis)
G. MIMICKING DENSITIES
  1. Fluid in interlobar fissure
  2. Mediastinal mass
  3. Pleural mass (mesothelioma)
  4. Chest wall density: nipple, rib lesion, skin tumor (mole, neurofibroma, lipoma)
  5. Artifacts (buttons, snaps)

DIFFERENTIAL DIAGNOSTIC FEATURES OF LUNG MASSES ON CXR
  √ corona radiata = spiculations strongly suggestive of primary malignancy
  √ lucencies / air bronchogram
    (a) cavitation
    (b) infiltrative spread with air bronchogram: bronchioloalveolar cell carcinoma, lymphoma, resolving pneumonia
  √ calcifications
    (a) central / complete: granuloma
    (b) peripheral   : granuloma, tumor
  √ decrease in size with time: benign lesion
  √ increase in size with time:
    masses with "doubling times" (refers to volume not diameter) of < 1 month / > 16 months are unlikely to be malignant
    (a) very rapid growth:
      osteosarcoma, choriocarcinoma, testicular neoplasm, organizing infectious process, infarct (thromboembolism, Wegener granulomatosis)
    (b) very slow growth:
      hamartoma, bronchial carcinoid, inflammatory pseudotumor, granuloma, low-grade adenocarcinoma, metastases from renal cell carcinoma
  √ lobulation
    (a) organizing mass
    (b) tumor with multiple cell types growing at different rates (e.g. hamartoma)
  √ vessel leading to mass: pulmonary varix, AVM

Multiple nodules and masses
  √ homogeneous mass with sharp border
  √ No air alveolo- / bronchogram
A. TUMORS
  (a) malignant
    1. Metastases:
      from breast, kidney, GI tract, uterus, ovary, testes, malignant melanoma, sarcoma, Wilms tumor
    2. Lymphoma (rare)
  (b) benign
    1. Hamartoma (rarely multiple)
    2. AV-malformations
    3. Amyloidosis
B. VASCULAR LESIONS
  1. Thromboemboli with organizing infarcts
  2. Septic emboli = organized infarcts
C. COLLAGEN-VASCULAR DISEASE
  1. Wegener granulomatosis: vasculitis with organizing infarcts
  2. Wegener variants
  3. Rheumatoid nodules: tendency for periphery, occasionally cavitating
D. INFLAMMATORY GRANULOMAS
  1. fungal: Coccidioidomycosis, Histoplasmosis, Cryptococcosis

2. bacterial: Nocardiosis, Tuberculosis
3. viral: Atypical measles
4. parasites: Hydatid cysts, Paragonimiasis
5. Sarcoidosis: large accumulation of interstitial granulomas
6. Inflammatory pseudotumors: fibrous histiocytoma, plasma cell granuloma, hyalinizing pulmonary nodules, pseudolymphoma

Small pulmonary nodules
mnemonic: "MALTS"
    Metastases (esp. thyroid)
    Alveolar cell carcinoma
    Lyphoma, **L**eukemia
    TBC
    Sarcoid

Pleural-based nodule
√ ill-defined/ sharply defined lesion mimicking a true pleural mass
√ associated linear densities in lung parenchyma
Causes:
1. Granuloma (fungus, tuberculosis)
2. Inflammatory pseudotumor
3. Metastasis
4. Rheumatoid nodule
5. Pancoast tumor
6. Lymphoma
7. Infarct: Hampton hump
8. Atelectatic pseudotumor

Cavitating nodules
A. NEOPLASM
  (a) Lung primary:
    1. Squamous cell carcinoma
    2. Adenocarcinoma
    3. Bronchioloalveolar carcinoma (rare)
    4. Hodgkin disease (rare)
  (b) Metastases (4% cavitate):
    1. Squamous cell carcinoma (2/3) nasopharynx (males), cervix (females), esophagus
    2. Adenocarcinoma
    3. Melanoma
    4. Sarcoma: Ewing sarcoma, Osteo-, Myxo-, Angiosarcoma
    6. Seminoma, Teratocarcinoma
    7. Wilms tumor
B. COLLAGEN-VASCULAR DISEASE
  1. Wegener granulomatosis + Wegener variant
  2. Rheumatoid nodules + Caplan syndrome
  3. SLE
  4. Periarteritis nodosa (rare)
C. GRANULOMATOUS DISEASE
  1. Histiocytosis X
  2. Sarcoidosis (rare)
D. VASCULAR DISEASE
  1. Pulmonary embolus with infarction
  2. Septic emboli (Staphylococcus aureus)

E. INFECTION
  (a) bacterial: pneumatoceles from staphylococcal / gram-negative pneumonia
  (b) mycobacterial: TB
  (c) fungal: Nocardiosis, Cryptococcosis, Coccidioidomycosis (in 10%), Aspergillosis
  (d) parasitic: Echinococcosis (multiple in 20 – 30%), Paragonimiasis
F. TRAUMA
  1. Traumatic lung cyst (after hemorrhage)
  2. Hydrocarbon ingestion (lower lobes)
G. BRONCHOPULMONARY DISEASE
  1. Infected bulla
  2. Cystic bronchiectasis
  3. Communicating bronchogenic cyst

mnemonic: "CAVITY"
  Carcinoma (squamous)
  Autoimmune disease (Wegener, Rheumatoid)
  Vascular (bland / septic emboli)
  Infection (abscess, fungal disease)
  Trauma
  Young = congenital (sequestration, diaphragmatic hernia, bronchogenic cyst)

cavitating metastases: "**S**quamous **C**ell **M**etastases **T**end to **C**avitate"
  Squamous cell carcinoma
  Colon
  Melanoma
  Transitional cell carcinoma
  Cervix

Intrathoracic mass of low attenuation
A. Cysts
  1. Bronchogenic / neurenteric / pericardial cyst
  2. Hydatid disease
B. Fatty substrate
  1. Hamartoma
  2. Lipoma
  3. Tuberculous lymph node
  4. Lymph adenopathy in Whipple disease
C. Necrotic masses
  1. Resolving hematoma
  2. Treated lymphoma
  3. Metastases from ovary, stomach, testes

Peripheral mass with air bronchogram
1. Bronchioloalveolar carcinoma
2. Lymphoma
3. Pseudolymphoma
4. Inflammatory pseudotumor

Pulmonary nodules + pneumothorax
1. Osteosarcoma
2. Wilms tumor
3. Histiocytosis

Pneumoconiosis with mass
Anthracosilicosis with:
1. Granuloma (Histoplasmosis, Tuberculosis, Sarcoidosis)
2. Bronchogenic carcinoma (incidence same as in general population)
3. Metastasis
4. Progressive massive fibrosis
5. Caplan syndrome (rheumatoid nodules)

Air-crescent sign
1. Invasive pulmonary aspergillosis
2. Noninvasive mycetoma
3. Septic emboli
4. Cavitating benign + malignant neoplasms
5. Echinococcal cyst
6. TB with Rasmussen aneurysms (most are too small to be identified on CXR)

Benign lung tumor
A. CENTRAL LOCATION
 1. Bronchial polyp
 2. Bronchlla papilloma
 3. **Granular cell myoblastoma**
  = cell of origin from neural crest
  Age: middle-aged, esp. black women
  √ endobronchial lesion in major bronchi
B. PERIPHERAL LOCATION
 1. Hamartoma
 2. Leiomyoma
  benign metastasizing leiomyoma, Hx of pelvic surgery (hysterectomy)
 3. Amyloid tumor
  not associated with amyloid of other organs / rheumatoid arthritis / myeloma
 4. Intrapulmonary lymph node
 5. Arteriovenous malformation
 6. Endometrioma, Fibroma, Neural tumor, Chemodectoma
C. CENTRAL / PERIPHERAL
 1. Lipoma: (a) subpleural (b) endobronchial
D. PSEUDOTUMOR
 1. Fibroxanthoma / Xanthogranuloma
 2. Plasma cell granuloma
 3. Sclerosing hemangioma
  middle-aged woman, RML / RLL (most commonly), may be multiple
 4. Pseudolymphoma
 5. Round atelectasis

LUCENT LUNG LESIONS
Hyperlucent lung
Bilateral hyperlucent lung
A. FAULTY RADIOLOGIC TECHNIQUE
 1. Overpenetrated film
B. DECREASED SOFT TISSUES
 1. Thin body habitus
 2. Bilateral mastectomy

C. CARDIAC CAUSE of decreased pulmonary blood flow
 1. Right-to-left shunt:
  Tetralogy of Fallot (small proximal pulmonary vessels), Pseudotruncus, Truncus type IV, Ebstein malformation, Tricuspid atresia
 2. Eisenmenger physiology of left-to-right shunt: ASD, VSD, PDA (dilated proximal pulmonary vessels)
D. PULMONARY CAUSE of decreased pulmonary blood flow
 (a) Decrease of vascular bed:
  1. Pulmonary embolism
   bilaterality is rare; localized areas of hyperlucency (Westermark sign)
 (b) Increase in air space:
  1. Air trapping (reversible changes): acute asthmatic attack, acute bronchiolitis (pediatric patient)
  2. Emphysema
  3. Bulla
  4. Bleb
  5. Interstitial emphysema

Unilateral hyperlucent lung
A. FAULTY RADIOLOGIC TECHNIQUE
 1. Rotation of patient
B. CHEST WALL DEFECT
 1. Mastectomy
 2. Absent pectoralis muscle (Poland syndrome)
C. INCREASED PULMONARY AIR SPACE
 with decreased pulmonary blood flow
 (a) Large airway obstruction with air trapping
  @ Bronchial compression:
   Hilar mass (rare), Cardiomegaly compressing LLL bronchus
  @ Endobronchial obstruction with air trapping (collateral air drift):
   Foreign body, Broncholith, Bronchogenic carcinoma, Carcinoid, Bronchial mucocele
 (b) Small airway obstruction
  1. Bronchiolitis obliterans
  2. Swyer-James / Macleod syndrome
  3. Emphysema (particularly bullous emphysema)
 (c) Pneumothorax (in supine patient)
D. PULMONARY VASCULAR CAUSE of decreased pulmonary blood flow
 1. Pulmonary artery hypoplasia
 2. Pulmonary embolism
 3. Congenital lobar emphysema
 4. Compensatory overaeration

Localized lucent lung defect
A. CAVITY = tissue necrosis with bronchial drainage
 (a) INFECTION
  Bacterial pneumonia
   1. Pyogenic infection = abscess = necrotizing pneumonia

Staphylococcus, Klebsiella, Pseudomonas, Anaerobes, beta-hemolytic Streptococcus, E. coli, mixed Gram-negative organisms
2. Aspiration pneumonia = gravitational pneumonia:
mixed Gram-negative organisms, anaerobes
Granulomatous infection
1. Tuberculosis
cavitation indicates active infectious disease with risk for hematogenous / bronchogenous dissemination
2. Fungal infection:
Nocardiosis (in immunocompromised), Coccidioidomycosis (any lobe, desert Southwest), Histoplasmosis, Blastomycosis, Mucormycosis, Sporotrichosis, Cryptococcosis, Aspergillosis
√ very thin-walled cavities less likely to follow apical distribution of TB / histoplasmosis
3. Sarcoidosis (stage IV, upper lobe predominance)
Parasitic infestation: Hydatid disease
(b) NEOPLASM
Primary lung tumor: 16% of peripheral lung cancers (in particular in squamous cell carcinoma (30%); also in bronchioloalveolar cell carcinoma)
Metastasis (usually multiple)
1. Squamous cell (nasopharynx, esophagus, cervix) in 2/3
2. Adenocarcinoma (lung, breast, GI)
3. Osteosarcoma (rare)
4. Melanoma
5. Lymphoma (rare): with adenopathy; cavities often secondary to opportunistic infection with nocardiosis + cryptococcosis
(c) VASCULAR OCCLUSION
1. Infarct (thromboembolic, septic)
2. Wegener granulomatosis
3. Rheumatoid arthritis
(d) INHALATIONAL
1. Silicosis with coal-worker's pneumoconiosis
— complicating tuberculosis
— ischemic necrosis of center of conglomerate mass (rare)
B. CYSTS
(a) Cystic bronchiectasis
1. Cystic fibrosis (more obvious in upper lobes)
2. Agammaglobulinemia (predisposed to recurrent bacterial infections)
3. Recurrent bacterial pneumonias
√ multiple thin-walled lucencies with air-fluid levels in lower lobes
4. Tuberculosis
5. Allergic bronchopulmonary aspergillosis (in asthmatic patients)
√ involvement of proximal perihilar bronchi

(b) Pneumatoceles
in area of previous pneumonia / posttraumatic hematoma
(c) Congenital lesions (rare)
1. Multiple bronchogenic cysts
2. Intralobar sequestration:
multicystic structure in lower lobes
3. Congenital cystic adenomatoid malformation (CCAM) Type I
4. Diaphragmatic hernia (congenital / traumatic)
(d) Centrilobular / bullous emphysema
(e) Honeycomb lung

Multiple lucent lung lesions
see causes of localized lucent defect
A. CAVITIES
(a) Infection
1. Bacterial pneumonia = necrotizing pneumonia
2. Granulomatous infection (TB, coccidioidomycosis)
3. Parasites (hydatid disease)
(b) Neoplasm
(c) Vascular
1. Thromboembolic + septic infarcts
2. Wegener granulomatosis
3. Rheumatoid arthritis
B. CYSTS
(a) Cystic bronchiectasis
1. Cystic fibrosis (more obvious in upper lobes)
2. Agammaglobulinemia (predisposed to recurrent bacterial infections)
3. Recurrent bacterial pneumonias
4. Tuberculosis
5. Allergic bronchopulmonary aspergillosis (in asthmatic patients)
(b) Pneumatoceles
(c) Congenital lesions (rare)
1. Multiple bronchogenic cysts
2. Intralobar sequestration:
multicystic structure in lower lobes
3. Congenital cystic adenomatoid malformation (CCAM) Type I
4. Diaphragmatic hernia (congenital / traumatic)
(d) Centrilobular / bullous emphysema
(e) Honeycomb lung
(f) Juvenile pulmonary polyposis

Mass within cavity
1. Mycetoma = aspergilloma
2. Tissue fragment within carcinoma
3. Necrotic lung within abscess
4. Disintegrating hydatid cyst
5. Intracavitary blood clot

Pulmonary cyst
A. CONGENITAL CYST
1. Cystic adenomatoid malformation
2. Congenital lobar emphysema

3. Bronchial atresia
4. Bronchogenic cyst
5. Sequestration
B. ACQUIRED CYST
   1. Pneumatocele (traumatic / infectious)
   2. Pseudocyst (from interstitial emphysema)
   3. Hydatid disease
   4. Bleb = cystic air collection within visceral pleura; mostly apical with narrow neck; associated with spontaneous pneumothorax
   5. Bulla = cystic air collection within lung parenchyma due to destruction of alveoli; associated with emphysema

Pneumothorax
Etiology:
1. Neonatal disease: Meconium aspiration, Respirator therapy for hyaline membrane disease
2. Malignancy: Primary lung cancer, Lung metastases (esp. osteosarcoma, pancreas, adrenal, Wilms tumor)
3. Pulmonary infections: Coccidioidomycosis, Hydatid disease, Acute bacterial pneumonia, Staphylococcal septicemia
4. Cx of honeycomb lung: Sarcoidosis, Histiocytosis X, Rheumatoid lung, Idiopathic pulmonary hemosiderosis, Pulmonary alveolar proteinosis
5. Marfan syndrome
6. Spasmodic asthma, diffuse emphysema
7. Pulmonary infarction
8. Catamenial pneumothorax = recurrent spontaneous pneumothorax during menstruation associated with endometriosis of the diaphragm; R >> L
9. Lymphangiomyomatosis + Tuberous sclerosis

Spontaneous Pneumothorax
result of rupture of subpleural bleb / bulla
Age: 3rd + 4th decade; M:F = 8:1, esp. in patients with tall thin stature
• chest pain (69%)
• dyspnea
Prognosis: recurrence in 30% on same side, in 10% on contralateral side

Traumatic Pneumothorax
(a) secondary to rib fractures / contusion / laceration
(b) iatrogenic: tracheostomy, central venous catheter, PEEP ventilator

Tension Pneumothorax
= intrapleural pressure exceeds atmospheric pressure in lung during expiration (check-valve mechanism)
√ displacement of mediastinum / anterior junction line
√ diaphragmatic inversion
√ total / subtotal lung collapse
√ collapse of SVC / IVC / right heart border (decreased systemic venous return)

RADIOGRAPHIC SIGNS OF PNEUMOTHORAX IN SUPINE POSITION
1. Anteromedial pneumothorax (earliest location)
   √ sharp delineation of mediastinal contours (SVC, azygos vein, left subclavian artery, anterior junction line, superior pulmonary vein, heart border, IVC, deep anterior cardiophrenic sulcus, pericardial fat pad)
   √ outline of medial diaphragm under cardiac silhouette
2. Subpulmonic pneumothorax (second most common location)
   √ hyperlucent upper abdominal quadrant
   √ deep lateral costophrenic sulcus
   √ visualization of anterior costophrenic sulcus
   √ visualization of inferior surface of lung
   √ sharply outlined diaphragm in spite of parenchymal disease
3. Apicolateral pneumothorax (least common location)
   √ visualization of visceral pleural line
4. Posteromedial pneumothorax (in presence of lower lobe collapse)
   √ lucent triangle with vertex at hilum
   √ V-shaped base delineating costovertebral sulcus
5. Pneumothorax outlines pulmonary ligament

MEDIASTINUM
Pneumomediastinum
A. SPONTANEOUS PNEUMOMEDIASTINUM (common)
   Age: neonates (0.05-1%), 2nd – 3rd decade
   Causes:
   (a) rupture of marginally situated alveoli from sudden rise in intraalveolar pressure (acute asthma, aspiration pneumonia, hyaline membrane disease, measles, giant cell pneumonia, coughing, vomiting, strenuous exercise, parturition, diabetic acidosis)
   (b) Tumor erosion of trachea / esophagus
   (c) Pneumoperitoneum / Retropneumoperitoneum
   Cx: air block = build-up of pressure impeding blood flow in low pressure veins particularly common in neonatal period

B. TRAUMATIC PNEUMOMEDIASTINUM (rare)
   1. Pulmonary interstitial emphysema
      = disruption of marginal alveoli with gas traveling toward mediastinum due to positive pressure ventilation
   2. Ruptured bronchus
      √ commonly associated with pneumothorax
   3. Ruptured esophagus (diabetic acidosis, alcoholic, Boerhaave syndrome)

Mediastinal shift
= displacement of heart, trachea, aorta, hilar vessels
Δ expiration film, lateral decubitus film (expanded lung down), fluoroscopy help to determine side of abnormality

A. DECREASED LUNG VOLUME
1. Atelectasis
2. Postoperative (lobectomy, pneumothorax)
3. Hypoplastic lung / lobe
√ small pulmonary artery + small hilum
√ decreased peripheral pulmonary vasculature
√ irregular reticular vascular pattern (bronchial origin) without converging on the hilum
4. Bronchiolitis obliterans = Swyer-James syndrome

B. INCREASED LUNG VOLUME = air trapping
@ Major bronchus
1. Foreign body obstructing mainstem bronchus (common in children) with ball valve mechanism + collateral air drift
√ contralateral mediastinal shift increasing with expiration
@ Emphysema
1. Bullous emphysema (localized form):
√ large avascular areas with thin lines
2. Congenital lobar emphysema: only in infants
3. Interstitial emphysema:
√ pattern of diffuse coarse lines;
Cx of positive pressure ventilation therapy
@ Cysts / Masses
1. Bronchogenic cyst: with bronchial connection + check valve mechanism
2. Cystic adenomatoid malformation = complex foregut anomaly
3. Large mass (pulmonary, mediastinal)

C. PLEURAL SPACE ABNORMALITY
1. Large unilateral pleural effusion:
opaque hemithorax through empyema, congestive failure, metastases
2. Tension pneumothorax:
not always complete collapse of lung
3. Large diaphragmatic hernia:
usually detected in neonatal period
4. Large mass

D. Partial absence of pericardium / pectus excavatum
√ shift of heart without shift of trachea, aorta, or mediastinal border

Mediastinal cysts
= 21% of all primary mediastinal tumors, mostly developmental
1. Pericardial cyst
2. Thymic cyst
3. FOREGUT CYST
(a) Bronchogenic cyst
(b) **Esophageal duplication cyst**
arise from foregut
Histo: contains no cartilage, lined by gastrointestinal tract epithelium
Location: adjacent to esophagus / within esophageal musculature at any level, posterior mediastinum in paraspinal position
Cx: peptic ulceration, perforation + bleeding (gastric mucosa)

(c) **Neurenteric cyst**
connected to meninges through midline defect
√ vertebral body anomalies (hemivertebrae, butterfly vertebrae, scoliosis) at the same level
√ air-fluid level (if communicating with GI-tract)
4. **Lateral meningocele**
= outpouching of leptomeninges through intervertebral foramen
Etiology: 75% in neurofibromatosis
√ spinal abnormalities (kyphoscoliosis, scalloping of dorsal vertebrae, enlargement of intervertebral foramen, pedicle erosion, thinning of ribs)
5. **Hydatid cyst**
Location: paravertebral gutter
√ erosion of ribs + vertebrae
6. **Thoracic duct cyst**
rare, filled with chyle
Etiology: degenerative / lymphangiomatous
7. Traumatic lymphocele
8. Parathyroid cyst
uncommon as mediastinal mass

Mediastinal fat
A. Mediastinal lipomatosis
B. Fat herniation
= omental fat herniating into chest
1. Foramen of Morgagni
= cardiophrenic angle mass, R >> L side
2. Foramen of Bochdalek
= costophrenic angle mass, almost always on left
3. Paraesophageal hernia = perigastric fat through phrenicoesophageal membrane
CT: √ fat with fine linear densities (= omental vessels)
C. Lipoma
un- / encapsulated with variable amount of fibrous septa
√ smooth + sharply defined boundaries
DDx: Liposarcoma, lipoblastoma (infancy), fat-containing teratoma, thymolipoma (inhomogeneous, higher CT numbers, poor demarcation, possibly invasion of surrounding structures)
D. Multiple symmetrical lipomatosis
rare entity without involvement of anterior mediastinal / cardiophrenic / paraspinal areas
√ compression of trachea
√ periscapular lipomatous masses

MEDIASTINAL MASS
(excluding hyperplastic thymus glands, granulomas, lymphoma, metastases)
1. Neurogenic tumors (28%) : malignant in 16%
2. Teratoid lesions (19%) : malignant in 15%
3. Enterogenous cysts (16%)
4. Thymomas (13%) : malignant in 46%
5. Pericardial cysts (7%)

Δ 75% of all mediastinal tumors are benign (in all age groups)

Δ 1/3 diagnosed on routine chest X-ray

Δ 2/3 found in association with symptoms (pain, cough, shortness of breath)

Δ 80% of malignant tumors are symptomatic

Inlet lesions from the neck

1. Thyroid mass
   1 – 3% of all thyroidectomies have a mediastinal component; 1/3 of goiters are intrathoracic
   Location: anterior (80%) / posterior (20%) mediastinum
   √ displacement of trachea posteriorly + laterally (anterior goiter)
   √ displacement of trachea anteriorly + esophagus posteriorly + laterally (posterior goiter)
   √ inhomogeneous density (cystic spaces, high-density iodine contents)
   √ focal calcifications are common
   √ marked + prolonged contrast enhancement
   √ connection to thyroid gland
   √ vascular compression
   NUC: (rarely helpful as thyroid tissue is nonfunctioning)
   √ may be nonfunctioning on I-123 scan
2. Cystic hygroma
   3 – 10% involve mediastinum; childhood
3. Lymphoma

Anterior mediastinal mass

mnemonic: "4 T's"
   Thymoma
   Teratoma
   Thyroid tumor / goiter
   Terrible lymphoma

A. SOLID THYMIC LESIONS
   1. Thymoma (benign, malignant): most common
   2. Normal thymus (neonate)
   3. Thymic hyperplasia (child)
   4. Thymolipoma
   5. Lymphoma
B. SOLID TERATOID LESIONS
   1. Teratoma
   2. Embryonal cell carcinoma
   3. Choriocarcinoma
   4. Seminoma
C. THYROID / PARATHYROID
   1. Substernal thyroid / goiter
   2. Thyroid adenoma / carcinoma
   3. Ectopic parathyroid adenoma
      ectopia in 10% (62% in anterior mediastinum, 30% within thyroid tissue, 8% in posterior superior mediastinum)
D. LYMPH NODES
   1. Lymphoma (Hodgkin, NHL): may arise in thymus, more common in young adults
   2. Metastases
   3. Benign lymph node hyperplasia
   4. Angioblastic lymph adenopathy

5. Mediastinal lymphadenitis: Sarcoidosis / granulomatous infection
E. CARDIOVASCULAR
   1. Tortuous brachiocephalic artery
   2. Aneurysm of ascending aorta
   3. Aneurysm of Sinus of Valsalva
   4. Dilated SVC
   5. Cardiac tumor
   6. Epicardial fat pad
F. CYSTS
   1. Cystic hygroma
   2. Bronchogenic cyst
   3. Extralobar sequestration
   4. Thymic cysts / Dermoid cysts
   5. Pericardial cyst: (a) true cyst
                          (b) pericardial diverticulum
   6. Pancreatic pseudocyst
G. OTHERS
   1. Neural tumor (vagus, phrenic nerve)
   2. Paraganglioma
   3. Hemangioma / Lymphangioma
   4. Mesenchymal tumor (fibroma, lipoma)
   5. Sternal tumors
      (a) Metastases from breast, bronchus, kidney, thyroid
      (b) Malignant primary (chondrosarcoma, myeloma, lymphoma)
      (c) Benign primary (chondroma, aneurysmal bone cyst, giant cell tumor)
   6. Primary lung / pleural tumor (invading mediastinum)
   7. Mediastinal lipomatosis: (a) Cushing disease
                                 (b) Corticosteroid therapy
   8. Morgagni hernia / Localized eventration
   9. Abscess

Middle mediastinal mass

A. LYMPH NODES
   90% of masses in the middle mediastinum are malignant
   (a) NEOPLASTIC ADENOPATHY
      1. Lymphoma (Hodgkin: NHL = 2 : 1)
      2. Leukemia (in 25%): lymphocytic > granulocytic
      3. Metastasis (bronchus, lung, upper GI, prostate, kidney)
      4. Angioimmunoblastic lymphadenopathy
   (b) INFLAMMATORY ADENOPATHY
      1. Tuberculosis / Histoplasmosis (may lead to fibrosing mediastinitis)
      2. Blastomycosis (rare) / Coccidioidomycosis
      3. Sarcoidosis (predominant involvement of paratracheal nodes)
      4. Viral pneumonia (particularly measles + cat scratch fever)
      5. Infectious mononucleosis / Pertussis pneumonia
      6. Amyloidosis
      7. Plague / Tularemia

8. Drug reaction
9. Giant lymph node hyperplasia
   = Castleman disease
10. Connective tissue disease (rheumatoid, SLE)
11. Bacterial lung abscess
(c) INHALATIONAL DISEASE ADENOPATHY
1. Silicosis (eggshell calcification also in
   sarcoidosis + tuberculosis)
2. Coal-worker's pneumoconiosis
3. Berylliosis
B. FOREGUT DUPLICATION CYST
1. Bronchogenic / respiratory cyst (cartilage,
   respiratory epithelium)
2. Enteric cyst
3. Extralobar sequestration (anomalous feeding
   vessel)
4. Hiatal hernia
C. PRIMARY TUMORS (infrequent)
1. Carcinoma of trachea
2. Bronchogenic carcinoma
3. Esophageal tumor:
   leiomyoma, carcinoma, leiomyosarcoma
4. Mesothelioma
5. Granular cell myoblastoma of trachea (rare)
D. VASCULAR LESIONS
1. Aneurysm
2. Distended veins (SVC, azygous vein)
3. Hematoma

Posterior mediastinal mass
A. NEOPLASM
1. Neurogenic tumor (largest group): 30% malignant
   (a) Ganglion series tumors (in children)
       √ 80% are elongated with tapered borders
       1. Neuroblastoma: highly malignant
          undifferentiated small round cell tumor
          originating in sympathetic ganglia,
          < 10 years of age
       2. Ganglioneuroma: benign tumor from mature
          ganglion cells
       3. Ganglioneuroblastoma: both features,
          spontaneous maturation possible
   (b) Nerve root tumors (in adults)
       √ 80% appear as round masses with sulcus
       1. Schwannoma: derived from sheath of
          Schwann without nerve cells
       2. Neurofibroma: contains Schwann cells +
          nerve cells, 3 + 4th decade
       3. Malignant schwannoma
   (c) Paraganglioma (rare)
       1. Chemodectoma
       2. Pheochromocytoma
   √ rib spreading, erosion, destruction
   √ enlargement of neural foramina (dumbbell
     lesion)
   √ scalloping of posterior aspect of vertebral body
   √ scoliosis
   CT: √ low density soft tissue mass (lipid contents)

2. Spine tumor: Metastases (e.g., bronchogenic
   carcinoma), ABC, chondrosarcoma, Ewing sarcoma
3. Lymphoma
4. Invasive thymoma
5. Mesenchymal tumor (fibroma, lipoma, leiomyoma)
6. Hemangioma
7. Lymphangioma
8. Thyroid tumor
B. INFLAMMATION
1. Paraspinous abscess (tuberculosis)
   √ destruction of endplates + disc space
2. Mediastinitis
3. Lymphoid hyperplasia
4. Sarcoidosis (in 2%, typically asymptomatic patient)
5. Pancreatic pseudocyst
C. VASCULAR MASS
1. Aneurysm of descending aorta (curvilinear
   calcification; elderly)
2. Enlarged azygos + accessory hemiazygos vein
3. Esophageal varices
D. TRAUMA
1. Traumatic aneurysm / Pseudoaneurysm
2. Hematoma
3. Loculated hemothorax
4. Traumatic pseudomeningocele
E. CONGENITAL
   √ cysts may demonstrate peripheral rimlike
     calcifications
1. Enteric cyst
2. Neurenteric cyst (hemi- / butterfly vertebra)
3. Bronchogenic cyst
4. Extralobar sequestration
F. OTHER
1. Loculated pleural effusion
2. Bochdalek hernia
3. Pancreatic pseudocyst
4. Lateral meningocele (neurofibromatosis; enlarged
   neural foramen)
5. Lipoma / lipomatosis
6. Extramedullary hematopoiesis (in chronic bone
   marrow deficiency) paraspinal area rich in RES-
   elements
   √ splenomegaly; widening of ribs
7. "Pseudomass" of the newborn
8. Teratoma (rare)

Enlargement of azygos vein
A. COLLATERAL CIRCULATION
1. Portal hypertension
2. SVC obstruction
3. IVC obstruction
4. Azygos continuation of IVC
B. HEART DISEASE
1. Right heart failure
2. Constrictive pericarditis
3. Pericardial effusion

Hilar mass

A. LARGE PULMONARY ARTERIES
√ enlargement of main pulmonary artery
√ abrupt change in vessel caliber
√ enlarged pulmonary artery compared with bronchus (in bronchovascular bundle)
√ cephalization
√ enlargement of right ventricle (RAO 45°, LAO 60°)
Cause:
  1. Chronic obstructive disease (emphysema)
  2. Chronic restrictive interstitial lung disease (idiopathic fibrosis, cystic fibrosis, rheumatoid arthritis, sarcoidosis)
  3. Pulmonary embolic disease (acute massive / chronic)
  4. Idiopathic pulmonary hypertension
  5. Left-sided heart failure + mitral stenosis
  6. Congenital heart disease with left-to-right shunt
    (a) acyanotic: ASD, VSD, PDA
    (b) cyanotic (admixture lesions): transposition of great vessels, truncus arteriosus

B. UNILATERAL HILAR ADENOPATHY
  (a) NEOPLASTIC
    1. Bronchogenic carcinoma (most common)
    2. Metastases (lack of mediastinal involvement exceptional)
    3. Lymphoma
  (b) INFLAMMATORY
    1. Tuberculosis (primary) in 80%
    2. Fungal infection: histoplasmosis, coccidioidomycosis, blastomycosis
    3. Viral infections (atypical measles)
    4. Infectious mononucleosis
    5. Drug reaction
    6. Sarcoidosis (in 1 – 3%)
    7. Bilateral lung abscess

C. BILATERAL HILAR ADENOPATHY
  (a) NEOPLASTIC
    1. Lymphomas (50% in Hodgkin disease)
    2. Metastases
    3. Leukemia
    4. Primary bronchogenic carcinoma
    5. Plasmacytoma
  (b) INFLAMMATORY
    1. Sarcoidosis (in 70 – 90%)
    2. Silicosis
    3. Histiocytosis X
    4. Idiopathic pulmonary hemosiderosis
    5. Chronic berylliosis
  (c) INFECTIOUS
    1. Rubella, ECHO virus, varicella, mononucleosis

D. DUPLICATION CYST

Egg shell calcification of nodes

A. Pneumoconiosis
  1. Silicosis (5%)
  2. Coalworker's pneumoconiosis (1.3-6%)
  not seen in: asbestosis, berylliosis, talcosis, baritosis

B. Sarcoidosis (5%)
C. Fungal + bacterial infection (rare):
  1. Tuberculosis
  2. Histoplasmosis
  3. Coccidioidomycosis
D. Lymphoma following radiation therapy

Right cardiophrenic angle mass

1. Epicardial fat pad / lipoma (most common cause)
  √ triangular opacity in cardiophrenic angle less dense than heart
  √ increase under corticosteroid treatment
2. Pericardial cyst
3. Aneurysm
4. Dilated right atrium
5. Diaphragmatic hernia
6. Diaphragmatic lymph node (esp. in Hodgkin disease + breast cancer)
7. Primary lung mass
8. Anterior mediastinal mass

THYMUS
Thymic mass

1. Thymoma
2. Thymolipoma
3. Thymic Cyst

Diffuse thymic enlargement

1. Thymic Hyperplasia
2. Thymic infiltration
by Leukemia, Hodgkin lymphoma, Non-Hodgkin lymphoma, Histiocytosis
  • presence of adenopathy elsewhere
  √ no pleural implants

PLEURA
Pleural Effusion

A. TRANSUDATE (protein level of 1.5 – 2.5 g/dl)
  (a) increased hydrostatic pressure
    1. Congestive heart failure (in 65%) bilateral (88%), right sided (8%), left sided (4%)
    2. Constrictive pericarditis (in 60%)
  (b) decreased colloid-oncotic pressure
    — decreased protein production
      1. Cirrhosis with ascites (in 6%): right-sided (67%)
    — protein loss / hypervolemia
      1. Nephrotic syndrome (21%), Overhydration, Glomerulonephritis (55%), Peritoneal dialysis
      2. Hypothyroidism
  (c) chylous effusion

B. EXUDATE (protein level > 3 g/dl)
  (a) Infection
    1. **Empyema** (anaerobic bacteria most frequent)
      • gross pus
      • WBC > 15, 000/ccm

- positive gram-stain
- pH < 7,2
- LDH > 1000 U/l
- glucose < 40 mg/dl
2. Parapneumonic (in 40%)
3. Tuberculosis (in 1%):
   high protein content (75 g/dl), lymphocytes > 70%, positive culture (only in 20-25%)
4. Fungi: actinomyces, nocardia
5. Parasites: amebiasis (secondary to liver abscess in 15-20%), echinococcus
6. Mycoplasma, Rickettsia (in 20%)

(b) Malignant disease (in 60%)
lung cancer (26 – 49%), breast cancer (8 – 24%), lymphoma (10 – 28%, in 2/3 chylothorax), ovarian cancer (10%), malignant mesothelioma (hyaluronic acid)
Pathogenesis:
- Δ pleural metastases (increase in permeability)
- Δ lymphatic obstruction (pleural vessels, mediastinal nodes, thoracic duct disruption)
- Δ bronchial obstruction (loss of volume + resorptive surface)
- Δ hypoproteinema (secondary to tumor cachexia)

(c) Vascular
Pulmonary emboli (in 15 – 30% of all embolic events): often serosanguinous

(d) Abdominal disease
1. Pancreatitis / Pseudocyst (in 2/3): usually left sided
2. Boerhaave syndrome: left-sided esophageal perforation
3. Subphrenic abscess
   √ pleural effusion (79%)
   √ elevation + restriction of diaphragmatic motion (95%)
   √ basal platelike atelectasis / pneumonitis (79%)
4. Abdominal tumor with ascites
5. **Meigs-Salmon syndrome**
   = primary pelvic neoplasms (ovarian fibroma, thecoma, granulosa cell tumor, Brenner tumor, cystadenoma, adenocarcinoma, fibromyoma of uterus) cause pleural effusion in 2 – 3%; ascites + hydrothorax resolve with tumor removal
6. Endometriosis
7. Bile fistula

(e) Collagen-vascular disease
1. Rheumatoid arthritis (in 3%):
   unilateral R > L (75%), recurrent alternating sides; relatively unchanged effusion for months, predominantly in men, LOW GLUCOSE content of 20 – 50 mg/dl (in 70 – 80%) without increase after I.V. infusion of glucose
   (DDx: TB, metastatic disease, parapneumonic effusion)

2. SLE (in 15 – 74%)
   most common collagenosis to give pleural effusion, bilateral in 50%;
   L > R;
   √ enlargement of cardiovascular silhouette (35 – 50%)
3. Wegener granulomatosis (in 50%)
4. Sjögren syndrome
5. Mixed connective tissue disease
6. Periarteritis nodosa
7. Postmyocardial infarct syndrome

(f) Traumatic
hemorrhagic, chylous, esophageal rupture, thoracic / abdominal surgery, intrapleural infusion, radiation pneumonitis

(g) Miscellaneous
1. Sarcoidosis
2. Uremic pleuritis (in 20% of uremic patients)
3. Drug-induced effusion

CXR:
√ first 300 ml not visualized on PA view (collect in posterior costophrenic sulcus)
√ lateral decubitus views may detect as little as 25 ml

CT:
√ fluid outside diaphragm
√ fluid elevating crus of diaphragm
√ indistinct fluid-liver interface
√ fluid posteromedial to liver (= bare area of liver)

CAVE: "central oval" sign of ascites may be seen in subpulmonic effusion with inverted diaphragm

Unilateral pleural effusion
1. Neoplasm
2. Infection (TB)
3. Collagen vascular disease
4. Subdiaphragmatic disease
5. Pulmonary emboli
6. Trauma
7. Chylothorax

Left-sided pleural effusion
1. Spontaneous rupture of the esophagus
2. Dissecting aneurysm of the aorta
3. Traumatic rupture of aorta distal to left subclavian artery
4. Transection of distal thoracic duct
5. Pancreatitis: left-sided (68%), right-sided (10%), bilateral (22%)
6. Pancreatic + gastric neoplasm

Right-sided pleural effusion
1. Congestive heart failure
2. Transection of proximal thoracic duct
3. Pancreatitis

Pleural effusion + large cardiac silhouette
1. Congestive heart failure (most common)

√ cardiomegaly
√ prominence of upper lobe vessels + constriction of lower lobe vessels
√ prominent hilar vessels
√ interstitial edema (fine reticular pattern, Kerley lines, perihilar haze, peribronchial thickening)
√ alveolar edema (perihilar confluent ill-defined densities, air bronchogram)
√ "phantom tumor" = fluid localized to interlobar pleural fissure (in 78% in right horizontal fissure)
2. Pulmonary embolus with right-sided heart enlargement
3. Myocarditis / Pericarditis with pleuritis
   (a) Viral infection
   (b) Tuberculosis
   (c) Rheumatic fever (poststreptococcal infection)
4. Tumor: metastatic, mesothelioma
5. Collagen-vascular disease
   (a) SLE (pleural + pericardial effusion)
   (b) Rheumatoid arthritis

Pleural effusion + subsegmental atelectasis
1. Postoperative (thoracotomy, splenectomy, renal surgery) secondary to thoracic splinting + small airway mucous plugging
2. Pulmonary embolus
3. Abdominal mass
4. Ascites
5. Rib fractures

Pleural effusion + lobar densities
1. Pneumonia with empyema
2. Pulmonary embolism
3. Neoplasm
   (a) bronchogenic carcinoma (common)
   (b) lymphoma
4. Tuberculosis

Pleural effusion + hilar enlargement
1. Pulmonary embolus
2. Tumor
   (a) bronchogenic carcinoma
   (b) lymphoma
   (c) metastasis
3. Tuberculosis
4. Fungal infection (rare)
5. Sarcoidosis (very rare)

Pleural solitary mass
= density with incomplete border and tapered superior + inferior borders, difficult to distinguish from chest wall mass (rib destruction reliable)
1. Loculated pleural effusion ("vanishing tumor")
2. Organized empyema
3. Metastasis
4. Local benign mesothelioma
5. Subpleural lipoma: may erode adjacent rib
6. Hematoma
7. Mesothelial cyst

8. Neural tumor (schwannoma, neurofibroma)
9. Fibrin bodies: 3 – 4 cm tumorlike concentrations of fibrin forming in serofibrinous pleural effusions; usually near lung base

Multiple pleural densities
√ diffuse pleural thickening with lobulated borders

1. Loculated pleural effusion: infectious, hemorrhagic, neoplastic
2. Metastasis (most common cause): predominantly adenocarcinoma
3. Diffuse malignant mesothelioma almost always unilateral, associated with asbestos exposure
4. Malignant thymoma (rare)
   √ contiguous spread, invasion of pleura, spreads around lung
   √ NO pleural effusion
5. **Thoracic splenosis**
   = autotransplantation of splenic tissue to pleural space following thoracoabdominal trauma; discovered 10 – 30 years later
   √ positive Tc-99m sulfur colloid scan

Pleural thickening
A. TRAUMA
   1. **Fibrothorax** (most common cause)
      = organizing effusion / hemothorax / pyothorax almost always on visceral pleura
      √ dense fibrous layer of approx. 2 cm thickness
      √ frequent calcification on inner aspect of pleural peel
B. INFECTION
   1. Chronic empyema: over bases; history of pneumonia; parenchymal scars
   2. Tuberculosis / Histoplasmosis: lung apex; associated with apical cavity
   3. Aspergilloma: in preexisiting cavity concomitant with pleural thickening
C. COLLAGEN-VASCULAR DISEASE
   1. Rheumatoid arthritis: pleural effusion fails to resolve
D. INHALATIONAL DISORDER
   1. Asbestos exposure: lower lateral chest wall; basilar interstitial disease (< 25%); thickening of parietal pleura with sparing of visceral pleura
   2. Talcosis
E. NEOPLASM
   (a) Metastases: often nodular appearance; may be obscured by effusion
   (b) Diffuse malignant mesothelioma
   (c) Pancoast tumor
F. OTHER
   1. **Pleural hyaloserositis**
      Path: hyaline sclerotic tissue = cartilagelike whitish sugar icing appearance (Zuckerguss) with occasional calcification

2. Mimicked by extrathoracic musculature, 1st + 2nd rib companion shadow, subpleural fat, focal scarring around old rib fractures

Pleural calcification
A. TRAUMA
1. Healed hemothorax = Fibrothorax:
   - Hx of significant chest trauma
   - √ irregular plaques of calcium usually in visceral pleura
   - √ healed rib fracture
2. Radiation therapy

B. INFECTION
1. Healed empyema
2. Tuberculosis (and Rx for TB: pneumothorax / oleothorax), histoplasmosis

C. PNEUMOCONIOSIS
1. Asbestos-related pleural disease (most common):
   - √ combination of basilar reticular interstitial disease (<1/3) + pleural thickening
   - √ calcifications of parietal pleura frequently diagnostic (diaphragmatic surface of pleura, bilateral but asymmetric)
2. Talcosis: similar to asbestos-related disease
3. Bakelite
4. Muscovite mica

D. HYPERCALCEMIA
1. Pancreatitis
2. Secondary hyperparathyroidism in chronic renal failure / scleroderma

E. MISCELLANEOUS
1. Mineral oil aspiration
2. Pulmonary infarction

mnemonic: "TAFT"
Tuberculosis
Asbestosis
Fluid (effusion, empyema, hematoma)
Talc

DIAPHRAGM
Bilateral diaphragmatic elevation
A. Shallow inspiration (most frequent)
B. Abdominal causes
   (1) Obesity (2) Pregnancy (3) Ascites (4) Large abdominal mass
C. Pulmonary causes
   (1) Bilateral atelectasis
   (2) Restrictive pulmonary disease (SLE)
D. Neuromuscular disease
   (1) Myasthenia gravis
   (2) Amyotrophic lateral sclerosis

Unilateral diaphragmatic elevation
1. Subpulmonic pleural effusion
   - √ dome of diaphragm migrates toward the costophrenic angle and flattens
2. Altered pulmonary volume

(a) Atelectasis
   - √ associated pulmonary density
(b) Postoperative lobectomy / pneumectomy
   - √ rib defects, metallic sutures
(c) Hypoplastic lung
   - √ small hemithorax (more often on the right), crowding of ribs, mediastinal shift, absent / small pulmonary artery, frequently associated with dextrocardia + anomalous pulmonary venous return
3. Phrenic nerve paralysis
   (a) Primary lung tumor
   (b) Malignant mediastinal tumor
   (c) Iatrogenic
   (d) Idiopathic
   - √ paradoxic motion on fluoroscopy (patient in lateral position sniffing)
4. Abdominal disease
   (a) Subphrenic abscess: history of surgery, accompanied by pleural effusion
   (b) Distended stomach / colon
   (c) Interposition of colon
   (d) Liver mass (tumor, echinococcal cyst, abscess)
5. Diaphragmatic hernia
6. Eventration of diaphragm
7. Traumatic rupture of diaphragm
   associated with rib fractures, pulmonary contusion, hemothorax
8. Diaphragmatic tumor
   mesothelioma, fibroma, lipoma, lymphoma, metastases

Chest wall lesions
A. EXTERNAL
1. Cutaneous lesion: moles, neurofibroma
2. Nipples
3. Artifact

B. NEOPLASTIC
1. Mesenchymal tumor
   muscle tumor, fibroma, desmoid tumor, lipoma (common; growing between ribs presenting as intrathoracic + subcutaneous mass; CT diagnostic)
2. Neural tumor
   Schwannoma, neurofibroma (may erode ribs inferiorly with sclerotic bone reaction), neuroblastoma
3. Vascular tumor
   hemangioma, hemangiopericytoma
4. Malignant bone tumor = Rib tumor
   Δ in adult: metastasis, multiple myeloma
   Δ in child: Ewing sarcoma, metastatic neuroblastoma, chondrosarcoma (calcified matrix), osteosarcoma (rare), fibrosarcoma
5. Benign bone tumor
   benign cortical defect, fibrous dysplasia, hemangioma of bone

C. TRAUMATIC
1. Hematoma

2. Rib fracture
D. INFECTIOUS
1. Actinomycosis (parenchymal infiltrate, pleural effusion, chest wall mass, rib destruction, cutaneous fistulas)
2. Aspergillosis, Nocardiosis, Blastomycosis, Tuberculosis (rare)

√ incomplete border sign
√ smooth tapering borders (tangential views)
√ rib destruction (metastases / small round cell tumors / aggressive granulomatous infections)
√ inferior rib erosion + sclerosis (neurofibroma, schwannoma)

Lung disease with chest wall extension
A. Infectious
1. Actinomycosis
2. Nocardia
3. Blastomycosis
4. Tuberculosis
B. Malignant tumor
1. Bronchogenic carcinoma
2. Lymphoma
3. Metastases
4. Mesothelioma
5. Breast carcinoma
6. Internal mammary node
C. Benign tumor
1. Capillary hemangioma of infancy
2. Cavernous hemangioma
3. Extrapleural lipoma
4. Abscess
5. Hematoma

Malignant tumors of chest wall in children
1. Ewing Sarcoma of a rib (most common)
(a) older child: rib involvement in 7%, predominant involvement of pelvis + lower extremity
(b) child < 10 years: rib involvement in 30%
2. Rhabdomyosarcoma
relatively common in children + adolescents
√ sclerosis / destruction / scalloping of cortex (local extension to contiguous bone)
√ may calcify
Metastases to: lung, occasionally lymph nodes
Prognosis: infiltrative growth with high risk of local recurrence
3. Neuroblastoma
10% present as chest wall mass
√ may calcify
4. **Askin tumor**
= uncommon tumor probably arising from intercostal nerves in young Caucasian females
Path: neuroectodermal small cell tumor containing neuron-specific enolase (may also be found in neuroblastoma)
√ rib destruction

√ pleural effusion
Metastases to: bone, CNS, liver, adrenal

PULMONARY MALFORMATION
= SEQUESTRATION SPECTRUM
1. Congenital lobar emphysema
2. Bronchogenic cyst
3. Congenital cystic adenomatoid malformation
4. Bronchopulmonary sequestration
5. Hypogenetic lung syndrome
6. Pulmonary arteriovenous malformation

NEONATAL LUNG DISEASE
Mediastinal shift + abnormal aeration
A. SHIFT TOWARD LUCENT LUNG
1. Diaphragmatic hernia
2. Chylothorax
3. Cystic adenomatoid malformation
B. SHIFT AWAY FROM LUCENT LUNG
1. Congenital lobar emphysema
2. Persistent localized pulmonary interstitial emphysema
3. Obstruction of mainstem bronchus (by anomalous or dilated vessel / cardiac chamber)

Reticulogranular densities in neonate
1. Respiratory distress syndrome (90%): premature infant, inadequate surfactant
2. Immature lung: premature infant, normal surfactant
3. Transient tachypnea of the newborn
4. Neonatal group-B streptococcal pneumonia
5. Idiopathic hypoglycemia
6. Congestive heart failure
7. Early pulmonary hemorrhage
8. Infant of diabetic mother

Hyperaeration in newborn
1. Fetal aspiration syndrome
2. Neonatal pneumonia
3. Pulmonary hemorrhage
4. Congenital heart disease
5. Transient tachypnea (mild)

Hyperinflation in child
mnemonic: "BUMP FAD"
Bronchiectasis
Upper airway obstruction
Mucoviscidosis
Pneumonia (esp. staph)
Foreign body (ball valve mechanism)
Asthma
Dehydration (diarrhea, acidosis)

Pulmonary Edema
transcapillary flow dependent on (1) hydrostatic pressure (2) colloid osmotic pressure (3) capillary permeability
A. INCREASED HYDROSTATIC PRESSURE

(a) CARDIOGENIC (most common)
= pulmonary venous hypertension
1. heart disease: left ventricular failure, mitral valve disease, left atrial myxoma
2. pulmonary venous disease: primary veno-occlusive disease, mediastinal fibrosis
3. pericardial disease: pericardial effusion, constrictive pericarditis (extremely rare)
4. drugs: antiarrhythmic drugs; drugs depressing myocardial contractility (beta-blocker)
(b) NONCARDIOGENIC
1. renal failure
2. IV fluid overload
3. hyperosmolar fluid (contrast medium)
(c) NEUROGENIC
? sympathetic venoconstriction in cerebrovascular accident, head injury, CNS tumor, postictal state
B. DECREASED COLLOID OSMOTIC PRESSURE
1. hypoproteinemia
2. transfusion of crystalloid fluid
3. rapid reexpansion of lung
C. INCREASED CAPILLARY PERMEABILITY
Endothelial injury from
(a) Physical trauma: parenchymal contusion, radiation therapy
(b) Aspiration injury:
1. Mendelson syndrome (gastric contents)
2. Near drowning in sea water / fresh water
3. Aspiration of hypertonic contrast media
(c) Inhalation injury:
1. nitrogen dioxide = silo-filler's disease
2. smoke (pulmonary edema may be delayed by 24 – 48 hours)
3. sulfur dioxide, hydrocarbons, carbon monoxide, beryllium, cadmium, silica, dinitrogen tetroxide, oxygen, chlorine, phosgene, ammonia, organophosphates
(d) Injury via blood stream
1. vessel occlusion: shock (trauma, sepsis, ARDS) or emboli (fat, amniotic fluid, thrombus)
2. circulating toxins: snake venom, paraquat
3. drugs: heroin, morphine, methadone, aspirin, phenylbutazone, nitrofurantoin, chlorothiazide
4. anaphylaxis: transfusion reaction, contrast medium reaction, penicillin
5. hypoxia: high altitude, acute large airway obstruction

Unilateral pulmonary edema
A. IPSILATERAL = on side of preexisting abnormality
1. Prolonged lateral decubitus position
2. Unilateral aspiration / pulmonary lavage
3. Pulmonary contusion
4. Rapid thoracentesis (rapid reexpansion)
5. Bronchial obstruction (drowned lung)
6. Unilateral venous obstruction
7. Systemic artery-to-pulmonary artery shunt (Waterston, Blalock-Taussig, Pott procedure)

B. CONTRALATERAL = opposite to side of abnormality
1. Congenital absence / hypoplasia of pulmonary artery
2. Unilateral arterial obstruction
3. Swyer-James syndrome
4. Thromboembolism
5. Unilateral emphysema
6. Lobectomy
7. Pleural disease

Interstitial pulmonary edema
Δ nothing differentiates it from other interstitial lesions
Δ does not necessarily develop before alveolar pulmonary edema
Δ often marked dissociation between clinical signs + symptoms + roentgenographic evidence
Δ NOT typical for bacterial pneumonia

PNEUMONIA
"Classic" pneumonia pattern
1. Lobar distribution : Streptococcus pneumoniae
2. Bulging fissure : Klebsiella
3. Pneumatocele : Staphylococcus
4. Pulmonary edema : Viral pneumonia, Pneumocystis pneumonia
5. Alveolar nodules : Varicella, bronchogenic spread of TB

Distribution:
A. SEGMENTAL / LOBAR
— Normal host: S. pneumoniae, Mycoplasma, Virus
— Compromised host: S. pneumoniae
B. BRONCHOPNEUMONIA
— Normal host: Mycoplasm, Virus, Streptococcus, Staphylococcus, S. pneumoniae
— Compromised host: Gram-negative, Streptococcus, Staphylococcus
— Nosocomial: Gram-negative, Pseudomonas, Klebsiella, Staphylococcus
— Immunosuppressed: Gram-negative, Staphylococcus, Nocardia, Legionella, Aspergillus, Phycomycetes
C. EXTENSIVE BILATERAL
— Normal host: Virus (e.g. influenza), Legionella
— Compromised host: Candidiasis, Pneumocystis, Tuberculosis
D. BILATERAL LOWER LOBE
— Normal host: Anaerobic (aspiration)
— Compromised host: Anaerobic (aspiration)

Transmission:
A. COMMUNITY-ACQUIRED PNEUMONIA
Organisms: Viruses, S. pneumoniae, Mycoplasma
B. NOSOCOMIAL PNEUMONIA
(a) gram-negative organisms (> 50%): Klebsiella pneumoniae, Ps. aeruginosa, E. coli, Enterobacter

(b) gram-positive organisms (10%): Staph. aureus, S. pneumoniae, H. influenzae

Lobar pneumonia
= ALVEOLAR PNEUMONIA
= pathogens reach peripheral air space, incite exudation of watery edema into alveolar space, centrifugal spread via small airways, pores of Kohn + Lambert into adjacent lobules + segments
√ nonsegmental sublobar consolidation
√ round pneumonia (=uniform involvement of contiguous alveoli)
  (a) Streptococcus pneumoniae
  (b) Klebsiella pneumoniae (more aggressive); in immunocompromised + alcoholics
  (c) any pneumonia in children
  (d) atypical measles
√ expansion of lobe with bulging of fissures
√ lung necrosis with cavitation
DDx: aspiration, pulmonary embolus

Lobular pneumonia
= BRONCHOPNEUMONIA
= inflammatory response in conducting airways + surrounding parenchyma
√ small fluffy ill-defined acinar nodules which enlarge with time
√ lobar + segmental densities with volume loss from airway obstruction secondary to bronchial narrowing + mucus plugging
Organisms:
Pseudomonas, Klebsiella pneumoniae, Bacillus proteus, E. coli, Anaerobes (Bacteroides + Clostridia), Legionnaires bacillus, Staphylococcus aureus, Nocardiosis, Actinomycosis

Acute interstitial pneumonia
initially predominantly affecting interstitial tissues
Organisms: Viruses, Mycoplasma, Pneumocystis
• often subacute atypical pneumonia
√ diffuse interstitial process with peribronchial thickening
√ segmental / lobar densities (mucus plugging + damage of surfactant producing type 2 alveolar cells)

Gram-negative pneumonia
in 50% cause of nosocomial necrotizing pneumonias (including staphylococcal pneumonia)
predisposed: elderly, debilitated, diabetes, alcoholism, COPD, malignancy, bronchitis, gram-positive pneumonia, treatment with antibiotics, respirator therapy
Organisms:
  1. Klebsiella   4. Proteus
  2. Pseudomonas   5. Hemophilus
  3. E. coli   6. Legionella
√ air-space consolidation (Klebsiella)
√ spongy appearance (Pseudomonas)

√ affecting dependent lobes (poor cough reflex without clearing of bronchial tree)
√ bilateral
√ cavitation common
Cx: (1) exudate / empyema (2) bronchopleural fistula

Mycotic infections of lung
(a) in healthy subjects
  1. Histoplasmosis
  2. Coccidioidomycosis
  3. Blastomycosis
(b) opportunistic infection
  1. Aspergillosis
  2. Candidiasis
  3. Mucormycosis (phycomycosis)
Growth: (a) mycelial form (b) yeast form (depending on environment)
Source of contamination:
(a) soil (b) growth in moist areas (apart from Coccidioides imitis) (c) contaminated bird / bat excreta

Cavitating pneumonia
1. Staphylococcus aureus
2. Haemophilus influenzae
3. S. pneumoniae
other Gram-negative organisms (e.g., Klebsiella)

Cavitating opportunistic infections
A. FUNGAL INFECTIONS
  1. Aspergillosis
  2. Nocardiosis
  3. Mucormycosis (= phycomycosis)
B. SEPTIC EMBOLI
  1. Anaerobic organisms
C. STAPHYLOCOCCAL ABSCESS
D. TUBERCULOSIS
nummular form

Repeated infections in same patient are not necessarily due to same organism !
DDx: (1) Metastatic disease in carcinoma / Hodgkin disease

Recurrent pneumonia in childhood
A. Immune problem
  1. Immune deficiency
  2. Chronic granulomatous disease of childhood (males)
  3. Alpha 1-antitrypsin deficiency
B. Aspiration
  1. Gastroesophageal reflux
  2. H-type tracheoesophageal fistula
  3. Disorder of swallowing mechanism
  4. Esophageal obstruction, impacted esophageal foreign body
C. Underlying lung disease
  1. Sequestration
  2. Bronchopulmonary dysplasia

3. Cystic fibrosis
4. Atopic asthma
5. Bronchiolitis obliterans
6. Sinusitis
7. Bronchiectasis
8. Ciliary dysmotility syndromes
9. Pulmonary foreign body

Hypersensitivity to organic dusts
A. TRACHEOBRONCHIAL HYPERSENSITIVITY
large particles reaching the tracheobronchial mucosa
(pollens, certain fungi, some animal / insect epithelial
emanations)
  1. Extrinsic Asthma
  2. Hypersensitivity Aspergillosis
  3. Bronchocentric Granulomatosis
  4. Byssinosis in cottonwool workers
B. ALVEOLAR HYPERSENSITIVITY
= HYPERSENSITIVITY PNEUMONITIS
= EXTRINSIC ALLERGIC ALVEOLITIS
small particles of < 5 μ reaching alveoli

Drug-induced pulmonary damage
A. CHEMOTHERAPEUTIC AGENTS
  1. BUSULFAN = Myleran® (for CML)
    dose-dependent toxicity after 3 – 4 years on the
    drug in 1 – 10%
    √ diffuse linear pattern (occasionally reticulonodular
      / nodular pattern)
    √ partial / complete clearing after withdrawal of
      drug
    DDx: pneumocystis pneumonia, interstitial
           leukemic infiltrate
  2. BLEOMYCIN (for squamous cell carcinoma,
    lymphoma, testicular tumor)
    Toxicity at doses > 300 mg (in 3 – 6%);
      increased toxicity with age + radiation therapy
      + high oxygen concentrations
    √ subpleural linear / nodular opacities in lower lung
      zones occuring after 1 – 3 months following
      beginning of therapy
  3. NITROSOUREAS = BCNU, CCNU (for glioma,
    lymphoma, myeloma)
    Incidence of 50% after doses > 1500 mg/sqm
    √ linear / finely nodular opacities (following
      treatment of 2-3 years)
    √ high incidence of pneumothorax
  4. METHOTREXATE, PROCARBAZINE (for AML,
    psoriasis, pemphigus)
    Not dose-related, usually self-limited despite
      continuation of therapy
    • blood eosinophilia (common)
    √ linear / reticulonodular process (time delay of 12
      days to 5 years, usually early)
    √ acinar filling pattern (later)
    √ transient hilar adenopathy + pleural effusion (on
      occasion)
    DDx: Pneumocystis pneumonia

B. NITROFURANTOIN (Macrodontin®)
  (a) acute disorder with fever + eosinophilia
      (commonest presentation)
  (b) chronic reaction with interstitial fibrosis (less
      common), may not be associated with peripheral
      eosinophilia
  • positive for ANA + LE cells
  √ bilateral basilar interstitial opacities
  √ prompt resolution after withdrawal from drug
C. HEROIN, PROPOXYPHENE, METHADONE
  overdose followed by pulmonary edema in 30 – 40%
  √ bilateral widespread air space consolidation
  √ aspiration pneumonia in 50 – 75%
D. SALICYLATES
  • asthma
  √ pulmonary edema (with chronic ingestion)
E. INTRAVENOUS CONTRAST AGENT
  √ pulmonary edema
F. AMIODARONE (for refractory ventricular arrhythmia)
  • pulmonary insufficiency after 1 – 12 months in
    14 – 18% on long-term therapy
  √ alveolar + interstitial infiltrates
  √ peripheral consolidation
  √ pleural thickening adjacent to consolidation

Diffuse pulmonary hemorrhage
1. Thrombocytopenia
2. Coagulopathy
3. Idiopathic pulmonary hemosiderosis
4. Goodpasture syndrome = antibasement membrane
   antibody disease
5. Collagen vascular disease + systemic vasculitides:
   SLE, Wegener granulomatosis, Polyarteritis nodosa,
   Henoch-Schönlein purpura, Behçet disease
6. Rapidly progressive glomerulonephritis ± immune
   complexes
7. Exogenous agents: D-penicillamine, lymphangiography

Hemoptysis
A. Tumor
  1. Carcinoma
  2. Bronchial adenoma
B. Bronchial wall injury
  1. Foreign body erosion
  2. Bronchoscopy / biopsy
C. Vascular
  1. COPD
  2. Pulmonary embolus with infarction
  3. Venous hypertension (most common)
  4. AV fistula
D. Infection
  1. Chronic bronchitis
  2. Bronchiectasis (mouthful)
  3. Tuberculosis (Rasmussen aneurysm)
  4. Aspergillosis

FUNCTION AND ANATOMY OF LUNG

Lung Volumes & Capacities

1. Tidal volume (**TV**)
   = amount of gas moving in and out with each respiratory cycle
2. Residual volume (**RV**)
   = amount of gas remaining in the lung after a maximal expiration
3. Total lung capacity (**TLC**)
   = gas contained in lung at the end of a maximal inspiration
4. Vital capacity (**VC**)
   = amount of gas that can be expired after a maximal inspiration without force
5. Functional residual capacity (**FRC**)
   = volume of gas remaining in lungs at the end of a quiet expiration

Changes in Lung Volumes

A. DECREASED VC:
   1. Reduction in functioning lung tissue due to
      (a) space-occupying process (pneumonia, infarction)
      (b) surgical removal of lung tissue
   2. Process reducing overall volume of the lungs (diffuse pulmonary fibrosis)
   3. Inability to expand lungs due to
      (a) muscular weakness (poliomyelitis)
      (b) increase in abdominal volume (pregnancy)
      (c) pleural effusion

B. INCREASED FRC and RV:
   characteristic of air trapping and overinflation (asthma, emphysema),
   associated with increased TLC
C. DECREASED FRC and RV:
   1. Process reducing overall volume of lungs (diffuse pulmonary fibrosis)
   2. Process that occupies volume within alveoli (alveolar microlithiasis)
   3. Process that elevates diaphragm (ascites, pregnancy), usually associated with decreased TLC

Flow Rates

A. Spirometric measurements:
   1. Forced expiratory volume (FEV)
      = amount of air expired during a time period (usually 1 + 3 sec);
      Normal values: FEV_1 = 83%; FEV_3 = 97%
   2. Maximal midexpiratory flow rate (MMFR)
      = amount of gas expired during the middle half of forced expiratory volume curve (largely effort independent)
      Indicator of small airway resistance
   3. Flow-volume loop
      = gas flow is plotted against the actual volume of lung at which this flow is occurring
      Useful in identifying obstruction in large airways

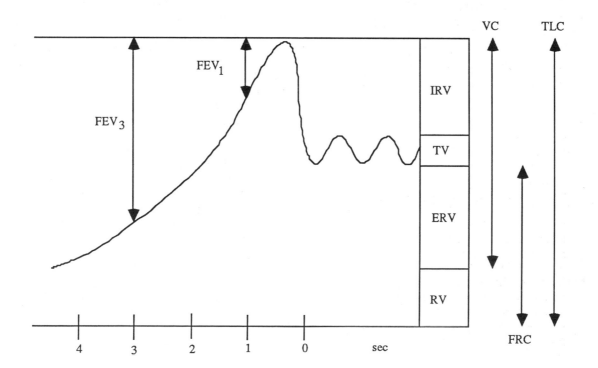

B. Resistance in small airways
Closing volume = lung volume at which dependent lung zones cease to ventilate because of airway closure in small airway disease or loss of lung elastic recoil
- decrease in FEV, MMFR, MBC:
    (a) expiratory airway obstruction (reversible as in spasmodic asthma / irreversible as in emphysema)
    (b) respiratory muscle weakness

Diffusing Capacity
= rate of gas transfer across the alveolocapillary membrane in relation to a constant pressure difference across it; measured by the carbon monoxide diffusion method
Reduction:
1. Ventilation / perfusion inequality: less CO is taken up by poorly ventilated or poorly perfused areas (emphysema)
2. Reduction of total surface area (emphysema, surgical resection)
3. Reduction in permeability from thickening of alveolar membrane (cellular infiltration, edema, interstitial fibrosis)
4. Anemia with lack of hemoglobin

Arterial Blood Gas Abnormalities
- decreased pulmonary arterial O_2:
    1. alveolar hypoventilation
    2. impaired diffusion
    3. abnormal ventilation/perfusion ratios
    4. anatomic shunting
- elevated pulmonary arterial CO_2:
    1. alveolar hypoventilation
    2. impaired ventilation / perfusion ratios

V/Q Inequality
A. normal:
    (a) blood flow decreases rapidly from base to apex
    (b) ventilation decreases less rapidly from base to apex
    Δ V/Q is low at base and high at apex;
    Δ pulmonary arterial O_2 is substantially higher at apex;
    Δ pulmonary arterial CO_2 is substantiallly higher at base
B. abnormal:
    chiefly resulting from non- / underventilated lung regions (non- /underperfused regions do not result in blood gas disturbances)

Compliance
= relationship of the change in intrapleural pressure to the volume of gas that moves into the lungs
A. Decreased compliance:
    edema, fibrosis, granulomatous infiltration
B. Increased compliance:
    emphysema (faulty elastic architecture)
√ height of diaphragm at TLC can provide some indication of lung compliance, particularly valuable in sequential roentgenograms for comparison in:
    1. Diffuse interstitial pulmonary edema
    2. Diffuse interstitial pulmonary fibrosis

THYMUS
Thymic weight increases from birth to age 11 – 12 years (22 ± 13 g in neonate, 34 ± 15 g at puberty); ratio of thymic weight to body weight decreases with age (involution after puberty, total fatty replacement after age 60)
√ measurement (perpendicular to axis of aortic arch):
    < 18 mm before age 20; < 13 mm after age 20
√ convex borders, triangular, vaguely bilobed with muscular density (before puberty)
√ flat / concave borders with abundant fat (after puberty)
Δ atrophies under stress (increase in endogenous steroids)

DISEASE ENTITIES OF CHEST DISORDERS

ACTINOMYCOSIS
Organism: Actinomyces israelii, gram-positive anaerobic pleomorphic small bacterium with proteolytic activity, superficially resembling the morphology of a hyphal fungus; closely related to mycobacteria
Histo: mycelial in tissue; rod-shaped bacterial form in oropharynx
Occurence: rod-shaped form in dental caries, gingival margins, tonsillar crypts, GI tract
predisposed: individuals with very poor dental hygiene, immunosuppressed
- "sulfur granules" in sputum / exudate = colonies of organisms arranged in circular fashion = mycelial clumps with thin hyphae 1 – 2 mm in diameter

Organ involvement: mandibulofacial > intestinal > lung
@ Mandibulofacial actinomycosis
   √ osteomyelitis of mandible
@ Abdominal actinomycosis
   √ fold thickening (resembling Crohn disease)
   √ rupture of abdominal viscus (usually appendix)
   √ fistula formation
@ Pleuropulmonary actinomycosis
   √ consolidation extending across interlobar fissures (acute air-space pneumonia rare)
   √ cavitary lesion (abscess)
   √ empyema
   √ osteomyelitis of ribs
   √ draining chest wall sinuses (spread through fascial planes)
Rx: surgical debridement + penicillin

AIDS
= Acquired Immune Deficiency Syndrome characterized by HIV seropositivity, specific opportunistic infections, specific malignant neoplasms (Kaposi sarcoma, Burkitt lymphoma, primary lymphoma of brain)

AIDS-RELATED COMPLEX (ARC)
= HIV seropositivity, generalized lymphadenopathy, CNS diseases other than those associated with AIDS

Organism: HIV (human immunodeficiency virus)
= HTLV III (human T-cell lymphotropic virus type III) = LAV (lymphadenopathy-associated virus)

Groups at risk:
1. Homosexual males (74%)
2. IV drug abusers (16%)
3. Contaminated blood products (3%)
4. Sexual partner of drug abuser + bisexual man
5. Infants born to woman infected with AIDS virus
Δ HIV antibodies present in > 50% of homosexuals + 90% of IV drug abusers

A. LYMPHADENOPATHY
   Cause: reactive follicular hyperplasia (50%), NHL (20%), mycobacterial infection (17%), Kaposi sarcoma (10%), metastatic tumor, opportunistic infection with multiple organisms, drug reaction
   Location: mediastinum, axilla, retrocrural
B. OPPORTUNISTIC INFECTION
   accounts for majority of pulmonary disease, recurrent in 20 – 40%
   1. Pneumocystis carinii pneumonia (up to 85%)
      > 60% develop at least 1 episode during disease
      - subacute insidious onset with malaise, minimal cough
      Prognosis: in 25% fatal
   2. CMV pneumonia
      most frequent infection found at autopsy
   3. Mycobacterium (20%): M. avium-intracellulare (83%), M. tuberculosis (9%)
   4. Nocardia pneumonia (< 5%)
      usually occurs in cavitating pneumonia
   5. Cryptococcal pneumonia (2 – 15%)
   6. Pyogenic bacteria (10%)
C. TUMOR
   1. Metastatic Kaposi sarcoma (25%)
      Location: widespread skin + organ involvement, lung (20%)
      √ numerous fluffy nodules of peribronchial distribution
      √ pleural effusion
   2. Lymphoma
      primarily immunoblastic NHL, occasionally Hodgkin disease
      Location: pulmonary involvement (< 9%), CNS, GI tract, liver, spleen, bone marrow
D. Lymphocytic interstitial pneumonitis (especially in children)
E. Septic emboli
F. Premature development of bullae (40%) with disposition to spontaneous pneumothorax

ALPHA-1 ANTITRYPSIN DEFICIENCY
= rare autosomal recessive disorder
Alpha-1 antitrypsin (glycoprotein) is synthesized in liver + released into serum
   Action: proteolytic inhibitor of trypsin, chymotrypsin, elastase, plasmin, thrombin, kallikrein, leukocytic + bacterial proteases; neutralizes circulating proteolytic enzymes
   Mode of injury from deficiency: PMNs + alveolar macrophages sequester into lung during recurrent bacterial infections + release elastase which digests basement membrane
Age: early age of onset (20 – 30 years); M:F = 1:1
- rapid + progressive deterioration of lung function

√ severe panacinar emphysema with basilar predominance

√ reduction in size + number of pulmonary vessels in lower lobes

√ redistribution of blood flow to unaffected upper lung zones

√ bullae at both lung bases

√ marked flattening of diaphragm

√ minimal diaphragmatic excursion

Cx: hepatic cirrhosis (in homozygotic individuals)

ALVEOLAR MICROLITHIASIS

= very rare disease of unknown etiology characterized by myriad of calco spher ites (= tiny calculi) within alveoli

Age peak: 30 – 50 years; begins in early life; has been identified in utero

M:F = 1:1; in 50% familial (restricted to siblings)

• usually asymptomatic (70%)

• dyspnea on exertion (reduction in residual volume)

• cyanosis, clubbing of fingers

• striking discrepancy between radiograph and clinical symptoms

• NORMAL serum calcium + phosphorus levels

√ very fine, sharply defined, sand-like micronodulations (<1mm)

√ diffuse involvement of both lungs

√ intense uptake on bone scan

Prognosis:

(a) late development of pulmonary insufficiency secondary to interstitial fibrosis

(b) disease may become arrested

(c) microliths may continue to form / enlarge

DDx: (1) "mainline" pulmonary granulomatosis = IV abuse of talc-containing drugs such as methadone (rarely as numerous + scarring + loss of volume)

ALVEOLAR PROTEINOSIS

= PULMONARY ALVEOLAR PROTEINOSIS (PAP)

= accumulation of PAS positive phospholipid material in alveoli (= surfactant)

Etiology: ?; associated with dust exposure (e.g. silicoproteinosis is histologically identical to PAP), immunodeficiency, hematologic + lymphatic malignancies, AIDS, chemotherapy

Pathophysiology: (a) overprodution of surfactant by granular pneumocytes

(b) defective clearance of surfactant by alveolar macrophages

Age peak: 30 – 50 years (age range 2 – 70 years); M:F = 3:1

• asymptomatic (10-20%)

• gradual onset of dyspnea + cough

• weight loss, weakness, hemoptysis

• defect in diffusing capacity

√ "bat-wing" consolidation of ground-glass pattern, predominant at bases

√ small acinar nodules + coalescence + consolidation

√ patchy peripheral / primarily unilateral infiltrates (rare)

√ reticular / reticulonodular / linear interstitial pattern with Kerley B lines (late stage)

√ slow clearing over weeks or months

√ slow progression (1/3), remaining stable (2/3)

√ NO adenopathy, NO cardiomegaly, NO pleural effusion

Cx: Infections (frequently secondary to poorly functioning macrophages + excellent culture medium): Nocardia asteroides (most common), mycobacterial, fungal, Pneumocystis, CMV

Prognosis:

Highly variable course with clinical and radiologic episodes of exacerbation + remissions

(a) 50% improvement / recovery

(b) 30% death within several years under progression

Rx: bronchopulmonary lavage

DDx:

(a) during acute phase: pulmonary edema, diffuse pneumonia, ARDS

(b) in chronic stage:

1. Idiopathic pulmonary hemosiderosis (boys, symmetric involvement of mid + lower zones, progression to nodular + linear pattern)

2. Hemosiderosis (bleeding diathesis)

3. Pneumoconiosis

4. Hypersensitivity pneumonitis

5. Goodpasture syndrome (more rapid changes, renal disease)

6. Desquamative interstitial pneumonia ("ground glass" appearance, primarily basilar + peripheral)

7. Pulmonary alveolar microlithiasis (widespread discrete intraalveolar calcifications primarily in lung bases, rare familial disease)

8. Sarcoidosis (usually with lymphadenopathy)

9. Lymphoma

10. Bronchioloalveolar cell carcinoma (more focal, slowly enlarging with time)

AMNIOTIC FLUID EMBOLISM

= most common cause of maternal peripartum death

• dyspnea

• shock during / after labor + delivery

Pathogenesis:

Amniotic debris enters maternal circulation resulting in (1) pulmonary embolization (2) anaphylactoid reaction (3) DIC

√ usually fatal before radiographs obtained

√ may demonstrate pulmonary edema

AMYLOIDOSIS

Histo: protein (immunoglobulin) / polysaccharide complex

• asthmalike symptoms

• hemoptysis

1. PRIMARY AMYLOIDOSIS

lung involvement in up to 70%

not associated with specific disease

2. SECONDARY AMYLOIDOSIS
 most common; lung involvement rare
 associated with: rheumatoid arthritis, multiple myeloma
@ Lung involvement
  A. Tracheobronchial type
   √ prominent bronchovascular markings
   √ destructive pneumonitis
  B. Nodular type
   √ hilar adenopathy
   √ parenchymal nodules
  C. Diffuse type
   √ multiple parenchymal masses

ANKYLOSING SPONDYLITIS
• bone manifestations obvious + severe
Location: apices / upper lung fields
√ bilateral, coarse, linear, shadows + cysts
√ bronchiectasis may be present
√ superinfection, especially with aspergillosis

ASBESTOS-RELATED DISEASE
Substances: fiber's length 100 μ
 (a) relatively benign:
  (1) Chrysotile (white asbestos) in Canada
  (2) Anthophyllite in Finland, North America
  (3) Tremolite
 (b) relatively malignant:
  (4) Crocidolite (blue / black asbestos) in South Africa, Australia
  (5) Amosite (brown asbestos)
 Δ very fine fibers (Crocidolite) associated with largest number of pleural disease
Occupational exposure:
 (a) asbestos mining + milling
 (b) insulation, textile manufacturing, construction, ship building, gaskets, brake linings

Pulmonary Asbestosis
= (term asbestosis reserved for) chronic progressive diffuse interstitial fibrosis
Incidence: in 49 – 52% of industrial asbestos exposure
Histo: interstitial fibrosis begins in peribronchiolar areas, then progresses to involve adjacent alveoli
Diagnostic criteria:
 1. reliable history of exposure
 2. appropriate time interval between exposure + detection
 3. CXR evidence
 4. restrictive pattern of lung impairment
 5. abnormal diffusing capacity
 6. bilateral crackles at posterior lung bases, not cleared by cough
• dyspnea
• restrictive pulmonary function tests
Location: more severe in lower subpleural zones (concentration of asbestos fibers under pleura)

√ small irregular opacities (NOT rounded as in coal / silica)
√ confined to lung bases, progressing superiorly
√ septal lines (= fibrous thickening around secondary lobules)
√ "shaggy" heart border = obscuration secondary to parenchymal + pleural changes
√ ill-defined outline of diaphragm
√ honeycombing (uncommon)
√ rarely massive fibrosis, predominantly at lung bases without migration toward hilum (DDx from silicosis / CWP)
√ NO hilar adenopathy
√ Ga-67 uptake gives a quantitative index of inflammatory activity
CT:
 √ curvilinear subpleural lines parallel to + within 1 cm of pleura (30%) = multiple subpleural dotlike reticulonodularities connected to the most peripheral branch of pulmonary artery
 √ parenchymal fibrous bands = linear opacities contacting pleural surface
 √ subpleural pulmonary arcades = branching linear structures most prominent posteriorly
 √ reticulation = network of linear densities, usually posteriorly at lung bases
 √ honeycombing = multiple cystic spaces < 1 cm in diameter with thickened wall
 √ thickened interlobular septal lines
 √ thickened intralobular lines

Asbestos-Related Pleural Disease
1. Focal Pleural Plaques (65%)
 = hyalinized collagen in submesothelial layer of parietal pleura
 Incidence: most common manifestation of exposure; 6% of general population will show plaques
 Latent period: in 10% after 20 years; in 50% after 40 years
 Location: bilateral; posterolateral midportion of chest wall between 7 – 10th rib; aponeurotic portion of diaphragm; mediastinum; following rib contours; visceral pleura + apices + costophrenic angles typically spared
 √ usually circumscribed thickening with edges thicker than central portions of plaque; in 48% alone; in 41% with parenchymal changes
 √ no hilar adenopathy
 √ usually not calcified
 DDx: chest wall fat, rib fractures, rib companion shadows

2. Diffuse Pleural Thickening (17%)
 = diffuse thickening of parietal ± visceral pleura (involved in 90%, but difficult to demonstrate)
 • may cause restriction of pulmonary function
 May be associated with rounded atelectasis

√ bilateral process with "shaggy heart" appearance (20%)
√ smooth; difficult to assess when viewed en face
√ thickening of interlobar fissures
√ commonly obliterates costophrenic angles

3. Pleural Calcification (21 – 50%)
   Overall incidence: 20%
   Latent period: 40% after 40 years
   √ dense lines paralleling the diaphragm (most common, PATHOGNOMONIC), chest wall, mediastinum, cardiac border
   √ calcium deposits may form within center of plaques
   DDx: talc exposure, hemothorax, empyema, therapeutic pneumothorax for TB (often unilateral, extensive sheet-like, on visceral pleura)

4. Benign Pleural Effusion (21%)
   Earliest asbestos related pleural abnormality
   Prevalence: 3% (increases with increasing levels of asbestos exposure)
   Latent period: 8 – 10 years after exposure
   Frequently followed by diffuse pleural thickening + rounded atelectasis
   • may be associated with chest pain (1/3)
   • usually small sterile, serous / hemorrhagic exudate
   √ recurrent bilateral effusions +/- plaque formation
   DDx: TB, mesothelioma

Atelectatic Asbestos Pseudotumor
= ROUNDED ATELECTASIS = 'FOLDED LUNG"
= infolding of redundant pleura accompanied by segmental / subsegmental atelectasis
Location: posteromedial / posterolateral lower lobe (most common); frequently bilateral
√ 2.5 – 8 cm subpleural mass related to a site of pleural abnormality
√ size + shape show little progression, occasionally decrease in size
CT:
   √ rounded / lentiform / wedge-shaped outline
   √ contiguous to areas of diffuse pleural thickening
   √ partial interposition of lung between pleura + mass
   √ volume loss in adjacent lung
   √ "crow's feet" = linear bands radiating from mass into lung parenchyma (54%)
   √ "comet tail" (= vessels + bronchi bundled together + converging toward mass)
   √ air bronchogram (18%)

Lung Cancer in Asbestos-Related Disease
Δ increased risk by factor of 5 (in smokers by factor of up to 90)
Δ up to 25% of asbestos workers who smoke may develop lung cancer
Occurrence related to:
   (a) cumulated dose of asbestos fibers
   (b) smoking (synergistic carcinogenic effect)
   (c) preexisting interstitial disease
   (d) occupational exposure to known carcinogen
Latent period: > 20 years
Associated with   increased incidence of gastric carcinoma
Histo: bronchogenic carcinoma (adenocarcinoma + squamous cell), bronchioloalveolar cell carcinoma
Location: at lung base / in any location if associated with smoking

ASPERGILLOSIS
Organism: Aspergillus fumigatus = ubiquitous soil fungus, commonly in sputum of normal persons, ability to invade arteries + veins facilitating hematogenous dissemination
M:F = 3:1
Predisposed:
   (a) preexisting lung disease (tuberculosis, bronchiectasis)
   (b) impairment of immune system (alcoholism, advanced age, malnutrition, concurrent malignancy, poorly controlled diabetes, cirrhosis, sepsis)
Cx: dissemination to heart, brain, kidney, GI tract, liver, thyroid, spleen

SAPROPHYTIC COLONIZATION
= commensal existence in upper respiratory tract

Noninvasive Aspergillosis
= noninvasive colonization of preexisting cavity / cyst [tuberculosis, bronchiectasis, sarcoidosis (common), bullous lung disease, carcinoma]
• sputum blood-streaked or severe hemoptysis (45 – 70%)
√ aspergilloma = solid round mass within spherical / ovoid thin-walled cavity
   Histo: mycetoma = intertwined hyphae matted together with fibrin, mucus, cellular debris
√ fungus ball moves with positioning
√ crescent-shaped air space separates fungus ball from cavity wall
√ fungus ball may calcify in scattered / rimlike fashion
√ pleural thickening, may be first sign of mycetoma in preexisting lung cyst / cavity

Semi-invasive Aspergillosis
= chronic cavitary slowly progressive disease in patients with preexisting lung injury (COPD, radiation therapy), mild immune suppression, or debilitation (alcohol, diabetes)
√ consolidation (usually upper lobe)
√ development of air crescent and fungus ball

Invasive Pulmonary Aspergillosis
= often fatal form in severely immunocompromised patients (most commonly in lymphoma / leukemia patients with prolonged granulocytopenia)

Histo: hemorrhagic infarction secondary to vascular invasion by aspergillus; thrombosis of pulmonary arterioles; fungus ball = devitalized sequestrum infiltrated by fungi
- Hx of series of bacterial infections + unremitting fever
- pleuritic chest pain (mimicking emboli)
- progression of pulmonary infiltrates despite broad spectrum antibiotics
(a) early signs:
  √ single / multiple nodules with halo of low attenuation
  √ patchy localized bronchopneumonia
(b) signs of progression
  √ enlargement of nodules into diffuse bilateral consolidation
  √ development into large wedge-shaped pleural-based lesions
  √ cavitation of existing nodules (air crescent between sequestrum and lung) 1 – 3 weeks after increase in white cell count
  Δ has better prognosis than consolidation without cavitation)

Allergic Bronchopulmonary Aspergillosis
= hypersensitivity towards aspergilli in patients with long-standing asthma
A. ACUTE ALLERGIC BRONCHOPULMONARY ASPERGILLOSIS
Type I reaction = immediate hypersensitivity (IgE-mediated)
Histo: alveoli filled with eosinophils
B. CHRONIC ALLERGIC BRONCHOPULMONARY ASPERGILLOSIS
Type III reaction = delayed immune complex response = Arthus reaction (IgG-mediated)
Histo: bronchial damage secondary to aspergillus antigen reacting with IgG antibodies, immune complexes activate complement leading to tissue injury
(a) PRIMARY DIAGNOSTIC CRITERIA:
  1. asthma (84%)
  2. blood eosinophilia
  3. immediate skin reaction to aspergillus
  4. precipitating antibodies against aspergillus (70%)
  5. elevated serum IgE
  6. proximal central bronchiectasis
  7. history of transient or fixed pulmonary infiltrates
(b) SECONDARY DIAGNOSTIC CRITERIA
  1. aspergillus mycelia in sputum
  2. expectoration of brown plugs in sputum (54%)
  3. late skin reactivity to aspergillus antigen

√ alveolar fleeting patchy subsegmental / lobar infiltrates: upper lobes (50%), lower lobes (20%), middle lobe (7%), both lungs (65%), may persist for > 6 months
√ "tram-like" bronchial walls (edema)
√ central bronchiectasis = 1 – 2 cm ring shadows around hilum + upper lobes

√ "finger-in-glove", "toothpaste shadows" = V- or Y-shaped central mucus plugs in 2nd order bronchi of 2.5 – 6 cm in length remaining for months + growing in size
√ lobar consolidation (32%)
√ atelectasis (14%) with collateral air drift
√ hyperinflation (due to bronchospasm)
√ cavitation in 14% (secondary to postobstructive abscess)
√ pulmonary fibrosis + retraction
√ NORMAL peripheral bronchi
unusual are mycetoma in cavity, empyema, pneumothorax
DDx: Tuberculosis, Lipoid pneumonia, Löffler syndrome, Bronchogenic carcinoma

Pleural Aspergillosis
= aspergillus empyema in patients with pulmonary tuberculosis, bacterial empyema, bronchopleural fistula
√ pleural thickening

ASPIRATION OF SOLID FOREIGN BODY
Age: in 50% < 3 years
Source: in 85% vegetable origin (peanut, barley grass)
Location: almost exclusively in lower lobes; R:L = 2:1
√ obstructive overinflation (68%) + reflex vasoconstriction
√ collapse (14-53%)
√ infiltrate (11%)
√ radiopaque foreign body (9%)
√ air trapping (expiratory / lateral decubitus film)
NUC: √ perfusion deficit
Cx: bronchiectasis (from long retention)
DDx: impacted esophageal foreign body

ASPIRATION PNEUMONIA
Predisposing conditions:
  (1) CNS-disorders / intoxication: alcoholism, mental retardation, seizure disorders, recent anesthesia
  (2) Swallowing disorders: esophageal motility disturbances, head + neck surgery
- low grade fever
- productive cough
- choking on swallowing
Location:
gravity-dependent portions of lung, posterior segments of upper lobes + lower lobes in bedridden patients, frequently bilateral, right middle + lower lobe with sparing of left lung is common
A. ACUTE ASPIRATION PNEUMONIA
Cause: mixed organisms (anaerobic) from GI tract
√ segmental consolidation in dependent portion
B. CHRONIC ASPIRATION PNEUMONIA
Cause: repeated aspiration of foreign material from GI tract over long time / mineral oil (laxatives)
Associated with: Zenker diverticulum, esophageal stenosis, achalasia, TE fistula, neuromuscular disturbances in swallowing

√ recurring segmental consolidation
√ progression to interstitial scarring (= localized honeycomb appearance)
√ bronchopneumonic infiltrates of variable location over months / years
√ residual peribronchial scarring
Upper GI:
    √ abnormal swallowing / aspiration

ASTHMA
= episodic reversible bronchoconstriction secondary to hypersensitivity to a variety of stimuli
A. INTRINSIC ASTHMA
    Age: middle age
    probably autoimmune phenomenon provoked by viral respiratory infections; no environmental antigen; often provoked by infection, exercise, pharmaceuticals
B. EXTRINSIC ASTHMA = ATOPIC ASTHMA
    Pathogenesis: secondary to antigens producing an immediate hypersensitivity response (type I); reagin sensitizes mast cells to release histamine followed by increased vascular permeability, edema, small muscle contraction; effects primarily bronchi causing airway obstruction
    Nonoccupational allergens: pollens, dog + cat fur, tamarind seed powder, castor bean, fungal spores, grain weevil
    Occupational allergens:
        (a) natural substances: wood dust, flour, grain, beans
        (b) pharmaceuticals: antibiotics, ASA
        (c) inorganic chemicals: nickel, platinum
    Path: bronchial plugging with large amounts of viscid tenacious mucus (eosinophils, Charcot-Leyden crystals), edematous bronchial walls, hypertrophy of mucous glands + smooth muscle

ACUTE SIGNS:
    • during asthmatic attack low values for FEV + MMFR and abnormal V/Q ratios
    • normal diffusing capacity
    √ hyperexpansion of lungs = severe overinflation + air trapping
        √ flattened diaphragmatic dome
        √ deepened retrosternal air space
    √ peribronchial cuffing

CHRONIC CHANGES:
    Normal chest x-ray in 73%, findings of abnormalities depend on
        (a) age of onset (< 15 years of age in 31%; > 30 years of age in 0%)
        (b) on severity of asthma
    √ central ring shadows = bronchiectasis
    √ scars (from recurrent infections)

Cx: (1) Pneumonia (2 x as frequent as in nonasthmatics)

√ peripheral pneumonic infiltrates (secondary to blocked airways)
(2) Atelectasis (5 – 15%) from mucoid impaction
(3) Pneumomediastinum (5%), pneumothorax, subcutaneous emphysema; predominantly in children
(4) Emphysema
(5) Mucous plugging with secondary aspergillosis

ATYPICAL MEASLES PNEUMONIA
= clinical syndrome in patients who have been previously inadequately immunized with killed rubeola vaccine and are subsequently exposed to the measles virus (= type III immune complex hypersensitivity); noted in children who have received live vaccine before 13 months of age
• 2 to 3-day prodrome of headache, fever, cough, malaise
• maculopapular rash beginning on wrists + ankles (sometimes absent)
• postinfectious migratory arthralgias
• history of exposure to measles
√ extensive nonsegmental consolidation, usually bilateral
√ hilar adenopathy (100%)
√ pleural effusion (0 – 70%)
√ nodular densities of 0.5–10 cm in diameter in peripheral location, may calcify and persist up to 30 months

ATYPICAL TUBERCULOSIS
Organisms:
    M. kansasii: lung infection in subjects with good immune status
    M. marinum: "swimming pool granuloma"
    M. ulcerans: "Buruli ulcer" in tropical areas
    M. scrofulaceum: cervical lymphadenitis in infants
    M. avium/intracellulare: esp. in AIDS
Histo: lesions indistinguishable from M. tuberculosis
Unfavorable response to antituberculous therapy is suspicious for atypical TB !
• weekly positive tuberculin skin test
Location: apicoposterior segment of LUL
√ multiple thin-walled cavities with little surrounding reaction
√ absence of significant pleural reaction
√ nodule formation infrequent
√ typically NO hilar elevation

BARITOSIS
= inhalation of nonfibrogenic barium sulfate
• asymptomatic
• normal pulmonary function (benign course)
√ bilateral nodular / patchy opacities, denser than bone (high atomic number)
√ similar to calcified nodules
√ NO cor pulmonale, NO hilar adenopathy
√ regression if patient removed from exposure

BEHÇET DISEASE
• mouth / genital ulceration

- iritis, arthritis, skin rashes, encephalitis, thrombophlebitis
- √ aneurysm of large arteries (e.g. pulmonary artery)
- √ large vein obstruction; may cause SVC syndrome

BERYLLIOSIS
= ? delayed hypersensitivity reaction after exposure to acid salts from extraction of beryllium oxide
Substance: one of the lightest metals (atomic weight 9), marked heat resistance, great hardness, fatigue resistance, no corrosion
Occupational exposure: fluorescent lamp factories
A. ACUTE BERYLLIOSIS (25%)
   √ pulmonary edema following an overwhelming exposure
B. CHRONIC BERYLLIOSIS
   widespread systemic disease of liver, spleen, lymph nodes, kidney, myocardium, skin, skeletal muscle; removed from lungs + excreted via kidneys
   Latent period: 5 – 15 years
   √ fine nodularity (granulomas similar to sarcoidosis)
   √ irregular opacities, particularly sparing apices + bases
   √ hilar + mediastinal adenopathy (may calcify)
   √ emphysema in upper lobes + interstitial fibrosis
   √ pneumothorax in 10%
DDx: (1) Nodular pulmonary sarcoidosis (indistinguishable)
      (2) Asbestosis without hilar adenopathy

BLASTOMYCOSIS
= NORTH AMERICAN BLASTOMYCOSIS
Organism: fungus Blastomyces dermatitides, most commonly found in upper Midwest, parts of Southeast, esp. in Carolinas (acquired through activities in woods)
- mouth ulcers
- √ alveolar consolidation
- √ multiple irregular nodules

BRONCHIAL ADENOMA
= misnomer secondary to locally invasive features, tendency for recurrence, and occasional metastasis to extrathoracic sites (10%) = low-grade malignancy
Incidence: 6 – 10% of all primary lung tumors
Age: mean age is 35-45 years (range 12 – 60 years); 90% occur < 50 years of age; most common primary lung tumor under age 16; M:F = 1:1; Whites:Blacks = 25:1
Path: arise from duct epithelium of bronchial mucous glands (predominant distribution of Kulchitsky cells at bifurcations of lobar bronchi)

Carcinoid	90%
Adenoid cystic carcinoma = Cylindroma	6%
Mucoepidermoid carcinoma	3%
Pleomorphic carcinoma	1%

Location: most commonly near / at bifurcation of lobar / segmental bronchi
central : peripheral = 4 : 1

— 48% on right: RLL (20%), RML (10%), RUL (7%), main right bronchus (8%), intermediate bronchus (3%)
— 32% on left : LLL (13%), LUL (12%), main left bronchus (6%), lingular bronchus (1%)
- hemoptysis (40 – 50%)
- atypical asthma
- persistent cough
- recurrent obstructive pneumonia
- asymptomatic (10%)
- √ complete obstruction / air trapping in partial obstruction (rare) / nonobstructive (10 – 15%)
- √ obstructive emphysema
- √ postobstructive infection: pneumonitis, bronchiectasis, abscess
- √ atelectasis / consolidation of a lung / lobe / segment (78%)
- √ collateral air drift may prevent atelectasis
- √ solitary round / oval slightly lobulated pulmonary nodule (19%) of 1-10 cm in size
- √ hilar enlargement / mediastinal widening
= central endo- / exobronchial mass
CT: √ well-marginated sharply defined mass
   √ in close proximity to an adjacent bifurcation with splaying of bronchus
   √ coarse peripheral calcifications in 1/3 (cartilaginous / bony transformation)
Biopsy: risky secondary to high vascularity of tumor
Prognosis: 95% 5-year survival rate, 75% 15-year survival rate after resection

Carcinoid
Carcinoid tumors of lung make up 12% of all carcinoid tumors in the body
Age peak: 5th decade
Path: Kulchitsky cells = argentaffine; neurosecretory production of serotonin, ACTH, and bradykinin; part of APUD (amine precursor uptake and decarboxylation) system = chromaffin paraganglioma; rarely found in bronchial carcinoids
Δ rarely cause for carcinoid syndrome or Cushing syndrome
Pathologic classification:
   (KCC = Kulchitsky Cell Carcinoma)
   KCC I = classic carcinoid; endobronchial growth; usually < 2.5 cm in size; younger patient; M:F = 1:10; Lnn metastases in 3%
   KCC II = atypical carcinoid (25% of carcinoid tumors); usually > 2.5 cm; older patient; M:F = 3:1; Lnn metastases in 40-50%
   KCC III = small cell carcinoma
- Carcinoid syndrome = flushing, fever, nausea + vomiting, diarrhea, hypotension, wheezing, respiratory distress, left-sided endocardial damage (cardiac valve fibrosis)
Location: 90% central, 10% peripheral; located in submucosa; endo- / exobronchial form

√ average size 2.2 cm
Malignant potential: low
Metastases:
    (a) regional lymph nodes in 25%
    (b) distantly in 5% (adrenals, liver, brain, skin,
          osteoblastic bone metastases)
Prognosis: 87% 10-year survival rate

Cylindroma
= ADENOID CYSTIC CARCINOMA (7%)
Second most common primary tumor of trachea
Path: mixed serous + mucous glands; resembles
             salivary gland tumor
Age peak: 4 – 5th decade
• typical Hx of refractory "asthma"
√ endotracheal mass with extratracheal extension
Malignant potential:
   more aggressive than carcinoid with propensity for
   local invasion + distant metastases in 25%

Mucoepidermoid Carcinoma
Path: squamous cells + mucus-secreting columnar
             cells; resembles salivary gland tumor
√ may involve trachea = locally invasive tumor
√ sessile / polyploid endobronchial lesion

Pleomorphic Adenoma
= MIXED TYPE = extremely rare

BRONCHIAL ATRESIA
= local obliteration of bronchial lumen from local
   interruption of bronchial arterial perfusion late in fetal life
• minimal symptoms, apparent later in childhood / adult
   life
Location: apicoposterior segment of LUL (>>RUL / ML)
√ decreased perfusion
√ overexpanded segment (collateral air drift with
   expiratory air-trapping)
√ finger-like opacity lateral to hilum (= mucous plug distal
   to atretic lumen) is CHARACTERISTIC for differentiation
   from congenital lobar emphysema

BRONCHIECTASIS
= localized irreversible dilatation of bronchial tree
Etiology:
   A. Congenital
      1. Structural defect of bronchi: Williams-Campbell
         syndrome (= bronchial cartilage deficiency),
         Bronchial atresia
      2. Abnormal mucociliary transport: Kartagener
         syndrome
      3. Abnormal secretions: Mucoviscidosis = Cystic
         fibrosis
   B. Congenital / acquired immune deficiency (usually
      IgG deficiency):
      Chronic granulomatous disease of childhood, Alpha
         1-antitrypsin deficiency

   C. Postinfectious: Measles, Whooping cough, Swyer-
      James syndrome, Allergic bronchopulmonary
      aspergillosis, Chronic granulomatous infection (TB)
   C. Bronchial obstruction: neoplasm, inflammatory
      nodes, foreign body
   D. Aspiration / Inhalation: gastric contents / inhaled
      fumes (late complication)

Classification:
   1. **Cylindrical / tubular / fusiform bronchiectasis**
      reversible if associated with pulmonary collapse
      √ 16 subdivisions of bronchi
      √ square abrupt ending with lumen of uniform
         diameter and same width as parent bronchus
      CT (thin-section CT is study of choice):
        √ "tramlines" (horizontal course)
        √ "signet ring" (vertical course with cross-section
          of dilated bronchus + branch of pulmonary
          artery)
   2. **Saccular / cystic bronchiectasis**
      Associated with   severe bronchial infection
      √ < 5 subdivisions of bronchi
      √ progressive ballooning dilatation toward periphery
        with diameter of saccules greater than parent
        bronchus
      √ dilatation of bronchi on inspiration, collapse on
        expiration
      CT:
        √ string of cysts (horizontal course) / cluster of
         cysts
        √ air-fluid level (frequent)
   3. **Varicose bronchiectasis**
      Rare, associated with Swyer-James syndrome
      √ 4 – 8 subdivisions of bronchi
      √ beaded contour with normal pattern distally

Age: predominantly pediatric disease
• cough + expectoration of purulent sputum
• shortness of breath
• hemoptysis (50%)
Location: posterior basal segments of lower lobes,
            bilateral (50%), middle lobe / lingula (10%),
            central bronchiectasis in bronchopulmonary
            aspergillosis
√ normal radiograph in 7%
√ increase in size of lung markings (retained secretions)
√ loss of definition of lung markings (peribronchial fibrosis)
√ crowding of lung markings (if associated with
   atelectasis)
√ cystic spaces ± air-fluid levels < 2 cm in diameter
   (dilated bronchi)
√ honeycomb pattern (in severe cases)
√ compensatory hyperinflation of uninvolved ipsilateral
   lung
√ increased background density
√ frequent exacerbations + resolutions (due to
   superimposed infections)
Cx: frequent respiratory infections

DDx of CT-appearance:
  (1) emphysematous blebs (no definable wall thickness)
  (2) "reversible bronchiectasis" = temporary dilatation during pneumonia

BRONCHIOLITIS OBLITERANS
Etiology: (1) 1 – 3 weeks after exposure to toxic fumes (phosgene, ammonia, sulfur dioxide, chlorine)
      (2) postinfectious: mycoplasma (children), virus (older individual)
      (3) connective tissue disorder
      (4) organ transplantation
      (5) idiopathic
Path: obliterative granulation tissue within lumen of small airways
Peak age: 40 – 60 years; M:F = 1:1
- flulike illness (fever, malaise, sore throat)
- no response to antibiotics
- persistent nonproductive cough
√ normal / hyperinflated lungs = limited disease with connective tissue plugs in airways
√ bilateral patchy alveolar infiltrates in lung periphery (organizing pneumonia)
DDx: (1) Bacterial / fungal pneumonia (response to antibiotics, positive cultures)
      (2) Chronic eosinophilic pneumonia (young female, eosinophilia in 2/3)
      (3) Usual interstitial pneumonia (irregular opacities, decreased lung volume)

BRONCHIOLOALVEOLAR CARCINOMA
= ALVEOLAR CELL CARCINOMA
20 – 25% of all primary lung cancers (increasing incidence)
Etiology: development from type II alveolar epithelial cells
Age: middle age; M:F = 1:1
Path: (a) cuboidal cells resembling alveolar type II pneumocytes
      (b) mucus-producing tall columnar cells similar to bronchial cells growing along alveolar walls + septa without disrupting lung architecture
Associated with: preexisting pulmonary scar, fibrosis, diffuse interstitial inflammation, scleroderma
- often asymptomatic
- cough (60%)
- abundant mucoid expectoration (25%) can produce hypovolemia + electrolyte depletion (bronchorrhea)
A. LOCAL FORM (60 – 90%)
    1. Single mass
      √ well-circumscribed focal mass at peripheral / subpleural location
      √ "rabbit ears" / pleural tags / triangular strand / "tail sign" (55%) = linear strands extending from nodule to pleura (desmoplastic reaction / scarring granulomatous disease / pleural indrawing)

√ irregular sunburst appearance
√ air bronchogram / pseudocavitation (= dilatation of intact air spaces from desmoplastic reaction / bronchiectasis / focal emphysema)
√ confined to single lobe
√ NO atelectasis
    2. Multinodular form
B. DIFFUSE FORM = Pneumonic form (10 – 40%)
√ acinar air space consolidation throughout both lungs (mucus secretion)
√ pleural effusion (8 – 10%)
Metastases: to local lymph nodes + distant sites
Prognosis: 4 – 15 years survival time with single nodule; worse with extensive form

BRONCHOGENIC CARCINOMA
Most frequent cause of cancer deaths in males (35%) and females (18%)
Prevalence (1982): 135:100,000 males;
                     61:100,000 females
Age at diagnosis: 55 – 60 years (range 40 – 80 years)
- asymptomatic (10 – 50%)
- cough (75%)
- hemoptysis (50%)
- dysphagia (2%)

TYPES
  1. **Adenocarcinoma** (25 – 35%)
    almost invariably develops in periphery, intermediate malignant potential (slow growth, high incidence of early metastases), frequently found in scars (tuberculosis, infarction, pneumoconiosis)
    √ solitary peripheral mass (52%) / alveolar infiltrate / multiple nodules
    √ upper lobe distribution (69%)
    √ calcification in periphery of mass (1%)
    √ desmoplastic reaction

  2. **Squamous cell carcinoma** = **epidermoid carcinoma** (30 – 35%)
    Most closely associated with smoking
    Slowest growth rate, lowest incidence of distant metastases
    (a) central location (2/3)
      √ airway obstruction with atelectasis (37%)
      √ postobstructive pneumonia
      √ large central mass
    (b) peripheral nodule (1/3)
      √ characteristic cavitation (7%)
      √ invasion of chest wall

  3. **Small cell undifferentiated carcinoma** = **oat cell cancer** (25%)
    Rapid growth + high metastatic potential (early metastases); should be regarded as systemic disease regardless of stage; virtually never resectable
    - hypoglycemia
    √ small lung lesion
    √ typically large hilar mass / mediastinal adenopathy

4. **Large cell undifferentiated carcinoma** (10 – 14%)
Intermediate malignant potential with distant metastases
√ large peripheral mass > 6 cm (50%)
√ pleural Involvement

Angio: √ bronchogenic carcinoma supplied by bronchial circulation
√ distortion / stenosis / occlusion of pulmonary arterial circulation

RISK FACTORS:
(1) cigarette smoking (squamous cell carcinoma + small cell carcinoma)
(2) industrial exposure: asbestos, uranium, arsenic, chlormethyl ether
(3) concomitant disease: tuberculous scar (in 10% develop adenocarcinoma)

PRESENTATION
√ solitary peripheral mass with corona radiata / pleural tail sign / satellite lesion
√ cavitation (16%): usually thick-walled with irregular inner surface; in 4/5 secondary to squamous cell carcinoma
√ central mass (38%): commonest for small cell carcinoma
√ unilateral hilar enlargement (secondary to primary tumor / enlarged lymph nodes)
   Nodes on CT: 0 – 10 mm negative, 10 – 20 mm indeterminate, > 20 mm positive
√ anterior + middle mediastinal widening (suggests small cell carcinoma)
√ segmental / lobar / lung atelectasis (37%) = "S sign of Golden" = secondary to airway obstruction, particularly in squamous cell carcinoma
√ rat tail bronchus
√ local hyperaeration
√ persistent peripheral infiltrate (30%) = postobstructive pneumonitis
√ NO air bronchogram
√ pleural effusion (8 – 15%)
√ bone erosion of ribs / spine (9%)
√ involvement of main pulmonary artery (18%); lobar + segmental arteries (53%)

PARANEOPLASTIC MANIFESTATIONS
1. Carcinomatous neuromyopathy (4 – 15%)
2. Migratory thrombophlebitis
3. Hypertrophic pulmonary osteoarthropathy (3 – 5%)
4. Endocrine manifestations (15%) usually with small cell carcinoma: Cushing syndrome, Inappropriate secretion of ADH, HPT, Excessive gonadotropin secretion

LOCATION
60 – 80% arise in segmental bronchi

— central: small cell carcinoma, squamous cell carcinoma (sputum cytology positive in 70%); arises in central airway often at points of bronchial bifurcation, infiltrates circumferentially, extends along bronchial tree
— peripheral: adenocarcinoma, large cell carcinoma
— upper lobe: lower lobe = right lung : left lung = 3 : 2
— most common site: anterior segment of RUL
— Pancoast tumor (4%) = superior pulmonary sulcus tumor, frequently squamous cell carcinoma
— SVC obstruction (5%): frequently small cell carcinoma

TNM STAGING
T 1 : < 3 cm in diameter, surrounded by lung / visceral pleura
T 2 : > 3 cm in diameter / invasion of visceral pleura / lobar atelectasis / obstructive pneumonitis / at least 2 cm from carina
T 3 : tumor of any size; less than 2 cm from carina / invasion of parietal pleura, chest wall, diaphragm, mediastinal pleura, pericardium; pleural effusion
T 4 : invasion of heart, great vessels, trachea, esophagus, vertebral body, carina / malignant effusion
N 1 : peribronchial / ipsilateral hilar nodes
N 2 : ipsilateral mediastinal nodes
N 3 : contralateral hilar / mediastinal nodes

LIMITED DISEASE:
1. Primary in one hemithorax
2. Ipsilateral hilar adenopathy
3. Ipsilateral supraclavicular adenopathy
4. Ipsi- and contralateral mediastinal adenopathy
5. Atelectasis
6. Paralysis of phrenic + laryngeal nerve
7. Small effusion without malignant cells

EXTENSIVE DISEASE:
1. Contralateral hilar adenopathy
2. Contralateral supraclavicular adenopathy
3. Chest wall infiltration
4. Carcinomatous pleural effusion
5. Lymphangitic carcinomatosis
6. Superior vena cava syndrome
7. Metastasis to contralateral lung
8. Distant metastases to liver, brain, bone, other lymph nodes

SPREAD
1. direct local extension
2. hematogenous (small cell ca.)
3. lymphatic spread (squamous cell ca.); tumor in 10% of normal sized lymph nodes
4. transbronchial spread – least common
DISTANT METASTASES
@ Bone
   (a) Marrow: in 40% at time of presentation

(b) Gross lesions in 10 – 35%:
   Location: vertebrae (70%), pelvis (40%),
      femora (25%)
   √ osteolytic metastases (3/4)
   √ osteoblastic metastases (1/4):
      in small cell carcinoma / adenocarcinoma
   √ occult metastases in 36% of bone scans
@ Adrenals: in 37% at time of presentation
@ Brain: asymptomatic metastases on brain scan in
      7% (30% at autopsy), in 2/3 multiple
@ Kidney, GI tract, liver, abdominal lymph nodes,
   contralateral lung

Cx:
1. Horner syndrome (Pancoast tumor)
2. Diaphragmatic elevation (phrenic nerve paralysis)
3. Hoarseness (laryngeal nerve involvement, left > right)
4. SVC obstruction (5%): cause of all SVC obstructions in 90%
5. Pleural effusion (10%): malignant, parapneumonic, lymphoobstructive
6. Dysphagia: enlarged nodes, esophageal invasion
Prognosis:
   mean survival time < 6 months; < 10% overall 5-year
   survival; Survival at 40 months: squamous cell 30% >
   large cell 16% > adenocarcinoma 15% > oat cell 1%

BRONCHOGENIC CYST
= budding / branching abnormality of primitive foregut
   (ventral segment = tracheobronchial tree; dorsal
   segment = esophagus)
Histo: thin-walled cyst filled with mucoid material, lined
      with columnar respiratory epithelium, mucous
      glands, cartilage, elastic tissue, smooth muscle
• contains mucus / clear fluid
√ sharply outlined round / oval mass
√ may contain air-fluid level
CT: √ water (50%) / higher density (50%) containing
      clear / turbid fluid

A. MEDIASTINAL BRONCHOGENIC CYST (86%)
   Associated with: spinal abnormalities
   M:F = 1:1
   • usually asymptomatic
   • stridor, dysphagia
   Location: posterior mediastinum (50%), pericarinal
         (35%), superior mediastinum (14%);
         usually on right
   √ may communicate with tracheal lumen
   √ may show esophageal compression
B. INTRAPULMONARY BRONCHOGENIC CYST (14%)
   M > F
   • infection (75%)
   • dyspnea, hemoptysis (most common)
   Location: LL:UL = 2:1; usually medial third
   √ 36% will eventually contain air
   DDx: solitary pulmonary nodule, cavitated neoplasm,
         cavitated pneumonia, lung abscess

C. INTRAMURAL ESOPHAGEAL CYST

BRONCHOPULMONARY DYSPLASIA
= RESPIRATOR LUNG = complication of prolonged
   respirator therapy of intermittent PEEP with high oxygen
   concentration = oxygentoxicity + barotrauma
Stage I   (2 – 3 days)   : √ RDS pattern of hyaline
                        membrane disease
Stage II (4 – 10 days) : √ complete opacification with
                        air bronchogram;
                        associated with congestive
                        failure from PDA
Stage III (10 – 20 days) : √ "spongy" / "bubbly" coarse
                        linear densities, esp. in upper
                        lobes;
                        √ hyperaeration of lung
                        √ lower lobe emphysema
Stage IV (after 1 month) : √ same pattern;
                        40% mortality if not resolved
                        by 1 month
Cx: (1) abnormal pulmonary function
      (2) increased frequency of lower respiratory tract
         infections
Prognosis:
      (1) complete clearing over months / years (1/3)
      (2) retained linear densities in upper lobe
         emphysema (29%)
DDx: (1) Diffuse neonatal pneumonia (2) Meconium
      aspiration (3) Total anomalous pulmonary venous
      return (4) Congenital pulmonary lymphangiectasia
      (5) Cystic fibrosis (6) Idiopathic pulmonary fibrosis
      (7) Pulmonary interstitial emphysema (8) Wilson-
      Mikity syndrome

BRONCHOPULMONARY FISTULA
= communication between the bronchial system + pleural
   space
Causes:
   A. Trauma
      1. Complication of resectional surgery
   B. Inflammation
      1. Putrid lung abscess
      2. Pneumonia: Klebsiella, H. influenza,
         Staphylococcus, Streptococcus, Tuberculosis
      3. Bronchiectasis (very rare)
   C. Tumor
      1. Carcinoma
Dx: (1) Introduction of methylene blue into pleural
         space, in 65% dye appears in sputum
      (2) Sinography (3) Bronchography

BRONCHOPULMONARY SEQUESTRATION
= congenital bronchopulmonary foregut malformation
   consisting of
   (1) nonfunctioning lung segment (2) no communication
   with the tracheobronchial tree (3) systemic artery supply

Etiology:
development of an accessory tracheobronchial foregut bud in which
(a) early appearance leads to incorporation forming intralobar sequestration
(b) late appearance leads to separate pleural investment
Incidence: 0.1 – 1.7%
Age of discovery: 1st decade (majority), occasionally in infants / in utero
Path: homogeneous bronchopulmonary mass
Location: LLL:RLL = 2:1; posterior basal segement of lower lobe; rarely upper lung / within fissure
• cough + sputum production
• hemoptysis, pain, infection
• respiratory distress + CHF in newborn (due to shunting of blood)
√ usually > 6 cm in size
√ round / oval, smooth, well-defined solid homogeneous mass near diaphragm
√ occasionally fingerlike appendage posteriorly + medially (anomalous vessel)
√ multiple / single air-fluid levels if infected
√ surrounding pneumonic consolidation = recurrent pulmonary consolidation in a lower lobe that never clears completely
√ may communicate with esophagus / stomach

A. INTRALOBAR SEQUESTRATION (75-86%)
= enclosed by visceral pleura of affected pulmonary lobe
Age at presentation: adulthood (50% > 20 years)
M:F = 1:1
• acute lower lobe pneumonia
Associated with congenital anomalies (14%):
skeletal deformities (4%), other foregut anomalies (4%), diaphragmatic anomaly (3%), cardiac, renal, cerebral anomalies
Location: posterobasal segments, L:R = 3:2
√ usually single large artery from distal thoracic aorta (65%) / proxima abdominal aorta (22%) coursing through pulmonary ligament
√ venous drainage via pulmonary veins to
(a) L atrium (L-to-L shunt) in 95%
(b) R atrium in 5%
√ communication with bronchial network (rare)
CT:
√ single / multiple cysts containing air / mucus / pus
√ emphysema bordering normal lung (37%)
√ homogeneous / inhomogeneous dense mass
√ irregular enhancement (rare)
√ one / two anomalous systemic arteries arising from aorta (2/3)(DDx: AVM, interrupted pulmonary artery, isolated anomaly, chronic infection / inflammation of lung or pleura, surgically created shunt)
√ premature atherosclerosis of anomalous arteries
OB-US:
√ spherical homogeneous highly echogenic mass

B. EXTRALOBAR SEQUESTRATION (14 – 25%)
= with own pleural sheath (prevents collateral air drift = airless round mass)
Age: neonatal presentation;   M:F = 8:1
Associated with congenital anomalies (60%):
diaphragmatic defect (28%), cystic adenomatoid malformation, lobar emphysema, anomalous pulmonary venous return, cardiac / pericardial anomalies (8%), epiphrenic diverticula (2%), TE fistula (1.5%), duplication of GI tract, renal anomaly
Location: L:R = 4:1, often in association with left hemidiaphragm; may be below diaphragm (5%) / within mediastinum
√ arterial supply variable from small aortic branches / pulmonary artery
√ venous drainage via systemic veins to R heart (IVC, azygos, hemiazygos, portal vein)
√ NO communication with bronchial tree, may connect with GI tract
OB-US:
√ conical / triangular highly echogenic homogeneous mass
√ fetal hydrops
DDx:
bronchiectasis, lung abscess, empyema, bronchial atresia, lobar emphysema, cystic adenomatoid malformation, intrapulmonary bronchogenic cyst, Swyer-James syndrome, pneumonia, arteriovenous fistula, primary / metastatic neoplasm, hernia of Bochdalek

CASTLEMAN DISEASE
= GIANT LYMPH NODE HYPERPLASIA
= ANGIOMATOUS LYMPHOID HAMARTOMA
= LYMPHOID HAMARTOMA = ANGIOFOLLICULAR LYMPH NODE HYPERPLASIA
= benign masses of lymphoid tissue of unknown etiology
Age: range of 8 – 66 years, < 30 years (70%); M:F = 1:1
TYPES
A. Hyaline-vascular type (80 – 90%)
Path: vascular proliferation + hyalinization with small follicle centers penetrated by capillaries, capillary proliferation in interfollicular areas
• cough, dyspnea, hemoptysis
• lassitude, weight loss, fever
• asymptomatic in 97%
• growth retardation
• refractory microcytic anemia
B. Plasma cell type (10 – 20%)
Path: sheets of plasma cells between normal / enlarged follicles
• fever, anemia, elevated sedimentation rate
• IgG, IgM, IgA hypergammaglobulinemia (50%)
Location:
@ Chest: middle / posterior mediastinum (70%), within lung (rare)
@ Extrathoracic: neck, axilla, shoulder, mesentery, pelvis, within muscle, retroperitoneum (rare)

Size: up to 16 cm in diameter
CT: √ well-defined mass of muscle density
√ spotty central calcification
√ enhancing rim (vascular capsule)
√ marked enhancement almost equal to aorta (in hyalin-vascular type)
√ slight enhancement (in plasma cell type)
Angio:√ mass with multiple feeding vessels
√ dense homogeneous blush (hyalin-vascular type)
√ some hypervascularity (plasma cell type)
DDx: indistinguishable from lymphoma

CHRONIC EOSINOPHILIC PNEUMONIA
= numerous eosinophils, macrophages, histiocytes, lymphocytes, PMNs within lung interstitium + alveolar sacs
Etiology: unknown
Age: middle-age; M < F
• common Hx of atopia (may occur during therapeutic desensitization procedure)
• adult onset asthma (wheezing)
• high fever, malaise, dyspnea (DDx to Löffler syndrome)
• peripheral blood eosinophilia (with rare exceptions)
√ homogeneous alveolar lung infiltrates with distribution at lung periphery = "photographic negative" of pulmonary edema
√ frequently bilateral nonsegmental
√ unchanged for many days / weeks (DDx to Löffler syndrome)
√ dramatic response to steroid therapy (within 3 – 10 days)
Rx: exquisite response to steroids

CHYLOTHORAX
= leakage of chyle from thoracic duct or its branches into pleural space secondary to obstruction / disruption of thoracic duct (in 2%)
Route of thoracic duct:
enters thorax through esophageal foramen, ascends in right prevertebral location (between azygos vein + descending aorta), swings to left at T4 – 6, terminates 3 – 5 cm above clavicle at venous angle
Etiology:
1. Neoplasm (54%): disruption by lymphoma
2. Trauma (25%): latent period of 10 days blunt /penetrating trauma, surgery, subclavian venous catheter
3. Esophageal / cardiovascular surgery (0.5%)
4. Inflammatory disease
5. Idiopathic (15%)
6. Lymphangiomatosis (rare): mediastinal / thoracic cystic hygroma of neck growing into mediastinum
7. Tuberous sclerosis
8. Filiariasis (rare)
Age: in full term infants; may be present in utero; M:F = 2:1
Incidence: 1:10,000 deliveries

May be associated with: Trisomy 21, TE-fistula, extralobar lung sequestration, Congenital pulmonary lymphangiectasia
• high in neutral fat + fatty acid (low in cholesterol)
√ usually unilateral pleural effusion, most commonly on right side
√ polyhydramnios (? result of esophageal compression)
Cx: (1) Pulmonary hypoplasia
(2) Hydrops (congestive heart failure secondary to impaired venous return)

COAL WORKER'S PNEUMOCONIOSIS
= CWP = ANTHRACOSIS = ANTHRACOSILICOSIS
= coal dust inhalation taken up by alveolar macrophages, in part cleared by mucociliary action (particle size > 5 μ), in part deposited around bronchioles + alveoli, coal dust in itself is inert, but admixed silica is fibrogenic

Simple CWP
= aggregates of coal dust = coal macules (usually < 3 mm)
NO progression in absence of further exposure
Histo: development of reticulin fibers associated with bronchiolar dilatation (focal emphysema) + bronchiolar artery stenosis (decreased capillary perfusion)
• poor correlation between symptoms, physiologic findings + roentgenogram
√ small round 1 – 5 mm opacities, frequently in upper lobes (radiographically only seen through superposition after an exposure > 10 years)
√ nodularity correlates with amount of collagen (NOT amount of coal dust)
Cx : (1) Chronic obstructive bronchitis
(2) Focal emphysema
(3) Cor pulmonale

COCCIDIOIDOMYCOSIS
Organism: soil fungus Coccidioides immitis, spores live in dry dust with spread by wind; endemic in southwest desert of USA (San Joaquin Valley, central Southern Arizona, western Texas, southern New Mexico) similar to histoplasmosis
A. PRIMARY COCCIDIOIDOMYCOSIS
• 60 – 80% asymptomatic
• arthralgias, erythema nodosum / multiforme (5 – 20%)
√ patchy infiltrates mainly in lower lobes (46- 80%)
√ hilar adenopathy (20%)
√ pleural effusion (10%)
B. DISSEMINATED COCCIDIOIDOMYCOSIS
Incidence: 1: 6,000 infections
√ meningeal spread
√ micronodular pattern
C. CHRONIC COCCIDIOIDOMYCOSIS
• hemoptysis in 50%
√ one / several well-defined nodules of 5 – 30 mm in size (5%)

√ "grape skin" thin-walled cavities (10 – 15%), in 90% solitary , 70% in anterior segment of upper lobes (DDx: TB), 3% rupture into pleural space due to subpleural location (pneumothorax / empyema)
√ mediastinal adenopathy (10 – 20%)

CONGENITAL LOBAR EMPHYSEMA
= progressive overdistension of one / multiple lobes; M:F = 3 :1
Etiology:
  (a) deficiency / dysplasia / immaturity of bronchial cartilage
  (b) endobronchial obstruction (mucosal fold / web, prolonged endotracheal intubation, inflammatory exudate, inspissated mucus)
  (c) bronchial compression (PDA, aberrant left pulmonary artery, pulmonary artery dilatation)
  (d) polyalveolar / macroalveolar hyperplasia
Associated with: CHD in 15% (PDA, VSD)

• respiratory distress (90%) + progressive cyanosis within first 6 months of life
Location: LUL (42 – 43%), RML (32 – 35%), RUL (20%), two lobes (5%)
√ hazy masslike opacity immediately following birth (delayed clearance of lung fluid in emphysematous lobe over 1 – 14 days)
√ air trapping
√ hyperlucent expanded lobe (after clearing of fluid)
√ compression collapse of adjacent lobes
√ contralateral mediastinal shift
√ widely separated vascular markings
Mortality: 10%
Rx: surgical resection

CONGENITAL LYMPHANGIECTASIA
  1. PRIMARY PULMONARY LYMPHANGIECTASIA (2/3)
    = abnormal development of lungs between 14 – 20th week of GA;
    Age: usually manifest at birth
    • respiratory distress
    Prognosis: invariably fatal at < 2 months of age
    √ marked prominence of interstitial markings (simulating interstitial edema)
    √ patchy areas of pneumonia + atelectasis
    √ focal overinflation
  2. SECONDARY LYMPHANGIECTASIA (1/3)
    Secondary to elevated pulmonary venous pressure in CHD (TAPVR)
  3. GENERALIZED LYMPHANGIECTASIA
    Systemic maldevelopment characterized by lymphangiomas of viscera + soft tissues and hemangiomas of bone

CRYPTOCOCCOSIS
= TORULOSIS = EUROPEAN BLASTOMYCOSIS
Organism: Cryptococcus neoformans, spherical single-budding yeast cell with thick capsule, stains with India ink, often in soil contaminated with pigeon excreta, opportunistic invader
Histo: granulomatous lesion with caseous necrotic center
predisposed: diabetics, immunocompromised
• low grade meningitis (affinity to CNS); M:F = 4:1
√ well-circumscribed mass (40%) of 2 – 10 cm in diameter, usually peripheral location
√ lobar / segmental consolidation (35%)
√ cavitation (15%)
√ hilar / mediastinal adenopathy (12%)
√ calcifications (extremely rare)

CYSTIC ADENOMATOID MALFORMATION
= CAM = hamartoma of lung characterized by an intralobar mass of disorganized pulmonary tissue communicating with bronchial tree secondary to arrest of normal bronchoalveolar differentiation between 4 – 10th week of gestation
Path:
  proliferation of bronchial structures at the expense of alveolar saccular development, modified by intercommunicating cysts of various size (adenomatoid overgrowth of terminal bronchioles, proliferation of smooth muscle in cyst wall, absence of cartilage)

TYPE I (50%):
  Histo: single / multiple large cyst(s) lined by ciliated pseudostratified columnar epithelium, mucus-producing cells in 1/3
  Prognosis: excellent following resection
TYPE II (40%):
  Histo: multiple cysts < 12 mm lined by ciliated cuboidal / columnar epithelium
  Prognosis: poor secondary to associated abnormalities
TYPE III (10%):
  Histo: solitary firm mass of bronchuslike structures lined by ciliated cuboidal epithelium with microscopic cysts
  Prognosis: poor secondary to pulmonary hypoplasia / hydrops

Age of detection: children, neonates, fetus; M:F = 1:1
• asymptomatic, incidental finding later in life (1/3)
• respiratory distress + severe cyanosis in first week of life (2/3)
Location: equal frequency in all lobes (middle lobe rarely affected); more than one lobe involved in 20%
CXR:
  √ proper position of abdominal viscera
  √ almost always unilateral mass with well-defined margins (80%)
  √ compression of adjacent lung
  √ contralateral shift of mediastinum (87%)
  √ multiple air-filled cysts / occasionally fluid-filled cysts
  √ hypoplastic ipsilateral lung

CT:
  √ solitary / multiple fluid or air-fluid filled cysts
  √ focal emphysematous changes
OB-US:
  √ single large cyst / multiple large cysts 2-10 cm in
    diameter (Type I)
  √ multiple small cysts < 12 mm in diameter (Type II)
  √ large homogeneously echogenic mass (Type III)
  √ polyhydramnios (66% — ? from esophageal
    compression) / normal fluid (28%) / oligohydramnios
    (6%)
  √ fetal ascites (71%)
  √ fetal hydrops in 8 – 47% (decreased venous return
    from compression)
Cx: Pulmonary hypoplasia
Prognosis: 50% premature, 25% stillborn,
            (polyhydramnios, ascites, hydrops indicate a
            poor outcome)
DDx: (1) Congenital lobar emphysema
      (2) Diaphragmatic hernia
      (3) Bronchogenic cyst (small solitary cyst near
          midline)
      (4) Sequestration (less frequently associated with
          polyhydramnios / hydrops)

CYSTIC FIBROSIS
  = MUCOVISCIDOSIS
  = autosomal recessive disease with (a) dysfunction of
    exocrine glands forming a thick tenacious material
    obstructing conducting system (b) reduced mucociliary
    transport
Incidence: 1:2000; almost exclusively in Caucasians
            (1:20 heterozygous); unusual in Blacks,
            Orientals, Polynesians
  • elevated concentrations of sodium + chloride in sweat
  @ Lung
  • chronic cough, recurrent pulmonary infections
  • progressive respiratory insufficiency
  • infertility in males
  √ "fingerlike" mucus plugging (mucoid impaction in
    dilated bronchi)
  √ subsegmental / segmental / lobar atelectasis with
    right upper lobe predominance (10%)
  √ cylindrical / cystic bronchiectasis (in 100% > 6
    months of age) ± air-fluid levels
  √ parahilar linear densities + peribronchial cuffing
  √ focal / generalized hyperinflation secondary to
    collateral air drift
  √ hilar adenopathy
  √ large pulmonary arteries (pulmonary arterial
    hypertension)
  √ recurrent local pneumonitis (Staphylococcus,
    Pseudomonas)
  NUC: √ matched patchy areas of decreased ventilation
         + perfusion
  Cx: (1) Pneumothorax (rupture of bulla / bleb),
             common + recurrent
         (2) Hemoptysis

      (3) Cor pulmonale
      (4) Hypertrophic pulmonary osteoarthropathy
          (rare)
  @ GI tract
  • steatorrhea + malabsorption (pancreatic insufficiency
    in 80 – 90%)
  • rectal prolapse (23%)
  • failure to thrive
  √ meconium ileus (10 – 15%), earliest finding
  √ meconium ileus equivalent
  √ fatty liver
  √ focal biliary cirrhosis with signs of portal hypertension
    (clinically rare, autoptic in up to 50%)
  √ gallstones
  √ echogenic pancreas (pancreatic cirrhosis due to
    recurrent acute pancreatitis)
  @ Skull
  √ sinusitis with opacification of well-developed maxillary,
    ethmoid, sphenoid sinuses
  √ hypoplastic frontal sinuses

DIAPHRAGMATIC HERNIA
Congenital Diaphragmatic Hernia
  = absence of closure of the pleuroperitoneal fold by 9th
    week of gestational age
Incidence: 1: 2,200 – 2,500 live births (0.04%);
            M:F = 2:1
  Δ delayed onset following Group B streptococcal
    infection
Etiology: insult that inhibits / delays normal migration
           of the gut + closure of the diaphragm
           between 8 – 12th week of embryogenesis
Associated anomalies (in 20% of liveborn, in 90% of
  stillborn fetuses):
  1. CNS (28%): neural tube defects
  2. Gastrointestinal (20%): particularly malrotation, oral
     cleft, omphalocele
  3. Cardiovascular (13 – 23%)
  4. Genitourinary (15%)
  5. Chromosomal abnormalities
  6. IUGR (concurrent major abnormality in 90%)
Location: L:R = 9:1

(1) Bochdalek Hernia (85 – 90%)
    = posterolateral defect caused by maldevelopment
      / defective fusion of the cephalic fold of the
      pleuroperitoneal membranes
    Location: left (80%), right (15%), bilateral (5%)
    Herniated organs:
      (a) on left: omental fat (6%), bowel, spleen,
            stomach (rare), kidney, pancreas
      (b) on right: part of liver
    mnemonic:
      Bochdalek
      Back (posterior location)
      Babies (age at presentation)
      Big (usually large)

(2) <u>Morgagni Hernia</u> (1 – 2%)
   = anteromedial parasternal defect (space of Larrey) caused by maldevelopment of septum transversum; R > L
   Often associated with pericardial deficiency
      (a) abdominal viscera / fat may herniate into pericardial sac
      (b) heart may herniate into upper abdomen
   mnemonic:
      Morgagni
      Middle (anterior + central location)
      Mature (present in older children)
      Minuscule (usually small)
(3) <u>Septum Transversum Defect</u> = defect in central tendon
(4) <u>Hiatal Hernia</u> = congenitally large esophageal orifice
(5) <u>Eventration</u> (5%) = upward displacement of abdominal contents secondary to a congenitally thin hypoplastic diaphragm
   Location: anteromedial on right, total involvement on left side; R:L = 5 :1
   √ small diaphragmatic excursions
   √ often lobulated contour
• respiratory distress in neonatal period (life-threatening deficiency of small airways + alveoli)
• scaphoid abdomen
Herniated organs:
   stomach (60%), small bowel (90%), large bowel (56%), spleen (54%), pancreas (24%), kidney (12%), adrenal gland, liver, gallbladder
√ bowel loops in chest as solid / multicystic mass
√ passage of nasogastric tube under fluoroscopic control
√ contralateral mediastinal shift
√ complete / partial abscence of diaphragm
√ absence of stomach, small bowel in abdomen
√ incomplete rotation + anomalous mesenteric attachment of bowel
OB-US (diagnosis possible by 18 wks.):
   √ peristalsis of bowel within fetal chest (inconsistent)
   √ scaphoid fetal abdomen with reduced abdominal circumference
   √ fetal stomach at level of fetal heart
   √ nonvisualization of fetal stomach (GI-obstruction / CNS abnormality)
   √ polyhydramnios (common, ? secondary to bowel obstruction) / oligohydramnios / normal fluid volume
   CT amniography (confirmation of diagnosis):
   √ swallowed fetal intestinal contrast appears in chest
Cx: (1) Bilateral pulmonary hypoplasia
         (2) Postsurgical pulmonary hypertension
Prognosis: (1) Stillbirth (35%)
               (2) Neonatal death (35%)
Mortality: in 10% death before surgery; 40 – 50% operative mortality; mortality of 60% with intrathoracic stomach, 6% with intraabdominal stomach

Traumatic Diaphragmatic Hernia

5% of all diaphragmatic hernias, but 90% of all strangulated diaphragmatic hernias
Etiology:
   (a) blunt trauma (5 – 50%) = marked increase in intraabdominal pressure: motor vehicle accident, fall from height, bout of hyperemesis
   (b) penetrating trauma (50%): knife, bullet, repair of hiatus hernia
Contents in order of frequency:
   stomach, colon, small bowel, omentum, spleen, kidney, pancreas
• may be asymptomatic for months / years following trauma, onset of symptoms may be so long delayed that traumatic event is forgotten
• virtually all become ultimately symptomatic, most in < 3 years
• **Bergqvist Triad:**
   (1) rib fractures (2) fracture of spine / pelvis (3) diaphragmatic hernia
Location: left side in 90 – 98%; central + posterior portion of diaphragm; 2 – 10% on right side
Size: most tears are > 10 cm in length
√ diaphragm cannot be traced / abnormal contour of hemidiaphragm
√ cephalad margin of bowel may simulate an elevated diaphragm (look for haustra)
√ lower lobe mass / consolidation (herniated solid organ / omentum / airless bowel loop)
√ inhomogeneous mass with air-fluid level in left hemithorax
√ displacement of mediastinum + lung
√ mushroomlike mass of herniated liver in right hemithorax
√ "hourglass" constriction of afferent + efferent bowel loops at orifice
√ hydrothorax / hematothorax indicates strangulation
√ nasogastric tube first dips below diaphragm (rent spares esophageal hiatus)
√ location of diaphragm may be documented by
   1. gas-filled bowel constricted at site of diaphragmatic laceration
   2. barium study
Associated injuries:
   √ fractures of lower ribs
   √ perforation of hollow viscus
   √ rupture of spleen
Cx: life-threatening strangulation occurs in majority (90% of strangulated hernias are traumatic in origin)
DDx: eventration, diaphragmatic paralysis

EMPHYSEMA

= increased air space size distal to terminal bronchiole with destruction of walls
A.CENTRILOBULAR EMPHYSEMA (more common)
   = abnormal enlargement of air spaces in central portion of secondary pulmonary lobule + destruction of respiratory bronchioles in center of lobe / eccentric

Predisposed: smokers
- blue bloater
Site: tendency for upper lobes
√ increased markings

B.PANACINAR / PANLOBULAR EMPHYSEMA
= destruction of lung distal to terminal bronchiole,
may be associated with alpha-1 antitrypsin deficiency
Age: older patients
- pink puffer
Site: panacinar emphysema more severe in bases
√ decreased markings
√ flattened diaphragm (most reliable sign)
√ centralization of pulmonary vasculature (pulmonary hypertension)
√ bullae

EOSINOPHILIC GRANULOMA
= variant of histiocytosis X localized to lung + bones
Path: granulomatous infiltration of alveolar septa + bronchial walls by foamy histiocytes, eosinophils with deposition of reticulin + collagen
Age: most frequently in 3rd – 4th decade; Caucasians >> Blacks
@ Lung involvement
- asymptomatic (1/3)
- nonproductive cough (2/3)
- fatigue, weight loss, fever (30%)
- dyspnea (40%)
- chest pain (25%)
- diabetes insipidus (10 – 25%)
Location: usually bilaterally symmetric, upper lobe predominance, sparing of costophrenic angles
√ diffuse fine reticulonodular pattern (cellular infiltrate)
√ nodules 3 – 10 mm (granuloma stage)
√ cavitation if nodules large (rare)
√ "honeycomb lung" = multiple 1 – 5 cm cysts + subpleural blebs (fibrotic stage)
√ recurrent pneumothoraces in 25% (from rupture of subpleural cysts) CHARACTERISTIC
√ emphysema
√ pleural effusions, hilar adenopathy (unusual)
√ thymic enlargement
@ Bone involvement
√ lytic bone lesions
√ vertebra plana
@ Other organs: lymph nodes, skin, endocrine glands
Prognosis: guarded with multisystem disease + organ dysfunction
Rx: chemotherapy (vincristine sulfate, prednisone, methotrexate, 6-mercaptopurine)

EOSINOPHILIC LUNG DISEASE
= PULMONARY INFILTRATION WITH BLOOD / TISSUE EOSINOPHILIA (PIE)
Classification:
1. IDIOPATHIC EOSINOPHILIC LUNG DISEASE
   (a) Transient pulmonary eosinophilia = Löffler syndrome

- peripheral eosinophilia
   (b) Chronic eosinophilic pneumonia
   - no peripheral eosinophilia
2. EOSINOPHILIC LUNG DISEASE OF SPECIFIC ETIOLOGY
   (a) drug induced: nitrofurantoin, penicillin, sulfonamides, ASA, tricyclic antidepressants, hydrochlorothiazide, cromolyn sodium, mephenesin
   (b) parasite induced: Tropical eosinophilia (ascariasis, schistosomiasis), Strongyloidiasis, Ancylostomiasis (hookworm), Filiarisis, Toxocara canis (visceral larva migrans), Dirofilaria immitis, Amebiasis (occasionally — in right lower + middle lobe)
   (c) fungus induced: Allergic bronchopulmonary Aspergillosis, Bronchocentric granulomatosis
   (d) Pulmonary eosinophilia with asthma
3. EOSINOPHILIC LUNG DISEASE ASSOCIATED WITH ANGIITIS ± GRANULOMATOSIS
   (a) Wegener granulomatosis
   (b) Polyarteritis nodosa
   (c) Allergic granulomatosis (Churg-Strauss) Variant of polyarteritis nodosa, strongly Associated with history of asthma
   - peripheral eosinophilia > 30%
   (d) Lymphomatoid granulomatosis may lead to lymphoma
   √ CXR similar to Wegener granulomatosis
   (e) Bronchocentric granulomatosis
   = granulomas forming around bronchi + vasculitis
   - often associated with long history of asthma
   √ bronchial obstruction
   (f) Necrotizing "sarcoidal" angiitis
   (g) Rheumatoid disease
   (h) Scleroderma
   (i) Dermatomyositis
   (j) Sjögren syndrome
   (k) CREST

EXTRAMEDULLARY HEMATOPOIESIS
= compensatory response to deficient bone marrow blood cell production
Etiology: (NO hematologic disease in 25%)
1. Thalassemia
2. Hereditary spherocytosis
3. Myelosclerosis
4. Carcinomatous / lymphomatous replacement of bone marrow
5. Iron deficiency anemia
6. Pernicious anemia
7. Acquired hemolytic anemia
- chronic anemia
Sites:
@ spleen, liver, lymph nodes
@ adrenal glands
@ cartilage, broad ligaments

@ thrombi, adipose tissue
@ mediastinum
√ frequently bilateral paraspinal lobulated masses in mid- to lower thorax
√ splenomegaly / absent spleen
√ lack of calcification / bone erosion

EXTRAMEDULLARY PLASMACYTOMA

Uncommon form; relatively benign course (dissemination may be found months / years later or not at all); question-able if precursor to multiple myeloma
Age : 35 – 40 years; M:F = 2:1
Location: air passages (50%) predominantly in upper nose and oral cavity; conjunctiva (37%); lymph nodes (3%)
• usually not associated with increased immunoglobulin titer or amyloid deposition
√ mass of 1 – several cm in size with well-defined lobulated border
DDx:
(1) MULTIPLE MYELOMA
= malignant course with soft tissue involvement in 50 – 73%:
(a) microscopic infiltration
(b) enlargement of organs
(c) formation of tumor mass (1/3)
• usually associated with protein abnormalities
• may have amyloid deposition
Age incidence: 50 – 85 years
Δ tends to occur late in the course of the disease and indicates a poor prognosis (0 – 6% 5-year survival)
Classification:
1. Medullary plasmocytoma
2. Multiple myeloma:
(a) scattered involvement of bone
(b) myelomatosis of bone
3. Extramedullary plasmacytoma

EXTRINSIC ALLERGIC ALVEOLITIS

= exposure to organic dust of < 5 μ particle size
• asymptomatic (10 – 40%)
• recurrent episodes of fever, chills, dry cough, dyspnea following exposure after 6-hour interval
• resolution of episodic symptoms after cessation of exposure, abate spontaneously over 1 – 2 days
• insidious onset of gradually progressive dyspnea
• reduction in vital capacity, diffusing capacity, arterial PO_2
• intracutaneous injection of antigen results in delayed hypersensitivity reaction
• presence of serum precipitins against antigen
• positive aerosol provocation inhalation test

Specific antigens for immune complex disease (Type III = Arthus reaction):
1. Farmer's lung from moldy hay (Thermoactinomyces vulgaris or Micropolyspora faeni)
2. Hypersensitivity pneumonitis from forced-air equipment = Pandora's pneumonitis with heating / humidifying / air conditioning systems (thermophilic actinomycetes)
3. Bird-fancier's lung, Pigeon breeder's lung from protein in bird serum / droppings / feathers
4. Mushroom worker's lung from mushroom compost (Thermoactinomyces vulgaris or Micropolyspora faeni)
5. Bagassosis from moldy sugar cane in sugar mill (contamination with Thermoactinomyces sacchari / vulgaris and Micropolyspora faeni)
6. Malt worker's lung from malt dust (Aspergillus claratus)
7. Maple bark disease from moldy maple bark in saw mill (Cryptostroma corticale)
8. Suberosis from moldy cork dust (Penicillium frequentans)
9. Sequoiosis from redwood dust (Graphium species)

A. ACUTE EXTRINSIC ALLERGIC ALVEOLITIS
√ No CXR abnormalities in 30 – 95%
√ diffuse acinar consolidative pattern (edema + exudate filling alveoli)
√ basilar distribution
√ lymph node enlargement (unusual, more common with recurrence)
B. CHRONIC EXTRINSIC ALLERGIC ALVEOLITIS
= HYPERSENSITIVITY PNEUMONITIS
Path: proliferation of epithelial cells + elaboration of reticulum fibers
√ interstitial reticulonodular pattern with basilar distribution
√ loss of lung volume (cicatrization atelectasis) in upper lobes
√ pleural effusion (rare)
√ lymph node enlargement may occur

FAT EMBOLISM

= obstruction of pulmonary vessels by fat globules followed by chemical pneumonitis from unsaturated plasma fatty acids producing hemorrhage / edema
Incidence: in necropsy series in 67 – 97% of patients with major skeletal trauma, however, symptomatic fat embolism syndrome in < 10% (M > F)
Onset: 24 – 72 hours after trauma
• dyspnea (progressive pulmonary insufficiency)
• fever
• systemic hypoxemia
• mentation changes
• petechiae (50%) from coagulopathy (release of tissue thromboplastin)
√ initial chest film usually negative
√ platelike atelectasis
√ diffuse alveolar infiltrates
√ consolidation

NUC: √ mottled perfusion defects (1 – 4 days after injury), later enlarging secondary to pneumonic infiltrates

FIBROSING MEDIASTINITIS
Etiology:
    (a) Granulomatous: histoplasmosis (most frequent), tuberculosis, actinomycosis
    (b) Sclerosing: autoimmune disease, methysergide-induced
May be associated with retroperitoneal fibrosis, orbital pseudotumor, Riedel struma
- cough, dyspnea, hemoptysis
- dysphagia
- superior vena cava syndrome
- cor pulmonale
√ increase in size of upper half of mediastinum, right > left
√ lobulated mediastinal / hilar fibrous masses, often calcified
√ lymphadenopathy (frequent)
NUC:
    √ decreased / absent perfusion with normal ventilation
Cx: (1) Compression of SVC (64%) + pulmonary veins (4%)
     (2) Chronic obstructive pneumonia (narrowing of trachea / central bronchi) in 5%
     (3) Esophageal stenosis (3%)
     (4) Pulmonary infarcts + fibrosis (narrowing of pulmonary artery)
     (5) Prominent intercostal arteries (narrowing of pulmonary artery)
DDx: (1) Swyer-James syndrome
     (2) Congenital absence of pulmonary artery
     (3) Embolus to main pulmonary artery
     (4) Bronchogenic carcinoma

FRACTURE OF TRACHEA / BRONCHI
Location: (a) main stem bronchus 1 – 2 cm distal to carina (80%); R > L
         (b) just above carina (20%)
√ fracture of first 3 ribs (53 – 91%), rare in children
√ pneumothorax (70%)
√ mediastinal ± subcutaneous emphysema
√ absence of pleural effusion
√ collapsed lung falling to dependent position (loss of anchoring support in bronchial transsection)
√ atelectasis (may be late development)
√ inadequate reexpansion of lung despite chest tube (due to large air leak)
Prognosis: 30% mortality (in 15% within 1 hour)

GOODPASTURE SYNDROME
= autoimmune disease characterized by
  (1) glomerulonephritis (2) circulating antibodies against glomerular + alveolar basement membrane
  (3) pulmonary hemorrhage
Pathogenesis:
  cytotoxic antibody-mediated disease = Type II hypersensitivity; alveolar basement membrane becomes

antigenic (perhaps viral etiology); IgG / IgM antibody with complement activation causes cell destruction + pulmonary hemorrhage, leads to hemosiderin deposition and pulmonary fibrosis
Age peak: 26 years (range 17 – 78 years); M:F = 7 : 1
- iron-deficiency anemia
- hepatosplenomegaly
- systemic hypertension
@ Lung
- preceding upper respiratory infection (in 2/3) + renal disease
- mild hemoptysis (72%) with hemosiderin-laden macrophages in sputum, commonly precedes the clinical manifestations of renal disease by several months
- cough, dyspnea, basilar rales
√ patchy alveolar filling pattern with predominance in perihilar area + lung bases
√ air bronchogram
√ consolidation at lung bases + central lung fields
√ gradually interstitial pattern (due to septal thickening) = organization of hemorrhage
√ hilar lymph nodes may be enlarged during acute episodes
@ Kidney
- Glomerulonephritis with IgG deposits in characteristic linear pattern in glomeruli
- hematuria
Prognosis: death within 3 years (average 6 months) because of renal failure
Rx: cytotoxic chemotherpay, plasmapheresis, bilateral nephrectomy
DDx: idiopathic pulmonary hemosiderosis

GRANULOMA OF LUNG
constitute the majority of solitary pulmonary solitary nodules
√ central nidus of calcification in a laminated / diffuse pattern
√ absence of growth for at least 2 years
CT: (most effective in nodules ≤ 3 cm of diameter with smooth discrete margins)
  √ 50 – 60% of pulmonary nodules demonstrate unsuspected calcification by CT
DDx: Carcinoma (in 10% eccentric calcification in preexisting scar / nearby granuloma / true intrinsic stippled calcification in larger lesion)

HAMARTOMA OF LUNG
= composed of tissues normally found in this location in abnormal quantity, mixture, and arrangement
Incidence: 0.25% in population (autopsy); 6 – 8% of all solitary pulmonary lesions; most common benign lung tumor
Etiology:
  1. congenital malformation of a displaced bronchial anlage
  2. hyperplasia of normal structures

3. cartilaginous neoplasm
4. response to inflammation

Path: columnar, cuboidal, ciliated epithelium, fat, bone, cartilage (predominates), muscle, vessels, fibrous tissue, calcifications, plasma cells originating in fibrous connective tissue beneath mucous membrane of bronchial wall

Age peak: 5th + 6th decade; M:F = 3:1
- mostly asymptomatic
- hemoptysis (rare)
- cough, vague chest pain, fever (with postobstructive pneumonitis)

Location: 2/3 peripheral; endobronchial in 10%; multiplicity (rare)
√ round smooth lobulated mass < 4 cm (averages 2.5 cm)
√ calcification in 15% (almost pathognomonic if of "popcorn" type)
√ fat in 50% (detection by CT)
√ cavitation (extremely rare)
√ growth patterns: slow / rapid / stable with later growth
√ usually 5 mm increase in diameter per year

CT: (thin-section)
  √ fat density alone in 34% (-80 to -120 HU); calcium + fat (19%)

DDx: Lipoid pneumonia (ill-defined mass / lung infiltrate)

HISTOPLASMOSIS OF LUNG

Organism: Histoplasma capsulatum, dimorphic fungus, widespread in soil of North America (Ohio, Mississippi, St. Lawrence river valleys)

A. PRIMARY HISTOPLASMOSIS
  - mostly subclinical
  √ bronchopneumonic pattern with tendency to clear in one area + appear in another
  √ multiple nodules changing into hundreds of punctate calcifications (3 – 4 mm)
  √ histoplasmoma (= one / several noncalcifying nodules < 3 cm)
  √ "target lesion" = central calcification is PATHOGNOMONIC
  √ hilar / mediastinal lymph node enlargement (DDx: acute viral / bacterial pneumonia)
  √ "popcorn" calcification of mediastinal lymph nodes

B. CHRONIC HISTOPLASMOSIS
  (reinfection / endogenous dispersion)
  - in individuals with chronic obstructive pulmonary disease
  √ upper lobe cavitation with considerable fibrosis (similar to TB)
  √ sclerosing mediastinitis with obstruction of SVC, pulmonary arteries + veins, esophageal narrowing, constrictive pericarditis

C. DISSEMINATED HISTOPLASMOSIS
  Predisposed: infants + elderly; massive inoculum
  - rapidly fatal / chronic illness

√ may show pulmonary consolidation
√ hilar + mediastinal adenopathy + hepatosplenomegaly
√ splenic calcifications (40%)

HYDATID DISEASE
= ECHINOCOCCOSIS
- asymptomatic
- eosinophilia (< 25%)
- cough, expectoration, fever
- positive Casoni skin test in 60%
- hypersensitivity reaction (if cyst rupture occurs)
√ solitary (75%) / multiple (25%) sharply circumscribed spherical / ovoid masses
√ size of 1 – 10 cm in diameter (16 – 20 weeks doubling time)
√ cyst communicating with bronchial tree
  √ "meniscus sign", "double arch sign", "moon sign", "crescent sign" (5%) = rupture of pericyst with air dissection between peri- and exocyst
  √ "water lily sign", "sign of the camalote" = collapsed cyst membrane floating on the fluid
  √ air-fluid level = rupture of all cyst walls
  √ hydropneumothorax
√ calcification of cyst wall (< 6%)
√ rib + vertebral erosion (rare)
√ mediastinal cyst: posterior (65%), anterior (26%), middle (9%) mediastinum

HYPOGENETIC LUNG SYNDROME
= PULMONARY VENOLOBAR SYNDROME
= SCIMITAR SYNDROME
= unique form of lung hypoplasia / aplasia affecting one / more lobes accompanied by partial anomalous pulmonary venous return; M:F = 1:1.4
Associated with:
  (1) Vascular anomalies: hypoplastic artery, anomalous venous return, systemic arterial supply
  (2) Anomalies of hemidiaphragm on affected side:
    √ retrosternal soft tissue density (= "accessory hemidiaphragm") on lateral view only due to mediastinal rotation
    √ phrenic cyst
    √ diaphragmatic hernia
  (3) Hemivertebrae + scoliosis
  (4) CHD: ASD, VSD, Tetralogy of Fallot, PDA, Coarctation of aorta, Persistent left SVC, Pulmonary stenosis
- asymptomatic (40%)
- may have dyspnea / recurrent infections
Location: right-sided predominance
√ hypoplasia / aplasia of one / more lobes of the lung with errors of lobation (bilateral left bronchial branching pattern / horseshoe lung)
√ "scimitar vein" (90%) = partial anomalous pulmonary venous return (commonly infradiaphragmatic into IVC / portal vein / hepatic vein / R atrium), on CXR seen only in 1/3

√ systemic arterial supply to abnormal segment may be present from thoracic aorta (bronchial, intercostal, transpleural) or abdominal aorta (celiac artery, transdiaphragmatic)
√ reticular densities (enlarged bronchial / transpleural arterial collaterals)
√ small hilus (absent / small pulmonary artery)
√ small right hemithorax + mediastinal shift
√ haziness of right heart border
√ cardiac dextroposition (in right lung hypoplasia)
√ anomalies of bony thorax / thoracic soft tissues
  √ absent inferior vena cava
  √ rib hypoplasia / malsegmentation
  √ rib notching
CT:
  √ small hemithorax + mediastinal shift
  √ abnormalities of bronchial branching
  √ anomalously located pulmonary fissure
  √ discontinuity of hemidiaphragm
  √ pulmonary arterial hypoplasia
  √ hyparterial right bronchus (instead of eparterial)
  √ one / more vessels increasing in diameter toward diaphragm
  √ lack of normal venous confluence of right lung
DDx: Meandering pulmonary vein, dextrocardia, hypoplastic lung, Swyer-James syndrome

HORSESHOE LUNG
= uncommon variant of hypogenetic lung syndrome in which RLL crosses midline between esophagus and heart + fuses with opposite lung
√ oblique fissure in left lower hemithorax (if both lungs separated by pleural layers)
√ pulmonary vessels + bronchi crossing midline

IDIOPATHIC PULMONARY HEMOSIDEROSIS
= IPH = probable autoimmune process with clinical + radiological remissions + exacerbations characterized by eosinophilia + mastocytosis, immunoallergic reaction, pulmonary hemorrhage, iron-deficiency anemia
Age: (a) Chronic form: most commonly < 10 years of age
        (b) Acute form (rare): in adults; M:F = 2:1
• iron deficiency anemia
• clubbing
• hepatosplenomegaly (25%)
• bilirubinemia
• recurrent episodes of severe hemoptysis
√ bilateral patchy alveolar-filling pattern (= blood in alveoli); initially for 2 – 3 days with return to normal in 10 - 12 days unless episode repeated
√ reticular pattern (= deposition of hemosiderin in interstitial space) later
√ moderate fibrosis after repeated episodes
√ hilar lymph nodes may be enlarged during acute episodes
Prognosis: death within 2 – 20 years (average survival 3 years)

DDx: SECONDARY PULMONARY HEMOSIDEROSIS caused by mitral valve disease
  √ septal lines (NOT in idiopathic form)
  √ ossifications (NOT in idiopathic form)

INTERSTITIAL PNEUMONIA
= ORGANIZING INTERSTITIAL PNEUMONIA
= CHRONIC DIFFUSE SCLEROSING ALVEOLITIS
= HAMMAN-RICH SYNDROME

Usual Interstitial Pneumonia
= UIP = IDIOPATHIC PULMONARY FIBROSIS (IPF)
= MURAL TYPE OF FIBROSING ALVEOLITIS
= commonest form of diffuse interstitial pneumonia
Etiology: 50% idiopathic; 25% familial; drug exposure (bleomycin, cyclophosphamide (Cytoxan®), busulfan, nitrofurantoin); serologic abnormalities associated with collagen vascular disease
Age peak: 5 – 6 th decade; M:F = 1:1
Path:
  proteinaceous exudate in interstitium + hyaline membrane formation in alveoli; necrosis of alveolar lining cells followed by cellular infiltration of mono- and lymphocytes + regeneration of alveolar lining; proliferation of fibroblasts + deposition of collagen fibers + smooth muscle proliferation; progressive disorganization of pulmonary architecture
• progressive dyspnea
• "Velcro" rales – crepitations
• clubbing of fingers (83%)
• lymphocytosis on lavage
√ occasionally ground glass pattern in early stage of alveolitis (alveolar wall injury, interstitial edema, proteinaceous exudate, hyaline membranes, infiltrate of monocytes + lymphocytes)
√ diffuse linear / small irregular reticulations (60%); predominance at bases
√ reticulonodular pattern = superimposition of linear opacities
√ heart border "shaggy"
√ honeycombing (numerous cystic spaces)
√ elevated diaphragm (progressive loss of lung volume)
√ pleural effusion (4%), pleural thickening (6%)
√ pneumothorax in 7% (in late stages)
Cx: bronchogenic carcinoma (more frequent occurrence)
Prognosis: average survival of 4 – 6 years; 87% mortality rate

Desquamative Interstitial Pneumonia
= DIP = DESQUAMATIVE TYPE OF FIBROSING ALVEOLITIS
= second commonest form of interstitial pneumonia with more benign course than UIP, may be self-limited disease or lead to UIP
Age: approximately 8 years younger than in UIP

Path: alveoli lined by large cuboidal cells + filled with heavy accumulation of mononuclear cells; preservation of normal lung architecture; minimal fibrosis
- asymptomatic
- weight loss
- dyspnea + nonproductive cough
- finger clubbing

√ normal chest X-ray (15 – 20%)
√ "ground-glass" alveolar pattern sparing costophrenic angles (20%)
√ linear irregular opacities (60%), predominantly at bases
√ progressive loss of lung volume (not as severe as in UIP)

Prognosis: better response to corticosteroid Rx than UIP; 16% mortality rate

KARTAGENER SYNDROME
= IMMOTILE / DYSMOTILE CILIA SYNDROME
Incidence: 1:40,000; high familial incidence
Etiology: abnormal mucociliary function secondary to generalized deficiency of dynein arms of cilia affecting respiratory epithelium, auditory epithelium, sperm
Triad: (1) Situs inversus (50%)
       (2) Sinusitis
       (3) Bronchiectasis
- deafness
- infertility (abnormal sperm tails)
Associated anomalies:
    Transposition of great vessels, Tri- / bilocular heart, Pyloric stenosis, Postcricoid web, Epispadia

KLEBSIELLA PNEUMONIA
Most common cause of Gram-negative pneumonias; community acquired
Incidence: responsible for 5% of adult pneumonias
Organism: Friedländer's bacillus = encapsulated, nonmotile, Gram-negative rod
Predisposed: elderly, debilitated, alcoholic, chronic lung disease, malignancy
- bacteremia in 25%

√ propensity for posterior portion of upper lobe / superior portion of lower lobe
√ dense lobar consolidation
√ bulging of fissure (large amounts of inflammatory exudate) CHARACTERISTIC but unusual
√ empyema (one of the most common causes)
√ patchy bronchopneumonia may be present
√ uni- / multilocular cavities (50%) appearing within 4 days
√ pulmonary gangrene = infarcted tissue (rare)

Cx: meningitis, pericarditis
Prognosis: mortality rate 25 – 50%
DDx: Acute pneumococcal pneumonia (bulging of fissures, abscess + cavity formation, pleural effusion / empyema frequent)

LEGIONELLA PNEUMONIA
Organism: Legionella pneumophila, Gram-negative, weekly acid-fast, silver-impregnation stain
Predisposed: middle-aged / elderly; immunosuppressed; alcoholism; chronic obstructive lung disease, diabetes, cancer, cardiovascular disease, chronic renal failure
Clue: involvement of other organs with
- diarrhea, myalgia, toxic encephalopathy, liver + renal disease

√ patchy bronchopneumonia
√ unilateral / bilateral (less frequent)
√ lobar / segmental
√ pleural effusion (rare)
√ cavitation (rare)

LIPOID PNEUMONIA
Etiology: aspiration of vegetable / animal / mineral oil (most common)
Predisposed: elderly, debilitated, neuromuscular disease, swallowing abnormalities
Path: pool of oil surrounded by giant cell foreign body reaction (mineral oil) / initially hemorrhagic bronchopneumonia (animal fat)
- mostly asymptomatic
- fever, constitutional symptoms
Location: predilection for right middle + lower lobes
√ homogeneous segmental consolidation (most common)
√ acinar alveolar consolidation
√ reticulonodular pattern (rare)
√ paraffinoma = circumscribed peripheral mass (granulomatous reaction + fibrosis)
√ slow progression / no change

LÖFFLER SYNDROME
= disorder of unknown etiology characterized by local areas of transient parenchymal consolidation associated with blood eosinophilia
Path: interstitial + alveolar edema containing a large number of lymphocytes
- no / mild symptoms
- eosinophilia
- history of atopia
√ single / multiple areas of homogeneous ill-defined consolidation
√ uni- or bilateral, nonsegmental distribution, predominantly in lung periphery
√ transient + shifting in nature (changes within one / several days)
Prognosis: may undergo spontaneous remission

LYMPHANGIOMYOMATOSIS
= rare disorder of women in child-bearing age characterized by (1) gradually progressive diffuse interstitial lung disease (2) recurrent chylous pleural effusions (3) recurrent pneumothoraces
Age: 17 – 50 years, exclusively in women

Histo: proliferation of atypical smooth muscle in pulmonary lymphatic vessels, blood vessels and airways

Pathogenesis:
proliferated muscle obstructs bronchioles (trapping of air, overinflation, formation of cysts, pneumothorax), venules (pulmonary edema, hemorrhage, hemosiderosis), lymphatics (thickening of lymphatics, chylothorax)

May be associated with: Tuberous sclerosis (lung involvement in 1%)
- increasing shortness of breath
- disease aggravated by birth control pills
- radiologic-physiologic discrepancy = severe airflow obstruction despite relatively normal findings on CXR

Classic signs:
√ coarse reticular interstitial pattern
√ recurrent large chylous pleural effusion (50 – 75%)
√ recurrent pneumothorax (40%)
√ increasing lung volume (only interstitial disease to develop increasing lung volumes)
√ Kerley-B lines
√ pulmonary cysts + honeycombing
√ occasionally chylous ascites
CT:
√ numerous randomly scattered thin-walled cysts of various sizes surrounded by normal lung parenchyma
√ bronchovascular bundles at periphery of cyst walls
Prognosis: death within 10 years
DDx:
(1) Histiocytosis (cyst walls more variable in thickness, nodularity common)
(2) Emphysema (lobular architecture preserved with bronchovascular bundle in central position, areas of lung destruction without arcuate contour)

LYMPHANGITIC CARCINOMATOSIS

= tumor cell accumulation within lymphatics (bronchovascular bundles, interlobular septa, pleura) from tumor embolization of blood vessels followed by lymphatic obstruction, interstitial edema, and collagen deposition (fibrosis from desmoplastic reaction)
Incidence: 7% of all pulmonary metastases
Tumor origin: bronchogenic carcinoma, carcinoma of breast (56%), stomach (46%), thyroid, pancreas, larynx, cervix
mnemonic: "Certain Cancers Spread By Plugging The Lymphatics"

Cervix
Colon
Stomach
Breast
Pancreas
Thyroid
Larynx

Path: (1) interstitial edema (2) interstitial fibrotic changes (3) lymphatic dilatation (4) tumor cells within connective tissue planes

- rarely cough + hemoptysis
- dyspnea (often preceding radiographic abnormalities)
Location: bilateral; unilateral if secondary to lung primary
CXR: (accuracy 23%)
√ reticular densities
√ coarsened bronchovascular markings
√ Kerley A + B lines
√ small lung volume
√ hilar adenopathy (20 – 50%)
CT:
√ circumferentially thickened linear irregular / nodular "beaded" densities forming a reticular network
√ well-defined polygonal lines (= interlobular septa)
Prognosis: death within 1 year

LYMPHOID INTERSTITIAL PNEUMONIA

= LIP = lymphocytic infiltration of pulmonary interstitium of unknown etiology with frequently chronic + progressive course
Histo: diffuse interstitial infiltrate of lymphocytes, histiocytes, plasma cells; difficult to distinguish from lymphoma
- dyspnea + cough
- cyanosis + clubbing (50%)
- enlargement of salivary glands (20%)
- NO lymphocytosis or Hx of atopia
- monoclonal gammopathy (usually IgM)
√ fine reticular changes in both lungs
√ resembling air space disease (in severe form)
√ nodular pattern

LOCALIZED FORM = PSEUDOLYMPHOMA
associated with: Sjögren syndrome
Prognosis: occasionally progression to Non-Hodgkin Lymphoma
Rx: most patients respond well to steroids initially

LYMPHOMA

HL: contiguous spread requires scanning of abnormal area only
NHL: noncontiguous spread requires scanning of chest, abdomen, pelvis
STAGES
Stage I = limited to one / two contiguous anatomic regions on same side of diaphragm
Stage Ie = single extralymphatic organ / site
Stage II = > 2 anatomic regions / two noncontiguous regions on same side of diaphragm
Stage IIe = with extralymphatic site
Stage III = on both sides of diaphragm, not extending beyond lymph nodes, spleen (Stage IIIe), Waldeyer's ring
Stage IV = organ involvement (bone marrow, bone, lung, pleura, liver, kidney, GI tract, skin)
Substage A = absence of systemic symptoms
Substage B = fever, night sweats, pruritus, ≥ 10% weight loss

@ Thorax
   Δ   Hodgkin lymphoma more common in thorax than NHL (esp. nodular sclerosing type)
   1.   Hilar + mediastinal adenopathy
      anteromediastinal, paratracheal, hilar, subcarinal, periesophageal, paracardiac lymph node groups
   2.   Lung parenchyma involvement (HL in 12%, NHL in 4%)
      commonly localized adjacent to outer limits of radiation field
   3.   Pleural + subpleural lymphoma (up to 30%)
@ Abdomen
   1.   Periaortic adenopathy   HL in 25%
                                     NHL in 49%
   2.   Mesenteric adenopathy   HL in 4%
                                       NHL in 51%
   3.   Liver involvement   HL in 8%
                                       NHL in 14%
      √   hepatomegaly with involvement   HL in < 30%
                                       NHL in 57%
   4.   Splenic involvement   HL in 37%
                                       NHL in 41%
      HL :   most common site of abdominal involvement
      NHL: 3rd most comon site of abdominal involvement; may be initial manifestation in large cell NHL
      Δ   Staging laparotomy necessary as 2/3 of tumor nodules < 1 cm in size
   5.   Gastrointestinal involvement
      in 10% of patients with abdominal lymphoma (uncommon in HL, common in histiocytic NHL); NHL accounts for 80% of all gastric lymphomas
   6.   Urinary tract involvement
      late manifestation, most commonly in NHL
   7.   Extranodal involvement
      more frequent with histologically diffuse forms of NHL

Hodgkin Lymphoma

   40% of all lymphomas; disease of t cells
   Age: bimodal distribution at 25 – 30 years + > 70 years
   •   asymptomatic unilateral cervical adenopathy
   Histo: Reed-Sternberg cell characteristic
   1.   lymphocyte predominance: uncommon, localized, excellent prognosis, majority < 35 years
   2.   nodular sclerosis: most common, localized, good prognosis; greatest adenopathy in anterior mediastinum
   3.   mixed cellularity: more commonly abdominal than mediastinal, less favorable prognosis
   4.   lymphocyte depletion: uncommon, disseminated, older patients, rapidly fatal

@ CHEST INVOLVEMENT
   at presentation: 67% with intrathoracic disease
   Sites of lymphoid aggregates:
     1.   Lymph nodes in mediastinum
     2.   Lymph nodes at bifurcation of 1st + 2nd order bronchi

     3.   Encapsulated lymphoid collections on thoracic surface deep to parietal pleura
     4.   Unencapsulated nodules at points of divisions of more distally situated bronchi, bronchioles, and pulmonary vessels
     5.   Unencapsulated lymphoid aggregates within peribronchial connective tissue
     6.   Small accumulations of lymphocytes in interlobular septa + lymphatic channels
(a)   INTRAPULMONARY MANIFESTATIONS
     In 15 – 40% during disease duration; most commonly in nodular sclerosing type; invariably subsequent to hilar adenopathy)
     1.   Bronchovascular Form (most common type of involvement):
        √   coarse reticulonodular pattern contiguous with mediastinum = direct extension from mediastinal nodes along lymphatics
        √   nodular parenchymal lesions
        √   miliary nodules
        √   endobronchial involvement
        √   lobar atelectasis secondary to endobronchial obstruction (rare)
        √   cavitation secondary to necrosis (rare)
     2.   Subpleural Form
        √   circumscribed subpleural masses
        √   pleural effusion (20 – 50%) from lymphatic obstruction
     3.   Massive Pneumonic Form
        √   diffuse nonsegmental infiltrate (pneumonic type)
        √   massive lobar infiltrates (30%)
        √   homogeneous confluent infiltrates with shaggy borders
        √   air bronchogram
(b)   EXTRAPULMONARY MANIFESTATIONS
     1.   Mediastinal + Hilar Lymphadenopathy
        Most common manifestation, present in 90 – 99%
        Location:
            anterior mediastinal + retrosternal nodes commonly involved (DDx: sarcoidosis); 20% with mediastinal nodes have hilar adenopathy also; enlargement of a single lymph node group in 5%, bilateral in 50%
        √   CXR: on initial film adenopathy identified in 50%
        √   lymph nodes may calcify following radiation / chemotherapy
     2.   Pleural Effusion (30%)
     3.   Pleural Masses + Plaques (direct invasion from mediastinum)
Cx:
   1.   Superimposed infection
      √   consolidation with bulging borders: necrotizing bacterial pneumonia
      √   multiple nodular foci: aspergillosis + nocardiosis

√ bilateral diffuse consolidation: pneumocystis carinii
√ rapidly developing cavitation within consolidation: anaerobics / fungus
    Dx: by culture, sputum cytology, lung biopsy
2. Drug toxicity

@ BONE INVOLVEMENT (15%)
√ frequently osteoblastic (28%) = e.g., ivory vertebrae
√ osteolysis of sternum / ribs (direct invasion)
Cx: increased risk for other malignancies from aggressive therapy (Acute leukemia, NHL, Radiation-induced sarcoma)

Non-Hodgkin Lymphoma
= NHL = disease of b cells
Modified Rappaport Classification:
A. Nodular
  (a) Poorly differentiated lymphocytic (PDL)
  (b) Mixed lymphocytic / histiocytic (mixed cell)
  (c) Large cell (histiocytic)
B. Diffuse
  (a) well-differentiated lymphocytic (WDL)
  (b) intermediate-differentiated lymphocytic (IDL)
  (c) poorly differentiated lymphocytic (PDL)
  (d) mixed lymphocytic / histiocytic large cell (histiocytic) (DLCL); undifferentiated Burkitt lymphoma; undifferentiated Non-Burkitt lymphoma (pleiomorphic); lymphoblastic (LBL); unclassified

√ hilar + mediastinal adenopathy (DDx: sarcoidosis; anterior nodes favor lymphoma)
√ lung nodules + air bronchograms
√ pleural effusion

MECONIUM ASPIRATION SYNDROME
= most common cause of neonatal respiratory distress in full term / postmature infants (hyaline membrane disease most common cause in premature infants)
Etiology: fetal circulatory accidents / placental insufficiency / postmaturity result in perinatal hypoxia + fetal distress with meconium defecated in utero
Pathogenesis: meconium produces bronchial obstruction + chemical pneumonitis
Incidence: 10% of all deliveries have meconium-stained amniotic fluid, 1% of all deliveries have respiratory distress
• cyanosis (rare)
√ large infant
√ bilateral diffuse grossly patchy opacities (atelectasis + consolidation)
√ hyperinflation with areas of emphysema (air trapping)
√ spontaneous pneumothorax + pneumomediastinum (25%), requiring NO therapy
√ small pleural effusions (20%)

√ No air bronchograms
√ rapid clearing usually within 48 hours
Cx: morbidity from anoxic brain damage is high

MEDIASTINAL LIPOMATOSIS
= excess unencapsulated fat deposition
Etiology:
  (a) Exogenous steroids (average daily dose of > 30 mg prednisone): (1) chronic renal disease, renal transplant (5%) (2) collagen vascular disease, vasculitis (3) hemolytic anemia (4) asthma (5) dermatitis (6) Crohn disease (7) myasthenia gravis
  (b) Endogenous steroid elevation: (1) adrenal tumor (2) pituitary tumor / hyperplasia (3) ectopic ACTH-production (carcinoma of the lung)
  (c) Obesity
• moon facies
• buffalo hump
• supraclavicular + episternal fat
Location: upper mediastinum (common), cardiophrenic angles + paraspinal areas (less common)
√ upper mediastinal widening
√ paraspinal widening
√ increase in epicardial fat pads
√ symmetric slightly lobulated extrapleural deposits extending from apex to 9th rib laterally
OTHER FEATURES:
√ osteoporosis
√ fractures
√ aseptic necrosis
√ increased rootcoacral distance

MESOTHELIOMA
A. BENIGN MESOTHELIOMA
No direct connection to asbestos; arises from visceral > parietal pleura
Age: greatest incidence > 40
Associated with hypertrophic osteoarthropathy
√ sharply circumscribed lobular mass of 2 – 15 cm in diameter
√ obtuse angle with chest wall
√ sessile (common) / predunculated (rare)
DDx: metastatic deposit
B. MALIGNANT MESOTHELIOMA
Δ occupational exposure of asbestos found in 80% of all cases
Δ 5 – 10% of occupationally exposed subjects will develop mesothelioma (risk factor of 300 compared with general population)
Δ No relation to duration / degree of exposure or smoking history
Carcinogenic potential: crocidolite > amosite > chrysotile > antophyllite
Latent period: 20 – 40 years
Peak age: 6 – 7th decade
Histo: (a) epithelial (b) mesenchymal (c) mixed; intracellular asbestos fibers in 25%

Associated with:　peritoneal mesothelioma
- dyspnea, chest pain
- √ extensive irregular lobulated bulky pleural-based masses / pleural thickening
- √ exudative / hemorrhagic pleural effusion without mediastinal shift (fixation by pleural rind of neoplastic tissue) in 80 – 100%
- √ associated with pleural plaques in 50%
- √ circumferential encasement = involvement of all pleural surfaces (mediastinum, pericardium, fissures) as late manifestation
- √ may show rib destruction
- √ ascites (peritoneum involved in 35%)

Metastases to:
　ipsilateral lung (60%), hilar + mediastinal nodes, contralateral lung + pleura (rare), extension through chest wall + diaphragm

Prognosis:　survival < 2 years

METASTASES TO LUNG

Pulmonary metastases occur in 30% of all malignancies; mostly hematogenous

Age:　> 50 years (in 87%)

FREQUENCY:

Origin of pulmonary mets		Probability of pulmonary mets	
1. Breast	22%	Kidney	in 75%
2. Kidney	11%	Osteosarcoma	in 75%
3. Head and Neck	10%	Choriocarcinoma	in 75%
4. Colorectal	9%	Thyroid	in 65%
5. Uterus	6%	Melanoma	in 60%
6. Pancreas	5%	Breast	in 55%
7. Ovary	5%	Prostate	in 40%
8. Prostate	4%	Head and Neck	in 30%
9. Stomach	4%	Esophagus	in 20%

Incidence of pulmonary metastases:
　mnemonic　"CHEST"

Choriocarcinoma	60%
Hypernephroma / Wilms tumor	30 / 20%
Ewing sarcoma	18%
Sarcoma (osteo- / rhabdomyosarcoma)	15 / 21%
Testicular tumor	12%

- √ multiple nodules (in 75%) of varying sizes (most typical), 82% subpleural
- √ cavitated nodules (4%): (75% are squamous cell carcinomas from head and neck + GU system)
- √ calcified nodules (< 1%): osteo- and chondrosarcoma, papillary carcinoma of thyroid, ovarian carcinoma, lung metastases following radiation / chemotherapy
- √ fine micronodular pattern: highly vascular tumor (renal cell, breast, thyroid, prostate carcinoma, bone sarcoma, choriocarcinoma)
- √ pneumothorax (2%): especially in children with bone tumors

CT:
- √ noncalcified multiple (> 10) round lesions > 2.5 cm likely to be metastatic

√ connection to pulmonary arterial branches

SOLITARY METASTATIC NODULE
- Δ a solitary lung nodule represents a primary lung tumor In 62% in patients with known Hx of neoplasm
- Δ 5% of all solitary nodules are metastatic; most likely origin: colon carcinoma (30 – 40%), osteosarcoma, renal cell carcinoma, testicular tumor, breast carcinoma

CALCIFYING METASTASES
　mnemonic:　"BOTTOM"
　Breast
　Osteosarcoma
　Thyroid
　Testicular
　Ovarian
　Mucinous adenocarcinoma

MUCORMYCOSIS
= PHYCOMYCOSIS = caused by a variety of phycomycetes (soil fungi)

Organisms:　Mucor (most common), Absidia, Rhizopus, cause severe vascular obstruction

Predisposed:　diabetics, immunocompromised (lymphoma, leukemia)

Opportunistic infection in:
1. Lymphoproliferative malignancies and leukemia
2. Acidotic diabetes mellitus
3. Immunosuppression through steroids, antibiotics, immunosuppressive drugs (rare)

A. RHINOCEREBRAL FORM
= involvement of paranasal sinuses (frontal sinus usually spared) with extension into:
　(a) orbit = orbital cellulitis
　(b) base of skull = meningoencephalitis + cerebritis

B. PULMONARY FORM
　Histo:　invasion of blood vessels
- √ segmental homogeneous consolidation
- √ cavitation
- √ nodules (from arterial thrombi + infarction)

DDx:　aspergillosis

MYCOPLASMA PNEUMONIA
= PRIMARY ATYPICAL PNEUMONIA (PAP) commonest cause of nonbacterial pneumonia with a mild course (only 2% require hospitalization), usually lasts 2 – 3 weeks; only 10% of infected subjects develop pneumonia

Incidence:　10 – 33% of all pneumonias; autumn peak

Organism:　Eaton agent = pleuropneumonia-like organism (PPLO)

Age:　most common in ages 5 – 20 years (esp. in closed populations)
- mild symptoms of cough + low fever, malaise, otitis
- mild leukocytosis (20%)
- most common respiratory cause of cold agglutinin production (60%)

√ radiologic findings often diverge from clinical condition
√ pulmonary infiltrates show a significant lag time
√ fine interstitial infiltration from hilum into lower lobe (earliest change)
√ alveolar infiltrates: unilateral (L > R) air-space consolidation in segmental lower lobe in 50%, bilateral in 10 – 40%,
√ small pleural effusions in 20%
√ hilar adenopathy (rare)
Cx: (1) Meningoencephalitis
   (2) Erythema nodosum, Erythema multiforme, Stevens-Johnson syndrome
Prognosis: 20% with recurrent symptoms of pharyngitis + bronchitis ± infiltrations

NEAR DROWNING
1. SEA WATER DROWNING
   • hemoconcentration, hypovolemia
2. FRESH WATER DROWNING
   • hemodilution, hypervolemia
   • hemolysis
3. SECONDARY DROWNING
   (a) pneumonia with toxic debris
   (b) progressive pulmonary edema
4. DRY DROWNING (20 – 40%)
   = laryngeal spasm prevents water from entering
   √ no roentgenographic abnormality
Similarities of all 4 types:
   • hypoxemia
   • metabolic acidosis
   √ pulmonary edema
   √ hyaline membrane formation = considerable loss of protein from blood

NEONATAL PNEUMONIA
Pathogenesis:
   (a) in utero infection (ascending from premature rupture of membranes or prolonged labor / transplacental route)
   (b) aspiration of infected vaginal secretions during delivery
   (c) infection after birth
Organism:
   (1) Group B Streptococcus (GBS): in low birth-weight premature infants; 50% mortality
      √ radiographic picture may be identical to RDS (in 52%)
      √ appearance suggesting retained lung fluid / focal infiltrates (35%)
      √ normal CXR (13%)
      √ cardiomegaly
      √ pleural effusions (in 2/3, but RARE in RDS)
      √ delayed onset diaphragmatic hernia (evidenced by clinical deterioration)
   (2) Pneumococci: RDS-like
   (3) Listeria: RDS-like
   (4) Candida: progressive consolidation + cavitation
   (5) Chlamydia: bronchopneumonic pattern

• afebrile
• lower ventilatory pressure requirements
√ bilateral focal / diffuse areas of opacities (may initially appear similar to fetal aspiration syndrome)
√ hyperaeration
√ may cause lobar atelectasis
√ may cause pneumothorax / pneumomediastinum
√ pleural effusion (exceedingly rare)

NOCARDIOSIS
Organism: Gram-positive acid fast bacterium resembling fungus
Predisposed: immunocompromised
√ multiple poorly / well-defined nodules ± cavitation
√ lobar consolidation
√ empyema without sinus tracts
√ SVC obstruction rare

PERICARDIAL CYST
secondary to defect in embryogenesis of coelomic cavities; M = F
Histo: lined by single layer of mesothelial cells
Location: 75% at cardiophrenic angle (R:L = 3:1), 25% higher; may extend into major fissure
√ mass of 3 – 8 cm (range 1 – 28 cm) in diameter
√ change in size + shape with respiration / body position

POLYARTERITIS NODOSA
= PERIARTERITIS NODOSA = systemic vasculitis of small + medium-sized arteries + arterioles characterized by necrotizing granulomas of all wall layers
usually in male adults
• associated with hepatitis B antigenemia
• systemic hypertension
@ Renal involvement (80%): aneurysms
@ Chest involvement (70%)
   √ cardiac enlargement / pericardial effusion (14%)
   √ pleural effusion (14%)
   √ pulmonary venous engorgement (21%)
   √ massive pulmonary edema (4%)
   √ linear densities / plate-like atelectasis (10%)
   √ wedge-shaped / round peripheral infiltrates of nonsegmental distribution (14%) (simulating thromboembolic disease with infarction)
   √ cavitation may occur
   √ interstitial lower lung field pneumonitis

PNEUMATOCELE
= cystic air collection within lung parenchyma due to obstructive overinflation
Δ does not indicate destruction of lung parenchyma
Δ occurs during healing phase
Δ appears to enlarge while patient improves
Δ frequently multiple
Developmental theories:
   (1) result of severe distension of small bronchioles secondary to check-valve endobronchial / peribronchial obstruction

(2) communication between ruptured peribronchial abscess + bronchus with check-valve obstruction
(3) subpleural collection of air formed by dissection of air from ruptured alveoli / bronchioles

A. PNEUMATOCELE ASSOCIATED WITH INFECTION
Organism: Pneumococci, E. coli, Klebsiella, Staphylococcus (in childhood)
√ appears within 1st week, disappears within 6 weeks
√ thin-walled + completely air-filled cavity
√ ± air-fluid level + wall thickening (during infection)
√ pneumothorax
√ spontaneous resolution (in most)

B. TRAUMATIC PNEUMATOCELE = PNEUMATOCYST
(a) appearance within hours after blunt chest trauma with lung hematoma
(b) hydrocarbon (furniture polish, kerosene) inhalation
√ single / multiple pneumatoceles
√ spontaneous resolution over several weeks to months

PNEUMOCOCCAL PNEUMONIA
Most common Gram-positive pneumonia
90% community-acquired, 10% nosocomial
Incidence: 15% of all adulthood pneumonias, uncommon in child; peaks in winter + early spring; increased during influenza epidemics
Organism: Streptococcus pneumoniae (formerly Diplococcus pneumoniae), Gram-positive, encapsulated, in pairs / chains, capsular polysaccharide responsible for virulence + serotyping
Susceptible: elderly, debilitated, alcoholics, CHF, COPD, multiple myeloma, hypogammaglobulinemia, functional / surgical asplenia
• rusty blood-streaked sputum
• left-shift leukocytosis
• impaired pulmonary function
Location: usually involves one lobe only; bias for lower lobes + posterior segments of upper lobes (bacteria flow under gravitational influence to most dependent portions as in aspiration)
√ extensive air-space consolidation abutting against visceral pleura (lobar / beyond confines of one lobe through pores of Kohn), CHARACTERISTIC
√ slight expansion of involved lobes
√ prominent air bronchograms (20%)
√ patchy bronchopneumonic pattern (in some)
√ pleural effusion (parapneumonic transsudate) uncommon with antibiotic therapy
√ cavitation (rare, with Type III)
Variations (modified by bronchopulmonary disease, e.g., chronic bronchitis, emphysema)
√ bronchopneumonia-like pattern
√ effusion may be only presentation (esp. in COPD)

√ empyema (with persistent fever)
Δ in children:
√ round pneumonia = sharply defined round lesion
Prognosis: prompt response to antibiotics (if without complications); 5% mortality rate
Dx: blood culture (positive in 30%)
Cx: meningitis, endocarditis, septic arthritis, empyema (now rarely seen)

PNEUMOCYSTOSIS
Most common cause of interstitial pneumonia in immuno-compromised patients which quickly leads to air space disease.
Organism: protozoan Pneumocystis carinii; often associated with simultaneous infection by CMV, mycobacterium avium-intracellulare, herpes simplex
Predisposed:
(1) debilitated premature infants, children with hypogammaglobulinemia (12%)
(2) immunocompromised patients: congenital immunodeficiency syndrome, AIDS (60 – 80%), lymphoproliferative disorders, organ transplant recipients (renal transplant patients in 10%), patients on long-term corticosteroid therapy (nephrotic syndrome, collagen vascular disease), patients on cytotoxic drugs [under therapy for leukemia (40%), lymphoma (16%)]
• severe dyspnea + cyanosis
• WBC slightly elevated (PMNs)
• lymphopenia (50%) heralds poor prognosis
√ bilateral + diffuse changes of perihilar + basilar distribution with sparing of apices (CHARACTERISTIC central location)
√ linear / reticular pattern (early changes)
√ "ground glass" = eventual progression to diffuse alveolar homogeneous consolidation (DDx: pulmonary edema)
√ air bronchogram
√ patchy localized consolidation (occasional presentation)
√ pleural effusion (uncommon)
√ No hilar lymphadenopathy
CT:
√ patchwork pattern (56%)
= bilateral asymmetric patchy mosaic appearance with sparing of segments / subsegments of pulmonary lobe
√ groundglass pattern (26%)
= bilateral diffuse symmetric airspace disease (fluid + inflammatory cells in alveolar space)
√ interstitial pattern (18%)
= bilateral symmetric / asymmetric, linear / reticular markings (thickening of lobular septa)
√ bullae + thin-walled cysts (38%)
√ pneumothorax (13%)
√ lymph adenopathy (18%)
√ pleural effusion (18%)
√ pulmonary nodules
usually due to malignancy (leukemia, lymphoma, Kaposi sarcoma, metastasis) / septic emboli

√ pulmonary cavities
usually due to superimposed fungal / mycobacterial infection

NUC:
√ Ga-67 uptake prior to roentgenographic changes

Dx: (1) sputum collection (2) bronchoscopy with lavage (3) transbronchial / transthoracic / open lung Bx

Prognosis: rapid fulminant disease; death within 2 weeks

PNEUMONECTOMY CHEST

Early signs (within 24 hours):
√ partial filling of thorax
√ ipsilateral mediastinal shift + diaphragmatic elevation

Late signs (after 2 months):
√ complete obliteration of space

N.B.: depression of diaphragm / shift of mediastinum to contralateral side indicates a bronchopleural fistula / empyema / hemorrhage !

POSTOBSTRUCTIVE PNEUMONIA

= chronic inflammatory disease distal to bronchial obstruction

Causes:
1. Bronchogenic carcinoma (most commonly)
2. Bronchial adenoma
3. Granular cell myoblastoma (almost always tracheal lesion)
4. Bronchostenosis

Histo: "golden pneumonia" = cholesterol pneumonia = endogenous lipid pneumonia = mixture of edema, atelectasis, round cell infiltration, bronchiectasis, liberation of lipid material from alveolar pneumocytes secondary to inflammatory reaction

√ frequently associated with some degree of atelectasis
√ persists unchanged for weeks
√ recurrent pneumonia in same region after antibiotic treatment

PROGRESSIVE MASSIVE FIBROSIS

= (PMF) = COMPLICATED PNEUMOCONIOSIS
= CONGLOMERATE ANTHRACOSILICOSIS

May develop / progress after cessation of dust exposure

Path: avascular amorphous central mass of insoluble proteins stabilized by cross-links + ill-defined bundles of coarse hyalinized collagen at periphery

Location: almost exclusively restricted to posterior segment of upper lobe / superior segment of lower lobe

√ large > 1 cm opacities initially in middle + upper lung zones at periphery of lung
√ discoid contour (44%) = mass flat from front to back (thin opacity on lateral view, large opacity on PA view), medial border often ill-defined, lateral borders sharp + parallel to rib cage
√ migration toward hila starting at lung periphery; bilateral symmetry

√ apparent decrease in nodularity (incorporation of nodules from surroundings)
√ cavitation (occasionally) due to ischemic necrosis / superimposed TB infection
√ bullous scar emphysema
√ pulmonary hypertension

PSEUDOLYMPHOMA

= reactive benign lesion resembling lymphoma histologically without lymph node involvement = localized form of lymphocytic interstitial pneumonitis (LIP); no progression to lymphoma
• mostly asymptomatic
√ well-demarcated dense infiltrate
√ infiltrate typically in central location extending to visceral pleura
√ prominent air bronchogram
√ NO lymphadenopathy

PSEUDOMONAS PNEUMONIA

= most dreaded nosocomial infection because of resistance to antibiotics in patients with debilitating diseases on multiple antibiotics + corticosteroids; rare in community

Organism: Pseudomonas aeruginosa, Gram-negative
• bradycardia
• temperature with morning peaks
√ widespread patchy bronchopneumonia (secondary to bacteremia; unlike other Gram-negative pneumonias)
√ predilection for lower lobes
√ extensive bilateral consolidation
√ "sponge-like pattern" with multiple nodules > 2 cm (= extensive necrosis with formation of multiple abscesses)
√ small pleural effusions

PULMONARY APLASIA

= rudimentary bronchus in blind pouch with absence of parenchyma + vessels

Agenesis = complete absence of tissue
Aplasia = bronchus without lung tissue
Hypoplasia = bronchus with rudimentary lung tissue

Incidence: 1:10,000; R:L = 1:1

Associated malformations:
1. hypoplasia of contralateral lung
2. diaphragmatic hernia
3. surrounding calcified pleura

• asymptomatic
√ dense small hemithorax with marked mediastinal shift + herniation of contralateral lung

CT:
√ absence of ipsilateral pulmonary artery + bronchus ending blindly
√ absence of ipsilateral pulmonary tissue

PULMONARY ARTERIAL MALFORMATION

= PAVM = PULMONARY ARTERIOVENOUS ANEURYSM = PULMONARY ARTERIOVENOUS

FISTULA = PULMONARY ANGIOMA = PULMONARY TELANGIECTASIA

= abnormal vascular communication between pulmonary artery and vein (95%) or systemic artery and pulmonary vein (5%)

Etiology:
(a) congenital defect of capillary structure
(b) acquired in cirrhosis (hepatogenic pulmonary angiodysplasia), cancer, trauma, surgery, actinomycosis, schistosomiasis

Path: hemangioma of cavernous type
Age: 3 – 4th decade; manifest in adult life, 10% in childhood

Occurrence:
(a) isolated abnormality (40%)
(b) associated with Osler-Weber-Rendu syndrome (in 30 – 88%) = Hereditary hemorrhagic telangiectasia; only 15% of patients with Osler-Weber-Rendu disease have pulmonary AVMs
  • family history
  • epistaxis
  • telangiectasia of skin / mucous membranes
  • GI bleeding

Types:
1. Simple type (79%)
   = single feeding artery empties into a bulbous nonseptated aneurysmal segment with a single draining vein
2. Complex type (21%)
   = more than one feeding artery empties into septated aneurysmal segment with more than one draining vein
• asymptomatic in 56% (until 3 – 4th decade) if AVM single and < 2 cm
• orthodeoxia (= increased hypoxemia with $PaO_2 < 85$ mmHg in erect position)
• cyanosis with normal-sized heart (R-to-L shunt) in 25 – 50%, clubbing
• bruit over lesion (increased during inspiration)
• dyspnea on exertion (60 – 71%)
• epistaxis (79%)
• palpitation, chest pain
• No CHF

Location: lower lobes (65 – 70%) > middle lobe > upper lobes; medial third of lung; often subpleural; bilateral (8 – 20%)
√ sharply defined, lobulated oval / round mass (90%) of 1 to several cm in size
√ cord-like bands from mass to hilum (feeding artery + draining veins)
√ 2/3 single, 1/3 multiple lesions
√ enlargement with advancing age
√ change in size with Valsalva / Mueller maneuver / erect vs. recumbent position (decrease with Valsalva maneuver)
√ phleboliths (occasionally)
√ increased pulsations of hilar vessels

CT:
√ vascular connection of mass with enlarged feeding artery + draining vein
√ rapid vascular enhancement pattern on dynamic CT
MRI: (contraindication to contrast / slow flow due to partial thrombosis / follow-up)
√ signal void on standard spin echo / high signal intensity on GRASS images
Cx: (1) Cerebrovascular accident: stroke (18%), transient ischemic attack (37%)
(2) Brain abscess (9%) secondary to loss of pulmonary filter function
(3) Hemoptysis in (13%) secondary to rupture of PAVM into bronchus, most common presenting symptom
(4) Hemothorax (9%) secondary to rupture of subpleural PAVM
(5) Polycythemia
Prognosis: 26% morbidity, 11% mortality
DDx: solitary / multiple pulmonary nodules
Rx: embolization with coils / detachable balloons

PULMONARY CONTUSION

= most common manifestation of blunt chest trauma, esp. deceleration trauma
Path: exudation of edema + blood into air space + interstitium
Time of onset: apparent within 6 hours after trauma
• clinically inapparent
• hemoptysis (50%)
Location: directly deep to site of impact / contrecoup
√ irregular patchy / diffuse homogeneous extensive consolidation
√ opacity may enlarge for 48 – 72 hours
√ rapid resolution beginning 24 – 48 hours, complete within 2 – 10 days
√ overlying rib fractures (frequent)
DDx: fat embolism (1 – 2 days after injury)

PULMONARY HYPOPLASIA

= completely formed but small bronchus affecting one lobe /entire lung with rudimentary parenchyma + small vessels
Causes:
(a) Extrathoracic compression
  1. Oligohydramnios
  2. Fetal ascites
  3. Membranous diaphragm
(b) Thoracic cage compression
  1. Thoracic dystrophies
  2. Muscular disease
(c) Intrathoracic compression
  1. Diaphragmatic defect
  2. Excess pleural fluid
  3. Large intrathoracic cyst / tumor
(d) Primary hypoplasia
  = idiopathic
• respiratory distress at birth

√ poorly expanded lungs
√ contralateral mediastinal shift (in unilateral process)

PULMONARY INTERSTITIAL EMPHYSEMA
= PIE = complication of respirator therapy with PEEP
Pathogenesis:
gas escapes from overdistended alveolus, dissects into perivascular sheath surrounding arteries, veins, and lymphatics, tracks into mediastinum forming clusters of blebs; AIRBLOCK = compression + obstruction of pulmonary veins + mediastinal structures by interstitial pulmonary emphysema / pneumomediastinum / pneumothorax (obstruction esp. during expiration)

• sudden deterioration in patient's condition during respiratory therapy
√ elongated lucencies following distribution of bronchovascular tree
√ circular densities
√ bilateral, symmetrical distribution
√ lobar overdistension (occasionally)
Cx: pneumomediastinum, pneumothorax, subcutaneous emphysema, pneumopericardium, intracardiac air, pneumoperitoneum, pneumatosis intestinalis

PULMONARY MAINLINE GRANULOMATOSIS
= pulmonary embolism in drug addicts from IV injection of oral medication
Drugs: amphetamines, methylphenidate hydrochloride ("Westcoast"), tripelenamine ("blue velvet"), methadone hydrochloride, dilaudid, meperidine, pentazocine, propylhexedrine, hydromorphone hydrochloride
Δ added talc (= magnesium silicate) particles incite a granulomatous foreign body reaction + subsequent fibrosis in perivascular distribution
• angiothrombotic pulmonary hypertension + cor pulmonale
√ widespread micronodularity of "pinpoint" size (1 mm) with perihilar / basilar predominance
√ loss of lung volume
√ coalescent opacities similar to progressive massive fibrosis (DDx: in silicosis away from hila)

PULMONARY THROMBOEMBOLIC DISEASE
= PULMONARY EMBOLISM (PE)
Incidence: 600,000 cases/year; in 9 – 56% of deep venous thrombosis; diagnosed in 1% of all hospitalized patients; in 12 – 64% at autopsy
Δ only 10 – 33% of patients with fatal PE are symptomatic for DVT
Δ DVT diagnosed ante mortem in < 30%
Δ clinically suspected diagnosis accurate in 26 – 45%
Δ 30% of patients with angiographically detected PE have negative bilateral venograms ("big bang" theory = clot embolizes in toto to lung leaving no residual in leg veins)

Age peak: > 70 years
Cause: deep vein thrombosis (DVT)
Pathophysiology:
Class 1 = < 20% of pulmonary arteries occluded
• asymptomatic
• normal arterial blood gas levels
• normal pulmonary + systemic hemodynamics
Class 2 = 20 – 30% of pulmonary arteries occluded
• anxiety, hyperventilation
• arterial PO_2 < 80 torr
• PCO_2 < 35 torr
Class 3 = 30 – 50% of pulmonary arteries occluded
• dyspnea, collapse
• arterial PO_2 < 65 torr
• arterial PCO_2 < 30 torr
• elevated central venous pressure
Class 4 = > 50% of pulmonary arteries occluded
• shock, dyspnea
• arterial PO_2 < 50 torr
• arterial PCO_2 < 30 torr
• elevated central venous pressure
• mean PA pressure > 20 mm Hg
• systolic blood pressure < 100 mm Hg
• Classic triad (< 33%):
(1) hemoptysis (25 – 34%) (2) pleural friction rub (3) thrombophlebitis
• may be asymptomatic
• false-positive clinical diagnosis in 62%
• dyspnea (81 – 86%)
• pleuritic chest pain (58 – 72%)
• apprehension (59%)
• cough (54 – 70%)
• tachycardia, tachypnea
• accentuated 2nd heart sound
• ECG changes (83%), mostly nonspecific
• bronchospasm (histamine-mediated), bronchial plugging, rales (loss of surfactant)
Sites of PE: lower lobes (> 50%), upper lobes (10%); bilateral (42%); multiple (65%)

RESOLUTION OF PE
(through thrombolysis + fragmentation):
in 8% by 24 hours, in 56% by 14 days, in 77% by 7 months; complete in 65%, partial in 23%, no resolution in 12%;
Δ resolution less favorable with increasing age + cardiac disease
Δ improved with urokinase > heparin within first week (after 1 year 80% for both)

A. EMBOLISM WITHOUT INFARCTION (90%)
Histo: hemorrhage + edema
√ normal chest film common (> 29%), abnormal CXR in 40 – 93%
√ platelike atelectasis
√ focal oligemia (vasoconstriction) distal to embolus (Westermark sign in 2%)
√ "knuckle sign" = abrupt tapering of an occluded vessel distally

√ local widening of artery by impaction of embolus
√ segmental / lobar consolidation
√ pleural effusion
B. EMBOLISM WITH INFARCTION (10 – 15%)
= any opacity developing as a result of thromboembolic disease; more likely to develop in presence of cardiopulmonary disease with obstruction of pulmonary venous outflow (diagnosed in retrospect)
Histo: (1) reversible hemorrhagic congestion
(2) hemorrhagic infarction with necrosis
√ segmentally distributed wedge-shaped consolidation (54%)
√ may cavitate
√ Hampton hump = pleural-based shallow consolidation in form of a truncated cone with base against pleural surface
√ pleural effusion (54%)
√ thoracentesis: bloody (65%), predominantly PMNs (61%), exudate (65%)
√ NO air-bronchogram (hemorrhage into alveoli)
√ "melting sign" = within few days to weeks regression from periphery toward center
√ Fleischner lines = long-line shadows (fibrotic scar) from invagination of pleura at the base of the collapse resulting in pseudofissure
√ platelike atelectasis (27%)
√ cardiomegaly / CHF (17%)
√ elevated hemidiaphragm (17%)
√ subsequent nodular / linear scar
CT:
√ pleural-based triangular appearance of lesion
√ vascular connection to a branch of pulmonary artery
√ peripheral rim-like contrast enhancement
NUC (V/Q scan = guide for angiographic evaluation)
Angio (indicated within 24 hours of indeterminate NUC scan):
√ intraluminal defect (94%)
√ abrupt termination of pulmonary arterial branch
√ pruning + attenuation of branches
√ wedge-shaped parenchymal hypovascularity
√ absence of draining vein in affected segment
√ tortuous arterial collaterals
Cx of pulmonary angiography (4%): arrhythmia, endocardial injury, cardiac perforation, cardiac arrest, contrast reaction
Mortality: 3:1,000 surgical procedures; 7% of all autopsies; 26% if untreated; 8% if treated; fatal if > 60% of pulmonary bed obstructed
Fatality rate: 0.2%

Acute thromboembolic pulmonary arterial hypertension
hypertension disappears as emboli lyse
• sudden onset of chest pain
• acute dyspnea
• hemoptysis occasionally

Prognosis: healthy patients may survive obstruction of 50 – 60% of vascular bed

Chronic thromboembolic pulmonary arterial hypertension
• Hx of previous embolic episodes
• may be clinically silent

PULMONARY VARIX
= abnormal tortuosity + dilatation of pulmonary vein just before entrance into left atrium
Etiology: congenital / associated with pulmonary venous hypertension
Location: medial third of either lung below hila
√ well-defined lobulated round / oval mass
√ change in size during Valsalva / Mueller maneuver

RADIATION PNEUMONITIS
= damage to lungs following radiation therapy dependent on:
(a) irradiated lung volume
(b) radiation dose: unusual < 2000 R given in 2 – 3 weeks; common > 6000 R given in 5 – 6 weeks
(c) number of fractions
(d) associated chemotherapy
Pathologic phases:
(1) Exudative phase = edema fluid + hyaline membranes
(2) Organizing phase
(3) Fibrotic phase = interstitial fibrosis
Time of onset: usually 4 – 6 months after treatment
Location: confined to radiation port

1. ACUTE RADIATION PNEUMONITIS
(1 month after radiation therapy)
Path: depletion of surfactant (1 week to 1 month later), plasma exudation, desquamation of alveolar + bronchial cells
• nonproductive cough, shortness of breath, weakness, fever (insidious onset)
√ changes usually within portal entry fields
√ patchy / confluent consolidation, may persist up to 1 month (exudative reaction)
√ atelectasis + air bronchogram
Prognosis: recovery / progression to death
Rx: steroids
2. CHRONIC RADIATION DAMAGE
(9 – 12 months after radiation therapy)
Histo: permanent damage of endothelial + type I alveolar cells
√ severe loss of volume
√ dense fibrous strands from hilum to periphery
√ thickening of pleura
√ pericardial effusion

RESPIRATORY DISTRESS SYNDROME OF NEW-BORN
= RDS = HYALINE MEMBRANE DISEASE

= immature surfactant production (usually begins at 24 weeks of gestational age) causing acinar atelectasis + dilatation of terminal airways

Predisposed:
   perinatal asphyxia, cesarean section, infants of diabetic mothers, premature infants (< 1000 g in 66%; 1000 g in 50%; 1500 g in 16%; 2000 g in 5%; 2500 g in 1%)
Onset: < 2 – 5 hours after birth, M:F = 1.8 : 1
• abnormal retraction of chest wall
• cyanosis
• expiratory grunting
• increased respiratory rate
√ hypoaeration with loss of lung volume (counteracted by respirator therapy)
√ reticulogranular pattern (coincides with onset of clinical signs)
√ prominent air bronchograms (distension of compliant airways)
√ bilateral + symmetrical distribution
Prognosis: spontaneous clearing within 7 – 10 days (mild course in untreated survivors)
ACUTE COMPLICATIONS
   (a) Barotrauma with air-block phenomena
      1. Parenchymal pseudocyst
      2. Pulmonary interstitial emphysema
      3. Pneumomediastinum, -thorax, -pericardium, -peritoneum, -retroperitoneum
      4. Subcutaneous emphysema
      5. Gas embolism
   (b) Diffuse opacity
      1. Worsening RDS
      2. Superimposed pneumonia
      3. Massive aspiration
      4. Pulmonary hemorrhage
      5. Congestive heart failure (PDA, fluid overload)
   (c) Persistent patency of ductus arteriosus
      oxygen stimulus is missing to close duct; gradual decrease in pulmonary resistance (by end of 1st week) leads to L-to-R shunt through PDA
   (d) Hemorrhage
      1. Pulmonary hemorrhage
      2. Intracranial hemorrhage
   (e) Necrotizing enterocolitis
   (f) Acute renal failure

CHRONIC COMPLICATIONS
   1. Lobar emphysema
   2. Localized interstitial emphysema
   3. Delayed onset of diaphragmatic hernia
   4. Recurrent inspiratory tract infections
   5. Hyperinflation
   6 Bronchopulmonary dysplasia
   7. Retrolental fibroplasia
   8. Subglottic stenosis (intubation)

RHEUMATOID LUNG
Type III hypersensitivity = delayed hypersensitivity
= immune complex disease

= formation of antigen-antibody complexes with complement fixation
Incidence: 2 – 54% of patients with rheumatoid arthritis; M >> F
                 (incidence of rheumatoid arthritis: M < F)
• rheumatoid arthritis
• subcutaneous nodules
• rheumatoid factor = IgM-antibody (positive in most) (DDx: In 5% of normals, in 25% of asbestos workers with fibrosing alveolitis)
• antinuclear antibodies (positive in many)
• LE cells (positive in some)

Stage 1:   multifocal ill-defined alveolar infiltrates
Stage 2:   fine interstitial reticulations (histio- and lymphocytes)
Stage 3:   honeycombing

A. Pleural abnormalities (most frequent manifestation)
   • Hx of pleurisy (21%)
   √ pleural effusion (3%): unilateral (92%), with little change over months; M:F = 9:1; most often without other pulmonary changes, may antedate rheumatoid arthritis
      • high in protein content (> 4 g/dl)
      • low in sugar content (< 30 mg/dl) without rise during glucose infusion (75%)
      • high in lymphocytes
      • positive for rheumatoid factor, LDH, RA cells
   √ pleural thickening, usually bilateral
B. Diffuse interstitial fibrosis (30%)
   • restrictive ventilatory defect
   Location: lower lung fields
   √ punctate / nodular densities (mononuclear cell infiltrates in early stage)
   √ reticulonodular densities
   √ medium to coarse reticulations (mature fibrous tissue in later stage)
   √ honeycomb lung (uncommon late stage)
C. Necrobiotic nodules (rare)
   = well-circumscribed nodular mass in lungs, pleura, pericardium identical to subcutaneous nodules associated with advanced rheumatoid arthritis
   Path: central zone of fibrinoid necrosis surrounded by palisading fibroblasts
   associated with interstitial lung disease
   √ well-circumscribed usually multiple nodules of 3 – 70 mm in size
   √ commonly located in lung periphery
   √ cavitation with thick symmetric walls + smooth inner lining (common)
D. Caplan syndrome
   = RHEUMATOID PNEUMOCONIOSIS
   = pneumoconiosis + rheumatoid arthritis in coal-workers with rheumatoid disease;
   = hypersensitivity reaction to irritating dust particles in lungs of rheumatoid patients
   Incidence: 2 – 6% of all men affected by pneumoconioses

Path: disintegrating macrophages deposit a
pigmented ring of dust surrounding the
central necrotic core + zone of fibroblasts
palisading the zone of necrosis
Δ NOT necessarily evidence of long-standing
pneumoconiosis
• concomitant with joint manifestation (most frequent)
/ may precede arthritis by several years
• concomitant with systemic rheumatoid nodules
√ rapidly developing well-defined nodules of 5 –
50 mm in size with a tendency to appear in crops
predominantly in upper lobes + in periphery of lung
√ nodules may remain unchanged / increase in
number / calcify
√ background of pneumoconiosis
√ pleural effusion (may occur)
E. Pulmonary arteritis
= fibroelastoid intimal proliferation of pulmonary
arteries
• pulmonary arterial hypertension
• cor pulmonale
F. Obliterative bronchitis – may be transient
G. Cardiac enlargement (pericarditis + carditis /
congestive heart failure)

ROUND PNEUMONIA
= NUMMULAR PNEUMONIA = fairly spherical pneumonia
caused by pyogenic organisms
Organism: Haemophilus influenzae, Streptococcus,
Pneumococcus
Age: children >> adults
• cough, chest pain, fever
Location: always posterior, usually in lower lobes
√ spherical infiltrate with slightly fluffy borders + air
bronchogram
√ triangular abutting a pleural surface (usually on lateral
view)
√ rapid change in size and shape

SARCOIDOSIS
= BOECK SARCOID = immunologically mediated
widespread formation of noncaseating granulomas of
unknown etiology
Prevalence: 1:10,000
Age peak: 20 – 40 years; M:F=1:3;
Blacks:Caucasians = 14:1
• Angiotensin-converting enzyme (ACE) elevated in 70%
• Hypercalcemia in 2 – 15% from enhanced sensitivity to
vitamin D
• Kveim test positive (70%), rarely used today
• Functional impairment: VC + FRC reduced, diffusing
capacity decreased, reduction in compliance (even with
NO radiographic abnormality)
A. ACUTE FORM = **Löfgren Syndrome**
bilateral hilar adenopathy + fever (17%), erythema
nodosum (13%), arthralgia of large joints
B. CHRONIC FORM
• asymptomatic (50%)

• fever, malaise, weight loss
• dry cough + shortness of breath (25%)
• hemoptysis in 4% (from endobronchial lesion /
vascular erosion / cavitation)
Prognosis:
75% complete resolution of hilar adenopathy
33% complete resolution of parenchymal disease
30% improve significantly
20% irreversible pulmonary fibrosis (may persist
unchanged for > 15 years)
10% mortality (cor pulmonale / CNS / lung fibrosis / liver
cirrhosis)
25% relapse (in 50% detected by CXR)
@ Bone (6 – 15%)   : √ phalangeal sclerosis of hands
√ lytic cystic lesions with lacelike
trabecular pattern
@ Liver   (25 – 70%)
@ Spleen (25 – 70%): splenomegaly
@ Skin   (10 – 60%): erythema nodosum, lupus pernio
(slightly raised purplish nodules)
@ Muscle (25%)   : myopathy
@ Eyes   (10 – 25%): uveitis
@ CNS   (9%)   : hypothalamus, basal
granulomatous meningitis, facial
nerve palsy
@ Myocardium (6 – 20%): paroxysmal arrhythmia, heart
block, cardiomyopathy
@ Salivary gland (4%): bilateral parotid enlargement
@ Involved peripheral lymph nodes (30%)
@ INTRATHORACIC DISEASE (90%)
Associated with tuberculosis in up to 13%
— adenopathy alone (43%)
— adenopathy + parenchymal disease (41%)
— parenchymal disease alone (16%)
√ Intrathoracic lymphadenopathy (80%)
Location:
(a) "1-2-3 sign" = Garland triad = right
paratracheal, right + left hilar groups most
frequent combination in 75 – 90%)
(b) unilateral hilar enlargement (3 – 8%)
(c) mediastinal nodes are regularly enlarged on
CT
Prognosis:
adenopathy commonly decreases as parenchymal
disease gets worse; subsequent parenchymal
disease in 32%; adenopathy does not develop
subsequent to parenchymal disease;
√ egg-shell calcification of lymph nodes (5%) in long-
standing sarcoidosis > 10 years
√ Parenchymal disease (60%); without adenopathy in
20%
Δ parenchymal granulomas are invariably present on
open lung biopsy
Site: predominantly mid-zone involvement
√ reticulonodular pattern (46%)
√ acinar pattern (20%) = ill-defined 6 – 7 mm
opacities/ coalescence

√ "alveolar / acinar sarcoidosis" = multiple large
nodules > 10 mm (2 – 10%) ± air bronchogram
(coalescence of numerous interstitial granulomas)
√ progressive fibrosis with upper lobe retraction +
bullae (20%)
√ end stage lung (11%)

ATYPICAL MANIFESTATIONS (25%):
√ pleural effusion (2%) = exudate with predominance
of lymphocytes
√ focal pleural thickening
√ solitary / multiple pulmonary nodule
√ cavitation of nodules (0.6%)
√ mycetoma formation (common complication of
advanced sarcoidosis)
√ isolated hilar / mediastinal nodal enlargement
√ bronchostenosis (2%) with lobar / segmental
atelectasis
√ pulmonary arterial hypertension (periarterial
granulomatosis without extensive pulmonary
fibrosis)
Cx: √ pneumothorax secondary to chronic lung
fibrosis (rare)
√ cardiomegaly from cor pulmonale (rare)

ASSESSMENT OF ACTIVITY
(1) ACE titer (= angiotensin I converting enzyme)
(2) Bronchopulmonary lavage: 20 – 50% lymphocytes
with number of T-suppressor lymphocytes 4 – 20
times above normal
(3) Gallium scan
√ uptake in lymph nodes + lung parenchyma +
salivary glands (correlates with alveolitis +
disease activity); monitor of therapeutic response
(indicator of macrophage activity)

SCLERODERMA
= PROGRESSIVE SYSTEMIC SCLEROSIS = PSS
= collagen disease characterized by atrophy + sclerosis of
many organ systems
Age: 4 – 6th decade; M:F = 1:3
• thickened inelastic waxy skin most prominent about face
+ extremities
• slightly productive cough + progressive dyspnea
• rheumatoid factor (35%)
• LE cells (5%)
• antinuclear antibodies (30 – 80%)
@ Pulmonary involvement (evident in 10 – 25%):
Path: thickening of basement membrane of alveoli +
small arteries and veins
• pulmonary function abnormalities in the absence of
frank roentgenographic changes (typical dissociation
of clinical, functional, and radiologic evidence)
Location: most prominent in lung bases (blood flow
greatest)
√ fine / coarse reticulations / diffuse interstitial infiltrates
√ alveolar changes (secondary to aspiration from
disturbed esophageal motility)

√ formation of subpleural fibrocystic spaces
(honeycombing)
√ progressive volume loss
√ air esophagogram (DDx: achalasia, mediastinitis)
√ pleural reaction / effusion distinctly uncommon
Cx: increased incidence of lung cancer
@ Gastrointestinal tract
√ esophageal dilatation + aperistalsis (> 50%)
√ hiatus hernia + GE reflux + esophagitis + distal
esophageal stricture
√ irregular dilatation + disturbed motility of small + large
bowel
√ pseudosacculations in colon
@ Musculoskeletal
• Arthralgia (50 – 80%)
• Raynaud phenomenon
√ resorption of distal phalanges of hand (63%)
√ arthritis of interphalangeal joints of hands (25%)
√ calcinosis of finger tips + over pressure areas
(elbows)
√ erosion of superior aspect of ribs
@ Heart: sclerosis of cardiac muscle ± cor pulmonale
@ Renal involvement (25%)

PROGRESSIVE SYSTEMIC SCLEROSIS (PSS) divided
into:
A.   DIFFUSE SCLERODERMA
interstitial pulmonary fibrosis common
B.   CREST: vasculitis with pulmonary arterial
hypertension; more common
Calcinosis of skin
Raynaud phenomenon
Esophageal dysmotility
Sclerodactyly
Telangiectasia
Prognosis: 50 – 67% 5-year survival rate

SEPTIC PULMONARY EMBOLI
= lodgement of an infected thrombus in a pulmonary
artery
Organism: Staph. aureus, Streptococcus
Predisposed: IV drug abusers, alcoholism,
immunodeficiency, CHD, dermal
infection (cellulitis, carbuncles)
Source:
(a) peripheral vein indwelling catheters, arteriovenous
shunts for hemodialysis, drug abuse producing
septic thrombophlebitis (heroin addicts), pelvic
thrombophlebitis, peritonsillar abscess,
osteomyelitis
(b) right side of heart acute bacterial endocarditis of
tricuspid valve
Age: majority < 40 years
• sepsis, cough, dyspnea, chest pain
• shaking chills, high fever, severe sinus tachycardia
√ multiple nondescript pulmonary infiltrates (initially)
√ migratory infiltrates (old ones heal, new ones appear)
√ cavitation (frequent), usually thin-walled

√ pleural effusion (rare)
CT: √ subpleural distribution of lesions
    √ triangular shape with apex of lesion directed toward pulmonary hilum
    √ vascular relationship to pulmonary arteries
    √ cavitation (esp. in staphylococcal emboli)

SIDEROSIS
= inert iron oxide / metallic iron deposits
Path: iron phagocytosed by macrophages in alveoli / respiratory bronchioles, elimination from lung by lymphatic circulation
Occupational exposure:
    arc welding, cutting / burning of steel, foundry workers, grinders, fettlers, polishers (jewelry industry)
√ reticulonodular pattern (may disappear after exposure discontinued)
√ small round opacities (indistinguishable from silica / coal)
√ NO secondary fibrosis + NO hilar adenopathy (unless mixed dust inhalation as in sidero-silicosis)

SILICOSIS
= inhalation of silicon dioxide; most prevalent silicosis of progressive nature after termination of exposure; similar to CWP (because of silica component in CWP)
Substance: Crystalline silica (quartz); one of most widespread elements on earth
Occupational exposure: tunneling, mining, quarrying, sandblasting, ceramic industry
Path: small particles engulfed by macrophages; liberation of silica results in cell death; 2 – 3 mm nodules with layers of laminated connective tissue around smaller vessels

A.   ACUTE SILICOPROTEINOSIS
    = acute silicosis of sandblasters; exposure may be < 1 year
    Associated with   increased risk to develop autoimmune disease
    √ diffuse air space disease
B.   CHRONIC SIMPLE SILICOSIS
    At least 10 – 20 years of dust exposure before appearance of roentgenographic abnormality
    √ small 1 – 10 mm rounded opacities, beginning in upper + middle lung zones
    √ may calcify centrally in 5 – 10% (rather typical for silicosis)
    √ hilar lymphadenopathy, may calcify in 5% ("egg shell pattern")
    √ ± reticulonodular pattern
C.   COMPLICATED SILICOSIS
    √ conglomerate masses of nonsegmental distribution in middle + upper lung zones
    √ progressive massive fibrosis = sausage-shaped masses with ill-defined margins (in advanced stages)
    √ compensatory emphysema in unaffected portion

√ slow change over years
√ may cavitate
D.   SILICOTUBERCULOSIS
    Doubtful synergistic relationship between silicosis + tuberculosis
    √ little change over years with intermittently positive sputa
E.   CAPLAN SYNDROME
    More common in coal worker's pneumoconiosis

Cx: predisposes to tuberculosis

SJÖGREN SYNDROME
= poorly understood chronic systemic inflammatory disorder of unknown etiology characterized by dryness of mucous membranes
A.   PRIMARY SJÖGREN SYNDROME
    without underlying systemic auto-immune disease
    (a) recurrent parotitis in children
    (b) SICCA SYNDROME = Mikulicz disease
        = xerophthalmia + xerostomia
B.   SECONDARY SJÖGREN SYNDROME
    associated with:
    (a) connective tissue diseases
       1. Rheumatoid arthritis (55%)
       2. Systemic lupus erythematosus (2%)
       3. Progressive systemic sclerosis (0.5%)
       4. Psoriatic arthritis, Primary biliary cirrhosis (0.5%)
    (b) lymphoproliferative disorders
       1. Lymphocytic interstitial pneumonitis (LIP)
       2. Pseudolymphoma
       3. Lymphoma (44 x increased risk)
       4. Waldenström macroglobulinemia
Mean age: 57 years; M:F = 1:9
Path: benign lymphoepithelioma = lymphoid infiltrates in lacrimal glands, mucous glands of conjunctivae, nasal cavity, pharynx, larynx, trachea, bronchi
• Xerophthalmia = dryness of eyes
= keratoconjunctivitis sicca = desiccation of cornea + conjunctiva
• Xerostomia = dryness of mouth + lips from diminished saliva
• Xerorhinia = dryness of nose
• Swelling of parotid gland: usually unilateral, recurrent
CXR:
    √ reticulonodular pattern (3 – 33%)
    √ patchy consolidation + atelectasis
    √ pneumonitis (secondary to dryness of respiratory tract)
    √ ± pleural effusion
Sialogram:
    √ nonobstructive punctate / globular / cavitary sialectasia (ducts + acini destroyed by lymphocytic infiltrates / infection)
US of parotid gland:
    √ multiple scattered cysts bilaterally

STAPHYLOCOCCAL PNEUMONIA
= most common cause of bronchopneumonia
- (a) common nosocomial infection (patients on antibiotic drugs most susceptible)
- (b) accounts for 5% of community-acquired pneumonias (esp. infants + elderly)

Δ secondary invader to influenza (commonest cause of death during influenza epidemics)

Organism: Staphylococcus aureus, Gram-positive, appears in clusters, coagulase-producing
- √ rapid spread through lungs
- √ empyema (esp. in children)
- √ pneumothorax, pyopneumothorax
- √ abscess formation
- √ bronchopleural fistula
- A. in CHILDREN:
  - √ rapidly developing lobar / multilobar consolidation
  - √ pleural effusion (90%)
  - √ pneumatocele (40 – 60%)
- B. in ADULTS:
  - √ patchy often confluent bronchopneumonia of segmental distribution, bilateral in > 60%
  - √ segmental collapse (air bronchograms absent)
  - √ late development of thick-walled lung abscess (25 – 75%)
  - √ pleural effusion / empyema (50%) (DDx from other pneumonias)
- *Cx:* Meningitis, Metastatic abscess to brain / kidneys, Acute endocarditis

STREPTOCOCCAL PNEUMONIA
Incidence: 1 – 5% of bacterial pneumonias (rarely seen); most common in winter months
Organism: Group A ß-hemolytic streptococcus = streptococcus pyogenes, Gram-positive cocci appearing in chains
Predisposed: newborns, following infection with measles
Associated with: delayed onset of diaphragmatic hernia (in newborns)
- • rarely follows tonsillitis + pharyngitis
- √ patchy bronchopneumonia
- √ lower lobe predominance (similar to staphylococcus)
- √ empyema
- *Cx:* (1) Residual pleural thickening (15%)
  - (2) Bronchiectasis
  - (3) Lung abscess
  - (4) Glomerulonephritis

SWYER-JAMES SYNDROME
= MACLEOD SYNDROME
= UNILATERAL LOBAR EMPHYSEMA
= IDIOPATHIC UNILATERAL HYPERLUCENT LUNG
Etiology: probably childhood adenoviral infection with acute obliterative bronchiolitis, bronchiectasis, distal air space destruction (develops in 7 – 30 months)
- • asymptomatic
- • dyspnea on exertion

- • history of repeated lower respiratory tract infections during childhood

Location: one / both lungs (usually entire lung, occasionally lobar / subsegmental)
- √ increased radiolucency of affected lung
- √ small hemithorax with decreased / normal volume (collateral airdrift)
- √ air trapping (expiration radiograph !)
  - *DDx:* no air trapping with proximal interruption of pulmonary artery (no hilum), hypogenetic lung syndrome, pulmonary embolus
- √ mild cylindrical bronchiectasis with paucity of bronchial subdivisions (cut-off at 4 – 5th generation = "pruned tree" bronchogram)
- √ small ipsilateral hilum (diminuted hilar vessels + attenuated arteries)
- √ diminutive pulmonary vasculature
- Angio: √ "pruned tree appearance"
- NUC: √ decreased perfusion
  - √ decreased ventilation + delayed washout

SYSTEMIC LUPUS ERYTHEMATOSUS
= most prevalent of the potentially grave collagen diseases characterized by involvement of vascular system, skin, serous + synovial membranes (type III immune complex phenomenon)
Incidence: 1:2,000; Blacks:Caucasians = 3:1
Age: women in child bearing age; M:F = 1:10
- • chronic false positive Wasserman test for syphilis (24%)
- • LE cells (= antigen-antibody complexes engulfed by PMNs) in 78%
- • Sjögren syndrome (frequent)
- • antinuclear-DNA-antibodies (87%)
- • hypergammaglobulinemia (77%)
- • positive rheumatoid factor (21%)
- • anemia (78%)
- • leukopenia (66%)
- • thrombocytopenia (19%)
- @ Skin changes (81%)
  - • "butterfly rash" (= facial erythema), discoid lupus erythematosus, alopecia, photosensitivity
  - • Raynaud phenomenon (15%)
- @ Thoracic involvement (30 – 70%)
  - • dyspnea, pleuritic chest pain (35%)
  - (a) Pulmonary changes
    - √ Lupus pneumonitis (acute form) = poorly defined patchy areas of increased density peripherally at lung bases (alveolar pattern) secondary to infection / uremia in 10%
    - √ interstitial reticulations in lower lung fields (chronic form) in 3%
    - √ fleeting platelike atelectasis in both bases (? infarction due to vasculitis)
    - √ cavitating nodules (vasculitis)
    - √ elevated sluggish diaphragms (progressive volume loss)
    - √ hilar + mediastinal lymphadenopathy (extremely rare)

(b) Pleural changes (most common manifestation)
  √ recurrent bilateral pleural effusions (70%)
    (pleuritis)
  √ pleural thickening
(c) Cardiovascular changes
  √ pericardial effusion (pericarditis)
  √ cardiomegaly (primary lupus cardiomyopathy)
@ Joints
  • arthralgia (95%)
  √ arthritis without deformity
@ Abdomen
  • renal failure (fibrinoid thickening of basement
    membrane)
  √ splenomegaly
Prognosis: 60 – 90% 10-year survival; death from renal
    failure / CNS involvement / myocardial
    infarction

DRUG-INDUCED LUPUS ERYTHEMATOSUS = DIL
(temporary):
  Agents: procainamide, hydralazine, isoniazid,
    phenytoin account for 90%
  √ pulmonary + pleural disease more common than in
    SLE

TALCOSIS
= prolonged inhalation of magnesium silicate dust
  containing amphibole fibers (tremolite and anthophyllite)
  and silica
Talcosis resembles:
  (1) Asbestosis (indistinguishable)
    √ massive and bizarre pleural plaques
    √ may encase lung with calcification
  (2) Silicosis
    √ small rounded + large opacities
    √ fibrogenic process (NO regression after removal
      of patient from exposure)

TERATOID TUMOR OF MEDIASTINUM
= GERM CELL NEOPLASM = arising from primordial
  germ cells
Age: 20 – 40 years, may be present at birth; M:F = 1:1.5
Incidence: 10 – 15% of all mediastinal tumors;
    16 – 28% of all mediastinal cysts
Δ occur in same frequency as the usually larger
  thymomas
Δ 1/3 of primary neoplasms in this area are in children
• sebaceous material, hair, teeth,
Location: 5% of all teratomas occur in mediastinum;
    mediastinum is 3rd most common site for
    teratoid lesions (after gonadal +
    sacrococcygeal location); posterior mediastinal
    location in only 1%
√ often inseparable from thymus gland
Physiologic activity:
  • thyroid hormone
  • alpha fetoprotein
  • HCG (may be associated with gynecomastia)

• amylase
• insulin
A. BENIGN TERATOID TUMOR (80 – 86%)
  1. Epidermoid = ectodermal derivatives (52%)
  2. Dermoid = ecto- + mesodermal derivatives (27%)
  3. Teratoma = ecto- + meso- + endodermal
    derivatives (21%)
  √ well demarcated smooth mass bulging into right /
    left hemithorax
  √ contains densities of fat, water, soft tissue, calcium,
    bone, teeth
  √ may be homogeneous (indistinguishable from
    lymphoma / thymoma)
  √ calcifications (25 – 40%); 4 x more common in
    benign lesions
  √ often inseparable from thymic gland
B. MALIGNANT (14 – 20%)
  1. Choriocarcinoma
  2. Seminoma (most common)
  3. Embryonal carcinoma
  4. Yolk sac / endodermal sinus tumor
  5. Mixed germ cell tumor
  6. Teratocarcinoma
  M > F
  √ lobulation suggests malignancy
  √ invasion of mediastinal structures (SVC obstruction
    is ominous)
  Δ absence of primary testicular tumor / retroperitoneal
    mass proves primary
Cx:
  (1) Hemorrhage
  (2) Pneumothorax (from bronchial obstruction with air
    trapping + alveolar rupture)
  (3) Respiratory distress (rapid increase in size from
    fluid production) with compression of trachea / SVC
  (4) Fistula formation to aorta, SVC, esophagus
  (5) Rupture into bronchus (trychoptysis in 5 – 14%),
    pericardium, pleural cavity

THYMIC CYST
Incidence: 1 – 2% of mediastinal tumors
Etiology:
  (1) congenital cyst (persistent tubular elements of 3rd
    pharyngeal pouch)
  (2) inflammatory cyst
  (3) neoplastic cyst (cystic teratoma, cystic
    degeneration within a thymoma), S/P radiation
    therapy for Hodgkin disease
Location: anterior mediastinum / lateral neck
√ multiloculated, may show partial wall calcification
√ low-density fluid (0 – 10 HU), may be higher depending
  on cyst contents

THYMIC HYPERPLASIA
Most common anterior mediastinal mass in pediatric age
group through puberty
Age: particular in young individual
Histo: numerous active lymphoid germinal centers

Etiology: Hyperthyroidism (most common), treatment of primary hypothyroidism, idiopathic thyromegaly, Graves disease, myasthenia gravis (65%), rebound growth in children recovering from stress (e.g. from burns), acromegaly, Addison disease

√ normal thymus visible in 50% of neonates 0 – 2 years of age
√ notch sign = indentation at junction of thymus + heart
√ sail sign = triangular density extending from superior mediastinum
√ wave sign = rippled border due to indentation from ribs
√ shape changes with respiration + position

THYMOLIPOMA

Incidence: 2 – 9% of thymic tumors; M > F
Histo: well-encapsulated benign adult adipose tissue interspersed with areas of normal / hyperplastic / atrophic thymus tissue

√ grows downward from cardiac base bilaterally, envelops heart
√ may be very large with enlargement of cardiac silhouette (68% > 500 g, may weigh up to 3000 g)
√ NO compression / invasion of adjacent structures

THYMOMA

Most common anterior mediastinal mass in adults; 50% benign, 50% malignant
Age: around 20 years
Associated with:
- MYASTHENIA GRAVIS:
  Δ 15 – 25% of patients with myasthenia gravis have a thymoma, (in 65% due to thymic hyperplasia)
  Δ 25 – 50% of patients with thymoma have myasthenia gravis; removal of thymic tumor often results in symptomatic improvement
- Pure red cell aplasia = aregenerative anemia
- Acquired hypogammaglobulinemia
- Paraneoplastic syndromes occur with thymic carcinoid (10%): e.g. Cushing syndrome (ACTH production)

Histo: (a) lymphocytic
(b) epithelial
(c) lymphoepithelial (mixed)
(d) spindle cell
Location: inferior mediastinum

(A) NONINVASIVE THYMOMA
Age peak: 5 – 6th decade, almost all are > 25 years of age
√ oval / round / lobulated sharply demarcated asymmetric homogeneous mass of soft tissue density, usually smaller than teratomas
√ displacement of heart + great vessels posteriorly
√ amorphous, flocculent, curvilinear calcification (5 – 20%)
(B) INVASIVE THYMOMA (in 30% of thymomas)
Stage I : intact capsule

Stage II : pericapsular growth into mediastinal fat
Stage III : invasion of surrounding organs, distant pleural implants (metastases to pleura + lung in 6%), rarely extrathoracic metastases
√ spread by contiguity along pleural reflections, extension along aorta reaching posterior mediastinum / crus of diaphragm / retroperitoneum
Prognosis: 67% 5-year survival; 53% 10-year survival

TRACHEOBRONCHOMEGALY

= MOUNIER-KUHN SYNDROME = primary atrophy / dysplasia of supporting structures of trachea + major bronchi with abrupt transition to normal bronchi at 4 – 5th division
Incidence: 0.5 – 1.5%
Age: discovered in 3rd – 5th decade
- cough with copious sputum
- shortness of breath on exertion
- long Hx of recurrent pneumonias
may be associated with: Ehlers-Danlos syndrome
√ marked dilatation of trachea (> 29 mm), right (> 20 mm) + left (> 15 mm) main stem bronchi
√ sacculated outline / diverticulosis of trachea on lateral CXR (= protrusion of mucous membrane between rings of trachea)
√ may have emphysema, bullae in perihilar region

TRANSIENT TACHYPNEA OF THE NEWBORN

= NEONATAL WET LUNG DISEASE = TRANSIENT RESPIRATORY DISTRESS OF THE NEWBORN
= RETAINED FETAL LUNG FLUID
Incidence: 6%; most common cause of respiratory distress in newborn
Causes: cesarean section, precipitous delivery, breech delivery, prematurity, maternal diabetes
Pathophysiology: delayed resorption of fetal lung fluid (normal clearance occurs through capillaries (40%), lymphatics (30%), thoracic compression during vaginal delivery (30%)
Onset: within 6 hours of life; peak at day 1 of age
- increasing respiratory rates during first 2 – 6 hours of life
- intercostal + sternal retraction
- normal blood gases during hyperoxygenation
√ linear opacities + perivascular haze + thickened fissures + interlobular septal thickening (interstitial edema)
√ mild hyperaeration
√ mild cardiomegaly
√ small amount of pleural fluid
Prognosis: resolving within 1 – 4 days (retrospective diagnosis)
DDx: (1) normal during first several hours of life (2) diffuse pneumonitis / sepsis (3) mild meconium aspiration syndrome (4) "drowned newborn syndrome" = clear amniotic fluid aspiration (5) alveolar phase of RDS (6) pulmonary venous

congestion (7) pulmonary hemorrhage
(8) hyperviscosity syndrome = thick blood
(9) immature lung syndrome

TRAUMATIC LUNG CYST
Age: children + young adults are particularly prone
√ thin-walled air-filled cavity (50%) ± air-fluid level
preceded by homogeneous well-circumscribed mass
(hematoma)
√ oval / spherical lesion of 2 – 14 cm in diameter
√ single / multiple / uni- or multilocular
√ usually subpleural under point of maximal injury
√ persistent up to 4 month + progressive decrease in size
(apparent within 6 weeks)

TUBERCULOSIS
Prevalence: 10 million people worldwide, active TB
develops in 5 – 10% of those exposed
Organism: mycobacterium = acid-fast aerobic rods
staining red with carbol-fuchsin;
M. tuberculosis (95%), other types
increasing: M. avium-intracellulare, M.
Kansasii, M. fortuitum
Susceptible: infants, pubertal adolescents, elderly,
alcoholics, blacks, diabetics, silicosis,
measles, AIDS, sarcoidosis (in up to 13%)
Outcome of primary infection:
1. Immunity prevents multiplication of organism
(delayed hypersensitivity)
2. Progressive primary TB (inadequate immune
mechanism)
3. Postprimary TB = Reactivation TB (reactivation after
asymptomatic years)
4. Superinfection overwhelms acquired immunity
Pathologic phases:
(a) exudative reaction (initial reaction, present for 1
month)
(b) caseous necrosis (after 2 – 10 weeks with onset of
hypersensitivity)
(c) hyalinization = invasion of fibroblasts (granuloma
formation in 1 – 3 week)
(d) calcification / ossification
(e) chronic destructive form in 10% (< 1 year of age,
adolescents, young adults)
Spread: regional lymph nodes, hematogenous
dissemination, pleura, pericardium, upper
lumbar vertebrae
Mortality: 1 : 100,000
Positive PPD test: 3 weeks after infection
Negative PPD test:
1. overwhelming tuberculous infection (miliary TB)
2. sarcoidosis
3. corticosteroid therapy
4. pregnancy
5. infection with atypical mycobacterium

ENDOBRONCHIAL TUBERCULOSIS
Path: ulceration of bronchial mucosa followed by
fibrosis leads to

(a) bronchial stenosis (lobar consolidation)
(b) bronchiectasis
(c) acinar nodules reflecting airway spread

TUBERCULOMA
= manifestation of primary / postprimary TB
√ round / oval smooth sharply defined mass
√ 0.5 – 4 cm in diameter remaining stable for a long
time
√ lobulated mass (25%)
√ satellite lesions (80%)
√ may calcify

CAVITARY TUBERCULOSIS
= hallmark of reactivation tuberculosis
= semisolid caseous material is expelled into bronchial
tree after lysis
√ moderately thick-walled cavity with smooth inner
surface
Cx:
(1) dissemination to other bronchial segments
√ multiple small acinar shadows remote from
massive consolidation
(2) colonization with aspergillus
√ aspergilloma

Primary Pulmonary Tuberculosis
Mode of infection: inhalation of infected airborne
droplets
Age: usually in childhood, becoming commoner in
adults
• asymptomatic (91%)
• symptomatic with complete recovery (5.3%)
Location: lower lobes, middle lobe, anterior segment of
upper lobes
√ one / more areas of homogeneous ill-defined air
space consolidation of 1 – 7 cm in diameter (requires
several weeks for complete clearing with
antituberculous therapy)
√ cavitation (rare in children, up to 29% in adults)
√ massive hilar (60%) / paratracheal (40%)
lymphadenopathy (particularly common in children),
in 80% unilateral
√ atelectasis (30%) esp. in right lung (anterior segment
of upper lobe / medial segment of middle lobe)
secondary to
(a) endobronchial tuberculosis
(b) bronchial / tracheal compression by enlarged
lymph nodes (68%)
√ pleural effusion (10% in childhood, 40% in
adulthood) most commonly 3 – 7 months after initial
exposure (from subpleural foci rupturing into pleural
space)
√ pneumonic reaction (mid or lower lung zones)
segmental / lobar consolidation
√ calcified lung lesion (17%) / parenchymal scar < 5 mm
= **Ghon lesion**
√ calcified lymph node (36%) in hilus / mediastinum

√ **Ranke complex** = Ghon lesion + calcified lymph node (22%)
√ **Simon focus** = healed site of primary infection in lung apex
CT:
√ tuberculous adenopathy may demonstrate necrotic center with low attenuation after enhancement
Prognosis: 3.6% mortality rate
Cx: (1) bronchopleural fistula + empyema
          (2) fibrosing mediastinitis

Postprimary Pulmonary Tuberculosis
= REACTIVATION TB = infection under the influence of acquired hypersensitivity and immunity secondary to longevity of bacillus + impairment of cellular immunity
Etiology: (a) reactivation of focus acquired in childhood
          (b) initial infection in individual vaccinated with BCG
          (c) continuation of initial infection
                = progressive primary tuberculosis (rare)
Path: foci of caseous necrosis with surrounding edema, hemorrhage, mononuclear cell infiltration; formation of tubercles
          = accumulation of epithelioid cells + Langhans giant cells; bronchial perforation leads to intrabronchial dissemination
Age: predominantly in adulthood
Site: 85% in apical + posterior segments of upper lobe, 10% in superior segment of lower lobe, 5% in mixed locations (anterior + contiguous segments of upper lobe)
          R > L
          (DDx: Histoplasmosis tends to affect anterior segment)
A. LOCAL EXUDATIVE TB
    √ chronic patchy / confluent ill-defined areas of acinar consolidation
    √ may show cavitation with smooth inner surface (present in more advanced disease), cavity under tension (air influx + obstructed efflux), no air-fluid level (most cavities are bronchiectatic in origin)
    √ accentuated drainage markings toward ipsilateral hilum
B. LOCAL FIBROPRODUCTIVE TB
    √ sharply circumscribed irregular + angular mass-like fibrotic lesion (in up to 7%)
    √ cavitation (secondary to expulsion of caseous necrosis into airways), esp. in apical / posterior segments of upper lobes
    √ reticular pulmonary scars
    √ cicatrization atelectasis = volume loss in affected lobe
    √ bronchiectasis in apical / posterior segments of upper lobes
    √ pleural thickening
    √ tuberculous lymphadenitis
    √ calcified hilar / mediastinal nodes
    √ Rasmussen aneurysm

Miliary Pulmonary Tuberculosis
= massive hematogenous dssemination of organisms any time after primary infection
Cause:
    (1) severe immunodepression during postprimary state of infection
    (2) impaired defenses during primary infection
          = PROGRESSIVE PRIMARY TB
Incidence: 2 – 3.5% of TB infections
√ chronic focus often not identifiable
√ radiographically recognizable after 6 weeks post hematogenous dissemination
√ generalized granulomatous interstitial small foci of pinpoint to 2 – 3 mm size
√ rapid complete clearing with appropriate therapy
CT (earlier detection than CXR):
√ diffusely scattered discrete 1 – 2 mm nodules
Cx: dissemination via bloodstream affecting lymph nodes, liver, spleen, skeleton, kidneys, adrenals, prostate, seminal vesicles, epididymis, Fallopian tubes, endometrium, meninges

UNILATERAL PULMONARY AGENESIS
= one-sided lack of primitive mesenchyme
• may be asymptomatic
• respiratory infections
√ complete opacity of hemithorax
√ ipsilateral absence of pulmonary artery + vein
√ absent ipsilateral mainstem bronchus
√ symmetrical chest cage with approximation of ribs
√ overdistension of contralateral lung
√ ipsilateral shift of mediastinum + diaphragm
Associated with
    anomalies in 60% (higher if right lung involved): PDA, anomalies of great vessels, Tetralogy of Fallot (left-sided pulmonary agenesis), bronchogenic cyst, congenital diaphragmatic hernia, bone anomalies

VARICELLA-ZOSTER PNEUMONIA
Incidence: 14% overall; 50% in hospitalized adults
Age: > 19 years (90%); 3rd – 5th decade (75%); contrasts with low incidence of varicella in this age group
• vesicular rash
√ patchy diffuse air space consolidation
√ tendency for coalescence near hila + lung bases
√ widespread nodules (30%) representing scarring
√ tiny 2 – 3 mm calcifications widespread throughout both lungs (2%)
Cx: unilateral diaphragmatic paralysis
Prognosis: 11% mortality rate

VIRAL PNEUMONIA
Organisms: Rhinovirus (43%), Respiratory syncitial virus (12%), Mycoplasma (10%), Parainfluenza virus, Adenovirus, Influenza virus

Path: necrosis of ciliated epithelial cells, goblet cells, bronchial mucous glands with frequent involvement of peribronchial tissues + interlobular septae
Age: most common cause of pneumonia in children under 5 years of age
Distribution: usually bilateral
√ hyperaeration + air trapping
√ "dirty chest" = peribronchial cuffing + opacification
√ perihilar linear densities (bronchial wall thickening)
√ interstitial pattern
√ air space pattern (from hemorrhagic edema) in 50%
√ pleural effusion (20%)
√ hilar adenopathy (3%)
√ striking absence of pneumatoceles, lung abscess, pneumothorax
√ radiographic resolution lags 2 – 3 weeks behind clinical
Cx: bronchiectasis; unilateral hyperlucent lung

Atypical measles pneumonia does NOT show the typical radiographic findings of viral pneumonias !

WEGENER GRANULOMATOSIS
= probably autoimmune disease characterized by systemic necrotizing granulomatous process with destructive angiitis
Path: peribronchial necrotizing granulomas + vasculitis not intimately related to arteries
Age peak: 5th decade (range of all ages); M:F = 2:1

@ Respiratory tract (100% involvement)
   (a) Upper respiratory tract (similar to midline granuloma)
      • rhinorrhea, sinusitis
      • bleeding mucosal ulcers of nose
      √ thickening of mucous membranes of paranasal sinuses
      √ may progress to destruction of cartilage + bone
   (b) Pulmonary disease
      • intractable cough, occasionally with hemoptysis
      √ patchy alveolar infiltrates (with acute air space pneumonia)
      √ widely distributed multiple irregular masses / nodules of varying sizes (up to 9 cm), especially in lower lung fields

√ thick-walled cavities with irregular shaggy inner lining (25 – 50%)
√ pleural effusion in 25%
√ lymphadenopathy exceedingly rare
@ Other organ involvement:
   (a) Urinary tract (83%): focal glomerulonephritis
   (b) Joints (56%): migratory polyarthropathy
   (c) Skin + muscle (44%): inflammatory skin lesions
   (d) Eyes + middle ear (29%): proptosis, otitis media
   (e) Heart + pericardium (28%): myocardial infarction (vasculitis)
   (f) CNS (22%): central / peripheral neuritis

Cx: (1) hypertension (2) uremia
Dx: lung / renal biopsy
Prognosis: death within 2 years from renal failure (83%) / respiratory failure
Rx: corticosteroids, cytotoxic drugs, renal transplantation

LIMITED WEGENER GRANULOMATOSIS
= Wegener granulomatosis WITHOUT renal involvement
MIDLINE GRANULOMA
= mutilating granulomatous + neoplastic lesions limited to nose + paranasal sinuses with very poor prognosis; considered a variant of Wegener granulomatosis WITHOUT the typical granulomatous + cellular components

WILSON-MIKITY SYNDROME
= PULMONARY DYSMATURITY = similarity to bronchopulmonary dysplasia in patients breathing room air; rarely encountered anymore
Predisposed: premature infants < 1500 g who are initially well
• gradual onset of respiratory distress between 10 – 14 days
√ hyperinflation
√ reticular pattern radiating from both hila
√ small bubbly lucencies throughout both lungs (identical to bronchopulmonary dysplasia)
Prognosis: resolution over 12 months

DIFFERENTIAL DIAGNOSIS OF BREAST DISEASE

Well-circumscribed breast lesion
1. Cysts (45%)
2. Fibroadenoma
3. Lipoma (9%)
3. Medullary / mucinous / intracystic / papillary carcinoma (5 – 9%)
4. Intramammary lymph node
5. Metastases to breast: melanoma, lymphoma / leukemia, lung cancer
6. Skin lesion: e.g., verrucae

Fat-containing breast lesion
1. Lipoma
   √ usually > 2 cm
2. Galactocele
   • during / shortly after lactation
3. Traumatic lipid cyst = fat necrosis = oil cyst
   • site of prior surgery / trauma
4. Focal collection of normal breast fat

MIXED FAT- AND WATER-DENSITY LESION
1. Intramammary lymph node
2. Hamartoma = lipofibroadenoma = fibroadenolipoma
   √ usually > 3 cm
3. Hematoma

Stellate lesion
1. Scirrhous carcinoma (infiltrating duct carcinoma)
   √ distinct central tumor mass
   √ length of spicules increase with tumor size
   √ localized skin thickening / retraction with extension to skin
   √ commonly associated with malignant-type calcifications
2. Sclerosing duct hyperplasia = Radial scar
   • absence of palpable lesion
   √ variable appearance in different projections
   √ oval / circular translucent areas at center
   √ radiolucent linear structures paralleling spicules
3. Traumatic fat necrosis
   √ translucent areas at center (in old lesions)
   √ fine spicules of low density varying with projection
   √ localized skin thickening / retraction possible
4. Hyalinized fibroadenoma with fibrosis
   √ changing pattern with different projections
   √ may be accompanied by typical coarse calcifications of fibroadenomas

Tumor-mimicking lesions
1. "Phantom breast tumor"
   = chance overlapping of glandular breast structures
   √ failure to visualize "tumor" on more than one view
2. Silicone injections

3. Skin lesions
   (a) Dermal nevi
       √ sharp halo / fissured appearance
   (b) Skin calcifications
       √ lucent center (clue)
       √ superficial location (tangential views)
   (c) Sebacious / epithelial inclusion cyst
   (d) Neurofibromatosis
   (e) Biopsy scar
4. Lymphedema
   Cause: (1) obstruction of lymphatic drainage to axilla (metastases, surgery)
            (2) congestive heart failure (may be unilateral if patient in lateral decubitus position)
5. Lymph nodes
   Location: axilla, subcutaneous tissue of axillary tail, lateral portion of pectoralis muscle, intramammary
   √ ovoid / bean-shaped mass with notch representing hilum
   √ central zone of radiolucency (fatty replacement of center) surrounded by "crescent" rim of cortex
   √ usually < 1.5 cm (up to 4 cm) in size

Calcifications
Indicative of focally active process + often requiring biopsy
Δ 75% of biopsied clusters of calcifications represent benign process
Δ 10 – 30% of microcalcifications in asymptomatic patients are associated with cancers

Ductal microcalcifications
√ 0.1 – 0.3 mm in size, irregular, sometimes mixed linear + punctate
Occurence: secretory disease, epithelial hyperplasia, atypical ductal hyperplasia, intraductal carcinoma

Lobular microcalcifications
√ smooth round, similar in size + density
Occurence: cystic hyperplasia, adenosis, sclerosing adenosis, atypical lobular hyperplasia, lobular carcinoma in situ
N.B.: lobular and ductal microcalcifications occur frequently in fibrocystic disease + breast cancer!

A. MALIGNANT CALCIFICATIONS
1. **granular calcifications**= resembling fine grains of salt
   √ amorphous, dotlike / elongated, fragmented
   √ grouped very close together
   √ irregular in form, size and density
2. **casting calcifications**= fragmented cast of calcifications within ducts

√ variable in size + length
√ great variation in density within individual particles + among adjacent particles
√ jagged irregular contour
√ ± Y-shaped branching pattern
√ clustered (> 5 per focus within an area of 1 cm²)

B. BENIGN CALCIFICATIONS
1. **lobular calcifications** = arise within a spherical cavity of cystic hyperplasia, sclerosing adenosis, atypical lobular hyperplasia
    √ sharply outlined, homogeneous, solid, spherical
    √ crescent-shaped on horizontal projection = "teacup-like" (milk of calcium settling in dependent portion)
    √ little variation in size
    √ uniform pearl-like density
    √ numerous + scattered
    √ associated with considerable fibrosis
    (a) adenosis
        √ diffuse calcifications involving both breasts symmetrically
    (b) periductal fibrosis
        √ diffuse / grouped calcifications + irregular borders, simulating malignant process
2. Arterial calcifications
    √ parallel lines of calcifications
3. Plasma cell mastitis = Periductal mastitis = Ductal ectasia
4. Sebaceous gland calcifications
    Site: occurs only within skin
    √ ring-shaped / oval calcifications with radiolucent center
    √ same size as skin pores
5. Small ring-like calcifications = liponecrosis microcystica calcificans
    = calcified microhematomas
    √ small egg-shell calcifications up to a few mm
    √ high uniform density in periphery
    √ usually subcutaneous
    √ no associated fibrosis
6. Large egg-shell calcifications
    (a) Liponecrosis macrocystica calcificans of oil cysts (= fatty acids precipitate as calcium soaps at capsular surface)
        √ spherical / oval up to several cm
        √ radiolucent center
    (b) Fibroadenoma
        √ radiodense center
7. Papillomatosis
    √ solitary raspberry configuration in size of duct
    √ central / retroareolar
8. Fibroadenoma
    √ bizarre, coarse, sharply outlined "popcorn-like" very dense calcification within dense mass (= myxoid degeneration)
    √ egg-shell type calcification
9. Cyst
    √ moderately radiolucent, rounded, nonclustered, peripheral in wall of cyst

Skin thickening of breast
A. Localized skin thickening
    1. Trauma (previous biopsy)
    2. Carcinoma
    3. Mastitis
    4. Infection
B. Generalized skin thickening
    (a) Axillary lymphatic obstruction
        1. Metastatic breast carcinoma
        2. Primary malignant lymphatic disease (e.g. Lymphoma)
        3. Advanced gynecological malignancies (ovarian, uterine)
        4. Advanced bronchial / esophageal carcinoma
    (b) Intradermal + intramammary obstruction of lymph channels
        1. Lymphatic spread of breast cancer from contralateral side
    (c) Inflammation
        1. Mastitis
        2. Retromamillary abscess
        3. Fat necrosis
        4. Radiation therapy
        5. Reduction mammoplasty
    (d) Right heart failure
        may be unilateral (R>L)
    (e) Nephrotic syndrome, anasarca
    (f) Subcutaneous extravasation of pleural fluid following thoracentesis

Nipple retraction
1. Positional
2. Relative to inflammation / edema of periareolar tissue
2. Congenital
3. Acquired (carcinoma, ductal ectasia)

Secretory disease
1. Retained lactiferous secretions
    result of incomplete / prolonged involution of lactiferous ducts
    √ branching pattern of fat density in dense breast (high lipid content)
2. Prolonged inspissation of secretion + intraductal debris
    √ duct dilatation
    √ calcifications with linear orientation towards subareolar area a few mm long: rod-shaped / sausage-shaped / spherical with hollow center
3. **Galactoceles**
    = retention of fatty material in areas of cystic duct dilatation appearing during / shortly after lactation
    • thick inspissated milky fluid
    Location: commonly retroareolar
    √ lucent lesion resembling lipoma / water-density / calcium-density
    √ fluid-calcium / fat-water level with horizontal beam
4. Plasma cell mastitis

DISEASE ENTITIES OF THE BREAST

BREAST CANCER
A. NONINVASIVE CARCINOMA (9%)
1. Intraductal carcinoma
   = entirely confined within ducts
   Histo: marked proliferation of atypical ductal epithelium with intraductal necrotic calcifying epithelium
   • may persist for years without palpatory abnormality
   √ clustered microcalcifications of similar size with irregular margins
2. Lobular carcinoma in situ
   = arises in epithelium of blunt ducts of mammary lobules
   Histo: monomorphous cell population filling + expanding lobule
   √ conglomerate round / streaky densities (similar in appearance to fibrocystic disease / ductal hyperplasia)
   √ clustered round microcalcifications with relatively smooth border + homogeneous appearance
B. INVASIVE CARCINOMA (90%)
1. Infiltrating ductal carcinoma = scirrhous (75%)
   • larger by palpation than on mammogram
   √ dense mass of variable size surrounded by spiculations
   √ malignant calcifications common
2. Invasive lobular carcinoma (5%)
   2nd most common type of breast cancer; 30 – 50% of patients will develop a second primary in same / opposite breast within 20 years
   Histo: single file of cells infiltrating the breast resulting in subtle changes in architecture
   √ difficult to detect mammographically (may be palpable)
   √ asymmetric density without definable margins (most frequent)
   √ dense tissue with radiating spicules
3. Mucinous / colloid carcinoma (< 1%)
4. Medullary carcinoma (5 – 10%)
5. Ductal papillary carcinoma = Comedocarcinoma in terminal portion of collecting ducts
   Histo: marked atypical ductal cells surrounding central calcifying necrosis
   • often soft + difficult to palpate
   √ irregular linear branching microcalcifications
   √ large typical sunburst calcification pattern
6. Tubular carcinoma (very uncommon)
7. Adenocystic carcinoma
8. Secretory (juvenile) carcinoma
9. Intracystic papillary carcinoma (0.5 – 2%)
   = rare form of ductal cancer
   Age: average of 51 years
   • well-circumscribed + freely movable
   • aspiration may yield bloody fluid (cytology negative in 80%)

√ pneumocystography only reliable way to establish diagnosis
√ solid appearing mass on US
√ benign appearing mass on mammography
Prognosis: favorable (if not yet invasive)
C. Paget carcinoma of the nipple (5%)
   • eczema-like crusting + erosion of nipple and areola
   • nipple discharge + itching
   associated with intraductal subareolar carcinoma

Epidemiology of Breast Cancer
Incidence: in USA > 180,000 new cases per year; 1 out of 10 women will develop breast cancer during her life
Mortality: 41,000 deaths per year

RISK FACTORS (increasing risk):
A. DEMOGRAPHIC FACTORS
   • increasing age (66% of cancers in women > 50 years)
   • whites > blacks after age 40
   • Jewish women + nuns
   • upper > lower social class
   • unmarried > married women
B. REPRODUCTIVE VARIABLES
   • nulliparous > parous
   • first full-term pregnancy after age 35
   • low parity > high parity
   • early age at menarche (< 12 years) + late age at menopause
   • bilateral oophorectomy under age 40 decreases risk
C. MULTIPLE PRIMARY CANCERS
   • 4 – 5 x increase in risk for cancer in contralateral breast
   • increased risk after ovarian + endometrial cancer
D. FAMILY HISTORY
   • breast cancer in first-degree relative
     — 2-fold increase if mother / sister had cancer
     — 3-fold increase if mother + sister had cancer
   • 25% of patients with carcinoma have a positive family history
   • carcinoma tends to affect successive generations approx. 10 years earlier
E. BENIGN BREAST DISEASE
   • 2 – 4 x increased risk in fibrocystic disease (atypical hyperplasia / epithelial hyperplasia
F. MAMMOGRAPHIC FEATURES
   • prominent duct pattern + extremely dense breasts
     N1 (0.14%), P1 (0.52%), P2 (1.95%), DY (5.22%)
G. RADIATION EXPOSURE
   excess risk of 3.5 – 6 cases per 1,000,000 women

per year per rad after a minimum latent period of
10 years (atomic bomb, fluoroscopy during
treatment of tuberculosis, irradiation for
postpartum mastitis)
  H. GEOGRAPHY
    • Western + industrialized nations (highest
      incidence)
    • Asia, Latin America, Africa (decreased risk)

Parenchymal breast pattern

N1   breast composed primarily of fat, prominent
     trabeculation is present which appears curvilinear
     and often branches, no ducts visible

P1   minor ducts occupy 1/4 or less of the breast
     volume, ducts have a definite cross-sectional
     diameter and often a nodular component

P2   severe ducting occupying more than 1/4 of the
     breast volume, strong tendency to form a central
     triangular density, ducts are coalescent

DY   severe mammary dysplasia, nearly completely
     homogeneous breasts without discernible
     linearity or nodularity, interspersed are irregular
     collections of fat

Breast cancer evaluation

A. PRIMARY SIGNS OF BREAST CANCER
  1. Dominant mass seen on two views with
    (a) spiculation = stellate / starburst appearance
         (= fine linear strands of tumor extension +
         desmoplastic response) "scirrhus" caused by:
         (1) infiltrating ductal carcinoma (75% of all
         invasive cancers) (2) invasive lobular
         carcinoma (occasionally)
         √ mass feels larger than its mammographic /
            sonographic size
    (b) ragged irregular border
         = asymmetric density with vague margins
    (c) smooth border (rare)
         "telltale" signs: lobulation, small comet tail,
         flattening of one side of the lesion, slight
         irregularity
         (1) intracystic carcinoma (rare): subareolar
              area; bloody aspiration
         (2) medullary carcinoma: soft tumor
         (3) mucinous / colloid carcinoma: soft tumor

    (d) lobulation
         Appearance similar to fibroadenoma (only
         characteristic calcifications may exclude
         malignancy)
         Δ the likelihood of malignancy increases with
            number of lobulations
         • clinical size of mass > radiographic size
            (Le Borgne's law)
  2. Diffuse increase in density (late finding)
      Cause: (1) plugging of dermal lymphatics with
              tumor cells (2) less flattening of sclerotic
              + fibrous elements of neoplasm in
              comparison with more compressible
              fibroglandular breast tissue
  3. Architectural distortion
  4. Microcalcifications
      Associated with malignant mass
      mammographically in 40%, pathologically with
      special stains in 60%, on specimen radiography
      in 86%
    (a) size: 100 – 300 μ (usually); rarely up to 2 mm
    (b) shape: punctate, rod-shaped, Y-shaped
         branching pattern, "salt and pepper" pattern,
         reticular pattern
    (c) number: >10 clustered together allows a
         somewhat confident diagnosis
    (d) grouping: tight cluster over on area of 1 cm
         or less is most suggestive; coursing along
         ductal system seen in ductal carcinoma with
         comedo elements
  5. Interval change
    (a) de novo developing density (in 6%
         malignant)
    (b) enlarging mass (malignant in 10 – 15%)

B. SECONDARY SIGNS OF BREAST CANCER
  1. Asymmetric thickening
  2. Asymmetric ducts, esp. discontinuous with
      subareolar area
  3. Skin changes
    (a) retraction of skin, nipple, areola
    (b) skin thickening secondary to blocked
         lymphatic drainage / tumor in lymphatics
         (peau d'orange)

RISK OF BREAST CANCER FOR VARIOUS PARENCHYMAL PATTERNS (patterns are important risk indicators in women < age 50)			
Designation	Risk	Recommended follow-up	% incidence of cancer
N1	lowest	2 – 5 years, based on age	20
P1	low	2 – 5 years, based on age	20
P2	high	every year	80
DY	highest	every year	80

(c) Paget disease = eczematoid appearance of nipple + areola in ductal carcinoma
Associated with ductal calcifications toward the nipple

4. <u>Increased vascularity</u> (not very important) venous diameter ratio of 1.4:1 in 75% of cancers
5. <u>Axillary nodes</u>: > 2.5 cm without fatty center; indistinguishable from reactive hyperplasia

LOCATION OF BREAST MASSES
benign + malignant masses are of similar distribution
@ upper outer quadrant (54%)
@ upper inner quadrant (14%)
@ lower outer quadrant (10%)
@ lower inner quadrant (7%)
@ retroareolar (15%)

METASTATIC BREAST CANCER
@ Axillary lymph adenopathy
   Incidence: 40 – 74 %
   risk for positive nodes: 30% if primary > 1 cm, 15% if primary < 1 cm
@ Bone
@ Liver
   Incidence: 48 – 60 %
   US: √ hypoechoic (83%) / hyperechoic (17%) masses

Screening of asymptomatic patients
Guidelines of American Cancer Society, American College of Radiology, American Medical Association, National Cancer Institute:
1. Self breast examination to begin at age 20
2. Breast examination by physician every 3 years between 20 – 40 years, in yearly intervals after age 40
3. Baseline mammogram between ages 35 – 40; follow-up screening based upon parenchymal pattern + family history
4. Initial screening at 30 years if patient has first-degree relative with breast cancer in premenopausal years; follow-up screening based upon parenchymal pattern
5. Mammography at 1 – 2 year intervals for women between 40 – 49 years
6. Mammography at yearly intervals after age 50
7. All women who have had prior breast cancer require annual followup

VALUE OF SCREENING MAMMOGRAPHY
1. <u>Health Insurance Plan (HIP) 1960's</u>
   Randomized controlled study
   • 25 – 30% reduction in mortality in women > 50 years
2. <u>Breast Cancer Detection Demonstration Project (BCDDP) 1973 – 1980</u>
   On 283,000 asymptomatic volunteers (4,443 cancers found)
   • 41.6% of cancers found by mammography alone (77% with negative nodes)
   • 8.7% of cancers found by physical examination alone
   • 59% of non-infiltrating cancers found by mammography alone
   • 25% of cancers were intraductal (vs. 5% in previous series)
   • 21% of cancers found in women aged 40 – 49 years (mammography alone detected 35.4%)
3. <u>Swedish study 1977 – 1984</u>
   randomized controlled study
   • 31% reduction in mortality in women > 50 years

OCCULT VERSUS PALPABLE CANCERS
27% are occult cancers (NO age difference)
Positive axillary nodes: occult cancers (19%);
                          palpable cancers (44%)
10-year survival: occult cancers (65%);
                          palpable cancers (25%)

PREDICTIVE VALUES OF RADIOGRAPHIC SIGNS FOR MALIGNANCY
1. classic mammographic findings of malignancy + palpable abnormality .... 100%   only 3 % of cancers present this way
2. classic mammographic findings of malignancy + NO palpable finding .... 74%   only 6 % of cancers present this way
3. indeterminate mammographic features + palpable mass 11%
4. indeterminate mass + no palpable finding 5%
5. mammographically benign mass 2%
6. Asymmetric density (mass questionable) + clinical finding 4%
7. Asymmetric density (mass questionable) + NO clinical finding 0%
8. Microcalcifications + clinical abnormality 25%
9. Microcalcifications + NO clinical abnormality .... 21%   (> 3 punctate irregular microcalcifications in area < 1 cm)
10. Vein dilatation 0%
11. Skin thickening 0%
12. Duct dilatation 0%

Role of mammography
MAMMOGRAPHY EQUIPMENT:
Optimal film-screen equipment and technique:
25 – 28 kVp with focal spot 0.1 – 0.4 mm (0.1 mm for magnification views); molybdenum target and filtration; grid if compressed breast > 5 cm / very dense breast; compression device

OVERALL DETECTION RATE:
58 – 69%; 8% if < 1 cm in size

MAMMOGRAPHIC ACCURACY:
88% correctly diagnosed by radiologist
27% only detected by mammography
8% misinterpretations
4% not detected

MAMMOGRAPHICALLY MISSED CANCERS
Incidence: approx. 10 – 30%
1. Technical error (5%): poor positioning, improper exposure technique
2. Observer error (30%): oversight, rushed interpretation, heavy caseload, extraneous distraction, eye fatigue
3. Unrecognized signs (33%): masked by dense / dysplastic breast parenchyma
4. Acute cancers (33%): cancers surfacing in screening interval

Role of breast ultrasound
Indications:
(1) principal role is to differentiate cystic from solid lesions
(2) peripheral lesions
(3) in pregnancy
(4) "radiophobic" patient
(5) bedridden patient
(6) evaluation of breast implants
(7) postmastectomy tissue
(8) dense breast, particularly in young patient
(9) ultrasound-guided cyst aspiration
Accuracy: 98% accuracy for cysts; 99% accuracy for solid masses; small carcinomas have the least characteristic features

Ultrasound pattern	Carcinoma	Fibroadenoma
smooth margin	1%	60%
ill-defined margin	84%	12%
echogenic halo	0%	71%
lateral shadowing	0%	45%
central shadowing	74%	5%
uniform internal echoes	21%	82%
nonuniform internal echoes	66%	17%
acoustic enhancement	7%	13%
broom-straw pattern	64%	0%
fir-tree pattern	24%	0%

CARCINOMA OF MALE BREAST
Incidence: 0.2 %
Peak age: 60 – 69 years
Associated with: high incidence of breast cancer in family members / radiation
√ resembles scirrhous carcinoma of female breast
√ usually located eccentrically
√ calcifications fewer + more scattered + more round + larger
√ enlarged axillary nodes

CHRONIC ABSCESS OF BREAST
= COLD ABSCESS usually seen in lactating women
• fever, pain, increased WBC (clinical diagnosis)
• rapid response to antibiotics
Location: most commonly in central / subareolar area
√ ill-defined / partially obscured mass of increased density
√ secondary changes common: architectural distortion, nipple + areolar retraction, skin thickening
US: √ anechoic / nearly anechoic area with posterior enhancement

CYSTOSARCOMA PHYLLOIDES
= GIANT FIBROADENOMA = usually benign giant form of intracanalicular fibroadenoma
Incidence: 1: 6,300 examinations; 0.3% of all breast tumors; 3% of all fibroadenomas
Mean age: 45 years
Histo: similar to fibroadenoma with anaplasia, fibroepithelial tumor with leaflike (phylloides) growth pattern = branching projections of tissue into cystic cavities; cystic degeneration + hemorrhage; cavernous structures containing mucus; cellular connective tissue stroma with wide variations in size, shape, differentiation
• rapidly enlarging breast mass
• sense of fullness
• firm, mobile, discrete, lobulated, smooth mass
√ mimics fibroadenoma with smooth polylobulated margins
√ rapid growth to large size (> 6 – 8 cm), may fill entire breast
Prognosis: limited invasion frequently seen; propensity for recurrence if not completely excised
Cx: malignant degeneration in < 5% with local invasion + hematogenous metastases to lung, pleura, bone

EDEMA OF BREAST
Etiology: (1) "Inflammatory" breast cancer (angiolymphatic spread)
(2) Post radiotherapy
(3) Infection / inflammatory causes
(4) Obstruction to lymphatic drainage in axilla
(5) Generalized edema from cardiac failure / hypoalbuminemia
(6) Complication of Coumadin therapy
(7) Accidental infusion of fluid into subcutaneous tissue

√ generalized increased density
√ skin thickening
√ reticular pattern in subcutis

FAT NECROSIS OF BREAST
= TRAUMATIC LIPID CYST = OIL CYST = aseptic saponification of fat by tissue lipase after local destruction of fat cells with release of lipids + hemorrhage
Incidence: 0.5% of breast biopsies
Histo: cavity with oily material surrounded by "foam cells" (= lipid-laden macrophages)
- Hx of trauma in 40% (e.g., prior surgery, radiation > 6 months ago, reduction mammoplasty, lumpectomy)
- firm slightly fixed mass
- skin retraction (50%)
- yellowish fatty fluid on aspiration
Location: anywhere; more common in areolar region
√ ill-defined irregular spiculated dense mass (indistinguishable from carcinoma if associated with distortion, skin thickening, retraction)
√ well-circumscribed mass with homogeneous fat density (oily cyst) surrounded by thin capsule near biopsy site / surgical scar
√ may calcify (= liponecrosis macrocystica calcificans)
  √ curvilinear / egg-shell calcification in wall (occasionally)
  √ branching configuration suggestive of malignancy
US:
  √ hypo- / anechoic mass with ill- / well-defined margins ± acoustic shadowing

Weber-Christian Disease
= nonsuppurative panniculitis with recurrent bouts of inflammation = areas of fat necrosis, involving subcutaneous fat + fat within internal organs
- accompanied by fever + nodules over trunk and limbs

FIBROADENOMA
= estrogen-induced benign tumor; pregnancy + lactation are growth stimulants; regression after menopause (mucoid degeneration, hyalinization, involution of epithelial components, calcification)
Incidence: 3rd most common type of breast lesion after fibrocystic disease + carcinoma, most common benign solid tumor in women of child-bearing age
Age: after puberty + before age 30; regresses after menopause
Histo: (a)   intracanalicular fibroadenoma
         (b)   pericanalicular fibroadenoma
         (c)   mixture
- firm, smooth, sometimes lobulated, freely moveable mass
- NO skin fixation
- may be tender / painful
- clinical size = radiographic size
Size: 1 – 5 cm (in 60%)

√ smooth, discrete margins (indistinguishable from cysts when small)
√ often with "halo" sign
√ nodular / lobulated contour when larger (areas with different growth rates)
√ multiple in 10 – 20%; bilateral in 4 %
√ calcifications in 3%; increase as soft tissue component regresses; ultimately "popcorn" calcification (PATHOGNOMONIC)
US: √ round uniformly hypoechoic mass with smooth margins + echogenic halo (capsule) with lateral shadowing
  √ posterior acoustic enhancement (25%)

JUVENILE FIBROADENOMA
= rapidly growing tumor in young girls during puberty
√ may grow to huge size, enlarging the breast

FIBROCYSTIC DISEASE
= Mazoplasia = Mastitis fibrosa cystica = Chronic cystic mastitis = Cystic disease = Generalized breast hyperplasia = Desquamated epithelial hyperplasia = Fibroadenomatosis = Mammary dysplasia = Schimmelbusch disease = Fibrous mastitis = Mammary proliferative disease
Incidence: most common diffuse breast disease; in 51% of 3,000 autopsies
Age: 35 – 55 years
Etiology: exaggeration of normal cyclical proliferation + involution of the breast
- asymptomatic
- fullness, tenderness, pain
- palpable nodules + thickening
- symptoms occur with ovulation; regression with pregnancy + menopause
Histo:
  (1)   overgrowth of fibrous connective tissue = stromal fibrosis, fibroadenoma
  (2)   cystic dilatation of ducts + cyst formation (in 100% microscopic, in 20% macroscopic)
  (3)   hyperplasia of ducts + lobules + acini = adenosis; ductal papillomatosis
√ individual round / ovoid cysts with discrete smooth margins
√ lobulated multilocular cyst
√ confluent + vaguely nodular pattern
√ thickening (= fibrous connective tissue overgrowth)
√ ill-defined fine / coarse nodular appearance (= duct proliferation)
√ linear / curvilinear thin calcifications with horizontal beam = milk of calcium (4%)
US: √ ductal pattern, ductectasia, cysts, ill-defined focal lesions

ADENOSIS
= increased number ± size of lobules
√ "snow-flake pattern" of widespread ill-defined nodular densities

SCLEROSING ADENOSIS
= adenosis + reactive fibrosis = proliferating acinar
structure maintaining a lobular configuration
√ adenosis + diffusely scattered calcifications
(calcifications in cystically dilated acinar structure)

FIBROSIS
√ round / oval clustered microcalcifications with smooth
contours + associated fine granular calcifications
filling lobules

ATYPICAL LOBULAR HYPERPLASIA
= proliferative cells not distending lobules (as in lobular
carcinoma in situ)
√ round dense microcalcifications in a loose cluster ,
some variability in size

INTRADUCTAL PAPILLOMATOSIS
= hyperplastic polypoid lesions within a duct
Age: perimenopausal
• spontaneous bloody / serous / serosanguinous nipple
discharge (most common cause of nipple discharge)
√ small retroareolar opacity (= dilated duct) extending 2
– 3 cm into breast
√ intraluminal filling defect on galactography

GRANULAR CELL MYOBLASTOMA OF BREAST
= tumor originating from ? Schwann cell, smooth muscle,
or undifferentiated mesenchymal cell
Age :   20 – 59 years; more common in blacks
Locations: tongue, skin, bronchial wall, subcutaneous
breast tissue (6%)
• asymmetric lump with slow growth, hardness, skin
fixation, ulceration
√ well-circumscribed mass with stellate extensions (tumor
insinuating itself into surrounding breast tissue)
√ may exhibit acoustic shadow

GYNECOMASTIA
= hypertrophy of male mammary gland
Causes:
(1) Hormonal
  (a) puberty: high estradiol levels
  (b) older men: decline in serum testosterone levels
  (c) Hypogonadism (Klinefelter syndrome, Testicular
  neoplasm)
  (d) Tumors: Adrenal carcinoma, Pituitary adenoma,
  Testicular tumor, Hyperthyroidism
(2) Systemic disorders
  Advanced alcoholic cirrhosis, Hemodialysis in
  chronic renal failure, Chronic pulmonary disease
  (emphysema, TB), Malnutrition
(3) Drug-induced
  estrogen treatment for prostate cancer, digitalis,
  cimetidine, thiazide, spironolactone, reserpine,
  isoniazid, ergotamine, marijuana
(4) Neoplasm: hepatoma (with estrogen production)
(5) Idiopathic
mnemonic: "CODES"
  Cirrhosis
  Obesity

Digitalis
Estrogen
Spironolactone

Incidence: 85% of all male breast masses
Age: adolescent boys (40%), men > 50 years (32%)
Histo: increased number of ducts, proliferation of duct
epithelium, periductal edema, fibroplastic stroma,
adipose tissue
• palpable firm mass > 2 cm in subareolar region
Location: bilateral (63%), left sided (27%), right sided
(10%)
Types: (a) focal type (b) diffuse type
DDx: Pseudogynecomastia (= fatty proliferation)

HAMARTOMA OF BREAST
= FIBROADENOLIPOMA = LIPOFIBROADENOMA
= ADENOLIPOMA
Incidence: 2 – 16 : 10,000 mammograms
Mean age: 45 (27 – 88) years
Histo: normal / dysplastic mammary tissue composed of
dense fibrous tissue + variable amount of fat,
delineated from surrounding tissue without a true
capsule
• soft, often nonpalpable (60%)
Location: retroareolar (30%),
upper outer quadrant (35%)
√ round / ovoid well-circumscribed mass
√ mixed density with mottled center (secondary to fat)
= "slice of sausage" pattern
√ smooth capsule (= thin layer of surrounding fibrous
tissue)
√ peripheral radiolucent zone
√ may contain calcifications

Cowden Disease = multiple hamartoma syndrome
1. Cutaneous + oral verrucous papules (lips, gingiva,
tongue)
2. Endodermal, ectodermal, mesodermal dysplasia with
tumors of skin, breast, GI tract, thyroid gland
3. Malignant tumors of breast + thyroid

HEMATOMA OF BREAST
Causes:
(1) surgery / biopsy (most common) (2) blunt trauma
(3) coagulopathy (leukemia, thrombocytopenia)
(4) anticoagulant therapy
√ well-defined mass (= hemorrhagic cyst)
√ ill-defined mass with diffuse increased density (edema +
hemorrhage)
√ adjacent skin thickening / prominence of reticular
structures
√ regression within several weeks leaving residual
scarring behind
√ calcifications (occasionally)
US: √ hypoechoic mass with internal echoes

INTRADUCTAL PAPILLOMA
Age: late reproductive years + postmenopause
Histo: hyperplastic proliferation of ductal epithelium; lesion may be pedunculated / broad-based; may cause duct obstruction + distension to form an Intracystic papilloma
- most common cause of serous / sanguinous nipple discharge
- √ usually NOT visualized on mammograms
- √ intraductal nodules in subareolar area / single dilated duct
- √ punctate calcifications in clusters (occasionally)
- √ galactography shows location of lesion
Cx: malignant degeneration rare but possible (increased risk of cancer in postmenopause)

LIPOMA OF BREAST
= usually solitary, asymptomatic, slow-growing lesion
Mean age: 45 years + postmenopause
- soft, freely moveable, well delineated
- √ radiolucent lesion easily seen in dense breast; almost invisible in fatty breast
- √ discrete thin radiopaque line (= capsule), seen in most of its circumference
- √ calcification (extremely rare)
DDx: fat lobule surrounded by trabeculae / suspensory ligaments

LYMPHOMA OF BREAST
A. Primary lymphoma: 0.3% incidence
B. Metastatic lymphoma
- axillary nodes involved in 35 %
Location: right-sided predominance; 13% bilateral
- √ round / oval mass
- √ infiltrate with poorly defined borders

PSEUDOLYMPHOMA
= lymphoreticular lesion as overwhelming response to trauma

MASTITIS
A. PUERPERAL MASTITIS
= usually interstitial infection during lactational period
  (a) through infected nipple cracks
  (b) hematogenous
  (c) ascending via ducts = galactophoritis
Organism: staphylococcus, streptococcus
- inflammation (DDx: inflammatory carcinoma)
- √ diffuse increased density
- √ diffuse skin thickening
- √ swelling of breast
- √ enlarged axillary lymph nodes
- √ rapid resolution under antibiotic therapy
B. NONPUERPERAL MASTITIS
  1. Infected cyst
  2. Purulent mastitis with abscess formation
  3. Plasma cell mastitis
  4. Nonspecific mastitis

C. GRANULOMATOUS MASTITIS
  1. Foreign body granuloma
  2. Specific disease (TB, Sarcoidosis, Leprosy, Syphilis, Actinomycosis, Typhus)
  3. Parasitic disease (Hydatid disease, Cysticercosis, Filiarisis, Schistosomiasis)

MEDULLARY CARCINOMA OF BREAST
Incidence: 5% of all breast carcinomas
Age: younger age group (11% of cancers diagnosed < 35 years of age)
Path: well-circumscribed mass with nodular architecture + lobulated contour; central necrosis is common in larger tumors; intense lymphoplasmocytic reaction (reflecting host resistance) propensity for syncytial growth, No glands
- √ uniformly dense round / oval noncalcified mass with lobulated margin
- √ may have partial / complete halo sign
US: √ hypoechoic mass + some degree of through transmission
  √ distinct / indistinct margins
Prognosis: 70% 10-year survival rate

METASTASES TO BREAST
Incidence: 1 %
Mean age: 43 years
Primaries: (1) Melanoma (2) Ovarian carcinoma
        (3) Leukemia / lymphoma
- √ solitary mass (85%), esp. in upper outer quadrant
- √ skin adherence (25%),
- √ axillary node involvement (40%)

PLASMA CELL MASTITIS
= rare aseptic inflammation of subareolar area
Age: elderly women
Histo: extravasation of intraductal secretions rich in fatty acids causing aseptic chemical mastitis followed by infiltration of plasma cells + giant cells + eosinophils
Location: subareolar, often bilateral + symmetric
- √ dense triangular mass with apex toward nipple
- √ distended ducts connecting to nipple
- √ periphery blending with normal tissue
- √ multiple often bilateral calcifications oriented towards nipple (very common)
  (a) periductal
   √ oval / elongated calcified ring around dilated ducts with very dense periphery (surrounding deposits of fibrosis + fat necrosis)
  (b) intraductal
   √ fairly uniform linear, often "needle-shaped" calcifications of wide caliber, occasionally branching (within ducts / confined to duct walls)
- √ nipple retraction / skin thickening may occur

SARCOMA OF BREAST
Incidence: 1% of malignant mammary lesions
Age: 45 – 55 years
Histo: Fibrosarcoma, Rhabdomyosarcoma, Osteogenic sarcoma, Mixed malignant tumor of the breast, Malignant fibrosarcoma and carcinoma, Liposarcoma

• rapid growth
√ smooth / lobulated large dense mass
√ well-defined outline
√ palpated size similar to mammographic size

DIFFERENTIAL DIAGNOSIS OF CARDIOVASCULAR DISORDERS

Classification of CHD

	acyanotic	cyanotic
Increased PBF + increased CT	*L-R shunts* VSD ASD PDA ECD PAPVR	*T-lesions* Transposition Truncus arteriosus TAPVR "Tingles" (single ventricle / atrium) Tricuspid atresia (without RVOT obstruction)
Normal PBF + normal CT	*LV outflow obstruction* AS Coarctation Interrupted aortic arch Hypoplastic left heart PS *LV inflow obstruction* Obstructed TAPVR Cor triatriatum Pulmonary vein atresia Congenital MV stenosis *Muscle Disease* Cardiomyopathy Myocarditis Anomalous LCA	
Decreased PBF + normal CT Cardiomegaly		*VSD present* Tetralogy of Fallot Tricuspid atresia (with PS + nonrestrictive ASD) Pulmonary atresia + VSD *Intact ventricular septum* Pulmonary atresia without VSD Ebstein anomaly Trilogy of Fallot Tricuspid atresia + PS + restrictive ASD Congenital tricuspid insufficiency

Incidence of CHD in live-born infants

Overall incidence: 8 – 9:1000 live births
- most common CHD: Mitral valve prolapse (5 – 20%), Bicuspid aortic valve (2%) [usually not recognized before late infancy / childhood]
- ASD + VSD + PDA account for 45% of all CHD
- 12 lesions account for 89% of all CHD

Ventricular septal defect	30.3%
Patent ductus arteriosus	8.6%
Pulmonary stenosis	7.4%
Septum secundum defect	6.7%
Coarctation of aorta	5.7%
Aortic stenosis	5.2%
Tetralogy of Fallot	5.1%
Transposition	4.7%
Endocardial cushion defect	3.2%
Hypoplastic right ventricle	2.2%
Hypoplastic left heart	1.3%
TAPVR	1.1%
Truncus arteriosus	1.0%
Single ventricle	0.3%
Double outlet right ventricle	0.2%

High risk pregnancy:
    (1) previous sibling with CHD: 2 – 5%
    (2) previous 2 siblings with CHD: 10 – 15%
    (3) one parent with CHD: 2 – 10%

Most common causes for CHF + PVH in neonate:
    1. left ventricular failure due to outflow obstruction
    2. obstruction of pulmonary venous return

CHD with relatively long life
Congenital lesions compatible with a relative long life are:
    1. Mild tetralogy: mild pulmonic stenosis + small VSD
    2. Valvar pulmonic stenosis: with relatively normal pulmonary circulation
    3. Transposition of great vessels: some degree of pulmonic stenosis + large VSD
    4. Truncus arteriosus: delicate balance between systemic + pulmonary circulation
    5. Truncus arteriosus type IV: large systemic collaterals
    6. Tricuspid atresia + transposition + pulmonic stenosis
    7. Eisenmenger complex
    8. Ebstein anomaly
    9. Corrected transposition without intracardiac shunt

Juxtaposition of atrial appendages
    1. Tricuspid atresia with transposition
    2. Complete transposition
    3. corrected transposition of great arteries
    4. DORV

Continuous heart murmur
    1. PDA
    2. AP window
    3. Ruptured sinus of Valsalva aneurysm
    4. Hemitruncus
    5. Coronary arteriovenous fistula

Neonatal cardiac failure
A. OBSTRUCTIVE LESIONS
    1. Coarctation of the aorta
    2. Aortic valve stenosis
    3. Asymmetrical septal hypertrophy / Hypertrophic obstructive cardiomyopathy
B. VOLUME OVERLOAD
    1. Congenital mitral valve incompetence
    2. Corrected transposition with left (= tricuspid) AV valve incompetence
    3. Congenital tricuspid insufficiency
    4. Ostium primum ASD
C. MYOCARDIAL DYSFUNCTION / ISCHEMIA
    1. Nonobstructive cardiomyopathy
    2. Anomalous origin of LCA from pulmonary trunk
    3. Primary endocardial fibroelastosis
    4. Glycogen storage disease (Pompe disease)
    5. Myocarditis
D. NONCARDIAC LESIONS
    1. AV fistulas: hemangioendothelioma of liver, AV fistula of brain, vein of Galen aneurysm, large pulmonary AV fistula
    2. Transient tachypnea of the newborn
    3. Intraventricular / subarachnoid hemorrhage
    4. Neonatal hypoglycemia (low birth weight, infants of diabetic mothers)
    5. Thyrotoxicosis (transplacental passage of LATS hormone)

Syndromes with CHD
5 p – (Cri-du-chat) syndrome
    Incidence of CHD: 20%

DiGeorge syndrome (thymic agenesis)
    1. Conotruncal malformation
    2. Interrupted aortic arch

Presenting age in CHD

AGE	SEVERE PVH	PVH + SHUNT VASCULARITY
0 – 2 days	Hypoplastic left heart Aortic atresia TAPVR below diaphragm Myocardiopathy in IDM	Hypoplastic left heart TAPVR above diaphragm Complete transposition
3 – 7 days		PDA in preterm infant
7 – 14 days	CoA + VSD / PDA Aortic valve stenosis Peripheral AVM Endocardial fibroelastosis Anomalous left coronary artery	Coarctation of aorta (CoA) AVM

Down syndrome = MONGOLISM = TRISOMY 21
1. Endocardial cushion defect (25%)
2. Membranous VSD
3. Ostium primum ASD
4. AV communis
5. Cleft mitral valve
6. PDA
7. 11 rib pairs (25%)
8. Hypersegmented manubrium (90%)

Ellis-van-Creveld syndrome
Incidence of CHD: 50%
• polydactyly
√ single atrium

Holt-Oram syndrome
= UPPER LIMB-CARDIAC SYNDROME
Incidence of CHD: 50%
1. ASD
2. VSD
3. Valvar pulmonary stenosis
4. Radial dysplasia

Hurler syndrome
Cardiomyopathy

Ivemark syndrome
Incidence of CHD: 100%
• asplenia
√ complex cardiac anomalies

Marfan syndrome = ARACHNODACTYLY
1. Aortic sinus dilatation
2. Aortic aneurysm
3. Aortic insufficiency
4. Pulmonary aneurysm

Noonan syndrome
Pulmonary stenosis, ASD, Hypertrophic cardiomyopathy

Postrubella syndrome
• Low birth weight
• Deafness
• Cataracts
• Mental retardation
1. Peripheral pulmonic stenosis
2. Valvar pulmonic stenosis
3. Supravalvar aortic stenosis
4. PDA

Turner syndrome (XO) = OVARIAN DYSGENESIS
Incidence of CHD: 35%
1. Coarctation of the aorta (in 15%)
2. Bicuspid aortic valve

Trisomy 16 – 18
VSD, PDA, DORV

Trisomy 13 – 15
VSD, Tetralogy of Fallot, DORV

William syndrome = IDIOPATHIC HYPERCALCEMIA
• peculiar elfin-like facies
• mental + physical retardation
• hypercalcemia (not in all patients)
1. Supravalvular aortic stenosis (33%)
2. ASD, VSD
3. Valvular + peripheral pulmonary artery stenosis
4. Aortic hypoplasia, stenoses of more peripheral arteries

SHUNT EVALUATION
Evaluation of L-to-R shunts
A. AGE
   Λ Infants:
   (1) isolated VSD
   (2) VSD with CoA / PDA / AV canal
   (3) PDA
   (4) Ostium primum
   Δ Children / adults:
   (1) ASD
   (2) Partial AV canal with   competent mitral valve
   (3) VSD / PDA with high pulmonary resistance
   (4) PDA without murmur
B. SEX
   99% chance for ASD / PDA in female patient
C. CHEST WALL ANALYSIS
   √ 11 pair of ribs + hypersegmented manubrium: Down syndrome
   √ pectus excavatum + straight back: prolapsing mitral valve
D. CARDIAC SILHOUETTE
   √ absent pulmonary trunk: corrected transposition with VSD; pink tetralogy
   √ left-sided ascending aorta: corrected transposition with VSD
   √ tortuous descending aorta: aortic valve incompetence + ASD
   √ enlarged left atrium: intact atrial septum; mitral regurgitation (endocardial cushion defect, prolapsing mitral valve + ASD)
   √ huge heart: Persistent complete AV canal (PCAVC); VSD + PDA; VSD + mitral valve incompetence

DIFFERENTIAL DIAGNOSIS OF L-R SHUNTS

	RA	RV	PA	LA	LV	Prox. Ao
ASD	inc	inc	inc	nl	nl	nl
VSD	nl	inc	inc	inc	inc	nl
PDA	nl	nl	inc	inc	inc	often inc

Shunt with normal left atrium
A. Precardiac shunt
 1. Anomalous pulmonary venous connection
B. Intracardiac shunt
 2. ASD (8%)
 3. VSD (25%)
C. Postcardiac
 4. PDA (12%)

Aortic size in shunts
A. Extracardiac shunts
 √ aorta enlarged + hyperpulsatile
 1. PDA
B. Pre- and intracardiac shunts
 √ aorta small but not hypoplastic
 1. Anomalous pulmonary venous return
 2. ASD
 3. VSD
 4. Common AV canal

Abnormal heart chamber dimensions
A. LEFT VENTRICULAR VOLUME OVERLOAD
 1. VSD
 2. PDA
 3. Mitral incompetence
 4. Aortic incompetence
B. LEFT VENTRICULAR HYPERTROPHY
 1. Coarctation
 2. Aortic stenosis
C. RIGHT VENTRICULAR VOLUME OVERLOAD
 1. ASD
 2. Partial APVR / total APVR
 3. Tricuspid insufficiency
 4. Pulmonary insufficiency
 5. Congenital / acquired absence of pericardium
 [6. Ebstein anomaly] – not truly RV
D. RIGHT VENTRICULAR HYPERTROPHY
 1. Pulmonary valve stenosis
 2. Pulmonary hypertension
 3. Tetralogy of Fallot
 4. VSD
E. Fixed subvalvar aortic stenosis
F. Hypoplastic left / right ventricle; Common ventricle
G. Congestive cardiomyopathy

CYANOTIC HEART DISEASE

A. OVERCIRCULATION VASCULARITY
 mnemonic: "5 T's + CAD"
 1. **T**ransposition, complete
 2. **T**ricuspid atresia with transposition
 3. **T**runcus arteriosus
 4. **T**APVR above diaphragm
 5. **T**ingle ventricle
 6. **C**ommon atrium
 7. **A**ortic atresia
 8. **D**ORV

B. DECREASED VASCULARITY (with R-to-L shunt)
 (a) at ATRIAL LEVEL
 1. Isolated pulmonary stenosis / atresia
 2. Tricuspid atresia without transposition with pulmonary stenosis
 3. Ebstein / Uhl malformation
 4. Congenital tricuspid regurgitation
 5. Pericardial effusion
 (b) at VENTRICULAR LEVEL
 1. Tetralogy of Fallot
 2. Single ventricle
 3. Tricuspid atresia without transposition without pulmonary stenosis
 4. DORV
 5. Asplenia syndrome
 6. Corrected transposition + VSD

C. PULMONARY VENOUS HYPERTENSION
 1. Atresia of common pulmonary vein
 2. TAPVR below diaphragm
 3. Aortic atresia
Nota bene: Tricuspid atresia = the great mimicker

Increased pulmonary blood flow with cyanosis
= ADMIXTURE LESIONS = bidirectional shunt with 2 components:
 (a) mixing of saturated blood (L-R shunt) and unsaturated blood (R-L shunt)
 (b) NO obstruction to pulmonary blood flow

Evaluation process:
 √ PA segment absent = Transposition
 √ PA segment present:
 (a) L atrium normal (= extracardiac shunt) = TAPVR
 (b) L atrium enlarged (= intracardiac shunt) = Truncus arteriosus

Nota bene: Overcirculation + cyanosis = complete transposition until proven otherwise!

ADMIXTURE LESIONS = T-LESIONS = *"5 T's plus CAD"*
Transposition of great vessels = complete TGV ± VSD (most common cause for cyanosis in neonate)
Tricuspid atresia with or without transposition + VSD (2nd most common cause for cyanosis in neonate)
Truncus arteriosus
Total anomalous pulmonary venous return (TAPVR) above diaphragm
 (a) supracardiac
 (b) cardiac (coronary sinus / right atrium)
"**T**ingle" = single ventricle
Common atrium
Aortic atresia
Double-outlet right ventricle (DORV type I) / Taussig-Bing anomaly (DORV type II)

Clues:
- √ skeletal anomalies: Ellis-van Creveld syndrome (truncus / common atrium)
- √ polysplenia: common atrium
- √ R aortic arch: persistent truncus arteriosus
- √ ductus infundibulum: aortic atresia
- √ pulmonary trunk seen: supracardiac TAPVR; DORV; tricuspid atresia; common atrium
- √ ascending aorta with leftward convexity: single ventricle
- √ dilated azygous vein: common atrium + polysplenia + interrupted IVC; TAPVR to azygous vein
- √ left-sided SVC: vertical vein of TAPVR
- √ "waterfall" right hilum: single ventricle + transposition
- √ large left atrium (rules out TAPVR)
- √ prominent L heart border: single ventricle with inverted rudimentary R ventricle; levoposition of R atrial appendage (tricuspid atresia + transposition)
- √ age of onset ≤ 2 days: aortic atresia

Decreased pulmonary blood flow with cyanosis

= two components of (a) impedance of blood flow through right heart due to obstruction / atresia at pulmonary valve / infundibulum (b) R-to-L shunt; pulmonary circulation maintained through systemic arteries / PDA

A. <u>SHUNT AT VENTRICULAR LEVEL</u>
1. Tetralogy of Fallot
2. Tetralogy physiology (associated with pulmonary obstruction):
   - Complete / corrected transposition
   - Single ventricle
   - DORV
   - Tricuspid atresia (PS in 75%)
   - Asplenia syndrome
- √ prominent aorta with L / R aortic arch; inapparent pulmonary trunk
- √ NORMAL R atrium (without tricuspid regurgitation)
- √ NORMAL-sized heart (secondary to escape mechanism into aorta)

Clues:
1. Skeletal anomaly (e.g. scoliosis): Tetralogy (90%)
2. Hepatic symmetry: Asplenia
3. Right aortic arch: Tetralogy, Complete transposition, Tricuspid atresia
4. Aberrant right subclavian artery: Tetralogy
5. Leftward convexity of ascending aorta: Single ventricle with inverted right rudimentary ventricle, Corrected transposition, Asplenia, JAA (tricuspid valve atresia)

B. <u>SHUNT AT ATRIAL LEVEL</u>
1. **P**ulmonary stenosis / atresia with intact ventricular septum
2. **E**bstein malformation + Uhl anomaly
3. **T**ricuspid atresia (ASD in 100%)
- √ moderate to severe cardiomegaly
- √ R atrial dilatation

- √ R ventricular enlargement (secondary to massive tricuspid incompetence)
- √ inapparent aorta
- √ left aortic arch

ACYANOTIC HEART DISEASE
Increased pulmonary blood flow without cyanosis

= indicates L-R shunt with increased pulmonary blood flow (> 40% shunt)

A. <u>WITH LEFT ATRIAL ENLARGEMENT</u>
Indicates shunt distal to mitral valve = increased volume without escape defect
1. VSD (25%): small aorta in intracardiac shunt
2. PDA (12%): aorta + pulmonary artery of equal size in extracardiac shunt
3. Ruptured sinus of Valsalva aneurysm (rare)
4. Coronary arteriovenous fistula (very rare)
5. Aortopulmonary window (extremely rare)

B. <u>WITH NORMAL LEFT ATRIUM</u>
Indicates shunt proximal to mitral valve = volume increased with escape mechanism through defect
6. ASD (8%)
7. Partial anomalous pulmonary venous return (PAPVR) + sinus venosus ASD
8. Endocardial cushion defect (ECD) (4%)

Normal pulmonary blood flow without cyanosis

A. <u>OBSTRUCTIVE LESION</u>
(a) Right ventricular outflow obstruction
1. at level of pulmonary valve: Subvalvar / valvar / supravalvar pulmonic stenosis
2. at level of peripheral pulmonary arteries: Peripheral pulmonary stenosis
(b) Left ventricular inflow obstruction
1. at level of peripheral pulmonary veins: Pulmonary vein stenosis / atresia
2. at level of left atrium: Cor triatriatum
3. at level of mitral valve: Supravalvar mitral stenosis, congenital mitral stenosis / atresia, "parachute" mitral valve
(c) Left ventricular outflow obstruction
1. at level of aortic valve: Anatomic subaortic stenosis, functional subaortic stenosis (IHSS), valvular aortic stenosis, hypoplastic left heart, supravalvar aortic stenosis
2. at level of aorta: Interruption of aortic arch, coarctation of aorta

B. <u>CARDIOMYOPATHY</u>
1. Endocardial fibroelastosis
2. Hypertrophic cardiomyopathy
3. Glycogen storage disease

C. <u>HYPERDYNAMIC STATE</u>
1. Noncardiac AVM (cerebral AVM, vein of Galen aneurysm, large pulmonary AVM, hemangioendothelioma of liver)
2. Thyrotoxicosis

3. Anemia
4. Pregnancy
D. MYOCARDIAL ISCHEMIA
   1. Anomalous left coronary artery
   2. Coronary artery disease (CAD)

PULMONARY VASCULARITY
Increased pulmonary vasculature
A. <u>Overcirculation</u> = shunt vascularity = arterial + venous overcirculation
   (a) Congenital heart disease (most common)
      (1) L-R shunts
      (2) Admixture lesions / cyanotic lesions
   (b) High-flow syndromes
      (1) Thyrotoxicosis (2) Anemia (3) Pregnancy
      (4) Peripheral arteriovenous fistula
   √ increased size of veins + arteries with size larger than accompanying bronchus (= "kissing cousin" sign), best seen just above hila on AP view
   √ enlarged hilar vessels (lateral view)
   √ diameter of right descending pulmonary artery larger than trachea just above aortic knob
   √ visualization of vessels below 10th posterior rib
B. <u>Pulmonary venous hypertension</u>
   √ redistribution of flow (not seen in younger children)
   √ indistinctness of vessels with Kerley lines (= interstitial edema)
   √ alveolar edema
   √ fine reticulated pattern
C. <u>Precapillary hypertension</u>
   √ enlarged main + right and left pulmonary arteries
   √ abrupt tapering of pulmonary arteries
D. <u>Prominent systemic / aortopulmonary collaterals</u>
   1. Tetralogy of Fallot with pulmonary atresia (= pseudotruncus)
   2. VSD + pulmonary atresia (single ventricle, complete transposition, corrected transposition)
   3. Pulmonary-systemic collaterals
   √ coarse vascular pattern with irregular branching arteries (from aorta / subclavian arteries)
   √ small central vessels despite apparent increase in vascularity

Decreased pulmonary vascularity
= obstruction to pulmonary flow
√ vessels reduced in size and number
√ hyperlucent lungs
√ small hilar vessels + pulmonary artery segment

Normal pulmonary vascularity + normal-sized heart
mnemonic: "MAN"
Myocardial ischemia
Afterload (= pressure overload problems)
Normal

Pulmonary arterial hypertension
= PAH = pulmonary arterial pressure in systole > 30 mmHg, in diastole > 15 mmHg, mean pressure > 20 mmHg
Pathogenesis:
A. PRIMARY PAH (rare) = plexogenic pulmonary arteriopathy = unknown cause / mechanism
B. SECONDARY PAH (more common)
   (a) Primary pleuropulmonic disease
      1. Parenchymal pulmonary disease = cor pulmonale: COPD, emphysema, chronic bronchitis, asthma, bronchiectasis, malignant infiltrate, granulomatous disease, cystic fibrosis, end-stage fibrotic lung, S/P lung resection, idiopathic hemosiderosis, alveolar proteinosis, Alveolar microlithiasis
      2. Pleural disease + chest deformity: Fibrothorax, thoracoplasty, kyphoscoliosis
      3. Alveolar hypoventilation = hypoxic pulmonary arterial hyperperfusion: Chronic high altitude, sleep apnea, hypoventilation due to neuromuscular disease / obesity
   (b) Primary vascular disease
      1. Congenital heart disease
         - increased flow: large L-R shunt (Eisenmenger syndrome)
         - decreased flow: Tetralogy of Fallot
      2. Capillary obliteration: Chronic pulmonary thromboembolism, persistent fetal circulation, arteritides (e.g., Takayasu)
      3. Venous obliteration: Pulmonary venoocclusive disease
   (c) Pulmonary venous hypertension

Histo:
Grade I = hypertrophy of media of muscular pulmonary arteries + arterioles
Grade II = hypertrophy of muscle cells + proliferation of intima cells in small muscular arteries + arterioles
Grade III = muscular hypertrophy + intimal thickening + subendothelial fibrosis
Grade IV = occlusion of vessels with progressive dilatation of small arteries nearby; muscular hypertrophy less apparent
Grade V = tortuous channels within proliferation of endothelial cells (= plexiform + angiomatoid lesions) + intraalveolar macrophages
Grade VI = thrombosis + necrotizing arteritis
√ dilatation of pulmonary trunk, main pulmonary arteries, intermediate arteries
√ rapid tapering of pulmonary arteries with narrowed peripheral pulmonary vessels
√ NO increase of pulsations in middle third of lung
√ calcification of central pulmonary vessels (PATHOGNOMONIC)
√ normal-sized heart / right heart enlargement

Pulmonary venous hypertension
= INCREASED VENOUS PULMONARY PRESSURE
= VENOUS CONGESTION
Causes:
  A. <u>LEFT VENTRICULAR INFLOW TRACT OBSTRUCTION</u>
   √ normal-sized heart with right ventricular hypertrophy
   √ prominent pulmonary trunk
   @ proximal to mitral valve:
    √ normal-sized left atrium
    1. TAPVR below the diaphragm
    2. Primary pulmonary veno-occlusive disease
    3. Stenosis of individual pulmonary veins
    4. Atresia of common pulmonary vein
    5. Cor triatriatum
    6. Left atrial tumor / clot
    7. Supravalvular ring of left atrium
    8. Fibrosing mediastinitis
    9. Constrictive pericarditis
   @ at mitral valve level
    √ enlarged left atrium
    1. Rheumatic mitral valve stenosis + regurgitation (99%)
     √ enlarged left atrial appendage
    2. Congenital mitral valve stenosis
    3. Parachute mitral valve (= single bulky papillary muscle)
  B. <u>LEFT VENTRICULAR FAILURE</u>
   (a) ABNORMAL PRELOAD with secondary mitral valve incompetence (= volume overload)
    1. Aortic valve regurgitation
    2. Eisenmenger syndrome (= R-to-L shunt in VSD)
    3. High-output failure:
     Noncardiac AVM (cerebral AVM, vein of Galen aneurysm, large pulmonary AVM, hemangioendothelioma of liver, iatrogenic), thyrotoxicosis, anemia, pregnancy
   (b) ABNORMAL AFTERLOAD (= pressure overload) = LV outflow tract obstruction
    1. Hypoplastic left heart syndrome
    2. Aortic stenosis (supravalvar, valvar, anatomic subaortic)
    3. Interrupted aortic arch
    4. Coarctation of the aorta
   (c) DISORDERS OF CONTRACTION AND RELAXATION
    1. Endocardial fibroelastosis
    2. Glycogen storage disease (Pompe disease)
    3. Cardiac aneurysm
    4. Cardiomyopathy
     (a) congestive (alcohol)
     (b) hypertrophic obstructive cardiomyopathy (HOCM), particularly in IDM
      — asymmetric septal hypertrophy (ASH)
      — idiopathic hypertrophic subaortic stenosis (IHSS)
   (d) MYOCARDIAL ISCHEMIA
    1. Anomalous left coronary artery
    2. Coronary artery disease (CAD)

AORTA
Enlarged aorta
  A. Increased volume load
    1. Aortic insufficiency
    2. PDA
  B. Poststenotic dilatation
    1. Valvular aortic stenosis
  C. Increased intraluminal pressure
    1. Coarctation
    2. Systemic hypertension
  D. Mural weakness / infection
    1. Cystic media necrosis: Marfan / Ehlers-Danlos syndrome
    2. Congenital aneurysm
    3. Syphilitic aortitis
    4. Mycotic aneurysm
    5. Atherosclerotic aneurysm (compromised vasa vasorum)
  E. Laceration of aortic wall
    1. Traumatic aneurysm
    2. Dissecting hematoma

Right aortic arch
Incidence: 1 – 2%
INCIDENCE OF RIGHT AORTIC ARCH IN CONGENITAL HEART DISEASE
  1. Truncus arteriosus   35%
  2. Tetralogy of Fallot   25%
  3. TGV   10%
  4. Tricuspid atresia   5%
  5. Large VSD   2%
  rare anomalies:
  1. Corrected transposition   50%
  2. Pseudotruncus   50%
  3. Asplenia   30%
  4. Pink tetralogy   15%

mnemonic: " TRUE TETRA TRICK"
TRUncus arteriosus
TEtralogy of Fallot
TRAnsposition
TRICuspid atresia

Right aortic arch with aberrant left subclavian artery
= interruption of embryonic left arch between left CCA and left subclavian artery; most common type of aortic arch anomaly: 35 – 72%
Incidence: 1:2,500
Associated with congenital heart disease in 12%:
  1. Tetralogy of Fallot   (2/3 = 8%)
  2. ASD ± VSD   (1/4 = 3%)
  3. Coarctation   (1/12 = 1%)

- usually asymptomatic (loose ring around trachea + esophagus)
- may be symptomatic in infancy / early childhood provoked by bronchitis + tracheal edema
- may be symptomatic in adulthood provoked by torsion of aorta
√ left common carotid artery is first branch of ascending aorta
√ retroesophageal aortic diverticulum (= diverticulum of Kommerell)
  √ small rounded density lateral to trachea
  √ impression on left side of esophagus simulating a double aortic arch
√ vascular ring (= left ductus extends from aortic diverticulum to left pulmonary artery)

√ right aortic arch impression on tracheal air shadow
√ broad posterior impression on esophagus (left subclavian artery)
√ small anterior impression on trachea
√ aorta descends on right side

Right aortic arch with mirror image branching
2nd most common aortic arch anomaly: 24 – 60%
= interruption of embryonic left arch between left subclavian artery and descending aorta; dorsal to left ductus arteriosus
(a) Type 1 = interruption of left aortic arch distal to ductus arteriosus (common)
  Associated with cyanotic congenital heart disease in 98%:

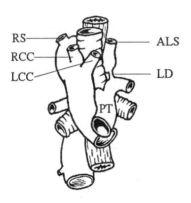

Right aortic arch with aberrant left subclavian

RS / LS   = right / left subclavian a.
LD   = left ductus arteriosus

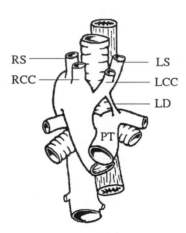

Right aortic arch with mirror image branching

RCC / LCC   = right / left common carotid a.
ALS   = aberrant left subclavian a.

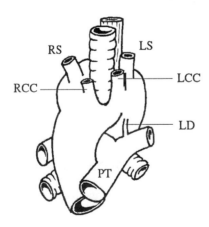

Double aortic arch

RS / LS   = Right / left subclavian a.
LD   = left ductus arteriosus
PT   = pulmonary trunk

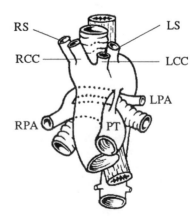

Aberrant left pulmonary artery

RCC / LCC   = right / left common carotid a.
RPA / LPA   = right / left pulmonary a.

1. Tetralogy of Fallot (87%)
2. Multiple defects (7.5%)
3. Truncus arteriosus (2 – 6%)
4. Transposition (1 – 10%)
5. Tricuspid atresia (5%)
6. ASD ± VSD (0.5%)
Δ 25% of patients with Tetralogy have right aortic arch
Δ 37% of patients with Truncus arteriosus have right aortic arch
√ NO vascular ring, NO retroesophageal component
√ NO structure posterior to trachea
√ R arch impression on tracheal air shadow
√ NORMAL barium swallow
(b) Type 2 = interruption of left aortic arch proximal to ductus arteriosus (rare)
true vascular ring (if duct persists)
rarely associated with CHD

Right aortic arch
with isolated left subclavian artery
3rd most common right aortic arch anomaly: 2%
= interruption of embryonic left arch between
(a) left CCA and left subclavian artery and
(b) left ductus and descending aorta
resulting in a connection of left subclavian artery with left pulmonary artery
Associated with: Tetralogy of Fallot
√ left common carotid artery arises as the first branch
√ left subclavian artery attaches to left pulmonary artery through PDA
√ NO vascular ring, NO retroesophageal component
• congenital subclavian steal syndrome

Right aortic arch
with aberrant left brachiocephalic artery
similar in appearance to R aortic arch + aberrant L subclavian artery

Left aortic arch
Left aortic arch
with aberrant right subclavian artery
= right subclavian artery arises as 4th branch from proximal descending aorta
Incidence: 1:200 (most common congenital vascular anomaly)
Associated with: (1) absent recurrent pharyngeal nerve
(2) CHD in 10 – 15%
Course: (a) behind esophagus (80%)
(b) between esophagus + trachea (15%)
(c) anterior to trachea (5%)
√ radiolucent band crossing the esophagus obliquely upward toward the right shoulder
√ unilateral L-sided rib notching (if aberrant R subclavian artery arises distal to coarctation)

Double Aortic Arch

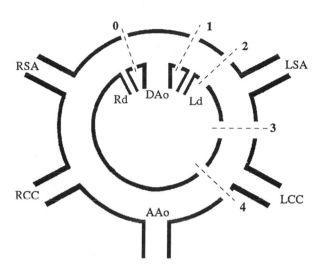

Anomalous innominate artery compression syndrome
= origin of R innominate artery to the left of trachea coursing to the right
√ anterior tracheal compression

Double Aortic Arch
common cause of vascular ring
• usually asymptomatic
• stridor, dyspnea, recurrent pneumonia
• dysphagia (less common than respiratory symptoms, more common after starting baby on solids)
Location: in 75% left descending aorta, in 25% right descending aorta; smaller arch anterior in 80%; right arch larger than left in 80%
√ impressions may be present on both sides of trachea: usually R > L
√ broad posterior impression on esophagus
√ small anterior impression on trachea
DDx: right arch with aberrant left subclavian artery (indistinguishable by esophagram when dominant arch on right side)

Pattern of vascular compression of esophagus and trachea
A. Large posterior impression on esophagus + anterior tracheal compression:
1. Double aortic arch
2. Right aortic arch with aberrant left subclavian + left ductus / ligamentum arteriosus
3. Left aortic arch with aberrant right subclavian + right ductus / ligamentum (extremely rare)
B. Anterior tracheal indentation
1. Compression by innominate artery with origin more distal along arch
2. Compression by left common carotid with origin more proximal on arch

3. Common origin of innominate and left common carotid artery
C. Small posterior indentation of esophagus
   1. Left aortic arch with aberrant right subclavian artery
   2. Right aortic arch with aberrant left subclavian artery (very rare)
D. Posterior indentation of trachea + anterior compression of esophagus:
   1. Aberrant left pulmonary artery

Symptomatic vascular rings

(a) Usually symptomatic lesions:
   1. Double aortic arch with R descending aorta + L ductus arteriosus
   2. R aortic arch with R descending aorta + aberrant L subclavian artery + persistent L ductus / ligamentum teres
   3. L arch with L descending aorta + R ductus / ligamentum
   4. Aberrant L pulmonary artery = "pulmonary sling"
(b) Occasionally symptomatic lesions:
   1. Anomalous innominate
   2. Anomalous L common carotid artery / common trunk
   3. R aortic arch with L descending aorta + L ductus / ligamentum
(c) Usually asymptomatic lesions:
   1. L aortic arch + aberrant R subclavian artery
   2. L aortic arch with R descending aorta

3. R aortic arch with R descending aorta + mirror image branching
4. R aortic arch with R descending aorta + aberrant L subclavian artery
5. R aortic arch with R descending aorta + isolation of L subclavian artery
6. R aortic arch with L descending aorta + L ductus / ligamentum

Abnormal left ventricular outflow tract

LVOT = area between IVS + aML from aortic valve cusps to mitral valve leaflets
1. Membranous subaortic stenosis
   = crescent-shaped fibrous membrane extending across LVOT + inserting at aML
   √ diffuse narrowing of LVOT
   √ abnormal linear echoes in LVOT space (occasionally)
2. Prolapsing aortic valve vegetation
3. Narrowed LVOT (< 20 mm)
   (a) Long-segment subaortic stenosis
      √ aortic valve closure in early systole with coarse fluttering
      √ high frequency flutter of mitral valve in diastole (aortic regurgitation)
      √ symmetric LV hypertrophy
   (b) ASH / IHSS
      √ asymmetrically thickened septum bulging into LV + LVOT
      √ systolic anterior motion of aML (SAM)

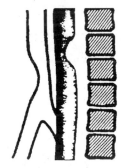

Pattern A

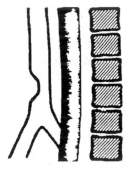

Pattern B

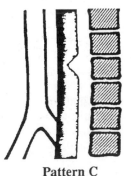

Pattern C

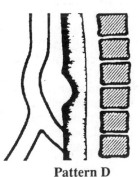

Pattern D

(c) Mitral stenosis
(d) Endocardial cushion defect

PULMONARY ARTERY
Unequal pulmonary blood flow
1. Tetralogy of Fallot
   √ diminished flow on left side (hypoplastic / stenotic pulmonary artery in 40%)
2. Persistent truncus arteriosus (esp., Type IV)
   √ diminished / increased blood flow to either lung
3. Pulmonary valvular stenosis
   √ increased flow to left lung secondary to jet phenomenon

Invisible main pulmonary artery
A. Underdeveloped = RVOT obstruction
   1. Tetralogy of Fallot
   2. Hypoplastic right heart syndrome (tricuspid / pulmonary atresia)
B. Misplaced pulmonary artery
   1. Complete transposition of great vessels
   2. Persistent truncus arteriosus

Dilatation of pulmonary trunk
1. Idiopathic dilatation of pulmonary artery
2. Pulmonic valve stenosis
   √ poststenotic dilatation of trunk + left pulmonary artery

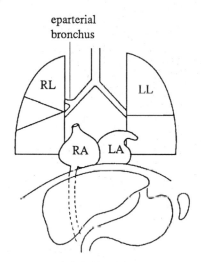

SITUS SOLITUS
anterior view

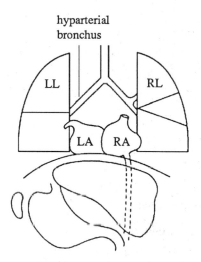

SITUS INVERSUS
anterior view

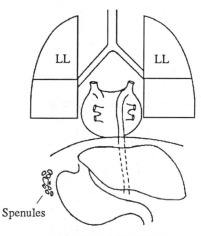

LEFT ISOMERISM
posterior view

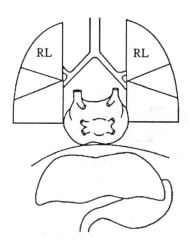

RIGHT ISOMERISM
posterior view

CARDIOSPLENIC SYNDROMES
= sporadic disorders with abnormal relationship between abdominal organs + tendency toward symmetric development of organs within trunk + associated cardiac anomalies

	Asplenia bilateral R sidedness	**Polysplenia** bilateral L sidedness
CLINICAL		
Presenting age	newborn / infant	infant / adult
Sex predominance	male	female
Cyanosis	severe	usually absent
Heart disease	severe	moderate / none
Howell-Jolly bodies	present	absent
Spleen scan	no spleen	multiple small spleens
Characteristic ECG	none	abnormal P wave vector
Prognosis	poor	good
Mortality	high	low
PLAIN FILM		
Lung vascularity	decreased	normal / increased
Aortic arch	right / left	right / left
Cardiac apex	right / left / midline	right / left
Bronchi	bilateral eparterial	bilateral hyparterial
Minor fissure	possibly bilateral	normal / none
Stomach	midline / right / left	right / left
Liver	symmetrical / R / L	in various positions
Malrotation of bowel	yes	yes
CARDIOGRAPHY		
Coronary sinus	usually absent	sometimes absent
Atrial septum	Common atrium (100%)	ASD (84%)
AV valve	atresia / common valve	normal / abnormal MV
Single ventricle	44%	infrequent
IVS	VSD	VSD common
Great vessels	d- / l-transposition (72%)	normal relationship
Pulmonary stenosis	the rule	frequent
Pulmonary veins	TAPVR	PAPVR (42%) TAPVR (6%)
Single coronary artery	19%	
SVC	bilateral (53%)	bilateral (33%)
IVC-aorta relationship	same side of spine	normal
IVC	normal	interrupted (84%) / normal
Azygos vein	inapparent	continuation R / L

3. Pulmonary regurgitation
   (a) severe pulmonic valve insufficiency
   (b) absence of pulmonic valve (may be associated with Tetralogy)

SITUS
= term describing the position of atria, tracheobronchial tree, pulmonary arteries, thoracic + abdominal viscera
A. SITUS SOLITUS = normal situs
   = position of anatomic LA is the same as that of the aortic arch + stomach bubble + hyparterial bronchus + bilobed lung; the position of the anatomic RA is the same as that of the eparterial bronchus + trilobed lung

Associated with:
   (a) levocardia   : < 1% chance for CHD
   (b) dextrocardia   : 95% chance for CHD
B. SITUS INVERSUS
   = mirror-image position of normal
Associated with:
   (a) dextrocardia = Situs inversus totalis (usual variant): 3 – 5% chance for CHD, e.g. Kartagener's syndrome
   (b) levocardia (extremely rare): 95% chance for CHD
C. SITUS INDETERMINATUS / INDETERMINUS / AMBIGUUS
   = ambiguous relationship

√ symmetrical liver + midline stomach
Associated with:
(a) bilateral right isomerism / sidedness
    = Asplenia syndrome
(b) bilateral left isomerism / sidedness
    = Polysplenia syndrome

Cardiac position
A. POSITION OF CARDIAC APEX
   1. Levocardia = L-sided heart
   2. Dextrocardia = R-sided heart
   3. Mesocardia = midline heart (usually with situs solitus)
B. CARDIAC DISPLACEMENT
   by extracardiac factors (e.g., lung hypoplasia, pulmonary mass)
   1. Dextroposition
      suggests hypoplasia of ipsilateral pulmonary artery (PAPVR implies scimitar syndrome)
   2. Levoposition
   3. Mesoposition
C. CARDIAC INVERSION
   = alteration of normal relationship of chambers
   1. D-bulboventricular loop
   2. L-bulboventricular loop
D. TRANSPOSITION
   = alteration of anterior-posterior relationship of great vessels

CARDIAC TUMOR
Malignant heart tumors
1. Angiosarcoma
2. Multiple cardiac myxomas
3. Metastatic disease: most commonly breast, lung, melanoma
4. Lymphoma
   Incidence: cardiac involvement in 29% on autopsy; pericardial involvement more frequent
   • intractable congestive heart failure
   • chest pain
   √ SVC obstruction

Benign heart tumor
1. Myxoma
2. Rhabdomyoma:
   associated with tuberous sclerosis
3. Hydatid Cyst (uncommon):
   √ localized bulge of left cardiac contour
   √ curvilinear / spotty calcifications (resembling myocardial aneurysm)
   Cx: may rupture into cardiac chamber / pericardium

Congenital cardiac tumor
Incidence: 1:10,000
1. Rhabdomyoma (58%)
   Associated with: tuberous sclerosis (in 50 – 86%)

• supraventricular tachycardia (accessory conductive pathways within tumor)
√ often mutliple
√ tendency to involve septum
2. Teratoma (20%): intrapericardiac, extracardiac
3. Fibroma (12%):
   √ may be pedunculated, may calcify
4. Myxoma, Hemangioma, Mesothelioma:
   √ mass-occupying lesion impinging upon cardiac cavities

PERICARDIUM
Cardiophrenic angle mass
A. Lesion of pericardium
   1. Pericardial cyst
   2. Intrapericardial bronchogenic cyst
   3. Benign intrapericardial neoplasm:
      teratoma, leiomyoma, hemangioma, lipoma
   4. Malignant neoplasm:
      mesothelioma, metastasis (lung, breast, lymphoma, melanoma)
B. Cardiac lesion: aneurysm
C. Others: masses arising from lung, pleura, diaphragm, abdomen

Pericardial effusion
= pericardial fluid > 50 ml
Etiology:
A. Serous fluid = transudate
   Congestive heart failure, Hypoalbuminemia, Irradiation
B. Blood
   (a) iatrogenic: Cardiac surgery, Cardiac catheterization, Anticoagulants, Chemotherapy
   (b) Trauma: penetrating / nonpenetrating
   (c) Acute myocardial infarction / rupture
   (d) Rupture of ascending aorta / pulmonary trunk
   (e) Coagulopathy
   (f) Neoplasm: Mesothelioma, Sarcoma, Teratoma, Fibroma, Angioma, Metastasis (lung, breast, lymphoma, leukemia, melanoma)
C. Lymph
   (a) Neoplasm (b) Congenital (c) Cardiothoracic surgery (d) Obstruction of hilum / SVC
D. Fibrin = exudate
   (a) Infection: viral, pyogenic, TB
   (b) Uremia: 18% in acute uremia; 51% in chronic uremia; dialysis patient
   (c) Collagen disease: Rheumatoid arthritis, SLE, Acute rheumatic fever
   (d) Hypersensitivity
CXR:
√ normal with fluid < 250 ml / in acute pericarditis
√ "water bottle configuration" = symmetrically enlarged cardiac silhouette
√ loss of retrosternal clear space
√ "fat pad sign" = separation of retrosternal from epicardial fat line > 2 mm (15%)

√ rapidly appearing cardiomegaly + normal pulmonary vascularity

√ "differential density sign" = increase in lucency at heart margin secondary to slight difference in contrast between perlcardlal fluid + heart muscle

√ diminished cardiac pulsations

ECHO: √ separation of epi- and pericardial echoes extending into diastole (rarely behind LA)
Volume estimates by M-mode:
(a) separartion only posteriorly = < 300 ml
(b) separation throughout cardiac cycle = 300 – 500 ml
(c) plus anterior separation = > 1000 ml

Vena cava anomalies

1. RETROCAVAL URETER = CIRCUMCAVAL URETER
2. DUPLICATED IVC
   Incidence: 0.2 – 3%
   Etiology: persistence of right + left supracardinal veins
   √ small / equal-sized left IVC formed by left iliac vein
   √ crossover to right IVC via left renal vein / or more inferiorly
   √ crossover usually anterior / rarely posterior to aorta
3. TRANSPOSITION OF IVC
   Incidence: 0.2 – 0.5%
   Etiology: persistence of left + regression of right supracardinal vein
   √ left IVC usually crosses over via left renal vein / or more inferiorly
   √ crossover usually anterior / rarely posterior to aorta
4. RETROAORTIC LEFT RENAL VEIN
   Incidence: 1.8 – 2.4%
   Etiology: persistence of posterior intersupracardinal anastomosis + regression of anterior intersubcardinal anastomosis
   √ crossover usually below / occasionally at level of right renal vein
5. CIRCUMAORTIC LEFT RENAL VEIN
   Incidence: 1.5 – 8.7%
   Etiology: persistence of anterior intersubcardinal + posterior intersupracardinal anastomosis
   √ venous collar encircling aorta
6. INTERRUPTED IVC WITH AZYGOS / HEMIAZYGOS CONTINUATION
   Incidence: 0.6%
   Etiology: failure to form subcardinohepatic anastomosis
   Associated with: congenital heart disease, indeterminate situs, polysplenia, asplenia (rare)
   √ drainage of hepatic veins directly into right atrium via posthepatic segment of IVC
   √ drainage of iliac + renal veins via azygos / hemiazygos vein
7. LEFT SVC
   Incidence: 0.3%
   Etiology: persistence of left anterior cardinal vein
   √ left SVC drains into coronary sinus

√ simultaneously present right SVC (82 – 90%) draining into right atrium

√ anastomosis between right + left anterior cardinal veins (in 35%)

IVC obstruction

INTRINSIC OBSTRUCTION
A. NEOPLASTIC (most frequent)
B. NON-NEOPLASTIC
   1. Idiopathic
   2. proximally extending thrombus from femoroiliac veins
   3. Systemic disorders: Coagulopathy, Budd-Chiari syndrome, Infection, Sepsis, CHF
   4. Postoperative / traumatic phlebitis, ligation, plication, clip, cava filter, severe exertion
   5. Congenital membrane

EXTRINSIC COMPRESSION
A. NEOPLASTIC
   1. Retroperitoneal lymphadenopathy (adults)
   2. Renal + adrenal tumors (children)
   3. Hepatic masses
   4. Pancreatic tumor
   5. Tumor-induced desmoplastic reaction (e.g., metastatic carcinoid)
B. NONNEOPLASTIC
   1. Hepatomegaly
   2. Tortuous aorta / aortic aneurysm
   3. Retroperitoneal hematoma
   4. Massive ascites
   5. Retroperitoneal fibrosis

FUNCTIONAL OBSTRUCTION
1. Pregnant uterus
2. Valsalva maneuver
3. Straining / crying (in children)
4. Supine position with large abdominal mass

Surgical procedures

AORTICOPULMONARY WINDOW SHUNT
= side-to-side anastomosis between ascending aorta and left pulmonary artery (reversible procedure)
Δ Tetralogy of Fallot

BLALOCK-HANLON PROCEDURE
= surgical creation of ASD
Δ Complete transposition

BLALOCK-TAUSSIG SHUNT
= end-to-side anastomosis of subclavian artery to pulmonary artery, performed ipsilateral to innominate artery / opposite to aortic arch
Δ Tetralogy, of Fallot Tricuspid atresia with pulmonic stenosis

FONTAN PROCEDURE
= (1) external conduit from right atrium to pulmonary trunk (= venous return enters pulmonary artery directly) (2) closure of ASD: floor constructed from flap of atrial wall and roof from piece of prosthetic material

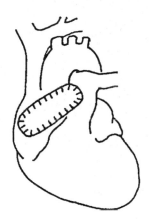

Fontan Procedure

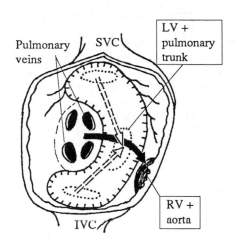

Mustard Procedure
(lateral view into opened right atrium)

Δ Tricuspid atresia
GLENN SHUNT
= end-to-side shunt between distal end of right
pulmonary artery and IVC; reserved for patients with
cardiac defects in which total correction is not
anticipated
Δ Tricuspid atresia
POTT SHUNT
= side-to-side anastomosis between descending aorta +
left pulmonary artery
Δ Tetralogy of Fallot
MUSTARD PROCEDURE
(1) removal of atrial septum (b) pericardial baffle placed
into common atrium such that systemic venous blood is
rerouted into left ventricle and pulmonary venous return
into right ventricle and aorta
Δ Complete transposition
RASHKIND PROCEDURE = balloon atrial septostomy
Δ Complete transposition
RASTELLI PROCEDURE
external conduit (Dacron) with porcine valve connecting
RV to pulmonary trunk
Δ Transposition
WATERSTON-COOLEY SHUNT
= side-to-side anastomosis between ascending aorta
and right pulmonary artery; (a) extrapericardial
(WATERSTON) (b) intrapericardial (COOLEY)
Δ Tetralogy of Fallot

Postoperative thoracic deformity
on RIGHT SIDE:
1. Systemic-PA shunt: Blalock-Taussig shunt,
Waterston-Cooley shunt,
Glenn shunt, Central conduit
shunt

2. Atrial septectomy: Blalock-Hanlon procedure
3. VSD repair: through RA
4. Mitral valve commissurotomy

on LEFT SIDE:
1. PDA
2. Coarctation
3. PA banding
4. Mitral valve commissurotomy
5. Systemic-PA shunt: Blalock-Taussig shunt, Pott
shunt

Heart valve prosthesis
1. Starr-Edwards
√   caged ball
Δ   predictable performance from large long-term
experience
2. Bjørk-Shiley / Lillehei-Kaster / St. Jude
√   tilting disc
Δ   excellent hemodynamics, very low profile, durable
3. Hancock / Carpentier-Edwards (= porcine xenograft)
Ionescu-Shiley (= bovine xenograft)
Δ   low incidence of thromboembolism, no hemolysis,
central flow, inaudible

Coronary artery calcification
= due to (1) arteriosclerosis of intima (2) Mönckeberg
medial sclerosis (exceedingly rare)
CXR: (detection rate up to 42%) indicating more severe
coronary artery disease
Fluoroscopy: (promoted as inexpensive screening test)
—   in 34% calcifications in asymptomatic male
individuals
—   in 54% of symptomatic patients with ischemic heart
disease

— in 35% of patients with calcifications exercise test will be positive (without calcifications only in 4% positive)
— calcifications indicate > 50% stenosis with 72 – 76% sensitivity, 78% specificity; frequency of coronary artery calcifications with normal angiogram increases with age; predictive values in population < 50 years as good as exercise stress test

Location:
   "coronary artery calcification triangle" = triangular area along mid left heart border, spine, and shoulder of LV containing left main coronary artery, proximal portions of LAD + LCX calcifications at autopsy:
      LAD (93%), LCX (77%), left main CA (70%), RCA (69%)
√ parallel calcified lines (lateral view)
Prognosis: 58% 5-year survival rate with and 87% without calcifications

CARDIAC ANATOMY AND ECHOCARDIOGRAPHY

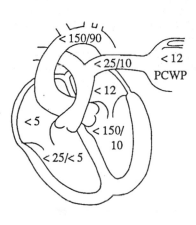

Normal Blood Pressures

PCWP = pulmonary capillary wedge pressure

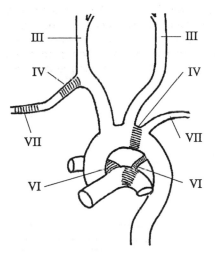

Development of Major Blood Vessels

numbers refer to embryologic aortic arche

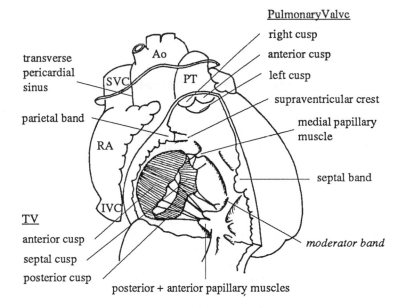

Right Ventricle Viewed From Front

Demarcation between posteroinferior inflow portion and anterosuperior outflow portion
by prominent muscular bands forming an almost circular orifice

— parietal band
— crista supraventricularis
— septomarginal trabeculae (= septal band + moderator band)

Anterior papillary muscle originates from moderator band!

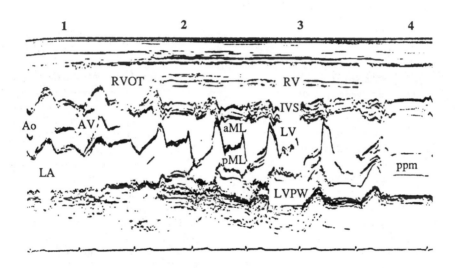

Sweep of transducer from aorta toward apex

Area 1: recognized by parallel motion of both aortic walls (a) toward the transducer during systole (b) away from the transducer during diastole. Left atrial posterior wall (LAPW) does not move because of mediastinal attachment by pulmonary veins

Aortic valve cusps (right coronary + noncoronary / left cusps) are positioned in middle of aorta during diastole, open abruptly during systole at onset of ventricular ejection in a "box-like" fashion.

Aortic + LA dimension are similar in most cases.

Area 2: Aortic-septal continuity = anterior aortic wall becomes interventricular septum

Aortic-mitral continuity = posterior aortic wall becomes anterior mitral valve leaflet

Mitral valve with typical "M" configuration during diastole; motion of aML toward transducer during systole secondary to movement of whole mitral valve apparatus

Area 3: posterior mitral valve leaflet (pML) = reciprocal "W-shaped" configuration; left ventricular posterior wall (PVPW) shows anterior motion during systole

Area 4: Chordae tendineae in continuity with mitral valve leaflets merge with a thick posterior band of echoes representing the posteromedial papillary muscle (ppm)

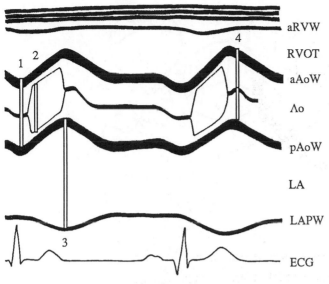

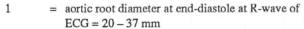

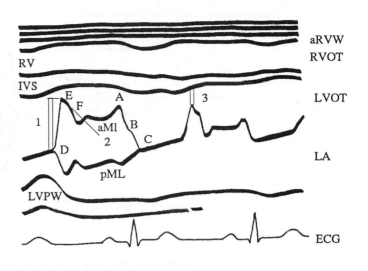

Echocardiogram of Aortic Root

1	=	aortic root diameter at end-diastole at R-wave of ECG = 20 – 37 mm
2	=	aortic cusp separation = 15 – 26 mm
3	=	left atrial dimension at moment of mitral valve opening = 15 – 40 mm
4	=	eccentricity index of aortic valve cusps = ratio of anterior to posterior dimension < 1.3 (rarely used)
aRVW	=	anterior right ventricular wall
RVOT	=	right ventricular outflow tract
aAoW	=	anterior aortic wall
Ao	=	aorta
pAoW	=	posterior aortic wall
LA	=	left atrium
LAPW	=	left atrial posterior wall
ECG	=	electrocardiogram

Echocardiogram of Mitral Valve

1	=	opening amplitude of anterior leaflet of mitral valve (DE amplitude) ≥ 16 mm
2	=	early diastolic posterior motion of anterior leaflet (EF slope) ≥ 75 mm/sec
3	=	E point septal separation ≤ 10 mm
RV	=	right ventricle
IVS	=	interventricular septum
LVPW	=	left ventricular posterior wall
aML	=	anterior mitral valve leaflet
pML	=	posterior mitral valve leaflet
aRVW	=	anterior right ventricular wall
RVOT	=	right ventricular outflow tract
LVOT	=	left ventricular outflow tract
LA	=	left atrium
ECG	=	electrocardiogram
A	=	point of atrial contraction
C	=	closure point
DE	=	opening secondary to passive ventricular filling
CD	=	systole with steady anterior drift of coapted leaflets (passive movement secondary to movement of entire heart toward chest wall)

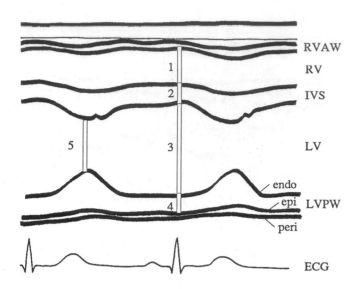

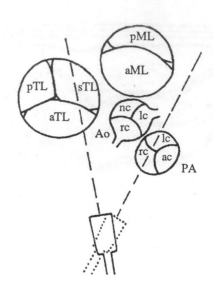

Echocardiogram of Right and Left Ventricle

1	=	RV end-diastolic dimension (RVEDD) at R-wave of ECG ≤ 30 mm
2	=	end-diastolic IVS thickness at R wave of ECG = 6 – 12 mm
3	=	LV end-diastolic dimension (LVEDD) at R-wave of ECG = 39 – 56 mm
4	=	end-diastolic LVPW thickness at R-wave of ECG = 6 – 12 mm
5	=	LV end-systolic dimension (LVESD)
RVAW	=	right ventricular anterior wall
RV	=	right ventricle
IVS	=	interventricular septum
LV	=	left ventricle
LVPW	=	left ventricular posterior wall
endo	=	endocardium
epi	=	epicardium
peri	=	pericardium

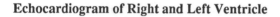

Fractional shortening (FS) = [(end-diastolic size - systolic size) / end-diastolic size] x 100

Δ	for LV	= 25 – 42%
Δ	for IVS	= 28 – 62%
Δ	for LVPW	= 36 – 70%

Diagram showing the relationship of the four cardiac valves in cross section

aTL, pTL, sTL = anterior, posterior, septal tricuspid valve leaflets
aML, pML   = anterior, posterior mitral valve leaflet
rc, lc, nc (Ao) = right, left, non-coronary cusp of aorta
rc, lc, ac (PA) = right, left, anterior cusp of pulmonary artery

Normal Echocardiographic Values in Adults

	range (mm)
Aortic root dimension (end-diastolic)	20 – 37
Aortic cusp separation	15 – 26
Left atrial dimension	15 – 40
Mitral valve excursion	≥ 16
E point septal separation	≤ 10
RV dimension (end-diastolic)	< 30
IVS thickness (end-diastolic)	6 – 12
LVPW thickness (end-diastolic)	6 – 12
IVS:LVPW thickness	< 1.3
Left ventricular dimension (end-diastolic)	39 – 56
Fractional shortening	0.25 – 0.42

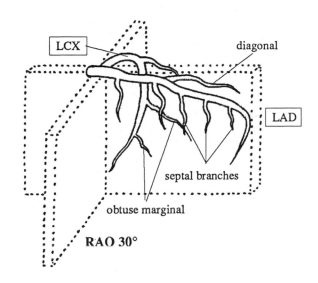

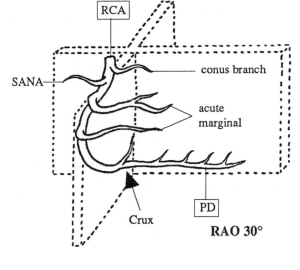

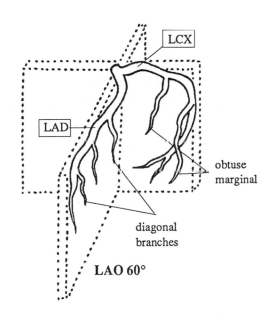

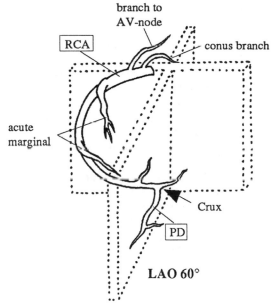

Anatomy of Left Coronary Artery

Marginals emanate from vessels in the AV groove (RCA, LXR)
— on left side called obtuse marginal arteries
— on right side called acute marginal arteries

Diagonals emanate from vessel in the interventricular groove
(LAD)
Note: **D**iagonals from LA**D**

Coronary Dominance
the dominant vessel is the one which supplies the
inferolateral wall of LV

AV-node branch from RCA (in 90%) = conus branch (1st
branch in 50%)

SA-node branch from RCA (in > 50%)

Anatomy of Right Coronary Artery

Arteries in atrioventricular plane:
RCA = right coronary artery
LCX = left circumflex artery

Arteries in interventricular plane:
LAD = left anterior descending artery
PD = posterior descending artery
SANA = sinoatrial node artery

CORONARY ARTERIES
Coronary arteriography
CONTRAST AGENTS:
1. Monomeric ionic contrast material:
   (a) negative inotropic = depression of myocardial contractility due to hyperosmolality of sodium + decrease in total calcium
   (b) peripheral vasodilatation
2. Meglumine diatrizoate (contains small quantities of sodium citrate + EDTA)
3. Nonionic contrast material = slight increase in LV contractility

Mortality: 0.05 %

Risk factors associated with death:
1. multiple ventricular premature contractions
2. congestive heart failure
3. systemic hypertension
4. severe triple-vessel coronary artery disease (highest risk)
5. LV ejection fraction < 30 %
6. Left main coronary artery stenosis

PROJECTIONS:
   (a) LAO + 20 – 30° caudocranial angulation
   proximal 1/3 of LAD + origin of first diagonal branch
   (b) LAO + 20 – 30° craniocaudal angulation = "spider view"
   Left main coronary artery, proximal LCX, first marginal / diagonal branches
   (c) RAO + 20 – 30° craniocaudal angulation
   Proximal 1/3 of LCX + origin of its branches
   (d) RAO + 20 – 30° caudocranial angulation
   Separation of LAD from diagonal branches

<u>False-negative interpretation</u>:
   (1) eccentric lesion in 75 %
   (2) foreshortening of vessel
   (3) overlap of other vessels remedied by angulated projections: improved diagnosis (50%), upgrade to more significant stenosis (30%), lesion unmasked (20%)

Coronary Collaterals
A. INTRACORONARY COLLATERALS
   = filling of a distal portion of an occluded vessel from the proximal portion
   √ tortuous course outside the normal path
B. INTERCORONARY COLLATERALS
   = between different coronary arteries / between branches of the same artery
   Location: on epicardial surface, in atrial / ventricular septum, in myocardium
   1. <u>proximal RCA to distal RCA</u>
      (a) by way of acute marginal branches
      (b) from sinoatrial node artery (SANA) to atrioventricular node artery (AVNA) = Kugel collateral
   2. <u>RCA to LAD</u>
      (a) between PDA and LAD through ventricular septum / around apex
      (b) conus artery (1st branch of RCA) to proximal part of LAD
      (c) acute marginals of RCA to right ventricular branches of LAD
   3. <u>distal RCA to distal LCX</u>
      (a) posterolateral segment artery of RCA to distal LCX (in AV groove)
      (b) AVNA of RCA to LCX (through atrial wall)
      (c) posterolateral branch of RCA to obtuse marginal branches of LCX (over left posterolateral ventricular wall)
   4. <u>proximal LAD to distal LAD</u>
      (a) proximal diagonal to distal diagonal artery of LAD
      (b) proximal diagonal to LAD directly
   5. <u>LAD to obtuse marginal of LCX</u>

DISEASE ENTITIES OF HEART AND GREAT VESSELS

ABERRANT LEFT PULMONARY ARTERY
= PULMONARY SLING = failure of development /
    obliteration of left 6th aortic arch followed by
    development of a collateral branch of right pulmonary
    artery to supply the left lung
Site: left PA passes above right mainstem bronchus +
    between trachea and esophagus on its way to left
    lung
Age at presentation: neonate / infant / child
Associated with:
    (1) "napkin-ring trachea" = absent pars membranacea
        (50%)
    (2) PDA (most common), ASD, Persistent left SVC
- stridor (most common), wheezing, apneic spells,
    cyanosis
- respiratory infection
- feeding problems
√ deviation of trachea to left
√ "inverted T" appearance of mainstem bronchi
    = horizontal course secondary to lower origin of right
    mainstem bronchus
√ anterior bowing of right mainstem bronchus
√ "carrot-shaped trachea" = narrowing of tracheal
    diameter in caudad direction resulting in functional
    tracheal stenosis
√ obstructive emphysema / atelectasis of RUL + LUL
√ low left hilum
√ separation of trachea + esophagus at hilum by soft
    tissue mass
√ anterior indentation on esophagogram

AMYLOIDOSIS
= extracellular deposits of insoluble fibrillar protein
- asymptomatic / CHF (restrictive cardiomyopathy),
    arrhythmia
CXR: √ normal / generalized cardiomegaly
        √ pulmonary congestion
        √ pulmonary deposits of amyloid
NUC: √ striking uptake of Tc-99m pyrophosphate
        greater than bone (50 – 90%)
ECHO: √ granular sparkling appearance of myocardium
        √ LV wall thickening
        √ decreased LV systolic + diastolic function

ANOMALOUS LEFT CORONARY ARTERY
= left coronary artery arises from pulmonary trunk (left
    sinus of Valsalva)
Hemodynamics: with postnatal fall in pulmonary arterial
    pressure perfusion of LCA drops (ischemic left coronary
    bed), collateral circulation from RCA with flow reversal in
    LCA
    —   adequate collateral circulation   = life-saving
    —   inadequate collateral circulation   = myocardial
    infarction

— large collateral circulation = L–R shunt with volume
    overload of heart
- episodes of sweating, ashen color (angina
    symptomatology)
- ECG: anterolateral infarction
- continuous murmur (if collaterals large)
√ dilatation of LV
√ enlargement of LA
√ normal pulmonary vascularity / redistribution
Rx:
    (1) Ligation of LCA at its origin from pulmonary trunk
    (2) Ligation of LCA + graft of left subclavian artery to
        LCA
    (3) Creation of an AP window + baffle from AP window
        to ostium of LCA
DDx: Endocardial fibroelastosis, Viral cardiomyopathy
    (NO shock-like Sx)

ANOMALOUS PULMONARY VENOUS RETURN
Total Anomalous Pulmonary Venous Return
= TAPVR = anomalous connection between pulmonary
    veins and systemic veins secondary to embryologic
    failure of the common pulmonary vein to join the
    posterior wall of the left atrium
Associated with: ASD (necessary for survival)

A. SUPRADIAPHRAGMATIC TAPVR
    Type I = SUPRACARDIAC TAPVR (52%)
            = drainage into left innominate vein / right
                + left persistent SVC / azygos vein;
                < 10% obstructed
    Type II = CARDIAC TAPVR (30%)
            = drainage into RA / coronary sinus
    Hemodynamics:
        — functional L-to-R shunt from pulmonary veins to
            right atrium
        — increased pulmonary blood flow
            (= overcirculation)
        — ASD restores oxygenated blood to left side
        — normal systemic venous pressure with
            increased flow through widened SVC
        — after birth CHF secondary to (a) mixture of
            systemic + pulmonary venous blood in RA
            (b) volume overload of RV
- neck veins undistended (shunt level distally)
- R ventricular heave (= increased contact of
    enlarged RV with sternum)
- systolic ejection murmur (large shunt volume)
√ "figure of 8" / "snowman" configuration of cardiac
    silhouette (= dilated SVC + left vertical vein)
√ pretracheal density on lateral film (= left vertical
    vein)
√ enlargement of RA + RV (= volume overload)
√ normal LA (= ASD acts as escape valve)

√ increased pulmonary blood flow
    (= overcirculation)
√ absent connection of pulmonary veins to LA

B. INFRACARDIAC TAPVR (12%) = Type III
    = drainage into IVC / portal vein / hepatic vein with
    constriction of descending pulmonary vein by
    diaphragm en route through esophageal hiatus
    leading to pulmonary venous hypertension + RV
    pressure overload; > 90% obstructed
    • intense cyanosis + respiratory distress (R-to-L
    shunt through ASD)
    Prognosis: death within a few days of life
    Associated with: asplenia syndrome (80%),
                           polysplenia
    √ unique appearance of pulmonary edema with
    normal-sized heart (DDx: hyaline membrane
    disease)
    √ low anterior indentation on barium-filled
    esophagus
C. MIXED TYPE = Type IV
    = with various connections to R side of heart (6%)
Overall Prognosis: 75% mortality rate within 1 year
                          of birth if untreated

Partial Anomalous Pulmonary Venous Return
= PAPVR
(a) RUL pulmonary vein enters SVC / RA
    frequently associated with: sinus venosus type
    ASD (90%)
    √ RUL vein courses in a horizontal direction
(b) LUL pulmonary vein enters innominate vein
    frequently associated with: ostium secundum
    type ASD
    √ vertical density along left upper border of
    mediastinum

AORTIC ANEURYSM
Causes:
1. Congenital (2%): post coarctation, ductus
    diverticulum
2. Atherosclerosis (73 – 80%): descending aorta
3. Posttraumatic (15 – 20%)
4. Syphilis: ascending aorta + arch
5. Mycotic
6. Arteritis (Takayasu, giant cell, relapsing
    polychondritis)
7. Cystic media necrosis (Marfan / Ehlers-Danlos
    syndrome, annuloaortic ectasia)

TRUE ANEURYSM   = all layers of wall intact
FALSE ANEURYSM   = all layers of wall disrupted
FUSIFORM ANEURYSM   = circumferential involvement
SACCULAR ANEURYSM   = involvement of portion of wall

Abdominal Aneurysm
= focal widening > 3 cm
Age: > 60 years; M:F = 5:1

Associated with:
(a) visceral + renal artery aneurysm (2%)
(b) isolated iliac + femoral artery aneurysm (16%):
    common iliac (89%), internal iliac (10%),
    external iliac (1%)
(c) stenosis / occlusion of celiac trunk / SMA (22%)
(d) stenosis of renal artery (22 – 30%)
(e) occlusion of inferior mesenteric artery (80%)
(f) occlusion of lumbar arteries (78%)
Growth rate of aneurysm of 3 – 6 cm in diameter:
    0.39 cm / year
• asymptomatic (30%)
• abdominal mass (26%)
• abdominal pain (37%)
Site: infrarenal (91%) with extension into iliac arteries
        (66%)
Plain film: √ mural calcification (86%)
CT: √ perianeurysmal fibrosis (10%), may cause
                  ureteral obstruction
US: √ > 98% accuracy in size measurement
Angio:
    √ focally widened aortic lumen > 3 cm
    √ normal-sized lumen secondary to mural thrombus
    (11%)
    √ mural clot (80%)
    √ slow antegrade flow of contrast medium
    Δ contained rupture = extraluminal hematoma / cavity
        √ absent parenchymal stain = avascular halo
        √ displacement + stretching of aortic branches
Cx:

(1) Rupture (25%)
    (a) into retroperitoneum: commonly on left
    (b) into GI tract: massive GI hemorrhage
    (c) into IVC: rapid cardiac decompensation
    Incidence: < 4 cm in 10%, 4 – 5 cm in 23%,
                       5 – 7 cm in 25%, 7 – 10 cm in
                       46%, > 10 cm in 60%
(2) Peripheral embolization
(3) Infection
(4) Spontaneous occlusion of aorta
Prognosis: 17% 5-year survival without surgery,
               50 – 60% 5-year survival with surgery
Postoperative Cx: (1) Left colonic ischemia (1.6%)
                           with 10% mortality
                      (2) Renal failure (14%)

Mycotic Aneurysm
Incidence: 2.6% of all abdominal aneurysms
A. PRIMARY MYCOTIC ANEURYSM (rare)
    unassociated with any demonstrable intravascular
    inflammatory process
B. SECONDARY MYCOTIC ANEURYSM
    Etiology:
    (1) IV drug abuse (2) bacterial endocarditis (12%)
    (3) immunocompromise (malignancy, alcoholism,
    steroids, chemotherapy, autoimmune disease,
    diabetes) (4) S/P aortic valve surgery / coronary
    artery bypass

Mechanism:
   (a) septicemia with abscess formation via vasa vasorum
   (b) septicemia with abscess formation via vessel lumen
   (c) direct extension of contiguous infection
   (d) preexisting intima laceration (trauma, atherosclerosis, coarctation)
Organism: S. aureus (53%), Salmonella (33-50%), Streptococcus, Mycobacterium
Site: ascending aorta > abdominal visceral artery > intracranial artery > lower / upper extremity vessel
√ saccular structure arising eccentrically from aortic wall, rapid enlargement
√ interrupted ring of aortic wall calcification
√ periaortic gas collection
√ adjacent vertebral osteomyelitis
√ adjacent reactive lymph node enlargement
Cx: life-threatening hemorrhage (75%)
Prognosis: 67% overall mortality

Thoracic Aneurysm

Normal size of thoracic aorta: 4 – 5 cm wide; most aneurysms rupture when > 10 cm in size
Associated with: hypertension, coronary artery disease, abdominal aneurysm
Mean age: 65 years; M:F = 3:1
• substernal / back / shoulder pain (26%)
• SVC syndrome (venous compression)
• dysphagia (esophageal compression)
• stridor, dyspnea (tracheobronchial compression)
• hoarseness (recurrent laryngeal nerve compression)
√ wide tortuous aorta
√ curvilinear peripheral calcifications
√ Angio: may show normal caliber secondary to mural thrombus
Prognosis: 1-year survival 57%, 3-year survival 26%, 5-year survival 19% (60% die from ruptured aneurysm, 40% die from other causes)
Surgical mortality: 10%

AORTIC DISSECTION

= hematoma developing in middle to outer third of aorta dissecting proximal + distally
Incidence: 3:1,000
Age: 30 – 85 years; M:F = 3:1
Path: hemorrhage of vasa vasorum leading to (a) tear in weakened intima (95 – 97%) if hematoma breaks into aortic lumen (b) no intimal tear (3 – 5%)
Predisposed: (cystic medial necrosis / disease of aortic wall)
1. Hypertension (60%)   5. S/P prosthetic valve
2. Marfan syndrome (16%)   6. Trauma (rare)
3. Coarctation   7. Pregnancy
4. Valvar aortic stenosis   NOT syphilis

TYPES:
DeBakey Type I   (29 – 34%)= dissection involving entire aorta
DeBakey Type II (12 – 21%)= dissection involving ascending aorta only
DeBakey Type III (50%)   = dissection involving descending aorta only
Stanford Type A   = ascending aorta involved
Stanford Type B   = ascending aorta NOT involved
Location of dissection:
— on lateral wall of ascending aorta
— on superior + posterior wall of aortic arch
— on posterior + left wall of descending aorta (involvement of left renal artery in 50%)
• sharp tearing intractable chest pain (75%)
• murmur, bruit (65%): aortic regurgitation
• asymmetric peripheral pulses (59%)
• absent femoral pulses (25%), reappearing after reentry
• hemodynamic shock (25%)
• neurologic deficits (25%): hemiplegia, paraparesis
• persistent oliguria
• congestive heart failure
• recurrent arrhythmias / right bundle branch block
• signs of pericardial tamponade

CXR: (best assessment from comparison with serial films)
√ mediastinal widening (40 – 80%) due to hemorrhage / large false channel
√ cardiac enlargement (LV hypertrophy / hemopericardium)
√ irregular wavy contour / indistinct outline of aorta
√ "calcification sign" = inward displacement of atherosclerotic plaque by 4 – 10 mm from outer aortic contour (7%), can only be applied to contour of descending aorta secondary to projection, may be misleading in presence of periaortic soft tissue mass / hematoma
√ left pleural effusion (27%)
√ atelectasis of lower lobe
√ displacement of trachea / endotracheal tube
Angio (1st choice because of contrast limitation):
√ abnormal catheter position outside anticipated aortic course
√ linear radiolucency within opacified aorta (= intimal / medial flap)
√ "double barrel aorta" (87%) = opacification of second channel
√ compression of true lumen by false channel (72 – 85%)
√ aortic valvular regurgitation (30%)
√ increase in aortic wall thickness > 6 – 10 mm
√ obstruction of aortic branches: left renal artery (25 – 30%)
√ slower blood flow in false lumen
CT: within 4 hours (if patient responds rapidly to medical Rx)

√ crescentic high-attenuation area along aortic wall
√ displaced intimal calcification
Cx: (1) aortic valve malfunction
     (2) rupture into pericardium / pleural cavity: 70%
          mortality
     (3) occlusion of major aortic branches:
          compromise of coronary artery (8%)
     (4) rupture of aorta
     (5) development of saccular aneurysm requiring
          surgery (15%)
Prognosis:
   immediate death (3%), death within 24 hrs. (20 – 30%),
   death by end of 1st week (50%), death by 3 weeks
   (60%), death at 3 months (80%), alive after 1 year
   (10 – 20%)
Rx:
   (1) Surgical reinforcement of aortic wall (Type I, II)
        preventing proximal extension
   (2) Reducing peak systolic pressure (Type III rarely
        progresses proximally)

AORTIC REGURGITATION
A. Intrinsic valve disease
    1. Congenital bicuspid valve
    2. Rheumatic endocarditis
    3. Bacterial endocarditis (perforation / prolapse of
        cusp)
    4. Myxomatous valve associated with cystic medial
        necrosis
    5. Prosthetic valve: mechanical break, thrombosis,
        paravalvular leak
B. Primary disease of ascending aorta
    (a) Dilatation of aortic annulus
        1. Syphilitic aortitis
        2. Ankylosing spondylitis (5 – 10%)
        3. Reiter disease
        4. Rheumatoid arthritis
        5. Cystic medial necrosis: Marfan syndrome
    (b) Laceration
        1. Decelerating trauma
        2. Hypertension
Pathogensis:
   progressive enlargement of diastolic + systolic LV
   dimensions results in increase in myocardial fiber length
   + increase in stroke volume; decompensation occurs if
   critical limit of fiber length is reached
• "water-hammer pulse" = twin-peaked pulse
• systolic ejection murmur + high-pitched diastolic murmur
• Austin Flint murmur = soft midiastolic or presystolic bruit
√ LV enlargement (cardiothoracic ratio > 0.55) + initially
   normal pulmonary vascularity (DDx: congestive
   cardiomyopathy, pericardial effusion)
√ normal aorta (in intrinsic valve disease)
√ dilatation ± calcification of ascending aorta (in aortic wall
   disease)
√ tortuous descending aorta
√ increased pulsations along entire aorta

ECHO:
   √ increased dimension of aortic root
   √ high frequency diastolic flutter of aML, IVS
      (uncommon)
   √ LV dilatation + large amplitude of LV wall motion
      (volume overload, increased ejection fraction)
   √ premature closure of mitral valve (high diastolic LV
      pressure)
Doppler:
   √ slope of peak diastolic to end-diastolic velocity
      decrease > 3 m/sec² in severe aortic regurgitation
   √ area of Color-Doppler regurgitant flow
   √ ratio of width of regurgitant beam to width of aortic
      root is good predictor of severity (Color-Doppler)

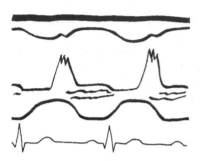

Mitral Valve in Severe Aortic Regurgitation
The valve is almost completely closed before onset of ventricular
systole. Atrial contraction has little effect in reopening the valve.
Complete closure occurs with ventricular systole. A high velocity
flutter of aML is present in diastole.

AORTIC STENOSIS
Aortic valve area decreased to < 0.8 cm² = 0.4 cm²/m²
BSA (normal 2.5 – 3.5 cm²)
A. Acquired
    1. Rheumatic valvulitis (almost invariably associated
        with mitral valve disease)
    2. Senile calcific valve degeneration
B. Congenital (most common)
    = most frequent CHD associated with IUGR
    1. Subvalvular AS (30%)
    2. Valvular AS (70%): degeneration of bicuspid valve
        most common cause
    3. Supravalvular AS
Pathogenesis:
   increased gradient across valve produces LV
   hypertrophy and diminished LV compliance; increased
   muscle mass may outstrip coronary blood supply
   (subendocardial myocardial ischemia with angina); LV
   decompensation leads to LV dilatation + pulmonary
   venous congestion
• asymptomatic for many years
• angina, syncope, heart failure
• systolic murmur
• carotid pulsus parvus et tardus
• diminished aortic component of 2nd heart sound

- sudden death in severe stenosis (20%) after exercise (diminished flow in coronary arteries causes ventricular dysrhythmias + fibrillation)
- √ poststenotic dilatation of ascending aorta (in 90% of acquired, in 70% of congenital AS)
- √ normal sized / enlarged LV (small LV chamber with thick walls)
- Δ in infancy:
  - √ left ventricular stress syndrome
- Δ in children / young adults
  - √ prominent ascending aorta
  - √ left ventricular heart configuration
- Δ in adults > 30 years
  - √ calcification of aortic valve (best seen on RAO); indicates gradient > 50 mmHg
  - √ discrete enlargement of ascending aorta (NO correlation with severity of stenosis)
  - √ "left ventricular configuration" = concavity along mid-left lateral + increased convexity along lower left lateral heart border
  - √ calcification of mitral annulus
- ECHO:
  - √ multiple dense cusp echoes throughout cardiac cycle; if thickened cusp echoes only in diastole then consider DDx of calcification of aortic annulus in elderly, calcified coronary artery ostium
  - √ decreased separation of leaflets in systole with reduced opening orifice (13 – 14 mm = mild AS; 8 – 12 mm = moderate AS; < 8 mm = severe AS)
  - √ dilated aortic root
  - √ increased thickness of LV wall (concentric LV hypertrophy)
  - √ hyperdynamic contraction of LV (in compensated state)
  - √ thickened + calcified aortic valve with restrictive motion ± doming in systole
  - √ increased aortic valve gradient (Doppler)
  - √ decreased aortic valve area by continuity equation
- *Prognosis:* depends on symptomatology (angina, syncope, CHF)

Subvalvular Aortic Stenosis

= SUBAORTIC STENOSIS
- (a) Anatomic / fixed subaortic stenosis
  Associated with cardiac defects in 50% (usually VSD)
  - Type I : thin 1 – 2 mm membranous diaphragmatic stenosis, usually located within 2 cm or less of valve annulus
  - Type II : thick collar-like stenosis
  - Type III : irregular fibromuscular stenosis
  - Type IV : "tunnel subaortic stenosis" = fixed tunnel-like narrowing of LVOT = excessive thickening of only upper ventricular septum with normal mitral valve motion
- (b) Functional / dynamic subaortic stenosis
  1. Asymmetric septal hypertrophy (ASH)

2. Idiopathic hypertrophic subaortic stenosis (IHSS)
3. Hypertrophic obstructive cardiomyopathy (HOCM)
   may occur in infants of diabetic mothers
- √ asymmetrically thicker ventricular septum than free wall of LV (95%)
- √ normal / small left + right ventricular cavities (95%)
- √ systolic anterior motion of mitral valve
- √ lucent subaortic filling defect in systole
- ECHO:
  - √ opening of leaflets followed by rapid inward move in mid-systole, leaflets may remain in partially closed position through latter portion of systole (to appose borders of the flow jet)
  - √ coarse systolic flutter of valve cusps
  - *Cx:* mitral regurgitation (secondary to abnormal position of anterolateral papillary muscle preventing complete closure of MV in systole)

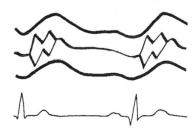

Aortic Valve in Hypertrophic Subaortic Stenosis
during midsystole the aortic valve closes secondary to subvalvular obstruction

Valvular Aortic Stenosis

= fusion of commissures between cusps
Congenital types:
- (a) bicuspid / unicuspid (in 95%): in 1 – 2% of population; M > F; commonly associated with coarctation of the aorta
- (b) tricuspid (5%)
- (c) dysplastic thickened aortic cusps
- √ valvar calcifications (in 60% of patients > 24 years of age)
- Δ IN INFANT with critical aortic stenosis:
  - intractable CHF in first days / weeks of life with severe dyspnea
  - may simulate neonatal sepsis
  Associated with L-R shunts (ASD, VSD)
  - √ marked cardiomegaly (thickened wall of LV)
  - √ pulmonary venous hypertension
  - √ decreased ejection fraction
  - √ doming of thickened valve cusps
  - √ dilated ascending aorta
  Rx: emergency surgical dilatation
- Δ IN CHILD:
  - asymptomatic until late in life
  - √ normal pulmonary vascularity
  - √ prominent ascending aorta

√ LV configuration with normal size of heart
√ large posterior noncoronary cusp, smaller fused
right + left cusps
√ doming of thickened valve cusps
√ eccentric jet of contrast
√ poststenotic dilatation of ascending aorta
ECHO:
√ increase in echoes from thickened deformed
leaflets (maximal during diastole)
√ decrease in leaflet separation

Supravalvular Aortic Stenosis
Types:
(a) localized hourglass narrowing just above aortic
sinuses
(b) discrete fibrous membrane above sinuses of
Valsalva
(c) diffuse tubular hypoplasia of ascending aorta +
branching arteries
Associated with: peripheral PS, valvar + discrete
subvalvar AS, Marfan syndrome, Williams syndrome
√ dilatation + tortuosity of coronary arteries (may
undergo early atherosclerotic degeneration secondary
to high pressure)
ECHO:
√ narrowing of supravalvular aortic area (normal root
diameter: 20 – 37 mm)
√ normal movement of cusps

AORTIC TRANSSECTION
= TRAUMATIC AORTIC RUPTURE = aortic laceration /
rupture from sudden horizontal deceleration injury
Site: (a) Aortic isthmus (88 – 95%)
brachiocephalic arteries + ligamentum
arteriosum fix aorta in this region
(b) Aortic arch with avulsion of brachiocephalic
trunk (4.5%)
(c) Ascending aorta immediately above aortic
valve (1%)
Cx: cardiac tamponade; NO mediastinal
hematoma
(d) Descending aorta (1.8%)
Extent of injury:
(a) transverse intimal tear
(b) tear of intima + media with subadventitial
accumulation of blood (40%) = false aneurysm
• interscapular severe chest pain, dyspnea
• hypertension in upper extremities = acute traumatic
coarctation
• alteration in peripheral pulses
• systolic murmur in 2nd left parasternal interspace
CXR:
√ mediastinal width > 8 cm at level of aortic knob (75%)
√ mediastinal width to chest width > 0.25
√ poorly defined irregular aortic contour (75%)
√ right / left "apical cap" sign = extrapleural hematoma
(37%)
√ opacification of aortopulmonary window

√ tracheal compression + displacement towards right
(61%)
√ depression of left mainstem bronchus anteroinferiorly
+ towards right (53%)
√ deviation of nasogastric tube to right of spinous
process at T4 (67%)
√ rapidly accumulating commonly left-sided hemothorax
without evident rib fracture (break in mediastinal
pleura)
√ fractures of 1st + 2nd rib (17%)
√ widening of right / left paraspinal line
√ widening of right paratracheal stripe > 5 mm
Angio (in survivors):
√ traumatic false aneurysm (common)
√ intimal tear (5 – 10%)
√ posttraumatic dissection (11%)
√ posttraumatic coarctation
DDx: ductus diverticulum (in 10% of normals)
Prognosis:
(a) no intervention: 80% dead within 1 hour; 85%
dead within 24 hours, 98% dead within 10 weeks;
chronic false aneurysm may develop in 5% at
isthmus / descending aorta
(b) with surgical repair: 15% survive

AORTOPULMONIC WINDOW
= defect in septation process characterized by large round
/ oval communication between left wall of ascending
aorta + right wall of pulmonary trunk
• clinically resembles PDA
CXR:
√ shunt vascularity
√ cardiomegaly (LA + LV enlargement)
√ diminutive aortic knob
√ prominent pulmonary trunk
Angio (left ventriculogram / aortogram in AP / LAO
projection):
√ defect several mm above aortic valve
√ pulmonary valve identified (DDx to truncus arteriosus)

ASPLENIA SYNDROME
= BILATERAL RIGHT-SIDEDNESS
= IVEMARK SYNDROME
Incidence: 1:1,750 to 1:40,000 live births; M > F
Associated with:
(a) CHD (in 50%):
TAPVR (almost 100%), endocardial cushion defect
(85%), single ventricle (51%), TGA (58%),
pulmonary stenosis / atresia (70%), dextrocardia
(42%), mesocardia, VSD, ASD, absent coronary
sinus, common atrium, bilateral right atrial
appendages, bilateral SVC, common hepatic vein
(b) GI anomalies:
Partial / total situs inversus, annular pancreas,
agenesis of gallbladder, ectopic liver, esophageal
varices, duplication + hypoplasia of stomach,
Hirschsprung disease, hindgut duplication,
imperforate anus

(c) GU anomalies (15%):
Horseshoe kidney, Double collecting system, Hydroureter, Cystic kidney, Fused / horseshoe adrenal, Absent left adrenal, Bilobed urinary bladder, Bicornuate uterus
(d) Cleft lip / palate, Scoliosis, Single umbilical artery, Lumbar myelomeningocele
• cyanosis in neonatal period / infancy (if severe cyanotic CHD)
• Howell-Jolly bodies = RBC inclusions in patients with absent spleen
√ absent spleen
@ Lung
√ bilateral trilobed lungs = bilateral minor fissures (SPECIFIC)
√ bilateral eparterial bronchi (tomogram)
√ diminished pulmonary vascularity / pulmonary venous hypertension (TAPVR below diaphragm)
√ bilateral SVC
√ right atrial isomerism
@ Abdomen
√ centrally located liver = hepatic symmetry
√ stomach on right / left side / in central position
√ abdominal aorta + IVC located on same side of spine (aorta usually posterior) (ALMOST PATHOGNOMONIC)
Prognosis: 80% mortality by end of 1st year of life

ATRIAL SEPTAL DEFECT
most common congenital cardiac defect in subjects > 20 years of age
Incidence: 8 – 14% of all CHD; M : F = 1 : 4
Age: presentation frequently > age 40 secondary to benign course
(a) mildly symptomatic (60%): dyspnea, fatigue, palpitations
(b) severely symptomatic (30%): cyanosis, heart failure

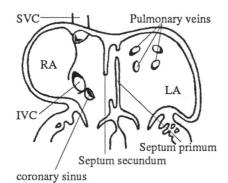

Normal Newborn Heart
atrial septum consists of two components
(a) right side: septum secundum (muscular, firm) with posterior opening = foramen ovale
(b) left side: septum primum (fibrous, thin) with anterior opening = ostium secundum

Embryology:
1. Septum primum = membrane growing from atrial walls toward endocardial cushion
2. Ostium primum = temporary orifice between septum primum + endocardial cushion which becomes obliterated by 5th week
3. Ostium secundum = multiple small coalescing perforations in septum primum
4. Septum secundum = membrane developing on right side of septum primum + covering part of ostium secundum
5. Foramen ovale = orifice limited by septum secundum + septum primum
6. Foramen ovale flap = lower edge of septum primum (foramen ovale patent in 6%, probe-patent in 25%; not considered an ASD)

1. OSTIUM SECUNDUM ASD (60 – 70%)
= absence / fenestration of the foramen ovale flap
Location: in the body of the atrial chamber at fossa ovalis
May be associated with:
Prolapsing mitral valve, Pulmonary valve stenosis, Tricuspid atresia, TAPVR, Hypoplastic left heart, Interrupted aortic arch

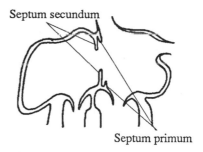

Ostium Secundum Defect

2. SINUS VENOSUS ASD (30%)
= defect of the superior inlet portion of the atrial septum

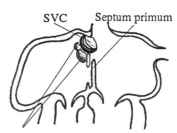

Anomalous
right upper lobe veins

Sinus Venosus Defect

Location: superior to fossa ovalis near entrance of
            superior vena cava (SVC straddles ASD)
Associated with:
    Partial anomalous pulmonary venous return (90%),
    Holt-Oram syndrome, Ellis-van Creveld syndrome

3. OSTIUM PRIMUM ASD (5%)
   = defect of atrioventricular endocardial cushion
   Location: inferior to fossa ovalis at outlet portion of
               atrial septum
   Almost always associated with   Endocardial cushion
   defects, Cleft mitral valve, Anteror fascicular block

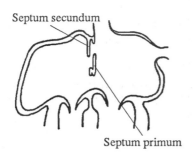

Septum secundum

Septum primum

Ostium Primum Defect

LUTEMBACHER SYNDROME = ASD + mitral stenosis

Hemodynamics:
    no hemodynamic perturbance in the fetus; after birth
    physiologic increase in LA pressure creates a L-R shunt
    (shunt volume may be 3 − 4 times that of systemic blood
    flow) with volume overload of RV leading to RV
    dilatation, right heart failure, pulmonary hypertension;
    diastolic pressure differences in atria determine direction
    of shunt; pulmonary pressure remains normal for
    decades before Eisenmenger syndrome sets in;
    pulmonary hypertension in young adulthood (6%)
- repeated respiratory infections
- feeding difficulties
- arrhythmias
- thromboembolism
- asymptomatic; occasionally discovered by routine CXR
- right ventricular heave
- fixed splitting of second heart sound with accentuation
  of pulmonary component
- ECG: right axis deviation + some degree of right bundle
  branch block
- exertional dyspnea after development of pulmonary
  arterial hypertension (= Eisenmenger syndrome)
- cyanosis may occur (shunt reversal to R-L shunt),
  typically during 3rd − 4th decade
- right heart failure in patients > 40 years
CXR:
    √ normal (if shunt < 2 x systemic blood flow)
    √ "hilar dance" = increased pulsations of central
      pulmonary arteries (DDx: other L-to-R shunts)
    √ overcirculation (if pulmonary-to-systemic blood flow ≥
      2 : 1)

√ loss of visualization of SVC (= clockwise rotation of
  heart due to RV hypertrophy)
√ small appearing aorta with normal aortic knob
√ normal sized LA after shunt reversal (due to
  immediate decompression into RA) in
  EISENMENGER SYNDROME
    √ enlargement of pulmonary trunk + arteries
    √ RV enlargement
ECHO:
    √ paradoxic interventricular septal motion (due to
      volume overload of RV)
    √ direct visualization of ASD (= lack of echoes of atrial
      septum) in subcostal view
    √ diastolic blood flow from interatrial septum crossing
      RA + tricuspid valve into RV observed by color
      Doppler
Angio:
    √ RA fills with contrast shortly after LA is opacified (on
      levophase of pulmonary angio in AP or LAO
      projection)
    √ injection into RUL pulmonary vein to visualize exact
      size + location of ASD (LAO 45° + C-C 45°)
Prognosis:
    (1) Mortality: 0.6% in1st decade; 0.7% in 2nd
         decade; 2.7% in 3rd decade; 4.5% in 4th decade;
         5.4% in 5th decade; 7.5% in 6th decade; median
         age of death is 37 years
    (2) Spontaneous closure: 22% in infants < 1 year;
         33% between ages 1 and 2 years; 3% in children
         > 4 years
Cx: (1) Tricuspid insufficiency (secondary to dilatation
              of AV ring)
         (2) Mitral valve prolapse
         (3) Atrial fibrillation (in 20% 1st presenting
              symptoms in patients > age 40)
Rx: (if vascular changes still reversible = resistance of
         pulmonary-to-systemic system ≤ 0.7); 1% surgical
         mortality
         1. Surgical patch closure
         2. Rashkind foam + stainless steel prosthesis

BENEFICIAL ASD
   = secundum type ASD serves an essential
     compensatory function in:
   1. Tricuspid atresia
      RA blood reaches pulmonary vessels via ASD +
      PDA; improvement through Rushkind procedure
   2. TAPVR
      significant shunt volume only available through ASD
      (VSD / PDA much less reliable)
   3. Hypoplastic left heart
      systemic circulation maintained via RV with
      oxygenated blood from LA through ASD into RA

AZYGOS CONTINUATION OF IVC
   = development failure of hepatic / infrahepatic segment of
     IVC
Incidence: 2% of CHD

Associated with: Asplenia syndrome, Polysplenia
syndrome
√ enlargement of arch of azygos
√ enlarged paraspinal + retrocrural azygos + hemiazygos
vein
√ absence of hepatic ± infrahepatic IVC

BACTERIAL ENDOCARDITIS
Predisposed:
1. Rheumatic valve disease
2. Mitral valve prolapse with mitral regurgitation
3. Aortic stenosis, Mitral stenosis, Aortic regurgitation,
   Mitral regurgitation
4. Most CHD (VSD, TOF) except ostium secundum
   ASD
5. Previous endocarditis
6. Drug addicts:
   endocarditis of tricuspid valve causes multiple septic
   pulmonary emboli
7. Bicuspid aortic valve:
   responsible for 50% of aortic valvular bacterial
   endocarditis
8. Prosthetic valve:
   4 % incidence of bacterial endocarditis
   √ exaggerated valve motion (= disintegration of
   suture line + regurgitation)

Valve Vegetations
ECHO:
√ usually discrete focal echodensities with sharp
edges; may show fuzzy / shaggy nonuniform
thickening of cusps (vegetations) in systole +
diastole
√ may appear as shaggy echoes that prolapse when
the valve is closed

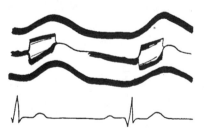

Aortic valve endocarditis

BUERGER DISEASE
= vasculitis of peripheral vessels
Etiology: cigarette smoking (95%)
Location: legs (80%), arms (10 – 20%)
√ thrombophlebitis (33%)
√ arterial occlusions, tapered narrowing, abundant
collaterals
√ relative absence of arteriosclerosis

CARDIAC TAMPONADE
= significant compression of heart by fluid contained within
pericardial sac causing compromise of diastolic filling of
ventricles
• pulsus paradoxus = exaggeration of normal pattern
= drop in systolic arterial pressure > 10 mmHg during
inspiration (secondary to increase in right heart filling
during inspiration at the expense of left heart filling)
• elevated jugular venous pressure
• distant heart sounds / friction rub
• ECG: reduced voltage, ST elevation, PR depression,
nonspecific T wave abnormalities
√ normal lung fields + normal pulmonary vascularity
√ rapid enlargement of heart size
ECHO: √ diastolic collapse of RV
√ cyclical collapse of either atrium

CARDIOMYOPATHY
Congestive Cardiomyopathy
= DILATED CARDIOMYOPATHY
Etiology:
(a) Myocarditis: viruses, bacteria
(b) Endocardial fibroelastosis = thickened
endocardium + reduced contractility
(c) Infants of diabetic mothers
(d) Inborn error of metabolism: glycogenosis,
mucolipidosis, mucopolysaccharidosis
(e) Coronary artery disease: Myocardial infarction,
Anomalous origin of left coronary artery,
Coronary calcinosis
(f) Muscular dystrophies
• tendency toward CHF
√ cardiomegaly + poor contractility of ventricular wall
√ global heart enlargement
√ LA enlargement without enlargement of LA
appendage
ECHO:
√ enlarged LV with global hypokinesis
√ IVS and LVPW of equal thickness with decreased
amplitude of motion
√ low profile / "miniaturized" mitral valve
√ mildly enlarged LA (elevated end-diastolic LV
pressure)
√ enlarged hypokinetic right ventricle

Hypertrophic Cardiomyopathy
= OBSTRUCTIVE CARDIOMYOPATHY
1. SYMMETRIC / CONCENTRIC HYPERTROPHY
   (uncommon)
   (a) midventricular (b) diffuse (c) apical
2. IDIOPATHIC HYPERTROPHIC SUBAORTIC
   STENOSIS (IHSS) = ASYMMETRIC SEPTAL
   HYPERTROPHY (ASH) is part of IHSS
   Etiology: autosomal dominant transmission
   √ prominent left midheart border (septal
   hypertrophy)
ECHO:
√ IVS > 14 mm thick; IVS : LVPW thickness > 1.3 : 1

√ systolic anterior movement of mitral valve (SAM) causing narrowed LVOT in systole
√ midsystolic closure of aortic valve
√ increased LVOT gradient with late systolic peaking on Doppler

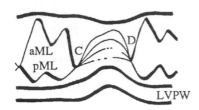

Systolic Anterior Motion (SAM) of MV in IHSS
mitral valve leaflets move abruptly toward septum at a rate greater than the endocardium of the posterior wall; responsible for obstruction to blood ejected from LV

Restrictive Cardiomyopathy
Etiology: (a) infiltrative disease: amyloid, glycogen, hemochromatosis
(b) constrictive pericarditis

COARCTATION OF AORTA
M:F = 4:1; rare in Blacks
A. LOCALIZED COARCTATION (former classification = ADULT / POSTDUCTAL / JUXTADUCTAL TYPE) (most common type)
= short discrete narrowing close to ligamentum arteriosum
Δ coexistent cardiac anomalies uncommon
Location: most frequent in juxtaductal portion of arch
• incidental finding late in life
• ductus usually closed
√ shelf-like lesion at any point along the aortic arch
√ narrow isthmus above the lesion
√ poststenotic aortic dilatation distally
B. TUBULAR HYPOPLASIA (former classification = INFANTILE / PREDUCTAL / DIFFUSE TYPE)
= hypoplasia of long segment of aortic arch after origin of innominate artery
Δ coexistent cardiac anomalies common
• CHF in neonatal period (in 50%)

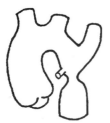 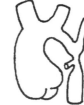

Localized coarctation   Tubular hypoplasia

Hemodynamics:
fetus   : no significant change because only 10% of cardiac output flows through aortic isthmus
neonate : determined by how rapidly the ductus closes; overload of LV without concurrent VSD leads to CHF in 2nd / 3rd week of life

Collateral circulation via subclavian artery and its branches:
— intercostals   — internal mammary
— anterior spinal artery   — scapular artery
— lateral thoracic   — transverse cervical artery

Associated with (in 50%):
1. Bicuspid aortic valve (in 25 – 50%) which may result in calcific aortic valve stenosis (after 25 years of age) + bacterial endocarditis
2. Intracardiac malformations:
PDA (33%), VSD (15%), Aortic stenosis, Aortic insufficiency, ASD, TGV, Ostium primum defect, Truncus arteriosus, Double outlet right ventricle
3. Noncardiac malformations (13%):
Turner syndrome (13 – 15%)
4. Cerebral berry aneurysms
5. Mycotic aneurysm distal to CoA
Prognosis: 11% mortality prior to 6 months of age

SYMPTOMATIC CoA
Second most common cause of CHF in neonate (after hypoplastic left heart)
Time: (a) toward the end of 1st week of life in "critical stenosis"
(b) more commonly presents in older child
• lower extremity cyanosis (in tubular hypoplasia)
• left ventricular failure (usually toward end of 1st week of life)
√ generalized cardiomegaly
√ increased pulmonary vasculature (L-to-R shunt through PDA / VSD)
√ pulmonary venous hypertension

ASYMPTOMATIC CoA
• headaches (from hypertension)
• claudication (from hypoperfusion)
√ "figure 3 sign" = indentation of lateral margin of aortic arch with poststenotic dilatation at site of coarctation
√ "reverse 3 sign" on barium esophagram
√ elevated left ventricular apex (secondary to hypertrophy)
√ linear wavy opacity behind sternum (= dilated internal mammary arteries)
√ dilatation of brachiocephalic vessels + aorta proximal to stenosis
√ rib notching in ribs 3 – 8 (in 75%, unusual before age 6)
√ bilateral
√ rib notching on L side: anomalous R subclavian artery

√ rib notching on R side: CoA proximal to L
subclavian artery

Rx: ages 3 – 5 years are ideal time for operation (late
enough to avoid restenosis + early enough before
irreversible hypertension occurs); surgical
correction past 1 year of age decreases operative
mortality drastically; 3 – 11% perioperative mortality

Procedures:
1. Resection + end-to-end anastomosis
2. Patch angioplasty
3. Subclavian flap (Waldhausen procedure) using left
   subclavian artery as a flap

Postsurgical Cx:
1. Residual coarctation (in 32%)
2. Subsequent obstruction (rare)
3. Mesenteric arteritis: 2 – 3 days after surgery
   secondary to paradoxical hypertension from
   increased plasma renin
   • abdominal pain, loss of bowel control
4. Chronic persistent hypertension

CONGENITAL ABSENCE OF PULMONARY VALVE

Massive regurgitation between pulmonary artery and RV
Associated with (in 90%):
VSD, Tetralogy of Fallot (50%)
• cyanosis (not in immediate newborn period)
• repeated episodes of respiratory distress
• continuous murmur
• ECG: right ventricular hypertrophy
√ prominent main, right, and left pulmonary artery
√ RV dilatation (increased stroke volume)
√ partial obstruction of right / left main stem bronchus
(compression by vessel)
√ right-sided aorta (33%)

CONSTRICTIVE PERICARDITIS

= fibrous thickening of pericardium interfering with filling of
ventricular chambers through restriction of heart motion
Age: 30 – 50 years; M:F = 3:1
Etiology:
1. Idiopathic (most common)
2. Viral (Coxsackie B)
3. Tuberculosis (formerly most common)
4. Chronic renal failure
5. Rheumatopid arthritis
6. Neoplastic involvement
7. Radiotherapy of mediastinum
• dyspnea
• abdominal enlargement (ascites + hepatomegaly)
• peripheral edema
• pericardial knock sound = loud early-diastolic sound
• neck vein distension
• Kussmaul sign = failure of venous pressure to fall with
inspiration
• prominent X and Y descent on venous pressure curve
√ linear / plaque-like pericardial calcifications (50%):
predominantly over RV, posterior surface of LV, in
atrioventricular groove

√ dilatation of SVC, azygos vein
√ small atria
√ normal / small-sized heart (enlargement only due to
preexisting disease)
√ normal pulmonary vascularity / pulmonary venous
hypertension
√ straightening of right + left heart borders
√ increase in ejection fraction (small EDV)
CT:
√ epicardium = visceral pericardium > 2 mm thick
√ dilatation of SVC + IVC
√ reflux of contrast into coronary sinus
√ flattening of right ventricle + curvature of
interventricular septum toward left
√ pleural effusion + ascites
ECHO (nonspecific features):
√ thickening of pericardium
√ rapid early filling motion followed by flat posterior wall
motion during diastasis period (= period between
early rapid filling and atrial contraction)
Cx: protein-losing enteropathy (increased pressure in
IVC + portal vein)
DDx: Cardiac tamponade, Restrictive cardiomyopathy
(e.g., amyloid)

CORONARY ARTERY FISTULA

= single / multiple fistulous connections between a
coronary artery (R > L) and other heart structures
(> 90% into right heart: RV > RA > pulmonary trunk
> coronary sinus > SVC)
Hemodynamics: L-R shunt; pulmonary:systemic blood
flow = < 1.5:1 (usually)
√ may have normal CXR (in small shunts)
√ cardiomegaly + shunt vascularity (in large shunts)
Angio:
√ dilated tortuous coronary artery with anomalous
connection

COR TRIATRIATUM

= rare congenital anomaly in which a fibromuscular
septum with a single stenotic / fenestrated / large
opening separates the embryologic common pulmonary
vein from the left atrium:
(1) proximal / accessory chamber lies posteriorly
receiving pulmonary veins
(2) distal / true atrial chamber lies anteriorly connected
to left atrial appendage + emptying into LV through
mitral valve
Etiology: failure of common pulmonary vein to
incorporate normally into left atrium
Associated with: ASD, PDA, Anomalous pulmonary
venous drainage, left SVC, VSD,
Tetralogy of Fallot, Atrioventricular canal
• dyspnea, heart failure, failure to thrive
• clinically similar to mitral valve stenosis
√ pulmonary venous distention + interstitial edema +
dilatation of pulmonary trunk and pulmonary arteries (in
severe obstruction)

√ enlarged RA + RV
√ mild enlargement of LA
Angio:
  √ dividing membrane on levophase of pulmonary
    arteriogram
Prognosis: usually fatal within first 2 years of life; 50%
                2-year survival; 20% 20-year survival (if
                untreated)
Rx: surgical excision of obstructing membrane

DEEP VEIN THROMBOSIS
  = DVT
  Incidence: 250 million new cases per year in USA;
                  600,000 deaths per year from pulmonary
                  embolism
  Risk factors:
    1. Surgery, esp. on legs / pelvis: orthopedic (45 –
       50%), gynecologic (7 – 35%), neurosurgery (18 –
       20%), urologic (15 – 35%), general surgery (20 –
       25%)
    2. Severe trauma
    3. Prolonged immobilization: hemiplegic extremity,
       paraplegia & quadriplegia, casting / orthopedic
       appliances
    4. Obesity
    5. Pregnancy
    6. Medication: birth control pills, estrogen
       replacement, tamoxifin
    7. Malignancy
    8. Congestive heart failure
    9. Varicose veins / Hx of previous DVT / PE
    10. Polycythemia
  Source of emboli:
    multiple sites (1/3), cryptogenic in 50%;
        (a) lower extremity   (46%)
        (b) inferior vena cava   (19%)
        (c) pelvic veins   (16%)
        (d) mural heart thrombus   (4.5%)
        (e) upper extremity   (2%)
    • Local symptoms due to obstruction / phlebitis usually
      only when (a) thrombus occlusive (b) clot extends into
      popliteal / more proximal vein : pain, warmth, swelling,
      tenderness
    Δ 2/3 of deep vein thrombosis are clinically silent
    Δ only in 50% present if clinically suspected
    Δ in 15 – 35% of patients DVT symptomatology due to
      other causes
    Δ 30% of patients with angiographically detected
      pulmonary emboli have negative bilateral venograms
      (big bang theory = clot embolizes in toto to the lung
      leaving no residual)
  Venography (89% sensitivity, 97% specificity):
    false negative in 11%, false positive in 5%;
    study aborted / nondiagnostic in 5%
    Risk: postvenography phlebitis, contrast reaction
  US (88 – 96% sensitivity, 96 – 100% specificity, > 90%
    accuracy for thigh and popliteal vein):
    √ lack of complete luminal collapse with compression

(DDx: deformity + scarring from prior DVT; technical
  difficulties in adductor canal + distal deep femoral
  vein)
  √ visualization of clot within vein (fresh thrombus
    anechoic, echogenicity increases with age of
    thrombus) (DDx: slow flowing blood; machine noise)
  √ >75% increase in diameter of common femoral vein
    during Valsalva
Doppler US:
  √ absence of spontaneity (= any waveform recording)
  √ continuous venous signal = absence of phasicity
    (= variation in flow velocity with respiration) is
    suspicious for proximal obstruction
  √ attenuation / absence of augmentation (= increase in
    flow velocity with distal compression) indicates
    thrombus / venous compression in intervening system
Cx: (1) Pulmonary embolism (50%): in 90% from
              lower extremity / pelvis
         (2) Postphlebitic syndrome (PPS) in 20% of cases
              with DVT (= recanalization to a smaller lumen,
              focal wall changes)
         (3) Phlegmasia cerulea / alba dolens (= severly
              impaired venous drainage resulting in
              gangrene)
Prognosis:
    Tibial / peroneal venous thrombi resolve spontaneously
    in 40%, stabilize in 40%, propagate into popliteal vein
    in 20%;
    Δ clinically significant pulmonary embolism is extremely
      uncommon in solated calf thrombosis

DOUBLE OUTLET RIGHT VENTRICLE
  = DORV = TAUSSIG-BING HEART = most of the aorta +
    pulmonary artery arise from the RV secondary to
    maldevelopment of conotruncus
  Type 1 = aorta posterior to pulmonary artery + spiraling
            course (most frequent)
  Type 2 = Taussig-Bing heart = aorta posterior to
            pulmonary artery + parallel course
  Type 3 = aorta anterior to pulmonary artery + parallel
            course
  Hemodynamics:
    Δ fetus   : no CHF in utero (in absence of obstructing
                  other anomalies)
    Δ neonate : ventricular work overload leads to CHF
  Associated with: VSD (100%), Pulmonary stenosis
                        (50%), PDA
  √ aorta overriding the interventricular septum with
    predominant connection to RV
  √ aorta posterior / parallel / anterior to pulmonary artery
  √ LV enlargement (volume overload)

EBSTEIN ANOMALY
  = downward displacement of septal + posterior leaflets of
    dysplastic tricuspid valve with ventricular division into
    (a) a large superior atrialized portion and
    (b) a small inferior functional chamber
  Etiology: chronic maternal lithium intake (10%)

Hemodynamics:
tricuspid valve insufficiency leads to tricuspid regurgitation ("ping-pong" volume); may be followed by CHF in utero / in neonate (50%); survival into adulthood if valve functions normally
Associated with: PDA, ASD (R-L shunt)
- cyanosis in neonatal period (R-L shunt), may improve / disappear postnatally with decrease in pulmonary arterial pressure
- systolic murmur (tricuspid insufficiency)
- Wolf-Parkinson-White syndrome (10%) = paroxysmal supraventricular tachycardia / right bundle branch block (responsible for sudden death)
√ "boxlike / funnellike" cardiomegaly (enlargement of RA + RV)
√ extreme RA enlargement (secondary to insufficient tricuspid valve)
√ IVC + azygos dilatation (secondary to tricuspid regurgitation)
√ hypoplastic aorta + pulmonary trunk (the ONLY cyanotic CHD to have this feature)
√ normal LA
√ calcification of tricuspid valve may occur
ECHO:
√ large "sail-like" tricuspid valve structure within dilated right heart
√ tricuspid regurgitation identified by Doppler ultrasound
Prognosis: 50% infant mortality;
13% operative mortality
Rx: 1. Digitalis + diuretics
2. Tricuspid valve prosthesis

EISENMENGER COMPLEX
= EISENMENGER DEFECT
= (1) high VSD ± overriding aorta with hypoplastic crista supraventricularis
(2) RV hypertrophy
and as consequence of increased pulmonary blood flow:
(3) dilatation of pulmonary artery + branches
(4) intimal thickening + sclerosis of small pulmonary arteries + arterioles
- cyanosis appears in 2nd + 3rd decade with shunt reversal

EISENMENGER SYNDROME
= EISENMENGER REACTION = development of high pulmonary vascular resistance after many years of increased pulmonary blood flow secondary to L-R shunt (ASD, PDA, VSD) which leads to a bidirectional = balanced shunt and ultimately to R-L shunt
Etiology:
pulmonary microscopic vessels undergo reactive muscular hypertrophy, endothelial thickening, in situ thrombosis, tortuosity + obliteration; once initiated pulmonary hypertension accelerates the vascular reaction, thus increasing pulmonary hypertension in a vicious cycle with RV failure + death

√ pronounced dilatation of central pulmonary arteries (pulmonary trunk, main pulmonary artery, intermediate branches)
√ pruning of peripheral pulmonary arteries
√ enlargement of RV
√ LA + LV return to normal size (with decrease of L-R shunt)
√ pulmonary veins NOT distended (NO increased blood flow)
√ NO redistribution of pulmonary veins (normal venous pressure)
Dx: measurement of pulmonary artery pressure + flow via catheter

ENDOCARDIAL CUSHION DEFECT
= ECD = ATRIOVENTRICULAR SEPTAL DEFECT
= PERSISTENT OSTIUM ATRIOVENTRICULARE COMMUNE = PERSISTENT COMMON ATRIOVEN-TRICULAR CANAL
= persistence of primitive atrioventricular canal + anomalies of AV valves
Associated with:
(1) Down syndrome:
in 25% of Trisomy 21 an ECD is present;
in 45% of ECD Trisomy 21 is present
(2) Asplenia, Polysplenia

A. INCOMPLETE / PARTIAL ECD
= (1) ostium primum ASD
(2) cleft in anterior mitral valve leaflet / trileaflet
(3) accessory short chordae tendineae arising from anterior MV leaflet insert directly into crest of deficient ventricular septum
√ "gooseneck" deformity secondary to downward attachment of anterior MV leaflet close to interventricular septum by accessory chordae tendineae
√ communication between LA–RA or LV–RA, occasionally LV–RV
√ right atrioventricular valve usually normal
√ left atrioventricular valve usually has 3 leaflets with a wide cleft between anterior + septal leaflet
B. TRANSITIONAL / INTERMEDIATE ATRIOVENTRICULAR CANAL
(uncommon)
= (1) ostium primum ASD
(2) high membranous VSD
(3) wide clefts in septal leaflets of both AV valves
(4) bridging tissue between anterior + posterior common leaflet of both AV valves
C. COMPLETE ECD = AV COMMUNIS = COMMON AV CANAL
= (1) ostium primum ASD above
(2) posterior VSD below
(3) one AV valve common to RV + LV with 5 – 6 leaflets
(a) anterior common "bridging" leaflet
(b) two lateral leaflets
(c) posterior common "bridging" leaflet

Type 1 = chordae tendineae of anterior bridging leaflet attached to both sides of ventricular septum

Type 2 = chordae tendineae of anterior leaflet attached medially to anomalous papillary muscle within RV, but unattached to septum

Type 3 = free floating anterior leaflet with chordae attachments to septum; only type becoming symptomatic in infancy !

√ common atrioventricular orifice
√ oval septal defect consisting of a low ASD + high VSD
√ atrial septum secundum usually spared ("common atrium" if absent)
√ frequently associated with mesocardia / dextrocardia

Hemodynamics:

Δ fetus   : atrioventricular valves frequently incompetent leading to regurgitation + CHF

Δ neonate : L-R shunt after decrease of pulmonary vascular resistance resulting in pulmonary hypertension

• incomplete right bundle branch block (distortion of conduction tissue)
• left-anterior hemiblock

CXR:
√ increased pulmonary vascularity (= shunt vascularity)
√ redistribution of pulmonary blood flow (mitral regurgitation)
√ enlarged pulmonary artery
√ diminutive aorta (secondary to L-R shunt)
√ cardiac enlargement out of proportion to pulmonary vascularity (L-R shunt + mitral insufficiency)
√ enlarged RV + LV
√ enlarged RA (LV blood shunted to RA)
√ normal-sized LA (secondary to ASD)

ECHO:
√ visualization of ASD + VSD + valve + site of insertion of chordae tindineae
√ paradoxical anterior septal motion (secondary to ASD)
√ atrioventricular insufficiency + shunts identified by Doppler ultrasound

Angio:
AP projection:
√ gooseneck deformity of LVOT (in diastole)
√ cleft in anterior leaflet of mitral valve (in systole)
√ mitral regurgitation

Hepatoclavicular projection in 45° LAO + C-C 45° (= 4 chamber view):
√ best view to demonstrate LV-RA shunt
√ best view to demonstrate VSD (inflow tract + posterior portion of interventricular septum in profile)

LAT projection:
√ irregular appearance of superior segment of anterior mitral valve leaflet over LVOT

Prognosis:
54% survival rate at 6 months, 35% at 12 months, 15% at 24 months, 4% at 5 years; 91% long-term survival with primary intracardiac repair, 4 – 17% operative mortality

ENDOCARDIAL FIBROELASTOSIS
= diffuse endocardial thickening of LV + LA from deposition of collagen + elastic tissue

Etiology:
(1) ? viral infection
(2) Secondary endocardial fibroelastosis
    = subendocardial ischemia in critical LVOT obstruction: Aortic stenosis, Coarctation, Hypoplastic left heart syndrome

• sudden onset of CHF during first 6 months of life
√ mitral insufficiency:
    (a) involvement of valve leaflets
    (b) shortening + thickening of chordae tendineae
    (c) distortion + fixation of papillary muscles
√ enlarged LV = dilatation of hypertrophied LV from mitral regurgitation
√ restricted LV motion
√ enlarged LA
√ pulmonary venous congestion + pulmonary edema
√ LLL atelectasis (= compression of left lower lobe bronchus by enlarged LA)

Prognosis: mortality almost 100% by 2 years of age

FLAIL MITRAL VALVE
Cause:
(1) ruptured chordae tendineae in rheumatic heart disease, ischemic heart disease, bacterial endocarditis
(2) rupture of head of papillary muscle in acute myocardial infarction, chest trauma

Location: chordae to leaflet from posteromedial papillary muscle (single vessel blood supply)

√ deep holosystolic posterior movement
√ random anarchic motion pattern of flail parts in diastole
√ excessively large amplitude of opening of aML

GIANT CELL ARTERITIS
= TEMPORAL / CRANIAL / GRANULOMATOUS ARTERITIS = POLYMYALGIA RHEUMATICA

Path: granulomatous inflammation with intimal proliferation, ± intimal necrosis with thrombosis

Age peak: 65 – 75 years; M:F = 35:65

• headache (50 – 90%)
• polymyalgia rheumatica (50%)
• synovitis
• scalp tenderness
• visual disturbances
• claudication of chewing + swallowing

Location: mainly medium-sized branches of aortic arch, any artery of the body

√ long smooth stenotic arterial segments with skip areas
√ smooth tapered occlusions
√ absence of atherosclerotic changes

GLYCOGEN STORAGE DISEASE
= POMPE DISEASE = abnormal metabolism with enlargement of myocardial cells due to glycogen deposition; similar to endocardial fibroelastosis
√ massive cardiomegaly with CHF
Prognosis: sudden death in 1st year of life (conduction abnormalities); survival rarely beyond infancy

HYPOPLASTIC LEFT HEART SYNDROME
= SHONE SYNDROME = AORTIC ATRESIA
= underdevelopment of left side of heart characterized by (a) aortic valve atresia (b) hypoplastic ascending aorta (c) hypoplastic / atretic mitral valve (d) endocardial fibroelastosis giving rise to small LA + small LV + small ascending aorta
Incidence: most common cause of CHF in neonate; responsible for 25% of all cardiac deaths in 1st week of life
Hemodynamics:
pulmonary venous return is diverted from LA to RA through herniated foramen ovale / ASD (L–R shunt); RV supplies (a) pulmonary artery (b) ductus arteriosus (c) descending aorta (antegrade flow) (d) aortic arch + ascending aorta + coronary circulation (retrograde flow) leading to RV work overload + CHF
• characteristically presents within first few hours of life
• ashen gray color (inadequate atrial L–R shunt with systemic underperfusion)
• myocardial ischemia (decreased perfusion of aorta + coronary arteries)
• cardiogenic shock, metabolic acidosis
• CHF (RV volume + pressure overload)

OB-US:
√ small left ventricular cavity (apex of LV and RV should be at same level)
√ hypoplastic ascending aorta + aortic arch
√ aortic coarctation (in 80%)
ECHO:
√ normal / enlarged LA
√ small LV
√ enlarged RA
√ herniation + prolapse of foramen ovale flap into RA
√ small / absent aortic root
√ absent / grossly distorted mitral valve echoes
Angio:
√ retrograde flow in ascending aorta + aortic arch + coronary arteries via PDA
√ string-like ascending aorta < 6 mm in diameter
√ massive enlargement of RV + RVOT
Prognosis: almost 100% fatal by 6 weeks
Rx: (1) Norwood procedure = palliative attempt
(2) Cardiac transplant

HYPOPLASTIC RIGHT VENTRICLE
= PULMONARY ATRESIA WITH INTACT VENTRICULAR SEPTUM
= underdeveloped right ventricle due to pulmonary atresia in the presence of an intact interventricular septum

Type I = small RV secondary to competent tricuspid valve (more common)
Type II = normal / large RV secondary to incompetent tricuspid valve
Hemodynamics:
Δ fetus : L–R atrial shunt through foramen ovale; retrograde flow through ductus arteriosus into pulmonary vascular bed
Δ neonate : closure of ductus results in cyanosis, acidosis, death

√ small right ventricular cavity (apex of RV + LV should be at same level)
√ atresia of pulmonary valve
√ hypoplastic proximal pulmonary artery
√ secundum atrial septal defect (frequently associated)
Rx: prostaglandin E1 infusion + valvotomy + systemic-pulmonary artery shunt

IDIOPATHIC DILATATION OF PULMONARY ARTERY
= CONGENITAL ANEURYSM OF PULMONARY ARTERY
Age: adolescence; M < F
• systolic ejection murmur (in most cases)
√ dilated main pulmonary artery
√ normal peripheral pulmonary vascularity
√ normal pulmonary arterial pulsations
√ NO lateralization of pulmonary flow
Dx per exclusion:
1. Absence of shunts, CHD, acquired disease
2. Normal RV pressure
3. No significant pressure gradient across pulmonic valve
DDx: (1) Marfan syndrome
(2) Takayasu arteritis

INTERRUPTION OF AORTIC ARCH
= rare congenital anomaly as a common cause of death in the neonatal period
Trilogy: 1. Interrupted aortic arch
2. VSD
3. PDA (pulmonary blood supplies lower part of body)
Associated with (in 1/3):
1. Transposition
2. Truncus arteriosus
3. Complete anomalous pulmonary venous return
• presents with CHF
Location:
Type A: distal to left subclavian artery (42%)
Type B: between left CCA and subclavian artery (53%)
Type C: between innominate and left CCA (4%)
√ dilatation of right atrium + ventricle
√ dilatation of pulmonary artery
√ ascending aorta much smaller than pulmonary artery
√ arch formed by pulmonary artery + ductus arteriosus gives the appearance of a low aortic arch

√ aortic knob absent

√ trachea in midline

√ NO esophageal impression

√ retrosternal clear space increased (small size of ascending aorta)

√ increased pulmonary vascularity (L-to-R shunt)

Prognosis: 76% dead at end of 1st month

INTERRUPTION OF PULMONARY ARTERY

= pulmonary trunk continues only as one large artery to one lung while systemic aortic collaterals supply the other side

Associated with   CHD (particularly if interruption on left side):

1.   Tetralogy of Fallot

2.   Scimitar syndrome = Congenital pulmonary venolobar syndrome

3.   PDA, VSD

4.   Pulmonary hypertension

Collateral supply:

1.   Arteries arising from arch + ascending aorta

2.   Bronchial vessels

3.   Intercostal vessels

4.   Branches from subclavian artery

Location: usually opposite from aortic arch;
              R + L pulmonary artery equally involved

CXR:

√ hypoplastic ipsilateral lung

√ mediastinal shift toward involved lung

√ hemidiaphragm may be elevated

√ small hyperlucent ipsilateral chest with narrowed intercostal spaces

√ "comma-shaped" small distorted hilar shadow

√ asymmetry of pulmonary vascularity

√ normal respiratory motion (normal aeration of hypoplastic lung)

NUC: √ absent perfusion with normal aeration

Angio: √ absent pulmonary artery

Rx: Surgical anastomosis between proximal + distal pulmonary artery (to prevent progressive pulmonary hypertension with dyspnea, cyanosis, hemoptysis, death)

DDx: (1)   Hemitruncus

        (2)   Swyer-James syndrome (ipsilateral air trapping, reduced ventilation + perfusion)

INTRAVENOUS DRUG ABUSE

Complications   secondary to:

(a)   direct toxic effects of drugs or drug combinations (e.g. heroin + cocaine / Talwin)

(b)   direct toxic effects of adulterants [e.g. heroin is mixed ("cut") with quinine, baking soda, sawdust]

(c)   septic preparation

(d)   injection technique

(e)   choice of injection site (e.g. "groin hit" into femoral vein; "pocket shot" into jugular, subclavian, brachiocephalic vein)

A.   Cardiovascular complications

1.   Arterial pseudoaneurysm may be folowed by rupture with exsanguination / loss of limb

2.   Arteriovenous fistula

3.   Arterial occlusion

(a)   at injection site due to intimal damage, thrombosis, spasm

(b)   distal to injection site due to embolization, spasm

4.   Venous thrombosis

5.   Intravenous migration of needle to heart / lungs

6.   Embolization of infectious agent / foreign body / air through inadvertent arterial injection ("hit the pink")

7.   Endocarditis (most commonly Staph. aureus)

B.   Soft tissue complications

1.   Hematoma / abscess

2.   Foreign bodies

3.   Lymphadenopathy

4.   Cellulitis

C.   Skeletal complications

1.   Osteomyelitis

(a)   direct contamination: e.g. pubic bone ("groin hit") / clavicle ("pocket shot")

(b)   hematogenous: spine most commonly affected

2.   Septic arthritis: sacroiliac, sternoclavicular, symphysis pubis, hip, knee, wrist

D.   Pleuropulmonary complications

1.   Pneumothorax ("pocket shot")

2.   Hemo-/ pyothorax

3.   Septic pulmonary emboli

E.   Gastrointestinal complications

1.   Severe colonic ileus

2.   Colonic pseudoobstruction

3.   Necrotizing enterocolitis

4.   Liver abscess

F.   Genitourinary complications

1.   Focal / segmental glomerulosclerosis (heroin abuser)

2.   Amyloidosis

G.   CNS complications

1.   Spinal epidural abscess in 5 – 18% (from vertebral osteomyelitis)

2.   Cord compression (from collapsed vertebral body)

3.   Cerebral infarction (from subacute bacterial endocarditis, toxic effect of drug, spasm, intimal damage from "pocket shot")

4.   Intracranial hemorrhage (from trauma, hypertension, injection of anticholinergic drugs, vasculitis, rupture of mycotic aneurysm)

5.   Meningitis, cerebral abscess

ISCHEMIC HEART DISEASE

CXR: √ often normal

√ coronary artery calcification

√ pulmonary venous hypertension following acute infarction (40%)

√ LV aneurysm

ECHO:
√ region of dilatation with disturbance of wall
movement
- (1) Akinesis = no wall motion
- (2) Hypokinesis = reduced wall motion
- (3) Dyskinesis = paradoxical systolic expansion
- (4) Asynchrony = disturbed temporal sequence of contraction

MARFAN SYNDROME
= autosomal dominant connective tissue disease with
variable penetrance, 15% new mutations
Cardiovascular abnormalities (60%):
affecting mitral valve, ascending aorta, pulmonary
artery, splenic + mesenteric arteries (occasionally)
@ Sinus of Valsalva + ascending aorta
√ "tulip bulb aorta" = dilatation of aortic sinuses of
Valsalva slightly extending into ascending aorta
√ fusiform aneurysm of ascending aorta, rarely
beyond innominate artery
Cx: (1) Aortic regurgitation:
in 81% if root diameter > 5 cm,
in 100% if root diameter > 6 cm
(2) Aortic dissection
@ Mitral valve
Myxomatous degeneration of valve leads to
redundancy + laxness
- mid-to-late systolic murmur + one / more clicks
√ prolapse of mitral valve + regurgitation
Cx: rupture of chordae tendineae (rare)
@ Coarctation (mostly not severe)
@ Cor pulmonale (secondary to chest deformity)
Prognosis: cardiovascular abnormalities are cause of
death in 93%; aortic disease is cause of
death in 55%

MITRAL REGURGITATION
Causes:
1. Rheumatic heart disease
   (a) isolated: frequently seen in children
   (b) uncommon in adults (mostly combined with
       stenosis)
2. Bacterial endocarditis
3. Myocardial infarction with involvement of papillary
   muscle
4. Congenital (short / abnormally inserted chordae
   tendineae)
5. Marfan syndrome
6. Corrected transposition with Ebstein-like anomaly
7. Idiopathic hypertrophic subaortic stenosis (IHSS)
8. Persistent ostium primum ASD with cleft mitral
   valve
9. Mitral valve prolapse syndrome
10. Functional / secondary
    (from dilatation of mitral ring in any condition with
    dilatation of LV)

Pathogenesis:
backward flow of blood from LV into LA during LV
systole; increased volume of blood under elevated
pressure causes dilatation of LA; marked increase in LV
diastolic volume with little increase in LV diastolic
pressure
√ mild pulmonary venous hypertension (less than with
mitral stenosis)
√ LA + LV enlargement (cardiothoracic ratio > 0.55)
√ enlarged LA appendage (with Hx of previous rheumatic
heart disease)
√ mitral annular calcification (frequent)
ECHO:
√ LA + LV enlargement
√ bulging of interatrial septum to the right
√ Doppler is diagnostic + allows assessment of severity

MITRAL STENOSIS
Acquired causes:
principal cause: rheumatic heart disease
rare cause: mass obstructing LV inflow (tumor,
myxoma thrombus)

Stages (according to degree of pulmonary venous
hypertension):
Stage 1 : √ loss of hilar angle, redistribution
Stage 2 : √ interstitial edema
Stage 3 : √ alveolar edema
Stage 4 : √ hemosiderin deposits + ossification
M:F = 1:8
Pathogenesis:
rise in left atrial + pulmonary vascular pressure
throughout systole and into diastole; development of
medial hypertrophy + intimal sclerosis in pulmonary
arterioles leads to pulmonary arterial hypertension, RV
hypertrophy, tricuspid regurgitation, RV dilatation, right
heart failure
- Hx of rheumatic fever (in 50%)
- atrial fibrillation
- systemic embolization from thrombosis of atrial
  appendage
√ calcification of valve leaflets (calcification of mitral
annulus is a feature of age)
√ prominent pulmonary artery segment (precapillary
hypertension)
√ small aorta (if forward cardiac output decreased)
√ enlarged LA ± wall calcification
√ "double density" seen through right upper cardiac
border (AP view)
√ bulge of superior posterior cardiac border below
carina (lateral view)
√ esophagus displaced toward right + posteriorly
√ dilated left atrial appendage (not present with retracting
clot)
√ hypertrophy of RV
√ dilatation of RV (tricuspid insufficiency / pulmonary
hypertension)
√ increase in cardiothoracic ratio

√ diminution of retrosternal clear space
√ IVC pushed backwards (lateral view)
√ redistribution of pulmonary blood flow to upper lobes (postcapillary pressure 16 – 19 mmHg)
√ interstitial pulmonary edema (postcapillary pressure 20 - 25 mm Hg)
√ alveolar edema (post-capillary pressure 25 – 30 mmHg)
ECHO:
  √ thickening of leaflets (fibrosis, calcification)
  √ commissural fusion
    √ restricted diastolic excursion of aML
    √ flattening of EF slope (early diastolic closing velocity) < 50 mm/sec in 90%
    √ anterior tracking of pML in 80% (secondary to pull by aML)
    √ doming in diastole possible
  √ restricted mobility
    √ DE opening amplitude reduced to < 16 mm (DDx: low cardiac output state)
    √ absent A-wave common (atrial fibrillation)
    √ slowed LV filling pattern
  √ dilatation of LA (> 5 cm increases risk of atrial fibrillation + left atrial thrombus)
  √ increase in valve gradient + pressure half-time on Doppler
  DDx: Cor triatriatum, Myxoma of LA (identical findings)

LUTEMBACHER SYNDROME = rheumatic mitral valve stenosis + ASD

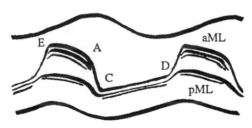

Classic mitral valve stenosis

MITRAL VALVE PROLAPSE
= "Floppy Mitral Valve" = elongation of cusps + chordae leading to redundant valve tissue which prolapses into LA during systole
Incidence: 2 – 6% of general population;
      5 – 20% of young women;
      ? autosomal dominant inheritance
Age: commonly 14 – 30 years
Associated with:
  (1) skeletal abnormalities: scoliosis, straightening of thoracic spine, narrow anteroposterior chest dimension, pectus excavatum deformity of sternum
    (a) Barlowe syndrome = straight back syndrome
    (b) Marfan syndrome
  (2) tricuspid valve prolapse
  (3) longstanding ASD
• arrhythmias, palpitation, chest pain, light-headedness, syncope

• responsible for midsystolic click + late systolic murmur (when associated with mitral regurgitation)
√ LA not enlarged (unless associated with significant mitral regurgitation)
ECHO:
  √ interruption of CD line with bulge toward left atrium
    √ abrupt mid-systolic posterior buckling of both leaflets (classic pattern)
    √ "hammocklike" pansystolic posterior bowing of both leaflets
  √ multiple scallops on leaflets
  √ valve leaflets may appear thickened (myxomatous degeneration + valve redundancy)
  √ amount of mitral valve leaflets passing posterior to plane of mitral annulus > 2 mm

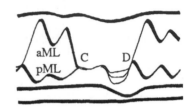

Mid-systolic mitral valve prolapse

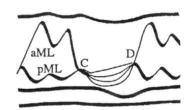

Holo-systolic mitral valve prolapse

MYOCARDIAL INFARCTION
• atrioventricular block (common with inferior wall infarction as AV nodal branch originates from RCA); complete heart block has worse prognosis because it indicates a large area of infarction
√ normal-sized heart (84 – 95%) in acute phase if previously normal
√ cardiomegaly: high incidence of congestive heart failure in anterior wall infarction, multiple myocardial infarctions, double- and triple-vessel CAD, LV aneurysm
Cx: (myocardium is prone to rupture during 3rd – 14th day post infarction)
  (1) LEFT VENTRICULAR FAILURE (60 – 70%)
    • "cardiac shock" = systolic pressure < 90 mmHg
    Δ signs of pulmonary venous hypertension are a good predictor of mortality (> 30% if present, < 10% if absent)
    √ progressive enlargement of heart
    √ haziness + indistinctness of pulmonary arteries
    √ increase in size of right descending pulmonary artery > 17 mm

√ pleural effusion
√ septal lines
√ perihilar ± peripheral parenchymal clouding
√ alveolar pulmonary edema
Mortality: 30 – 50% with mild LV failure; 44% with pulmonary edema; 80 – 100% with cardiogenic shock; (8% with absence of LV failure)
(2) ANEURYSM (12 – 15% of survivors)
(3) MYOCARDIAL RUPTURE (3.3%)
  • occurs usually on 3rd – 5th day post MI
  √ enlargement of heart (slow leakage of blood into pericardium)
  Prognosis: cause of death in 13% of all infarctions; almost 100% mortality
(4) RUPTURE OF PAPILLARY MUSCLE (1%)
  from infarction of posteromedial papillary muscle in inferior MI (common) / anterolateral papillary muscle in anterolateral MI (uncommon)
  • sudden onset of massive mitral insufficiency
  • unresponsive to medical management
  √ abrupt onset of severe persistent pulmonary edema
  √ minimal LV enlargement / normal-sized heart
  √ NO dilatation of LA (immediate decompression into pulmonary veins)
  Prognosis: 70% mortality within 24 hours; 80 – 90% within 2 weeks
(5) RUPTURE OF INTERVENTRICULAR SEPTUM (0.5 – 2%)
  • occurs usually within 4 – 21 days with rapid onset of L–R shunt
  • Swan-Ganz catheterization: increase in oxygen content of RV, capillary wedge pressure may be within normal limits
  √ right-sided cardiac enlargement
  √ engorgement of pulmonary vasculature
  √ NO pulmonary edema (DDx to ruptured papillary muscle)
  Prognosis: 24% mortality within 24 hours; 87% within 2 months; > 90% in 1 year
(6) DRESSLER SYNDROME (< 4%)
  = POSTMYOCARDIAL INFARCTION SYNDROME
  Etiology: autoimmune reaction
  • onset 2 – 3 weeks (range 1 week – several months) following infarction
  • relapses occur as late as 2 years after initial episode
  • fever
  √ pericarditis + pericardial effusion
  √ pleuritis + pleural effusion
  √ pneumonitis

Right Ventricular Infarction
right ventricle involved in 33% of left inferior myocardial infarction
√ decreased RV ejection fraction

√ accumulation of Tc-99m pyrophosphate
Prognosis: in 50% RV ejection fraction returns to normal within 10 days
Cx: (1) cardiogenic shock (unusual)
     (2) elevation of RA pressure
     (3) decrease of pulmonary artery pressure

MYXOMA
Most common benign primary intracardiac tumor in adults, 40% of all cardiac tumors
Age: 30 – 60 years
Location: LA:RA = 4:1; ventricles (exceptional); attached to atrial septum by small stalk; may protrude into ventricle causing partial obstruction of atrioventricular valve
• short Hx + rapid progression
• weight loss
• murmur (change with position)
• syncope
• fever
• anemia
√ generalized cardiac enlargement
√ atrial obstruction
√ persistent defect in atrium / diastolic defect in ventricle

A. LEFT ATRIAL MYXOMA
   with obstruction of mitral valve:
   √ enlargement of LA
   √ pulmonary venous hypertension
   √ ossific lung nodules
   √ NO enlarged atrial appendage
   Cx: systemic emboli (27%)
B. RIGHT ATRIAL MYXOMA
   with obstruction of tricuspid valve:
   √ enlargement of RA
   √ prominent SVC, IVC, azygos vein
   √ decreased pulmonary vascularity
   Cx: pulmonary emboli
ECHO: (2D-ECHO is study of choice)
   M-mode findings only of historical interest !

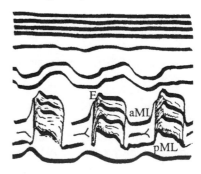

Atrial Myxoma Prolapsing into Mitral Valve Orifice
Note the interval between the opening of aML and pML and the moment that the tumor reaches its maximal anterior excursion at point E when a slight additional opening of the aML results; aML stays open during entire diastole as a result of obstruction to left atrial emptying.

√ dense echoes appearing posterior to aML soon after onset of diastole

√ pML obscured

√ tumor echoes can be traced into LA

√ dilated LA

√ reduced E-F slope

DDx: (1) Thrombus (most commonly in LA + LV)
(2) Other cardiac tumors: sarcoma, malignant mesenchymoma, metastasis

PATENT DUCTUS ARTERIOSUS

= PDA = persistence of left 6th aortic arch

Incidence: 9% of all CHD; M:F = 1:2

Associated with:
Prematurity, Birth asphyxia, High altitude births, Rubella syndrome, Coarctation, VSD, Trisomy 18 + 21

Normal physiology in mature infant:
increase in arterial oxygen pressure leads to constriction + closure of duct

Δ functional closure due to muscular contraction within 10 – 15 hours

Δ anatomic closure due to subintimal fibrosis + thrombosis: in 35% by 2 weeks; in 90% by 2 months; in 99% by 1 year

- mostly asymptomatic
- congestive heart failure (rare) usually by 3 months of age (in large L–R shunts)
- continuous murmur
- bounding peripheral pulses (intraaortic pressure run-off through PDA)

CXR (mimicks VSD):

√ LA enlargement

√ enlarged pulmonary artery segment

√ increase of pulmonary vasculature (less flow directed to LUL)

√ enlarged RV + LV

√ enlarged ascending aorta + aortic arch (thymus may obscure this)

√ prominent ductus infundibulum (diverticulum)
= prominence between aortic knob + pulmonary artery segment

√ obscured aortopulmonary window

√ "railroad track" = calcified ductus arteriosus

ECHO:

√ LA:Ao ratio = > 1.2:1 (signalizes significant L–R shunt)

Angio:

√ catheter course from RA to RV, main pulmonary artery, PDA, descending aorta

√ communication from aorta (distal to left subclavian artery) to left pulmonary artery on AP / LAT / LAO aortogram

PDA IN PREMATURE INFANT

Premature infant not subject to medial muscular hypertrophy of small pulmonary artery branches (which occurs in normal infants subsequent to progressive hypoxia in 3rd trimester)

- CHF

Cause:
(a) pulmonary artery pressure remains low without opposing any L–R shunts (PDA / VSD)
(b) ductus arteriosus remains open secondary to hypoxia in RDS

√ recurrence of alveolar air space filling after resolution of RDS

√ granular pattern of hyaline membrane disease becomes more opaque

√ enlargement of heart (masked by positive pressure ventilation)

Rx:
(a) Medical therapy:
(1) supportive oxygen, diuretics, digitalis
(2) avoid fluid overload (not to increase shunt volume)
(3) antiprostaglandins = indomethacine opposes prostaglandins which are potent duct dilators
(b) Surgical ligation

BENEFICIAL PDA = compensatory effect of PDA in:

1. Tetralogy of Fallot
cyanosis occurs during closure of duct shortly after birth

2. Eisenmenger pulmonary hypertension
PDA acts as escape valve shunting blood to descending aorta

3. Interrupted aortic arch
supply of lower extremity via PDA

NONBENEFICIAL PDA
in L–R shunts (VSD, aorticopulmonary window) a PDA increases shunt volume

PERICARDIAL CYST

M:F = 3:2

- asymptomatic

Location: (a) Costophrenic angles, R:L = 3:2
(b) Mediastinum (rare)

√ round / ovoid cyst, usually 3 – 8 cm in diameter

√ attenuation values of 20 – 40 HU, occasionally higher

PERICARDIAL DEFECT

= failure of pericardial development secondary to premature atrophy of the left duct of Cuvier (cardinal vein) which fails to nourish the left pleuropericardial membrane

Incidence: 1:13,000; M:F = 3:1

Age at detection: newborn – 81 years (mean 21 years)

Location:
(a) foraminal defect on left side (35%)
(b) complete absence on left side (35%)
(c) diaphragmatic pericardial aplasia (17%)
(d) total bilateral absence (9%)
(e) foraminal defect on right side (4%)

Associated with (in 30%):
(a) Bronchogenic cyst (30%)
(b) VSD, PDA, Mitral stenosis
(c) Diaphragmatic hernia, Sequestration

- mostly asymptomatic
- ECG: right axis deviation, right bundle branch block
- palpitations, tachycardia, dyspnea, dizziness, syncope
- positional discomfort while lying on left side
- nonspecific intermittent chest pain (lack of pericardial cushioning, torsion of great vessels, tension on pleuropericardial adhesions, pressure on coronary arteries by rim of pericardial defect)
√ size: Δ small foraminal defect = no abnormality
          Δ large defect   = herniation of cardiac structures / lung
          Δ complete absence   = levoposition of heart
√ absence of left pericardial fat pad
√ levoposition of heart with lack of visualization of right heart border
√ prominence / focal bulge in the area of RVOT, main pulmonary artery, left atrial appendage
√ sharp margination + elongation of left heart border
√ insinuation of lung between heart + left hemidiaphragm
√ insinuation of lung between aortic knob + pulmonary artery
√ increased distance between heart + sternum secondary to absence of sternopericardial ligament (cross-table lateral projection)
√ pneumopericardium following pneumothorax
√ NO tracheal deviation
Rx: Foraminal defect requires surgery because of
      (a) herniation + strangulation of left atrial appendage (b) herniation of LA / LV
      (1) closure of defect with pleural flap
      (2) resection of pericardium

PERSISTENT FETAL CIRCULATION
= PERSISTENT PULMONARY HYPERTENSION OF THE NEWBORN
= delay in transition from intra- to extrauterine pulmonary circulation
Cause: primary disorder related to birth asphyxia, concurrent parenchymal lung disease (meconium aspiration, pneumonia, pulmonary hemorrhage, hyaline membrane disease, pulmonary hypoplasia), concurrent cardiovascular disease, hypoxic myocardial injury, hyperviscosity syndromes)
- labile PO_2
√ structurally normal heart

POLYARTERITIS NODOSA
= PERIARTERITIS NODOSA = necrotizing vasculitis of medium-sized arteries
Etiology: ? immune complex phenomenon
Associated with: hepatitis B antigen
- fever, arthralgias, malaise
- painless hematuria
Location: all organs may be involved, kidney (85%), heart (65%), liver (50%)
√ focal narrowing of arteries
√ small aneurysms

√ arterial occlusions + small tissue infarctions
Cx: hypertension, renal failure

POLYSPLENIA SYNDROME
= BILATERAL LEFT-SIDEDNESS
Age: presentation in infancy / adulthood; M < F
Associated with:
  (a) Low incidence of CHD:
      APVR (70%), dextrocardia (37%), ASD (37%), ECCD (43%), pulmonic valvular stenosis (23%), TGA (13 – 17%), DORV (13 – 20%)
  (b) GI abnormalities:
      esophageal atresia, TE fistula, gastric duplication, preduodenal portal vein, duodenal webs + atresia, short bowel, mobile cecum, malrotation, semiannular pancreas, biliary atresia, absent gallbladder
  (c) GU anomalies (15%): renal agenesis, renal cysts, ovarian cysts
  (d) Vertebral anomalies, common celiac trunk–SMA
- heart murmur, CHF, occasional cyanosis
- leftward / superiorly directed P wave vector
- extrahepatic biliary obstruction
@ Lung
  √ bilateral morphologic left lungs (68%), normal (18%), bilateral R-sided lungs (7%)
  √ bilateral hyparterial bronchi
  √ normal / increased pulmonary vascularity
  √ bilateral SVC (50%)
  √ azygos / hemiazygos continuation with interruption of hepatic segment of IVC (70%)
  √ large azygos vein (MOST SPECIFIC sign) may mimic aortic arch
@ Abdomen
  √ presence of > 2 spleens (usually two major + indefinite number of splenules) located on both sides of the mesogastrium (esp. greater curvature of stomach)
  √ hepatic symmetry
  √ stomach on right / left side
  √ malrotation of bowel (80%)
OB-US:
  √ interrupted IVC
  √ aorta anterior to spine in midline
  √ azygos vein on left / right side of spine
Prognosis: 50 – 60% mortality within 1st year of life; 75% mortality by 5 years; 90% mortality by midadolescence

PRIMARY PULMONARY HYPERTENSION
= PLEXOGENIC PULMONARY ARTERIOPATHY
Diagnosis per exclusion:
  clinically unexplained progressive pulmonary arterial hypertension without evidence for thromboembolic disease + pulmonary venoocclusive disease
Histo: plexiform + angiomatoid lesions = tortuous channels within proliferation of endothelial cells
Age: 3rd decade; M < F

- dyspnea on exertion, syncope
- easy fatiguability
- hyperventilation
- chest pain
- hemoptysis

PSEUDOCOARCTATION
= AORTIC KINKING = variant of coarctation without a pressure gradient
Age: 12 – 64 years
Associated with:
  Bicuspid aortic valve, PDA, VSD, Aortic / subaortic stenosis, Single ventricle, ASD, Anomalies of aortic arch branches
- asymptomatic
- ejection murmur
- NO pressure gradient across the buckled segment
√ mediastinal widening (elongation of ascending aorta + aortic arch)
√ anteromedial deviation of aorta
√ "chimney shaped" high aortic arch (in children)
√ rounded / oval mass in left upper mediastinum above aortic arch (in adults)
√ anterior displacement of esophagus
√ NO rib notching / dilatation of brachiocephalic arteries / LV enlargement / poststenotic dilatation
Angio:
  √ high position of aortic arch
  √ "figure 3 sign" = notch in descending aorta at attachment of short ligamentum arteriosum
DDx: true coarctation, aneurysm, mediastinal mass

PULMONARY ATRESIA
= CONGENITAL ABSENCE OF PULMONARY ARTERY
= atretic pulmonary valve with underdeveloped pulmonary artery distally
√ small hemithorax of normal radiodensity
√ mediastinal shift to affected side
√ elevation of ipsilateral diaphragm
√ rib notching from prominence of intercostal arteries

PULMONARY ATRESIA WITH INTACT INTERVEN-TRICULAR SEPTUM
Associated with ASD (R-L shunt)
Type I : no remaining RV, No tricuspid regurgitation
  √ moderately enlarged RA (depending on size of ASD)
Type II : normal RV with tricuspid regurgitation
  √ massive enlargement of RA
√ cardiomegaly (LV, RA)
√ concave / small pulmonary artery segment
√ diminished pulmonary vascularity

PULMONARY VENOOCCLUSIVE DISEASE
= fibrous narrowing of intrapulmonary veins in the presence of a normal left heart characterized by pulmonary arterial hypertension, pulmonary edema, normal wedge pressures

Age: children, adolescents; M:F = 1:1
Histo: fibrous narrowing + thrombosis in up to 95% of pulmonary veins
√ pulmonary edema
√ pleural effusions
√ delayed filling of normal main pulmonary veins + left heart
Prognosis: poor (no effective therapy)

PULMONIC STENOSIS
Pulmonary stenosis without VSD = 8% of all CHD
- mostly asymptomatic
- cyanosis / heart failure
- loud systolic ejection murmur
√ systolic doming of pulmonary valve (= incomplete opening)
√ normal / diminished / increased pulmonary vascularity (depending on presence + nature of associated malformations)
√ enlarged pulmonary trunk + left pulmonary artery (poststenotic dilatation)
√ prominent left pulmonary artery + normal right pulmonary artery
√ hypertrophy of RV with reduced size of RV chamber
  √ elevation of cardiac apex
  √ increased convexity of anterior cardiac border on LAO
  √ diminution of retrosternal clear space
√ cor pulmonale
√ mild enlargement of LA (reason unknown)
√ calcification of pulmonary valves in older adults (rare)
Prognosis: 21 years mean age at death if untreated

Subvalvular Pulmonary Stenosis
A. INFUNDIBULAR PULMONARY STENOSIS
   typically in Tetralogy of Fallot
B. SUBINFUNDIBULAR PULMONARY STENOSIS
   = hypertrophied anomalous muscle bundles crossing portions of RV
   Associated with: VSD (73 – 85%)
   (a) Low type:
       courses diagonally from low anterior septal side to crista posteriorly
   (b) High type:
       horizontal defect across RV below infundibulum

Valvular Pulmonary Stenosis
1. CLASSIC / TYPICAL PULMONARY VALVE STENOSIS (95%)
   = commissural fusion of pulmonary cusps
   Age of presentation: childhood
   - pulmonic click
   - ECG:hypertrophy of RV
   √ thickened dome-shaped valve
   √ dilated main + left pulmonary artery
   √ jet of contrast
   Rx: balloon valvuloplasty

2. DYSPLASTIC PULMONARY VALVE STENOSIS
(5%)
= thickened redundant distorted cusps, immobile secondary to myxomatous tissue
- NO click
√ NO poststenotic dilatation
Rx: surgical resection of redundant valve tissue

CXR: √ normal pulmonary vascularity
√ normal-sized heart
Angio: √ increase in trabecular pattern of RV
√ hypertrophied crista supraventricularis (lateral projection)

TRILOGY OF FALLOT (infantile presentation)
(1) severe pulmonary valvular stenosis
(2) hypertrophy of RV
(3) ASD with R-L shunt (increased pressure in RA forces foramen ovale open)

Supravalvular Pulmonary Stenosis
60% of all pulmonary valve stenoses
Site of narrowing: pulmonary trunk, pulmonary bifurcation, one / both main pulmonary arteries, lobar pulmonary artery, segmental pulmonary artery
Shape of narrowing:
(a) localized with poststenotic dilatation
(b) long tubular hypoplasia
May be associated with:
(1) Valvular pulmonary stenosis, supravalvular aortic stenosis, VSD, PDA, systemic arterial stenoses
(2) Familial peripheral pulmonary stenoses + supravalvular aortic stenosis
(2) Williams-Beuren Syndrome: PS, supravalvular AS, peculiar facies
(3) Ehlers-Danlos Syndrome
(4) Postrubella Syndrome: peripheral pulmonary stenoses, valvular pulmonary stenosis, PDA, low birth weight, deafness, cataract, mental retardation
(5) Tetralogy of Fallot / Critical valvular pulmonary stenosis

SINGLE VENTRICLE
= UNIVENTRICULAR HEART
= DOUBLE INLET SINGLE VENTRICLE
= failure of development of interventricular septum ± absence of one atrioventricular valve (mitral / tricuspid atresia) ± aortic / pulmonic stenosis
- conduction defect (aberrant anatomy of conduction system)
√ two atrioventricular valves connected to a main ventricular chamber
√ the single ventricle may be a LV (85%) / RV / undetermined
√ a second rudimentary ventricular chamber may be present which is located anteriorly (in left univentricle) / posteriorly (in right univentricle)

√ rudimentary chamber ± connection to one great artery
√ may be associated with tricuspid / mitral atresia

SINUS OF VALSALVA ANEURYSM
= deficiency between aortic media + annulus fibrosis of aortic valve resulting in distension + eventual aneurysm formation
Age: puberty to 30 years of age
Site: right sinus / noncoronary sinus (> 90%)
Δ right sinus usually ruptures into RV, occasionally into RA
Δ noncoronary sinus ruptures into RA
- sudden retrosternal pain, dyspnea, continuous murmur
√ shunt vascularity
√ cardiomegaly
√ prominent ascending aorta

SUBCLAVIAN STEAL SYNDROME
= stenosis / obstruction of subclavian artery near its origin with flow reversal in ipsilateral vertebral artery at the expense of the cerebral circulation
Incidence: 2.5% of all extracranial arterial occlusions
Age: 40 – 60 years; M:F = 3:1
Etiology:
(a) congenital: interruption of aortic arch, preductal infantile coarctation, hypoplasia of left aortic arch, hypoplasia / atresia / stenosis of an anomalous left subclavian artery with right aortic arch, coarctation with aberrant subclavian artery arising distal to the coarctation
(b) atherosclerosis (most common), dissecting aneurysm, chest trauma, embolism, tumor thrombosis, inflammatory arteritis (Takayasu, syphilitic), ligation of subclavian artery in Blalock-Taussig shunt, complication of coarctation repair, radiation fibrosis

- Signs of vertebrobasilar insufficiency (40%)
  - syncopal episodes initiated by exercising the ischemic arm
  - headaches, nausea, vertigo, ataxia
  - mono-, hemi-, para-, quadriparesis, paralysis
  - diplopia, dysphagia, dysarthria, paresthesias around mouth
  - uni-/ bilateral homonymous hemianopia
- Signs of brachial insufficiency (3 – 10%)
  - intermittent / constant pain in affected arm precipitated by increased activity of that arm
  - paresthesia, weakness, coolness, numbness, burning in fingers + hand
  - fingertip necrosis
  - difference in systolic blood pressure > 20 – 40 mmHg between arms
  - weak / absent pulse in ipsilateral extremity
Location: L:R = 3:1
Angio:
√ subclavian stenosis / occlusion (aortic arch injection)

√ reversal of vertebral artery flow (Doppler US, selective injection of contralateral subclavian / vertebral artery)

CAVE: may appear falsely positive in high pressure injection causing transient retrograde flow in contralateral vertebral artery

Rx: surgery, PTA (good long-term results)

SUPERIOR VENA CAVA SYNDROME

= obstruction of SVC with development of collateral pathways

Etiology:
- (a) Malignant lesion (80 – 90%)
  1. Bronchogenic carcinoma (> 50%)
  2. Lymphoma
- (b) Benign lesion
  1. Granulomatous mediastinitis (usually histoplasmosis, sarcoidosis, TB)
  2. Substernal goiter
  3. Ascending aortic aneurysm
  4. Pacer wires / central venous catheters (23%)
  5. Constrictive pericarditis

Collateral routes:
1. Esophageal venous plexus = "downhill varices" (predominantly upper 2/3)
2. Azygous + hemiazygous veins
3. Accessory hemiazygos + superior intercostal veins = "aortic nipple" (visualization in normal population in 5%)
4. Lateral thoracic veins + umbilical vein
5. Vertebral veins

- head and neck edema (70%)
- cutaneous enlarged venous collaterals
- headache, dizziness, syncope
- with benign etiology: slower onset + progression, both sexes 25 – 40 years
- with malignancy: rapid progression within weeks, mostly males 40 – 60 years
- proptosis, tearing
- dyspnea, cyanosis, chest pain
- hematemesis (11%)

√ superior mediastinal widening (64%)
√ encasement / compression / occlusion of SVC
√ dilated cervical + superficial thoracic veins (80%)
√ SVC thrombus

NUC:
√ increased tracer uptake in caudate lobe (umbilical pathway toward liver when injected in upper extremity)

SYPHILITIC AORTITIS

Incidence: in 10 – 15% of untreated patients (accounts for death in 1/3)

Path: periaortitis (via lymphatics), mesaortitis (via vasa vasorum)

Site: ascending aorta (36%), aortic arch (24%), descending aorta (5%), sinus of Valsalva (1%), pulmonary artery

√ thick aortic wall (fibrous + inflammatory tissue)

√ saccular (75%) / fusiform (25%) dilatation of ascending aorta
√ small saccular aneurysms often protrude from fusiform aneurysm
√ fine pencil-like calcifications of intima (15%) in ascending aorta, late in disease

Cx: (1) Stenosis of coronary ostia (intimal thickening)
(2) Aortic regurgitation (syphilitic valvulitis), rare

TAKAYASU ARTERITIS

Incidence: 2.2% (at autopsy)

Age: 15 – 25 years; M > F

- (a) Acute stage
- (b) Fibrotic stage (weeks to years)

Location: ascending + abdominal aorta, brachiocephalic artery, renal arteries, pulmonary arteries

√ long + diffuse / short + segmental narrowing / occlusion of arteries
√ frequent skip areas
√ abundant collateralization
√ aneurysm

TETRALOGY OF FALLOT

= underdevelopment of pulmonary infundibulum secondary to unequal partitioning of the conotruncus

Incidence: 8% of all CHD; most common CHD with cyanosis after 1 year of life

TETRAD:
1. Obstruction of right ventricular outflow tract: usually at pulmonary infundibulum, occasionally at pulmonary valve
2. VSD
3. Right ventricular hypertrophy
4. Aorta overriding the interventricular septum

Hemodynamics:

Δ fetus: pulmonary blood flow supplied by retrograde flow through ductus arteriosus with absence of RV hypertrophy / IUGR

Δ neonate: R–L shunt bypassing pulmonary circulation with decrease in systemic oxygen saturation (cyanosis); pressure overload + hypertrophy of RV secondary to pulmonic-infundibular stenosis

Associated with:
1. Bicuspid pulmonic valve (40%)
2. Stenosis of left pulmonary artery (40%)
3. R aortic arch (25%)
4. TE fistula
5. Down syndrome
6. Forked ribs, scoliosis
7. Anomalies of coronary arteries in 10% (single RCA / LAD from RCA)

- cyanosis by 3 – 4 months of age (concealed at birth by PDA)
- dyspnea on exertion, clubbing of fingers and toes
- "squatting position" when fatigued (increases pulmonary blood flow)
- "episodic spells" = loss of consciousness

- polycythemia, lowered PO_2 values, systolic murmur in pulmonic area

√ pronounced concavity in region of pulmonary artery trunk (small / absent PA)
√ coeur en sabot (boot-shaped heart) = enlargement of right ventricle
√ right-sided aortic arch in 25%
√ marked reduction in caliber + number of pulmonary vessels
√ asymmetric pulmonary vascularity
√ reticular pattern with horizontal course usually in periphery (= prominent collateral circulation of pleuropulmonary connections)

OB-US:
√ dilated aorta overriding the interventricular septum
√ usually perimembranous VSD
√ mildly stenotic RV outflow tract
√ NO RV hypertrophy in midtrimester

ECHO:
√ discontinuity between anterior aortic wall + interventricular septum (= overriding of the aorta)
√ small left atrium
√ RV hypertrophy with small right ventricular outflow tract
√ widening of the aorta
√ thickening of right ventricular wall + interventricular septum

Prognosis: spontaneous survival without surgical correction in 50% up to age 7; in 10% up to age 21
Rx: Surgery in early childhood
(a) Palliative
  1. Blalock-Taussig shunt = end-to-side anastomosis of subclavian to pulmonary artery opposite aortic arch (64% survival rate at 15 years, 55% at 20 years)
  2. Potts operation on left = anastomosis of left PA with descending aorta
  3. Waterston-Cooley procedure = anastomosis between ascending aorta + right pulmonary artery
  4. Central shunt = Rastelli procedure = tubular synthetic graft between ascending aorta + pulmonary artery
(b) Corrective open cardiac surgery = VSD-closure + reconstruction of RV outflow tract by excision of obstructing tissue (82% survival rate at 15 years)
Operative mortality: 3 – 10%

PINK TETRALOGY = infundibular hypertrophy in VSD (3%)
PENTALOGY OF FALLOT = tetralogy + ASD
TRILOGY OF FALLOT = pulmonary stenosis + RV hypertrophy + patent foramen ovale

THORACIC OUTLET SYNDROME
Causes:
A. CONGENITAL
  1. Cervical rib (0.5%)
    = elevation of floor of scalene triangle with decrease of costoclavicular space
    - < 50% of complete cervical ribs are symptomatic
    - 70% of symptomatic patients have a responsible cervical rib
  2. Scalenus minimus muscle (rare) extending from transverse process of 7th cervical vertebra to 1st rib with insertion between brachial plexus + subclavian artery
  3. Anterior scalene muscle = Scalenus anticus syndrome (most common) =wide / abnormal insertion / hypertrophy of muscle
  4. Anomalous 1st rib = unusually straight course with narrowing of costoclavicular space
B. ACQUIRED
  1. Muscular body habitus = arterial compression in pectoralis minor tunnel
  2. Slender body habitus with long neck, sagging shoulders
  3. Fracture of clavicle / 1st rib (34%) with nonanatomical alignment / exuberant callus
  4. Supraclavicular tumor / lymphadenopathy
- pain in hand with increase on elevation of arm
- hyperabduction maneuver with obliteration of radial pulse (34%)
- numbness of hand + fingers, paresthesias
- intermittent claudication, ischemia of fingers
- decreased skin temperature
- Raynaud phenomenon (40%): episodic constriction of small vessels

Angio:
√ abnormal course of distal subclavian artery
√ focal stenosis / occlusion
√ poststenotic dilatation of distal subclavian artery
√ aneurysm
√ stress test: band-like / concentric compression
√ mural thrombus ± distal embolization
√ venous thrombosis / obstruction

TRANSPOSITION OF GREAT ARTERIES
Complete Transposition of Great Arteries
= TGA = D-TRANSPOSITION = failure of the aorticopulmonary septum to follow a spiral course characterized by (1) aorta originating from RV (2) pulmonary artery originating from LV (3) normal position of atria + ventricles
Incidence: 10% of all CHD
VARIATIONS:
1. Complete TGA + intact interventricular septum
2. Complete TGA + VSD: CHF due to VSD
3. Complete TGA + VSD + PS: PS prevents CHF = longest survival

Hemodynamics:
Δ fetus: no hemodynamic compromise with
            normal birth weight
Δ neonate: mixing of the 2 independent circulations
            necessary for survival
Admixture of blood from both circulations via:
    (1) PDA + patent foramen ovale (when PDA closes
        worst prognosis)
    (2) VSD (in 50%)
• cyanosis (most common cause for cyanosis in
  neonate) 2nd most common cause of cyanosis after
  Tetralogy
• symptomatic 1 – 2 weeks following birth
CXR:
    √ "egg-on-its-side" appearance of heart = narrow
      superior mediastinum secondary to hypoplastic
      thymus + hyperaeration + abnormal relationship of
      great vessels
    √ cardiac enlargement beginning 2 weeks after birth
    √ right heart enlargement
    √ enlargement of LA (with VSD)
    √ absent pulmonary trunk (99%) = PA located
      posteriorly in midline
    √ increased pulmonary blood flow (if not associated
      with PS)
    √ midline aorta (30%) / ascending aorta with
      convexity to the right
    √ right aortic arch in 3% (difficult assessment due to
      midline position + small size)
OB-US:
    √ great arteries arise from ventricles in a parallel
      fashion
    √ aorta anterior + to right of pulmonary artery (in
      60%; rarely side by side)
Prognosis: overall 70% survival rate at 1 week, 50%
                at 1 month, 11% at 1 year by natural
                history

Rx:
    (1) Prostaglandin E1 administration to maintain
        ductal patency
    (2) Rashkind procedure = balloon septostomy to
        create ASD
    (3) Blalock-Hanlon procedure = surgical creation of
        ASD
    (4) Mustard operation (corrective) = removal of atrial
        septum + creation of intraatrial baffle directing the
        pulmonary venous return to RV + systemic
        venous return to LV; 79% 1-year survival rate;
        64 – 89% 5-year survival

Corrected Transposition of Great Arteries
= CONGENITALLY CORRECTED TRANSPOSITION
= L-TRANSPOSITION
= anomalous looping of the primordial ventricles
  associated with lack of spiral rotation of truncoconal
  septum characterized by
    (1) transposition of great arteries
    (2) inversion of ventricles (LV on right side, RV on left
        side):
        Δ   RA connected to morphologic LV
        Δ   LA connected to morphologic RV
    (3) AV valves + coronary arteries follow their
        corresponding ventricles
Hemodynamics: functionally corrected abnormality
Associated with:
    (1) usually perimembranous VSD (in > 50%)
    (2) pulmonic stenosis (in 50%)
    (3) anomaly of left (= tricuspid) atrioventricular valves
        (Ebstein-like)
    (4) dextrocardia (high incidence)
• atrioventricular block (malalignment of atrial +
  ventricular septa)
CXR:
    √ abnormal convexity / straightening in upper portion
      of left heart border (ascending aorta arising from
      inverted RV)
    √ inapparent aortic knob + descending aorta
      (overlying spine)
    √ inapparent pulmonary trunk (rightward posterior
      position) = PREMIER SIGN
    √ humped contour of lower left heart border with
      elevation above diaphragm (anatomic RV)
    √ apical notch (= septal notch)
    √ increased pulmonary blood flow (if shunt present)
    √ pulmonary venous hypertension (if left-sided AV
      valve incompetent)
    √ LA enlargement
Angio:
    √ original LV on right side: smooth-walled, cylinder- /
      cone-shaped with high recess emptying into aorta
      (= venous ventricle)
    √ original RV on left side: bulbous, triangular shape,
      trabeculated chamber with infundibular outflow tract
      into pulmonary trunk (= arterial ventricle)

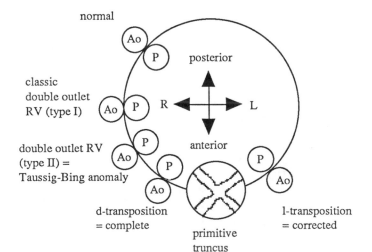

normal

Ao
P
posterior

classic
double outlet
RV (type I)

Ao P   R ←→ L

double outlet RV
(type II) =
Taussig-Bing anomaly

P
Ao
P
Ao   anterior   P
                  Ao

d-transposition   l-transposition
= complete   = corrected

primitive
truncus

OB-US:
- √ great arteries arise from ventricles in a parallel fashion
- √ aortic valve separated from tricuspid valve by a complete infundibulum
- √ fibrous continuity between pulmonic valve + mitral valve

Prognosis: (unfavorable secondary to additional cardiac defects) 40% 1-year survival rate, 30% 10-year survival rate

TRICUSPID ATRESIA

2nd most common cause of pronounced neonatal cyanosis (after transposition) characterized by absent tricuspid valve, ASD, and small VSD (in most patients)

Incidence: 1.5% of all CHD

1. TRICUSPID ATRESIA WITHOUT TRANSPOSITION (80%)
   (a) without PS (b) with PS (c) with pulmonary atresia
2. TRICUSPID ATRESIA WITH TRANSPOSITION
   (a) without PS (b) with PS (most favorable combination) (c) with pulmonary atresia

Δ usually small VSD + PS (75%) restrict pulmonary blood flow

- progressive cyanosis from birth on, increasing with crying = OUTSTANDING FEATURE (inverse relationship between degree of cyanosis + volume of pulmonary blood flow)
- pansystolic murmur (VSD)
- ECG: left-axis deviation

Prognosis: may survive well into early adulthood

CXR: (typical cardiac contour)
- √ left rounded contour = enlargement + hypertrophy of LV
- √ right rounded contour = enlarged RA
- √ flat / concave pulmonary segment
- √ normal / decreased pulmonary vascularity
- √ typical flattening of right heart border with transposition (in 15%)

Rx:
1. Blalock-Taussig procedure (if pulmonary blood flow decreased in infancy)
2. Glenn procedure = shunt between IVC + right PA (if total correction not anticipated)
3. Fontan procedure = external conduit from RA to pulmonary trunk + closure of ASD (if pulmonary vascular disease has not developed)

TRUNCUS ARTERIOSUS

= PERSISTENT TRUNCUS ARTERIOSUS
= SINGLE OUTLET OF THE HEART
= abnormal septation of the conotruncus characterized by
   (1) one great artery arising from the heart giving rise to the coronary, pulmonary, and systemic arteries, straddling
   (2) large VSD

Incidence: 2% of all CHD

Types:

Type I	(50%)	= main PA + aorta arise from common truncal valve
Type II	(25%)	= both pulmonary arteries arise from back of trunk
Type III	(10%)	= both pulmonary arteries arise from side of trunk
Type IV		= "Pseudotruncus" = absence of pulmonary arteries; pulmonary supply from systemic collaterals arising from descending aorta
Type A		= infundibular VSD present
Type B		= VSD absent

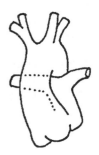 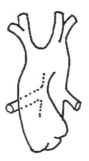

Type I   **Type II**

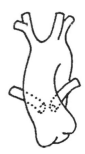 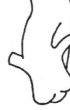

Type III   **Type IV**

Associated with:
(1) right aortic arch (in 35%)
   Cyanosis + Shunt vascularity + Right aortic arch = TRUNCUS
(2) forked ribs

Hemodynamics:
Δ fetus: CHF only with incompetent valve secondary to massive regurgitation from truncus to ventricles
Δ neonate: L–R shunt after decrease in pulmonary resistance (massive diversion of flow to pulmonary district) leads to CHF (ventricular overload) / pulmonary hypertension with time

- moderate cyanosis, apparent with crying
- severe CHF within first days / months of life (in large R–L shunt)
- systolic murmur

CXR:
√ cardiomegaly (increased LV volume)
√ enlarged LA (50%) secondary to increased pulmonary blood flow
√ large "aortic shadow" = truncus arteriosus
√ "waterfall / hilar comma sign" = elevated right hilum (30%); elevated left hilum (10%)
√ concave pulmonary segment (50%) (Type I has left convex pulmonary segment)
√ markedly increased pulmonary blood flow, may be asymmetric

ECHO:
√ single arterial vessel overriding the interventricular septum (DDx: Tetralogy of Fallot)
√ frequently dysplastic + incompetent single semilunar valve with 3 – 6 leaflets (most commonly 3 leaflets)

Prognosis: 40% 6-months survival rate,
                20% 1-year survival rate

Rx: Rastelli procedure (30% no longer operable at 4 years of age) = (a) artificial valve placed high in RVOT and attached via a dacron graft to main pulmonary artery (b) closure of VSD

Hemitruncus
= rare anomaly characterized by
(a) one pulmonary artery (commonly right PA) arising from trunk
(b) one pulmonary artery arising from RV / supplied by systemic collaterals
Associated with: PDA (80%), VSD, Tetralogy (usually isolated to left PA)
• acyanotic

Pseudotruncus Arteriosus
= TRUNCUS TYPE IV = severe form of tetralogy of Fallot with atresia of the pulmonary trunk; entire pulmonary circulation through bronchial collateral arteries (NOT a form of truncus arteriosus in its true sense); characterized by (1) pulmonary atresia (2) VSD with R–L shunt (3) RV hypertrophy
Associated with: right aortic arch in 50%
• cyanosis
√ concavity in area of pulmonary segment
√ comma-like abnormal appearance of pulmonary artery
√ absent normal right and left pulmonary artery (lateral chest film)
√ esophageal indentation posteriorly (due to large systemic collaterals)
√ prominent hilar + intrapulmonary vessels (= systemic collaterals)
√ "coeur en sabot" = RV enlargement
√ prominent ascending aorta with hyperpulsations

VENTRICULAR ANEURYSM
A. CONGENITAL LEFT VENTRICULAR ANEURYSM
    rare, young black adult
    (a) Submitral type: √ bulge at left middle / upper cardiac border

(b) Subaortic type: √ small + not visualized
                        √ heart greatly enlarged (from aortic insufficiency)

B. ACQUIRED LEFT VENTRICULAR ANEURYSM
    = complication of myocardial infarction, Chagas disease
    • may be asymptomatic + well tolerated for years
    • occasionally associated with persistent heart failure, arrhythmia, peripheral embolization

True Aneurysm
= circumscribed noncontractile outpouching of ventricular cavity with broad mouth + localized dyskinesis
Cause: sequela of transmural myocardial infarction
Location:
(a) left anterior + anteroapical: readily detected (anterior + LAO views)
(b) inferior + inferoposterior: less readily detected (steep LAO + LPO views)
Detection rate: 50% by fluoroscopy; 96% by radionuclide ventriculography; frequently not visible on CXR
√ localized bulge of heart contour = "squared-off" appearance of mid left lateral margin of heart border
√ localized paradoxical expansion during systole (CHARACTERISTIC)
√ rim of calcium in fibrotic wall (chronic), rare
√ akinetic / severely hypokinetic segment
√ left ventriculography in LAO, RAO is diagnostic
√ wide communication with heart chamber (no neck)
Cx: wall thrombus with embolization
Prognosis: rarely ruptures

Pseudoaneurysm
= FALSE ANEURYSM = left ventricular rupture contained by fused layers of visceral + parietal pericardium / extracardiac tissue
(a) cardiac rupture with localized hematoma contained by adherent pericardium; typically in the presence of pericarditis
(b) subacute rupture with gradual / episodic bleeding
Etiology: trauma, myocardial infarction
Location: typically at posterolateral / diaphragmatic wall of LV
√ left retrocardiac double density
√ diameter of mouth smaller than the largest diameter of the globular aneurysm
√ delayed filling
Cx: high risk of delayed rupture (infrequent in true aneurysms)

VENTRICULAR SEPTAL DEFECT
most common CHD (25 – 30%): (a) isolated in 20% (b) with other cardiac anomalies in 5%;
Δ Acyanotic L-R shunt + right aortic arch (in 2 – 5%) = VSD

1. MEMBRANOUS = PERIMEMBRANOUS VSD
   (75 – 80%)
   Location: posterior + inferior to crista supraventricularis
               near commissure between right and
               posterior (= noncoronary) aortic valve cusps
   May be associated with small aneurysms of
      membranous septum commonly leading to decrease
      in size of membranous VSD (their presence does not
      necessarily predict eventual complete closure)

2. SUPRACRISTAL = CONAL VSD (5 – 8%)
   Δ   crista supraventricularis = inverted U-shaped
       muscular ridge posterior + inferior to pulmonary
       valve
   (a) on RV side = VSD just beneath pulmonary valve with
       valve forming part of superior margin of defect
   (b) on LV side = VSD just below commissure between R
       + L aortic valve cusps
   Cx: right aortic valve cusp may herniate into VSD
           (= aortic insufficiency)

3. MUSCULAR VSD (5 – 10%)
   May consist of multiple VSDs; bordered entirely by
      myocardium
   Location: (a) inlet portion (b) trabecular portion
               (c) infundibular / outlet portion

4. ATRIOVENTRICULAR CANAL TYPE
   = ENDOCARDIAL CUSHION TYPE
   = POSTERIOR VSD (5 – 10%)
   Location: adjacent to septal + anterior leaflet of mitral
               valve; rare as isolated defect
   Hemodynamics:
      small bidirectional shunt during fetal life (similar
      pressures in RV + LV); after birth a decrease in
      pulmonary arterial pressure + increase in systemic
      arterial pressure occurs with development of L-R shunt
   (a) small VSD: little / no hemodynamic significance
   (b) large VSD: pulmonary vascular disease +
       hypertension will increase RV pressure; eventually
       leads to shunt reversal (L-R shunt)
   (c) very large VSD: gross right ventricular overload
       creates CHF soon after birth

NATURAL HISTORY OF VSD causing reduction in
pulmonary blood flow:
   1. Spontaneous closure
      in 40% within first 2 year years of life; 60% by 5
      years (65% with muscular VSD, 25% with
      membranous VSD); with large VSD in 10%; with
      small VSD in 50%
   2. Eisenmenger syndrome
      = progressive increase in pulmonary vascular
      resistance through intima + medial hyperplasia;
      occurs in 10% of large VSDs by 2 years of age
   3. RVOT obstruction
      infundibular hypertrophy in 3% = pink tetrad

4. Prolapse of right aortic valve cusp
   = aortic valve insufficiency

CLASSIFICATION:
Group I: "maladie de Roger" = small shunt with defect
           < 1 cm; normal pulmonary artery pressure,
           normal pulmonary vascular resistance;
           spontaneous closure
           • asymptomatic
           • heart murmur
           √ normal plain film
Group II: moderate shunt with defect of 1 – 1.5 cm;
           intermediate pulmonary artery pressure;
           normal pulmonary vascular resistance;
           spontaneous closure in large percentage
           • respiratory infections, mild dyspnea
           √ slight prominence of pulmonary vessels
             (45% shunt)
           √ slight enlargement of LA
Group III: nonrestrictive large shunt with size equal to
           aortic valve orifice; pulmonary artery pressure
           approaching systemic levels; slightly increased
           pulmonary vascular resistance; pulmonary
           blood flow 2 – 4 x systemic flow
           • bouts of respiratory infections
           • feeding problems, failure to thrive
           √ prominent pulmonary segment + vessels
             (= shunt vascularity)
           √ enlargement of LA + LV
           √ normal / small aorta
Group IV: Eisenmenger syndrome with shunt reversal
           into R–L shunt; irreversible increase in
           pulmonary vascular resistance (when
           pulmonary vascular resistance > 0.75 of
           systemic vascular resistance)
           • cyanotic, but less symptomatic; CHF rare
           √ decrease of pulmonary vessel caliber
           √ decrease in size of LA + LV

CXR (with increase in size of VSD):
   √ enlargement of LA
   √ enlargement of pulmonary artery segment
   √ enlargement of LV
   √ RV hypertrophy
   √ increase in pulmonary blood flow (= > 45% of
     pulmonary blood flow from systemic circulation)
   √ Eisenmenger reaction
ECHO:
   √ lack of echoes in region of interventricular septum
     with sharp edges (DDx: artifactual drop out with
     sound beam parallel to septum); muscular VSD
     difficult to see
   √ LA enlargement
   √ prolapse of aortic valve cusp (in supracristal VSD)
   √ deformity of aortic cusp (in membranous VSD)

Angio:
  Projections:
    (a) LAO 60° C-C 20° for membranous + anterior muscular VSD
    (b) LAO 45° C-C 45 ° (hepatoclavicular) for posterior endocardial cushion + posterior muscular VSD
    (c) RAO for supracristal VSD + assessment of RVOT
  √ RVOT / pulmonary valve fill without filling of RV chamber (in supracristal VSD)

Rx:
  (a) Large VSD + left heart failure at 3 months of age: aim is to delay closure until child is 18 months of age; pulmonary-to-systemic blood flow > 2:1 requires surgery before pulmonary hypertension becomes manifest
    1. Digitalis + diuretics
    2. Pulmonary artery banding
    3. Patching of VSD: surgical approach through RA / through RV for supracristal VSD
  (b) Small VSDs without increase in pulmonary arterial pressure are followed

DIFFERENTIAL DIAGNOSIS OF HEPATIC, BILIARY, PANCREATIC, AND SPLENIC DISORDERS

LIVER
Diffuse hepatic enlargement
NORMAL LIVER SIZE (in midclavicular line):
- < 13 cm = normal
- 13.0 – 15.5 cm = indeterminate (in 25% of patients)
- > 15.5 cm = hepatomegaly (accuracy of 87%)

A. METABOLIC
  1. Fatty infiltration
  2. Amyloid
  3. Wilson disease
  4. Gaucher disease
  5. Von Gierke disease
  6. Niemann-Pick disease
  7. Weber-Christian disease
  8. Galactosemia
B. MALIGNANCY
  1. Lymphoma
  2. Diffuse metastases
  3. Diffuse HCC
  4. Angiosarcoma
C. INFLAMMATION / INFECTION
  1. Hepatitis
  2. Mononucleosis
  3. Miliary TB, histoplasmosis, sarcoid
  4. Malaria
  5. Syphilis
  6. Leptospirosis
  7. Chronic granulomatous disease of childhood
D. VASCULAR
  1. Passive congestion
E. OTHERS
  1. Early cirrhosis
  2. Polycystic liver disease

Increased liver attenuation
Abnormal deposits of substances with high atomic numbers
1. IRON
   (a) Primary hemochromatosis (b) Transfusional hemosiderosis (c) Bantu siderosis = excessive dietary iron from food preparation in iron containers (Kaffir beer)
2. COPPER
   Wilson disease = hepatolenticular degeneration = increased copper deposits in liver + basal ganglia
3. IODINE
   Amiodarone (= antiarrhythmic drug with 37% iodine by weight)
   √ 95 – 145 HU (normal range 30 – 70 HU)
4. GOLD
   Colloidal form of gold for therapy of rheumatoid arthritis

5. THOROTRAST
   Alpha-emitter with atomic number of 90; previously used for cerebral angiography and liver spleen imaging; > 100,000 people injected; intravascular injected colloidal thorium dioxide is deposited in liver (70%), spleen (30%), bone marrow, abdominal lymph nodes (20%); biologic half-life of 400 years; hepatic dose in 20 years: 1000 – 3000 rads
   Cx: angiosarcoma (50%), cholangiocarcinoma, hepatocellular carcinoma (latency period of 3 – 40 years; mean 26 years)
6. THALLIUM
   Accidental / suicidal ingestion of rodenticides (lethal dose is 0.2 – 1.0 gram)
7. ACUTE MASSIVE PROTEIN DEPOSITS
8. GLYCOGEN STORAGE DISEASE

Generalized increased liver echogenicity
1. Fatty infiltration
2. Cirrhosis
3. Chronic hepatitis
4. Vacuolar degeneration

Focal liver lesions
A. SOLITARY
  (a) benign
      1. Simple cyst / echinococcal cyst
      2. Cavernous hemangioma
      3. Abscess
      4. Hematoma / traumatic cyst
      5. Adenoma
      6. Focal nodular hyperplasia
      7. Fatty change
  (b) malignant
      1. Hepatoma
      2. Metastasis
      3. Peripheral cholangiocarcinoma
B. MULTIPLE
  (a) benign
      1. Simple cysts
      2. Cavernous hemangioma
      3. Polycystic disease
      4. Multiple abscesses
      5. Caroli disease
      6. Adenoma
      7. Regenerating hepatic nodules
  (b) malignant
      1. Metastases (most common malignant liver tumor)
      2. Multifocal hepatoma
      3. Lymphoma

Solitary echogenic liver mass
1. Hemangioma
2. Focal fatty infiltration
3. Hepatoma
4. Adenoma
5. Focal nodular hyperplasia
6. Hepatic lipoma

Hepatic lesion with central scar
1. Focal nodular hyperplasia
2. Hepatic adenoma
3. Giant cavernous hemangioma
4. Fibrolamellar hepatocellular carcinoma

Primary benign liver tumors
A. EPITHELIAL TUMORS
    (a) hepatocellular
       1. Nodular transformation
       2. Focal nodular hyperplasia
       3. Hepatocellular adenoma
    (b) cholangiocellular
       1. Bile duct adenoma
       2. Biliary cystadenoma
B. MESENCHYMAL TUMORS
    (a) tumors of adipose tissue
       1. Lipoma
       2. Myelolipoma
       3. Angiomyolipoma
    (b) tumors of muscle tissue
       1. Leiomyoma
    (c) tumors of blood vessels
       1. Infantile hemangioendothelioma
       2. Hemangioma
    (d) mesothelial tumors
       1. Benign mesothelioma
C. MIXED TISSUE TUMORS
    1. Mesenchymal hamartoma
    2. Benign teratoma
D. MISCELLANEOUS
    1. Adrenal rest tumor
    2. Pancreatic rest

Primary malignant liver tumors
A. EPITHELIAL TUMORS
    (a) hepatocellular
       1. Hepatoblastoma (7%)
       2. Hepatocellular carcinoma (75%)
    (b) cholangiocellular (6%)
       1. Cholangiocarcinoma
       2. Cystadenocarcinoma
B. MESENCHYMAL TUMORS
    (a) tumors of blood vessels
       1. Angiosarcoma
       2. Hemangioendothelioma
    (b) other tumors
       1. Embryonal sarcoma
       2. Fibrosarcoma

C. TUMORS OF MUSCLE TISSUE
    1. Leiomyosarcoma
    2. Rhabdomyosarcoma
D. MISCELLANEOUS
    1. Carcinosarcoma
    2. Teratoma
    3. Yolk sac tumor
    4. Carcinoid
    5. Squamous carcinoma
    6. Primary lymphoma

Low-density mass in porta hepatis
1. Choledochal cyst
2. Hepatic cyst
3. Pancreatic pseudocyst
4. Enteric duplication
5. Hepatic artery aneurysm
6. Biloma

Low-density hepatic mass with enhancement
1. Hepatoma
2. Hypervascular metastases (lesions that may be obscured after contrast injection: pheochromocytoma, carcinoid, melanoma)
3. Cavernous hemangioma
4. Focal nodular hyperplasia with central fibrous scar
5. Hepatic adenoma

Portal venous gas
Etiology:
    (1) bowel infarction
    (2) ulcerative colitis
    (3) necrotizing enterocolitis
    (4) small bowel obstruction
    (5) intraabdominal abscess
    (6) gastric ulcer
    (7) pneumonia
√ branching linear gas densities in periphery of liver
√ gas in mesenteric vessels
√ gas in intestinal wall

Hepatic calcifications
A. INFECTION
    1. Tuberculosis (48%), Histoplasmosis, Gumma, Brucellosis
    2. Echinococcal cyst (in 33%)
    3. Chronic granulomatous disease of childhood
    4. Old pyogenic / amebic abscess
B. VASCULAR
    1. Hepatic artery aneurysm
    2. Portal vein thrombosis
C. BILIARY
    1. Intrahepatic calculi
D. BENIGN TUMORS
    1. Congenital cyst
    2. Cavernous hemangioma
    3. Capsule of regenerating nodules
    4. Infantile hemangioendothelioma

E. PRIMARY MALIGNANT TUMORS
    1. Hepatoblastoma (10 – 20%)
    2. Cholangiocellular carcinoma
F. METASTATIC TUMOR
    1. Mucinous carcinoma of colon, breast, stomach
    2. Ovarian carcinoma (psammomatous bodies)
    3. Melanoma, Pleural mesothelioma, Osteosarcoma, Carcinoid, Leiomyosarcoma

PANCREAS
Pancreatic calcifications
1. CHRONIC PANCREATITIS
    Numerous irregular stippled calcifications of varying size; predominantly intraductal
    (a) Alcoholic pancreatitis (in 20 – 50%): limited to head / tail in 25%
    (b) Biliary pancreatitis (in 2%)
    (c) Hereditary pancreatitis (in 35 – 60%): round calcifications throughout gland
    (d) Idiopathic pancreatitis
    (e) Pancreatic pseudocyst
2. NEOPLASM
    (a) Microcystic adenoma (in 33%): "sunburst" appearance
    (b) macrocystic cystadenoma: rounded cystic areas
    (c) Adenocarcinoma (in 2%): with "sunburst" pattern
    (d) Cavernous lymphangioma / hemangioma: multiple phleboliths
    (e) Metastases from colon cancer
3. INTRAPARENCHYMAL HEMORRHAGE
    (a) Old hematoma / abscess / infarction
    (b) Rupture of intrapancreatic aneurysm
4. HYPERPARATHYROIDISM (in 20%):
    50% of patients develop chronic pancreatitis, concomitant nephrocalcinosis
    indistinguishable from alcoholic pancreatitis
5. CYSTIC FIBROSIS
    Fine granular calcifications imply advanced pancreatic fibrosis
6. HEMOCHROMATOSIS
7. KWASHIORKOR = tropical pancreatitis: indistinguishable from alcoholic pancreatitis

Pancreatic masses
A. NEOPLASTIC
    1. Adenocarcinoma
    2. Islet cell tumor
    3. Cystadenoma / -carcinoma
    4. Solid and papillary neoplasm
    5. Lymphoma
B. INFLAMMATORY
    1. Acute pancreatitis
    2. Pseudocyst
    3. Pancreatic abscess

Pancreatic cyst
1. Pseudocyst (90%): secondary to obstructive tumor /

trauma / acute pancreatitis (in 2 – 4%), chronic pancreatitis (in 10 – 15%) [develop within 10 – 20 days, consolidated after 6 – 8 weeks]
2. Cystic neoplasm (10%):
    < 5% of all pancreatic tumors
    (a) microcystic adenoma
    (b) mucinous cystic neoplasm
3. Congenital cyst (rare)
    (a) solitary
    (b) multiple (when associated with cystic disease of the liver / other organs):
        Adult polycystic kidney disease (hepatic cysts in 90% at autopsy); von Hippel-Lindau disease (72% at autopsy; in only 25% on CT)
4. Acquired cyst: retention cyst (= exudate within bursa omentalis), parasitic cyst

Pancreatic neoplasm
A. EPITHELIAL ORIGIN
    1. Ductal adenoma, Intraductal papilloma
        < 1% of epithelial cell neoplasms
    2. Serous cystadenoma
    3. Mucinous cystadenoma
    4. **Ductectatic mucinous tumor**
        √ mass usually in uncinate portion of pancreatic head = cystic dilatation of pancreatic duct + branches
        √ grape-like clusters of cysts containing thick mucinous secretions
        √ surrounded by thin rim of normal pancreatic parenchyma
    5. Solid and papillary neoplasm
B. ACINAR CELL ORIGIN
    1. Solid and papillary neoplasm of pancreas
    2. **Acinar cell carcinoma**
        in elderly patients
        • increased serum lipase ± amylase
        • disseminated subcutaneous + intraosseous fat necrosis
        √ lobulated mass of 2 – 15 cm in diameter
        √ moderately vascular tumor + neovascularity + arterial and venous encasement
        Prognosis: median survival of 7 months
C. NONEPITHELIAL ORIGIN
    1. Lymphoma
        (a) Primary lymphoma:
            < 1% of pancreatic neoplasms
        (b) Secondary lymphoma
            √ large homogeneous solid mass, infrequently with central cystic area
            √ peripancreatic nodal masses
            √ peripancreatic vessels displaced + stretched
    2. Metastases
        melanoma, lung cancer, breast cancer, ovarian cancer, hepatocellular carcinoma, renal cell carcinoma, sarcoma

Hypervascular pancreatic tumors
A. PRIMARY
Islet cell tumor
B. METASTASES from
angiosarcoma, leiomyosarcoma, melanoma, carcinoid, renal cell carcinoma, adrenal carcinoma, thyroid carcinoma

Hyperamylasemia
A. PANCREATIC
1. Acute / chronic pancreatitis
2. Pancreatic trauma
3. Pancreatic carcinoma
B. GASTROINTESTINAL
1. Perforated peptic ulcer
2. Intestinal obstruction
3. Peritonitis
4. Acute appendicitis
5. Afferent loop syndrome
6. Mesenteric infarction
C. TRAUMA
1. Burns
2. Cerebral trauma
3. Postoperative
D. OBSTETRICAL
1. Pregnancy
2. Ectopic
E. RENAL
1. Transplantation
2. Renal insufficiency
F. METABOLIC
1. Diabetic ketoacidosis
2. Drugs
G. PNEUMONIA
H. SALIVARY GLAND LESION
1. Facial trauma

BILE DUCTS
Obstructive jaundice in adult
Etiology:
A. BENIGN DISEASE (76%)
1. Traumatic / operative stricture (44%)
2. Calculi (21%)
3. Pancreatitis (8%)
4. Sclerosing cholangitis (1%)
5. Recurrent pyogenic cholangitis
6. Parasitic disease (ascariasis)
7. Liver cysts
8. Aortic aneurysm
B. MALIGNANCY (24%)
1. Pancreatic carcinoma (18%)
2. Ampullary / duodenal carcinoma (8%)
3. Cholangiocarcinoma (3%)
4. Metastatic disease (2%)
from stomach, pancreas, lung, breast, colon, lymphoma

INCIDENCE OF INFECTED BILE IN BILE DUCT OBSTRUCTION
(a) incomplete / partial obstruction in 64%
(b) complete obstruction in 10%
Δ infection twice as high with biliary calculi than with malignant obstruction
Organisms: E. coli (21%), Klebsiella (21%), Enterococci (18%), Proteus (15%)

TEST SENSITIVITY OF COMMON BILE DUCT OBSTRUCTION
1. Intravenous cholangiography
depends on level of bilirubin: < 1 mg/dl in 92%; < 2 mg/dl in 82%; < 3 mg/dl in 40%; > 4 mg/dl in < 10%
False negative rate: 45%
Cx: adverse reactions in 4 – 10%
2. US
88 – 90% sensitivity with dilatation of CBD
Δ in 27 – 95% correct level of obstruction determined by US
Δ in 23 – 81% correct cause of obstruction determined by US
False-negative: not dilated in acute obstruction (in 70%), sclerosing cholangitis, intermittent obstruction from choledocholithiasis
√ "double channels" = dilated intrahepatic bile ducts
√ "Swiss cheese sign" = abundance of fluid-filled structures in liver sections
3. CT
100% visualization in tumerous obstruction, 60% in non-tumerous obstruction
4. NUC
√ delayed / nonvisualization of biliary system (93% specificity)
√ vicarious excretion of tracer through kidneys

Neonatal obstructive jaundice
= severe persistent jaundice in a child beyond 3 – 4 weeks of age
Causes:
A. INFECTION
(a) bacterial: E. coli, Syphilis, Listeria monocytogenes
(b) viral: TORCH, Hepatitis B, Coxsackie, Echovirus, Adenovirus
B. METABOLIC
(a) inherited: Alpha 1-antitrypsin deficiency, Cystic fibrosis, Galactosemia, Hereditary tyrosinemia
(b) acquired: Inspissated bile syndrome (= cholestasis due to erythroblastosis); Cholestasis due to total parenteral nutrition
C. BILIARY TRACT ABNORMALITIES
(a) extrahepatic: Biliary obstruction / hypoplasia / atresia, Choledochal cyst, Spontaneous perforation of bile duct, "Bile plug" syndrome

(b) intrahepatic: Ductular hypoplasia / atresia
D.   IDIOPATHIC NEONATAL HEPATITIS
mnemonic: "CAN"
   Choledochal cyst
   Atresia
   Neonatal hepatitis

NUC – imaging regimen:
   (1) premedication with phenobarbital (5 mg/kg/day) over 5 days to induce hepatic microsomal enzymes which enhance uptake and excretion of certain compounds and increase bile flow
   (2) IDA scintigraphy (50 mµCi/kg; minimum of 1 mCi)
   (3) Imaging at 5 minute intervals for 1 hour + at 2, 4, 6, 8, 24 hours

Large nonobstructed CBD
   1. passage of stone (return to normal after days to weeks)
   2. common duct surgery (return to normal in 30 – 50 days)
   3. post-cholecystectomy dilatation (in up to 16%)
   4. intestinal hypomotility
   5. normal variant (aging)
   Fatty-meal sonography (to differentiate from obstruction)
   Method: peroral Lipomul (1.5 ml/kg) followed by 100 ml of water [cholecystokinin causes contraction of gallbladder, relaxation of sphincter of Oddi, increase in bile secretion], CBD measured before and 45 / 60 minutes after stimulation
   √   little change / decrease in size = normal response
   √   increase in size > 2 mm = partial obstruction

Filling defects in bile ducts
   A.   ARTIFACTS
      1. Pseudocalculus = contracted sphincter of Boyden + Oddi with smooth arcuate contour
      2. Air bubble: confirmed by positional changes
      3. Blood clot: spheroid configuration, spontaneous resolution with time
   B.   BILIARY CALCULI
   C.   MIRIZZI SYNDROME
   D.   NEOPLASM
      1. Cholangiocarcinoma: irregular stricture, intraluminal polypoid mass
      2. Others: ampullary carcinoma, hepatoma, villous tumor, hamartoma, carcinoid, adenoma, papilloma, fibroma, lipoma, neuroma, cystadenoma, granular cell myoblastoma, sarcoma botryoides
   E.   PARASITES
      1. Ascaris lumbricoides: long linear filling defect / discrete mass if coiled
      2. Liver flukes (clonorchis sinensis, fasciola hepatica): intrahepatic epithelial hyperplasia, periductal fibrosis, cholangitis, liver abscess, hepatic duct stones, common duct obstruction

   3. Hydatid cyst: after erosion into biliary tree

Gas in biliary tree
   mnemonic: "SITS"
   Stone
   Inflammation (emphysematous cholecystitis)
   Tumor with fistula
   Surgery

Bile duct narrowing
   A.   BENIGN STRICTURE (44%)
      (a) Inflammation
         1. Sclerosing cholangitis
         2. Recurrent pyogenic cholangitis
         3. Acute / chronic pancreatitis
         4. Pancreatic pseudocyst
         5. Perforated duodenal ulcer
         6. Erosion by biliary calculi
         7. Gallstones + cholecystitis
         8. Abscess
         9. Radiation therapy
         10. Papillary stenosis
      (b) Congenital
         1. Choledochal cyst
      (c) Trauma
         1. Postoperative stricture (99%)
         2. Blunt / penetrating trauma
         3. Hepatic artery embolization
         4. Infusion of chemotherapeutic agents
   B.   MALIGNANT STRICTURE
      1. Pancreatic carcinoma
      2. Ampullary carcinoma
      3. Cholangiocarcinoma
      4. Compression by enlarged lymph node

Congenital cystic dilatation of bile ducts
   1. Choledochal cyst (87%)
   2. Choledochocele (6%)
   3. Choledochal diverticulum (3%)
   4. Caroli disease
   5. Multiple hepatic cysts

   TYPE A = anomalous pancreaticobiliary duct system causing cystic dilatation of CBD, involving papilla of Vater = CHOLEDOCHAL CYST (most common type)
   TYPE B = true diverticulum of CBD
   TYPE C = true diverticulum of hepatic duct
   TYPE D = CHOLEDOCHOCELE = intraduodenal portion of CBD analogous to ureterocele

   Classification of Biliary Tree Anomalies:
   I.   Common bile duct
      A.   Choledochal cyst
      B.   Segmental dilatation
      C.   Diffuse dilatation
   II.   Diverticulum of extrahepatic ducts
   III.   Choledochocele

IV. Multiple cysts
   A. in intra- and extrahepatic ducts
   B. in extrahepatic ducts
V. Intrahepatic cysts

Nonvisualization of gallbladder on OCG
Peak opacification of gallbladder: 14 – 19 hours (13 – 35% of dose excreted in urine)

A. EXTRABILIARY CAUSES
   1. Failure to ingest contrast
   2. Fasting
   3. Failure to reach absorptive surface of bowel
      (a) vomiting, nasogastric suction
      (b) esophageal / gastric obstruction
      (c) hiatal, umbilical, inguinal hernias
      (d) Zenker, epiphrenic, gastric, duodenal, jejunal diverticula
      (e) gastric ulcer, gastrocolic fistula
      (f) malabsorption, diarrhea
      (g) postoperative ileus, severe trauma
      (h) inflammation: acute pancreatitis, acute peritonitis
   4. Deficiency of bile salts
      Crohn disease, surgical resection of terminal ileum, liver disease, cholestyramine therapy, abnormal communication between biliary system and gastrointestinal tract
B. INTRINSIC GALLBLADDER DISEASE
   1. Cholecystectomy
   2. Anomalous position
   3. Obstruction of cystic duct
   4. Chronic cholecystitis

ORAL CHOLECYSTOGRAM (OCG)
Dose: 6 x 0.5 g tablets 2 hours after evening meal
A. PATIENT SELECTION
   • bilirubin < 5 mg% (not necessary if due to hemolysis)
   • contraindicated in serious liver disease
   • relative contraindications in peritonitis, postoperative ileus, acute pancreatitis
B. TOXICITY
   1. Nausea + vomiting (also noted in 29% on placebo)
   2. Immediate anaphylactic response
   3. Delayed hypotensive reaction (increased risk in cirrhosis)
   4. Renal failure
   5. Precipitation of hyperthyroidism

High density bile
1. Hemorrhagic cholecystitis
2. Hemobilia
3. Prior contrast administration
   (a) vicarious excretion of urographic agent
   (b) cholecystopaque
4. Milk of calcium bile

Displaced gallbladder
A. NORMAL IMPRESSION
   by duodenum / colon, (positional change)
B. HEPATIC MASSES
   Hepatoma, Hemangioma, Regenerating nodule, Metastases, Intrahepatic cyst, Polycystic liver, Hydatid disease, Hepar lobatum (tertiary syphylis), Granuloma, Abscess
C. EXTRAHEPATIC MASSES
   1. Retroperitoneal tumors (renal, adrenal)
   2. Polycystic kidney
   3. Lymphoma
   4. Lymph node metastases to porta hepatis
   5. Pancreatic pseudocyst

Alterations in gallbladder size
A. ENLARGED GALLBLADDER
   = CHOLECYSTOMEGALY
   (a) OBSTRUCTION
      1. Cystic duct obstruction (40%)
         (a) Hydrops: chronic cystic duct obstruction + distension with clear sterile mucus (white bile)
         (b) Empyema: acute / chronic obstruction with superinfection of bile
      2. Cholelithiasis causing obstruction (37%)
      3. Cholecystitis with cholelithiasis (11%)
      4. Courvoisier phenomenon (10%) = secondary to neoplastic process in pancreas / duodenal papilla / ampulla of Vater / common bile duct
      5. Pancreatitis
   (b) UNOBSTRUCTED (mostly neuropathic)
      1. S/P vagotomy
      2. Diabetes mellitus
      3. Alcoholism
      4. Appendicitis (in children)
      5. Narcotic analgesia
      6. WDHA syndrome
      7. Hyperalimentation
      8. Acromegaly
      9. Kawasaki syndrome
      10. Anticholinergics
      11. bedridden patient with prolonged illness
      12. AIDS (in 18%)
   (c) NORMAL (2%)
B. SMALL GALLBLADDER
   1. Chronic cholecystitis
   2. Cystic fibrosis: in 30 – 50% of patients
   3. Congenital hypoplasia / multiseptate gallbladder

Focal gallbladder wall thickening
A. METABOLIC
   1. Metachromatic sulfatides
   2. Hyperplastic cholecystoses
B. BENIGN TUMORS
   1. Adenoma: glandular elements (0.2%)
   2. Papilloma: fingerlike projections (0.2%)
   3. Fibroadenoma

4. Cystadenoma: ? premalignant
5. Neurinoma, Hemangioma
6. Carcinoid tumor
C. MALIGNANT TUMORS
 1. Carcinoma of gallbladder: adenocarcinoma /
  squamous cell carcinoma
 2. Leiomyosarcoma
 3. Metastases: from malignant melanoma (15%),
  lung, kidney, esophagus
D. INFLAMMATION / INFECTION
 1. Inflammatory polyp: in chronic cholecystitis
 2. Parasitic granuloma: ascaris lumbricoides,
  paragonimus westermanii, clonorchis, filariasis,
  schistosoma, fasciola
 3. Intramural epithelial cyst / mucinous retention cyst
 4. Xanthogranulomatous cholecystitis
E. WALL-ADHERENT GALLSTONE = embedded
 calculus
F. HETEROTOPIC MUCOSA
 1. Ectopic pancreatic tissue
 2. Ectopic gastric glands
 3. Ectopic intestinal glands
 4. Ectopic hepatic tissue
 5. Ectopic prostatic tissue

FIXED FILLING DEFECTS IN GALLBLADDER
 mnemonic: "PANTS"
 Polyp
 Adenomyosis
 Neurinoma
 Tumor, primary / secondary
 Stone, wall-adherent

Diffuse gallbladder wall thickening
= anterior wall of gallbladder > 3 mm
A. INTRINSIC
 1. Acute cholecystitis
 2. Chronic cholecystitis (10 – 25%)
 3. Hyperplastic cholecystosis
 4. GB perforation
 5. Sepsis
 6. Gallbladder carcinoma
 7. AIDS (average of 9 mm in up to 55%)
B. EXTRINSIC
 1. Hepatitis (in 80%)
 2. Hypoalbuminemia
 3. Renal failure
 4. Right heart failure
 5. Ascites
 6. Multiple myeloma
 7. Portal node lymphatic obstruction
 8. Cirrhosis
 9. Acute myelogenous leukemia
 10. Brucellosis
 11. Graft-versus-host disease
 12. Systemic venous hypertension
C. PHYSIOLOGIC
 = contracted gallbladder after eating

SPLEEN
Splenomegaly
Normal size: (in children)
 Formula for length = 5.7 + 0.31 x age (in years)
Normal weight: 150 g

A. CONGESTIVE SPLENOMEGALY
 Heart failure, Portal hypertension, Cirrhosis, Cystic
 fibrosis, Portal / splenic vein thrombosis
B. NEOPLASM
 Leukemia, Lymphoma, Metastases, Primary
 neoplasm
C. STORAGE DISEASE
 Gaucher disease, Niemann-Pick disease,
 Amyloidosis, Diabetes mellitus, Histiocytosis,
 Hemochromatosis, Gargoylism
D. INFECTION
 Hepatitis, Malaria, Infectious mononucleosis,
 Leishmaniosis, Brucellosis, TB, Typhoid, Syphilis,
 Echinococcus
E. HEMOLYTIC ANEMIA
 Hemoglobinopathy, Hereditary spherocytosis, Primary
 neutropenia, Thrombotic thrombocytopenic Purpura
F. EXTRAMEDULLARY HEMATOPOIESIS
 Osteopetrosis, Myelofibrosis
G. COLLAGEN VASCULAR
 Systemic lupus erythematosus, Rheumatoid arthritis,
 Felty syndrome
H. TRAUMA
 Intrasplenic laceration / fracture, Subcapsular
 hematoma
I. OTHERS
 Sarcoidosis, Hemodialysis

Small spleen
1. Hereditary hypoplasia
2. Irradiation
3. Infarction
4. Polysplenia syndrome
5. Atrophy

Splenic calcifications
A. DISSEMINATED
 1. Phleboliths
 2. Granulomas: histoplasmosis, TB, brucellosis
B. CAPSULAR & PARENCHYMAL
 1. Pyogenic / tuberculous abscess
 2. Infarction (multiple)
 3. Hematoma
C. VASCULAR
 1. Splenic artery calcification
 2. Splenic artery aneurysm
 3. Splenic infarcts
D. CALCIFIED CYST WALL
 1. Congenital cyst
 2. Posttraumatic cyst
 3. Echinococcal cyst
 4. Cystic dermoid
 5. Epidermoid

E. GENERALIZED INCREASED DENSITY
    1. Sickle cell anemia (in 5% of sicklers)
    2. Hemochromatosis
    3. Thorotrast
    4. Lymphangiography

mnemonic: "HITCH"
    Histoplasmosis (most common)
    Infarcts (sickle cell)
    Tuberculosis
    Cyst (echinococcus)
    Hematoma

Cystic splenic lesions
A. CONGENITAL
    1. Epidermoid cyst = Epithelial cyst = Primary cyst
B. VASCULAR
    1. Splenic laceration / fracture
    2. Hematoma
    3. Posttraumatic cyst
    4. Cystic degeneration of infarct (embolic / local thrombosis)
C. INFECTION / INFLAMMATION
    1. Abscess: incidence of 0.1 – 0.7%; sickle cell disease predisposes
    2. Parasitic cyst
    3. Pancreatic pseudocyst
D. CYSTIC NEOPLASM
    1. Cavernous hemangioma
        Most common benign splenic tumor; autopsy
        Incidence: 0.03 – 14%
        Age: 20 – 50 yrs.
    2. Lymphangiomatosis
    3. Necrotic metastasis

Solid splenic lesions
A. MALIGNANT TUMOR
    1. Metastases (7%)
        melanoma (34%), breast carcinoma (12%), bronchogenic carcinoma (9%), colon carcinoma (4%), renal cell carcinoma (3%), ovary, prostate, stomach, pancreas, endometrium
    2. Lymphoma (Hodgkin disease, Non-Hodgkin lymphoma)
        Spleen involved in 70%
        √ splenomegaly (from diffuse infiltration)
        √ miliary nodules
        √ large 2 – 10 cm nodules (10 – 25%)
        √ nodes in splenic hilum (50%) in NHL; uncommon in Hodgkin disease
    3. Angiosarcoma
        May be associated with liver angiosarcoma
        Age: 50 – 60 years; poor survival rate
B. BENIGN TUMOR
    1. Hamartoma = SPLENOMA
    2. Hemangioma
    3. Hematopoietic
    4. Sarcoidosis
C. SPLENIC INFARCTION

ANATOMY OF LIVER AND BILE DUCTS

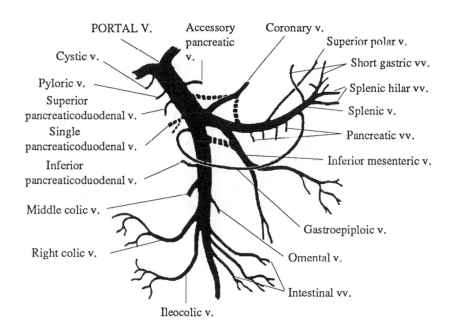

PORTAL V.
Accessory pancreatic v.
Coronary v.
Cystic v.
Superior polar v.
Pyloric v.
Short gastric vv.
Superior pancreaticoduodenal v.
Splenic hilar vv.
Single pancreaticoduodenal v.
Splenic v.
Inferior pancreaticoduodenal v.
Pancreatic vv.
Middle colic v.
Inferior mesenteric v.
Right colic v.
Gastroepiploic v.
Omental v.
Intestinal vv.
Ileocolic v.

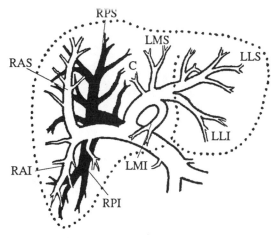

RAI	= right anterior inferior
RAS	= right anterior superior
RPS	= right posterior superior
RPI	= right posterior inferior
C	= caudate lobe
LMI	= left median inferior
LMS	= left median superior
LLS	= left lateral superior
LLI	= left lateral inferior

Normal size of bile ducts
- @ CBD at point of maximum diameter:
  ≤ 5 mm = normal; 6 – 7 mm = equivocal;
  ≥ 8 mm = dilated
- @ CHD at porta hepatis + CBD in head of pancreas:
  5 mm
- @ right intrahepatic duct just proximal to CHD:
  2 – 3 mm
- @ Cystic duct diameter: 1.8 mm
  average length of 1 – 2 cm
  distal cystic duct posterior to CBD (in 95%),
  anterior to CBD (in 5%)

Biliary tract anomalies
Incidence: 2.4% of autopsies;
in 5 – 13% of operative cholangiograms
1. ABERRANT INTRAHEPATIC DUCT
   may join CHD, CBD, cystic duct, right hepatic duct, gallbladder
   Cx: postoperative bile leak if severed
2. CYSTIC DUCT ENTERING RIGHT HEPATIC DUCT
3. DUPLICATION OF CYSTIC DUCT / CBD
4. CONGENITAL TRACHEOBILIARY FISTULA
   = fistulous communication between carina and left hepatic duct
   • infants with respiratory distress
   • productive cough with bilious sputum
   √ pneumobilia

Gallbladder

Size: 7 – 10 cm in length; 2 – 3.5 cm in width
Capacity: 30 – 50 ml
Wall thickness: 2 – 3 mm

Congenital gallbladder anomalies

Hypoplastic Gallbladder
(a) congenital
(b) associated with cystic fibrosis

Agenesis of Gallbladder
Incidence: 0.04 - 0.07 % (autopsy)
Associated with:
Δ (common): Rectovaginal fistula, Imperforate anus, Hypoplasia of scapula + radius, Intracardiac shunt
Δ (rare): Absence of corpus callosum, Microcephaly, Atresia of external auditory canal, Tricuspid atresia, TE fistula, Dextroposition of pancreas + esophagus, Absent spleen, High position of cecum, Polycystic kidney

Septations of Gallbladder
A. LONGITUDINAL SEPTA
1. Duplication of gallbladder
    Incidence: 1:3000 to 1:12000
    = two separate lumens + two cystic ducts
2. Bifid gallbladder = double gallbladder
    = two separate lumens with one cystic duct
3. Triple gallbladder (extremely rare)
B. TRANSVERSE SEPTA
1. Isolated transverse septum
2. PHRYGIAN CAP (2 – 6 % of population)
    = kinking / folding of fundus ± septum
3. Multiseptated gallbladder (rare)
    = multiple cyst-like compartments connected by small pores
    Cx: stasis + stone formation
C. GALLBLADDER DIVERTICULUM
    = persistence of cystohepatic duct

Gallbladder Ectopia
Most frequent locations:
(1) beneath the left lobe of the liver > (2) intrahepatic > (3) retrohepatic
Rare locations:
(4) within falciform ligament (5) within interlobar fissure (6) suprahepatic (lodged between superior surface of right hepatic lobe + anterior chest wall) (7) within anterior abdominal wall (8) transverse mesocolon (9) retrorenal (10) near posterior spine + IVC (11) intrathoracic GB (inversion of liver
Associated with   eventration of diaphragm
"Floating GB"
= gallbladder with loose peritoneal reflections, may herniate through foramen of Winslow into lesser sac
"Torqued GB"
= results in hydrops

DISEASE ENTITIES OF LIVER, BILIARY TRACT, PANCREAS, AND SPLEEN

ACCESSORY SPLEEN
= failure of coalescence of several small mesodermal buds in the dorsal mesogastrium which comprise the spleen
Incidence: 10 – 30% of population; multiple in 10%
Δ undergoes hypertrophy after splenectomy + is responsible for recurrence of hematologic disorders (idiopathic thrombocytopenic purpura, hereditary spherocytosis, acquired autoimmune hemolytic anemia, hypersplenism)
Location: splenic hilum (most common), gastrosplenic ligament, other suspensory ligaments of spleen, rare in pancreas / pelvis
NUC (Tc-99m sulfur colloid scan):
√ usually < 1 cm in diameter
√ < 10% identified when normal spleen present

ANNULAR PANCREAS
= uncommon congenital anomaly wherein a ring of normal pancreatic tissue encircles the duodenum secondary to abnormal migration of ventral pancreas (head + uncinate); most common congenital anomaly of pancreas
Age at discovery: childhood (50%); adulthood (50%)
Associated with other congenital anomalies (in 75%): Esophageal atresia; TE fistula; duodenal atresia / stenosis; duodenal diaphragm; imperforate anus; malrotation; Down syndrome
Location: 2nd portion of duodenum (85%); 1st / 3rd portion of duodenum (15%)
• neonate : persistent vomiting
• adult : nausea, vomiting (60%), abdominal pain (70%), hematemesis (10%), jaundice (50%)
√ polyhydramnios (in utero)
√ "double bubble" = dilated duodenal bulb + stomach
√ eccentric narrowing with lateral notching + medial retraction of duodenal sweep
√ reverse peristalsis, pyloric incompetency
√ enlargement of pancreatic head
√ pancreatic duct originates on anterior left + passes posteriorly around duodenum
√ periampullary ulcers

ASCARIASIS
Organism: Ascaris lumbricoides, 25 – 35 cm long as adult worm; life span of 1 year
Country: 644 million humans harbor the roundworm; 70 – 90% in America; in United States endemic in: Appalachian range, southern + Gulf coast states
Incidence: in blacks (12%), in whites (1%)
Cycle:
ingestion of contaminated soil / vegetable; larvae penetrate intestinal wall; migrate into mesenteric lymphatics + veins; reach lung via right heart +

pulmonary artery; mature in pulmonary capillary bed to 2 – 3 mm length; burrow into alveoli; ascend in respiratory tract; are swallowed and remain in GI tract
Cx: (1) Intestinal obstruction
(2) Intermittent biliary obstruction
(3) Liver abscess (rare)
(4) Granulomatous stricture of extrahepatic bile ducts (rare)
√ barium study
√ cholangiography (49%)
√ plain film

BILIARY CYSTADENOMA
= BILE DUCT CYSTADENOMA
= rare benign tumor resembling mucinous cystic neoplasms of the pancreas; < 5% of all intrahepatic cysts of bile duct origin
Age: > 30 years (82%); M:F = 1:4
Histo: single layer of biliary-type epithelium with papillary projections, subepithelial stroma resembles that of the ovary
Location: intrahepatic bile ducts (85%); extrahepatic bile ducts (15%); right lobe (50%); both lobes (30%); left lobe (20%)
√ mass of 1.5 – 30 cm in size
√ papillary excrescences + mural nodules
US: √ ovoid complex mass with irregular margins + single / multiple septations
√ may contain fluid-fluid levels
CT: √ multiloculated mass of near water density with septations
Angio:√ avascular mass with small clusters of peripheral abnormal vessels
√ stretching + displacement of vessels
√ thin subtle blush of neovascularity in septa + wall
Aspirated fluid: mucinous, serous, containing hemosiderin / cholesterol / necrosis
Cx: malignant transformation into cystadenocarcinoma
DDx: Echinococcal cyst, Necrotic hepatic metastasis, Cystic hamartoma, Hepatic abscess

BILIARY-ENTERIC FISTULA
Incidence: 5% at cholecystectomy; 0.5% at autopsy
Etiology:
cholelithiasis (90%), acute / chronic cholecystitis, biliary tract carcinoma, regional invasive neoplasm, diverticulitis, inflammatory bowel disease, peptic ulcer disease, echinococcal cyst, trauma, congenital communication
Communication with:
duodenum (70%), colon (26%), stomach (4%), jejunum, ileum, hepatic artery, portal vein (caused death of Ignatius Loyola), bronchial tree, pericardium, renal pelvis, ureter, urinary bladder, vagina, ovary

A. CHOLECYSTODUODENAL FISTULA (51 – 70%)
1. Perforated gallstone (90%):
associated with gallstone Ileus in 20%
2. Perforated duodenal ulcer (10%)
3. Surgical anastomosis
4. Gallbladder carcinoma
B. CHOLECYSTOCOLIC FISTULA (13 – 21%)
C. CHOLEDOCHODUODENAL FISTULA (13 – 19%)
due to perforated duodenal ulcer disease
D. MULTIPLE FISTULAE (7%)

√ branching tubular radiolucencies, more prominent centrally
√ barium filling of biliary tree
√ multiple hyperechoic foci with dirty shadowing
DDx: Patulous sphincter of Oddi, Ascending cholangitis, Surgery (choledochoduodenostomy, cholecystojejunostomy, sphincterotomy)

BUDD-CHIARI SYNDROME
= global / segmental obstruction of hepatic venous outflow
Causes:
A. IDIOPATHIC (66%)
B. THROMBOSIS
(a) Hypercoagulable state: (1) Polycythemia rubra vera (1/3) (2) Oral contraceptives (3) Pregnancy + postpartum state (4) Paroxysmal nocturnal hemoglobulinuria (successive thrombosis of small veins)
(b) Injury to vessel wall: (1) Phlebitis (2) Tumor compression (liver, kidney, adrenal)
B. NONTHROMBOTIC OCCLUSION
(a) Tumor growth into IVC / hepatic veins (renal cell carcinoma, hepatoma, adrenal carcinoma, metastasis)
(b) IVC membrane / diaphragm (= congenital web), common cause in Oriental + Indian population
(c) Right atrial tumor
(d) Constrictive pericarditis
(e) Right heart failure
M < F
• insidious onset of intractable ascites
• abdominal pain (liver congestion)
• hepatomegaly without derangement of liver function
Location:
Type I : occlusion of IVC ± hepatic veins
Type II : occlusion of major hepatic veins ± IVC
Type III: occlusion of small centrilobar veins

ACUTE STAGE
√ globally enlarged liver
√ NECT: diffuse hypodensity
√ CECT: central patchy enhanced areas with poor peripheral enhancement, hypodense lumina of hepatic veins

CHRONIC STAGE
√ nonvisualization of hepatic veins (75%)

√ enlargement + hypodensity of hepatic veins (18%)
√ enlargement of caudate lobe (88%)
√ hypodensity in atrophic areas / periphery (82%) with inversion of portal blood flow
√ patchy enhancement (85%) with normal portal blood flow
√ ascites (97%)
CT:
√ enhancement of enlarged caudate lobe
√ infarcted hypodense nonenhancing regions
US:
√ enlargement of caudate lobe + atrophy of rest of liver
√ hepatic veins nonvisualized / reduced in size / filled with thrombus
NUC:
√ central region of normal activity (hot caudate lobe) surrounded by greatly diminished activity (venous drainage of hypertrophied caudate lobe into IVC)
√ colloid shift to spleen + bone marrow
√ wedge-shaped focal peripheral defects
Angio:
√ absence of main hepatic veins
√ spider weblike appearance of collaterals + small hepatic veins
√ stretching + draping of intrahepatic arteries with hepatomegaly
√ inhomogeneous prolonged intense hepatogram with fine mottling
√ large lakes of sinusoidal contrast accumulation
√ bidirectional / hepatofugal portal vein flow

CANDIDIASIS OF LIVER
= almost exclusively seen in immunocompromised patients (leukemia, chronic granulomatous disease of childhood, renal transplant, chemotherapy for myeloproliferative disorders)
√ hepatomegaly
US: √ "target" / "bull's eye" sign = multiple small hypoechoic masses with echogenic centers
NUC: √ uniform uptake / focal photopenic areas
√ diminished Ga-67 uptake
DDx: Metastases, Lymphoma, Leukemia, Septic emboli

CAROLI DISEASE
= COMMUNICATING CAVERNOUS ECTASIA OF INTRAHEPATIC DUCTS
= segmental saccular cystic dilatation of major intrahepatic bile ducts
Etiology: (a) ? perinatal hepatic artery occlusion; may be autosomal recessive
(b) ? hypoplasia / aplasia of fibromuscular wall components
Age: childhood + 2nd – 3rd decade, occasionally in infancy; M:F = 1:1
Associated with: Medullary sponge kidney (in 80%), Infantile polycystic kidney disease, Renal tubular ectasia, Choledochal cyst (rare), Congenital hepatic fibrosis

- recurrent cramplike abdominal pain
- NO cirrhosis / portal hypertension
- √ multiple cystic structures converging toward porta hepatis as either localized / diffusely scattered cysts communicating with bile ducts
- √ segmental saccular / beaded appearance of intrahepatic bile ducts extending to periphery of liver
- √ frequent ectasia of extrahepatic ducts + CBD
- √ sludge / calculi in dilated ducts
- *Cx:* (1) Bile stasis with recurrent cholangitis (2) Biliary calculi (3) Liver abscess (4) Septicemia (5) Increased risk for cholangiocarcinoma

CHOLANGIOCARCINOMA

Intrahepatic Cholangiocarcinoma

= CHOLANGIOCELLULAR CARCINOMA
Incidence: 1/3 of all malignancies originating in the liver; 8 – 13% of all cholangiocarcinomas; 2nd most common primary hepatic tumor after hepatoma

Types:
(1) Massive / nodular type
(2) Diffuse (sclerosing cholangitis) type
Δ cannot be depicted by crosssectional imaging (CT / US)
- abdominal pain (47%)
- palpable mass (18%)
- weight loss (18%)
- jaundice (12%)
Spread: (1) local extension along duct (2) local infiltration of liver substance (3) metastatic spread to regional lymph nodes (in 15%)
- √ size of mass 5 – 20 cm in diameter
- √ satellite nodules in 65%
- √ punctate / chunky calcifications in 18%
- √ calculi in biliary tree
NUC:
- √ cold lesion on sulfur colloid / IDA scans
- √ segmental biliary obstruction
- √ may show uptake on gallium scan
US:
- √ dilated biliary tree
- √ predominantly homo- / heterogeneous mass
- √ hyper- (75%) / iso- / hypoechoic (14%) mass
CT:
- √ single predominantly homogeneous round/oval hypodense mass with irregular borders
- √ no / peripheral / central enhancement
Angiography:
- √ avascular / hypo- / hypervascular mass
- √ stretched / encased arteries
- √ neovascularity in 50%
- √ lack of venous invasion
Prognosis: < 20% resectable; 30% 5-year survival

Extrahepatic Cholangiocarcinoma

= BILE DUCT CARCINOMA
Age peak: 6 – 7th decade, M:F = 3:2

Incidence: < 0.5% of autopsies; 90% of all cholangiocarcinomas; more frequent in Far East
Histo: well-differentiated sclerosing adenocarcinoma (2/3), anaplastic carcinoma (11%), cystadenocarcinoma, adenoacanthoma, malignant adenoma, squamous cell = epidermoid carcinoma, leiomyosarcoma
Predisposed:
(1) Inflammatory bowel disease (10 x increased risk); incidence of 0.4 – 1.4% in ulcerative colitis; latent period of 15 years; tumors usually multicentric + predominantly in extrahepatic sites; GB involved in 15% (simultaneous presence of gallstones is rare)
(2) Sclerosing cholangitis (10%)
(3) Caroli disease
(4) Clonorchis sinensis infestation (Far East); most common cause worldwide
(5) Thorotrast exposure
(6) history of other malignancy (10%)
(7) Previous surgery for choledochal cyst / congenital biliary atresia
(8) Alpha-1-antitrypsin deficiency
(9) Cholecystolithiasis (20 – 50%), probably coincidental
(10) Papillomatosis of bile ducts
- gradual onset of fluctuating painless jaundice
- cholangitis (10%)
- weight loss, fatigability
- intermittent epigastric pain
- elevated bilirubin + alkaline phosphatase
- enlarged tender liver
Growth pattern:
(1) Obstructive Type (70 – 85%)
√ U- / V-shaped obstruction with nipple, rattail, smooth/irregular termination
(2) Stenotic Type (10 – 25%)
√ strictured rigid lumen with irregular margins + prestenotic dilatation
(3) Polypoid / papillary Type (5 – 6%)
√ intraluminal filling defect with irregular margins
Spread:
(a) lymphatic spread: cystic + CBD nodes (> 32%), celiac nodes (> 16%), peripancreatic nodes, superior mesenteric nodes
(b) infiltration of liver (23%)
(c) peritoneal seeding (9%)
(d) hematogenous (extremely rare): liver, peritoneum, lung
Location:

left / right hepatic duct	in 8 – 13%
confluence of hepatic ducts (Klatskin tumor)	in 10 – 26%
common hepatic duct	in 14 – 37%
proximal CBD	in 15 – 30%
distal CBD	in 30 – 50%
cystic duct	in 6%

UGI:
√ infiltration / indentation of stomach / duodenum
Cholangiography (PTC or ERC best modality to depict
bile duct neoplasm):
√ exophytic intraductal tumor mass (46%), 2 – 5 mm
in diameter
√ frequently long / rarely short concentric focal
stricture in infiltrating sclerosing cholangitic type
with wall irregularities
√ prestenotic diffuse / focal biliary dilatation (100%)
√ progression of ductal strictures (100%)
US / CT:
√ mass within / surrounding the ducts at point of
obstruction
√ dilatation of intrahepatic ducts without extrahepatic
duct dilatation
√ failure to demonstrate the confluence of L + R
hepatic ducts
√ small low-density mass
Angiography:
√ hypervascular tumor with neovascularity (50%)
√ arterioarterial collaterals along the course of bile
ducts associated with arterial obstruction
√ poor / absent tumor stain
√ displacement / encasement / occlusion of hepatic
artery + portal vein
Cx: (1) Obstruction (biliary cirrhosis, intrahepatic
abscess)
(2) Hepatomegaly
(3) Intrahepatic abscess (subdiaphragmatic,
perihepatic, septicemia)
(4) Biliary peritonitis
Prognosis: median survival of 5 months; 1.6% 5-year
survival; 39% 5-year survival for
carcinoma of papilla of Vater
DDx: Benign stricture, Chronic pancreatitis, Sclerosing
cholangitis, Edematous papilla, Idiopathic
inflammation of CBD

CHOLANGITIS
Acute Cholangitis
Causes:
A. Benign disease:
(1) Stricture from prior surgery (36%) (2) Calculi
(30%) (3) Sclerosing cholangitis (4) Obstructed
drainage catheter (5) Parasitic infestation
B. Malignant disease: Ampullary carcinoma

Types:
1. ACUTE NONSUPPURATIVE ASCENDING
CHOLANGITIS
• bile remains clear
• patient nontoxic
2. ACUTE SUPPURATIVE ASCENDING
COLANGITIS (14%)
Associated with   obstructing biliary stone or
malignancy

• septicemia, CNS depression, lethargy, mental
confusion, shock (50%)
√ purulent material fills biliary ducts
Organisms: E. coli > Klebsiella > Pseudomonas >
Enterococci
• recurrent episodes of sepsis + RUQ pain
• Charcot triad (70%) : fever + chills + jaundice
• bile cultures for infection positive in 90%
Cx: miliary hepatic abscess formation
Prognosis: 100% mortality if not decompressed;
40 – 60% mortality with treatment; overall
mortality rate 13 – 16%

Recurrent Pyogenic Cholangitis
= PRIMARY CHOLANGITIS = RECURRENT
PYOGENIC HEPATITIS = ORIENTAL
CHOLANGIOHEPATITIS = ORIENTAL CHOLANGITIS
= HONG KONG DISEASE = INTRAHEPATIC PIGMENT
STONE DISEASE
Etiology: ? clonorchis infestation; endemic to
Indochina, South China, Taiwan, Japan,
Korea
Incidence: 3rd most common cause of an acute
abdomen in Hong Kong after appendicitis
and perforated ulcer
Age: 20 – 50 years; M:F = 1:1
• recurrent attacks of fever, chills, abdominal pain,
jaundice
Location: particularly in lateral segment of L lobe +
posterior segment of R lobe
√ marked dilatation of proximal intrahepatic ducts
(3 – 4 mm) in 100%
√ decreased arborization of intrahepatic radicles
√ intrahepatic bile ducts filled with pigment stones +
sludge (64%)
√ dilatation of CBD (68%) + choledocholithiasis (30%)
√ bile duct strictures (22%)
√ pneumobilia (3 – 52%)
√ segmental hepatic atrophy (36%)
Cx: Liver abscess (18%), Splenomegaly (14%),
Biloma (4%), Pancreatitis (4%)
DDx: complication of Caroli disease

Sclerosing Cholangitis
= insidious progressive disease affecting the intra- and
extrahepatic bile ducts
Histo: chronic obliterative fibrotic inflammation
(pericholangitis)
Age: < 45 years (2/3); range 21 – 67 years;
M:F = 2:1
• chronic / intermittent obstructive jaundice (most
frequent)
• history of previous biliary surgery (53%) + chronic /
recurrent pancreatitis (14%)
• fatigability, abdominal pain, pruritus
• fever (1/3)
Location:
1. CBD almost always involved

2. intra- and extrahepatic ducts (68 – 89%)
3. cystic duct involved in 18%
4. intrahepatic ducts only (1 – 25%)
5. extrahepatic ducts only (3%)
US:
  √ brightly echogenic portal triads
CT:
  √ dilatation, stenosis, pruning, beading of intrahepatic bile ducts (80%)
  √ dilatation, stenosis, wall nodularity, duct wall thickening, mural contrast enhancement of extrahepatic bile ducts (100%)
  √ hepatic metastases + lymph nodes in porta hepatis
Cholangiography:
  √ multifocal strictures with predilection for bifurcations + skip lesions (uninvolved duct segments of normal caliber)
  √ "pruned tree" appearance (= opacification of central ducts + diffuse obstruction of peripheral smaller radicles)
  √ "cobblestone" appearance (= coarse nodular mural irregularities) in 50%
  √ small saccular outpouchings (diverticula / pseudodiverticula) = PATHOGNOMONIC
  √ uncommonly "beaded appearance" (= alternating segments of dilatation + focal circumferential stenoses)
  √ new strictures + lengthening of strictures between 6 months and 6 years (< 20%)
  √ marked ductal dilatation (24%)
  √ polypoid mass (7%)
  √ gallbladder irregularities uncommon
NUC (Tc99m-IDA scan):
  √ multiple persistent focal areas of retention in distribution of intrahepatic biliary tree
  √ marked prolongation of hepatic clearance
  √ gallbladder visualized only in 70%
Cx: (1) Biliary cirrhosis
     (2) Portal hypertension
     (3) Cholangiocarcinoma (12%)
DDx:
  (1) Sclerosing cholangiocarcinoma (progressive cholangiographic changes within 0.5 – 1.5 years of initial diagnosis, marked ductal dilatation upstream from a dominant stricture, intraductal mass > 1 cm in diameter)
  (2) Acute ascending cholangitis (history)
  (3) Primary biliary cirrhosis (disease limited to intrahepatic ducts, strictures less pronounced, pruning + crowding of bile ducts, normal AMA titer)

Primary Sclerosing Cholangitis
Etiology: idiopathic, ? hypersensitivity reaction (speculative)
CRITERIA:
  (1) progressive jaundice of obstructive type
  (2) diffuse generalized involvement of extrahepatic ducts
  (3) exclusion of prior biliary tract surgery, gallstones, bile duct carcinoma
  (4) exclusion of primary biliary cirrhosis, Crohn disease, ulcerative colitis, retroperitoneal fibrosis, Riedel struma
Path: fibrosis + nonspecific inflammation with poorly defined aggregates of lymphocytes + plasma cells; sclerosing form resembles bile duct carcinoma

Secondary Sclerosing Cholangitis
Associated with:
  (1) Inflammatory bowel disease (ulcerative colitis in 66%, occasionally Crohn disease);
      Δ 1% of patients with inflammatory bowel disease develop sclerosing cholangitis
  (2) Cirrhosis, Chronic active hepatitis, Pericholangitis, Fatty degeneration
  (3) Pancreatitis
  (4) Retroperitoneal / mediastinal fibrosis
  (5) Peyronie disease
  (6) Riedel thyroiditis, hypothyroidism
  (7) Retroorbital pseudotumor
NO association with gallstones

CHOLECYSTITIS
Acute Cholecystitis
Etiology: (a) in 80 – 95% cystic duct obstruction by impacted calculus; 85% disimpact spontaneously
           (b) in 10% acalculous cholecystitis
Pathogenesis: chemical irritation from concentrated bile, bacterial infection, reflux of pancreatic secretions
Age peak: 5 – 6th decade; M:F = 1:3
• Murphy sign = inspiratory arrest upon palpation of GB area (falsely positive in 6% of patients with cholelithiasis)
Oral cholecystography:
  √ nonvisualization / poor visualization of gallbladder
US (sensitivity 85 – 95%, specificity 64 – 100%):
  √ GB wall thickening > 3 mm (mean 9 mm)
  √ hazy delineation of GB wall
  √ "halo sign" = GB wall lucency (in 70%) = 3-layered configuration with sonolucent middle layer
  √ striated wall thickening (62%) = several alternating irregular discontinuous lucent + echogenic bands within GB wall (positive predictive value of 100%)
  √ GB hydrops = distension with AP diameter > 5 cm
  √ sonographic Murphy sign in 85% (sensitivity 63%, specificity 93%)
  √ pericholecystic fluid
  √ presence of pseudomembranes
  √ coarse nonshadowing nondependent echodensities

NUC (sensitivity 95 – 97%, specificity 74 – 94%, accuracy 95%):
√ visualization of biliary tract + bowel
√ nonvisualization of GB during 1st hour (in 83%)
√ nonvisualization of GB + CBD (in 13%)
√ increased activity in GB fossa conforming to inferior hepatic edge (= sign of gangrenous / perforated GB in 75%)
False-positive scans (10 – 12%): Congenital absence of GB, Carcinoma of GB, Chronic cholecystitis, Biliary pancreatitis, Alcoholic liver disease, Hepatocellular disease, Severe intercurrent illness, Hyperalimentation, Prolonged fasting, Inadequate fasting < 4 – 6 hours prior to study
Reduction to 2% false-positive scans through:
(1) delayed images at 4 hours
(2) cholecystokinin injection 15 minutes prior to study
(3) morphine IV at 40 minutes + reimaging after 20 minutes (contraction of sphincter of Oddi)
False-negative scan: Dilated cystic duct
Cx:
(1) Gangrene of gallbladder
√ shaggy, irregular, asymmetric wall (mucosal ulcers, intraluminal hemorrhage, necrosis)
√ hyperechoic foci within GB wall (microabscesses in Rokitansky-Aschoff sinuses)
√ intraluminal membranes (gangrene)
(2) Perforation of gallbladder (in 5 – 10%)
Location: most commonly in fundus
√ gallstone lying free in peritoneal cavity
√ sonolucent / complex collection surrounding GB
(3) Empyema of gallbladder
√ multiple medium / coarse highly reflective intraluminal echoes without shadowing / layering / gravity dependence (purulent exudate / debris)

Chronic Cholecystitis
Most common form of gallbladder inflammation
√ gallstones
√ smooth / irregular GB wall thickening (mean of 5 mm)
√ mean volume of 42 ml
NUC:
√ normal GB visualization in majority of patients
√ delayed GB visualization
√ absent GB visualization by 4 hours (99% specificity)
√ visualization of bowel prior to GB (sensitivity 45%, specificity 90%)
√ noncontractility / decreased response after CCK injection

Acalculous Cholecystitis
Frequency: 5 – 10%
Etiology: (probably caused by decreased blood flow through cystic artery)

(1) depressed motility / starvation in trauma, burns, surgery, total parenteral nutrition, anesthesia, mechanical ventilation, narcotics, shock, congestive heart failure, arteriosclerosis, polyarteritis nodosa, SLE, diabetes mellitus
(2) obstruction of cystic duct by extrinsic inflammation, lymphadenopathy, metastases
(3) infection from Salmonella, Cholera, Kawasaki syndrome

Emphysematous Cholecystitis
Age: > 50 years;   M:F = 5:1
Predisposed: diabetics (22 – 50%)
Etiology: ? calculous / acalculous cystic duct obstruction with inflammatory edema resulting in cystic artery occlusion
Organism: clostridium perfringens, clostridium Welchii, E. coli, staphylococcus, streptococcus
• WBC count may be normal (1/3)
• point tenderness rare (diabetic neuropathy)
Plain film: (gas appears 24 – 48 hours after onset of symptoms)
√ air-fluid level in GB lumen, air in GB wall within 24 – 48 hours after acute episode
√ pneumobilia (rare)
US: √ high-level echoes outlining GB wall
Cx: gangrene (75%); perforation (20%)
Mortality: 15%
DDx: 1. Enteric fistula
2. Incompetent sphincter of Oddi
3. Air-containing periduodenal abscess
4. Periappendiceal abscess in malpositioned appendix
5. Lipomatosis of gallbladder

CHOLEDOCHAL CYST
= CYSTIC DILATATION OF EXTRAHEPATIC BILE DUCT
= segmental aneurysmal dilatation of common bile duct; most common congenital lesion of bile ducts
Etiology: anomalous junction of pancreatic duct and CBD proximal to duodenal papilla, higher pressure in pancreatic duct and absent ductal sphincter allows free reflux of enzymes into CBD resulting in weakening of CBD wall

Kimura Type I = pancreatic duct enters the proximal / mid CBD
Kimura Type II = CBD drains into pancreatic duct
Incidence: 0.2 – 0.5:1,000,000; high incidence in Japanese
Age: < 10 years (50%) + young adulthood, (occasionally up to 7th decade); M:F = 1:3
Histo: fibrous cyst wall without epithelial lining
Associated with:
(1) dilatation, stenosis or atresia of other portions of the biliary tree (2%)
(2) gallbladder anomaly (aplasia, double GB)

  (3) failure of union of left + right hepatic ducts
  (4) pancreatic duct + accessory hepatic bile ducts may drain into cyst
  (5) congenital hepatic fibrosis
  (6) polycystic liver disease
  (7) gallbladder carcinoma, bile duct carcinoma (increasing with age, up to 40% in adulthood)

Classic Triad (30%):
- intermittent jaundice (50%)
- recurrent RUQ colicky pain (> 75%), back pain
- intermittent palpable RUQ abdominal mass
- recurrent fever

Location: (a) extra- and intrahepatic ducts (73%)
         (b) dilatation of L + R main intrahepatic ducts (45%)
             — unilateral (42%) involving only left lobe
             — bilateral (58%)
         (c) extrahepatic ducts only (27%) (= below entry of cystic duct)

√ Size: diameter of 2 cm up to 15 cm (largest contained 13 liters)
√ abrupt change in caliber at site of cyst
√ rounded smooth extrinsic compression of CBD
√ NO / mild peripheral intrahepatic bile duct dilatation
√ may contain stones / sludge

US:
√ large fluid-filled structure beneath porta hepatis separate from gallbladder, communication with hepatic ducts need to be demonstrated
√ abrupt change of caliber at junction of dilated segment to normal ducts
√ intrahepatic bile duct dilatation (16%) secondary to stenosis

OB-US:
√ right-sided cyst in fetal abdomen + adjacent dilated hepatic ducts
    DDx: Duodenal atresia; Cyst of ovary, mesentery, omentum, pancreas, liver

NUC:
(excludes effectively DDx of hepatic cyst, pancreatic pseudocyst, enteric duplication, spontaneous loculated biloma)
√ late filling with stasis of tracer within cyst
√ some dilatation of proximal intrahepatic biliary system

UGI:
√ soft tissue mass in RUQ
√ anterior displacement of 2nd portion of duodenum + distal portion of stomach / inferior displacement of duodenum / widening of C-loop

Cx: 1. Rupture with bile peritonitis (1.8%)
      2. Secondary infection (cholangitis)
      3. Malignant transformation into cholangiocarcinoma (3.2%)
      4. Bleeding
      5. Biliary cirrhosis + portal hypertension
      6. Calculus formation (8%)
      7. Recurrent pancreatitis (occasionally)

Rx: extensive resection to avoid possibility of malignant transformation

CHOLEDOCHOCELE
= DUODENAL DUPLICATION CYST
  = ENTEROGENOUS CYST OF AMPULLA OF VATER / DUODENUM = INTRADUODENAL CHOLEDOCHAL CYST = DIVERTICULUM OF COMMON BILE DUCT
= herniation of CBD into duodenum with dilatation of the intraduodenal portion of the CBD (similar to ureterocele)
Etiology: originates from tiny bud / diverticulum of distal CBD (found in 5.7% of normal population)
Age: 33 years
Types: (a) CBD terminates in cyst, cyst drains into duodenum (common)
        (b) cyst drains into adjacent intramural portion of CBD (less common)
- biliary colic, episodic jaundice, pancreatitis
√ stones / sludge are frequently present

UGI:
√ smooth well-defined intraluminal duodenal filling defect at region of papilla
√ change in shape with compression / peristalsis

Cholangiography:
√ smooth clublike / saclike dilatation of intramural segment of CBD

CHOLELITHIASIS
Composition:
  A. CHOLESTEROL STONE
      = main component of most calculi (80%)
      √ slightly hypodense compared with bile
      (a) pure cholesterol stones (10%): yellowish, soft
         √ buoyancy in contrast-enhanced bile
         √ density of < 100 HU
      (b) mixture of cholesterol + calcium carbonate / bilirubinate (70%)
         √ laminated appearance
         √ radiopaque (15 – 20%)
  B. PIGMENT STONE (20%)
      from deconjugation of bilirubin by beta-glucoronidase from E. coli organisms; contains < 25% cholesterol: black / brown in color
      √ multiple tiny faceted / spiculated stones
Predisposing factors: "female, forty, fair, fat, fertile, flatulent"
  (a) Hemolytic disease
      Sickle cell disease (7 – 37%), hereditary spherocytosis (43 – 85%), pernicious anemia (16 – 20%), prosthetic cardiac valves + mitral stenosis (hemolysis), cirrhosis (hemolysis secondary to hypersplenism)
  (b) Metabolic
      Diabetes mellitus, obesity, pancreatic disease, cystic fibrosis, hypercholesterolemia, hemosiderosis (20%), hyperparathyroidism, hypothyroidism, prolonged use of estrogens / progesterone, pregnancy

(c) Hepatobiliary disease
    Hepatitis, Caroli disease, parasitic infection, benign
    / malignant strictures, foreign bodies (sutures,
    Ascariasis)
(d) Inflammatory bowel disease
    (10 x increased risk of stone formation); Crohn
    disease (28 – 34%)
(e) Genetic predisposition
    Navaho, Pima, Chippewa indians
(e) Others
    Muscular dystrophy

FLOATING STONES (20 – 25%)
(a) relatively pure cholesterol stones
(b) gas-containing stones
(c) rise in specific gravity of bile (1.03) from oral
    cholecystopaques (1.06) causing stones (1.05) to
    float

GAS-CONTAINING STONES
Mechanism: dehydration of older stones leads to
               internal shrinkage + dendritic cracks +
               subsequent gas-filling from negative
               internal pressure
√ "crow-foot" = "Mercedes-Benz" sign = radiating
  streaklike lucencies within stone, also responsible for
  buoyancy

SLUDGE
= calcium-bilirubinate granules + cholesterol crystals
  associated with biliary stasis secondary to prolonged
  fasting, hyperalimentation, hemolysis, cystic duct
  obstruction, acute + chronic cholecystitis
√ non-shadowing echogenic homogeneous mass
  shifting position slowly
√ "sludge ball" = tumefactive sludge (DDx: gallbladder
  cancer)
DDx: Hemobilia, Blood clot, Parasitic infestation

Cholecystolithiasis
Incidence: 10% of population; M:F = 1:3;
               in 3rd decade M:F = 2%:4%;
               in 7th decade M:F = 10%:25%
Peak age: 5th – 6th decade
• asymptomatic (60 – 65%)
• biliary colic (at a rate of 2% per year)

√ high-level intraluminal echoes + acoustic shadowing
  (100% diagnostic)
√ reverberation artifact
√ nonvisualization of GB + collection of echogenic
  echoes with acoustic shadowing (15 – 25%)
√ "double-arc shadow" = 2 echogenic curvilinear parallel
  lines separated by sonolucent rim (i.e., GB wall + GB
  lumen + stone with acoustic shadowing)
√ focal nonshadowing opacities < 5 mm in diameter (in
  70% gallstones)
√ infrequently adherent to wall

Cx: cholangitis, pancreatitis, fistula; cancer of GB +
        biliary ducts (2 – 3 x more frequent)

Cholangiolithiasis
A. CHOLEDOCHOLITHIASIS
   Etiology: (a) passed stones originating in GB
                 (b) primary development in intra- /
                      extrahepatic ducts
   Incidence: in 15% of cholecystectomy patients; in
                 3 – 4% of postcholecystectomy
                 patients; in 75% of patients with
                 chronic bile duct obstruction
   • recurrent episodes of jaundice, chills, fever
     (25 – 50%)
   • elevated transaminase (75%)
   • spontaneous passage with stones < 6 mm size
   Cholangiography (most specific technique):
     √ stone visualization in 92%
   US:
     √ stone visualization in 13 – 75% (more readily
       with CBD dilatation + good visibility of
       pancreatic head)
     √ dilated ducts in 64 – 77% / normal-sized duct in
       36%
     √ no stone in gallbladder (11%)
   CT:
     √ stone visualization in 50 – 90%
     √ intraluminal mass with crescentic ring (= stone
       of soft-tissue density) in 85%
B. STONE IN CYSTIC DUCT REMNANT:
   retained in 0.4% after surgery for choledocholithiasis

CHRONIC GRANULOMATOUS DISEASE OF CHILDHOOD
= recessive sex-linked polymorphonuclear leukocyte
  dysfunction characterized by a defect in microbicidal
  activity causing prolonged intracellular survival of
  phagocytized bacteria
Path: chronic infection with granuloma formation /
          caseation / suppuration
Age: onset in childhood; M > F (more severe in boys)
• recurrent chronic infections: suppurative lymphadenitis,
  pyoderma
√ chronic pneumonia
√ hilar lymphadenopathy
√ pleural effusions
√ hepatosplenomegaly
√ hepatic abscess
√ liver calcifications
√ osteomyelitis

CIRRHOSIS
= chronic liver disease characterized by diffuse
  parenchymal destruction, fibrosis, and nodular
  regeneration with abnormal reconstruction of preexisting
  lobular architecture

Etiology:
A. TOXIC: (1) Alcoholic liver disease (2) Drug-induced (prolonged methotrexate, oxyphenisatin, alpha-methyldopa, nitrofurantoin, isoniazid) (3) Iron overload (hemochromatosis, hemosiderosis)
B. INFLAMMATION: Viral hepatitis
C. BILIARY OBSTRUCTION: (1) Cystic fibrosis (2) Inflammatory bowel disease (3) Primary biliary cirrhosis (4) Obstructive infantile cholangiopathy
D. VASCULAR: (1) Prolonged CHF (2) Hepatic venoocclusive disease
E. NUTRITIONAL: (1) Intestinal bypass (2) Severe steatosis (3) Abetalipoproteinemia
F. HEREDITARY: (1) Wilson disease (2) Alpha-1-antitrypsin deficiency (3) Juvenile polycystic kidney disease (4) Galactosemia (5) Type IV glycogen storage disease (6) Hereditary fructose intolerance (7) Tyrosinemia (8) Hereditary tetany (9) Osler-Weber-Rendu syndrome (10) Familial cirrhosis

Morphology: nodular regeneration
(1) Micronodular (1 – 5 mm): usually due to alcoholism
(2) Macronodular (up to several cm): usually due to hepatitis B
(3) Mixed: usually following bile duct obstruction

√ enlarged (early stage) / normal / shrunken liver
√ caudate lobe hypertrophy + shrinkage of right lobe
  ratio of caudate to right lobe > 0.65 on transverse images (sensitivity 43 – 84%, least sensitive in alcoholic cirrhosis, most sensitive in cirrhosis caused by hepatitis B; specificity 100%; 26% sensitivity; 04% accuracy) (DDx: Budd-Chiari syndrome)
√ thickening of fissures + porta hepatis
√ surface nodularity + indentations (regenerating nodules)
√ signs of portal hypertension
√ splenomegaly
√ ascites (failure of albumin synthesis, portal hypertension)
√ associated with fatty infiltration (in early cirrhosis)
US:
(sensitivity 65 – 80%; DDx: chronic hepatitis, fatty infiltration)
Hepatic signs:
√ hepatomegaly (63%)
√ hypertrophy of caudate lobe (26%)
√ surface irregularity (88 sensitivity, 95% specificity)
√ increased echogenicity in 66% (as a sign of superimposed fatty infiltration)
√ increased sound attenuation (9%)
√ heterogeneous coarse (usually) / fine echotexture (7%)
√ decreased / normal definition of walls of portal venules (sign of associated fatty infiltration NOT of fibrosis)
√ occasional depiction of isoechoic regenerating nodules
√ dilatation of hepatic arteries (increased arterial flow)

with demonstration of intrahepatic arterial branches (DDx: dilated biliary radials)
Extrahepatic signs:
√ splenomegaly
√ ascites
√ signs of portal hypertension
CT:
√ parenchymal inhomogeneity
√ decreased attenuation (steatosis) in early cirrhosis
√ occasionally depiction of isodense regenerating nodules
MRI:
√ no alteration of liver parenchyma
√ regenerating nodules may have increased signal intensity
Angio:
√ stretched hepatic artery branches (early finding)
√ enlarged tortuous hepatic arteries = "corkscrewing" (increase in hepatic arterial flow)
√ shunting between hepatic artery and portal vein
√ mottled parenchymal phase
√ delayed emptying into venous phase
√ pruning of hepatic vein branches (normally depiction of 5th order branches) = postsinusoidal compression by developing nodules
NUC:
√ high blood pool activity secondary to slow clearance
√ colloid shift to bone marrow + spleen
√ shrunken liver with little or no activity + splenomegaly
√ mottled hepatic uptake (pseudotumors) on colloid scan with normal activity on IDA scans
√ displacement of liver + spleen from abdominal wall by ascites
Cx: (1) Ascites
(2) Portal hypertension
(3) Hepatocellular carcinoma (in 44% associated with macronodular cirrhosis, in 6% associated with micronodular cirrhosis)

Primary Biliary Cirrhosis
= CHRONIC NONSUPPURATIVE DESTRUCTIVE CHOLANGITIS
Histo: idiopathic progressive destructive cholangitis of interlobar and septal bile ducts, portal fibrosis, nodular regeneration, shrinkage of hepatic parenchyma
Age: 35 – 55 years; M:F = 1:9
• fatigue, pruritus
• xanthelasma / xanthoma (25%)
• hyperpigmentation (50%)
• insidious onset of pruritus (60%)
• IgM increased (95%)
• positive antimitochondrial antibodies (AMA) in 85 – 100%
√ normal extrahepatic ducts
√ cholelithiasis in 35 – 39%
√ hepatomegaly (50%)

√ tortuous intrahepatic ducts with narrowing + caliber variation / decreased arborization = "tree-in-winter" appearance
NUC:
   √ marked prolongation of hepatic Tc-99m IDA clearance
   √ uniform hepatic isotope retention
   √ normal visualization of GB and major bile ducts in 100%
DDx: (1) Sclerosing cholangitis (young men)
      (2) CBD obstruction
Prognosis: mean survival 6 (range 3 – 11) years after onset of cholestatic symptoms

CLONORCHIASIS
Rarely of clinical significance
Country: Japan, Korea, Central + South China, Taiwan, Indochina
Organism: Chinese liver fluke = Clonorchis sinensis
Cycle: parasite cysts digested by gastric juice, larvae migrate up the bile ducts, remain in small intrahepatic ducts until maturity (10 – 30 mm in length), travel to larger ducts to deposit eggs
Infection: snail + fresh-water fish serve as intermediate hosts; infection occurs by eating raw fish; hog, dog, cat, man are definite hosts
Path: (a) desquamation of epithelial bile duct lining with adenomatous proliferation of ducts + thickening of duct walls (inflammation, necrosis, fibrosis)
     (b) bacterial superinfection with formation of liver abscess
• remittent incomplete obstruction + bacterial superinfection
√ multiple crescent- / stilett-shaped filling defects within bile ducts
Cx: (1) Bile duct obstruction (conglomerate of worms / adenomatous proliferation)
     (2) Calculus formation (stasis / dead worms / epithelial debris)
     (3) Jaundice in 8% (stone / stricture / tumor)
     (4) Generalized dilatation of bile ducts (2%)

CONGENITAL BILIARY ATRESIA
Etiology: ? variation of same infectious process as in neonatal hepatitis with additional component of sclerosing cholangitis or vascular injury
Histo: proliferation of bile ducts in all portal triads
In 15% associated with: polysplenia, trisomy 18
NUC (sensitivity 90 – 97%, specificity 82 – 85%):
   √ good hepatic activity within 5 min
   √ delayed clearance from cardiac blood pool
   √ NO visualization of bowel on delayed images at 24 hours
   √ increased renal excretion
US:
   √ normal (visualization of gallbladder in 20%)
Rx: Kasai procedure (= portoenterostomy)

   (a) child < 60 days of age: 90% success rate
   (b) child between 60 and 90 days of age: 50% success rate
   (c) child > 90 days of age: 17% success rate

CONGENITAL HEPATIC FIBROSIS
= congenital cirrhosis with rapid + fatal progression
Histo: fibrous tissue within hepatic parenchyma with excess numbers of distorted terminal interlobular bile ducts + cysts which rarely communicate with bile ducts
Age: usually present in childhood resulting in early death
Associated with: autosomal recessive type of polycystic kidney disease, medullary sponge kidney (80%)
• hepatosplenomegaly, portal hypertension
• predisposed to cholangitis + calculi
√ "lollipop-tree" = ectasia of peripheral biliary radicles
√ hepatosplenomegaly
√ periportal fibrosis + portosystemic collaterals
Cx: Portal hypertension, Hepatocellular carcinoma, Cholangiocellular carcinoma

CYSTIC FIBROSIS
= autosomal recessive multisystem disorder with widespread abnormalities of mucus secreting exocrine glands
Incidence: 1:1,500 live births in Caucasians
Histo: increased pancreatic lobulation, fibrosis, replacement by fat, pancreatic atrophy, progressive dilatation of acini + ductules
• acute pancreatitis
• diabetes mellitus
• abnormal loss of electrolytes in sweat
• growth failure
• cirrhosis + portal hypertension
• rectal prolapse
• pancreatic insufficiency with malabsorption (90%)
• obstructive lung disease
• chronic pulmonary infection (pseudomonas colonization)
√ meconium peritonitis (50%) (intraperitoneal meconium may calcify within 24 hours)
@ Liver
   Histo: focal biliary cirrhosis from inspissated bile (33%); mucus-containing cysts in gallbladder wall
   √ portal hypertension + hepatosplenomegaly + hypersplenism
   √ fatty infiltration of liver (if malabsorption untreated)
   √ "microgallbladder" + cholecystolithiasis (rare)
@ Pancreas
   √ increased pancreatic echogenicity
   √ occasionally macroscopic pancreatic cysts (= dilated acini + ducts)
   √ fatty replacement of pancreas (-90 to -120 HU)
   √ pancreatic calcifications
@ Small bowel
   √ meconium ileus (10 – 15%) = obstruction usually at level of distal ileum

√ meconium ileus equivalent = episodes of low-grade obstruction later in life

√ thickened folds, dilatation, mucosal redundancy of duodenum

√ dilatation of Brunner glands

@ Colon

√ "microcolon" = colon of normal length but diminished caliber

√ "jejunization of colon" = coarse redundant + hyperplastic colonic mucosa (distended crypt goblet cells)

√ rectal prolapse between 6 months and 3 years in untreated patients

ECHINOCOCCAL DISEASE

Echinococcus granulosus

= E. cysticus = Hydatid disease (more common); man is accidental host

(a) pastoral form: dog is definite host; intermediate hosts are cattle, sheep, horses, hogs; endemic in sheep-raising countries: East Africa, USSR, Mediterranean, Middle East countries, Argentina, Chile, Uruguay

(b) sylvatic form: wolf is definite host; intermediate hosts are deer, moose; endemic in northern - Canada, Alaska

Cycle: ingestion of contaminated material; eggs hatch in duodenum; penetration of intestinal wall + mesenteric venules; larvae carried through body + deposited in capillary filters at various sites

Organs: liver (73%); lung (14%); peritoneum (12%); kidney (6%); spleen (4%); spinal cord; brain, bladder; thyroid; prostate; heart; eye; bone

Histo:

(1) ENDOCYST (parasitic component of capsule)

   (a) inner GERMINATIVE LAYER (resembling wet tissue paper) giving rise to brood - capsules which may remain attached to cyst wall harboring up to 400,000 scolices / may detach + form sediment in cyst fluid = "hydatid sand" / may break up into numerous self-contained daughter cysts

   (b) CYST MEMBRANE = laminated chitin-like substance

(2) PERICYST / ECTOCYST = highly vascularized adventitial layer (resembling egg white), organized host granulation tissue replacing tissue necrosis from compression of expanding cyst, marginal vascular rim of 0.5 – 4 mm

• pain
• recurrent jaundice + biliary colic (transient obstruction by membrane fragments + daughter cysts expelled into biliary tree)
• urticaria + anaphylaxis (following rupture)
• blood eosinophilia (20 – 50%)

• Tests: 1. Casoni (60% sensitivity; may be falsely positive)
2. Complement fixation double diffusion (65% sensitivity)
3. Immunoelectrophoresis (most specific)
4. Indirect hemagglutination (85% sensitivity)

Time to diagnosis: 11 – 81 (mean 51) years

Location: right lobe > left lobe of liver; multiple cysts in 20%

Size: up to 50 cm (average size of 5 cm), up to 16 liters of fluid

Plain film:

√ may have crescentic / ring-shaped / polycyclic calcifications (10 – 33%)

√ pneumohydrocyst (infection / communication with bronchial tree)

US:

√ complex heterogeneous mass (most common)

√ well-defined anechoic cyst (common)

√ "racemose" appearance = multiseptated cyst = daughter cysts internally and tangent to mother cyst (characteristic, but rare)

√ mass with egg-shell calcification

√ floating undulating membrane / vesicles (characteristic, but rare)

CT:

√ well-demarcated low-density round mass ± internal septations

√ enhancement of cyst wall + septations

Angio:

√ avascular area with splaying of arteries

√ halo of increased density around cyst (inflammation / compressed liver)

Cholangiography:

√ cyst may communicate with bile ducts: right hepatic duct (55%), left hepatic duct (29%), CHD (9%), gallbladder (6%), CBD (1%)

Percutaneous aspiration:

Δ risk of anaphylactic shock (0.5%); asthma (3%)

Δ fluid analysis positive for hydatid disease in 70% (fragments of laminated membrane in 54%; scolices in 15%; hooklets in 15%)

Cx: (1) Compression of vital structures
(2) Infection
(3) Rupture

Echinococcus multilocularis

= E. alveolaris = less common but more aggressive form of echinococcal disease definite hosts are rodents (moles, lemmings, wild mice) + domestic cat

Path: larvae proliferate by exogenous extension + penetration of surrounding tissue (= diffuse + infiltrative process resembling malignancy); chronic granulomatous reaction with central necrosis, cavitation, calcification

Location: widespread hematogenous dissemination is not uncommon

√ faint / dense punctate calcifications (dystrophic calcifications scattered throughout necrotic + granulomatous tissue)

US:
√ echogenic ill-defined single / multiple masses
√ propensity of spread to liver hilum

CT:
√ heterogeneous hypodense poorly marginated masses
√ pseudocystic necrotic regions of near water density surrounded by hyperdense solid component

Angio:
√ intrahepatic arterial tapering + obstruction

EPIDERMOID CYST OF SPLEEN

Histo: (1) mesothelial lining (2) squamous epithelial lining = epidermoid cyst
Age: 2nd – 3rd decade
May be associated with polycystic kidney disease
(a) unilocular + solitary (80%)
(b) multiple + multilocular (20%)
√ average size of 10 cm
√ curvilinear calcification in wall (9 – 25%)
√ may contain cholesterol crystals, fat, blood
Cx: trauma, rupture, infection

FATTY LIVER

= FATTY INFILTRATION OF THE LIVER = HEPATIC STEATOSIS
Causes:
(a) Metabolic derangement: Diabetes mellitus (50%), obesity, hyperlipidemia, acute fatty liver of pregnancy, protein malnutrition, IV hyperalimentation, malabsorption (ileojejunal bypass), glycogen storage disease, glycogen synthetase deficiency, cystic fibrosis, Reye syndrome, corticosteroids, severe hepatitis, trauma
(b) Hepatotoxins: alcohol (> 50%), carbonchlorides, phosphorus, chemotherapy
Histo: hepatocytes with large cytoplasmatic fat vacuoles filled with triglycerides; > 5% fat of total liver weight
Types: uniform / nonuniform / focal – multifocal

Diffuse Fatty Infiltration

√ hepatomegaly (75 – 80%) / normal sized liver
√ rapid change with time (after improved nutrition)

Plain film:
√ radiolucent liver sign = enlarged radiolucent liver
US: sensitivity > 90%, accuracy 85 – 97%
√ increased sound attenuation (scattering of sound beam) = poor definition of posterior aspect of liver
√ fine (more typical) / coarsened hyperechogenicity (compared with kidney)
√ impaired visualization of borders of hepatic vessels
√ attenuation of sound beam (feature of fat, NOT fibrosis)

CT:
√ areas of lower attenuation than normal portal vein / IVC density
√ reversal of liver-spleen density relationship (normally spleen is 6 – 12 HU below liver)
√ hyperdense intrahepatic vascular structures

NUC:
√ diffuse heterogeneous uptake (68%)
√ reversal of liver-spleen uptake (41%)
√ increased bone marrow uptake (41%)
√ increased activity during wash-out phase of Xe-133 scintigraphy (38%)

MRI:
√ increased signal on T1 + T2 weighted images; relative insensitive (10% fat by weight will alter SE signal intensities only by 5 – 15%)
√ fat turns black with Dixon technique

FAT-SPARED AREA in Diffuse Fatty Infiltration
√ hypoechoic ovoid / spherical / sheet-like mass
Location: (a) quadrate lobe (anterior to portal vein bifurcation)
            (b) next to gallbladder bed
            (c) subcapsular skip areas
√ NO mass effect (undisplaced course of vessels)
DDx: tumor mass

Focal Fatty Infiltration

√ fan-shaped lobar / segmental distribution with angulated / interdigitating geographic margins
√ multiple / rarely single echogenic nodules simulating metastases (rare)
√ NO mass effect (undisplaced course of vessels)
US:
√ discrete hyperechoic area
CT:
√ patchy areas of decreased attenuation (DDx: liver tumor)
MRI:
√ high signal on T1W, low / isointense signal on T2W
DDx: Primary / secondary hepatic tumor

FOCAL NODULAR HYPERPLASIA

= benign congenital hamartomatous malformation or reparative process in areas of focal injury; twice as common as hepatocellular adenoma; associated with oral contraceptives in 11%
Histo: composed of abnormally arranged hepatocytes, numerous bile ducts, fibrous bands, Kupffer cells (the only tumor that contains Kupffer cells); difficult differentiation from regenerative nodules of cirrhosis + hepatocellular adenoma; frequently central fibrous scar
Age peak: 3rd – 5th decade (range: 7 months – 75 years); M:F = 1:2
• initially asymptomatic
• vague abdominal pain (20%)
√ size < 5 cm (in 85%); right lobe:left lobe = 2:1

√ well-circumscribed, non-encapsulated nodular cirrhotic-like mass in an otherwise normal liver
√ "central stellate scar" = central fibrous core with radiating fibrous septa (15%) (DDx: fibrolamellar HCC)
√ NO calcifications
√ pedunculated mass (in 5 – 20%)
√ multiple masses (in 20%)
NECT:
   √ homogeneous mass of slightly decreased attenuation
CECT:
   √ isodense / hyperdense on bolus injection
US:
   √ hypo- / hyper- / rarely isoechoic homogeneous mass
MRI:
   √ usually nearly isointense with liver on T1WI + T2WI
   √ central scar hypointense on T1WI + hyperintense on T2WI (bile stasis ± slow flowing blood)
NUC:
   sulfur colloid scan:
      √ normal (30 – 55%), cold spot (40%),
      √ hot spot (10%), only reported in FNH
   Tc-HIDA:
      √ normal / increased uptake (40 – 70%), cold spot (60%)
Angio:
   √ hypervascular mass (90%) with intense capillary blush / hypovascular (10%)
   √ enlargement of main feeding artery with central blood supply (= "spoke wheel" pattern in 33%)
   √ decreased vascularity in central stellate fibrous scar
MRI:
   √ homogeneous isointense tumor on T1WI + T2WI
   √ central scar hypointense on T1WI, hyperintense on T2WI
Rx: Resection for pedunculated mass; biopsy for extensive tumor
Cx: Rupture with hemoperitoneum (increased incidence in patients on oral contraceptives — 14%)

GALLBLADDER CARCINOMA

Most common biliary cancer (9 x more common than extrahepatic bile duct cancer);
5th most common gastrointestinal malignancy (after colorectal, pancreatic, gastric, esophageal carcinoma);
3% of all intestinal neoplasms
Incidence: 0.4 – 4.6% of biliary tract operations; 6,500 deaths / year in United States
Peak age: 6 – 7th decade;   M:F = 1:3
Histo: (a) well differentiated adenocarcinoma of scirrhous type (80 – 90%)
   (b) anaplastic carcinoma, squamous cell carcinoma, adenoacanthoma (10 – 20%)
   (c) carcinoid, sarcoma, basal cell carcinoma, lymphoma (extremely rare)
Predisposed: patients with porcelain gallbladder (14%)
Associated with:
   (a) gallstones in 70 – 98% (in only 1% of all patients with gallstones)

   (b) porcelain gallbladder (in 25 – 60%)
   (c) inflammatory bowel disease (predominantly - ulcerative colitis, less common in Crohn disease
   (d) familial polyposis coli
   (e) chronic cholecystitis
• history of past GB disease (50%)
• malaise, vomiting, weight loss
• RUQ pain (76%)
• jaundice (50%)
• abnormal liver function tests (20 – 75%)
Location: usually in body / fundus; rarely in cystic duct
√ replacement of gallbladder by mass (40 – 65%)
√ focal / diffuse asymmetric irregular thickening of GB wall (20 – 30%)
√ polypoid / fungating intraluminal mass with wide base (15 – 25%)
√ bulky tumor involving gallbladder fossa + adjacent liver + hepatoduodenal ligament
√ dilatation of biliary tree
√ liver metastases
√ enlarged regional lymph nodes (peripancreatic / in porta hepatis)
√ fine granular / punctate flecks of calcification (mucinous adenocarcinoma)
OCG:
   √ non-visualization of gallbladder (2/3)
Metastases: in 77% at time of diagnosis
   (a) local invasion of liver (50 – 70%), duodenum (12%), colon (9%), stomach, bile duct, pancreas, right kidney, abdominal wall
   (b) lymphatic spread (50 – 63%): cystic duct node, CBD nodes, lesser omental nodes, superior + posterior pancreaticoduodenal nodes, periaortic nodes
   (c) intraperitoneal seeding (common)
   (d) hematogenous spread (less common): liver, lung, bones
   (e) neural spread (frequent): associated with more aggressive tumors
   (f) intraductal spread (least common): particularly in papillary adenocarcinoma
Prognosis: 75% unresectable at presentation; average survival is 6 months; 5% 1-year survival rate; 6% 5-year survival rate
DDx: (1) Xanthogranulomatous cholecystitis (lobulated mass filling gallbladder + stones)
   (2) Chronic cholecystitis (generalized gallbladder wall thickening)
   (3) Liver tumor invading gallbladder fossa
   (4) Tumors from adjacent organs (pancreas, duodenum)
   (5) Metastases (melanoma, leukemia, lymphoma)

GALLSTONE ILEUS

1 – 3% of all intestinal obstructions (20% of obstruction in patients > 65 years; 24% of obstructions in patients > 70 years);
Age: average 65 – 75 years;   M:F = 1:7

Incidence: develops in < 1% of patients with
             cholelithiasis, in 1 of 6 perforations; risk
             increases with age; stones are commonly
             > 2.5 cm in diameter
- acute colicky abdominal pain (20 – 30%)
- nausea, vomiting, fever, distension, obstipation

Rigler triad on plain film:
√ 1. Partial / complete intestinal obstruction (usually
     small bowel), "string of rosary beads" = multiple
     small amounts of air trapped between dilated +
     stretched valvulae conniventes
√ 2. Air in biliary tree
√ 3. Ectopic calcified gallstone
√ change in position of previously identified gallstone

UGI / BE:
√ well-contained localized barium collection lateral to
  first portion of duodenum (barium-filled collapsed GB
  + possibly biliary ducts)
  Fistulous communication:
    cholecystoduodenal (60%), choledochoduodenal,
    cholecystocolic, choledochocolic, cholecystogastric
√ identification of site of obstruction: terminal ileum
  (60 – 70%), proximal ileum (25%), distal ileum (10%),
  pylorus, sigmoid, duodenum (Bouveret syndrome)
Cx: recurrent gallstone ileus in 5 – 10% (additional
       silent calculi more proximally)
Prognosis: high mortality

GLYCOGEN STORAGE DISEASE
= autosomal recessive diseases with varying severity and
  clinical syndromes
A. VON GIERKE (TYPE I)
    Etiology: defect in glucose-6-phosphatase with
                 excess deposition of glycogen in liver,
                 kidney, intestines
    Dx: failure of rise in blood glucose after glucagon
           administration
    Age at presentation: infancy
    √ hepatomegaly
    US:
    √ increased echogenicity (glycogen / fat)
    CT:
    √ increased (glycogen) / normal / decreased (fat)
      parenchymal attenuation
    Prognosis: death in infancy, may survive into
                  adulthood with early therapy
    Cx: (1) Hepatic adenoma
           (2) Hepatocellular carcinoma
B. CORI DISEASE (TYPE III)
C. ANDERSON DISEASE (TYPE IV)
D. HERS DISEASE (TYPE VI)

HEMOCHROMATOSIS
= excess iron deposition in various parenchymal organs
  (liver, pancreas, spleen, kidneys) leading to cirrhosis
  with portal hypertension [HEMOSIDEROSIS =
  increased iron deposition without organ damage]

Path: iron deposition occurs initially in RES, eventually
         within hepatocytes, produces periportal fibrosis
         resulting ultimately in cirrhosis
Types:
A. PRIMARY / IDIOPATHIC HEMOCHROMATOSIS
    genetically determined mucosal defect in intestinal
    wall / increased absorption of intestinal iron
B. SECONDARY HEMOCHROMATOSIS
    result of multiple blood transfusions (usually > 100
    units)
    Age for secondary hemochromatosis:
      4 – 5th decade; M:F = 10:1
- hyperpigmentation (90%)
- hepatomegaly (90%)
- arthralgias (50%)
- diabetes mellitus (30%)
- CHF + arrythmias (15%)
- loss of libido, impotence, amenorrhea, testicular
  atrophy, loss of body hair
CT:
√ diffuse / rarely focal increase in liver density (up to 75
  – 130 HU)
√ depiction of hepatic veins on NECT
√ dual energy CT (at 80 + 120 kVp) can quantitate
  amount of iron deposition
MRI:
√ significant signal loss from liver on T2W
Cx: hepatocellular carcinoma (in 14%)

HEPATIC ABSCESS
Etiology:
(1) Obstructive biliary tract disease with cholangitis
(2) Portal pyemia (suppurative appendicitis, diverticular
    disease, colitis)
(3) Infarction from embolism
(4) Indwelling arterial catheters
(5) Direct spread from contiguous organ (cholecystitis,
    peptic ulcer, subphrenic sepsis)
(6) Trauma (rupture / laceration with direct
    contamination)
(7) Cryptogenic (invasion of cysts / dead tissue by
    pyogenic intestinal flora)
Types: pyogenic (88%), amebic (10%), fungal (2%)
Location: multiple in 50%
√ hepatomegaly
√ elevation of right hemidiaphragm
√ pleural effusion
√ right lower lobe atelectasis / infiltration
√ gas within abscess (esp. Klebsiella)
Cx: (1) Septicemia (2) Rupture into right subphrenic
       space (3) Rupture into abdominal cavity (4) Rupture
       into pericardium (5) Empyema (6) Common hepatic
       duct obstruction
Mortality: 100% if unrecognized / untreated

Pyogenic Liver Abscess
Organisms: E. coli, aerobic streptococci, St. aureus,
              anaerobic bacteria (45%)

Incidence: 0.016%

Etiology: (1) ascending cholangitis (2) portal phlebitis (3) trauma (penetrating wounds, biopsy) (4) direct spread from contiguous infection

Age: 6 – 7th decade; M > F

- pyrexia (79%)
- abdominal pain (68%)
- nocturnal sweating (43%)
- vomiting / malaise (39%)
- jaundice (0 – 20%)
- positive blood culture (50%)

Location: right lobe affected in 75%; multiple abscesses in 50 – 67%

US:
- √ hypoechoic round lesion with well-defined mildly echogenic rim
- √ distal acoustic enhancement
- √ coarse clumpy debris / low-level echoes / fluid-debris level
- √ intensely echogenic reflections with reverberations (from gas) in 20%

CT:
- √ inhomogeneous hypodense single / multiloculated cavity
- √ "double target sign" = wall-enhancement + surrounding hypodense zone (30%)

NUC:
- √ photon-deficient area on sulfur colloid + IDA scan
- √ Ga-67 citrate uptake in 80%
- √ In-111 tagged WBC uptake is highly specific

Mortality: 20 – 80%

Amebic Abscess

Organism: Entamoeba histolytica

Etiology: spread of viable amebae from colon to liver via portal system

Incidence: in 1 – 25% of intestinal amebiasis

Age: 3rd – 5th decade; M:F = 4:1

- amebic dysentery
- amebic hepatitis (15%)

Location: liver abscess (right lobe) in 2 – 25%; systemic dissemination by invasion of lymphatics / portal system (rare) liver:lung:brain = 100:10:1

Size: 2 – 12 cm; multiple liver abscesses in 25%

- √ nodularity of abscess wall (60%)
- √ internal septations (30%)
- √ not gas-containing (unless hepatobronchial / hepatoenteric fistula present)

NUC:
- √ sensitivity of sulfur colloid scan is 98%
- √ photon-deficient area surrounded by rim of uptake on Ga-67 scan

Aspiration:
typically opaque reddish / dirty brown / pink material ("anchovy paste / chocolate sauce"), usually sterile, parasite confined to margin of abscess

Cx: (1) Diaphragmatic disruption (rare) is strongly suggestive of amebic abscess
(2) Fistulization into colon, right adrenal gland, bile ducts, pericardium

Rx: conservative treatment with chloroquine / metronidazole (Flagyl®)

HEPATIC ADENOMA
= HEPATOCELLULAR ADENOMA = most frequent hepatic tumor in young women several months to years after use of contraceptive steroids; not seen in males unless on anabolic steroids

Histo: solitary spherical benign growth of hepatocytes, high incidence of hemorrhage and necrosis ± fibrotic scars if large; sheets of hepatocytes without portal veins, central veins; scattered thin-walled vascular channels + bile canaliculi; decrease in number of abnormally functioning Kupffer cells; hepatocytes contain increased amounts of glycogen ± fat

Predisposed: Type I glycogen storage disease (von Gierke)

- asymptomatic / RUQ pain
- hepatomegaly
- √ round well-circumscribed mass; between 6 – 30 cm in size
- √ pedunculated (in 10%)

CT:
- √ round mass of decreased density; areas of necrosis (30 – 40%)
- √ hyperdense areas of fresh intratumoral hemorrhage (22 – 50%)
- √ variable patterns of enhancement, does not enhance to the same degree as normal liver

US:
- √ usually small well-demarcated solid echogenic / complex hyper- and hypoechoic heterogeneous mass with anechoic areas (if large)

MRI:
- √ inhomogeneous on all pulse sequences (indistinguishable from HCC)
- √ may have hyperintense areas on T1WI (due to presence of fat)
- √ isointense (sheets of hepatocytes) and hyperintense areas (necrosis, hemorrhage) on T2WI

NUC:
- √ focal photopenic lesion on sulfur colloid scan surrounded by rim of increased uptake; may rarely show increased uptake
- √ NO gallium uptake

Angio:
- √ usually hypervascular mass
- √ homogeneous but not intense stain in capillary phase
- √ enlarged hepatic artery with feeders at tumor periphery (50%)
- √ hypo- / avascular regions (secondary to hemorrhage / necrosis)
- √ neovascularity

Cx: spontaneous hemorrhage with subcapsular
         hematoma / hemoperitoneum (41%)
Rx: surgical resection

HEPATIC ANGIOSARCOMA
= HEMANGIOENDOTHELIAL SARCOMA = KUPFFER
  CELL SARCOMA = HEMANGIOSARCOMA
= extremely rare tumor (0.2 per million) with rapid
  metastatic spread
Etiology: (a) thorotrast (latent period of 15 – 24 years)
               (b) arsenic
               (c) polyvinyl chloride (latent period of 4 – 28
                    years)
Age: 6 – 7th decade
Metastases to:
   lung, spleen, porta hepatis nodes, portal vein, thyroid,
   peritoneal cavity, bone marrow (rapid metastatic spread)
√ areas of increased density in RES (liver, spleen, lymph
  nodes)
√ portal vein invasion
NUC:
   √ cold defect on sulfur colloid scan
US:
   √ solid / mixed mass with anechoic areas (hemorrhage /
     necrosis)
CT:
   √ hypodense masses with high density regions
     (hemorrhage / necrosis)
   √ striking peripheral enhancement
Angio:
   √ hypervascular stain around tumor periphery, NO
     arterial encasement
Prognosis: death within 1 year

HEPATIC CYST
= second most common benign hepatic lesion (22%)

A. ACQUIRED HEPATIC CYST
    secondary to trauma, inflammation, parasitic
    infestation, neoplasia

B. CONGENITAL HEPATIC CYST
    = defective development of aberrant intrahepatic bile
      ducts
    Incidence: liver cysts detected at autopsy in 50%;
                    in 22% detected during life
    Age of detection: 5th – 8th decade
    Histo: cysts surrounded by fibrous capsule + lined
                by columnar epithelium, related to bile ducts
                within portal triads
    Associated with:
       (1) Tuberous sclerosis
       (2) Polycystic kidney disease (25 – 33% have liver
            cysts)
       (3) Polycystic liver disease: autosomal dominant;
            M:F = 1:2; (50% have polycystic kidney
            disease)
    • hepatomegaly (40%); pain (33%); jaundice (9%)

Size of cyst:
   range from microscopic to huge (average 1.2 cm; in
   25% largest cyst < 1 cm; in 40% largest cyst
   > 4 cm; maximal size of 20 cm); multiple cysts
   spread throughout liver (in 60%) / solitary cyst
√ "cold spot" on IDA, Ga-68, Tc-99m sulfur colloid scans
√ echo-free cyst, may show fluid-fluid interface

HEPATIC HEMANGIOMA
Cavernous Hemangioma of Liver
most common benign liver tumor (78%); second most
common liver tumor after metastases
Incidence: 4%; autopsy incidence 0.4 – 7.3% ;
                increased with multiparity
Age: rarely seen in young children; M:F = 1:5
Histo: large vascular channels filled with slowly
            circulating blood; lined by single layer of
            mature flattened endothelial cells separated by
            thin fibrous septa; no bile ducts; common
            thrombosis of vascular channels resulting in
            fibrosis + calcifications
Associated with: (1) Hemangiomas in other organs
                      (2) Focal nodular hyperplasia
                      (3) Rendu-Osler-Weber disease
• asymptomatic if tumor small (50 – 70%)
• may present with hemorrhage if large (5%)
• hepatomegaly
• abdominal discomfort + pain (from thrombosis in large
  hemangioma)
• **Kasabach-Merritt syndrome** (= hemangioma +
  thrombocytopenia) rare
Location: frequently peripheral / subcapsular;
             posterior right lobe of liver; 20% are
             pedunculated; multiple in 10%
Size: < 4 cm (90%); giant cavernous hemangioma
       (10%)
√ may have central area of fibrosis = areas of
  nonenhancement / nonfilling / cystic space
  (occurrence increases with age)
√ calcifications (phleboliths / septal calcifications) are
  extremely uncommon
US:
   √ hyperechoic (80%), hypoechoic (20%) mass with
     discrete margins
   √ hypoechoic center possible
   √ may show acoustic enhancement
   √ unchanged in size / appearance (82%) on 1 – 6
     year follow-up
   √ no Doppler signals
CT (scanning guidelines: precontrast, good bolus,
    dynamic scanning):
   √ well-circumscribed spherical / ovoid low-density
     mass
   √ may have areas of higher / lower density within
     mass
   √ typical pattern of low-density on NECT + peripheral
     enhancement + complete fill-in on delayed images
     3 – 30 minutes post IV bolus (55 – 89%)

√ peripheral (72%) / central (in 8%) / diffuse dense (in 8%) enhancement

√ complete (75%) / partial (24%) / no (2%) fill-in to isodensity in delayed phase

Angio (historical gold standard):

√ dense opacification of well-circumscribed, dilated, irregular, punctate vascular lakes / puddles in late arterial + parenchymal phase starting at periphery

√ normal-sized feeders; No AV shunting

√ contrast persistence late into venous phase

NUC:

√ delayed filling on Tc-99m labeled RBC scans with increased activity on delayed images at 1 – 2 hours (detectable > 2 cm in size)

√ cold defect on sulfur colloid scans

MRI (accuracy 90%):

√ well-defined mass with regular contour; homogeneous internal architecture if < 4 cm, hypointense internal inhomogeneities if > 4 cm

√ hypo- / isointense on T1WI; hyperintense "light bulb" appearance on T2WI (due to slow flowing blood) (DDx: hepatic cyst, hypervascular tumor, necrotic tumor, cystic neoplasm)

√ peripheral enhancement with subsequent fill-in toward center after gadolinium-DTPA

Bx: may be biopsied safely with small needles (< 20 gauge)

√ nonpulsatile blood (73%)

√ endothelial cells without malignancy (27%)

Cx (rare): (1) Spontaneous rupture (4.5%)
(2) Abscess formation
(3) Kasabach Merritt syndrome (platelet sequestration)

Infantile Hemangioendothelioma of Liver

= CAPILLARY HEMANGIOMA = most common benign hepatic tumor in infants

Histo: thick-walled endothelium-lined vascular spaces similar to cavernous hemangioma but with multiple layers and scattered bile ducts; involutional changes (infarction, hemorrhage, necrosis, scarring)

Age at presentation: < 6 months (in 85%)
M:F = 2:1

• abdominal mass secondary to hepatomegaly

• cutaneous hemangiomas (45%)

• may present with high-output CHF secondary to AV shunts (15%)

Size: several mm up to 15 cm

√ diffuse involvement of entire liver, rarely focal; single / multiple

Plain film:

√ fine speckled / fibrillary calcifications (DDx: hepatoblastoma, hamartoma, metastatic neuroblastoma)

US:

√ predominantly hypoechoic / complex / hyperechoic lesion

√ multiple sonolucent areas (= enlarging vascular channels secondary to initial rapid growth) (DDx: mesenchymal hamartoma)

CT:

√ focal areas of low attenuation with early peripheral enhancement + variable delayed central enhancement (similar to cavernous hemangioma)

MRI:

√ inhomogeneous on T1WI + T2WI (hemorrhage, necrosis, scarring)

√ varying degrees of hyperintensity on T2WI (resembling hemangioma)

NUC:

√ early appearance of tracer in liver

√ marked delay in tracer clearance

√ multiple defects on static images

Angio:

√ enlargement of celiac + hepatic arteries

√ rapid decrease in aortic caliber below celiac trunk

√ enlarged, tortuous feeding arteries and stretched intrahepatic vessels

√ hypervascular tumor with inhomogeneous stain; clusters of small abnormal vessels

√ pooling of contrast material in sinusoidal lakes with rapid clearing through early venous drainage (AV shunting)

Prognosis: tendency to involute within 6 – 8 months; reduction in size with steroids / radiotherapy

Cx: (1) Congestive heart failure
(2) Disseminated intravascular coagulopathy
(3) Thrombocytopenia (platelet trapping)

HEPATITIS

A. ACUTE HEPATITIS

US:

√ decreased parenchymal echogenicity

√ increased brightness of portal venule walls ("starry sky" pattern) = centrilobular pattern (DDx: leukeumic infiltrate, diffuse lymphomatous involvement, toxic shock syndrome)

B. CHRONIC HEPATITIS

US:

√ increased liver echogenicity

√ coarsening of parenchymal texture

√ silhouetting of portal vein walls = loss of definition of portal venules

√ NO sound attenuation

HEPATOBLASTOMA

Incidence: 3rd most common abdominal tumor in children; most frequent malignant hepatic tumor in children (51%)

Incidence increased with: hemihypertrophy, Beckwith syndrome

Histo: small cells resembling embryonal / fetal liver + mesenchymal cells (osteoid, cartilagenous, fibrous tissue)

Age: < 3 years; < 18 months (In 50%); range from
newborn to 15 years; M:F = 2:1 (DDx:
hepatocellular carcinoma > 5 years)
- upper abdominal mass, weight loss, nausea, vomiting
- precocious puberty (production of endocrine
substances)
- persistently + markedly elevated alpha-fetoprotein
(66%)
Location: right lobe of the liver
√ coarse calcifications / osseous matrix (12-30%) (DDx:
hemangioendothelioma with fine granular calcifications,
hepatoma has no calcifications)
US:
√ large heterogeneous echogenic mass, sometimes
with calcifications, occasionally cystic areas (necrosis
/ extramedullary hematopoiesis)
CT:
√ hypointense tumor with peripheral rim enhancement
MRI:
√ inhomogeneously hypointense on T1WI with
hyperintense foci (hemorrhage)
√ inhomogeneously hyperintense with hypointense
bands (fibrous septae) on T2WI
NUC:
√ photopenic defect
Angio:
√ hypervascular mass with dense stain
√ marked neovascularity; NO AV-shunting
√ vascular lakes may be present
√ avascular areas (secondary to tumor necrosis)
√ may show caval involvement (= unresectable)
Prognosis: 60% resectable; 75% mortality; better
prognosis than hepatoma
DDx: Hemangioendothelioma, Metastatic neuroblastoma,
Mesenchymal hamartoma, Hepatocellular
carcinoma

HEPATOCELLULAR CARCINOMA

= HEPATOMA = most frequent primary visceral
malignancy in the world; 90% of all primary liver
malignancies; 2nd most frequent malignant hepatic
tumor in children (39%) after hepatoblastoma
Incidence: (a) in industrialized world: 0.2 – 0.8%
            (b) in Africa, Southeast Asia, Japan,
                Greece, Italy: 5.5 – 20%
Peak age:
(a) industrialized world: 6th – 7th decade; M:F = 2.5:1
fibrolamellar subtype (in 3 – 10%) below age 40
years
(b) high incidence areas: 30 – 40 years; M:F = 5:1
(c) in children: > 5 years of age; M:F = 4:3
Etiology:
1. Cirrhosis (80%); 5% of alcoholic cirrhotics develop
HCC
   Latent period: 8 months – 14 years from onset
                    of cirrhosis
   Most frequently found in macronodular
   (=postnecrotic) cirrhosis due to hepatitis B virus and
   hemochromatosis

(a) alcohol   (e) metabolic
(b) hemochromotosis   (f) Wilson disease
(c) cardiac   (g) alpha-1-antitrypsin
(d) biliary   deficiency
2. Chronic hepatitis B; 12% develop HCC
3. Carcinogens
   (a) aflatoxin
   (b) siderosis
   (c) oral contraceptives / anabolic androgens
   (d) thorotrast
4. Inborn errors of metabolism
   (a) tyrosinosis
   (b) galactosemia
   (c) type I glycogen storage disease (von Gierke)
   (d) biliary atresia
mnemonic: "CASH"
   Cirrhosis, post-necrotic
   Administration of thorotrast
   Schistosomiasis
   Hemochromatosis
Histo: HCC cells resemble hepatocytes in appearance +
structural pattern (trabecular, pseudoglandular,
compact, scirrhous);
   (a) expansive encapsulated HCC: collapsed
        portal vein branches at capsule
   (b) infiltrative nonencapsulated HCC: portal
        venules communicate with tumoral sinusoids
        = often invasion of portal ± hepatic veins
GROWTH PATTERN:
(1) Multicentric nodular (22%):
     small foci up to 5 cm in both hepatic lobes
(2) Solitary massive (27%):
     bulk in one (most often right) lobe involved with
     satellite nodules
(3) Diffuse microscopic (51%):
     tiny indistinct nodules closely resembling cirrhosis
- elevated alpha-fetoprotein (90%), negative in
cholangiocarcinoma
- elevated liver function tests
- persistent RUQ pain, hepatomegaly, ascites
- fever, weight loss, malaise
- Paraneoplastic syndromes :
  (a) sexual precocity / gynecomastia
  (b) hypercholesterolemia
  (c) erythrocytosis (tumor produces erythropoietin)
  (d) hypoglycemia
  (e) hypercalcemia
  (f) carcinoid syndrome
Metastases to: lung (most common = 8%), adrenal,
             lymph nodes, bone

√ portal vein invasion (25 – 40%)
√ invasion of hepatic vein (16%) / IVC (= Budd-Chiari
syndrome)
√ occasionally invasion of bile ducts
√ NO calcifications in usual HCC; however, common in
fibrolamellar HCC (40%) and in sclerosing HCC
√ hepatomegaly and ascites

NUC:
√ Sulfur colloid scan: single cold spot (70%), multiple defects (15 – 20%), heterogeneous distribution (10%)
√ Tc-HIDA scan: cold spot / atypical uptake in 4% (delayed images)
√ Gallium-scan: avid accumulation in 70 – 90%
CT (accuracy > 80%):
√ hypodense mass / rarely isodense / hyperdense in fatty liver
√ circular zone of radiolucency surrounding the mass
CECT:
√ enhancement during arterial phase (80%)
√ isodensity on delayed scans (10%)
CT with intraarterial ethiodol injection:
√ hyperdense mass detectable as small as 0.5 cm
US (sensitivity 86 – 99%; specificity 90 – 93%; accuracy 65 – 94%):
√ hyperechoic large tumor (59%) / hypoechoic small tumors (26%) / mixed echogenicity in diffuse form (15%)
MRI:
√ iso- / hyperintense (50%), hyperintense (50%) on T1WI
√ well-defined capsule hypointense on T1WI (24 – 44%), double layer of inner hypointensity (fibrous tissue) + outer hyperintensity (compressed blood vessels + bile ducts) on T2WI in expansive-type of HCC
√ hyperintense on T2W
√ Gd-DTPA enhancement peripherally (21%) / centrally (7%) / mixed (10%) / no enhancement (21%)
Angio:
√ "thread and streaks" = linear parallel vascular channels coursing along portal venous radicles seen with portal venous involvement
√ in differentiated HCC: enlarged arterial feeders, coarse neovascularity, vascular lakes, dense tumor stain, arterioportal shunts
√ in anaplastic HCC: vascular encasement, fine neovascularity, displacement of vessels + corkscrew-like vessels of cirrhosis

FIBROLAMELLAR HEPATOCELLULAR CARCINOMA
NO underlying cirrhosis or known risk factors
• alpha-fetoprotein negative
Age: 5 – 35 (mean 23) years
Path: well-circumscribed strikingly desmoplastic tumor with calcifications + fibrous central scar
√ partially / completely encapsulated solitary mass 4 – 17 cm in diameter
√ prominent depressed central fibrous scar
√ central stellate / trabecular calcifications (40%)
MRI:
√ heterogeneously hypointense on T1WI; hyperintense on T2WI
√ central scar hypointense on T1WI + T2WI (DDx: hyperintense scar on T2WI in FNH)

Prognosis:
Δ overall mortality: > 90%
Δ resectability rate: 17% (48% for fibrolamellar subtype)
Δ average survival time: 6 months (32 months for fibrolamellar subtype)
Δ 5-year survival time: 30% (63% for fibrolamellar subtype)
Cx: spontaneous rupture (in 8%)
Rx: (1) resection (2) I-131 antiferritin IgG (remission rate > 40% up to 3 years)

HYPOSPLENISM
= NO uptake of Tc-99m sulfur colloid

A. ANATOMIC ABSENCE OF SPLEEN
   1. Congenital asplenia = Ivemark syndrome
   2. Splenectomy
B. FUNCTIONAL ASPLENIA
   = spleen anatomically present without uptake of Tc-99m sulfur colloid
   1. Circulatory disturbances:
      Occlusion of splenic artery / vein, Hemoglobinopathies (sickle cell disease, hemoglobin-SC disease, thalassemia), Polycythemia vera, Idiopathic thrombocytopenic purpura
   2. Altered RES activity:
      Thorotrast irradiation, Combined splenic irradiation + chemotherapy, Replacement of RES by tumor / infiltrate, Splenic anoxia (cyanotic congenital heart disease), Sprue
   3. Autoimmune disease
      Cx: children at risk for pneumococcal pneumonia (liver partially takes over immune response later in life)
C. FUNCTIONAL ASPLENIA + SPLENIC ATROPHY
   Ulcerative colitis, Crohn disease, Celiac disease, Tropical sprue, Dermatitis herpetiformis, Thyrotoxicosis, Idiopathic thrombocytopenic purpura, Thorotrast
D. FUNCTIONAL ASPLENIA + NORMAL / LARGE SPLEEN
   Sarcoidosis, Amyloidosis, Sickle cell anemia (if not infarcted)

• RBC (acanthocytes, siderocytes)
• lymphocytosis, monocytosis
• Howell-Jolly bodies (intraerythrocytic inclusions)
• thrombocytosis
√ spleen not visualized on Tc-99m sulfur colloid
√ Tc-99m heat-damaged RBCs / In-111 labeled platelets may demonstrate splenic tissue if Tc-99m sulfur colloid does not
Cx: increased risk of infection (pneumococcus, meningococcus, influenza)

HYPERPLASTIC CHOLECYSTOSIS

= variety of degenerative + proliferative changes of gallbladder wall characterized by hyperconcentration, hyperexcitability, and hyperexcretion
Incidence: 30 – 50% of all cholecystectomy specimens; M:F = 1:6

Cholesterolosis

= abnormal deposits of cholesterol esters in macrophages within lamina propria (foam cells) + in mucosal epithelium

1. STRAWBERRY GALLBLADDER = LIPID CHOLECYSTITIS = CHOLESTEROSIS
   = planar form = seedlike patchy / diffuse thickening of the villous surface pattern (disseminated micronodules)
   Associated with cholesterol stones in 50 – 70%
   • not related to serum cholesterol level
   √ radiologically not demonstrable

2. CHOLESTEROL POLYP (90%) = polypoid form
   = abnormal deposit of cholesterol ester producing a villouslike structure covered with a single layer of epithelium and attached via a delicate stalk
   Location: commonly in middle 1/3 of gallbladder
   √ multiple small filling defects < 10 mm in diameter
   Δ most common fixed filling defect of GB
   DDx: papilloma, adenopapilloma, inflammatory granuloma

Adenomyomatosis of Gallbladder

= increase in number + height of mucosal folds
Histo: hyperplasia of epithelial + muscular elements with mucosal outpouching of epithelial-lined cystic spaces through thickened muscular layers as tubules / crypts / saccules (= intramural diverticula = Rokitansky-Aschoff sinus)
Incidence: 5% of all cholecystectomies
Age: > 35 years;   M:F = 1:3
Associated with: (1)   gallstones in 25 – 75%
                           (2)   cholesterolosis in 33%

(a) generalized form = ADENOMYOMATOSIS
    √ "pearl necklace gallbladder" = tiny extraluminal extensions of contrast on OCG (enhanced after contraction)
(b) segmental form
    compartmentalization most often in neck / distal 1/3
(c) localized form in fundus = ADENOMYOMA
    √ smooth sessile fundal mass in GB fundus
    = solitary adenomyoma + extraluminal diverticulalike formation
(d) annular form
    √ "hourglass" configuration of GB with transverse congenital septum

KAWASAKI SYNDROME

= MUCOCUTANEOUS LYMPH NODE SYNDROME
Histo: vasculitis
Age: < 5 years of age; M > F
• fever, mucosal reddening
• cervical adenopathy
• rash on palms + soles with desquamation
• polyarthritis
• myocarditis
√ coronary artery aneurysm
√ intestinal pseudoobstruction
√ transient gallbladder hydrops
Prognosis: 1 – 2% mortality (from coronary thrombosis)

LIPOMA OF LIVER

extremely rare
• asymptomatic
May be associated with tuberous sclerosis
US:
    √ echogenic mass
    √ striking acoustic refraction (sound velocity in soft tissue 1,540 m/sec, in fat 1,450 m/sec)
Prognosis: no malignant potential

LYMPHOMA OF LIVER

A. Primary Lymphoma (rare)
   √ solid solitary mass
B. Secondary Lymphoma (common)
   Autoptic incidence of liver involvement:
       60% in Hodgkin disease
       50% in Non-Hodgkin lymphoma
Pattern:
   (1)   Infiltrative diffuse (most common): no alteration in hepatic architecture
   (2)   Focal nodular: detectable by cross-sectional imaging
   (3)   Combination of diffuse + nodular (3%)
DETECTION RATE (for CT, MRI):   < 10%

MACROCYSTIC ADENOMA OF PANCREAS

= MUCINOUS CYSTIC NEOPLASM
= thickwalled uni- / multilocular benign tumor composed of large cystic spaces
Mean age: 50 years; in 50% between 40 – 60 years; M:F = 1:9
Histo: cysts lined by columnar, mucin-producing cells often in papillary arrangement, lack of cellular glycogen
Location: often in pancreatic tail (85%) / tail, infrequently in head
√ well-demarcated thick-walled mass of 5 – 33 (mean 12) cm in diameter
√ large cysts > 2 cm, uni- / multilocular with septations
√ curvilinear peripheral mural calcifications (15%)
√ hypovascular mass with sparse neovascularity
√ vascular encasement and splenic vein occlusion may be present

√ solid papillary excrescences protrude into the interior of tumor (sign of malignancy)

Metastases: √ round thick-walled cystic lesions in liver

Prognosis: invariable transformation into cystadenocarcinoma

MESENCHYMAL HAMARTOMA OF LIVER

= rare developmental cystic liver tumor

Histo: disordered arrangement of primitive mesenchyme, bile ducts, hepatic parenchyma; stromal / cystic predominance with cysts of a few mm up to 14 cm in size; no capsule

Age peak: 15 – 22 months (range from newborn to 19 years); M:F = 2:1

Location: right lobe:left lobe = 6:1; 20% pedunculated

√ 16 cm average tumor size (range of 5 – 29 cm)

√ grossly discernible cysts in 80%

US:
  √ multiple rounded cystic areas on an echogenic background
  √ may appear solid in younger infant (when cysts are still small)

CT:
  √ multiple lucencies of variable size + attenuation

NUC:
  √ one / more areas of diminished uptake on sulfur colloid scan

Angio:
  √ hypovascular mass
  √ may show patchy areas of neovascularity
  √ enlarged irregular tortuous feeding vessels

METASTASES TO LIVER

Incidence:
liver is most common metastatic site after regional lymph nodes; incidence of metastatic carcinoma 20 x greater than primary carcinoma; metastases represent 22% of all liver tumors in patients with known malignancy; most common malignant lesion of the liver

Organ of origin: colon (42%), stomach (23%), pancreas (21%), breast (14%), lung (13%)
• hepatomegaly (70%)
• abnormal liver enzymes (50 – 75%)

Location :   both lobes (77%), right lobe (20%), left lobe (3%)

Number :   multiple (98%), solitary (2%)

√ involvement of liver + spleen typical in lymphoma + melanoma

US: most sensitive imaging modality

NUC: sensitivity 90 – 95% in lesions > 1.5 cm; lesions < 2 cm are frequently missed

CT: sensitivity 88 – 90%; specificity 99%; lesions of approx. 1 cm can usually be detected

CECT:
  √ no (35%), peripheral (37%), mixed (20%), central (8%) enhancement
  √ complete isodense fill-in on delayed scans (5%)

CT-Angiography:
(additional lesions detected in 40 – 55%)
  (1) CT arteriography = angiography catheter in hepatic artery, detects lesions by virtue of increased enhancement
  (2) CT arterial portography = angiography catheter in SMA, detects hypodense lesions on a background of increased enhancement of normal surroundings in portal venous phase

CT-delayed iodine scanning:
= CT performed 4 – 6 hours following administration of 60 mg iodine results in detection of additional lesions in 27%

CALCIFIED LIVER METASTASES
Incidence: 2 – 3%
1. Mucinous carcinoma of GI tract (colon, rectum, stomach)
2. Endocrine pancreatic carcinoma
3. Leiomyosarcoma, osteosarcoma
4. Malignant melanoma
5. Papillary serous ovarian cystadenocarcinoma
6. Lymphoma
7. Pleural mesothelioma
8. Neuroblastoma
9. Breast cancer
10. Medullary carcinoma of the thyroid
11. Renal cell carcinoma
12. Lung carcinoma
13. Testicular carcinoma

HYPERVASCULAR LIVER METASTASES
1. Renal cell carcinoma
2. Carcinoid tumor
3. Colonic carcinoma
4. Choriocarcinoma
5. Breast carcinoma
6. Melanoma
7. Pancreatic islet cell tumor
8. Ovarian cystadenocarcinoma
9. Sarcomas
10. Pheochromocytoma

ECHOGENIC LIVER METASTASES
Incidence: 25%
1. Colonic carcinoma (mucinous adenocarcinoma) 54%
2. Hepatoma 25%
3. Treated breast carcinoma 21%

LIVER METASTASES OF MIXED ECHOGENICITY
Incidence: 37.5%
1. Breast cancer   31%
2. Rectal cancer   20%
3. Lung cancer   17%
4. Stomach cancer   14%
5. Anaplastic cancer   11%
6. Cervical cancer   5%
7. Carcinoid   1%

CYSTIC LIVER METASTASES
1. Mucinous ovarian carcinoma
2. Colonic carcinoma
3. Sarcoma
4. Melanoma
5. Lung carcinoma
6. Carcinoid tumor

ECHOPENIC LIVER METASTASES
Incidence: 37.5%
1. Lymphoma   44%
2. Pancreas   36%
3. Cervical cancer   20%
4. Lung (adenocarcinoma)
5. Nasopharyngeal cancer

MICROCYSTIC ADENOMA OF PANCREAS
= SEROUS CYSTADENOMA = GLYCOGEN-RICH
  CYSTADENOMA
= benign lobulated neoplasm composed of innumerable
  small cysts (1 – 20 mm) containing proteinaceous fluid
  separated by thin connective tissue septa
Incidence: approximately 50% of all cystic pancreatic
                neoplasms
Histo: cyst walls lined by cuboidal / flat glycogen-rich
            epithelial cells derived from centroacinar cells of
            pancreas (DDx: lymphangioma), thin fibrous
            pseudocapsule
Age: 34 – 88 years; mean age 65 years;
          82% over 60 years of age;   M:F = 1:4
Associated with: von Hippel-Lindau syndrome
• pain, weight loss, jaundice
• palpable mass
Location: any part of pancreas affected, slight
            predominance for head
√ well-demarcated lobulated mass 4 – 25 (mean 13) cm
  in diameter
√ innumerable small < 2 cm cysts; uncommonly larger
  cyst up to 8 cm in diameter
√ prominent central stellate scar
√ amorphous central calcifications (in 33% on plain film) in
  dystrophic area of scar ("sunburst")
√ pancreatic duct + CBD may be displaced, encased or
  obstructed
US:
  √ solid predominantly echogenic mass with mixed
    hypoechoic + echogenic areas
CT:
  √ attenuation values close to water
  √ contrast enhancement
Angio:
  √ hypervascular mass with dilated feeding arteries,
    dense tumor blush, prominent draining veins,
    neovascularity, occasional AV shunting, NO vascular
    encasement
Prognosis: no malignant potential
Rx: surgical excision / follow-up examinations

MILK OF CALCIUM BILE
= LIMY BILE = CALCIUM SOAP = precipitation of
  particulate material with high concentration of calcium
  carbonate, calcium phosphate, calcium bilirubinate
Associated with: chronic cholecystitis + gallstone
                    obstruction of cystic duct
√ diffuse opacification of GB lumen with dependent
  layering
√ usually functionless GB on oral cholecystogram
US: √ intermediate features between sludge + gallstones

MIRIZZI SYNDROME
= extrinsic right-sided compression of common hepatic
  duct by large gallstone impacted in cystic duct /
  gallbladder neck / cystic duct remnant; accompanied by
  chronic inflammatory reaction
Frequently associated with   formation of fistula between
  gallbladder and common hepatic duct
√ normal CBD
TRIAD:
  √ stone impacted in GB neck
  √ dilatation of intrahepatic ducts + CHD
  √ smooth curved segmental stenosis of CHD
DDx: lymphadenopathy, neoplasm of GB / CHD

NEONATAL HEPATITIS
Etiology: CMV, hepatitis A/B, rubella, toxoplasmosis,
              spirochetes, idiopathic
Path: multinucleated giant cells, bile ducts relatively
           free of bile
NUC:
  √ normal / decreased hepatic tracer accumulation
  √ prolonged clearance of tracer from blood pool
  √ bowel activity faint / delayed (best seen on lateral
    view) usually by 24 hours
  √ gallbladder may not be visualized
Prognosis: spontaneous remission

PANCREAS DIVISUM
= failure of fusion of the ventral and dorsal anlage at 8th
  week of fetal life
  (a) dorsal anlage: develops into tail, body, and cranial
      portion of pancreatic head; drains to the minor
      papilla through accessory duct of Santorini
  (b) ventral anlage: arises between duodenum and liver
      bud; forms the caudal portion of the pancreatic
      head, uncinate process and CBD; the ventral duct
      of WIRSUNG drains with the CBD through ampulla
      of Vater and becomes the major drainage pathway
      for the entire pancreas after fusion with the duct of
      SANTORINI
Incidence: 4 – 14% in autopsy series;
                1.3 – 6.7% in ERCP series;
                3 – 4% in normal population;
                12 – 26% in patients with idiopathic recurrent
                pancreatitis
Hypothesis: relative / actual stenosis of minor papilla
             predisposes to pancreatitis in dorsal
             segment

Pancreatography: ONLY reliable means for diagnosis
CT:
√ oblique fat cleft between ventral + dorsal pancreas (25%)
√ failure to see union of dorsal + ventral pancreatic ducts (rare)

PANCREATIC DUCTAL ADENOCARCINOMA
= DUCT CELL ADENOCARCINOMA

Incidence: 80% of nonendocrine pancreatic neoplasms, 4th – 5th leading cause of cancer death in the United States

Etiology: alcohol abuse (4%), diabetes (2 x more frequent than in general population, particularly in females), hereditary pancreatitis (in 40%); cigarette smoking (risk factor 2 x)

Path: scirrhous infiltrative adenocarcinoma

Mean age at onset: 55 years; peak age in 7th decade; M:F = 2:1

Origin: - in 99% exocrine ductal epithelium
- in 1% acinar portion of pancreatic glands
- in 0.1% malignant ampullary tumor with better prognosis

STAGE I   = confined to pancreas
     II   = + regional lymph node metastases
     III   = + distant spread

Extension:
(a) local extension beyond margins of organ (68%): posteriorly (96%), anteriorly (30%), into porta hepatis (15%), into splenic hilum (13%)
(b) invasion of adjacent organs (42%): duodenum > stomach > left adrenal gland > spleen > root of small bowel mesentery

Metastases:
liver (30 – 36%), regional lymph nodes > 2 cm (15 – 28%), ascites from peritoneal carcinomatosis (7 – 10%), lungs (pulmonary nodules / lymphangitic), pleura, bone

- weight loss, anorexia, fatigue
- abdominal pain radiating to back
- obstructive jaundice (75%): most frequent cause of malignant biliary obstruction
- new onset diabetes (25 – 50%)

Location: pancreatic head (56 – 62%); body (26%); tail (12%)

√ Size: 2 – 10 cm (in 60% between 4 – 6 cm)

UGI:
√ "antral padding" = extrinsic indentation of the posteroinferior margin of antrum
√ "Frostberg 3" sign = inverted 3 contour to the medial portion of the duodenal sweep
√ spiculated duodenal wall + traction + fixation (neoplastic infiltration of duodenal mucosa / desmoplastic response)
√ irregular / smooth nodular mass with ampullary carcinoma

BE:
√ localized haustral padding / flattening / narrowing with serrated contour at inferior aspect of transverse colon / splenic flexure
√ diffuse tethering throughout peritoneal cavity (intraperitoneal seeding)

CT (for dynamic CT detection rate of 99%; 100% in predicting unresectability):
√ pancreatic mass (95%) / diffuse enlargement (4%) / normal scan (1%)
√ mass with central zone of diminished attenuation (75 – 83%)
√ pancreatic + bile duct obstruction without detectable mass (4%)
√ duct dilatation (58%): 3/4 biductal, 1/10 isolated to one duct; dilated pancreatic duct (67%); dilated bile ducts (38%)
√ atrophy of pancreatic body + tail (20%)
√ calcifications (2%)
√ postobstructive pseudocyst (11%)
√ obliteration of retropancreatic fat (50%)
√ thickening of celiac axis / SMA in 60% (invasion of perivascular lymphatics)
√ dilated collateral veins (12%)
√ thickening of Gerota fascia (5%)
√ local tumor extension posteriorly, into splenic hilum, into porta hepatis (68%)
√ contiguous organ invasion (duodenum, stomach, mesenteric root (42%)

US:
√ hypoechoic pancreatic mass
√ focal / diffuse (10%) enlargement of pancreas
√ contour deformity of gland; rounding of uncinate process
√ dilatation of pancreatic ± biliary duct

Angiography (accuracy 70%):
√ hypovascular tumor / neovascularity (50%)
√ arterial encasement: SMA (33%), splenic artery (14%), celiac trunk (11%), hepatic artery (11%), gastroduodenal artery (3%), left renal artery (0.6%)
√ venous obstruction: splenic vein (34%), SMV (10%)
√ venous encasement: SMV (23%), splenic vein (15%), portal vein (4%)

Cholangiography:
√ occlusion of CBD in configuration of "rattail / nipplelike"
√ nodular mass / meniscus-like occlusion in ampullary tumors

Pancreatography: (abnormal in 97%)
√ irregular, nodular, rattailed, eccentric obstruction
√ localized encasement with prestenotic dilatation
√ acinar defect

Prognosis:
1-year survival in 10%, 3-year survival in 2%, 5-year survival < 1%; medial survival after curative resection is 14 months, after palliative resection 8 months, without treatment 5 months, tumors resectable in only 8 – 15% at presentation, 5% 5-year survival rate after surgery

DDx: focal pancreatitis, islet cell carcinoma, metastasis, lymphoma, normal variant

PANCREATIC ISLET CELL TUMORS
Origin: embryonic neuroectoderm, derivatives of APUD (amino precursor and uptake decarboxylation) cell line arising from islet of Langerhans (APUDOMA)
Prevalence: 1:100,000; isolated or part of MEN I syndrome
Average time from onset of symptoms to diagnosis is 2.7 years
Classification: (a) functional (85%)
             (b) nonfunctional (below threshold of detectability) / hypofunctional
Metastases: in 60 – 90% to liver ± regional lymph nodes
√ calcifications highly suggestive of malignancy

Insulinoma
most common functioning islet cell tumor
Age: 4th – 6th decade; M:F = 2:3
Associated with: MEN Type I
Path: (a) single benign adenoma (80 – 90%)
      (b) multiple adenomas / microadenomatosis (5 – 10%)
      (c) islet cell hyperplasia (5 – 10%)
      (d) malignant adenoma (5 – 10%)
• Whipple triad: starvation attack + hypoglycemia (fasting glucose < 50 mg/dl) + relief by IV dextrose
• obesity
Location: anywhere within pancreas (head = body = tail), 2 – 5% in ectopic location; 10% multiple
√ average tumor size 1 – 2 cm; < 1.5 cm in 70%
√ solid homogeneous hypoechoic mass
√ hypervascular tumor (66%): accurate angiographic localization in 60 – 90%
√ pancreatic venous sampling (correct localization in 95%)
Prognosis: malignant transformation in 5 – 10%

Gastrinoma
2nd most common islet cell tumor; in alpha-cells / delta-cells
Age: 8% in patients < 20 years; M > F
Path: (a) solitary adenoma (25%)
      (b) multiple adenomas (20%)
      (c) ectopic (7 – 33%) in duodenal wall / peripancreatic nodes / stomach / omentum
Associated with: MEN Type I (in 20 – 40%)
• Zollinger-Ellison syndrome: peptic ulcers, malabsorption, hypokalemia, gastric hypersecretion, hyperacidity / occasionally hypoacidity, diarrhea
• GI bleeding
Location: 50% solitary in head / tail; 10% diffuse hyperplasia; rarely ectopic
√ average tumor size 3.4 cm (up to 10 cm)
√ successful angiographic localization in 70% (hypervascular lesion)

√ homogeneous hypoechoic mass (sonographic detection rate 50%)
Prognosis: 60% malignant transformation

Glucagonoma
uncommon tumor; derived from alpha cells;
Associated with MEN
M < F
• necrolytic erythema migrans (erythematous macules / papules on lower extremity, groin, buttocks, face)
• diarrhea, diabetes, glossitis, weight loss, anemia
Location: predominantly in pancreatic body / tail
√ tumor size 2.5 – 25 cm (mean 6.4 cm)
√ hypervascular in 90%; successful angiographic localization in 15%
Prognosis: in 80% malignant transformation (liver metastases at time of diagnosis in 50%)

Vipoma
= **v**asoactive **i**ntestinal **p**eptides, from delta cells
Histo: adenoma / hyperplasia
• WDHA syndrome = watery diarrhea + hypokalemia + achlorhydria ("pancreatic cholera") = Verner-Morrison syndrome
Location: predominantly in pancreatic body / tail
√ average size 5 – 10 cm
√ mostly hypervascular tumor
√ dilatation of gallbladder
Prognosis: in 60% malignant transformation

Somatostatinoma
Somatostatin function: suppresses release of growth hormone, TSH, insulin, glucagon, gastric acid, pepsin, secretin
— from delta cells
• diabetes, cholelithiasis, dyspepsia
Location: predominantly in pancreatic head
√ tumor size 0.6 – 20 cm (average > 4 cm)
Prognosis: 90% malignant transformation

Nonfunctioning Islet Cell Tumors
Incidence:
3rd most common islet cell tumor after insulinoma + gastrinoma; 15 – 25% of all islet cell tumors
— either from alpha or beta cells
Age: 24 – 74 (mean 57) years
• mostly asymptomatic
• palpable mass, gastric outlet obstruction, jaundice, GI-bleeding
Location: predominantly in pancreatic head
√ tumor size 6 – 20 cm (> 5 cm in 72%)
√ coarse nodular calcifications (22%)
√ CT contrast enhancement in 83%
√ hypoechoic mass
√ late dense capillary stain
√ large irregular pathological vessels with early venous filling
Prognosis: in 80 – 90% malignant transformation; 60% 3-year survival; 44% 5-year survival

PANCREATIC LIPOMATOSIS
Etiology:
1. Atherosclerosis of elderly
2. Obesity
3. Steroid therapy
4. Cushing syndrome
5. Main pancreatic duct obstruction
6. Cystic fibrosis
7. Malnutrition
8. Hemochromatosis
9. Viral infection
10. Schwachman-Diamond syndrome

US:
√ increased pancreatic echogenicity
CT:
√ "marbling" of pancreatic parenchyma / total fatty replacement / lipomatous pseudohypertrophy

PANCREATIC PSEUDOCYST
Etiology: (a) acute pancreatitis ; pseudocysts mature in 6 – 8 weeks
(b) chronic pancreatitis
(c) posttraumatic
(d) pancreatic cancer
Incidence: 2 – 4% in acute pancreatitis
10 – 15% in chronic pancreatitis

Location: 2/3 within pancreas
Atypical location (can dissect along tissue planes in 1/3):
1. intraperitoneal: mesentery of small bowel / transverse colon / sigmoid colon
2. retroperitoneal: along psoas muscle; may present as groin mass / in scrotum
3. intraparenchymal: liver, spleen, kidney
4. mediastinal (through esophageal hiatus > aortic hiatus > foramen of Morgagni > erosion through diaphragm): may present as neck mass

Plain film / contrast radiograph:
√ smooth extrinsic indentation of posterior wall of stomach / inner duodenal sweep (80%)
√ indentation / displacement of splenic flexure / transverse colon (40%)
√ downward displacement of duodenojejunal junction
√ gastric outlet obstruction
√ splaying of renal collecting system / ureteral obstruction

US (pseudocyst detectable in 50 – 92%; 92 – 96% accuracy):
√ usually single + unilocular cyst
√ multilocular in 6%
√ fluid-debris level / internal echoes (may contain sequester, blood clot, cellular debris from autolysis)
√ septations (rare; sign of infection / hemorrhage)
√ may increase in size (secondary to hypertonicity of fluid, communication with pancreatic duct, hemorrhage, erosion of vessel)
√ obstruction of pancreatic duct / CBD

CT:
√ fluid in pseudocyst (0 – 30 HU)
√ cyst wall calcification (extremely rare)
Pancreatography:
√ communication with pancreatic duct in 50%
Cx (in 40%):
1. Rupture into abdominal cavity, stomach, colon, duodenum
2. Hemorrhage / formation of pseudoaneurysm
3. Infection
√ gas bubbles (DDx: fistulous communication to GI tract)
√ increase in attenuation of fluid contents
4. Intestinal obstruction
Prognosis: spontaneous resolution (in 20 – 50%) secondary to rupture into GI tract / pancreatic / bile duct
DDx: Pancreatic cystadenoma, Cystadenocarcinoma, Necrotic pancreatic arcinoma, Fluid-filled bowel loop, Fluid-filled stomach, Duodenal diverticulum, Aneurysm

PANCREATITIS
Etiology:
A. IDIOPATHIC (20%)
B. ALCOHOLISM: acute pancreatitis (15%); chronic pancreatitis (70%)
C. CHOLELITHIASIS: acute pancreatitis (75%); chronic pancreatitis (20%)
D. METABOLIC DISORDERS
1. <u>Hypercalcemia</u> in hyperparathyroidism (10%), multiple myeloma, amyloidosis, sarcoidosis
2. <u>Hereditary pancreatitis</u>: autosomal dominant, only Caucasians affected, most common cause of large spherical pancreatic calcifications in childhood, recurrent episodes of pancreatitis, development into pancreatic carcinoma in 20 – 40%; pronounced dilatation of pancreatic duct; pseudocyst formation (50%); associated with type I hypercholesterolemia
3. <u>Hyperlipidemia</u> Types I and V
4. <u>Kwashiorkor</u> = Tropical Pancreatitis
E. INFECTION / INFESTATION
1. Viral infection (mumps, hepatitis, mononucleosis)
2. Parasites (ascariasis, clonorchis)
F. TRAUMA
1. Penetrating ulcer
2. Surgery, Blunt / penetrating trauma
G. STRUCTURAL ABNORMALITIES
1. Pancreas divisum
2. Choledochocele
H. DRUGS
azathioprine, thiazide, furosemide, ethacrynic acid, sulfonamides, tetracycline, phenformin, procainamide, steroids (e.g. renal transplant)
I. MALIGNANCY
Pancreatic carcinoma (in 1%), metastases, lymphoma

Acute Pancreatitis
= inflammatory disease of pancreas producing temporary changes with restoration of normal anatomy + function following resolution

Path:
1. EDEMATOUS PANCREATITIS:
   edema, congestion, leukocytic infiltrates; mortality rate of 4%
2. NECROTIZING PANCREATITIS:
   proteolytic destruction of pancreaticparenchyma; mortality rate of 80 – 90%
   (a) HEMORRHAGIC PANCREATITIS:
       + fat necrosis and hemorrhage
   (b) SUPPURATIVE PANCREATITIS:
       + bacterial infection

A. Diffuse form (52%)
B. Focal form (48%): location of head:tail = 3:2
- abdominal pain, nausea, vomiting
- raised pancreatic amylase + lipase in blood + urine
- increased amylase-creatinine clearance ratio

√ NO findings on US / CT in 29%

Abdominal film:
√ "colon cutoff" sign = dilated transverse colon with abrupt change to a gasless descending colon (inflammation via phrenicocolic ligament causes spasm + obstruction at the splenic flexure impinging on a paralytic colon)
√ "sentinel loop" (10 – 55%) = localized segment of gas-containing bowel in duodenum (in 20 – 45%) / terminal ileum / cecum
√ "renal halo" sign = water-density of inflammation in anterior pararenal space contrasts with perirenal fat; more common on left side
√ mottled appearance of peripancreatic area (secondary to fat necrosis in pancreatic bed, mesentery, omentum)
√ intrapancreatic gas bubbles (from acute gangrene / suppurative pancreatitis)
√ "gasless abdomen" = fluid-filled bowel associated with vomiting
√ ascites

CXR (findings in 14 – 71%):
√ pleural effusion (in 5%), usually left-sided, with elevated amylase levels (in 85%)
√ diaphragmatic elevation, atelectasis (20%), pulmonary infiltrates, ARDS

UGI:
√ esophagogastric varices (from splenic vein obstruction)
√ enlarged tortuous edematous rugal folds along antrum + greater curvature (20%)
√ widening of retrogastric space (from pancreatic enlargement / inflammation in lesser sac)
√ diminished duodenal peristalsis + edematous folds
√ widening of duodenal sweep + downward displacement of ligament of Treitz
√ Poppel sign = edematous swelling of papilla

√ Frostberg inverted 3 sign = segmental narrowing with fold thickening of duodenum
√ jejunal + ileal fold thickening (proteolytic spread along mesentery)

BE:
√ narrowing, nodularity, fold distortion along inferior haustral row of transverse colon ± descending colon

Cholangiography:
√ long gently tapered narrowing of CBD
√ prestenotic biliary dilatation
√ smooth / irregular mucosal surface

Bone films (findings in 6%):
secondary to metastatic intramedullary lipolysis + fat necrosis
√ punched out / permeative destruction of cancellous bone + endosteal erosion
√ aseptic necrosis of femoral / humeral heads
√ metaphyseal infarcts, predominantly in distal femur + proximal tibia

US (pancreatic visualization in 62 – 78%):
√ hypoechoic diffuse / focal enlargement of pancreas
√ dilatation of pancreatic duct (if head focally involved)
√ extrapancreatic hypoechoic mass with good acoustic transmission = phlegmonous pancreatitis)
√ fluid collection: lesser sac (60%), L > R anterior pararenal space (54%), posterior pararenal space (18%), around left lobe of liver (16%), in spleen (9%), mediastinum (3%)
√ pseudocyst formation (52%): extension into lesser sac, transverse mesocolon, around kidney, mediastinum, lower quadrants of abdomen

CT (pancreatic visualization in 98%):
√ no detectable change in size / appearance (29%)
√ hypodense (5 – 20 HU) mass in phlegmonous pancreatitis; may persist long after complete recovery
√ hyperdense areas (50 – 70 HU) in hemorrhagic pancreatitis for 24 – 48 hours
√ enlargement with convex margins + indistinctness of gland with parenchymal inhomogeneity
√ thickening of anterior pararenal fascia
√ non-contrast-enhancing parenchyma during bolus injection (= pancreatic necrosis)

Angiography: (may be normal)
√ hypovascular areas (15 – 56%)
√ hypervascularity + increased parenchymal stain (12 – 45%)
√ venous compression secondary to edema
√ formation of pseudoaneurysms (in 10% with chronic pancreatitis): splenic artery (50%), pancreatic arcades, gastroduodenal artery

Cx:
1. Phlegmon (18%): extension into lesser sac, anterior pararenal space, transverse mesocolon, small bowel mesentery, retroperitoneum, pelvis
2. Pseudocyst formation (10%)

3. Hemorrhage (3%)
4. Abscess (2 – 10%): 2 – 4 weeks after severe acute pancreatitis; most common due to E. coli; DDx: air secondary to intestinal fistula
5. Pancreatic ascites
6. Biliary duct obstruction
7. Pseudoaneurysm
   (a) rupture into preexisting pseudocyst
   (b) digestion of arterial wall by enzymes
   Incidence: in up to 10% of severe pancreatitis
   Location: splenic artery (most common)
   Mortality: 37% for rupture, 16 – 50% for surgery
8. Thrombosis of splenic vein / SMV

Chronic Pancreatitis

= continuing inflammatory disease of pancreas characterized by irreversible damage to anatomy + function
A. CHRONIC CALCIFYING PANCREATITIS:
   √ protein plugs / calculi within ductal system
B. CHRONIC OBSTRUCTIVE PANCREATITIS:
   secondary to slow growing tumor / surgical duct ligation / ampullary stenosis
   √ dilatation of pancreatic duct
   √ normal sized / focally or diffusely enlarged / small atrophic gland
   √ calcifications uncommon
- acute exacerbation of epigastric pain / painless
- steatorrhea, diabetes mellitus (80%)
- secretin test with decreased amylase + bicarbonate in duodenal fluid
Plain films:
   √ numerous irregular calcifications (in 20 – 50% of alcoholic pancreatitis)
UGI:
   √ displacement of stomach / duodenum by pseudocyst
   √ shrinkage / fold induration of stomach (DDx: linitis plastica)
   √ stricture of duodenum
Cholangiopancreatography (most sensitive imaging modality):
   √ slight ductal ectasia / clubbing of side branches (minimal disease)
   √ "nipping" = narrowing of the origins of side branches
   √ dilatation > 2 mm, tortuosity, wall rigidity, main ductal stenosis (moderate disease)
   √ "beading, chain of lakes, string of pearls" = dilatation, stenosis, obstruction of main pancreatic duct + side branches (severe disease)
   √ intraductal protein plugs / calculi
   √ prolonged emptying of contrast material
   √ may have stenosis / obstruction + prestenotic dilatation of CBD
US/ CT:
   √ irregular (73%) / smooth (15%) / beaded (12%) pancreatic ductal dilatation (in 41 – 68%)

√ small atrophic gland (in 10 – 54%)
√ pancreatic mostly intraductal calcifications (4 – 68%)
√ inhomogeneous gland with increased echogenicity (62%)
√ irregular pancreatic contour (45 – 60%)
√ focal (12 – 30%) / diffuse (27 – 45%) pancreatic enlargement
√ mostly mild biliary ductal dilatation (29%)
√ intra- / peripancreatic pseudocysts (20 – 25%)
√ segmental portal hypertension (= splenic vein thrombosis + splenomegaly)
√ arterial pseudoaneurysm formation
√ peripancreatic fascial thickening + blurring of organ margins (16%)
Angiography:
   √ increased tortuosity + angulation of pancreatic arcades + intrahepatic arteries (88%)
   √ luminal irregularities / focal fibrotic arterial stenoses (25 – 75%) / smooth beaded appearance
   √ irregular parenchymal stain
   √ venous compression / occlusion (20 – 50%)
   √ portoportal shunting + gastric varices without esophageal varices
   Cx: pancreatic carcinoma (4%)

PAPILLARY STENOSIS

Etiology:
A. PRIMARY PAPILLARY STENOSIS (10%)
   1. Congenital malformation of papilla
   2. Sequelae of acute / chronic inflammation
   3. Adenomyosis
B. SECONDARY PAPILLARY STENOSIS (90%)
   1. Mechanical trauma of stone passage (choledocholithiasis in 64%; cholecystolithiasis in 26%)
   2. Functional stenosis: associated with pancreas divisum, history of pancreatitis
   3. Reflex spasm
   4. Previous surgical manipulation
   5. Periampullary neoplasm

√ prestenotic dilatation of CBD
√ increase in pancreatic duct diameter (83%)
√ long smooth narrowing / beak (fibrotic stenosis)
√ prolonged bile-to-bowel transit time > 45 minutes on Tc-IDA scintigraphy

PORCELAIN GALLBLADDER

= calcium incrustation of gallbladder wall
Incidence: 0.6 – 0.8% of cholecystectomy patients
M:F = 1:5
Histo:
1. Flakes of dystrophic calcium within chronically inflamed + fibrotic muscular wall
2. Microliths scattered diffusely throughout mucosa, submucosa, glandular spaces, Rokitansky-Aschoff sinuses

Associated with gallstones in 90%
- minimal symptoms
√ curvilinear (muscularis) / granular (mucosal) calcifications in segment / entire wall
√ nonfunctioning GB on oral cholecystogram
√ highly echogenic shadowing curvilinear structure in GB fossa (DDx: stone-filled contracted GB)
√ echogenic GB wall with little acoustic shadowing (DDx: emphysematous cholecystitis)
√ scattered irregular clumps of echoes with posterior acoustic shadowing
Cx: 10 – 20% develop carcinoma of gallbladder

PORTAL HYPERTENSION
- normal hepatic blood flow of 1.5 l/min (= 25% of cardiac output) passes through portal sytem (2/3) + through hepatic artery (1/3)

Classification:
A. PRESINUSOIDAL
   (a) EXTRAHEPATIC
      1. Portal Vein Obstruction
         — extrinsic compression (tumor, lymphadenopathy, fibrosis, pseudocyst, trauma)
         — occlusion (portal phlebitis, oral contraceptives, coagulopathy, neoplastic invasion, pancreatitis, neonatal omphalitis)
      2. Dynamic Portal Hypertension
         traumatic / neoplastic arterioportal fistula
      3. Segmental Portal Hypertension
         splenic vein occlusion / superior mesenteric vein occlusion
   (b) INTRAHEPATIC (= obstruction of portal venules)
      1. Congenital hepatic fibrosis
      2. Idiopathic noncirrhotic fibrosis
      3. Primary biliary cirrhosis
      4. Wilson disease
      5. Sarcoid liver disease
      6. Toxic fibrosis (arsenic, copper, PVC vapors)
      7. Reticuloendotheliosis
      8. Myelofibrosis
      9. Felty syndrome
      10. Schistosomiasis
      11. Chronic malaria
B. SINUSOIDAL
   (1) Cirrhosis (most frequent): Laennec cirrhosis, Postnecrotic cirrhosis from hepatitis
   (2) Sclerosing cholangitis
C. POSTSINUSOIDAL
   (1) Budd-Chiari syndrome
   (2) Constrictive pericarditis
   (3) Congestive heart failure
- elevated hepatic wedge pressure (HWP) = portal venous pressure; (normal < 10 mmHg); normal values seen in presinusoidal portal hypertension
- caput medusae
√ portal vein > 13 mm (57% sensitivity, 100% specificity)
√ portal vein aneurysm

√ portal vein thrombosis
√ SMV + splenic vein > 10 mm; coronary vein > 4 mm; recanalized umbilical vein > 3 mm (size of vessels not related to degree of portal hypertension or presence of collaterals)
√ loss of respiratory increase of splanchnic vein diameters (80% sensitivity, 100% specificity)
√ serpentine tubular rounded structures = porto-systemic collaterals: coronary, esophageal, splenorenal, omental, gastrosplenic, hemorrhoidal, retroperitoneal shunting veins (in up to 88%)
√ esophageal / gastric / sigmoid / rectal varices
√ hypoechoic channel in ligamentum teres
   (a) size < 2 mm (in 97% of normal subjects; in 14% of patients with portal hypertension)
   (b) size ≥ 2 mm (86% sensitivity for portal hypertension)
√ arterial signal on Doppler US in 38%
√ Cruveilhier-von Baumgarten syndrome (26%) = recanalized paraumbilical vein
√ hepatofugal venous flow (82% sensitivity, 100% specificity for portal hypertension)
√ cavernous transformation of portal vein
√ splenomegaly (absence does not rule out portal hypertension)
√ increased echogenicity + thickening of portal vein walls
√ ascites
Cx: Acute gastrointestinal bleeding (mortality of 30 – 50% during 1st bleeding)

PORTAL VEIN THROMBOSIS
Etiology:
   A. idiopathic (mostly): ? neonatal sepsis
   B. secondary:
      (1) tumor invasion by HCC, cholangiocarcinoma, pancreatic carcinoma, gastric carcinoma / extrinsic compression by tumor

      (2) trauma; blood dyscrasia; clotting disorder; estrogen therapy; Cx of splenectomy for myeloproliferative disease, severe dehydration
      (3) intraabdominal sepsis with phlebitis; pancreatitis; ascending cholangitis
      (4) cirrhosis + portal hypertension (5%)
Age: predominantly children, young persons
- abdominal pain
- portal systemic encephalopathy
- hematemesis (esophageal varices)
√ nonvisualization of portal vein
√ calcification within clot / wall of portal vein
√ splenomegaly
√ ascites
US:
   √ echogenic material within vessel lumen (67%)
   √ increase in diameter (57%)
   √ cavernous transformation = **cavernoma** (19%)
   √ portal vein collateral circulation (48%)
   √ enlargement of thrombosed segment > 15 mm (38%)

CECT:
√ low-density center in portal vein surrounded by
peripheral enhancement
√ portal vein density 20 – 30 HU less than aortic
density after contrast
Angio:
√ "thread and streaks" sign of tumor thrombus (streaky
contrast opacification of tumor vessels)
Cx: (1) Hepatic infarction
(2) Bowel infarction

POSTCHOLECYSTECTOMY SYNDROME
= symptoms recurring / persisting after cholecystectomy
Incidence:
mild recurrent symptoms in 9 – 25%; severe symptoms
in 2.6 – 32% result of 1,930 cholecystectomies:
— completely cured (61%)
— satisfactory improvement with
(a) persistent mild dyspepsia (11%)
(b) mild attacks of pain (24%)
— failure with
(a) occasional attacks of severe pain (3%)
(b) continuous severe distress (1.7%)
(c) recurrent cholangitis (0.7%)
Causes:
A. BILIARY CAUSES
(a) Incomplete surgery:
1. Gallbladder / cystic duct remnant
2. Retained stone in cystic duct remnant
3. Overlooked CBD stone
(b) Operative trauma
1. Bile duct stricture
2. Bile peritonitis
(c) Bile duct pathology
1. Fibrosis of sphincter of Oddi
2. Biliary dyskineasia
3. Biliary fistula
(d) Residual disease in neighboring structures
1. Pancreatitis
2. Hepatitis
3. Cholangitis
(e) Overlooked bile duct neoplasia
B. EXTRABILIARY CAUSES (erroneous preoperative
diagnosis)
(a) Other GI tract disease
1. Inadequate dentition
2. Hiatus hernia
3. Peptic ulcer
4. Spastic colon
(b) Anxiety state, Air swallowing
(c) Abdominal angina
(d) Carcinoma outside gallbladder
(e) Coronary artery disease

RICHTER SYNDROME
= development of large cell / diffuse histiocytic lymphoma
in patients with CLL
Etiology: transformation / dedifferentiation of CLL
lymphocytes

Incidence in CLL patients: 3 – 10%
Median age: 59 years
Medium time interval after diagnosis of CLL: 24 months
Median survival time: 4 months from diagnosis of
lymphoma; remission rate: 14%
• fever (65%) without evidence of infection
• increasing lymphadenopathy + hepatosplenomegaly
(46%)
• weight loss (26%)
• abdominal pain (26%)
Location: bone marrow, lymph nodes, liver, spleen,
bowel, lung, pleura, kidney, dura

SCHISTOSOMIASIS
worldwide major cause of portal hypertension: 200 million
people affected
Types:
A. SCHISTOSOMA HAEMATOBIUM
in Africa, Mediterranean, Southwest Asia
B. SCHISTOSOMA MANSONI
in parts of Africa, Arabia, West Indies, northern part
of South America
C. SCHISTOSOMA JAPONICUM
coastal areas of China, Japan, Formosa, Philippines,
Celebes
Cycle:
cercariae enter lymphatics + blood system via thoracic
duct; larvae are transported into mesenteric capillaries;
mature in portal system + liver into worms; worms live in
pairs in copula within portal vein + tributaries for 10 – 15
years; female swims against bloodflow to reach venules
of urinary bladder (S. haematobium) or intestine +
rectum (S. mansoni, S. japonicum); deposits eggs in
wall of urinary bladder or intestines, eggs pass with
urine + feces; hatch within water to release miracidia
which infect snail hosts; cercariae emerge after
maturation from snails
Infection: cercaria penetrate human skin / buccal mucosa
from contaminated water (slow-moving
streams, irrigation canals, paddy fields, lakes)
Histo: granulomatous reaction + fibrosis along portal
vein branches
@ Liver
√ marked diffuse thickening + echogenicity of walls of
portal venules
√ hepatosplenomegaly
√ portal vein dilatation in 73% (portal hypertension)
√ normal parenchymal echogenicity
@ GI tract
√ gastric + esophageal varices
√ polypoid bowel wall masses (esp. in sigmoid)
√ granulomatous colitis
√ strictures with extensive pericolic inflammation
Cx: ileus

SCHWACHMAN-DIAMOND SYNDROME
= rare congenital absence of pancreatic exocrine tissue,
2nd most frequent cause of exocrine pancreatic
insufficiency in childhood

- pancreatic insufficiency
- recurrent respiratory and skin infections (secondary to bone marrow hypoplasia)
- dwarfism (metaphyseal dysostosis)
- normal electrolytes in sweat
- tends to improve with time
√ total fatty replacement of pancreas

SOLID AND PAPILLARY NEOPLASM OF PANCREAS

= SOLID AND CYSTIC TUMOR = PAPILLARY-CYSTIC NEOPLASM = SOLID AND PAPILLARY EPITHELIAL NEOPLASM
= rare, low-grade malignant tumor; often misclassified as nonfunctioning islet cell tumor, cystadenoma, cystadenocarcinoma of pancreas
Mean age: 27 (range 10 – 46) years ; M:F = 1:9
Path: large well-encapsulated mass with considerable hemorrhagic necrosis + cystic degeneration
- gradually enlarging abdominal mass
√ sharply defined inhomogeneous round / lobulated pancreatic mass with solid + cystic portions
√ mean diameter of 10 cm (range 3 – 15 cm)
√ may calcify
√ hypovascular with no contrast enhancement / enhancement of solid tissue projecting toward center of mass
US:
  √ echogenic mass with necrotic center
Prognosis: excellent after excision; metastases in 4%
DDx:
  (1) microcystic adenoma (innumerable tiny cysts, older age group)
  (2) mucinous cystic neoplasm (large uni- / multilocular cysts, older age group)
  (3) nonfunctioning islet cell tumor (hypervascular)

SPLENIC INFARCTION

most common cause of focal defects
Cause:
  bacterial endocarditis (responsible in 50%), atheromatous plaque, cardiac thrombus, valve vegetation, sickle cell disease (leading to functional asplenia), myeloproliferative / lymphoproliferative disorders (CML most common), polycythemia vera, myelofibrosis with myeloid metaplasia + splenomegaly, Gaucher disease, metastatic carcinoma, local inflammatory process (e.g. pancreatitis), periarteritis nodosa

mnemonic: "PSALMS"
  Pancreatic carcinoma, **P**ancreatitis
  Sickle cell disease / trait
  Adenocarcinoma of stomach
  Leukemia
  Mitral stenosis with emboli
  Subacute bacterial endocarditis
√ wedge-shaped peripheral defect

SPLENOSIS

= autotransplantation of splenic tissue to other sites following trauma
Age: young men with history of trauma / splenectomy
Time of detection: mean of 10 years (range of 6 months – 32 years) after trauma
Location: diaphragmatic surface, liver, omentum, - mesentery, peritoneum, pleura
√ multiple small encapsulated sessile implants (mm – 3 cm)
√ demonstrated by Tc-99m sulfur colloid; In-111 labeled platelets; Tc-99m heat-damaged RBC (best detection rate)
DDx: accessory spleen

UNDIFFERENTIATED SARCOMA OF LIVER

= EMBRYONAL SARCOMA = 4th most frequent hepatic tumor in childhood
Age: < 2 months (5%); 6 – 10 years (52%); by 15 years (90%); up to 30 years
Histo: stellate / spindle-shaped sarcomatous cells arranged in whorls + sheets with foci of hematopoiesis (50%)
- RUQ mass
- mild anemia + leukocytosis (50%)
- elevated liver enzymes (33%)
- fever (5%)
Location: right lobe (75%); left lobe (10%); both lobes (15%)
√ 10 – 20 cm in size
NUC:
  √ photodefect on sulfur colloid scan
US+CT:
  √ large intrahepatic masses with cystic regions (necrosis + hemorrhage)
Angio:
  √ hyper- / hypovascular with stretching of vessels
  √ scattered foci of neovascularity
DDx: mesenchymal hamartoma
Prognosis: mostly results in death within 12 months

DIFFERENTIAL DIAGNOSIS OF GASTROINTESTINAL DISORDERS

ABNORMAL AIR
Abnormal air collection

1. Abnormally located bowel
    Chilalditi syndrome, Inguinal hernia
2. Pneumoperitoneum
3. Retropneumoperitoneum
    Perforation of duodenum / rectum / ascending +
    descending colon, Diverticulitis, Ulcerative disease,
    Endoscopic procedure
4. Gas in bowel wall
    Gastric pneumatosis, Phlegmonous gastritis,
    Endoscopy, Rupture of lung bulla
5. Gas within abscess
    located in subphrenic, renal, perirenal, hepatic,
    pancreatic space, lesser sac
6. Gas in biliary system
    Hepatobiliary fistula, Surgery, Duodenal ulcer,
    Duodenal diverticulum, Cancer, Stone, Patulous
    ampulla, Emphysematous cholecystitis
    √   gas outlines choledochus ± gallbladder
    √   peripheral branches of bile ducts not filled
7. Gas in portal venous system
    generally associated with intestinal necrosis (air
    leakage) / infection with gas-forming organisms in:
    Vascular accidents, Superior mesenteric artery
    syndrome, Diabetes, Imperforate anus, Duodenal
    atresia, Esophageal atresia, Diarrhea, Dead fetus
    √   branching air within 2 cm of liver periphery

Pneumoperitoneum in infants
Etiology:
A. Diseases of GI tract
    1. Necrotizing enterocolitis with perforation
    2. Perforated peptic / stress ulcer
    3. Ruptured Meckel diverticulum / sigmoid
        diverticulum
    4. Perforated appendix
    5. Obstruction (imperforate anus, Hirschsprung
        disease, meconium ileus)
    6. Perforated foreign body (e.g., thermometer
        injury to rectum)
    7. Ruptured pneumatosis cystoides intestinalis
B. Dissection from pneumomediastinum
C. Iatrogenic perforation:
    diagnostic pneumoperitoneum, laparoscopy /
    laparotomy (for 1 – 3 days), leaking surgical
    anastomosis
D. Idiopathic gastric perforation = spontaneous
    perforation in premature infants
•   history of perinatal asphyxia
•   acute shock
√   abdominal distension, no gastric air-fluid level
√   "saddlebag / mustache sign" = gas under the
    hemidiaphragm

√   "wall sign" = "Rigler sign" = outline of inner + outer wall
    of intestine
√   "football sign" = large pneumoperitoneum outlining
    entire abdominal cavity
√   "telltale triangle sign" = triangular air pocket between
    loops of bowel
√   "inverted V sign" = outline of both lateral umbilical
    ligaments
√   "urachal sign" = outline of middle umbilical ligament
√   outline of falciform ligament (medial RUQ); most
    common structure outlined
√   gas bubble lateral to right edge of liver
√   gas in scrotum (through open processus vaginalis)

Pneumoretroperitoneum
Causes:
(1) Traumatic rupture (usually duodenum)
(2) Perforation of duodenal ulcer
(3) Gas abscess of pancreas (usually extends into
     lesser sac)
(4) Urinary tract gas (trauma, infection)
(5) Dissected mediastinal air
√   kidney outline
√   outline of psoas margin ± streaks in muscle bundles

Pneumatosis intestinalis
=   multiple thin-walled, noncommunicating, gas-filled cysts
    located in subserosa ± submucosa with a normal
    mucosa + muscularis
1. PRIMARY PNEUMATOSIS INTESTINALIS (15%)
2. SECONDARY PNEUMATOSIS INTESTINALIS (85%)
    Causes:
    A. ISCHEMIA
        1. Necrotizing enterocolitis
        2. Mesenteric vascular disease
    B. TRAUMA
        1. Ingestion of corrosives
        2. Gastrointestinal endoscopy
        3. Jejunoileal bypass surgery
    C. INFECTION
        1. Primary infection of bowel wall
        2. Intestinal parasites
        3. Perforated jejunal diverticulum
    D. INFLAMMATION
        1. Pyloric / duodenal ulcer
        2. Inflammatory bowel disease
        3. Connective tissue disease
        4. Whipple disease
    E. PULMONARY CAUSES
        1. Emphysema
        2. Bullous disease of lung
        3. Chronic bronchitis
        4. Asthma
    F. COLONIC OBSTRUCTION

- asymptomatic
√ radiolucent clusters of cysts along contour of bowel wall
√ polypoid defects in barium column
√ ± pneumoperitoneum

Soap bubble appearance in abdomen of neonate
1. Feces in infant fed by mouth
2. Meconium ileus:
   gas mixed with meconium, usually RLQ
3. Meconium plug:
   gas in and around plug, in distribution of colon
4. Necrotizing enterocolitis: submucosal pneumatosis
5. Atresia / severe stenosis: pneumatosis
6. Hirschsprung disease:
   impacted stool, sometimes pneumatosis

ABDOMINAL CALCIFICATIONS
Diffuse abdominal calcifications
1. Cystadenoma of ovary
   √ granular, sandlike psammomatous calcifications
2. Pseudomyxoma peritonei
   (a) pseudomucinous adenoma of ovary
   (b) mucocele of appendix
3. Undifferentiated abdominal malignancy
4. Tuberculous peritonitis
   √ mottled calcifications, simulating residual barium
5. Meconium peritonitis
6. Oil granuloma: √ annular, plaquelike

Focal alimentary tract calcifications
A. ENTEROLITHS
   1. Appendicolith: in 10 – 15% of acute appendicitis
   2. Stone in Meckel diverticulum
   3. Diverticular stone
   4. Rectal stone
   5. Proximal to partial obstruction
B. MESENTERIC CALCIFICATIONS
   1. Dystrophic calcification of omental fat deposits +
      appendices epiploicae (secondary to infarction /
      pancreatitis / TB)
   2. Cysts: mesenteric cyst, hydatid cyst
C. INGESTED FOREIGN BODIES
   trapped in appendix, diverticula, proximal to stricture
   1. calcified seeds + pits
   2. birdshot
D. TUMOR
   1. Mucocele of appendix:
      √ crescent-shaped / circular calcification
   2. Mucinous adenocarcinoma of stomach / colon
      = COLLOID CARCINOMA
      √ small mottled / punctate calcifications in
         primary site ± in regional lymph node
         metastases, adjacent omentum, metastatic
         liver foci
   3. Gastric / esophageal leiomyoma: calcifies in 4%
   4. Lipoma

Abdominal wall calcifications
A. IN SOFT TISSUES
   1. Hypercalcemic states
   2. Idiopathic calcinosis
B. IN MUSCLE
   (a) Parasites:
      1. Cysticercosis = taenia solium
         √ round / slightly elongated calcifications
      2. Guinea worm = dracunculiasis
         √ stringlike calcifications up to 12 cm long
   (b) Injection sites
      from quinine, bismuth, calcium gluconate,
      calcium penicillin
   (c) Myositis ossificans
C. IN SKIN
   1. Soft-tissue nodules: papillomas, neurofibromas,
      melanomas, nevi
   2. Scars: √ linear density
   3. Colostomy / ileostomy
   4. Tattoo markings

Abdominal vascular calcifications
A. ARTERIES
   1. Atheromatous plaques
   2. Arterial calcifications in diabetes mellitus
B. VEINS
   Phleboliths = calcified thrombus, generally seen
   below interspinous line
   (a) in normal / varicose veins
   (b) in hemangioma
C. LYMPH NODES
   1. Histoplasmosis / tuberculosis
   2. Chronic granulomatous disease
   3. Residual lymphographic contrast
   4. Silicosis

ABNORMAL FLUID
Ascites
A. TRANSUDATE:
   (1) Hypoproteinemia (2) CHF (3) Constrictive
   pericarditis (4) Chronic renal failure (5) Cirrhosis
   (6) Budd-Chiari syndrome
B. EXUDATE:
   (1) Carcinomatosis (2) Polyserositis (3) TB peritonitis
   (4) Pancreatitis (5) Meig syndrome
C. Hemorrhagic / chylous fluid

Early signs (accumulation in pelvis):
   √ round central density in pelvis + ill-defined bladder top
   √ thickening of peritoneal flank stripe
   √ space between properitoneal fat and gut > 3 mm
Late signs:
   √ Hellmer sign = medial displacement of lateral liver
      margins
   √ medial displacement of ascending + descending colon
   √ obliteration of hepatic + splenic angles
   √ bulging flanks
   √ gray abdomen

√ floating centralized loops
√ separation of loops

Neonatal ascites
A. Gastrointestinal
(a) perforation of hollow viscus: meconium peritonitis
(b) inflammatory lesions: Meckel diverticulum, appendicitis
(c) ruptured mesenteric / omental / choledochal cyst
(d) bile leakage (biliary obstruction / perforation)
B. Portohepatic
(a) extrahepatic portal vein obstruction: atresia of veins, compression by mass
(b) intrahepatic portal vein obstruction: portal cirrhosis (neonatal hepatitis), biliary cirrhosis (biliary atresia)
C. Urinary tract
urine ascites (most common cause) from lower urinary tract obstruction + upper urinary tract rupture: posterior / anterior urethral valves, ureterovesical / ureteropelvic junction obstruction, renal / bladder rupture, anterior urethral diverticulum, bladder diverticula, neurogenic bladder, extrinsic bladder mass
D. Genital
ruptured ovarian cyst, hydrometrocolpos
E. Hydrops fetalis
immune hydrops, nonimmune hydrops (usually cardiac causes)
F. Miscellaneous
chylous ascites, lymphangiectasia, congenital syphilis, trauma, idiopathic

Chylous ascites

IN ADULTS:	1. Inflammatory process	(35%)
	2. Tumor	(30%)
	3. Idiopathic	(23%)
	4. Trauma	(11%)
	5. Congenital	(1%)
IN CHILDREN:	1. Congenital	(39%)
	2. Inflammatory process	(15%)
	3. Trauma	(12%)
	4. Tumor	(3%)
	5. Idiopathic	(33%)

Fluid collection
mnemonic: "BLUSCHINGS"
Biloma
Lymphocele, **L**ymphoma (almost anechoic)
Urinoma
Seroma
Cyst (pseudocyst, peritoneal inclusion cyst)
Hematoma (aneurysm, AVM)
Infection, **I**nfestation (empyema, abscess, echinococcus)
Neoplasm (necrotic)
GI tract (dilated loops, ileus, duplication)
Serosa (ascites, pleural fluid, pericardial effusion)

DILATED BOWEL
Bowel distension
A. Colon obstruction
B. Small bowel obstruction
C. Adynamic distension:
postoperative ileus, hypoelectrolytemia, peritonitis, trauma to spine, neurogenic disease
√ large + small bowel ± gastric distension
√ decreased small bowel distension on serial films
√ delayed but free passage on contrast material

Paralytic Ileus
= derangement impairing proper distal propulsion of intestinal contents, nonamenable to surgical correction
Cause: metabolic, chemical, idiopathic
• intestinal sounds decreased / absent
• abdominal distension

Localized ileus
= isolated distended loop of small / large bowel
= SENTINEL LOOP
Often associated with an adjacent acute inflammatory process
Etiology:
1. Acute pancreatitis: duodenum, jejunum, transverse colon
2. Acute cholecystitis: hepatic flexure of colon
3. Acute appendicitis: terminal ileum, cecum
4. Acute diverticulitis: descending colon
5. Acute ureteral colic: GI tract along course of ureter

Pseudoobstruction
A. Transient pseudoobstruction:
1. Electrolyte imbalance
2. Renal failure
3. Congestive failure
B. Chronic pseudoobstruction
1. Scleroderma
2. Amyloidosis
C. Idiopathic pseudoobstruction in young women
no apparent cause

ESOPHAGUS
Esophageal contractions
NORMAL PERISTALSIS = orderly propagation of bolus
1. PRIMARY CONTRACTIONS
= centrally mediated (medulla) swallow reflex via glossopharyngeal + vagal nerve; initiated by swallowing
√ rapid wave of inhibition followed by slower wave of contraction
√ longitudinal stripping wave interrupted by repetitive swallowing
2. SECONDARY CONTRACTIONS
(a) normal
local peristaltic wave elicited through esophageal distension = sensorimotor stretch reflex

(b) pathologic
peptic esophagitis, esophageal ulcer, long-lasting achalasia
√ in erect position, rarely observed
√ originate in inferior / middle third of esophagus during resting stage
√ "hourglass" = contraction spreads simultaneously up- and downward
3. TERTIARY CONTRACTIONS
√ "curling" = erratic segmental peristalsis

Abnormal esophageal peristalsis
A. PRIMARY CAUSES
  1. Idiopathic achalasia
  2. Intestinal pseudoobstruction
  3. Congenital TE fistula
  4. Diffuse esophageal spasm
  5. Presbyesophagus
  6. Chalasia
B. SECONDARY CAUSES
  (a) Connective Tissue Disorders
    1. Scleroderma
    2. SLE
    3. Rheumatoid arthritis
    4. Polymyositis
    5. Dermatomyositis
    6. Muscular dystrophy
  (b) Chemical / Physical Disorders
    1. Reflux / peptic esophagitis
    2. S/P vagotomy
    3. Caustic esophagitis
    4. Radiotherapy
  (c) Infectious Diseases
    Fungal: candidiasis
    Parasitic: Chagas disease
    Bacterial: TB, diphtheria
    Viral: herpes simplex
  (d) Metabolic Disorders
    1. Diabetes mellitus
    2. Amyloidosis
    3. Alcoholism
    4. Electrolyte disturbances
  (e) Endocrine Disease
    1. Myxedema
    2. Thyrotoxicosis
  (f) Neoplasm
  (g) Pharmacologic Action
    atropine, propantheline, curare
  (h) Muscular Disease
    1. Myotonic dystrophy
    2. Muscular dystrophy
    3. Oculopharyngeal dystrophy
    4. Myasthenia gravis
  (i) Neurologic Disease
    1. Parkinsonism
    2. Multiple sclerosis
    3. CNS neoplasm
    4. Amyotrophic lateral sclerosis
    5. Bulbar poliomyelitis
    6. Cerebrovascular disease
    7. Huntington chorea
    8. Ganglioneuromatosis
    9. Wilson disease
    10. Friedreich ataxia
    11. Familial dysautonomia (Riley-Day)
    12. Stiff-man syndrome

Achalasia pattern
= MEGAESOPHAGUS
1. Idiopathic achalasia
2. Chagas disease: patients commonly from South America; often associated with megacolon + cardiomegaly
3. Infiltrating lesion of distal esophagus / gastric cardia (e.g., carcinoma)
4. Amyloidosis: associated with macroglossia, thickened small bowel folds
5. Idiopathic intestinal pseudoobstruction
= degeneration of innervation
6. Presbyesophagus
7. Ehlers-Danlos syndrome
8. Postvagotomy syndrome
9. Scleroderma

Air esophagram
1. Normal variant
2. Scleroderma
3. Distal obstruction
tumor, stricture, achalasia
4. Thoracic surgery
5. Mediastinal inflammatory disease
6. S/P total laryngectomy (esophageal speech)
7. Endotracheal intubation + PEEP

Tracheo-broncho-esophageal fistula
A. CONGENITAL
  1. Congenital tracheoesophageal fistula
B. MALIGNANT
  1. Lung cancer
  2. Metastases to mediastinal lymph nodes
C. TRAUMATIC
  1. Instrumentation (esophagoscopy, bouginage, pneumatic dilatation)
  2. Blunt ("crush injury") / penetrating chest trauma
  3. Surgery
  4. Foreign body perforation
  5. Corrosives
  6. Postemetic rupture = Boerhaave syndrome
D. INFECTIOUS / INFLAMMATORY
  — TB, syphilis, histoplasmosis, actinomycosis, Crohn disease
  — Perforated diverticulum
  — Pulmonary sequestration / cyst

Esophageal diverticulum
1. ZENKER DIVERTICULUM (pharyngoesophageal)
2. INTERBRONCHIAL DIVERTICULUM
   = traction diverticulum
   Response to pull from fibrous adhesions following lymph node infection (TB), contains all 3 esophageal layers
   Location: usually on right anterolateral wall of interbronchial segment
   √ calcified mediastinal nodes
3. INTERAORTICO-BRONCHIAL DIVERTICULUM
   = thoracic pulsion diverticulum
   Location: on left anterolateral wall between inferior border of aortic arch + upper margin of left main bronchus
4. EPIPHRENIC DIVERTICULUM (rare)
   Location: usually on lateral esophageal wall, right > left, in distal 10 cm
   √ often associated with hiatus hernia
5. Intramural esophageal pseudodiverticulosis
   √ outpouching from mucosal glands

Esophageal inflammation
A. CONTACT INJURY
   (a) reflux related:
      1. Peptic ulcer disease
      2. Barrett esophagus
      3. Scleroderma (patulous LES)
      4. Nasogastric Intubation
   (b) caustic:
      1. Foreign body
      2. Corrosives
   (c) thermic: habitual ingestion of excessively hot meals / liquids
B. RADIATION INJURY
C. INFECTION
   1. Candidiasis
   2. Herpes simplex virus / CMV
   3. Diphtheria
D. SYSTEMIC DISEASE
   (a) dermatologic disorders: pemphigoid, epidermolysis bullosa
   (b) others:
      1. Crohn disease
      2. Graft-versus-host disease
      3. Behçet disease
      4. Eosinophilic gastroenteritis

Esophageal ulceration
A. PEPTIC
   1. Reflux esophagitis: scleroderma
   2. Barrett esophagus
   3. Crohn disease: aphthous ulcer
   4. Dermatologic disorders: pemphigoid, epidermolysis bullosa, Behçet disease
B. INFECTIOUS
   1. Candidiasis
   2. Herpes

C. CONTACT INJURY / EXTERNAL INJURY
   1. Corrosives: alkali, strictures in 50%
   2. Drug-induced:
      antibiotics, quinidine, potassium chloride
   3. Radiotherapy: smooth stricture > 4500 rads
   4. Nasogastric tube:
      elongated stricture in middle + distal 1/3
D. MALIGNANT
   1. Esophageal carcinoma
Location:
@ Upper esophagus = Barrett ulcer in islets of gastric mucosa
@ Lower esophagus
   √ esophagus of normal length
   √ usually associated with gastric / duodenal ulcers (peptic)
   √ narrowed segment + proximal dilatation
   √ secondary contractions + retroperistalsis
   DDx: achalasia, neoplastic infiltration
@ Esophagogastric junction
   √ associated with hiatal hernia
   √ "frontier ulcer" = at junction of esophageal + gastric mucosa
   √ esophageal shortening (part of stomach pulled into thorax)
   √ esophageal dilatation + slow emptying

Long smooth esophageal narrowing
1. Congenital esophageal stenosis
   √ at junction between middle + distal third
   √ web-like / tubular stenosis of 1 cm in length
2. Surgical repair of esophageal atresia
   √ interruption of primary peristaltic wave at anastomosis
   √ secondary contractions may produce retrograde flow with aspiration
   √ impaction of food
3. Caustic burns = alkaline burns
   Corrosive agents:
      lye (sodium hydroxide), washing soda (sodium carbonate), household cleaners, iodine, silver nitrate, household bleaches, clinitest tablets (tend to be neutralized by gastric acid)
   Location: middle + lower thirds of esophagus (esophageal injury frequent); gastric injury in 7 – 8%
   √ mucosal blurring (edema)
   √ ulceration + pseudomembranes
   √ dilated atonic esophagus
   √ long segmental stricture after 10 days when acute edema subsides (7 – 30%)
   Cx: increased incidence of malignancy
4. Gastric acid: reflux, hyperemesis gravidarum
5. Intubation: reflux + compromise of circulation
6. Radiotherapy
7. Post infection: moniliasis (rare)

LOWER ESOPHAGEAL NARROWING
    mnemonic: "SPADE"
      Scleroderma
      Presbyesophagus
      Achalasia; **A**nticholinergics
      Diffuse esophageal spasm
      Esophagitis

Double-barrel esophagus

1. Dissecting intramural hematoma from emetogenic injury
2. Mallory-Weiss tear
   trauma, esophagoscopy (in 0.25%), bougiage (in 0.5%), ingestion of foreign bodies, spontaneous (bleeding diathesis)
3. Intramural abscess
4. Intraluminal diverticulum
5. Esophageal duplication (if communication with esophageal lumen present)

Esophageal filling defect

A. BENIGN TUMORS
    < 1% of all esophageal tumors
    (a) Submucosal tumor (75%)
       = nonepithelial, intramural
       1. Leiomyoma (> 50% of all benign tumors)
       2. Lipoma, fibroma, lipoma, fibrolipoma, myxofibroma, hamartoma, hemangioma, lymphangioma, neurofibroma, schwannoma, granular cell myoblastoma
         √ primary wave stops at level of tumor
         √ proximal esophageal dilatation + hypotonicity
         √ rigid esophageal wall at site of tumoral implant
         √ disorganized / altered / effaced mucosal folds around defect
         √ tumor shadow on tangential view extending beyond esophageal margin
    (b) Mucosal tumor (25%) = epithelial, intraluminal
       1. Fibrovascular / inflammatory polyp; adenomatous polyp
       2. Squamous papilloma, fibropapilloma
       3. Villous adenoma, fibroadenoma
         √ no interruption of primary peristalsis
         √ well-circumscribed central radiolucent defect
         √ symmetrical ampullary distension of esophagus around defect
         √ no change of mucosal pattern at periphery of defect

B. MALIGNANT TUMORS
    1. Esophageal cancer, varicoid squamous cell carcinoma
    2. Gastric cancer
    3. Leiomyosarcoma, carcinosarcoma, pseudosarcoma
    4. Metastases: malignant melanoma, lymphoma (< 1% of gastrointestinal lymphomas), stomach, lung, breast

C. VASCULAR
    varices
D. INFECTION / INFLAMMATION
    candida / herpes esophagitis, drug-induced inflammatory reaction
E. CONGENITAL / NORMAL VARIANT
    prolapsed gastric folds, esophageal duplication cyst
F. FOREIGN BODIES
    chicken bone, fish bone, pins, coins, small toys, meat, air bubble

Fine nodular esophageal lesions

1. **Leukoplakia** = epithelial hyperplasia; mid 1/3 of esophagus
2. Superficial spreading esophageal carcinoma
3. **Glycogen acanthosis**
   Histo: hyperplasia + hypertrophy of squamous mucosal cells secondary to increased glycogen; premalignant lesion
4. Candida esophagitis: earliest morphologic abnormality
5. Reflux esophagitis
6. Corrosive esophagitis
7. Tuberculous esophagitis

Extrinsic esophageal impression
Cervical causes of esophageal impression
    A. OSSEOUS LESIONS
       1. Anterior marginal osteophyte / DISH
       2. Anterior disk herniation
       3. Cervical trauma + hematoma
       4. Osteomyelitis
       5. Bone neoplasm
    B. ESOPHAGEAL WALL LESIONS
       (a) muscle
         1. Cricopharyngeus
         2. Esophageal web
       (b) vessel
         1. Pharyngeal venous plexus
         2. Lymph node enlargement
    C. ENDOCRINE ORGANS
       1. Thyroid / parathyroid enlargement (benign / malignant)
       2. Fibrotic traction after thyroidectomy
    D. Retropharyngeal / mediastinal abscess

Thoracic causes of esophageal impression
    A. NORMAL INDENTATIONS
       aortic arch, left main stem bronchus, left inferior pulmonary vein
    B. ABNORMAL VASCULATURE
       Right-sided aortic arch, cervical aortic arch, aortic unfolding, aortic tortuosity, aortic aneurysm, double aortic arch ("reverse S"), coarctation of aorta ("reverse figure 3"), aberrant right subclavian artery = arteria lusoria (semilunar / bayonet-shaped imprint upon posterior wall of esophagus), aberrant left pulmonary artery (between trachea + esophagus), anomalous pulmonary venous return (anterior), persistent truncus arteriosus (posterior)

C.   CARDIAC CAUSES
   (a)   Enlargement of chambers:
      Left atrial / left ventricular enlargement:
         Mitral disease (esophageal displacement
         backwards + to the right)
   (b)   Pericardial masses:
      Pericardial tumor / cyst / effusion
D.   MEDIASTINAL CAUSES
   Mediastinal tumor, lymphadenopathy (metastatic,
   tuberculous), inflammation, cyst
F.   PULMONARY CAUSES
   Pulmonary tumor, bronchogenic cyst, atypical
   pulmonary fibrosis (retraction)
E.   ESOPHAGEAL ABNORMALITIES
   1.   Esophageal diverticulum
   2.   Paraesophageal hernia
   3.   **Esophageal duplication:**   R:L = 2:1, mostly
      tubular shape, almost never communicating;
      intramural / paraesophageal, 60% at lower
      esophagus

STOMACH
Gastric pneumatosis
A.   TRAUMA
   (a)   Iatrogenic
      1.   Recent gastroduodenal surgery
      2.   Endoscopy (1.6%)
   (b)   Ingested material:
      1.   Corrosive gastritis
      2.   Acid ingestion
B.   ISCHEMIA
   1.   Gastric ulcer disease with intramural perforation
   2.   Severe necrotizing gastroenteritis
   3.   Gastric carcinoma
   4.   Volvulus
   5.   Gastric infarction
C.   INFECTION
   1.   Emphysematous gastritis
D.   OVERDISTENSION (increased intraluminal pressure)
   1.   Gastric outlet obstruction
   2.   Volvulus
   3.   Overinflation during gastroscopy
   4.   Profuse vomiting
E.   DISSECTING AIR
   1.   Pulmonary bulla rupturing along esophageal wall /
      mediastinum
F.   IDIOPATHIC
   1.   Nonbacterial gastric emphysema = intramural
      gastric emphysema

√ thin discrete sharply defined streaks of gas in
   submucosa ± subserosa
√ irregular radiolucent band of innumerable small bubbles
   with constant relationship to each other
√ bulging of mucosa
√ gas within portal venous system

Gastric outlet obstruction
A.   CONGENITAL LESION
   1.   Antral mucosal diaphragm = antral web
   2.   Annular pancreas
   3.   Gastric duplication: usually along greater
      curvature, abdominal mass in infancy
   4.   Hypertrophic pyloric stenosis
B.   INFLAMMATORY NARROWING
   1.   Peptic ulcer disease: cause in adults in 60 – 65%
   2.   Corrosive gastritis
   3.   Crohn disease, sarcoidosis, syphilis, tuberculosis
   4.   Pancreatitis, cholecystitis
C.   MALIGNANT NARROWING
   1.   Antral carcinoma: cause in adults in 30 – 35%
   2.   Scirrhous carcinoma of pyloric channel
D.   OTHERS
   1.   Prolapsed antral polyp / mucosa
   2.   Bezoar
   3.   Gastric volvulus

Gastric atony
= gastric retention in the absence of mechanical
   obstruction
Pathophysiology: reflex paralysis
A.   ACUTE GASTRIC ATONY
   (may develop within 24 – 48 hours)
   1.   Acute gastric dilatation: secondary to decreased
      arterial perfusion (ischemia, congestive heart
      failure) in old patients, usually fatal
   2.   Postsurgical atony, ureteral catheterization
   3.   Immobilization: body cast, paraplegia,
      postoperative state
   4.   Abdominal trauma: especially back injury
   5.   Severe pain: renal / biliary colic, migraine
      headaches, severe burns
   6.   Infection: peritonitis, pancreatitis, appendicitis,
      subphrenic abscess, septicemia
B.   CHRONIC GASTRIC ATONY
   1.   Neurologic abnormalities: brain tumor, bulbar
      poliomyelitis, vagotomy, tabes
   2.   Muscular abnormalities: scleroderma, muscular
      dystrophy
   3.   Drug-induced atony: atropine, morphine, heroin,
      ganglionic blocking agents
   4.   Electrolyte imbalance: diabetic ketoacidosis,
      hypercalcemia, hypocalcemia, hypokalemia,
      hepatic coma, uremia, myxedema
   5.   Diabetes mellitus = gastroparesis diabeticorum
      (0.08% incidence)
   6.   Emotional distress
   7.   Lead poisoning
   8.   Porphyria
•   abdominal distension
•   vascular collapse (decreased venous return)
•   vomiting
√ large stomach filled with air + fluid (up to 7,500 ml)
√ retention of barium
√ absent / diminished peristaltic activity

√ patulous pylorus
√ frequently dilated duodenum
DDx: gastric volvulus, pyloric stenosis

Narrowing of stomach
=   linitis plastica type of stenosis
A. MALIGNANCY
1. Scirrhous gastric carcinoma (involving portion / all of stomach)
2. Hodgkin lymphoma, NHL
3. Metastatic involvement (carcinoma of breast, pancreatic carcinoma, colonic carcinoma)
B. INFLAMMATION
1. Chronic gastric ulcer disease with intense spasm
2. Pseudobillroth-I pattern of Crohn disease
3. Sarcoidosis
√   polypoid appearance, pyloric hypertrophy
√   gastric ulcers, duodenal deformity
4. Eosinophilic gastritis
5. Polyarteritis nodosa
6. Stenosing antral gastritis / hypertrophic pyloric stenosis
C. INFECTION
1. Tertiary stage of syphilis
√   absent mucosal folds + peristalsis
√   no change over years
2. Tuberculosis (rare)
√   hyperplastic nodules / ulcerative lesion / annular lesion
√   pyloric obstruction, may cross into duodenum
3. Histoplasmosis
4. Actinomycosis
5. Strongyloidiasis
6. Phlegmonous gastritis
D. TRAUMA
1. Corrosive gastritis
2. Radiation injury
3. Gastric freezing
4. Hepatic arterial chemotherapy infusion
E. OTHERS
1. Perigastric adhesions (normal mucosa, no interval change, normal peristalsis)
2. Amyloidosis
3. Pseudolymphoma
4. Exogastric mass (hepatomegaly, pancreatic pseudocyst)

Widened retrogastric space
A. PANCREATIC MASSES (most common cause)
1. Acute + chronic pancreatitis
2. Pancreatic pseudocyst
3. Pancreatic cystadenoma + carcinoma
B. OTHER RETROPERITONEAL MASSES
Sarcoma, renal tumor, adrenal tumor, lymph node enlargement, abscess, hematoma
D. GASTRIC MASSES
1. Leiomyoma, leiomyosarcoma

C. OTHERS
1. Aortic aneurysm
2. Choledochal cyst
3. Obesity
4. Postsurgical disruptions + adhesions
5. Ascites
6. Gross hepatomegaly + enlarged caudate lobe
7. Hernia involving omentum

Intramural-extramucosal lesions of stomach
√ sharply delineated marginal / contour defect
√ stretched folds over intact mucosa
√ acute angle at margins
√ may ulcerate centrally
√ may become pedunculated and acquire polypoid appearance over years
A. NEOPLASTIC
1. Leiomyoma   (48%)
2. Neurogenic tumors   (14%)
3. Heterotopic pancreas   (12%)
4. Fibrous tumor   (11%)
5. Lipoma   (7%)
6. Hemangioma   (7%)
7. Glomus tumor   (rare)
8. Carcinoid
9. Metastatic tumor
B. INFLAMMATION / INFECTION
1. Granuloma: (1) Foreign body granuloma (2) Sarcoidosis (3) Crohn disease (4) Tuberculosis (5) Histoplasmosis
2. Eosinophilic gastritis
3. Tertiary syphilis: infiltrative / ulcerative / tumorous type
4. Echinococcal cyst
C. PANCREATIC ABNORMALITIES
1. Ectopic pancreas
2. Annular pancreas
3. Pancreatic pseudocyst
D. DEPOSITS
1. Amyloid
2. Endometriosis
3. Localized hematoma
E. OTHERS
1. Varices (i.e., fundal)
2. Duplications (4% of all GI tract duplications)

Gastric filling defects
A. INTRINSIC WALL LESIONS
(a) BENIGN (most common)
1. Polyps: hyperplastic, adenomatous, villous, hamartomatous (Peutz-Jeghers syndrome, Cowden disease)
2. Leiomyoma
3. Granulomatous lesions:
(a) Eosinophilic granuloma (b) Crohn disease (c) Tuberculosis (d) Sarcoidosis
4. Pseudolymphoma = benign reactive proliferation of lymphoid tissue

5. Extramedullary hematopoiesis
6. Ectopic pancreas
7. Gastric duplication cyst
8. Intramural hematoma
9. Esophagogastric herniation
  (b) MALIGNANT
    1. Gastric carcinoma, lymphoma
    2. Gastric sarcoma: leiomyosarcoma, liposarcoma, leiomyoblastoma
    3. Gastric metastases: melanoma, breast, pancreas, colon
B. EXTRINSIC IMPRESSIONS ON STOMACH
in 70% nonneoplastic (extrinsic pseudotumors in 20%)
  (a) normal organs: organomegaly, tortuous aorta, heart, cardiac aneurysm
  (b) benign masses: cysts of pancreas, liver, spleen, adrenal, kidney; gastric duplication, postoperative deformity (e.g., Nissen fundoplication)
  (c) malignant masses: enlarged celiac nodes
  (d) inflammatory lesion: left subphrenic abscess / hematoma
  — lateral displacement: enlarged liver, aortic aneurysm, enlarged celiac nodes
  — medial displacement: splenomegaly, mass in colonic splenic flexure, cardiomegaly, subphrenic abscess
C. INTRALUMINAL GASTRIC MASSES
  1. Bezoar
  2. Foreign bodies: food, pills, blood clot, gallstone
D. TUMORS OF ADJACENT ORGANS
Pancreatic carcinoma + cystadenoma, liver carcinoma, carcinoma of gallbladder, colonic carcinoma, renal carcinoma, adrenal carcinoma, lymph node involvement
E. THICKENED GASTRIC FOLDS

Bull's eye lesions
A. PRIMARY NEOPLASMS
  1. Leiomyoma, leiomyosarcoma
  2. Lymphoma
  3. Carcinoid
  4. Primary carcinoma
B. HEMATOGENOUS METASTASES
  1. Malignant melanoma
    √ usually spares large bowel
  2. Breast cancer (15%)
    √ scirrhous appearance in stomach
  3. Cancer of lung
  4. Renal cell carcinoma
  5. Kaposi sarcoma
  6. Bladder carcinoma
C. ECTOPIC PANCREAS
to duodenum / stomach
D. EOSINOPHILIC GRANULOMA
most frequently in stomach

Lesions involving stomach and duodenum
1. Lymphoma: in < 33% of patients with lymphoma

2. Gastric carcinoma: in < 5%, but 50 x more common than lymphoma
3. Peptic ulcer disease
4. Tuberculosis: in 10% of gastric TB
5. Crohn disease: pseudo-Billroth-I pattern
6. Strongyloidiasis
7. Eosinophilic gastroenteritis

Thickened gastric folds
A. INFLAMMATION / INFECTION
  1. Inflammatory gastritis
    alcoholic, hypertrophic, antral, corrosive, postirradiation, gastric cooling
  2. Crohn disease
  3. Sarcoidosis
  4. Infectious gastritis
    bacterial invasion, bacterial toxins from botulism, diphtheria, dysentery, typhoid fever, anikasiasis, TB, syphilis
  5. Pseudolymphoma
B MALIGNANCY
  1. Lymphoma
  2. Gastric carcinoma
C. INFILTRATIVE PROCESS
  1. Eosinophilic gastritis
  2. Amyloidosis
D. PANCREATIC DISEASE
  1. Pancreatitis
  2. Direct extension from pancreatic carcinoma
E. OTHERS
  1. Zollinger-Ellison syndrome
  2. Menetrier disease
  3. Gastric varices

Gastric Ulcer
A. HORMONAL
  1. Zollinger-Ellison syndrome
  2. Hyperparathyroidism (in 1.3 – 24%)
    duodenum:stomach = 4:1; M:F = 3:1
    Δ duodenal ulcers predominantly in females,
    Δ gastric ulcers in males
    • absence of gastric hypersecretion
  3. Steroid-induced ulcer
    Gastric > duodenal location; frequently multiple + deep ulcers
    Commonly associated with erosions
    • bleeding (in 1/3)
  4. Curling ulcer (burn) (in 0.09 – 2.6%)
  5. Retained gastric antrum
B. INFLAMMATION
  1. Peptic ulcer disease
  2. Gastritis
  3. Radiation-induced ulcer
C. BENIGN MASS
  1. Leiomyoma
  2. Granulomatous disease
  3. Pseudolymphoma (lymphoid hyperplasia)
D. MALIGNANT MASS
  1. Gastric carcinoma

2. Lymphoma (2% of all gastric neoplasms)
   √ multiple ulcers with aneurysmal appearance
3. Leiomyosarcoma, neurogenic sarcoma, fibrosarcoma, liposarcoma
4. Metastases
   (a) hematogenic: malignant melanoma, breast cancer, lung cancer
   (b) per continuum: pancreas, colon, kidney
E. DRUGS
   ASA: greater curvature

Metastases to stomach

Organ of origin: malignant melanoma, breast, lung, colon, prostate, leukemia, secondary lymphoma
• GI bleeding + anemia (40%)
• epigastric pain
√ solitary mass (50%)
√ multiple nodules (30%)
√ linitis plastica (20%): especially breast
√ multiple umbilicated nodules: melanoma

Complications of postoperative stomach

1. Filling defect of gastric remnant
2. Retained gastric antrum
3. Dumping syndrome
4. Afferent loop syndrome
5. Stomal obstruction
   (a) temporary reversible: edema of suture line, abscess / hematoma, potassium deficiency, inadequate electrolyte replacement, hypoproteinemia, hypoacidity
   (b) late mechanical: stomal ulcer (75%)

mnemonic: "LOBULATING"
   Leaks (early)
   Obstruction (early)
   Bezoar
   Ulcer (especially marginal)
   Loop (afferent loop syndrome)
   Anemia (macrocytic secondary to decreased intrinsic factor)
   Tumor (increased incidence)
   Intussusception
   Not feeling well after meals (dumping syndrome)
   Gastritis (bile reflux)

Filling defect of gastric remnant

A. IATROGENIC
   Surgical deformity / plication defect, suture granuloma
B. INFLAMMATORY
   Bile reflux gastritis, hyperplastic polyps
C. INTUSSUSCEPTION
   1. **Jejunogastric intussusception**
      (efferent loop in 75%, afferent loop in 25%)
      (a) acute form: high intestinal obstruction, left hypochondriac mass, hematemesis

(b) chronic / intermittent form: may be self-reducing
   √ "coil spring" appearance of gastric filling defect
2. Gastrojejunal / gastroduodenal mucosal prolapse
   • often asymptomatic
   • bleeding, partial obstruction

D. NEOPLASTIC
   1. Gastric stump carcinoma = > 5 years after resection for benign disease; 15% within 10 years; 20% after 20 years
   2. Recurrent carcinoma (10%) secondary to incomplete removal of gastric cancer
   3. Malignancy at anastomosis (incomplete resection)
E. INTRALUMINAL MATTER: Bezoar

Gastric surgical procedures

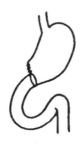

Billroth I

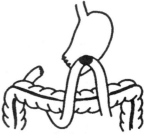

Billroth II

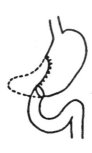

Shoemaker

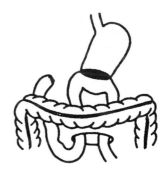

retrocolic (Polya)

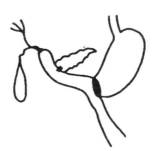

Whipple

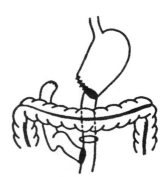

Roux-en-Y

SMALL BOWEL
Enlargement of papilla of Vater
A. Normal variant
identified in 60% of UGI series; atypical location in 3rd portion of duodenum in 8%; 1.5 cm in diameter in 1% of normals
B. Papillary edema
   1. Impacted stone
   2. Pancreatitis (Poppel sign)
   3. Acute duodenal ulcer disease
   4. Papillitis
C. Perivaterian neoplasms
   = tumor mass + lymphatic obstruction
   1. Adenocarcinoma
   2. Adenomatous polyp (premalignant lesion)
   √ irregular surface + erosions
D. Lesions simulating enlarged papilla
   1. Benign spindle cell tumor
   2. Ectopic pancreatic tissue

Thickened duodenal folds
A. INFLAMMATION
   (a) within bowel wall: Peptic ulcer disease, Zollinger-Ellison syndrome, regional enteritis, lymphoid hyperplasia, uremia
   (b) surrounding bowel wall: Pancreatitis, cholecystitis
B. INFECTION: Giardiasis, TB, strongyloidiasis, nontropical sprue
C. NEOPLASIA: Lymphoma, metastases to peripancreatic nodes
D. DIFFUSE INFILTRATIVE DISORDER: Whipple disease, amyloidosis, mastocytosis, eosinophilic enteritis, intestinal lymphangiectasia
E. VASCULAR DISORDER: Duodenal varices, mesenteric arterial collaterals, intramural hemorrhage, chronic duodenal congestion (congestive heart failure, portal venous hypertension)
F. GLANDULAR ENLARGEMENT: Brunner gland hyperplasia, cystic fibrosis

mnemonic: "BAD HELP"
Brunner gland hyperplasia
Amyloidosis
Duodenitis (Z-E syndrome, peptic)
Hemorrhage
Edema, **E**ctopic pancreas
Lymphoma
Pancreatitis, **P**arasites

Duodenal filling defect
A. EXTRINSIC
   Gallbladder impression, CBD impression, gas-filled diverticulum
B. INTRINSIC TO WALL
   (a) NON-NEOPLASTIC MASS
       Papilla of Vater, choledochocele, duplication cyst, pancreatic pseudocyst, duodenal varix, mesenteric artery collaterals, intramural hematoma, adjacent abscess, stitch abscess, ectopic pancreas, heterotopic gastric mucosa, prolapsed antral mucosa, Brunner gland hyperplasia, benign lymphoid hyperplasia
   (b) BENIGN NEOPLASTIC MASS
       Adenoma, leiomyoma, lipoma, hamartoma (Peutz-Jeghers syndrome), prolapsed antral polyp, Brunner gland adenoma, villous adenoma, islet cell tumor
   (c) MALIGNANT NEOPLASTIC MASS
       Carcinoid tumor, adenocarcinoma, ampullary carcinoma, lymphoma, sarcoma, metastasis (stomach, pancreas, gallbladder, colon, kidney, melanoma), retroperitoneal lymph node involvement
C. INTRALUMINAL
   Blood clot, foreign body (fruit pit, gallstone, feeding tube)

Extrinsic pressure effect on duodenum
A. BILE DUCTS
   Normal impression, dilated CBD, choledochal cyst
B. GALLBLADDER
   Normal impression, gallbladder hydrops, Courvoisier phenomenon, gallbladder carcinoma, pericholecystic abscess
C. LIVER
   Hepatomegaly, hypertrophied caudate lobe, anomalous hepatic lobe, hepatic cyst, hepatic tumor
D. RIGHT KIDNEY
   Bifid collecting system, hydronephrosis, multiple renal cysts, polycystic kidney disease, hypernephroma
E. RIGHT ADRENAL
   Adrenal carcinoma, enlargement in Addison disease
F. COLON
   Duodenocolic apposition due to anomalous peritoneal fixation, carcinoma of hepatic flexure
G. VESSELS
   Lymphadenopathy, duodenal varices, dilated arterial collaterals, aortic aneurysm, intramural / mesenteric hematoma

Widened duodenal sweep
A. Normal variant
B. Pancreatic lesions
   1. Acute pancreatitis
   2. Chronic pancreatitis
   3. Pancreatic pseudocyst
   4. Pancreatic carcinoma
   5. Metastasis to pancreas
   6. Pancreatic cystadenoma
C. Vascular lesion
   1. Lymph node enlargement: lymphoma, metastasis, inflammation
   2. Cystic lymphangioma of the mesentery
D. Retroperitoneal mass
   1. Aortic aneurysm
   2. Choledochal cyst

Duodenal narrowing
A. DEVELOPMENTAL ANOMALIES
 1. Duodenal atresia
 2. Congenital web / duodenal diaphragm
 3. Intraluminal diverticulum
 4. Duodenal duplication cyst
 5. Annular pancreas
 6. Midgut volvulus, peritoneal bands (Ladd bands)
B. INTRINSIC DISORDERS
 (a) INFLAMMATION / INFECTION
  1. Postbulbar ulcer
  2. Crohn disease
  3. Sprue
  4. Tuberculosis
  5. Strongyloidiasis
 (b) TUMOR
  Duodenal / ampullary malignancy
C. DISEASE IN ADJACENT STRUCTURES
 1. Pancreatitis, pseudocyst, pancreatic carcinoma
 2. Cholecystitis
 3. Contiguous abscess
 4. Metastases to pancreaticoduodenal nodes
  (lymphoma, lung cancer, breast cancer)
D. TRAUMA
 1. Duodenal rupture
 2. Intramural hematoma
E. VASCULAR
 1. Superior mesenteric artery syndrome
 2. Aorticoduodenal fistula
 3. Preduodenal portal vein (anterior to descending
  duodenum)

Postbulbar ulceration
1. Benign postbulbar peptic ulcer
 √ medial aspect of upper 2nd portion
 √ incisura pointing to ulcer
 √ occasionally barium reflux into CBD
 √ ring stricture
 √ stress- and drug-induced ulcers heal without
 deformity
2. Zollinger-Ellison syndrome
 √ multiple ulcers distal to duodenal bulb
 √ thickening of folds + hypersecretion
3. Leiomyoma
4. Malignant tumors:
 (a) Primaries:
  adenocarcinoma, lymphoma, sarcoma
 (b) Contiguous spread:
  pancreas, colon, kidney, gallbladder
 (c) Hematogenous spread:
  melanoma, Kaposi sarcoma
 (d) Lymphogenic spread:
  metastases to periduodenal lymph nodes
5. Granulomatous disease: Crohn disease, TB
6. Aorticoduodenal fistula
7. Mimickers: ectopic pancreas, diverticulum

Benign duodenal tumors
1. Leiomyoma	(27%)
2. Adenomatous polyp	(21%)
3. Lipoma	(21%)
4. Brunner gland adenoma	(17%)
5. Angiomatous tumor	(6%)
6. Ectopic pancreas	(2%)
7. Duodenal cyst	(2%)
8. Neurofibroma	(2%)
9. Hamartoma	(2%)

Malignant duodenal tumors
1. Adenocarcinoma (73%)
 Location: 40% in duodenum, most often in 2nd + 3rd
   portion = periampullary neoplasm
 (a) suprapapillary: apt to cause obstruction + bleeding
 (b) peripapillary: extrahepatic jaundice
 (c) intrapapillary: GI bleeding
 May be associated with Peutz-Jeghers syndrome
 √ annular / polypoid / ulcerative
 Regional lymph node metastases (2/3)
 DDx: (1) Primary bile duct carcinoma
   (2) Ampullary carcinoma
2. Leiomyosarcoma (14%)
 most often beyond 1st portion of duodenum
 √ up to 20 cm in size
 √ frequently ulcerated exophytic mass
3. Carcinoid (11%)
4. Lymphoma (2%)
 √ marked wall thickening
 √ bulky periduodenal lymphadenopathy

Small bowel obstruction
A. EXTRINSIC BOWEL LESIONS
 1. Fibrous adhesions (in 75%) from previous surgery /
  peritonitis
 2. Hernias (inguinal, femoral, umbilical, paraduodenal,
  foramen of Winslow, incisional, Spigelian, obturator)
 3. Masses: neoplasm, abscess
 4. Volvulus
 5. Congenital bands (e.g., Ladd bands)
 6. Enteric duplication: located on antimesenteric side
 7. Mesenteric cyst: located on mesenteric side
B. LUMINAL OCCLUSION
 1. Foreign body, bezoar, gallstone
 2. Meconium ileus: √ microcolon in cystic fibrosis
 3. Intussusception (tumor, Meckel diverticulum,
  chronic ulcers, adhesions)
 4. Tumor
C. INTRINSIC BOWEL WALL LESION
 1. Strictures from neoplasm, Crohn disease,
  tuberculous enteritis, parasitic disease, potassium
  chloride tablets, surgical anastomosis, irradiation,
  massive deposition of amyloid
 2. Vascular insufficiency: arterial / venous occlusion
 3. Congenital atresia / stenosis (jejunum, ileum)

ACQUIRED SMALL BOWEL OBSTRUCTION IN CHILDHOOD
  mnemonic: "AAIIMM"
  Adhesions
  Appendicitis
  Intussusception
  Incarcerated hernia
  Malrotation
  Meckel diverticulum

MECHANICAL SMALL BOWEL OBSTRUCTION IN ADULT
  mnemonic: "SHAVIT"
  Stone (gallstone ileus)
  Hernia
  Adhesion
  Volvulus
  Intussusception
  Tumor

DUODENAL OBSTRUCTION
  mnemonic: "VA BADD TU BADD"

child	adult
Volvulus	Tumor
Atresia	Ulcer
Bands	Bands
Annular pancreas	Annular pancreas
Duplication	Duplication
Diverticulum	Diverticulum

√ "candy cane" appearance in erect position = distended small loops with gas-fluid levels (> 3 – 5 hours after onset of obstruction)
√ disparity in size between contiguous small bowel loops with normal caliber of small bowel beyond site of obstruction
√ small bowel positioned in center of abdomen
√ little / no gas in small bowel = fluid-distended loops
√ little / no gas in colon with complete mechanical obstruction
√ "stretch sign" = erectile valvulae conniventes completely encircle bowel lumen
√ "stepladder appearance" in low obstruction
√ "string-of-beads" indicate peristaltic hyperactivity
√ hyperactive peristalsis / aperistalsis = fatigued small bowel
√ "snakes head" appearance = active peristalsis forms bulbous head of barium column in an attempt to overcome obstruction

STRANGULATED OBSTRUCTION:
  √ "coffee-bean" appearance
  √ featureless bowel wall with flattening of valvulae (from edema / hemorrhage)
  √ "pseudotumor" in unchanged position (from closed loop obstruction)
  √ separation of bowel loops (from exudate / free fluid)
  √ free intraperitoneal gas (from frank perforation)

Small bowel diverticula
A. TRUE DIVERTICULA
  (a) Duodenum
    1. Racemose diverticula: bizarre, lobulated
    2. Giant diverticula
    3. Intraluminal diverticula: result of congenital web / diaphragm
  (b) Jejunal diverticulosis
      blind loop syndrome with bacterial overgrowth (steatorrhea, diarrhea, malabsorption, anemia, weight loss) leading cause of pneumoperitoneum without peritonitis
  (c) Meckel diverticulum
B. PSEUDODIVERTICULA
  1. Scleroderma
  2. Crohn disease
  3. Lymphoma
  4. Communicating ileal duplication
  5. Giant duodenal ulcer

Small bowel ulcer
Aphthous ulcers of small bowel
A. INFECTION
  1. Yersinia enterocolitis (25%)
  2. Salmonellosis
  3. Tuberculosis
  4. Rickettsiosis
B. INFLAMMATION
  1. Crohn disease (22%)
  2. Behçet syndrome
  3. Reiter syndrome
  4. Ankylosing spondylitis

Large nonstenotic ulcers of small bowel
1. Primary nonspecific ulcer	47% incidence
2. Yersiniosis	33%
3. Crohn disease	30%
4. Tuberculosis	18%
5. Salmonellosis / Shigellosis	7%
6. Meckel diverticulum	5%

Cavitary small bowel lesions
1. Lymphoma (exoenteric form)
2. Leiomyosarcoma (exoenteric form)
3. Primary adenocarcinoma
4. Metastases (especially malignant melanoma)

Separation of bowel loops
A. INFILTRATION OF BOWEL WALL / MESENTERY
  (a) INFLAMMATION / INFECTION
    1. Crohn disease
    2. TB
    3. Radiation injury
    4. Retractile mesenteritis
    5. Intraperitoneal abscess
  (b) DEPOSITS
    1. Intestinal hemorrhage / mesenteric vascular occlusion

        2.   Whipple disease
        3.   Amyloidosis
    (c) TUMOR
        1.   Carcinoid tumor: local release of serotonin
             responsible for muscular thickening +
             fibroplastic proliferation = desmoplastic
             reaction
        2.   Primary carcinoma of small bowel (unusual
             presentation)
        3.   Lymphoma
        4.   Neurofibromatosis
B. ASCITES
    Hepatic cirrhosis (75%), peritonitis, peritoneal
    carcinomatosis, congestive heart failure, constrictive
    pericarditis, primary / metastatic lymphatic disease
C. EXTRINSIC MASS
    1.   Peritoneal mesothelioma, mesenteric tumors
         (fibroma, lipoma, fibrosarcoma, leiomyosarcoma,
         malignant mesenteric lymphoid tumor,
         metastases)
    2.   Intraperitoneal abscess
    3.   Retractile mesenteritis (fibrosis, fatty infiltration,
         panniculitis)

Dilatated small bowel & normal folds

mnemonic: "SOS"
    Sprue
    Obstruction
    Scleroderma

A. EXCESSIVE FLUID
    (a) Mechanical obstruction
    (b) Malabsorption syndromes
        1.   Sprue
        2.   Lactase deficiency
B. VASCULAR COMPROMISE
    1.   Mesenteric ischemia (atherosclerosis)
    2.   Amyloidosis
    3.   SLE
C. BOWEL WALL PARALYSIS
    1.   Surgical vagotomy
    2.   Chemical vagotomy: atropine-like substances,
         morphine, L-DOPA, glucagon
    3.   Chagas disease
    4.   Adynamic ileus, Diabetes with hypokalemia
    5.   Chronic idiopathic pseudo-obstruction
D. BOWEL WALL DESTRUCTION
    1.   Lymphoma
    2.   Scleroderma (smooth muscle atrophy)
    3.   Dermatomyositis

Normal small bowel folds & diarrhea

1.   Pancreatic insufficiency
2.   Lactase deficiency
3.   Lymphoma / pseudolymphoma

Abnormal small bowel folds
Thickened folds of stomach + small bowel
    1.   Lymphoma

        2.   Crohn disease
        3.   Eosinophilic gastroenteritis
        4.   Zolinger-Ellison syndrome
        5.   Menetrier disease
        6.   Cirrhosis = gastric varices + hypoproteinemia
        7.   Amyloidosis
        8.   Whipple disease

Thickened regular folds ± dilatation
A . HEMORRHAGE
    (a) Vessel injury
         Ischemia, infarction, trauma
    (b) Vasculitis
         Connective tissue disease, Henoch-Schönlein
         purpura, thrombangitis obliterans
    (c) Hypocoagulability
         Hemophilia, anticoagulant therapy,
         hypofibrinogemia, circulating anticoagulants,
         fibrinolytic system activation, idiopathic
         thrombocytopenic purpura, coagulation
         defects (leukemia, lymphoma, multiple
         myeloma, metastatic carcinoma),
         hypoprothrombinemia
B. EDEMA
    (a) Hypoproteinemia
         Cirrhosis, Nephrotic syndrome, Protein-losing
         enteropathy (Celiac disease, Whipple disease)
    (b) Increased capillary permeability
         Angioneurotic edema
    (c) Increased hydrostatic pressure
         Portal venous hypertension
C. LYMPHATIC BLOCKAGE
    1.   Tumor infiltration: Lymphoma, pseudolymphoma
    2.   Irradiation
    3.   Mesenteric fibrosis
    4.   Intestinal lymphangiectasia
    5.   Whipple disease
D. DEPOSITS
    1.   Eosinophilic enteritis
    2.   Pneumatosis intestinalis
    3.   Amyloid vasculitis
    4.   Abetalipoproteinemia
    5.   Crohn disease
    6.   Graft-versus-host disease

Thickened irregular folds ± dilatation
A. INFLAMMATION
    1.   Crohn disease
B. NEOPLASTIC
    1.   Lymphoma
C. INFECTION
    (a) Protozoan: giardiasis, strongyloidiasis
    (b) Bacterial: yersinia enterocolica, typhoid fever,
         tuberculosis
    (c) Fungal: histoplasmosis
D. IDIOPATHIC
    (a) Lymphatic dilatation:
        1.   Inflammatory process, tumor growth,
             irradiation fibrosis

2. Whipple disease
(b) Cellular infiltration:
1. Eosinophilic enteritis
2. Mastocytosis
(c) Deposits
1. Amyloidosis
2. Alpha chain disease: defective secretory IGA system
3. Abetalipoproteinemia: recessive, retinitis pigmentosa, neurologic disease
4. Fibrocystic disease of the pancreas

Tethered folds
= indicative of desmoplastic reaction
√ kinking, angulation, tethering, separation of bowel loops
1. Carcinoid
2. Postoperative in Gardner syndrome
3. Retractile mesenteritis
4. Hodgkin disease
5. Peritoneal implants
6. Endometriosis
7. Tuberculous peritonitis
8. Mesothelioma
9. Postoperative adhesions

Atrophy of folds
1. Celiac disease
2. Chronic radiation injury

Multiple stenotic lesions of small bowel
1. Crohn disease
2. End-stage radiation enteritis
3. Metastatic carcinoma
4. Endometritis
5. Eosinophilic gastroenteritis
6. Tuberculosis
7. Drug-induced (e.g., potassium chloride tablets)

Delayed small bowel transit
= transit time > 6 hours
mnemonic: "SPATS DID"
Scleroderma
Potassium (hypokalemia)
Anxiety
Thyroid (hypothyroidism)
Sprue
Diabetes (poorly controlled)
Idiopathic
Drugs (opiates, atropine, phenothiazine)

Small bowel filling defects
Solitary filling defect
A. INTRINSIC TO BOWEL WALL
(a) Benign neoplasm: Leiomyoma (97%), adenoma, lipoma, hemangioma, neurofibroma

(b) Malignant primary: Adenocarcinoma, lymphoma (desmoplastic response), sarcoma, carcinoid
(c) Metastases: from melanoma, lung, kidney, breast
(d) Inflammation: Inflammatory pseudotumor
(e) Infection: Parasites
B. EXTRINSIC TO BOWEL WALL
1. Duplication cyst
2. Endometrioma
C. INTRALUMINAL
1. Gallstone ileus
2. Parasites (ascariasis, strongyloidiasis)
3. Inverted Meckel diverticulum
4. Blood clot
5. Foreign body, bezoar, pills, seeds

Multiple filling defects of small bowel
A. POLYPOSIS SYNDROMES
1. Peutz-Jeghers syndrome
2. Gardner syndrome
3. Disseminated gastrointestinal polyposis
4. Generalized gastrointestinal juvenile polyposis
5. Cronkhite-Canada syndrome
B. BENIGN TUMORS
1. Multiple simple adenomatous polyps
2. Hemangioma
3. Leiomyoma, neurofibroma
4. Nodular lymphoid hyperplasia
= normal terminal ileum in children + adolescents; may be associated with dysgammaglobulinemia
√ symmetric fairly sharply demarcated filling defects
5. Varices (multiple phlebectasia in jejunum, oral mucosa, tongue, scrotum)
C. MALIGNANT TUMORS
1. Carcinoid tumor
2. Lymphoma
(a) primary lymphoma (rarely multiple)
(b) secondary lymphoma: gastrointestinal involvement in 63% of disseminated disease; 19% in small intestine
3. Metastases: melanoma > lung > breast > choriocarcinoma > kidney > stomach, uterus, ovary, pancreas
D. INTRALUMINAL
1. Foreign bodies, food particles, seeds, pills
2. Gallstones
3. Parasites: ascariasis, strongyloidiasis, hookworm, tapeworm

Sandlike lucencies of small bowel
1. Waldenström macroglobulinemia
2. Mastocytosis
3. Histoplasmosis
4. Nodular lymphoid hyperplasia
5. Intestinal lymphangiectasia

6. Eosinophilic gastroenteritis
7. Lymphoma
8. Crohn disease
9. Whipple disease
10. Yersinia enterocolitis
11. Cronkhite-Canada syndrome
12. Cystic fibrosis
13. Food particles / gas bubbles
14. Strongyloides stercoralis

Acute small bowel hemorrhage
1. Crohn disease
2. Meckel diverticulum
3. Leiomyoma
4. Metastatic tumor

SMALL BOWEL TUMORS
   Incidence: 1:100,000; 1.5 – 6% of all neoplasms in the
                   GI tract;
   Malignant:benign = 1:1
   Symptomatic malignant:symptomatic benign = 3:1
   Location of small bowel primaries:
      ileum (41%), jejunum (36%), duodenum (18%)
   ROENTGENOGRAPHIC APPEARANCE:
   (1) pedunculated intraluminal tumor, usually originating
        from mucosa
        √ smooth / irregular surface without visible mucosal
          pattern
        √ moves within intestinal lumen twice the length of
          the stalk
   (2) sessile intraluminal tumor without stalk, usually from
        tissues outside mucosa
        √ smooth / irregular surface without visible mucosal
          pattern
   (3) intra- / extramural tumor
        √ base of tumor greater than any part projecting
          into the lumen
        √ mucosal pattern visible, may be stretched
   (4) serosal tumor
        √ displacement of adjacent loops
        √ small bowel obstruction (rare)
        √ coilspring pattern of intussusceptum

Benign small bowel tumors
   • asymptomatic (80%)
   • melena, pain, weakness
   • palpable abdominal mass (20%)
   Types:
      1. Leiomyoma   (36 – 49%)
      2. Adenoma   (15 – 20%)
      3. Lipoma   (14 – 16%)
         Location: duodenum (32%), jejunum (17%),
                   ileum (51%)
      4. Hemangioma   (13 – 16%)
      5. Lymphangioma   (5%)
         Location: duodenum > jejunum > ileum
      6. Neurogenic tumor   (1%)

Malignant small bowel tumors
   • asymptomatic (10 – 30%)
   • pain / obstruction (80%)
   • weight loss (66%)
   • blood loss (50%)
   • palpable abdominal mass (50%)
   1. Carcinoid (46 – 48%)
   2. Adenocarcinoma (25 – 26%)
      may arise in villous tumors / de novo
      Location: duodenum (48%), jejunum (44%),
                ileum (8%)
      √ annular stricture (60%)
      √ lobulated / ovoid polypoid sessile mass (41%)
      √ ulceration (27%)
   3. Lymphoma (16 – 17%)
   4. Leiomyosarcoma (9 – 10%)
   5. Vascular malignancy (1%)
   6. Fibrosarcoma (0.3%)
   7. Metastatic tumor

Mesenteric masses
   1. Fibromatous tumors (most common)
   2. Fibrous histiocytoma
   3. Smooth muscle tumor
   4. Neural tumor
   5. Hemangioma
   6. Lipoma (uncommon)
   7. Mesenteric cyst
   8. Hematoma
   9. Lipomatosis
   10. Lipodystrophy / panniculitis
   11. Desmoid tumor
   12. Liposarcoma

Ileocecal valve abnormalities
   A. Lipomatosis: > 40 years of age, female
      √ stellate / rosette pattern
   B. NEOPLASM
      1. Lipoma, adenomatous polyp, villous adenoma
      2. Carcinoid tumor
      3. Adenocarcinoma: 2% of all colonic cancers
      4. Lymphoma: often involving terminal ileum
   C. INFLAMMATION
      1. Crohn disease
      2. Ulcerative colitis
         √ patulous valve, fixed in open position
      3. Tuberculosis
         √ "Fleischner sign" = wide gaping ileocecal valve
           associated with narrowing of the immediately
           adjacent ileum
      4. Amebiasis: terminal ileum not involved (in United
         States)
      5. Typhoid fever, anisakiasis, schistosomiasis,
         actinomycosis
      6. Cathartic abuse
   D. PROLAPSE
      (a) Antegrade: indistinguishable from lipomatosis /
          prolapsing mucosa / neoplasm

(b) Retrograde
E. INTUSSUSCEPTION
F. LYMPHOID HYPERPLASIA

Malabsorption
= deficient absorption of any essential food materials within small bowel
(1) PRIMARY MALABSORPTION
  = the digestive abnormality is the only abnormality present
  1. Celiac disease = nontropical sprue
  2. Tropical sprue
  3. Disaccharidase deficiencies
(2) SECONDARY MALABSORPTION
  = occurring during course of gastrointestinal disease
  (a) Enteric
    1. Whipple disease
    2. Parasites: hookworm, giardia, fish tapeworm
    3. Mechanical defects: fistulas, blind loops, adhesions, volvulus, short circuits
    4. Neurological: diabetes, functional diarrhea
    5. Inflammatory: enteritis (viral, bacterial, fungal, nonspecific)
    6. Endocrine: Zollinger-Ellison syndrome
    7. Drugs: neomycin, phenindione, cathartics
    8. Collagen disease: scleroderma, lupus, polyarteritis
    9. Lymphoma
    10. Benign + malignant small bowel tumors
    11. Vascular disease
    12. CHF, agammaglobulinemia, amyloid, abetalipoproteinemia, intestinal lymphangiectasia
  (b) Gastric
    Vagotomy, gastrectomy, pyloroplasty, gastric fistula (to jejunum, ileum, colon)
  (c) Pancreatic
    Pancreatitis, pancreatectomy, pancreatic cancer, cystic fibrosis
  (d) Hepatobiliary
    Intra- and extrahepatic biliary obstruction, acute + chronic liver disease

ROENTGENOGRAPHIC SIGNS IN MALABSORPTION
√ SMALL BOWEL WITH NORMAL FOLDS + FLUID
  1. Maldigestion (deficiency of bile salt / pancreatic enzymes)
  2. Gastric surgery
  3. Alactasia
√ SMALL BOWEL WITH NORMAL FOLDS + WET
  1. Sprue
  2. Dermatitis herpetiformis
√ DILATED DRY SMALL BOWEL
  1. Scleroderma
  3. Dermatomyositis
  4. Pseudoobstruction: no peristaltic activity

√ DILATED WET SMALL BOWEL
  1. Sprue
  2. Obstruction
  3. Blind loop
√ THICKENED STRAIGHT FOLDS + DRY SMALL BOWEL
  1. Amyloidosis (malabsorption is unusual)
  2. Radiation
  3. Ischemia
  4. Lymphoma (rare)
  5. Macroglobulinemia (rare)
√ THICKENED STRAIGHT FOLDS + WET SMALL BOWEL
  1. Zollinger-Ellison syndrome
  2. Abetalipoproteinemia: rare inherited disease characterized by CNS damage, retinal abnormalities, steatorrhea, acanthocytosis
√ THICKENED NODULAR IRREGULAR FOLDS + DRY SMALL BOWEL
  1. Lymphoid hyperplasia
  2. Lymphoma
  3. Crohn disease
  4. Whipple disease
  5. Mastocytosis
√ THICKENED NODULAR IRREGULAR FOLDS + WET SMALL BOWEL
  1. Lymphangiectasia
  2. Giardiasis
  3. Whipple disease (rare)

SMALL BOWEL NODULARITY WITH MALABSORPTION
  mnemonic: "**Wh**at **Is** **H**is **M**ain **A**im? **L**eave **E**arly, **B**y **G**eorge"
  Whipple disease
  Intestinal lymphangiectasia
  Histiocytosis
  Mastocytosis
  Amyloidosis
  Lymphoma, **L**ymphnodular hyperplasia
  Edema
  Blood
  Giardiasis

COLON
Colon cutoff sign
= abrupt cutoff of gas column at splenic flexure
Causes:
  1. Acute pancreatitis (inflammatory exudate along transverse mesocolon)
  2. Colonic obstruction
  3. Mesenteric thrombosis
  4. Ischemic colitis

Coned cecum
A. INFLAMMATION
  1. Crohn disease
    √ involvement of ascending colon + terminal ileum

2. Ulcerative colitis
   √ backwash ileitis (in 10%)
   √ gaping ileocecal valve
3. Appendicitis
4. Typhlitis
5. Perforated cecal diverticulum

B. INFECTION
1. Tuberculosis
   √ colonic involvement more prominent than that of terminal ileum
   √ Stierlin sign = terminal ileum empties directly into stenotic ascending colon with nonopacification of the fibrotic + contracted cecum
2. Amebiasis
   √ involvement of cecum in 90% of amebiasis
   √ thickened ileocecal valve fixed in open position
   √ reflux into normal terminal ileum
   √ skip lesions in colon
3. Actinomycosis
   • palpable abdominal mass
   • indolent sinus tracts in abdominal wall
4. Blastomycosis
5. Anisakiasis
   from ingestion of raw fish with ascaris-like nematode
6. Typhoid, Yersinia

C. TUMOR
1. Carcinoma of the cecum
2. Metastasis to cecum

Colonic thumbprinting
= sharply defined fingerlike marginal indentations at contours of wall
1. ISCHEMIA = Ischemic colitis
   Occlusive vascular disease, hypercoagulability state, hemorrhage into bowel wall (bleeding diathesis, anticoagulants), traumatic intramural hematoma
2. INFLAMMATION
   Ulcerative colitis, Crohn colitis
3. INFECTION
   Acute amebiasis, schistosomiasis, strongyloidiasis, cytomegalovirus (in renal transplant recipients), pseudomembranous colitis
4. MALIGNANT LESIONS
   Localized primary lymphoma, hematogenous metastases
5. MISCELLANEOUS
   Endometriosis, amyloidosis, pneumatosis intestinalis, diverticulosis, diverticulitis, hereditary angioneurotic edema

Colonic urticaria pattern
A. OBSTRUCTION
1. Obstructing carcinoma
2. Cecal volvulus
3. Colonic ileus
B. ISCHEMIA

C. INFECTION / INFLAMMATION
1. Yersinia enterocolitis
2. Herpes
3. Crohn disease
D. URTICARIA

Colonic ulcers
A. IDIOPATHIC
1. Ulcerative colitis
2. Crohn colitis
B. ISCHEMIC
1. Ischemic colitis
C. TRAUMATIC
1. Radiation injury
2. Caustic colitis
D. NEOPLASTIC
1. Primary colonic carcinoma
2. Metastases (prostate, stomach lymphoma, leukemia)
E. INFLAMMATORY
1. Pseudomembranous colitis
2. Pancreatitis
3. Diverticulitis
4. Behçet syndrome
5. Solitary rectal ulcer syndrome
6. Nonspecific benign ulceration
F. INFECTION
   (a) PROTOZOAN
      1. Amebiasis
      2. Schistosomiasis
      3. Strongyloidiasis
   (b) BACTERIAL
      1. Shigellosis, salmonellosis
      2. Staphylococcal colitis
      3. Tuberculosis
      4. Gonorrheal proctitis
      5. Yersinia colitis
      6. Campylobacter fetus colitis
   (c) FUNGAL
      Histoplasmosis, mucormycosis, actinomycosis, candidiasis
   (d) VIRAL
      1. Lymphogranuloma venereum
      2. Herpes zoster
      3. Cytomegalovirus (transplants)

APHTHOUS ULCERS
1. Crohn disease
2. Amebic colitis
3. **Yersinia enterocolitis**
   Location: terminal ileum
   √ thickened folds + ulceration
   √ lymphoid nodular hyperplasia
4. Behçet syndrome
5. Lymphoma
6. Ischemia

Double tracking of colon
= longitudinal extraluminal tracks paralleling the colon
1. Diverticulitis: generally 3 – 6 cm in length
2. Crohn disease: generally > 10 cm
3. Primary carcinoma: wider + more irregular

Colonic narrowing
A. CHRONIC STAGE OF ANY ULCERATING COLITIS
   (a) Inflammatory : Ulcerative colitis, Crohn colitis, solitary rectal ulcer syndrome, nonspecific benign ulcer
   (b) Infectious: Amebiasis, schistosomiasis, bacillary dysentery, TB, fungal disease, lymphogranuloma venereum, herpes zoster, cytomegalovirus, strongyloides
   (c) Ischemic: Ischemic colitis
   (d) Traumatic: Radiation injury, cathartic colon, caustic colitis
B. MALIGNANT LESION
   (a) Primary: Colonic carcinoma (annular / scirrhous); complication of ulcerative colitis + Crohn colitis
   (b) Metastatic from prostate, cervix, uterus, kidney, stomach, pancreas, primary intraperitoneal sarcoma
      — hematogenous (e.g., breast)
      — lymphangitic spread
      — peritoneal seeding
C. EXTRINSIC PROCESS
   (a) Inflammation: Retractile mesenteritis, diverticulitis, pancreatitis
   (b) Deposits: Amyloidosis, endometriosis, pelvic lipomatosis
D. POSTSURGICAL
   Adhesivie bands, surgical anastomosis
E. NORMAL
   Cannon point

Rectal narrowing
1. Pelvic lipomatosis + fibrolipomatosis
2. Lymphogranuloma venereum
3. Radiation injury of rectum
4. Chronic ulcerative colitis

Enlarged presacral space
Normal width < 5 mm in 95%; abnormal width > 10 mm
A. RECTAL INFLAMMATION / INFECTION
   Ulcerative colitis, Crohn colitis, idiopathic proctosigmoiditis, radiation therapy
B. RECTAL INFECTION
   1. Proctitis (TB, amebiasis, lymphogranuloma venereum, radiation, ischemia)
   2. Diverticulitis
C. BENIGN RECTAL TUMOR
   1. Developmental cyst (dermoid, enteric cyst, tail gut cyst)
   2. Lipoma, neurofibroma, hemangioendothelioma
D. MALIGNANT RECTAL TUMOR
   1. Adenocarcinoma, cloacogenic carcinoma
   2. Lymphoma, sarcoma, lymph node metastases
   3. Prostatic carcinoma, bladder tumors, cervical cancer, ovarian cancer
E. BODY FLUIDS / DEPOSITS
   1. Hematoma: Surgery, sacral fracture
   2. Pus: Perforated appendix, presacral abscess
   3. Serum: Edema, venous thrombosis
   4. Deposits of fat: Pelvic lipomatosis, Cushing disease
   5. Deposit of amyloid: Amyloidosis
F. SACRAL TUMOR
   1. Sacrococcygeal teratoma, anterior sacral meningocele
   2. Chordoma, metastasis to sacrum
G. MISCELLANEOUS
   1. Inguinal hernia containing segment of colon
   2. Colitis cystica profunda
   3. Pelvic lipomatosis

Colonic obstruction
A. INTRALUMINAL
   Fecal impaction, fecaloma, intussusception, meconium plug
B. BOWEL WALL LESION
   (a) malignant: 70% of obstructions, predominantly in sigmoid
   (b) inflammatory: Crohn disease, ulcerative colitis, mesenteric ischemia, diverticulitis (15%)
   (c) infectious: Infectious granulomatous process (actinomycosis, tuberculosis, lymphogranuloma venereum), parasitic disease (amebiasis, schistosomiasis)
   (d) congenital: Aganglionosis, imperforate anus
C. EXTRINSIC
   (a) MASS IMPRESSION: Endometriosis, large tumor mass, abscess, hugely distended bladder, mesenteritis
   (b) SEVERE CONSTRICTION: volvulus (3rd most common cause), hernia, adhesion

RADIOLOGIC PATTERNS:
   (a) dilated colon only = competent ileocecal valve
   (b) dilated small bowel (25%) = incompetent ileocecal valve
   (c) dilated colon + dilated small bowel = ileocecal valve obstruction secondary to cecal overdistension
   Δ cecum most dilated portion (in 75% of cases); critical at 8 cm diameter
The lower the obstruction the more the proximal distension !

Colonic filling defects
Single colonic filling defect
A. BENIGN TUMORS
   1. Polyps (hyperplastic, adenomatous, villous adenoma, villoglandular); most common benign tumor

2. Lipoma
Most common intramural tumor, 2nd most common benign tumor; M < F
Location: ascending colon + cecum > left side of colon
3. Carcinoid: 10% metastasize
4. Spindle cell tumors (leiomyoma, fibroma, neurofibroma); 4th most common benign tumor; rectum > cecum
5. Lymphangioma, hemangioma

B. MALIGNANT TUMORS
1. Primary tumors: Carcinoma, sarcoma
2. Secondary tumors:
Metastases (breast, stomach, lung, pancreas, kidney female genital tract), lymphoma, invasion by adjacent tumors

C. INFECTION
1. Ameboma
2. Polypoid granuloma: schistosomiasis, TB

D. INFLAMMATION
1. Inflammatory pseudopolyp: ulcerative colitis, Crohn disease
2. Periappendiceal abscess
3. Diverticulitis
4. Foreign body perforation

E. NONSESSILE INTRALUMINAL BODY
1. Fecal impaction
2. Foreign body
3. Gallstone
4. Bolus of ascaris worms

F. MISCELLANEOUS
1. Endometriosis:
3rd most common benign tumor
Location: sigmoid colon, rectosigmoid junction (at level of cul-de-sac)
   • may cause bleeding (after invasion of mucosa)
2. Localized amyloid deposition
3. Suture granuloma
4. Intussusception
5. Pseudotumors (adhesions, fibrous bands)
6. Colitis cystica profunda

Multiple colonic filling defects
A. NEOPLASMS
1. Polyposis syndrome: Familial polyposis, Gardner syndrome, Peutz-Jeghers syndrome, Turcot syndrome, juvenile polyposis syndromes, disseminated gastrointestinal polyps, multiple adenomatous polyps
2. Hematogenous metastases from breast, lung, stomach, ovary, pancreas, uterus
3. Multiple tumors
(a) benign: Neurofibromatosis, colonic lipomatosis, multiple hamartoma syndrome (Cowden disease)
(b) malignant: Lymphoma, leukemia, adenocarcinoma

B. INFLAMMATORY PSEUDOPOLYPS
Ulcerative colitis, Crohn colitis, ischemic colitis, amebiasis, schistosomiasis, strongyloidiasis, trichuriasis

C. ARTIFACTS
Feces, air bubbles, oil bubbles, mucus strands, ingested foreign body (e.g. corn kernels)

D. MISCELLANEOUS
Nodular lymphoid hyperplasia, lymphoid folicular pattern, hemorrhoids, diverticula, pneumatosis intestinalis, colitis cystica profunda, colonic urticaria, submucosal colonic edema secondary to obstruction, cystic fibrosis, amyloidosis, ulcerative pseudopolyps, proximal to obstruction

Cecal filling defect
A. ABNORMALITIES OF THE APPENDIX
1. Acute appendicitis / appendiceal abscess
2. Crohn disease
3. Inverted appendiceal stump / appendiceal intussusception
4. Mucocele
5. Myxoglobulosis
6. Appendiceal neoplasm: carcinoid tumor (90%), leiomyoma, neuroma, lipoma, adenocarcinoma, metastasis

B. COLONIC LESION
1. Ameboma
2. Primary cecal neoplasm
3. Ileocolic intussusception
4. Lipomatosis of ileocecal valve

C. UNUSUAL ABNORMALITIES
1. Ileocecal diverticulitis (in 50% < age 30 years)
2. Solitary benign ulcer of the cecum
3. Adherent fecolith (e.g., in cystic fibrosis)
4. Endometriosis
5. Burkitt lymphoma

mnemonic: "MACALIFT"
Mucocele
Abscess (periappendiceal)
Carcinoid
Ameboma
Lymphoma
Inflammation (Crohn diseas, ulcerative colitis, TB)
Feces
Tumor (adenocarcinoma, villous adenoma)

Carpet lesions of colon
= flat lobulated lesions with alteration of surface texture + little / no protrusion into lumen
Location: rectum > cecum > ascending colon
Causes:
A. Neoplasms:
1. Tubular / tubulovillous / villous adenoma
2. Familial polyposis
3. Adenocarcinoma
4. Submucosal tumor spread (from adjacent carcinoma)

	Single Polyp	Multiple Polyps
Neoplastic (10 %) — epithelial	1. Tubular adenoma 2. Tubulovillous adenoma 3. Villous adenoma 4. Turcot syndrome	1. Familial adenomatosis coli 2. Adenomatosis of GI tract 3. Gardner syndrome
— nonepithelial	1. Carcinoid 2. Leiomyoma 3. Lipoma 4. Hem-, lymphangioma 5. Fibroma, neurofibroma	
Nonneoplastic (90 %) — unclassified	1. Hyperplastic polyp	1. Hyperplastic polyposis
— hamartomatous	1. Juvenile polyp 2. Peutz-Jeghers syndrome	1. Juvenile polyposis
— inflammatory	1. Ulcerative colitis 2. Benign lymphoid polyp 3. Fibroid granulation polyp	1. Cronkhite-Canada syndrome 2. Ulcerative colitis

B. Miscellaneous
  1. Nonspecific follicular proctitis
  2. Biopsy site
  3. Endometriosis
  4. Rectal varices
  5. Colonic urticaria

Colonic polyps
Histologic Classification
  ADENOMATOUS POLYPS
    1. Familial polyposis
    2. Gardner syndrome
    3. Peutz-Jeghers syndrome (some in SB + colon)
    4. Turcot syndrome
  INFLAMMATORY POLYPS
    1. Juvenile polyposis
    2. Cronkhite-Canada syndrome
  HAMARTOMATOUS POLYPS
    1. Peutz-Jeghers syndrome (most in small bowel)
  POLYPOSIS LOOK-ALIKES
    1. Inflammatory polyposis
    2. Lymphoid hyperplasia
    3. Lymphoma
    4. Metastases
    5. Pneumatosis coli

Polyposis Syndromes
= more than 100 polyps in number
Mode of Transmission
  A. HEREDITARY
    (a) Autosomal dominant
      1. Familial polyposis

      2. Gardner syndrome
      3. Peutz-Jeghers syndrome
    (b) Autosomal recessive
      1. Turcot syndrome
  D. NONHEREDITARY
    1. Cronkhite-Canada syndrome
    2. Juvenile polyposis

Mesenteric masses
  1. Round solid masses
    Δ benign primary tumors are more common than malignant primary tumors
    (a) Metastases especially from colon, ovary (most frequent neoplasm of mesentery),
    (b) Lymphoma
    (c) Leiomyosarcoma (more frequent than leiomyoma)
    (d) Neural tumor (neurofibroma, ganglioneuroma)
    (e) Lipoma (uncommon), lipomatosis
    (f) Fibrous histiocytoma
    (g) Hemangioma
  2. Ill-defined masses
    metastases (ovary), lymphoma, fibromatosis, fibrosing mesenteritis (associated with Gardner syndrome), lipodystrophy, panniculitis
  3. Loculated cystic masses
    lymphangioma (most common), pseudomyxoma peritonei, mesenteric cyst, hematoma
  4. Omental cake
    lymphoma, tuberculosis, mesothelioma
  5. Stellate masses
    mesothelioma, metastases, fibrosing mesenteritis, tuberculous peritonitis, desmoid tumor

Intramural hemorrhage
Causes:
1. Trauma
2. Leukemia, lymphoma
3. Multiple myeloma
4. Metastatic carcinoma
5. Hemophilia
6. Anticoagulant therapy
7. Schönlein-Henoch purpura
8. Idiopathic thrombocytopenic purpura
- abdominal pain
- melena

Site: submucosal / intramural / mesenteric
√ "stacked coin" / "picket fence" appearance of mucosal folds
√ separation + uncoiling of bowel loops
√ narrowing of lumen + localized filling defects (asymmetric hematoma)
√ no spasm / irritability
√ mechanical obstruction + proximal distension of loops
√ resolution within 2 – 6 weeks

Gastrointestinal bleeding
Mortality: approx. 10%
  barium examination should be avoided in acute bleeders !
Sources:
A. UPPER GASTROINTESTINAL HEMORRHAGE
  = bleeding site proximal to ligament of Treitz
  @ Esophagogastric junction
    1. Esophageal varices (17%): 50% mortality
    2. Mallory-Weiss syndrome (7 – 14%): very low mortality
  @ Stomach
    1. Acute hemorrhagic gastritis (17 – 27%)
    2. Gastric ulcer (10%)
    3. pyloroduodenal ulcer (17 – 25%)
      Mortality: < 10% if under age 60; > 35% if over age 60
  @ Other causes (14%): visceral artery aneurysm, vascular malformation, neoplasm, vascular-enteric fistula
    Average mortality: 8 – 10%
B. LOWER GASTROINTESTINAL HEMORRHAGE
  @ Small intestine
    Tumor, ulcers, diverticula, inflammatory bowel disease, vascular malformation, visceral artery aneurysm, aortoenteric fistula
  @ Colorectal (70%)
    1. Diverticula (most common): hemorrhage in 25% of patients with diverticulosis; spontaneous cessation of bleeding in 80%; recurrent bleeding in 25%
    2. Colonic angiodysplasia = dilated submucosal arteries + veins overlying mucosal thinning (? secondary to mucosal ischemia)
    3. Colitis, tumors, mesenteric varices

INFANTILE GASTROINTESTINAL BLEEDING
(1) Peptic ulcer (2) Varices (3) Ulcerated Meckel diverticulum

GI abnormalities in chronic renal failure and renal transplantation
@ Esophagus
  1. Esophagitis
    Cause: candida, CMV, herpes
@ Stomach & duodenum
  1. Gastritis
    √ thickened gastric folds (38%)
    √ edema + erosions
      Cause:
      (a) imbalance of gastrin levels + gastric acid secretion due to (1) reduced removal of gastrin from kidney with loss of cortical mass (2) impaired acid feedback mechanism (3) hypochlorhydria
      (b) opportunistic infection (e.g., CMV)
  2. Gastric ulcer (3.5%)
  3. Duodenal ulcer (2.4%)
  4. Duodenitis (47%)
@ Colon
  More severely + frequently affected after renal transplantation
  1. Progressive distention + pseudoobstruction
    Contributing factors: dehydration, alteration of diet, inactivity, nonabsorbable antacids, high-dose steroids
  2. Ischemic colitis
    (a) primary disease responsible for end-stage renal disease (e.g., diabetes, vasculitis)
    (b) trauma of renal transplantation
  3. Diverticulitis
    Contributing factors: chronic obstipation, steroids, autonomic nervous dysfunction
  4. Pseudomembranous colitis
  5. Uremic colitis = nonspecific colitis
  6. Spontaneous colonic perforation
    Cause: nonocclusive ischemia, diverticula, duodenal + gastric ulcers
@ Pancreas
  1. Pancreatitis
    Cause: hypercalcemia, steroids, infection, immunosuppressive agents, trauma
@ General
  1. GI hemorrhage
    Cause:
    gastritis, ulcers, colonic diverticula, ischemic bowel, infectious colitis, pseudomembranous colitis, nonspecific cecal ulceration
  2. Bowel perforation (in 1 – 4% of transplant recipients)
  3. Opportunistic infection
    Organisms: candida, herpes, CMV, strongyloides
  4. Malignancy
    (a) skin tumors
    (b) lymphoma

ANATOMY AND FUNCTION OF GASTROINTESTINAL TRACT

Gastrointestinal hormones

Cholecystokinin

= CCK = 33 amino acid residues (former name: Pancreozymin); the 5 C-terminal amino acids are identical to those of gastrin causing similar effects as gastrin

Produced in: duodenal + upper intestinal mucosa

Released by: fatty acids, some amino acids (phenylalanine, methionine), hydrogen ions

Effects:

@ Stomach
  (1) weakly stimulates HCl secretion
  (2) given alone: inhibits gastrin which leads to decrease in HCl production
  (3) stimulates pepsin secretion
  (4) stimulates gastric motility

@ Pancreas
  (1) stimulates secretion of pancreatic enzymes (= Pancreozymin)
  (2) stimulates bicarbonate secretion (weakly by direct effect; strongly through potentiating effect on secretin)
  (3) stimulates insulin release

@ Liver
  (1) stimulates water + bicarbonate secretion

@ Intestine
  (1) stimulates secretion of Brunner glands
  (2) Increases motility

@ Gallbladder
  (1) strong stimulator of contraction
  (2) relaxation of sphincter of Oddi

Gastrin

= 17 amino acid peptide amide; PENTAGASTRIN = acyl derivative of the biologic active C-terminal tetrapeptide amide

Produced in: antral cells + G-cells of pancreas

Released by: mediated by neuroendocrine cholinergic reflexes
  (a) vagal stimulation, gastric distension
  (b) short-chain alcohol (ethanol, propanol)
  (c) amino acids (glycine, ß-alanine)
  (d) caffeine
  (e) hypercalcemia

Inhibited by: drop in pH of antral mucosa < 3.5

Effects:

@ Stomach:
  (1) stimulation of gastric HCl secretion from parietal cells which in turn
  (2) increases pepsinogen production by chief cells through local reflex
  (3) increased antral motility

  (4) trophic effect on gastric mucosa (parietal cell hyperplasia)

@ Pancreas
  (1) strong increase in enzyme output
  (2) weakly stimulates fluid + bicarbonate output
  (3) stimulates insulin release

@ Liver
  (1) water + bicarbonate secretion

@ Intestine
  (1) stimulates secretion of Brunner glands
  (2) increases motility

@ Gallbladder
  (1) stimulates contraction

@ Esophagus
  (1) increases resting pressure of LES

Secretin

Produced in: duodenal mucosa

Released by: hydrogen ions providing a pH < 4.5

Effects:

@ Stomach
  (1) inhibits gastrin activity which leads to decrease in HCl secretion
  (2) stimulates pepsinogen secretion by chief cells (potent pepsigogue)
  (3) decreases gastric and duodenal motility + contraction of pyloric sphincter

@ Pancreas
  (1) increases alkaline pancreatic secretions ($NaHCO_3$)
  (2) weakly stimulates enzyme secretion
  (3) stimulates insulin release

@ Liver
  (1) stimulates water + bicarbonate secretion (most potent choleretic)

@ Intestine
  (1) stimulates secretion of Brunner glands
  (2) inhibits motility

@ Esophagus
  (1) opens LES

Small bowel peristalsis

A. INCREASED
  1. Vagal stimulation
  2. Acetylcholine
  3. Anticholinesterase (e.g., neostigmine)
  4. Cholecystokinine

B. DECREASED
  1. Atropine (e.g., probanthine)
  2. Bilateral vagotomy

Effect of bilateral vagotomy

= cholinergic denervation
(1) decreased MOTILITY of stomach + intestines

(2) decreased GASTRIC SECRETION
(3) decreased TONE OF GALLBLADDER + bile ducts
(4) increased TONE OF SPHINCTERS (Oddi + lower esophageal sphincter)

Esophageal rings
A. Esophageal Vestibule
= saccular termination of lower esophagus with upper boundary at tubulovestibular junction + lower boundary at esophagogastric junction
√ collapsed during resting state
√ assumes bulbous configuration with swallowing
(a) tubulovestibular junction = A-level = junction between tubular and saccular esophagus
(b) phrenic ampulla = bell-shaped part above diaphragm (term should be discarded because of dynamic changes of configuration)
(c) submerged segment = infrahiatal part of esophagus
√ widening / disappearance is indicative of GE reflux disease
B. Gastroesophageal Junction
Site: at upper level of gastric sling fibers straddling cardiac incisura demarcating the left lateral margin of GE junction
C. Z-line = B-level = squamocolumnar junction line
not acceptable criterion for locating GE junction
Site: 1 – 2 cm above gastric sling fibers
D. Lower Esophageal Sphincter
= physiologic 2 – 4 cm high pressure zone corresponding to esophageal vestibule
√ tightly closed during resting state
√ assumes bulbous configuration with swallowing

Muscular rings of esophagus
A Ring
= contracted / hypertrophied muscles in response to incompetent GE sphincter
• rarely symptomatic / dysphagia
Location: at tubulovestibular junction = superior aspect of vestibule
√ usually 2 cm proximal to GE junction at upper end of vestibule
√ varies in caliber during the same examination, may disappear on maximum distension
√ broad smooth narrowing with thick rounded margins
√ visible only if tubular esophagus above + vestibule below are distended

B Ring
= sling fibers representing a U-shaped thickening of inner muscle layers with open arm of U toward lesser curvature = inferior aspect of vestibule
Location: < 2 cm from hiatal margins
√ only visible when esophagogastric junction is above hiatus
√ thin ledge-like ring just below the mucosal junction (Z-line)

Pylorus
= fan-shaped specialized circular muscle fibers with:
(a) distal sphincteric loop = right canalis loop
√ corresponds to radiologic pyloric sphincter
(b) proximal sphincteric loop = left canalis loop
√ 2 cm proximal to distal sphincteric loop on greater curvature (seen during complete relaxation)
(c) torus = fibers of both sphincters converge on the lesser curvature side to form a muscular prominence; prolapse of mucosa between sphincteric loops produces a niche simulating ulcer
√ pyloric channel 5 –10 mm long, wall thickness of 4 – 8 mm
√ concentric indentation of the base of the duodenal bulb

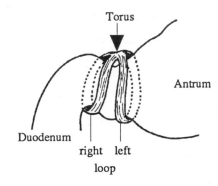

Small bowel folds
A. NORMAL FOLD THICKNESS
@ jejunum 1.7 – 2.0 mm   > 2.5 mm pathologic
@ ileum   1.4 – 1.7 mm   > 2.0 mm pathologic
B. NORMAL NUMBER OF FOLDS
@ jejunum 4 – 6 / inch
@ ileum   3 – 5 / inch
C. NORMAL FOLD HEIGHT
@ jejunum 3.5 – 7.0 mm
@ ileum   2.0 – 3.5 mm
D. NORMAL LUMEN DIAMETER
@ upper jejunum 3.0 – 4.0 cm > 4.5 cm pathologic
@ lower jejunum 2.5 – 3.5 cm > 4.0 cm pathologic
@ ileum   2.0 – 2.8 cm > 3.0 cm pathologic

RULE OF 3's:
Δ wall thickness < 3 mm
Δ valvulae conniventes < 3 mm
Δ diameter < 3 cm
Δ air-fluid levels < 3

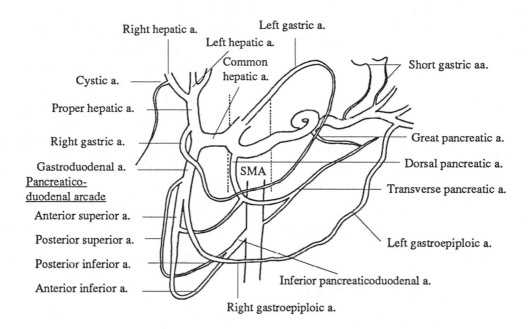

Blood Supply of Stomach, Duodenum, and Pancreas

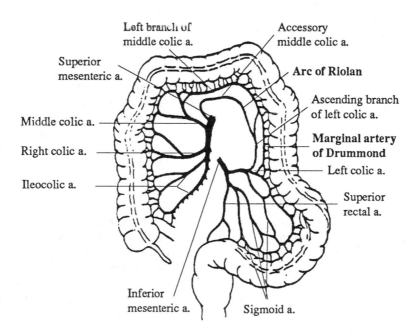

Blood Supply of Large Intestine

DISEASE ENTITIES OF GASTROINTESTINAL TRACT

ACHALASIA
= failure of organized peristalsis + relaxation at level of lower esophageal sphincter

Etiology:
(a) idiopathic: ? neurotropic virus, ? gastrin hypersensitivity
(b) Chagas Disease

√ megaesophagus = dilatation of esophagus beginning in upper 1/3, ultimately entire length

√ small / absent gastric air bubble

√ stasis in thoracic esophagus filled with alimentary residue

√ absence of primary peristalsis below level of cricopharyngeus

√ nonperistaltic contractions

√ "bird beak" / "rat tail" deformity = V-shaped conical + symmetric tapering of stenotic segment with most marked narrowing at GE junction

√ Hurst phenomenon = temporary transit through cardia provoked by hydrostatic pressure of barium column reaching above a critical level

√ sudden esophageal emptying after ingestion of carbonated beverage (e.g., coke)

Cx: esophageal carcinoma in 7% (usually midesophagus)

DDx: (1) Neoplasm (separation of gastric fundus from diaphragm; normal peristalsis; asymmetric tapering)
         (2) Peptic stenosing esophagitis

ADENOMA OF SMALL BOWEL
Location: duodenum (21%), jejunum (36%), ileum (43%) — ileocecal valve

Path: (1) hamartomatous polyp (77%), multiple in 47%, 1/3 of multiple lesions associated with Peutz-Jeghers syndrome
        (2) adenomatous polyp (13%), may have malignant potential
        (3) polypoid gastric heterotopic tumor (10%)

ADENOMATOUS COLONIC POLYP
= EPITHELIAL POLYP
most common benign colonic tumor (68 – 79%)

Predisposed:
previously detected polyp / cancer; family history of polyps / cancer; idiopathic inflammatory bowel disease; Peutz-Jeghers syndrome; Gardner syndrome; familial polyposis

Incidence: 3% in 3rd decade; 10% in 7th decade; 26% in 9th decade

Location: rectum (21 – 34%); sigmoid (26 – 38%); ascending colon (9 – 12%); transverse colon (12 – 13%); descending colon (6 – 18%)

Histo:
1. Tubular adenoma (75%)
   = cylindrical glandular structure lined by stratified columnar epithelium
   malignant potential: < 10 mm (1%); 10 – 20 mm (10%); > 20 mm (35%)
2. Tubulovillous adenoma (15%)
   = mixture between tubular + villous adenoma
   malignant potential: < 10 mm (4%); 10 – 20 mm (7%); > 20 mm (46%)
3. Villous adenoma (10%)
   = infolding of papillary projections of glandular structure ("villous fronds")
   malignant potential: < 10 mm (10%); 10 – 20 mm (10%); > 20 mm (53%)
   • potassium depletion

Size & Malignancy:
< 5 mm in 0%; 5 – 9 mm in 1%; 10 – 20 mm in 10%; > 20 mm in 46% malignant

• asymptomatic (75%)
• diarrhea, abdominal pain
• peranal hemorrhage (67%) correlating with size + location

Colonoscopy (incomplete in 16 – 43%)

BE (rate of detection of polyps < 10 mm higher with double contrast; false negative rate of 7%):

√ sessile flat / round polyp

√ pedunculated polyp: stalk > 2 cm in length almost always indicative of a benign polyp

√ suggestive of malignancy: irregular lobulated surface, broad base = width of the base greater than height, retraction of colonic wall = dimpling / indentation / puckering at base of tumor, interval growth

DDx:
(1) Nonneoplastic: hyperplastic polyp, inflammatory pseudopolyp, lymphoid tissue, ameboma, tuberculoma, foreign body granuloma, malakoplakia, heterotopia, hamartoma
(2) Neoplastic subepithelial: lipoma, leiomyoma, neurofibroma, hemangioma, lymphangioma, endothelioma, myeloblastoma, sarcoma, lymphoma, enteric cyst, duplication, varix, pneumatosis, hematoma, endometriosis

AFFERENT LOOP SYNDROME
= PROXIMAL LOOP SYNDROME = BLIND LOOP SYNDROME
= partial intermittent obstruction of afferent loop leading to overdistension of loop by gastric juices after Billroth II gastrojejunostomy

Cause:
gastrojejunostomy with left-to-right anastomosis (= proximal jejunal loop attached to greater curvature instead of lesser curvature), mechanical factors

(intussusception, adhesion, kinking), inflammatory
disease, neoplastic infiltration of local mesentery or
anastomosis, idiopathic motor dysfunction
- postprandial epigastric fullness relieved by bilious
vomiting
- Vitamin B_{12} deficiency with megaloblastic anemia
- afferent loop with abnormal bacterial flora (Gram
negative, resembling colon in quality + quantity)
UGI:
√ preferential emptying of stomach into proximal loop
√ proximal loop stasis
√ regurgitation
CT:
√ rounded water-density masses adjacent to head + tail
of pancreas forming a U-shaped loop
√ oral contrast material may not enter loop
√ may result in biliary obstruction (increased pressure at
ampulla)
Rx: antibiotic therapy

AIDS
Organisms: CMV, mycobacterium avium intracellulare,
cryptosporidium, candida, pneumocystis
1. AIDS-related cholangitis
Organism: CMV, cryptosporidium
- RUQ pain, fever, jaundice, abnormal LFT
√ irregular dilatation of intra- and extrahepatic bile
ducts similar to sclerosing cholangitis
2. Liver abscess
3. Splenomegaly (very common)
4. Splenic infarction (septic emboli)
5. CMV esophagitis
6. Cryptosporidium antritis
√ area of focal gastric thickening + ulceration
7. CMV gastritis
frequently affects GE junction + prepyloric antrum
8. AIDS enteritis
(a) **Cryptosporidiosis enteritis**
Location: proximal small bowel
√ small bowel dilatation of proximal jejunal loops
√ small bowel thickening (mimicking sprue)
√ thickening + effacement of mucosal folds
√ "toothpaste" appearance of small bowel
(b) **Mycobacterium avium intracellulare enteritis**
√ dilatation of distal small bowel
√ mucosal fold thickening + nodularity
√ mesenteric + retroperitoneal lymphadenopathy
√ splenomegaly
9. AIDS colitis
— ischemic bowel
— acute appendicitis
— neutropenic colitis
— pseudomembranous colitis
— infectious colitis / ileitis
CMV colitis / ileitis
- hematochezia, crampy abdominal pain, fever
Path: small vessel vasculitis resulting in
hemorrhage, ischemic necrosis,
ulceration

Location: terminal ileum
√ marked bowel wall thickening
√ double-ring / target sign (due to increased
submucosal edema)
√ ascites
√ inflammation of pericolonic fat + fascia
10. Bowel obstruction
(a) infectious
(b) intussusception (Kaposi sarcoma, lymphoma)

AMEBIASIS
= primary infection of the colon by protozoan entamoeba
histolytica
Countries: worldwide distribution, most common in warm
climates; South Africa, Egypt, India, Asia,
Central + South America (20%); United States
(5%)
Route: contaminated food / water (human cyst carriers);
cyst dissolved in small bowel; trophozoites settle
in colon; proteolytic enzymes + hyaluronidase
lyse intestinal epithelium; may embolize into
portal venous + systemic blood system
Histo: amebic invasion of mucosa + submucosa
causing tiny ulcers which spread beneath
mucosa + merge into larger areas of necrosis;
mucosal sloughing; secondary bacterial infection
- asymptomatic for months / years
- acute attacks of diarrhea (loose mucoid blood-stained
stools)
- fever, headache, nausea
Location: (areas of relative stasis) right colon + cecum
(90%) > hepatic + splenic flexures > recto
sigmoid
√ loss of normal haustral pattern with granular
appearance (edema, punctate ulcers)
√ "collar-button" ulcers
√ cone-shaped cecum
√ several cm long stenosis of bowel lumen in transverse
colon, sigmoid colon, flexures (result of healing +
fibrosis); in multiple segments
√ ameboma = hyperplastic granuloma with bacterial
invasion of amebic abscess; usually annular +
constricting / intramural mass / cavity continuous with
bowel lumen; shrinkage under therapy in 3 – 4 weeks
√ ileocecal valve thickened + fixed in open position with
reflux
√ involvement of distal ileum (10%)
Dx: stool examination / rectal biopsy
Cx: (1) Toxic megacolon with perforation
(2) Amebic abscess in liver (2%), brain, lung
(transdiaphragmatic spread of infection),
pericolic, ischiorectal, subphrenic space
(3) Intussusception in children (due to ameboma)
(4) Fistula formation (colovesical, rectovesical,
rectovaginal, enterocolic)

AMYLOIDOSIS

= deposition of a protein-polysaccharide material in various organs leads to hypoxia, mucosal edema, hemorrhage, ulceration, mucosal atrophy, muscle atrophy

Histo: amorphous eosinophilic material deposited around terminal blood vessels, stains with Congo red + Crystal violet

A. PRIMARY AMYLOIDOSIS
probably autosomal dominant inheritance with immunologically determined dysfunction of plasma cells
- idiopathic amyloid deposition in liver, spleen, kidneys, adrenals, bowel

B. SECONDARY AMYLOIDOSIS
following prolonged infectious / inflammatory process: rheumatoid arthritis (in 20%), multiple myeloma (in 10%), lymphoreticular malignancy, chronic infection (TB), paraplegia, old age

Δ GI involvement in primary more common than in secondary amyloidosis
- macroglossia
- occult GI bleeding

@ Esophagus
√ loss of peristalsis
√ megaesophagus

@ Stomach
- postprandial epigastric pain + heartburn
- acute erosive hemorrhagic gastritis
(a) diffuse infiltrative form
√ small-sized stomach with rigidity + loss of distensibility simulating linitis plastica (from thickening of gastric wall)
√ effaced rugal pattern
√ diminished / absent peristalsis
√ marked retention of food
(b) localized infiltration (often located in antrum)
√ irregularly narrowed + rigid antrum
√ thickened rugae
√ superficial erosions / ulcerations
(c) Amyloidoma = well-defined submucosal mass

@ Small bowel
(a) diffuse form (more comon)
√ diffuse uniform thickening of valvulae conniventes in entire small bowel
√ broadened flat undulated mucosal folds (mucosal atrophy)
√ "jejunalization" of ileum
√ impaired intestinal motility
√ small bowel dilatation
(b) localized form (less common)
√ multiple pea- / marble-sized deposits
√ pseudoobstruction = physical + plain film findings suggesting mechanical obstruction with patent large + small bowel on barium examination
Cx: ·   small bowel infarction
@ Colon: √ pseudopolyps in colon
@ Bone: √ bone cysts

Dx: by oral / rectal biopsy

ANGIODYSPLASIA OF COLON

= VASCULAR ECTASIA = ARTERIOVENOUS MALFORMATION

Acquired lesion

Associated with: aortic stenosis (20%)

Incidence at autopsy: 2%

Age: majority > 55 years

Location: (a) cecum + ascending colon (majority)
(b) descending = sigmoid colon (25%)
- chronic intermittent low-grade bleeding
- occasionally massive bleeding
√ "vascular tufts" = cluster of vessels during arterial phase along antimesenteric border
√ early opacification of ileocolic vein
√ densely opacified dilated tortuous ileocolic vein into late venous phase
√ contrast extravasation (unusual)

ANORECTAL ATRESIA

= first trimester embryologic event

Incidence: 1:5,000 live births

A. LOW ANOMALY: bowel has passed through levator sling; anal opening in abnormal location (perineal fistula)

B. HIGH ANOMALY: bowel ends above levator sling; opening into vagina / posterior urethra (air in bladder in males; air in vagina in females)

√ distance between rectal air and skin will not accurately outline the extent of atretic rectum and anus (varying length during crying with increase in abdominal pressure + contraction of levator ani muscle)

OB-US: (earliest GA at diagnosis by 26 – 28 weeks
√ dilated colon + normal amniotic fluid

Associated with: (part of VACTERL syndrome)
(1) Duodenal atresia / stenosis (20%)
(2) Esophageal atresia (20%)
(3) Spinal anomalies (50%): defective sacral segmentation
(4) Arrest of descent of urorectal septum (50%) (most commonly when rectum ends above levator sling)
(5) GU anomalies: M > F
more common in supralevator than infralevator termination
(6) Cardiac anomalies
(7) Caudal regression syndrome (anorectal atresia, sacral agenesis, renal agenesis / dysplasia, lower limb hypoplasia, sirenomelia)

ANTRAL MUCOSAL DIAPHRAGM

= antral web

Age range: 3 months – 80 years

Associated with: gastric ulcers (30 – 50%)

- symptomatic if opening < 1 cm

Location: usually 1.5 cm from pylorus (range 0 – 7 cm)

√ constant symmetrical band of 2 – 3 mm thickness traversing the antrum perpendicular to long axis of stomach
√ "double bulb" appearance (in profile)
√ concentric / eccentric orifice
√ normal peristaltic activity

APPENDICITIS
Etiology: obstruction of appendiceal lumen by fecolith, lymphoid hyperplasia, foreign bodies, parasite; Crohn disease (in 25%)
• classic signs + symptoms not present in 20 – 30% (32 – 45% misdiagnosis rate in women between ages 20 – 40)
• fever (56%)
• nausea + vomiting (40%)
• RLQ pain (72%)
• leukocytosis (88%)
Abdominal plain film (abnormalities seen in < 50%):
√ usually laminated calcified appendicolith in RLQ (in 7 – 15%)
√ paucity of intestinal gas in RLQ
√ "cecal ileus" = gas-fluid level in cecum in gangrene (= local paralysis)
√ small bowel dilatation with air-fluid level in terminal ileum + cecum (= signs of mechanical obstruction) (infrequent)
√ distortion of psoas margin + flank stripes
√ focal increase in thickness of lateral abdominal wall (in 32%) = edema between properitoneal fat line + cecum
√ loss of properitoneal fat line
√ thickening of cecal wall
√ loss of definition of right inferior hepatic outline = free peritoneal fluid
√ fluid / pus in cul-de-sac
√ pneumoperitoneum (rare)
BE / UGI (accuracy 50 – 84%):
√ failure to fill appendix with barium (normal finding in 10%)
√ indentation on medial wall of cecum (= edema at base of appendix / matted omentum / periappendiceal abscess)
US: (75 – 89% sensitivity, 90 – 93% overall accuracy; nondiagnostic study in 4% due to inadequate compression of RLQ); useful in ovulating women (false-negative appendectomy rate in males 15%, in females 35%)
√ visualization of noncompressible appendix (seen only in 2% of normals) as a blind-ending tubular aperistaltic structure
√ target appearance of ≥ 6 mm in total diameter on cross section / mural wall thickness ≥ 3 mm
√ lumen may be distended with anechoic / hyperechoic material
√ visualization of appendicolith (6%)
√ localized periappendiceal fluid collection
CT: (appendix rarely visualized)
√ circumferential symmetrical thickening of wall of appendix
√ linear streaky densities in pericecal / mesenteric / pelvic fat
√ phlegmon = pericecal soft-tissue mass
√ appendicolith = homogeneous / ringlike calcification (25%)
√ pericecal / mesenteric / pelvic abscess = poorly encapsulated single / multiple fluid collection with air / extravasated contrast material
DDx: colitis, mesenteric lymphadenitis, ovarian torsion, pelvic inflammatory disease
Rx: finding of appendicolith is sufficient evidence to perform prophylactic appendectomy in asymptomatic patients (50% have perforation / abscess formation at surgery)

ASCARIASIS
= most common parasitic infection in world; cosmopolitan occurrence; endemic along Gulf Coast, Ozark Mountains, Nigeria, Southeast Asia
Organism: ascaris lumbricoides = roundworm parasite, 15 – 35 cm in length; production of 200,000 eggs daily
Cycle: infection by contaminated soil, eggs hatch in duodenum, larvae penetrate into venules / lymphatics, carried to lungs, migrate to alveoli and up the bronchial tree, swallowed, maturation in jejunum within 2.5 months
Age: children age 1 – 10 years
• colic
• eosinophilia
• appendicitis
• hematemesis / pneumonitis
• jaundice (if bile ducts infested)
Location: jejunum > ileum (99%), duodenum, stomach, CBD, pancreatic duct
√ 15 – 35 cm long tubular filling defects
√ barium-filled enteric canal outlined within Ascaris
√ whirled appearance, occasionally in coiled clusters ("bolus of worms")
Cx: (1) perforation of bowel (2) mechanical obstruction

BARRETT ESOPHAGUS
= replacement of squamous epithelium with columnar metaplasia in lower esophagus
Incidence: in 2 – 10% of patients with reflux esophagitis
Associated with gastroesophageal reflux
√ large deep ulceration ± stricture at distal / midesophagus
√ fine reticular pattern
√ commonly reflux
√ columnar epithelium secretes Tc-99m pertechnetate
Cx: adenocarcinoma in 8 – 10%

BEHÇET SYNDROME
= multisystem inflammatory disorder with relapsing course

Age at onset: 3rd decade; M:F = 2:1
@ Mucocutaneous: aphthous stomatitis, papules,
                      pustules, vesicles, folliculitis,
                      erythema nodosum-like lesions
@ Genital : ulcers on penis + scrotum / vulva + vagina
@ Ocular : relapsing iridocyclitis, hypopyon, chorioditis,
                      papillitis, retinal vasculitis
@ Articular: mild nondestructive arthritis
@ Vascular: migratory thrombophlebitis
@ CNS   : chronic meningoencephalitis
@ Colon   : multiple discrete deep ulcers in normal
                      mucosa
DDx: Reiter syndrome, Steven-Johnson syndrome, SLE,
          ulcerative colitis, ankylosing spondylitis

BEZOAR
= intragastric mass composed of accumulated ingested
  material
(a) Phytobezoar (fruit / vegetable): 55% of all bezoars;
     most commonly due to unripened persimmons
(b) Trichobezoar (hair): 80% are < age 30, almost
     exclusively in females; associated with gastric ulcer in
     24 – 70%

BOERHAAVE SYNDROME
= complete transmural disruption of esophageal wall with
  extrusion of gastric content into mediastinum / pleural
  space secondary to food bolus impaction
• forceful vomiting with sudden onset of pain (substernal,
  left chest, in neck, pleuritic, abdominal)
• dyspnea
• NO hematemesis (blood escapes outside esophageal
  lumen)
√ rent 2 – 5 cm in length, 2 – 3 cm above GE junction,
  predominantly on anterior right side
√ pleural effusion on left >> right side /
  hydropneumothorax
√ mediastinal emphysema (single most important plain
  film finding)
√ "V-sign of Naclerio" = air between lower thoracic aorta +
  diaphragm
√ extravasation of contrast medium into mediastinum /
  pleura

BRUNNER GLAND HYPERPLASIA
Etiology: hyperplasia secondary to hyperacidity
Physiology: secrete a clear viscous alkaline substance
                 into crypts of Lieberkühn
MORPHOLOGIC TYPES:
  1. Diffuse nodular hyperplasia
  2. Circumscribed nodular hyperplasia:
     in suprapapillary portion
  3. Single adenomatous hyperplastic polyp:
     in duodenal bulb
Location: duodenal glands begin in vicinity of pylorus
           extending distally within proximal 2/3 of
           duodenum

√ multiple nodular filling defects (usually limited to 1st
  portion of duodenum
√ "cobblestoning" (most common finding)
√ occasionally single large mass ± central ulceration

BURKITT LYMPHOMA
= most common type of Non-Hodgkin lymphoma in
  children
Etiology: tumor from undifferentiated B-cell-derived
             lymphocytes; associated with Epstein-Barr
             virus
Age: children + young adults
Histo: characteristic "starry sky" plattern
Location: salivary glands, thyroid, ovary, small bowel,
            bone marrow; often multicentric in origin
• jaw mass
• abdominal mass
• paraplegia
• NO peripheral leukemia
√ usually intraabdominal extranodal involvement with
  sparing of spleen
A. ENDEMIC FORM (Africa, New Guinea)
    50% of all childhood cancers in central Africa
    Age: 6 – 8 years
B. NONENDEMIC FORM
    Age: 10 – 12 years
    √ higher incidence of intraabdominal tumors +
      peripheral lymph node enlargement
    √ pleural effusion (most common chest abnormality)

CANDIDIASIS OF ESOPHAGUS
= MONILIASIS
Predisposed:
   individuals with depressed immunity (hematologic
   disease, renal transplant, leukemia, chronic debilitating
   disease, diabetes mellitus, antibiotics, steroids,
   chemotherapy, radiotherapy, AIDS), scleroderma,
   strictures, achalasia, S/P fundoplication
Path: patchy, creamy-white plaques covering a friable
            erythematous mucosa
• dysphagia (= difficult swallowing)
• odynophagia (= painful swallowing from segmental
  spasm)
• intense retro- / substernal pain
• associated with thrush (= oral moniliasis) in 20 – 80%
Location: predilection for lower 1/2 of esophagus
√ involvement of long esophageal segments
√ tiny 1 – 2 mm nodular filling defects with linear
  orientation (plaques)
√ "cobble stone" apearance = mucosal nodularity in early
  stage (from growth of colonies on surface)
√ shaggy / fuzzy / serrated contour (from
  pseudomembranes, erosions, ulcerations, intramural
  hemorrhage)
√ narrowed lumen (from spasm, pseudomembranes,
  marked edema)
√ "intramural diverticulosis" = multiple tiny indentations +
  protrusions

√ sluggish / absent primary peristalsis
√ strictures (rare)
Diagnostic sensitivity:
   endoscopy (97%), double contrast (88%), single
   contrast (55%)
Cx: Systemic candidiasis
Rx: Mycostatin
DDx:
   reflux esophagitis, herpes esophagitis, acute caustic
   ingestion, intramural pseudodiverticulosis, squamous
   papillomatosis, glycogen acanthosis, Barrett esophagus,
   superficial spreading carcinoma, epidermolysis bullosa,
   varices

CARCINOID
= most common tumor of small bowel + appendix;
M:F = 2:1
Path: arising from argentophil Kulchitsky cells in the
      crypts of Lieberkühn; invasion into mesentery
      incites an intense fibrotic reaction
Biochemistry:
   tumor elaborates (1) ACTH (2) histamine (3) bradykinin
   (4) kallikrein (5) serotonin = 5-hydroxytryptamine (from
   tryptophan over 5-hydroxytryptophan) which is
   metabolized in liver by monamine oxidase into
   5-hydroxyindole acetic acid (5-HIAA) and excreted in
   urine; 5-hydroxytryptophan is destroyed in pulmonary
   circulation
- asymptomatic (66%)
- pain / obstruction (19%)
- weight loss (16%)
- palpable mass (14%)
- **Carcinoid syndrome** (7% of small bowel carcinoids)
   requires that serotonin metabolism (to 5-HIAA in liver) is
   bypassed
   (a) with liver metastases: in 90% liver metastases are
       present
   (b) with primary pulmonary / ovarian carcinoids
   - recurrent diarrhea (70%)
   - right-sided endocardial fibroelastosis (35%) resulting
     in tricuspid regurgitation + pulmonary valve stenosis +
     right heart failure
   - attacks precipitated by ingestion of food / alcohol
   - asthmatic wheezing (15%)
   - desquamative skin lesions (5%)
   - cutaneous flushing (rare)
Metastases:
   to lymph nodes + liver (in 90% of patients with carcinoid
   syndrome)
   (a) incidence versus tumor size

tumor of	< 1 cm	(in 75%)	metastasizes in 2%
tumor of	1 – 2 cm	(in 20%)	metastasizes in 50%
tumor of	> 2 cm	(in 5%)	metastasizes in 85%

   (b) incidence versus location

tumor in ileum	(in 28%)	metastasizes in 35%
tumor in appendix	(in 46%)	metastasizes in 3%
tumor in rectum	(in 17%)	metastasizes in 1%

Location:
   @ GI tract: between gastric cardia and anus
     (a) appendix (60%): commonly benign; surgical
        incidence of 0.03 – 0.7%
     (b) small bowel (25%): 91% in ileum (in 1/3
        multiple); 7% in jejunum, 2% in duodenum
     (c) rectum (10%): rarely metastasize
     (d) remainder of colon (5%); rare in stomach
   @ Others: bronchus, thyroid, pancreas, biliary tract,
     teratomas (ovarian, sacrococcygeal, testicular)
UGI:
√ small smooth submucosal mass impinging
   eccentrically on lumen
√ angulation + kinking of loops leading to obstruction
   (DIAGNOSTIC)
√ spiculated / tethered appearance of mucosal folds
   (desmoplastic reaction)
√ separation of loops due to large mesenteric
   metastases
CT:
√ stellate radiating pattern of mesenteric neurovascular
   bundles
√ displacement + kinking of adjacent bowel loops
√ segmental thickening of adjacent bowel loops
   (encasement of mesenteric vessels leads to chronic
   ischemia)
√ liver metastases may become isodense following slow
   contrast infusion
Angio:
√ thickening + foreshortening of mesenteric vessels
√ kinking of small- and medium-sized vessels with
   stellate configuration
√ venous occlusion / mesenteric varices
√ encasement of medium-sized vessels
√ simulated hypervascularity secondary to fibrotic
   retraction of mesenteric vessels
Cx: second primary malignant neoplasm in other
      location (36% at necropsy)
Rx: Somatostatin / SMS 201-995
DDx: oat-cell carcinoma, pancreatic carcinoma,
       medullary thyroid carcinoma, retractile mesenteritis,
       desmoplastic carcinoma / lymphoma

CATHARTIC COLON
= prolonged use of stimulant-irritant cathartics (> 15
   years) resulting in neuromuscular incoordination from
   chronically increased muscular activity + tonus
Agents: castor oil, senna, phenolphthalein, cascara,
         podophyllum, aloin
Location: involvement of colon proximal to splenic flexure
√ effaced mucosa with flattened smooth surface
√ diminished / absent haustrations
√ "pseudostrictures" = smoothly tapered areas of ---
   narrowing are typical (sustained tonus of circular-
   muscles)
√ poor evacuation of barium
√ flattened + gaping ileocecal valve
√ shortened but distensible ascending colon

DDx: "burned out" ulcerative colitis with right-sided predominance (very similar)

CHAGAS DISEASE

= damage of ganglion cells by neurotoxin liberated from protozoa trypanosoma cruzi resulting in aperistalsis of GI tract + dilatation

Endemic to Central + South America (esp. eastern Brazil)

Histo: decreased number of cells in medullary dorsal motor nucleus + Wallerian degeneration of vagus + decrease / loss of argyrophilic cells in myenteric plexus of Auerbach

Peak age: 30 – 50 years; M:F = 1:1
- intermittent / persistent dysphagia
- odynophagia (= fear of swallowing)
- foul breath, regurgitation
- aspiration
- Mecholyl test: abnormal response indicative of deficient innervation; 2.5 – 10 mg methacholine subcutaneously followed by severe tetanic nonperistaltic contraction 2 – 5 minutes after injection, commonly in distal half of esophagus, accompanied by severe pain
- @   Dilatative cardiomyopathy (myocarditis)
- @   Megacolon (bowels move at intervals of 8 days to 5 months)
    Cx: Impacted feces, Sigmoid volvulus
- @   Esophagus: changes as in achalasia

CHALASIA

= continuously relaxed sphincter with free reflux in the absence of a sliding hernia

Etiology: elevated submerged segment

Causes: (1)   delayed development of esophagogastric region in newborns
(2)   scleroderma, Raynaud disease
(3)   S/P forceful dilatation / myotomy for achalasia

√ free / easily induced reflux

CHRONIC IDIOPATHIC INTESTINAL PSEUDOOBSTRUCTION

= nonpropulsive intestine without definable cause; ? autosomal dominant

Age: all ages, M:F = 1:1
- recurrent attacks of abdominal distension, periumbilical pain, nausea, vomiting, constipation

√ mild to marked gaseous distension of duodenum + proximal small bowel

√ esophageal dilation + hypoperistalsis (lower third)

√ excessive duodenal dilation (DDx: megaduodenum, superior mesenteric artery syndrome)

√ ligament of Treitz may be placed lower than usual

√ delayed transit of barium through affected segments

COLITIS CYSTICA PROFUNDA

= rare benign condition characterized by submucosal mucus-containing cysts lined by normal colonic epithelium

Etiology: probably related to chronic inflammation

Age: primarily disease of young adults
- brief periods of bright red rectal bleeding
- mucous / bloody discharge
- intermittent diarrhea

Location: (a)   localized to rectum (most commonly) / sigmoid
(b)   generalized colonic process (less common)

√ nodular polypoid / cauliflower-like lesions < 2 cm in size, containing no gas

√ spiculations mimicking ulcers (barium-filled clefts between nodules)

DDx: Pneumatosis (rarely affects rectum)

COLON CARCINOMA

most common cancer of GI tract; 2nd most common cause of death from malignancy after lung cancer (in men) + breast cancer (in women)

Incidence: 140,000 new cases / year

Predisposed: socioeconomic status, diet, obesity (in men), asbestos worker, Peutz-Jeghers syndrome

Risk factors:
1. Colonic adenoma
   Δ 93% of colorectal carcinomas arise from adenomatous polyp
   Δ 5% of adenomas 5 mm in size develop into invasive cancers
   Δ a patient with one adenoma has a 9% chance of having a colorectal carcinoma by 15 years
2. Family history of benign / malignant colorectal tumors
3. Chronic ulcerative colitis
4. Prominent lymphoid follicular pattern
5. History of endometrial / breast cancer

Age: peak age 50 – 70 years

Histo: (1)   adenocarcinoma with varied degrees of differentiation
(2)   mucinous carcinoma (uncommon)
(3)   squamous cell carcinoma + adenoacanthoma (rare)

Staging:
Dukes A : limited to bowel wall (15%)
Dukes B : extension through bowel wall into serosa / mesenteric fat (35%)
Dukes C : lymph node metastases (50%)
  C_1: growth limited to bowel wall
  C_2: growth extending into adipose tissue
Dukes D : distant metastases

Location: rectum (15 – 41%), sigmoid (20 – 37%), descending colon (10 – 11%), transverse colon (12%), ascending colon (8 – 16%), cecum (8 – 10%); "aging gut" = right-sided lesions increasing with age

Metastases:
1. liver (25%)
2. retroperitoneal + mesenteric nodes (15%)
3. hydronephrosis (13%)

4. adrenal (10%)
5. ovarian metastases
6. psoas muscle tumor deposits
7. ascites

BE (90 – 95% rate of detection: single contrast 95%, double contrast 93%):
√ fungating polypoid carcinoma
√ annular ulcerating carcinoma = "saddle lesion" / "apple-core lesion"
√ scirrhous carcinoma: rare variant with circumferential + longitudinal spread; often seen in ulcerative colitis
√ curvilinear / mottled calcifications (rare)

CT: staging accuracy of 48 – 90%, for lymph node metastases of 25 – 73%

CT staging (poor accuracy compared with Duke classification):
Stage 1 intramural polypoid mass
Stage 2 thickening of bowel wall
Stage 3 slight invasion of surrounding tissues
Stage 4 massive invasion of surrounding tissue + adjacent organs / distant metastases
√ low density mass + low density lymph nodes in mucinous adenocarcinoma
√ psammomatous calcifications in mucinous adenocarcinoma

MRI: staging accuracy of 73%, 40% sensitivity for lymph node metastases

Prognosis: 40 – 50% overall 5-year survival rate; 80 – 90% with Dukes A; 70% with Dukes B; 33% with Dukes C; 5% with Dukes D; recurrence at line of anastomosis (11%) within 2 years after resection in 1/3

Risk:
of 1% for synchronous colon cancer
of 14% with "sentinel polyp"
of 3% for metachronous colon cancer
of 3.8% for extracolonic malignancy

Cx: (1) obstruction (frequently in descending + sigmoid colon)
(2) perforation
(3) intussusception
(4) pneumatosis cystoides intestinalis

DDx: (1) Prolapsing ileocecal valve (change on palpation)
(2) Spasm (intact mucosa, released by propantheline bromide)
(3) Diverticulitis

COLONIC VOLVULUS

= most common form of volvulus

A. VOLVULUS OF CECUM
Associated with malrotation + long mesentery
Age peak: 20 – 40 years; M > F
√ "kidney-shaped" distended cecum, usually positioned in LUQ
√ tapered end of barium column points toward torsion

B. VOLVULUS OF SIGMOID
= sigmoid twists on mesenteric axis

Usually in elderly / psychiatrically disturbed
Degree of torsion: 360° (50%), 180° (35%), 540° (10%)
√ greatly distended paralyzed loop with fluid-fluid levels, mainly on left side, extending toward diaphragm (erect film)
√ "coffee bean sign" = distinct midline crease corresponding to mesenteric root in largely gas-distended loop (supine)
√ "bird-of-prey sign" = tapered hooklike end of barium column

CT:
√ "whirl sign" = tightly torsioned mesentery formed by twisted afferent + efferent loop

CONGENITAL INTESTINAL ATRESIA

Incidence: 1:300 live births
Location: jejunum + ileum (70%), duodenum (25%), colon (5%)
√ "triple bubble sign" = intraluminal gas in stomach + duodenal bulb + proximal jejunum as pathognomonic sign for jejunal atresia
√ gasless lower abdomen (gut usually air-filled by 4 hours after birth)
√ meconium peritonitis
√ polyhydramnios (in 50% if obstruction with duodenal / proximal jejunal atresia; rarely in ileal / colonic atresia)

CORROSIVE GASTRITIS

Agents:
(a) acid, formaldehyde
· clinically usually silent
Location: esophagus usually unharmed, severe gastric damage, duodenum may be involved (newer potent materials cause atypical distribution)
(b) alkaline
Location: pylorus + antrum most frequently involved

A. ACUTE CHANGES (edema + mucosal sloughing)
√ marked enlargement of gastric rugae + erosions / ulceration
√ complete cessation of motor activity
√ gas in portal venous system
Cx: perforation

B. CHRONIC CHANGES
√ firm thick non-pliable wall
√ stenotic / incontinent pylorus (if involved)
√ gastric outlet obstruction (cicatrization) after 3 – 10 weeks

CRICOPHARYNGEAL ACHALASIA

= hypertrophy of cricopharyngeus muscle (= upper esophageal sphincter) with failure of complete relaxation
Etiology:
1. Normal variant without symptoms: seen in 5 – 10% of adults

2. Compensatory mechanism to gastroesophageal reflux
3. Neuromuscular dysfunction of deglutition
    (a) Primary neural disorders
        Brainstem disorder (bulbar poliomyelitis, syringomyelia, multiple sclerosis, amyotrophic lateral sclerosis); central / peripheral nerve palsy; cerebrovascular occlusive disease; Huntington chorea
    (b) Primary muscle disorder
        Myotonic dystrophy; polymyositis; dermatomyositis; sarcoidosis; myopathies secondary to steroids / thyroid dysfunction; oculopharyngeal myopathy
    (c) Myoneural junction disorder
        Myasthenia gravis; Diphtheria; Tetanus
- mostly asymptomatic
- dysphagia
Cineradiography / videotape recording required for demonstration !
√ distension of proximal esophagus + pharynx
√ smoothly outlined shelf- / liplike projection at level of cricoid (= pharyngoesophageal junction) from posteriorly = level of C5/6
√ barium may overflow into larynx + trachea
Cx: Zenker diverticula
Rx: cricopharyngeal myotomy

CROHN DISEASE
= REGIONAL ENTERITIS = disease of unknown etiology with prolonged + unpredictable course characterized by discontinuous + asymmetric involvement of entire GI tract
Path: transmural inflammation (noncaseating granuloma with Langhans giant cells and epitheloid cells, edema, fibrosis); obstructive lymphedema + enlargement of submucosal lymphoid follicles; ulceration of mucosa overlying lymphoid follicles
Age: onset between 15 – 30 years; M:F = 1:1
- recurrent episodes of diarrhea
- colicky / steady abdominal pain
- low-grade fever
- weight loss, anorexia
- occult blood + anemia
- perianal abscess / fistulas (40%)
- malabsorption (30%)
Associated with   erythema nodosum, pyoderma gangrenosum
INTESTINAL MANIFESTATIONS
  @ Esophagus (rare)
  @ Stomach (2 – 20%) = granulomatous gastritis
     √ pseudo-post Billroth-I appearance
     √ "ramshorn sign" = poorly distensible, smooth, tubular narrowed antrum + widened pylorus + narrow duodenal bulb
     √ aphthous ulcers (= pinpoint erosions)
     √ cobblestone mucosa
     √ antral-duodenal fistula

  @ Duodenum (4 – 10%)
     almost always associated with gastric involvement
     Location: duodenal bulb + proximal half of duodenum
     √ superficial erosions / aphthoid ulcers (early lesion)
     √ thickened duodenal folds
  @ Small bowel (80%) = regional enteritis
     terminal ileum (alone / in combination in 95%); jejunum / ileum (15%)
     √ thickening + slight nodularity of circular folds
     √ aphthous ulcers
     √ cobblestone mucosa / ulceration
     √ commonly associated with medial cecal defect
  @ Colon (22 – 55%) = granulomatous colitis
     particularly on right side with rectum + sigmoid frequently spared
     √ tiny 1 – 2 mm nodular filling defects (lymphoid follicular pattern)
     √ aphthous ulcers with "target / bull's-eye" appearance
     √ "transverse stripe sign" = 1 cm long straight stripes representing contrast medium within deep grooves of coarse mucosal folds
     √ long fistulous tracts parallel to bowel lumen
  @ Rectum (35 – 50%)
     √ deep / collar-button ulcers
     √ rectal sinus tracts
Phases:
  (a) Nonstenotic phase
     √ blunting / flattening / distortion / straightening / thickening of mucosal folds (early event from obstructive lymphedema)
     √ aphthous ulcers = nodules with shallow central ulceration
     √ "cobble stoning" = serpiginous longitudinal + transverse ulcers separated by areas of edema
     √ pseudopolyps = islands of hyperplastic mucosa between denuded mucosa
     √ inflammatory polypoid masses
     √ sessile / pedunculated / filiform postinflammatory polyps
     √ straightening + rigidity of loops with luminal narrowing (spasm + submucosal edema)
     √ separation + displacement of small bowel loops (from increase in mesenteric fat / enlarged mesenteric lymph nodes / perforation with abscess formation)
     √ "skip lesions" (90%) = discontinuous involvement with intervening normal areas
     √ pseudodiverticula = bulging area of normal wall opposite affected scarred wall, mostly on antimesenteric side
  (b) Stenotic phase
     √ "string sign" = strictures (most frequently in terminal ileum) / marked narrowing of rigid loops
     √ normal proximal loops may be dilated with stasis ulcers + fecoliths

CT:
- √ skip areas of asymmetrical bowel wall thickening of 10 - 20 mm (82%)
- √ homogeneous density of thickened bowel wall
- √ "double halo configuration" (50%) = intestinal lumen surrounded by inner ring of low attenuation (= edematous mucosa) + outer ring of soft-tissue density (= thickened fibrotic muscularis + serosa) (DDx: radiation enteritis, ischemia, mesenteric venous thrombosis, acute pancreatitis)
- √ luminal narrowing + proximal dilatation
- √ "creeping fat" = massive proliferation of mesenteric fat (40%) with mass effect separating small bowel loops
- √ mesenteric adenopathy (18%)
- √ abscess (DDx: postoperative blind loop)

US:
- √ thickening of bowel wall (65%) about 8 mm (DDx: ulcerative colitis)
- √ inflammatory mass (14%), abscess (4%)
- √ distended fluid-filled loops (12%)

Prognosis: recurrence rate of up to 39% after resection (commonly at the site of the new terminal ileum, most frequently during first 2 years after resection); mortality rate of 7% at 5 years, 12% at 10 years after 1st resection

Cx:
- (1) Fistula (33%):
  - (a) enterocolic: most frequent between ileum and cecum
  - (b) enterocutaneous: rectum-to-skin; rectum-to-vagina
  - (c) perineal fistula + sinus tracts
  - Crohn disease is 3rd most common cause of fistula / sinus tracts (*DDx:* iatrogenic [most common cause], diverticula [2nd most common cause])
- (2) Intramural sinus tracts
- (3) Abscess
- (4) Free perforation (rare)
- (5) Toxic megacolon
- (6) Small bowel obstruction (15%)
- (7) Hydronephrosis (generally on right side from ureteric compression)
- (8) Adenocarcinoma in ileum / colon

DDx:
- (1) Yersinia (in terminal ileum, resolution within 3 – 4 months)
- (2) Tuberculosis (more severe involvement of cecum, pulmonary TB)
- (3) Segmental infarction (acute onset, elderly patient)
- (4) Radiation ileitis (appropriate history)
- (5) Lymphoma (no spasm, luminal narrowing is uncommon, tumor nodules)
- (6) Carcinoid tumor (tumor nodules)
- (7) Eosinophilic gastroenteritis
- (8) Potassium stricture

EXTRAINTESTINAL MANIFESTATIONS
1. Fatty infiltration of liver
2. Gallstones (incidence 28 – 34%) risk 3-5 x higher than expected interrupted enterohepatic circulation secondary to malabsorption of bile salts in terminal ileum; correlates with length of diseased ileum, resected ileum, duration of disease
3. Sclerosing cholangitis
4. Bile duct carcinoma
5. Amyloidosis
6. Urolithiasis: oxalate / uric acid stones
7. Migratory arthritis (5 – 20%); sacroiliitis; ankylosing spondylitis
8. Erythema nodosum, uveitis

CRONKHITE-CANADA SYNDROME
= non-neoplastic nonhereditary inflammatory polyps (as in juvenile polyposis)

Path: inflammatory polyps = multiple cystic spaces filled with mucin secondary to degenerative changes

Age: 62 years (range 42 – 75 years); M < F
- exudative protein-losing enteropathy, diarrhea
- severe weight loss
- abdominal pain
- nail atrophy
- brownish hyperpigmentation of skin
- alopecia
- √ multiple polyps

Location: stomach (100%); small bowel (> 50%); colon (100%)

Prognosis: rapidly fatal in women within 6 – 18 months (cachexia); tendency toward remission in men

CYSTIC FIBROSIS
= MUCOVISCIDOSIS = FIBROCYSTIC DISEASE
= autosomal disorder characterized by mucous plugging of exocrine glands secondary to Increased viscosity of secreted mucus; heterozygous in 5%; more common in Caucasians
- high sweat chlorides
- chronic obstipation
- infertility
- decreased urinary PABA excretion
- sinusitis
- exocrine pancreatic insufficiency (endocrine function not affected)
- √ large distended colon with mottled appearance (retained bulky dry stool)
- √ rectal prolapse
- √ meconium ileus (10 – 15%)
- √ microcolon
- √ thickened folds in duodenum, small bowel, colon
- √ calcific chronic pancreatitis
- √ increased pancreatic echogenicity
- √ cirrhosis
- √ bronchiectasis

DISACCHARIDASE DEFICIENCY
= enzyme deficiencies for any of the disaccharides (maltose, lactose, etc.)
A. PRIMARY
B. SECONDARY to other diseases (e.g., Crohn disease)
Pathophysiology:
  (a) unabsorbed disaccharides produce osmotic - diarrhea
  (b) bacterial fermentation produces short chain volatile fatty acids causing further osmotic + irritant diarrhea
√ normal small bowel series without added lactose
√ abnormal small bowel series done with lactose (50 g added to 600 ccm of barium suspension)
√ small + large bowel distension
√ dilution of barium
√ shortening of transit time

DIVERTICULAR DISEASE OF COLON
= overactivity of smooth muscle causing herniation of mucosa + submucosa through muscle layers
Incidence: 5 – 10% in 5th decade; 33 – 48% over age 50; 50% past 7th decade; M:F = 1:1; most common affliction of colon in developed countries
Cause: decreased fecal bulk (diet high in refined fiber + low in roughage)
Location: in 80% in sigmoid (= narrowest colonic segment with highest pressure);
in 17% distributed over entire colon;
in 4 – 12% isolated to cecum / ascending colon

Prediverticular Disease of Colon
= longitudinal + circular smooth muscle thickening with redundancy of folds secondary to myostatic contracture
√ "saw-tooth sign" = crowding + thickening of haustral folds (shortening of colonic segment)
√ plump marginal indentations
√ superimposed muscle spasm (relieved by antispasmodics)
DDx: Hemorrhage; ischemia; radiation changes; pseudomembranous colitis

Colonic Diverticulosis
= acquired herniations of mucosa + muscularis mucosae through the muscularis propria with wall components of mucosa, submucosa, serosa = false diverticula of pulsion type
Site:
  (a) lateral diverticula arise between mesenteric + antimesenteric teniae on opposite sides
  (b) antimesenteric intertenial diverticula opposite of mesenteric side = intramural type vasa recta = nutrient arteries pass through the circular muscle (weakness in muscular wall) and are carried over the fundus of the diverticula as it enlarges

√ Size: tiny V-shaped protrusion up to several cm in diameter (usually 3 – 10 mm)
√ bubbly appearance of air-containing diverticula
√ residual barium within diverticula from previous study
√ spiky irregular outline (antimesenteric intertenial ridge is typical site for intramural diverticula)
√ smooth dome-shaped appendages with a short neck
√ may be pointed, attenuated, irregular with variable filling
√ circular line with sharp outer edge + fuzzy blurred inner edge (en face view in double contrast BE)
√ **Giant Sigmoid Diverticulum** = large gas-containing cyst (air entrapment secondary to ball-valve mechanism) arising in left iliac fossa
CT:
  √ diverticula
  √ distorted luminal contour + muscular hypertrophy

Colonic Diverticulitis
= perforation of diverticulum with intramural / localized pericolic abscess
Incidence: in 20 – 25% of diverticular disease
• pain + local tenderness + mass in LLQ
• fever, leukocytosis
√ localized ileus / bowel obstruction (kinking / edema)
√ gas in abscess / fistula
√ pneumoperitoneum (rare)
√ eccentric external pressure on bowel lumen by inflammatory mass
√ extraluminal contrast = PERIDIVERTICULITIS
  √ "double-tracking" = pericolonic longitudinal sinus tract
  √ pericolonic collection = peridiverticular abscess
  √ fistula to bladder / small bowel / vagina
CT:
  √ inflammation of pericolic fat (98%)
  √ diverticula (84%)
  √ circumferential bowel wall thickening of 4 – 12 mm (70%)
  √ abscess (47%)
  √ fluid ± air of peritonitis (16%)
  √ fistula (14%)
  √ colonic obstruction (12%)
  √ intramural sinus tracts (9%)
  √ ureteral obstruction (7%)
Prognosis:
  (a) self-limiting (usually)
  (b) transmural perforation
  (c) superficial ulceration
  (d) chronic abscess
DDx:
  (1) Colonic neoplasm (shorter segment, heaped-up margins, ulcerated mucosa)
  (2) Crohn colitis (double-tracking longer than 10 cm)

Colonic Diverticular Hemorrhage
not related to diverticulitis
Incidence: in 3 – 47% of diverticulosis

Location: 75% located in ascending colon (larger neck + dome of diverticula)
- massive rectal hemorrhage without pain
√ extravasation of radionuclide tracers
√ angiographic contrast pooling in bowel lumen
Rx: (1) transcatheter infusion of vasoconstrictive agents (Pitressin)
(2) embolization with Gelfoam

DUMPING SYNDROME
= early postprandial vascular symptomatology of sweating, flushing, palpitation, feeling of weakness and dizziness
Pathophysiology:
rapid entering of hypertonic solution into jejunum resulting in fluid shift from blood compartment into small bowel
Incidence: 1 – 5% ; M:F = 2:1
Roentgenologic findings not diagnostic !
√ rapid emptying of barium into small bowel (= loss of gastric reservoir function)
Rx: (1) lying down (2) diet
DDx: Late postprandial hypoglycemia (90 – 120 minutes after eating)

DUODENAL ATRESIA
= most common cause of congenital duodenal obstruction; second most common site of gastrointestinal atresias after ileum
Incidence: 1:10,000; M:F = 1:1
Etiology: defective vacuolization of duodenum between 6th – 11th weeks of fetal life; rarely from vascular insult (extent of obstruction usually involves larger regions with vascular insult)
Age at presentation: first few days of life
- persistent bilious vomiting a few hours after birth / following 1st feeding
- rapid deterioration secondary to loss of fluids + electrolytes
— isolated sporadic anomaly (30 – 52%)
Associated anomalies (in 60%):
(1) Down syndrome (20 – 33%);
Δ 25% of fetuses with duodenal atresia have Down syndrome
Δ < 5% of fetuses with Down syndrome have duodenal atresia
(2) CHD (8 – 50%): endocardial cushion defect, VSD
(3) Gastrointestinal anomalies (26%): esophageal atresia, biliary atresia, duodenal duplication, imperforate anus, small bowel atresia, intestinal malrotation, Meckel diverticulum, transposed liver, annular pancreas (20%)
(4) Urinary tract anomalies (8%)
(5) Vertebral + rib anomalies (37%)
Location: (a) usually distal to ampulla of Vater (80%)
(b) proximal duodenum (20%)
√ "double bubble sign" = gas-fluid levels in duodenal bulb + gastric fundus

√ total absence of intestinal gas in small / large bowel
√ colon of normal caliber
OB-US (usually not identified prior to 24 weeks GA):
√ double bubble sign = simultaneous distension of stomach + 1st portion of duodenum, continuity must be demonstrated
√ increased gastric peristalsis
√ polyhydramnios (100%)
DDx: (1) Prominent incisura angularis causing bidissection of stomach
(2) Choledochal cyst
Cx: Prematurity (40%) secondary to preterm labor related to polyhydramnios

DUODENAL DIVERTICULUM
Incidence: 1 – 5% of GI studies; 22% of autopsies
A. PRIMARY DIVERTICULUM
= mucosal prolapse through muscularis propria
Location: 2nd portion (62%), 3rd portion (30%), 4th portion (8%)
Site: medial wall in region of papilla (88%), posteriorly (8%), lateral wall (4%)
B. SECONDARY DIVERTICULUM
= all layers of duodenal wall = true diverticulum as complication of duodenal / periduodenal inflammation
Location: almost invariably in 1st portion of duodenum
- mostly asymptomatic
Cx: (1) perforation + peritonitis (2) bowel obstruction
(3) biliary obstruction (4) bleeding (5) diverticulitis

DUODENAL ULCER
Incidence: 200,000 cases / year; 2 – 3 x more frequent than gastric ulcers; M:F = 3:1
Pathophysiology:
too much acid in duodenum from (a) abnormally high gastric secretion (b) inadequate neutralization
Predisposed: cortisone therapy, severe cerebral injury, post surgery, chronic obstructive pulmonary disease
Location:
(a) bulbar (95%):
anterior wall (50%), posterior wall (23%), inferior wall (22%), superior wall (5%)
(b) postbulbar (3 – 5%):
majority on medial wall of supraampullary region; tendency for hemorrhage in 66%, M:F = 7:1
√ frequently small round / ovoid / linear ulcer niche
√ "kissing ulcers" = ulcers opposite from each other on anterior + posterior wall
√ giant duodenal ulcer > 3 cm (rare) with higher morbidity + mortality; may be overlooked by simulating a normal / deformed duodenal bulb
√ "clover-leaf deformity, hourglass stenosis" (healed stage) with prestenotic dilatation of recesses
Cx: (1) obstruction (5%)
(2) perforation (< 10%): anterior > posterior wall; fistula to gallbladder

(3) penetration (< 5%) = sealed perforation
(4) hemorrhage (15%):   melena > hematemesis

DUODENAL VARICES
= dilated collateral veins secondary to portal hypertension
(posterior superior pancreaticoduodenal vein)
√ lobulated filling defects (best demonstrated in prone
position, maximal luminal distension will obliterate them)
√ commonly associated with fundal + esophageal varices

ECTOPIC PANCREAS
= submucosal nodule located at distal greater curvature of
antrum or pylorus (80%), duodenal bulb, jejunum; may
be multiple; M:F = 2:1
√ smooth cone- / nippleshaped mass 1 – 5 cm in size
√ central umbilication representing orifice of filiform duct

EOSINOPHILIC GASTROENTERITIS
Histo: fibrous tissue + eosinophilic infiltrate
A.   LOCALIZED FORM / circumscribed type
     = EOSINOPHILIC GRANULOMA
     = FIBROUS POLYPOID LESION
     = INFLAMMATORY PSEUDOTUMOR
     Location: almost exclusively in stomach (most
                common in antrum + pylorus)
     √ submucosal polypoid mass / pedunculated polyp
B.   diffuse type = EOSINOPHILIC GASTROENTERITIS
     = eosinophilic infiltration of mucosa, submucosa, and
       muscular layers of small intestine ± stomach by
       mature eosinophils (? gastric pendant to Löffler
       syndrome)
Types: (a) mucosal (b) muscular (c) serosal (rare)
• abdominal pain, diarrhea, vomiting
• weight loss
• hematemesis (from ulceration)
• peripheral eosinophilia, anemia
• history of systemic allergy / food allergy
• hypoalbuminemia
• malabsorption + hypoproteinemia
• protein-losing enteropathy
Location: entire small bowel (particularly jejunum),
            stomach, omentum, mesentery
@ Stomach (almost always limited to antrum)
   √ enlarged gastric rugae / cobblestone nodules / polyps
     (= mucosal type)
   √ rigid wall with narrowed gastric antrum / pylorus
   √ bulky intraluminal mass up to 9 cm in size (= muscular
     type)
   √ "wet stomach"
   √ ulcers are rare
   √ may have ascites
   Cx: pyloric obstruction
   DDx: hypertrophic gastritis, lymphoma, carcinoma
@ Small bowel
   √ thickening + distortion of folds (predominantly
     jejunum) (mucosal type)
   √ distorted valvulae + irregular angulation
   √ effacement of mucosal pattern + narrowing of lumen
     (muscular type)

Prognosis: tendency toward spontaneous remission
Rx: steroids / removal of sensitizing agent

ESOPHAGEAL CANCER
Incidence: < 1% of all cancers; 4 – 10% of all GI
                malignancies; 9000 cases / year (United
                States); M:F = 4:1; Blacks:Whites = 2:1
High-risk regions: Iran, parts of Africa, Italy, China
Predisposing factors:
   achalasia (risk factor of 1000 x), asbestosis, Barrett
   esophagus, celiac disease, ionizing radiation, lye
   stricture (risk factor of 1000 x), Plummer-Vinson
   syndrome, tannins, alcohol, tobacco, history of oral /
   pharyngeal cancer, tylosis palmaris et plantaris
Histo:
(1) Squamous cell carcinoma (95%)
(2) Adenocarcinoma (4%) arising from mucosal /
     submucosal glands or heterotopic gastric mucosa
     or columnar-lined epithelium (Barrett)
     (a) in 70% from Barrett esophagus
     (b) at gastroesophageal junction
(3) Carcinosarcoma = pseudosarcoma = spindle-cell
     squamous carcinoma
     Location: usually middle third of esophagus
     √ large bulky polypoid smooth, lobulated, scalloped
       intraluminal mass, may be pedunculated
(4) Mucoepidermoid carcinoma, adenoid cystic
     carcinoma
Cancer Staging:
   TNM-system:
      T_1 tumor < 5 cm in length without circumferential
              involvement
      T_2 tumor > 5 cm in length / circumferential or
              obstructive lesion
      T_3 extraesophageal spread
   CT-staging (Moss):
      Stage 1 intraluminal tumor / localized wall thickening
               of 3 – 5 mm
      Stage 2 localized / circumferential wall thickening
               > 5 mm
      Stage 3 contiguous spread into adjacent
               mediastinum (trachea, main stem bronchi,
               aorta, pericardium)
               √ loss of fat planes (nonspecific, often still
                 resectable)
               √ mass in contact with aorta > 90 ° (in 20 –
                 70% still resectable)
               √ displacement / compression of airway (50
                 – 100% accuracy for invasion)
               √ esophagotracheal / -bronchial fistula
                 (unresectable)
      Stage 4 distal metastases
               √ enlarged abdominal lymph nodes > 10 mm
                 (12 – 85% accuracy)
               √ hepatic, pulmonary, adrenal metastases
               √ direct erosion of vertebral body
• dysphagia (87 – 95%)
• weight loss (71%)

- retrosternal pain (46%)
- regurgitation (29%)

Location: upper 1/3 (15 – 20%); middle 1/3 (37 – 44%);
lower 1/3 (38 – 43%)

RADIOLOGIC TYPES:
(1) Polypoid / fungating form (most common)
√ sessile / pedunculated tumor with lobulated surface
√ protruding, irregular, polycyclic, overhanging, steplike "applecore" lesion
(2) Ulcerating form
√ large ulcer niche within bulging mass
(3) Infiltrating form
√ gradual narrowing with smooth transition (DDx: benign stricture)
(4) Varicoid form = superficial spreading carcinoma (DDx: varices)
√ thickened nodular tortuous longitudinal folds

Metastases:
(a) lymphogenic: anterior jugular chain + supraclavicular nodes (primary in upper 1/3); paraesophageal + subdiaphragmatic nodes (primary in middle 1/3); mediastinal + paracardial + celiac trunk nodes (primary in lower 1/3)
(b) hematogenous: lung, liver, adrenal gland

Cx: Fistula formation to trachea / bronchi / mediastinum

Prognosis: 3 – 20% 5-year survival rate

ESOPHAGEAL INTRAMURAL PSEUDODIVERTICULOSIS

= dilated excretory ducts of esophageal glands

Incidence: about 100 cases in world literature

Site: diffuse / segmental involvement

In 90% associated with:
any severe esophagitis (most often reflux / candida), esophageal stenosis
√ multiple rounded / flask-shaped barium collections outside esophageal lumen
√ commonly associated with strictures

ESOPHAGEAL PERFORATION

Cause:
(1) Emetogenic injuries of the esophagus from sudden increase in intraabdominal pressure + relaxation of distal esophageal sphincter in the presence of a moderate to large amount of gastric contents
(2) Closed chest trauma
(3) Complication of endoscopy, dilatation of stricture, bougie, disruption of suture line following surgical anastomosis, attempted itubation
(4) Esophageal carcinoma

- rapid onset of overwhelming sepsis

Plain film: (normal in 12%)
√ pneumomediastinum
√ subcutaneous emphysema of the neck
√ delayed widening of the mediastinum (secondary to mediastinitis)

√ hydrothorax (after rupture into pleural cavity), usually unilateral
√ hydropneumothorax (often initially not seen)
√ confirmation with contrast study

A. UPPER ESOPHAGEAL LACERATION:
√ widening of upper mediastinum
√ right-sided hydrothorax

B. DISTAL ESOPHAGEAL LACERATION:
√ left-sided hydrothorax
√ little mediastinal changes

Cx: (1) Acute mediastinitis (2) Obstruction of SVC
(3) Mediastinal abscess

ESOPHAGEAL VARICES

A. UPHILL VARICES
= collateral blood flow from portal vein via azgos vein into SVC (usually lower esophagus drains via left gastric vein into portal vein)
Cause:
(a) intrahepatic obstruction from cirrhosis
(b) splenic vein thrombosis (usually gastric varices)
(c) obstruction of hepatic veins
(d) IVC obstruction below hepatic veins
(e) IVC obstruction above hepatic vein entrance / CHF
(f) marked splenomegaly / splenic hemangiomatosis (rare)
√ varices in lower half of esophagus

B. DOWNHILL VARICES
= collateral blood flow from SVC via azygos vein into IVC / portal venous system (upper esophagus usually drains via azygos vein into SVC)
Cause: obstruction of superior vena cava distal to entry of azygos vein; most comon cause: lung cancer, lymphoma, retrosternal goiter, thymoma, mediastinal fibrosis
√ varices in upper 1/3 of esophagus

EXAMINATION TECHNIQUE
(a) small amount of barium (not to obscure varices)
(b) relaxation of esophagus (not to compress varices): refrain from swallowing because succeeding swallow initiates a primary peristaltic wave which lasts for 10 – 30 seconds; sustained Valsalva maneuver precludes from swallowing
(c) horizontal position in LAO projection

Plain film:
√ paraspinal widening (in 5% of patients with portal hypertension)

UGI:
√ thickened sinuous interrupted mucosal folds (earliest sign)
√ tortuous radiolucencies of variable size + location
√ "worm-eaten" smooth lobulated filling defects

CT:
√ right- / left-sided soft-tissue masses (= paraesophageal varices)

√ marked enhancement following dynamic CT
Cx: bleeding in 28% within 3 years; exsanguination in
       10 – 15%

ESOPHAGEAL WEB
= ringlike constriction covered by squamous epithelium on
    superior + inferior surfaces
Age: middle-aged females
? association with:
    Plummer-Vinson syndrome = Paterson-Kelley syndrome
    (iron deficiency anemia, stomatitis, glossitis, dysphagia,
    spoon-shaped nails)
Location: in cervical esophagus near cricopharyngeus
             (most common); may be multiple
√ visualized during maximal distension (in one tenth of a
    second)
√ arises at right angles from anterior esophageal wall
√ thin delicate membrane of uniform thickness of < 3 mm
Cx: high risk of upper esophageal + hypopharyngeal
       carcinoma
DDx: stricture (circumferential + thicker)

ESOPHAGITIS
Acute Esophagitis
√ thickened > 3 mm wide folds with irregular lobulated
    contour
√ mucosal nodularity (= multiple ulcerations +
    intervening edema)
√ erosions
√ vertically oriented ulcers usually 3 – 10 mm in length
√ inflammatory esophagogastric polyp = proximal
    gastric fold extending across esophagogastric
    junction (rare)
√ abnormal motility

Chronic Esophagitis
√ luminal narrowing with tapered transition to normal +
    proximal dilatation
√ circumferential / eccentric stricture
√ pseudodiverticula

FAMILIAL ADENOMATOUS POLYPOSIS
= FAMILIAL MULTIPLE POLYPOSIS = autosomal
    dominant disease with 80% penetrance; sporadic
    occurrence in 1/3
Incidence: 1:7,000 to 1:24,000 live births
Histo: tubular / villotubular adenomatous polyps;
          usually about 1000 adenomas

Age: 20 years at onset (range 5 – 55 years)
• family history of colonic polyps (66%)
• clinical symptoms during 3rd – 4th decade
• vague abdominal pain, weight loss
• diarrhea, bloody stools
• protein-losing enteropathy (occasionally)
Associated with:
    (1) hamartomas of stomach in 49%
    (2) adenomas of duodenum in 25%
    (3) periampullary carcinoma
@ Colon (100%):   especially descending colon + rectum
@ Stomach (5%)
@ Small bowel (< 5%)
√ "carpet of polyps" = myriads of 2 – 3 mm (up to 2 cm)
    polypoid lesions
√ more numerous in distal colon; always affecting rectum
√ normal haustral pattern
Cx: malignant transformation: colon > stomach > small
       bowel (in 12% by 5 years; in 30% by 10 years;
       in 100% by 20 years after diagnosis; age at
       carcinomatous development usually 20 – 40 years;
       multiple carcinomas in 48%)
Rx: prophylactic total colectomy in late teens / early
       twenties
DDx: other polyposes, lymphoid hyperplasia,
       lymphosarcoma, ulcerative colitis with
       inflammatory pseudopolyps

FIBROSING MESENTERITIS
= RETRACTILE MESENTERITIS = MULTIFOCAL
    SUBPERITONEAL SCLEROSIS = MESENTERIC
    PANNICULITIS = LIPOSCLEROTIC MESENTERITIS
    = MESENTERIC LIPODYSTROPHY
Histo: components of inflammation, fibrosis, fatty
          infiltration
Associated with:
    (1) Gardner syndrome
    (2) Fibrosing mediastinitis
√ separation of bowel loops with kinking + angulation
√ mesenteric thickening with fine stellate pattern
√ single mesenteric soft tissue mass (fibroma)
√ multiple nodules throughout mesentery (fibromatosis)

GALLSTONE ILEUS
0.4 – 5% of all small bowel obstructions in elderly;
M:F = 1:4
• previous history of gallbladder disease
• intermittent episodes of abdominal cramps, nausea,
  vomiting

Prognostic Parameters of Gastric Carcinoma			
Tumor size	Metastases	Limited to Submucosa	5-year Survival Rate
1 cm	11%		87%
2 cm	25%	70%	67%
3 cm	45%		35%
4 cm	59%	60%	33%
> 4 cm	72%	33%	

TRIAD:
√ mechanical small bowel obstruction (in 86%)
√ gas within biliary tree (in 69%)
√ ectopic gallstone (in 25%)

GARDNER SYNDROME
= autosomal dominant disease (? variant of familial polyposis) characterized by a triad of (1) colonic polyposis (2) osteomas (3) soft tissue tumors
Histo: adenomatous polyps
Age: 15 – 30 years
Associated with: ? MEA complex
  (1) periampullary carcinoma (12%)
  (2) thyroid carcinoma
  (3) adrenal adenoma / carcinoma
  (4) parathyroid adenoma
  (5) pituitary chromophobe adenoma
  (6) carcinoid, adenoma of small bowel
  (7) retroperitoneal leiomyoma
• skin pigmentation
@ Polyposis
  Location: colon (100%), stomach (5 – 68%), duodenum (90%), small bowel (< 5%)
  √ multiple colonic polyps appearing during teens, increasing in number during 3rd – 4th decade
  √ lymphoid hyperplasia of terminal ileum
  √ hamartomas of stomach
@ Soft tissue tumors
  (a) sebaceous / epidermoid inclusion cysts (scalp, back, face, extremities)
  (b) fibroma, lipoma, leiomyoma, neurofibroma
  (c) desmoid tumors (5 – 6%); peritoneal adhesions (desmoplastic tendency); mesenteric fibrosis, retroperitoneal fibrosis, mammary fibromatosis, marked keloid formation, hypertrophied scars (anterior abdominal wall) arise 1 – 3 years after surgery
    • GI / urinary tract obstruction
@ Osteomatosis of membranous bone (50%)
  Location: calvarium, mandible (81%), maxilla
@ Long bones
  √ localized wavy cortical thickening / exostoses
  √ slight shortening + bowing
@ Teeth
  √ odontoma, unerupted supernumerary teeth, hypercementosis
  √ tendency toward numerous caries (dental prosthesis at early age)
Cx: malignant transformation in 100% (average age at death is 41 years if untreated)
Rx: prophylactic total colectomy at about 20 years of age

GASTRIC CARCINOMA
3rd most common GI-malignancy after colorectal + pancreatic cancer, 6th leading cause of cancer deaths
Prevalence declining; 24 000 cases / year in USA

Predisposed:
  pernicious anemia (risk factor of 2), chronic atrophic gastritis, adenomatous + villous polyp (7 – 27% are malignant), gastrojejunostomy, Billroth II > Billroth I
Histo: adenocarcinoma (95%); rarely squamous cell carcinoma / adenoacanthoma
Staging:
T_1 tumor limited to mucosa / submucosa
T_2 tumor involves muscle / serosa
T_3 tumor penetrates through serosa
T_{4a} invasion of adjacent contiguous tissues
T_{4b} invasion of adjacent organs, diaphragm, abdominal wall
N_1 involvement of perigastric nodes within 3 cm of primary along greater / lesser curvature
N_2 involvement of regional nodes > 3 cm from primary along branches of celiac axis
N_3 paraaortic, hepatoduodenal, retropancreatic, mesenteric nodes
M_1 distant metastases
Location: mostly distal third of stomach + cardia; 60% on lesser curvature, 10% on greater curvature; esophagogastric junction in 30%
Probability of malignancy of an ulcer: at lesser curvature 10 – 15%, at greater curvature 70%, in fundus 90%

MORPHOLOGY
  1. Polypoid / fungating carcinoma
  2. Ulcerating / penetrating carcinoma (70%)
  3. Infiltrating / scirrhous carcinoma = linitis plastica
    Histo: frequently signet ring cell type + increase in fibrous tissue
    √ firmness, rigidity, reduced capacity of stomach, aperistalsis in involved area
    √ granular / polypoid folds with encircling growth
  4. Superficial spreading carcinoma
    = confined to mucosa / submucosa; 5-year survival of 90%
    √ patch of nodularity
    √ little loss of elasticity
  5. Advanced carcinoma

EARLY GASTRIC CANCER (20%)
  = invasion limited to mucosa + submucosa
  Type I Protruded type = eminent protrusion into gastric lumen (10 – 20%)
  Type II Superficial type
    IIa slightly elevated surface (10 – 20%)
    IIb flat / almost unrecognizable (2%)
    IIc slightly depressed surface (50 – 60%)
  Type III Excavated type (5 – 10%)

ADVANCED GASTRIC CANCER
  UGI:
  √ rigidity
  √ filling defect
  √ amputation of folds ± ulceration ± stenosis
  √ calcifications (mucinous adenocarcinoma)

CT:
- √ irregular nodular luminal surface
- √ asymmetric thickening of folds
- √ mass of uniform density / varying attenuation
- √ wall thickness > 3 mm with gas distension + 13 mm with positive contrast material distension
- √ increased density in perigastric fat
- √ enhancement exclusively in linitis plastica type
- √ nodules of serosal surface (= dilated surface lymphatics)
- √ diameter of esophagus at gastroesophageal junction larger than adjacent aorta (DDx: hiatal hernia)
- √ lymphadenopathy below level of renal pedicle (3%)

Metastases:
1. along peritoneal ligaments
   (a) gastrocolic lig.: transverse colon, pancreas
   (b) gastrohepatic + hepatoduodenal lig.: liver
2. local lymph nodes
3. hematogenous: liver (most common), adrenals, ovaries, bone (1.8%), lymphangitic carcinomatosis of lung (rare)
4. peritoneal seeding:
   rectal wall = Blumer shelf
5. left supraclavicular lymph node = Virchow node

Prognosis:
overall 5-year survival rate of 5 – 18%, mean survival time of 7 – 8 months;
- — 85% 5-year survival in stage T_1
- — 52% 5-year survival in stage T_2
- — 47% 5-year survival in stage T_3
- — 17% 5-year survival in stage N_{1-2}
- — 5% 5-year survival in stage N_3

GASTRIC DIVERTICULUM
stomach is least common site of diverticula
Incidence: 1:600 – 2,400 of UGI studies
Etiology: (a) traction secondary to scarring / periantral inflammation = true diverticulum
   (b) pulsion (less common) = false diverticulum
Age: beyond 40 years
Location: juxtacardia on posterior wall (75%), prepyloric (15 – 22%), greater curve (3%)
Often associated with aberrant pancreas in antral location
- √ pliability + varying degrees of distension
- √ NO mass, edema or rigidity of adjacent folds
DDx: small ulcer in intramural-extramucosal mass

GASTRIC DUPLICATION CYST
= intramural cyst lined with secretory epithelium (may grow)
Age: in 75% detected before age 12
Location: frequently on greater curvature (65%)
- √ seldom communicates with main gastric lumen at one / both ends
- √ may ulcerate
- √ up to 12 cm in size

GASTRIC EMPHYSEMA
= relatively benign condition of mucosal disruption
Cause:
(1) severe vomiting
(2) gastroscopic manipulation
(3) increased intraluminal pressure in gastric outlet obstruction
(4) rupture + dissection of subpleural blebs in bullous emphysema
(5) cystic pneumatosis = benign idiopathic round submucosal air lucencies

GASTRIC POLYP
Incidence: 1.5 – 5%, most common benign gastric tumor
Associated with: hyperacidity + ulcers, chronic atrophic gastritis, gastric carcinoma
Prognosis: low incidence of malignant transformation

1. HYPERPLASTIC POLYP (75 – 90%)
   = REGENERATIVE POLYP = INFLAMMATORY POLYP
   Histo: proliferated gastric mucosa + acute and chronic inflammatory infiltrates in lamina propria
   Associated with: chronic atrophic gastritis, pernicious anemia
   Location: random distribution within stomach
   - √ sharply delineated polyp with smooth circular border
   - √ "Mexican hat sign" = stalk seen en face overlying the head of polyp
   - √ sessile / pedunculated, usually multiple polyps
   - √ usually < 1 cm in diameter without progression
   - √ no contour defect of stomach
2. ADENOMATOUS POLYP (10 – 20%)
   = true neoplasm with malignant potential (as high as 51%)
   Associated with: Gardner syndrome, coexistent gastric carcinoma
   Location: more commonly in antrum (antrum spared in Gardner syndrome)
   - √ elliptical / mushroom-shaped; often single
   - √ usually > 1.5 cm in diameter
   - √ smooth / irregular lobulated contour
3. HAMARTOMATOUS POLYP (rare)
   Histo: densely packed gastric glands
   Associated with: Peutz-Jeghers syndrome
   - √ usually < 2 cm in diameter
4. RETENTION POLYP (rare)
   Histo: dilated cystic glands + stroma
   Associated with: Cronkhite-Canada syndrome
5. VILLOUS POLYP (rare)
   - √ trabeculated / lobulated slightly irregular contour
   Cx: malignant transformation
DDx:
(1) Menetrier disease (antrum spared)
(2) Eosinophilic polyps (peripheral eosinophilia, linitis plastica appearance, small bowel changes)

(3) Lymphoma
(4) Carcinoma

GASTRIC ULCER
Benign Gastric Ulcer
95% of all gastric ulcers
Causes:
(1) stress (2) burns = Curling ulcer (3) cerebral disease = Cushing ulcer (4) uremia (5) severe prolonged illness (6) gastritis (7) steroid therapy (8) intubation (9) stasis ulcer proximal to pyloric / duodenal obstruction (10) HPT (25% with ulcer disease)
Pathophysiology:
disrupted mucosal barrier with vulnerability to acid + secretion of large volume of gastric juice containing little acid
Incidence: 5:10,000; 100,000 / year (United States)
Age peak: 55 – 65 years; M:F = 1:1
Multiplicity:
   (a) multiple in 2 – 8% (17 – 24% at autopsy), especially with aspirin
   (b) coexistent duodenal ulcer in 5 – 64% gastric:duodenal = 1:3 (adults) = 1:7 (children)
Location: lesser curvature at junction of corpus + antrum within 7 cm from pylorus; proximal half of stomach in older patients (geriatric ulcer); adjacent to GE junction within hiatal hernia
- abdominal pain: in 30% at night, in 25% precipitated by food
√ ulcer size usually < 2 cm (range 1 – 250 mm); in 4% > 40 mm
√ Haudek niche = conical / collar button-shaped barium collection projecting outside gastric contour (profile view)
√ Hampton line = 1 mm thin straight lucent line traversing the orifice of the ulcer niche (seen on profile view + with little gastric distension) = ledge of touching overhanging gastric mucosa of undermined benign ulcer
√ ulcer collar = smooth thick lucent band interposed between the niche and gastric lumen (thickened rim of edematous gastric wall) in well distended stomach
√ ulcer mound = smooth, sharply delineated, gently sloping extensive tissue mass surrounding a benign ulcer (edema + lack of wall distensibility) in well distended stomach
√ ulcer crater = round / oval barium collection with smooth border on dependent side (en face view)
√ halo defect = wide lucent band symmetrically surrounding ulcer resembling extensive ulcer mound (viewed en face)
√ ring shadow : ulcer on nondependent side (en face view)
√ radiating thick folds extending directly to crater edge fusing with the effaced marginal fold of the ulcer collar / halo of ulcer mound

√ incisura defect = smooth, deep, narrow, sharp indentation on greater curvature opposite a niche on lesser curvature at / slightly below the level of the ulcer (spastic contraction of circular muscle fibers)
Prognosis:
healing in 50% by 3 weeks, in 100% by 6 – 8 weeks; slower healing in older patients; only complete healing proves benignancy
Cx: bleeding, perforation

Malignant Gastric Ulcer
Incidence: 5% of ulcers are malignant
Prognosis: partial healing may occur
Location: anywhere within stomach; fundal ulcers above level of cardia are usually malignant
√ ulcer location within gastric lumen, i.e., not projecting beyond expected margin of stomach (profile view)
√ eccentrically located ulcer within the tumor
√ irregularly shaped ulcer
√ shallow ulcer with width greater than depth
√ nodular ulcer floor
√ abrupt transition between normal mucosa + abnormal tissue at some distance (usually 2 – 4 cm) from ulcer edge
√ rolled / rounded / shouldered edges surrounding ulcer
√ nodular irregular folds approaching ulcer with fused / clubbed / amputated tips
√ rigidity / lack of distensibility
√ associated large irregular mass
√ **Carman meniscus sign** = curvilinear lens-shaped intraluminal form of crater with convexity of crescent toward gastric wall and concavity toward gastric lumen (profile view, usually under compression) found in specific type of ulcerating carcinoma, seen only infrequently; wall aspect can also be concave / flat
√ **Kirklin meniscus complex** = Carman sign (appearance of crater) + radiolucent slightly elevated rolled border

GASTRIC VOLVULUS
= abnormal degree of rotation of one part of stomach around another part, usually requires > 180° twisting to produce complete obstruction
Etiology: (a)   abnormality of suspensory ligaments (hepatic, splenic, colic, phrenic)
          (b)   unusually long gastrohepatic + gastrocolic mesenteries
Usually associated with diaphragmatic abnormality:
(1) paraesophageal hiatus hernia in 33%
(2) eventration
Types:
   (a) ORGANOAXIAL VOLVULUS
      rotation around a line extending from cardia to pylorus
   (b) MESENTEROAXIAL VOLVULUS
      rotation around an axis extending from lesser to greater curvature
- severe epigastric pain

- vigorous attempts to vomit without results
- inability to pass tube into stomach
√ massively distended stomach in LUQ extending into chest
√ incomplete / absent entrance of barium into stomach
√ barium demonstrates area of twist
Cx: (1) intramural emphysema (2) perforation
DDx: (1) gastric atony (2) acute gastric dilatation (3) pyloric obstruction

GASTRITIS
Emphysematous Gastritis
= rare but severe form of widespread phlegmonous gastritis subsequent to mucosal disruption characterized by gas in wall of stomach
Cause of mucosal disruption:
ingestion of toxic / corrosive substances (most common), alcohol abuse, trauma, gastric infarction, necrotizing enterocolitis, ulcer
Histo: bacterial invasion of submucosa + subserosa
Organism: Hemolytic streptococcus, Clostridia welchii, E. coli, S. aureus
- explosive onset of abdominal pain, nausea, chills, fever, leukocytosis
- bloody foul smelling emesis
√ linear small gas bubbles within grossly thickened gastric wall
√ may be associated with gas in portal vein
Cx: leads to cicatricial stenosis / sinus tract formation
Prognosis: 60 – 80% mortality

Erosive Gastritis
= HEMORRHAGIC GASTRITIS
Incidence: 0.5 – 10% of GI studies
Etiology (in 50% without causative factors):
(1) Emotional stress, alcohol, acid, corrosives, severe burns, antiinflammatory agents (aspirin, steroids, phenylbutazone, indomethacin)
(2) Crohn disease
(3) Herpes simplex virus, CMV, candidiasis
Histo: epithelial defect not penetrating beyond muscularis mucosae
- 10 – 20% of all GI hemorrhage
- vague dyspepsia, ulcerlike symptoms
Location: antrum, rarely extending into fundus
√ varioliform erosion = tiny fleck of barium surrounded by radiolucent halo ("target lesion") < 5 mm, usually multiple
√ nodularity / scalloping of prominent antral folds
√ incomplete erosion = linear streaks / dots of barium
√ contiguous duodenal disease may be present
√ limited distensibility, poor peristalsis / atony, delayed gastric emptying

Phlegmonous Gastritis
Etiology: septicemia, local abscess, postoperative stomach, complication of gastric ulcer / cancer

Organism: Streptococcus
Path: multiple gastric wall abscesses which may communicate with lumen
- severe fulminating illness
- patient may vomit pus
Location: usually limited to stomach not extending beyond pylorus; submucosa most severely affected gastric layer
√ barium dissection into submucosa + serosa

GIARDIASIS
= overgrowth of commensal parasite Giardia lamblia
Organism: Giardia lamblia (flagellated protozoan); often harmless contaminant of UGI tract; capable of pathogenic behavior with invasion of gut wall
Incidence: infests 4 – 16% of inhabitants of tropical countries, found in 3 – 20% of children in parts of Southern United States
Predisposed: altered immune mechanism (dysgammaglobulinemia, nodular lymphoid hyperplasia of ileum)
- abdominal pain, weight loss, failure to thrive (especially in children)
- spectrum from asymptomatic to severe debilitating diarrhea, steatorrhea
- reduced fat absorption (simulating celiac disease)
- stool shows trophozoites or cysts
Location: most pronounced in duodenum + jejunum
√ thickened distorted mucosal folds in duodenum + jejunum with normal ileum (mucosal edema)
√ marked spasm + irritability with rapid change in direction + configuration of folds
√ hypersecretion with blurring + indistinctness of folds
√ ± lymphoid hyperplasia
√ hyperperistalsis
Dx: duodenal aspirate / jejunal biopsy
DDx: Strongyloides infection
Rx: quinacrine (Atabrine®)

HEMANGIOMA OF SMALL BOWEL
Increased incidence in: Turner syndrome, tuberous sclerosis, Osler-Weber-Rendu disease
Location: duodenum (2%), jejunum (55%), ileum (42%)
√ multiple sessile compressible intraluminal filling defects
√ nodular segmental mucosal abnormality
√ phleboliths in intestinal wall

HIATAL HERNIA
Associated with: diverticulosis (25%), esophagitis (25%), duodenal ulcer (20%), gallstones (18%)
A. SLIDING HIATAL HERNIA (99%)
= AXIAL HERNIA = CONCENTRIC HERNIA
= portion of peritoneal sac forms part of wall of hernia
Etiology: rupture of phrenicoesophageal membrane due to repetitive stretching with swallowing
Incidence: increasing with age

√ reducible in erect position
√ epiphrenic bulge = entire vestibule + sleeve of stomach are intrathoracic
√ distance between B ring and hiatal margin > 2 cm
√ tortuous esophagus having an eccentric junction with hernia
√ gastroesophageal reflux
√ numerous coarse thick gastric folds within suprahiatal pouch (> 6 longitudinal folds)
CT:
  √ dehiscence of diaphragmatic crura > 15 mm
  √ pseudomass within / above esophageal hiatus
  √ increase in fat surrounding distal esophagus (= herniation of omentum through phrenicoesophageal ligament)

B. PARAESOPHAGEAL HERNIA (1%)
= ROLLING HIATAL HERNIA = PARAHIATAL HERNIA = portion of stomach superiorly displaced into thorax with esophagogastric junction remaining in subdiaphragmatic position
√ cardia in normal position
√ herniation of portion of stomach anterior to esophagus
√ frequently nonreducible
√ may be associated with gastric ulcer of lesser curvature at level of diaphragmatic hiatus

C. TOTALLY INTRATHORACIC STOMACH
= defect in central tendon of diaphragm in combination with slight volvulus in transverse axis of stomach behind heart
√ cardia may be intrathoracic (usually) / subdiaphragmatic
√ great gastric curvature either on right / left side

D. CONGENITALLY SHORT ESOPHAGUS
(not true hernia, very rare)
= gastric ectopy by lack of lengthening of esophagus
√ nonreducible intrathoracic gastric segment (in erect / supine position)
√ cylindrical / round intrathoracic segment with large sinuous folds
√ short straight esophagus
√ circular narrowing at gastroesophageal junction, frequently with ulcer
√ gastroesophageal reflux

HIRSCHSPRUNG DISEASE
= AGANGLIONOSIS OF THE COLON = AGANGLIONIC MEGACOLON
= absence of parasympathetic ganglia in muscle + submucosal layers (Meissner + Auerbach plexi) secondary to an arrest of craniocaudal migration of neuroblasts before 12th week leading to relaxation failure of the aganglionic segment
Incidence: 1:5,000 – 8,000 live births; usually sporadic; familial in 4%
Age: fulll-term infant during first 6 weeks of life (70 – 80%); M:F = 4 – 9:1; extremely rare in premature infants

Associated with: Trisomy 21 (2%)
Location: over varying distances proximal to anus, usually rectosigmoid
  (a) short segment disease   (80%)
  (b) long segment disease   (15%)
  (c) total colonic aganglionosis (5%)
  (d) skip aganglionosis = sparing of rectum (very rare)
• failure to pass meconium within first 24 hours of life
• intermittent constipation + paradoxical diarrhea (25%)
• rectal manometry with absence of spike activity
√ "transition zone" = aganglionic segment appears normal in size
√ dilatation of large + small bowel aborally from transition zone
√ marked retention of barium on delayed films after 24 hours
√ normal appearing rectum in 33%
√ 10 – 15 cm segment of persistent corrugated / convoluted rectum (= abnormal uncoordinated contractions of the aganglionic portion of colon) in 31% (DDx: colitis, milk allergy, normal intermittent spasm of rectum)
√ avoid digital exam / cleansing enema prior to radiographic studies
OB-US: √ dilated small bowel / dilated colon
Cx: (1) Necrotizing enterocolitis
    (2) Cecal perforation (secondary to stasis, distension, ischemia)
    (3) Obstructive uropathy
Dx: suction mucosal biopsy of rectum (increased acetylcholinesterase activity)
Rx: (1) Swenson pull-through procedure
    (2) Duhamel operation
    (3) Soave procedure

HODGKIN DISEASE
Incidence: 0.75% of all cancers diagnosed each year
Age: bimodal peaks at age 25 – 30 years and 75 – 80 years
Histo: Reed-Sternberg cell = binucleate cell with prominent centrally located nucleolus
  (1) Lymphocyte predominance (5%)
= abundance of normal-appearing lymphocytes + relative paucity of abnormal cells; often diagnosed in younger people; frequently early stage; systemic symptoms are uncommon; most favorable natural history
  (2) Nodular sclerosis (78%)
= lymph nodes traversed by broad bands of birefringent collagen separating nodules which consist of normal lymphocytes, eosinophils, plasma cells, and histiocytes; most common subtype; typically mediastinal involvement; 1/3 with systemic symptoms
  (3) Mixed cellularity (17%)
= diffuse effacement of lymph nodes with lymphocytes, eosinophils, plasma cells + relative abundance of atypical mononuclear and Reed-

Sternberg cells; more commonly advanced stage at presentation and older age
(4) <u>Lymphocyte depletion</u> (1%)
= paucity of normal appearing lymphocytes + abundance of abnormal mononuclear and Reed-Sternberg cells; least common subtype with worst prognosis; associated with advanced stage and systemic symptoms

STAGE
I   involvement of single lymph node region
II   involvement of ≥ 2 lymph node regions on same side of diaphragm
III lymph node involvement on both sides of diaphragm
IV   diffuse / disseminated involvement of ≥ 1 extralymphatic organs / tissues ± associated lymph node involvement
E   = extralymphatic site
S   = splenic involvement
A   = absence of fever, night sweats, > 10% weight loss in past 6 months
B   = presence of fever, night sweats, > 10% weight loss in past 6 months
• painless lymphadenopathy
• alcohol-induced pain
• unexplained fevers, night sweat, weight loss
• generalized pruritus
Location: intestinal involvement uncommon (10 – 15%); duodenum + jejunum (67%); terminal ileum (20%)
√ narrow rigid obstructive lesion
√ abundance of desmoplastic reaction (DDx from NHL)
√ infiltrating (60%); polypoid (26%); ulcerated (14%)
Prognosis: excellent for isolated / localized disease

HYPERPLASTIC POLYP OF COLON
= intestinal metaplasia consisting of mucous glands lined by a single layer of columnar epithelium; NO malignant potential
Path: infolding of epithelium into the glandular lumen
Location: rectum
√ usually < 5 mm in diameter

HYPERTROPHIC PYLORIC STENOSIS
= idiopathic hypertrophy and hyperplasia of circular muscle fibers of pylorus with proximal extension into gastric antrum
Incidence: 3:1,000;   M:F = 5:1
Etiology: inherited as a dominant polygenic trait; increased incidence in first-born boys
A. INFANTILE FORM
Age: manifestation at 2 – 8 weeks of life; M:F = 4:1
• nonbilious projectile vomiting (sour formula / clear gastric contents) with progression over a period of several weeks after birth
• positive family history
• olive-shaped mass

Barium:
Precautions: (1) empty stomach via nasogastric tube before study
                (2) remove contrast at end of study
√ pyloric wall thickness >10 mm
√ elongation + narrowing of pyloric canal (2 – 4 cm in length)
√ "double / triple track sign" = crowding of mucosal folds in pyloric channel
√ "string sign" = passing of small barium streak through pyloric channel
√ Twining recess = "diamond sign" = transient triangular tentlike cleft / niche in midportion of pyloric canal with apex pointing inferiorly secondary to mucosal bulging between two separated hypertrophied muscle bundles on the greater curvature side within pyloric channel
√ "pyloric teat" = outpouching along lesser curvature due to disruption of antral peristalsis
√ "antral beaking" = mass impression upon antrum with streak of barium pointing toward pyloric channel
√ Kirklin sign = "mushroom sign" = indentation of base of bulb (in 50%)
√ gastric distension + fluid
√ active gastric hyperperistalsis
√ "caterpillar sign" = appearance of peristaltic gastric wave
US:
√ "target sign" = hypoechoic ring of hypertrophied pyloric muscle around echogenic central mucosa on cross section
√ pyloric transverse diameter ≥ 13 – 15 mm; transverse muscle wall thickness ≥ 3 – 4 mm
√ "cervix sign" = longitudinal section of the elongated narrowed pyloric channel with indentation of muscle mass on fluid-filled antrum
√ pyloric canal length ≥ 15 – 17 mm
√ exaggerated peristaltic waves, failure of fluid to pass into duodenum
Cx: hypochloremic metabolic alkalosis
DDx: Infantile pylorospasm (variable caliber of antral narrowing, antral peristalsis, resolves in several days)

mushroom sign / diamond sign / teat sign / caterpillar sign / double / triple track sign / shoulder sign / beak sign

B. ADULT FORM (secondary to mild infantile form)
- acute obstructive symptoms uncommon
- nausea, intermittent vomiting
- postprandial distress, heartburn

Associated with:
- (1) peptic ulcer disease (in 50 – 74%) (prolonged gastrin production secondary to stasis of food)
- (2) chronic gastritis (54%)

√ persistent elongation (2 – 4 cm) + concentric narrowing of pyloric channel
√ parallel + preserved mucosal folds
√ antispasmodics show no effect on narrowing
√ proximal benign ulcer (74%), usually near incisura

TORUS HYPERPLASIA = FOCAL PYLORIC HYPERTROPHY
= localized muscle hypertrophy on the lesser curvature (= torus)
= milder atypical form of HPS
√ flattening of distal lesser curvature

INFLAMMATORY COLONIC POLYP
Etiology: ulcerative colitis (10 – 20%); granulomatous colitis (less frequent); schistosomiasis (endemic); amebic colitis (occasionally)
√ sessile + frondlike appearance
√ filiform polyposis = multiple fingerlike postinflammatory polyps
√ most common in left hemicolon

INTERNAL HERNIA
= responsible for < 1% of mechanical small bowel obstruction

Classification of hernias:
- (a) Retroperitoneal: usually congenital containing a hernial sac
  1. paraduodenal
  2. foramen of Winslow
  3. intersigmoid
  4. pericecal / ileocolic
  5. supravesical
- (b) Anteperitioneal:
  small group of hernias without a peritoneal sac
  1. transmesenteric
  2. transomental
  3. pelvic (including broad ligament)

A. PARADUODENAL HERNIA (53%)
- (a) through fossa of Landzert on left side (3/4)
  √ lateral to 4th portion of duodenum and behind descending + transverse mesocolon
- (b) through fossa of Waldeyer on right side (1/4)
  √ caudal to SMA and inferior to 3rd portion of duodenum

B. LESSER SAC HERNIA (< 10%)
through foramen of Winslow in retrogastric location invaginated gut:

ileum > jejunum, cecum, appendix, ascending colon, Meckel diverticulum, gallbladder, greater omentum

C. HERNIA THROUGH BROAD LIGAMENT (very rare)
after laceration / fenestration from surgery or during pregnancy

D. SPIGELIAN HERNIA
through spontaneous defect in anterior abdominal wall along semilunar line lateral margin of rectus muscle)

INTESTINAL LYMPHANGIECTASIA
A. CONGENITAL LYMPHANGIECTASIA = PRIMARY PROTEIN-LOSING ENTEROPATHY
= generalized congenital malformation of lymphatic system with congenital atresia of the thoracic duct + gross dilatation of lymphatics of small bowel

Age: presentation in childhood
- asymmetrical lymphedema in various parts of the body
- chylous pleural effusions (45%)
- diarrhea (60%), steatorrhea (20%)
- vomiting (15%)
- abdominal pain (15%)
- decreased albumin + globulin
- lymphocytopenia (90%)
- decreased serum fibrinogen, transferrin, ceruloplasmin

B. ACQUIRED LYMPHANGIECTASIA
Causes leading to dilatation of intestinal lymphatics:
1. diffuse small bowel lymphoma
2. mesenteric adenitis
3. pericardial effusion with obstruction of thoracic duct
4. retroperitoneal fibrosis
5. pancreatitis

- massive edema, chylous + serous effusion
- diarrhea, vomiting, abdominal pain, malabsorption, steatorrhea
- hypoproteinemia secondary to protein loss into intestinal lumen

Path: dilatation of lymph vessels in mucosa + submucosa + abundance of foamy fat-staining macrophages (negative for PAS)
√ diffuse symmetrical marked enlargement of folds in jejunum + ileum
√ slight separation + rigidity of folds
√ dilution of barium column (considerable increase in fluid)
√ no / mild dilatation of bowel

Lymphangiogram:
√ hypoplasia of lower extremity lymphatics
√ occlusion of thoracic duct / large tortuous thoracic duct
√ obstruction of cisterna chyli with reflux into mesenteric lymphatics
√ hypoplastic lymph nodes

Dx: small bowel biopsy (dilated lymphatics in lamina propria + vascular core)
Rx: low-fat diet

DDx: (1) Whipple disease (more segmentation + fragmentation, wild folds)
(2) Amyloidosis (edema + secretions usually absent)
(3) Hypoalbuminemia (less pronounced symmetrical thickening of folds, less prominent secretions)

INTRALUMINAL DUODENAL DIVERTICULUM
= congenital lesion secondary to elongation of an incomplete duodenal diaphragm
Age at presentation: in young adult
• easy satiety
• vomiting
• upper abdominal cramping pain
Location: 2nd – 3rd portion of duodenum
√ barium-filled sac within duodenal lumen (pathognomonic picture) = "windsock, comma, teardrop" appearance
√ anchored to the lateral wall of the duodenum
√ "halo" sign = duodenal mucosa covers outer + inner wall of diverticulum

INTRAMURAL ESOPHAGEAL RUPTURE
= DISSECTING INTRAMURAL HEMATOMA = mucosal tear with dissecting hemorrhage into submucosa and involvement of venous plexus
• hematemesis
√ intramural hematoma simulates retained solid material within lumen
√ "mucosal stripe sign" = dissected mucosa floating within lumen

INTUSSUSCEPTION
= invagination or prolapse of a segment of intestinal tract (= intussusceptum) into the lumen of adjacent intestine (= intussuscipiens)
A. IN CHILDREN (94%)
   most common abdominal emergency of early childhood, leading cause of acquired bowel obstruction in childhood
   Etiology:
     (1) idiopathic (over 95%): ileocecal valve
     (2) leadpoint (5%): Meckel diverticulum, lymphosarcoma, polyp, lymphoid hyperplasia secondary to viral infection, enterogenous cyst, duplication, suture granuloma, appendiceal inflammation, Henoch-Schönlein purpura, inspissated meconium (usually > 6 years)
   Age: 3 – 9 months (40%); < 1 year (50%); < 2 years (75%); > 3 years (< 10%); M:F = 2:1
   • abrupt onset of violent pain (90%), vomiting (85%)
   • abdominal mass (60%)
   • "currant jelly" bloody stools (60%)
   Location: ileocolic (90%) > ileoileal (4%) > colocolonic
   Cx: vascular compromise secondary to incorporation of mesentery (hemorrhage, infarction, acute inflammation)

B. IN ADULTS (6%)
   Etiology:
     (1) specific cause (80%): benign tumor (1/3), malignant tumor (1/5), lipoma, Meckel diverticulum, prolapsed gastric mucosa, aberrant pancreas, adhesions, foreign bodies, tubes, chronic ulcer (TB, typhoid), prior gastroenteritis, sprue, scleroderma, gastroenterostomy, trauma, fasting, anxiety, agonal state
     (2) idiopathic (20%)
   • recurrent episodes of colicky pain, nausea, vomiting
   Location: ileoileal (40%) > ileocolic (13%)

Plain film: no abnormality (in 25%)
   √ soft-tissue mass
   √ small bowel obstruction pattern (50 – 60%) with nipplelike termination of gas shadow
Antegrade barium study:
   √ "coiled spring" pattern
   √ beaklike abrupt narrowing of barium column demonstrating a central channel
Retrograde barium study:
   √ convex intracolic mass + "coil spring" pattern
CT:
   √ "multiple concentric rings" = 3 concentric cylinders (central cylinder = canal + wall of intussusceptum; middle cylinder = crescent of mesenteric fat; outer cylinder = returning intussusceptum + intussuscipiens)
   √ proximal obstruction
US:
   √ "doughnut sign" (on transverse sections); "pseudokidney sign" on longitudinal sections = targetlike dense central echoes surrounded by peripheral rim of hypoechogenicity (edema)

HYDROSTATIC / PNEUMATIC REDUCTION
Mortality is < 1% if reduction occurs < 24 hours after onset
Overall success rate: 18 – 90%
Contraindications to barium enema:
   pneumoperitoneum, peritonitis, hypovolemic shock
Technique:
   (1) sedation with morphine sulfate (0.2 mg/kg IM) / fentanyl citrate IV
   (2) barium enema container between 24 – 36 inches above level of anus
   (3) maximum of 3 attempts for 3 minutes each
   (4) reduction should be accomplished within 10 minutes
   (5) extensive reflux into small bowel desirable to exclude residual ileoileal intussusception
"RULE OF THREES" = Δ 3 feet above table
                              Δ no more than 3 attempts
                              Δ 3 minutes per attempt
Cx: perforation (0.4%); reduction of nonviable bowel; incomplete reduction; missed lead point; recurrence (3.5 – 10%)

ISCHEMIC COLITIS

Precipitating factors:
Volvulus, carcinoma, history of cardiovascular disease with spontaneous thrombosis, history of aortoiliac reconstruction (2%) with ligation of IMA

Age: > 50 years
- abrupt onset of lower abdominal pain + rectal bleeding
- abdominal tenderness, diarrhea

Location: splenic flexure (80%) + rectosigmoid
("watershed areas")

BE: single contrast preferable as lesions may become effaced by double contrast
- √ serrated mucosa = inflammatory edema + superficial ulceration
- √ transverse ridging = markedly enlarged mucosal folds (spasm)
- √ pseudopolyposis = intraluminal masses with smooth surface (submucosal edema + hemorrhage)
- √ "thumbprinting" = marginal indentations on mesenteric side
- √ some wall pliability is preserved
- √ deep penetrating ulcers

CT:
- √ symmetrical / lobulated segmental thickening of colonic wall
- √ irregular narrowed atonic lumen (= thumbprinting)
- √ curvilinear collection of intramural gas
- √ portal + mesenteric venous air
- √ blood clot in SMA / SMV

Angio: (similar to inflammatory disease)
- √ normal / slightly attenuated arterial supply
- √ mild acceleration of arteriovenous transit time
- √ small tortuous ectatic draining veins

Prognosis: (1) complete resolution
(2) stricture: √ narrowed foldless segment
(3) gangrene with necrosis + perforation

JEJUNAL DIVERTICULUM

= acquired mucosal herniation, frequently multiple
Incidence: 0.1% on UGI, 1% of autopsy series; M > F
Site: on mesenteric border near entrance of blood vessels
- upper abdominal pain
- indigestion, malabsorption
- macro- / microcytic anemia

Plain film:
- √ slight dilatation of jejunal loops

BE:
- √ may not fill (narrow neck / stagnant secretions)
- √ trapped barium on delayed film after 24 hours

Cx: (1) hemorrhage (2) diverticulitis (3) intestinal obstruction (4) free perforation

JUVENILE POLYPOSIS

= retention / inflammatory polyp = polyps with inflammatory changes secondary to chronic irritation
Δ most common familial / nonfamilial colonic polyp in children (75%)

Histo: hyperplasia of mucous glands; retention cysts develop with obstruction of gland orifices (multiple mucin-filled spaces)

Peak age: 4 – 6 years (range 1 – 10 years); M:F = 3:2
- rectal bleeding (95%) most commonly as intermittent bright red hematochezia
- anemia, pain
- diarrhea, constipation
- abdominal pain (from intussusception)
- rectal prolapse (rare)

Location: rectosigmoid (80%); rare in small bowel + stomach
- √ solitary polyp (75%); multiple polyps (1/3) of smooth round contour
- √ variable size of pinpoint lesion to several cm in size
- √ invariably on stalk of variable length
- √ autoamputation / regression with time

LADD BANDS

= congenital peritoneal bands extending from cecum / hepatic flexure over anterior surface of 2nd / 3rd portion of duodenum causing duodenal obstruction at its 2nd portion (even without volvulus)
Associated with   malrotation

LEIOMYOMA

Leiomyoma of Esophagus

most common benign tumor of esophagus
- asymptomatic
- dysphagia, hematemesis if large (rare)

Age: young males
Site: frequently lower 1/3 of esophagus, intramural
- √ may have coarse calcifications (the only calcifying esophageal tumor)
- √ ulceration uncommon
- √ smooth well-defined mass causing excentric thickening of wall + deformity of lumen

CT: √ uniform soft-tissue density
√ diffuse contrast enhancement

Leiomyoma of Small Bowel

most common benign tumor of small bowel
Location: duodenum (21%), jejunum (48%), ileum (31%); single in 97%
Site: mainly serosal (50%), mainly intraluminal (20%), intramural (10%)
Size: < 5 cm (50%), 5 – 10 cm (25%), > 10 cm (25%)
- √ small ulcer + large barium-filled cavity (central necrosis + communication with lumen)
- √ hypervascular

Leiomyoma of Stomach

2nd most common benign gastric tumor, most common of calcified benign tumors
Location: pars media (39%), antrum (26%), pylorus (12%), fundus (12%), cardia (10%)

Site: intraluminal submucosal (60%), exophytic
        subserosal (35%), combined intramural
        extramural dumbbell type (5%)
√ average size: 4.5 cm
√ ovoid mass with smooth margin + smooth surface
  (most frequently)
√ forms right angle with gastric wall
√ ulcerated in 50%
√ pedunculated intraluminal tumor (rare) = submucosal
  growth
√ "iceberg phenomenon" = large extraluminal
  component in subserosal growth
√ calcifies in 4%
Cx: (1) Hemorrhage (acute / chronic)
      (2) Obstruction (tumor bulk / intussusception)
      (3) Infection
      (4) Fistulization / perforation
      (5) Malignant degeneration (benign:malignant =
           3:1)

LEIOMYOSARCOMA

Leiomyosarcoma of Small Bowel
Location: duodenum (26%), jejunum (34%),
            ileum (40%)
√ usually > 6 cm
√ nodular mass: intraluminal (10%), intraluminal
  pedunculated (5%), intramural (15%), chiefly extrinsic
  (66%)
√ mucosa may be stretched + ulcerated (50%)
√ may show central ulcer pit / fistula communicating
  with a large necrotic center
√ intussusception

Leiomyosarcoma of Stomach
Incidence: 0.1 – 1.5% of all gastric malignancies
Age: 10 – 73 years; M > F
Histo: pleomorphism, hypercellularity, mitotic figures,
         necrosis
Location: anterior / posterior wall of body of stomach
Metastases:
   (1) direct extension into surrounding tissues
   (2) liver, omentum, retroperitoneum
   (3) lymph nodes (rare)
√ average size of 12 cm
√ intramural mass
√ may be pedunculated
√ large masses tend to be exogastric
√ very frequently ulcerated
CT:
   √ lobulated irregular outline
   √ central zones of low density (necrosis with
     liquefaction)
   √ air / positive contrast within tumor (= ulceration)
   √ dystrophic calcifications

Carney Syndrome
Triad of (1) gastric leiomyosarcoma
          (2) functioning extraadrenal paraganglioma

          (3) pulmonary chondromas
Incidence: 24 patients; M:F = 1:11

LIPOMA
Most common submucosal tumor in colon
Incidence: in colon in 0.25% (autopsy)
Location: colon (particularly in cecum + ascending colon)
            > duodenum > ileum > stomach > jejunum >
            esophagus
• asymptomatic
• crampy pain
√ smooth, sharply outlined, round / ovoid intramural mass
  of 1 – 3 cm
√ pedunculated in 1/3 (prone to intussuscept)
√ marked radiolucency
√ softness causing change in shape + size on
  compression
√ "squeeze sign" = sausage-shaped mass on
  postevacuation films
√ ulceration (rare); mucosa usually intact
CT: √ sharply defined intramural mass of fat density
Cx: intussusception (rare)

LYMPHOGRANULOMA VENEREUM
= LGV = sexually transmitted disease caused by virus
  Chlamydia trachomatis producing a nonspecific
  granulomatous inflammatory response in infected
  mucosa (mononuclear cells + macrophages), perirectal
  lymphatic invasion
Location: rectum, may extend to sigmoid + descending
            colon
M:F = 3.4:1
√ narrowing + straightening of rectum
√ widening of retrorectal space
√ irregularity of mucosa + ulcerations
√ progression to long narrow rectal stricture + obstruction
√ shortening + straightening of sigmoid
√ paracolic abscess + rectovaginal fistula
Rx: Tetracyclines effective in acute phase before
      scarring has occurred

LYMPHOID HYPERPLASIA
Histo: hyperplastic lymph follicles in lamina propria
         (Peyer patches), probably compensatory attempt
         for immunoglobulin deficiency
Etiology: (1) self-limiting local / systemic inflammation /
                 infection / allergy
            (2) immunodeficiency /
                 dysgammaglobulinemia
Age: (a) generally in children < 2 years
       (b) in adult invariably associated with late onset
            immunoglobulin deficiency (IgA, IgM)
Associated with: splenomegaly, large tonsils,
                   eczematous dermatitis, achlorhydria,
                   pernicious anemia, acute pancreatitis,
                   colonic carcinoma

At risk for
   (1) **Good syndrome** (10%)
       = gastric carcinoma + benign thymoma + lymphoid hyperplasia
   (2) Respiratory infections
   (3) Giardia lamblia infection (90%)
   (4) Functional thyroid abnormalities
Location: primarily jejunum, may involve entire small bowel
- malabsorption (diarrhea + steatorrhea)
- low serum concentrations of IgA, IgG, IgM
√ mucosa studded with innumerable small 1 – 3 mm uniform polypoid lesions
√ lesions may be umbilicated

LYMPHOMA
Incidence: 10% of patients with abdominal lymphoma have bowel involvement
Histo: predominantly NHL (lymphosarcoma, reticulum cell sarcoma); in 15% Hodgkin disease
Types:
   (a) polypoid (47%)
       √ enlarged nodular folds
   (b) ulcerative (42%)
       √ ulcerative lesions, may be complicated by perforation
       √ aneurysmal configuration
   (c) diffuse (11%)
       √ diffuse hoselike thickening of bowel wall
       √ decreased / absent peristalsis
CT-staging:
   Stage I   tumor confined to bowel wall
   Stage II   limited to local nodes
   Stage III widespread nodal disease
   Stage IV   disseminated to bone marrow, liver, other organs
Location: 10 – 25% of NHL are extranodal; stomach > small bowel > colon > esophagus; multicentric in 10 – 50%
√ enlargement of spleen
√ enlargement of regional lymph nodes
May be associated with enlargement of extraabdominal lymph nodes, malabsorption
Prognosis:
   (a) 71 – 82% 2-year survival rate in isolated bowel lymphoma
   (b) 0% 2-year survival rate in stage IV disease with bowel involvement
Cx during chemotherapy: perforation (9 – 40%), hemorrhage
@ Esophagus
   least common site of GI involvement (in < 1%)
@ Stomach
   1 – 5% of all gastric malignancies; most common site of extranodal Hodgkin disease; 25% of extranodal lymphoma; mostly NHL with histiocytic cell type
   Site: lower 2/3 of stomach
   √ flexibility of gastric wall preserved

√ crossing of lesion into duodenum
√ circumscribed mass with endogastric / exogastric (25%) growth
√ broad tortuous mucosal folds over large portions of stomach (diffuse form)
√ large irregular ulcers
CT:
   √ diffuse involvement > 50% of stomach (77%)
   √ segmental involvement (15%)
   √ ulcerated mass (8%)
   √ average wall thickness of 4 – 5 cm
   √ luminal irregularity (66%)
   √ hyperrugosity (58%)
Prognosis: 55% 5-year survival rate after resection
@ Small bowel
1/5 of all small bowel malignancies; most common malignant small bowel tumor; multiple sites of involvement in 1/5; most common cause of intussusception in children > 6 years
Location: ileum (51%), jejunum (47%), duodenum (2%),
Site: arising from lymphoid patches of Peyer
Types:
   (1) infiltrating lymphoma with plaquelike involvement of wall > 5 cm in length (80%) / > 10 cm in length (20%) (DDx: Crohn disease)
       √ ulceration (considerable excavation) + cicatrization may occur
       √ thickened valvulae with corrugated appearance
       √ aneurysmal dilatation (secondary to tumor necrosis + muscle destruction)
   (2) single / multiple polypoid mucosal / submucosal masses
       √ cobblestone defects due to lymphomatous polyps
       √ nodules may ulcerate
       √ may cause intussusception
       √ sprue pattern
   (3) endoexoenteric mass
       √ large mass with only small intramural component
       √ ± ulcer + fistulae + aneurysmatic dilatation
   (4) mesenteric / retroperitoneal adenopathy
       √ single / multiple extraluminal masses displacing bowel
       √ ill-defined confluent mass engulfing + encasing multiple loops of adjacent bowel
       √ "sandwich configuration" = mass surrounding mesenteric vessels which are separated by perivascular fat
       √ conglomerate mantle of retroperitoneal + mesenteric mass
@ Colon
colon less commonly involved than stomach / small bowel; 1.5% of all abdominal lymphomas frequently resembles inflammatory disease / polyposis
Location: cecum most commonly involved (85%)

√ single mass > diffuse infiltration > polypoid lesion
√ paradoxical dilatation
√ gross mural circumferential / focal soft-tissue thickening (average 5 cm)
√ slight enhancement
√ massive regional + distant mesenteric + retroperitoneal adenopathy

MALIGNANT MELANOMA
= develops from melanocytes derived from neural crest cells, arising in preexisting benign nevi
Incidence: 1% of all cancers
Clark Staging:
   Level I   all tumor cells above basement membrane (in situ lesion)
   Level II   tumor extends to papillary dermis
   Level III   tumor extends to interface between papillary + reticular dermis
   Level IV   tumor extends between bundles of collagen of reticular dermis
   Level V   tumor invasion of subcutaneous tissue (in 87% metastatic)
Breslow staging:
   thin   < 0.75 mm depth of invasion
   intermediate   0.76 – 3.99 mm depth of invasion
   thick   > 4 mm depth of invasion
METASTASES:
latent period of 2 – 20 years after initial diagnosis (most commonly 2 – 5 years)
Primary site: head + neck (79%), eye (77%), GU system (67%)
   @ Lymphadenopathy
     — in 23% with level II + IV
     — in 75% with level V
   @ Bone (11 – 17%)
     • often initial manifestation of recurrence
     • poor prognosis
     axial skeleton (80%), ribs (38%)
   @ Lung (70% at autopsy)
     most common site of relapse
     respiratory failure most common cause of death
   @ Liver (17 – 23%; 58% at autopsy)
     √ single / multiple lesions 0.5 – 15 cm in size
     √ larger lesion often necrotic
     √ may be partially calcified
   @ Spleen (1 – 5%)
     √ single / multiple lesions of variable size
     √ solid / cystic
   @ Bowel + mesentery (8%)
     most common site is small bowel
   @ Kidney (up to 35% at autopsy)
   @ Adrenal (11%, up to 50% at autopsy)
   @ Subcutis
Prognosis: 30 – 40% die eventually of this tumor

MALLORY-WEISS SYNDROME
= mucosal + submucosal tear with involvement of venous plexus

Pathophysiology: violent projection of gastric content against lower esophagus
Age: 30 – 60 years; M > F
predisposed: alcoholics
• history of repeated vomiting prior to hematemesis
• massive painless hematemesis
Location: at / above / below (76%) esophagogastric junction
√ longitudinal single tear in 77%, in 23% multiple
√ extravasation of barium
Angio: √ bleeding site at gastric cardia
DDx: peptic ulcer / ulcerative gastritis

MASTOCYTOSIS
= systemic disease with mast cell proliferation in skin + RES (lamina propria of small bowel; bone; lymph nodes; liver; spleen) associated with eosinophils + lymphocytes
Age: < 6 months old (in 50%)
• nausea, vomiting, diarrhea, steatorrhea
• urticaria pigmentosa
• abdominal pain, anorexia
• alcohol intolerance
• tachycardia, asthma, flushing, headaches, pruritus (histamine liberation)
@ Small bowel
   √ generalized irregular distorted thickened folds ± wall thickening
   √ diffuse pattern of sandlike nodules
   √ urticaria-like lesions of gastric + intestinal mucosa
@ Liver & spleen
   √ hepatosplenomegaly
@ Bone
   √ sclerotic bone lesions
Dx: jejunal biopsy demonstrates an excess of mast cells
Cx: (1) peptic ulcer disease (histamine-mediated acid secretion)
     (2) leukemia
Rx: antihistamines, histamine decarboxylase inhibitors, sodium chromoglycase

MECKEL DIVERTICULUM
= persistence of the omphalomesenteric duct (= vitelline duct) which usually obliterates by 5th embryonic week, most common anomaly of the GI tract
Incidence: 2 – 3% of population
Age: majority in children < 10 years of age; M:F = 3:1
Histo: contains heterotopic tissue in 12 – 16%: gastric / pancreatic / colonic mucosa; frequency of ectopic gastric mucosa: 30% overall; 60% in symptomatic children; in > 95% with GI hemorrhage
Location: within terminal 6 feet of ileum; in 94% on antimesenteric border
RULE OF 2's: Δ in 2% of population
     Δ symptomatic usually before age 2
     Δ located within 2 feet of ileocecal valve
     Δ length of 2 inches

NUC (> 85% sensitivity, > 95% specificity, > 88% accuracy):
Δ Tc-99m pertechnetate is excreted by mucoid cells of gastric mucosa, excretion is not dependent on presence of parietal cells
Preparation:
(1) no irritative measures for 48 hours (contrast studies, endoscopy, cathartics, enemas, drugs irritating GI tract)
(2) fasting for 3 – 6 hours (results in decreased gastric secretion + diminished bowel peristalsis)
(3) evacuation of bowel + bladder prior to study

Dose: 5 – 20 mCi (100 µCi / kg) Tc-99m pertechnetate
Radiation dose: 0.54 rad/2 mCi for thyroid;
0.3 rad/2 mCi for large intestine;
0.2 rad/2 mCi for stomach
Imaging: serial in 5 – 10 minute-intervals for 1 hour
√ improved visualization through
(a) pentagastrin = stimulates uptake (6 µg/kg SC 20 min prior to pertechnetate)
(b) cimetidine = inhibits secretion (maximum 300 mg/dose IV 1 hour prior)
(c) glucagon = decreases peristalsis (50 µg/kg IM 5 – 10 minutes prior)
√ poor visualization with perchlorate + atropin (= depressed uptake)
False-positive results:
(1) Ectopic gastric mucosa in gastrogenic cyst, enteric duplication, normal small bowel, Barrett esophagus
(2) Increased blood pool in AVM, hemangioma, hypervascular tumor, aneurysm
(3) Duodenal ulcer, ulcerative colitis, Crohn disease, appendicitis, laxative abuse
(4) Intussusception, intestinal obstruction, volvulus
(5) Urinary tract obstruction, calyceal diverticulum
(6) Anterior meningomyelocele, poor technique
False-negative results:
(1) Insufficient mass of ectopic gastric mucosa
(2) Dilution of intraluminal activity (hemorrhage / hypersecretion)
Cx (in 20%):
(1) GI bleeding secondary to ulceration
(2) Acute diverticulitis
(3) Intestinal obstruction secondary to intussusception / fibrous bands / volvulus (when attached to umbilicus)
(4) Malignant tumor (rare): carcinoma, sarcoma, carcinoid
(5) Chronic abdominal pain

MECONIUM ILEUS
= low small bowel obstruction secondary to inspissated meconium which impacts in distal ileum
Age: may develop in utero (in 15%)

Associated with:
mucoviscidosis (= cystic fibrosis) with thick + sticky meconium due to deficiency of pancreatic secretions (in almost 100%)
Δ 10 – 15% of infants with cystic fibrosis present with meconium ileus
√ numerous dilated small bowel loops with paucity of air-fluid levels
√ "bubbly" / "frothy" appearance of intestinal contents
√ "soap bubble" / "applesauce" in RLQ
√ multiple round / oval filling defects in distal ileum
√ microcolon (unused colon)
OB-US:
√ small bowel dilatation
√ usually polyhydramnios
√ unusual echogenic intraluminal areas (DDx: normal transient inspissated meconium)
Cx (in 40 – 50%): volvulus, ischemia, necrosis, perforation, meconium peritonitis, atresia
Rx: (1) gastrografin enema (attention to fluid + electrolyte balance)
(2) acetylcysteine enema

MECONIUM PERITONITIS
= sterile chemical peritonitis secondary to perforation of bowel proximal to high-grade / complete obstruction which seals in utero due to inflammatory response
Incidence: 1:35,000 live births
Age: antenatal perforation after 3rd month of gestation
Cause:
(1) Atresia (secondary to ischemic event) (50%)
(a) of small bowel (usually ileum or jejunum)
(b) of colon (uncommon)
(2) Bowel obstruction (46%)
(a) meconium ileus
(b) volvulus, internal hernia
(c) intussusception, congenital bands, Meckel diverticulum
(3) Hydrometrocolpos
Δ meconium peritonitis diagnosed in utero due to cystic fibrosis in 8%
Δ meconium peritonitis diagnosed at birth due to cystic fibrosis in 15 – 40%
Types:
(a) Fibroadhesive type:
= intense chemical reaction of peritoneum which seals off the perforation
√ dense mass with calcium deposits
(b) Cystic type:
= cystic cavity formed by fixation of bowel loops surrounding the perforation site which continues to leak meconium
√ cyst outlined by calcific rim
√ intra-abdominal calcifications (conspicuously absent in cystic fibrosis)
√ small flecks of calcifications scattered throughout abdomen

√ larger aggregates of calcifications along inferior
surface of liver / flank /processus vaginalis / scrotum
√ obstructive roentgen signs following birth
√ microcolon = "unused colon"
OB-US:
√ polyhydramnios (64 – 71%)
√ fetal ascites (54 – 57%)
√ bowel dilatation (27 – 29%)
√ intraabdominal bright echogenic mass
√ multiple linear / clumped foci of calcifications (84%);
may develop within 12 hours after perforation
√ meconium pseudocyst = well-defined hypoechoic
mass surrounded by an echogenic calcified wall
(contained perforation)
DDx: (1) Intraabdominal teratoma (2) Fetal gallstones
Mortality: up to 62%

MECONIUM PLUG SYNDROME

= local inspissation of meconium leading to low colonic
obstruction secondary to colonic inertia (functional); not
related to meconium ileus
Age: newborn infant, many of diabetic mothers
• abdominal distension
• vomiting
• failure to pass meconium
√ distended transverse + ascending colon + dilated small
bowel (proximal to obstruction)
√ occasionally bubbly appearance in colon
√ presacral pseudotumor (no gas in rectum)
√ double-contrast effect = barium between meconium plug
+ colonic wall
Rx: water-soluble enema
DDx: Hirschsprung disease

MELANOSIS COLI

= benign brown-black discoloration of colonic mucosa
Incidence: 10% of autopsies
Cause: ? chronic anthracene cathartic usage
• asymptomatic
Prognosis: no malignant potential

MENETRIER DISEASE

= GIANT HYPERTROPHIC GASTRITIS
= HYPERPLASTIC GASTROPATHY characterized by
excessive mucus production and TRIAD of (1) giant
mucosal hypertrophy (2) hypoproteinemia
(3) hypochlorhydria
Histo: hyperplasia of glandular tissue + microcyst
formation, mucosal thickness up to 6 mm (normal
range: 0.6 -1.0 mm)
Age: 20 – 70 years; M:F = 2:1
Associated with   benign gastric ulcer (13 – 72%)
• protein-losing enteropathy with hypoproteinemia +
peripheral edema
• weight loss
• gastrointestinal bleeding
• absent / decreased acid secretion (> 50%)
• epigastric pain, vomiting

Location: throughout fundus + body, particularly
prominent along greater curvature, antrum
usually spared (DDx to lymphoma: usually in
antrum)
√ markedly enlarged + tortuous gastric folds in spite of
adequate gastric distension
√ relatively abrupt demarcation between normal +
abnormal areas
√ marked hypersecretion (mucus)
√ preserved pliability
CT:
√ wall thickening of proximal stomach
√ nodular symmetric folds
DDx:· lymphoma, polypoid variety of gastric carcinoma,
acute gastritis, chronic gastritis, gastric varices

MESENTERIC / OMENTAL CYST

= lymphatic hamartomas lined by mesothelial cells with
serous, chylous, (occasionally) hemorrhagic fluid
contents
Location: small bowel mesentery (78%)
• asymptomatic
√ single multilocular cyst up to several cm in size
√ omental cysts may be pedunculated
CT:
√ density near water / soft tissue
√ ± fluid levels related to fatty + water-density
components
Cx: torsion, hemorrhage, intestinal obstruction

MESENTERIC ISCHEMIA

Etiology:
(a) arterial: older patient, usually complication of
arteriosclerosis
— **"abdominal angina"** = intermittent mesenteric
ischemia in severe arterial stenosis with
inadequate collateralization provoked by food
ingestion
— **occlusive mesenteric infarction** = thrombosis
at atherosclerotic site / embolus; 90% mortality
rate
— **nonocclusive mesenteric ischemia**
= preexisting atherosclerosis with systemic low-
flow state (cardiac failure / intraoperative
hypotension)
(b) venous: young patient, often following abdominal
surgery
(c) incarceration of hernia, volvulus, constriction by
adhesive bands, intussusception, disseminated
intravascular coagulation, endotoxic shock
Pathophysiology: mucosa is most sensitive area to
anoxia from arterial / venous occlusion with early
ulcerations leading to formation of strictures
Spectrum:
1. Asymptomatic in spite of vascular occlusion
secondary to abundant collaterals
2. Angina abdominalis
3. Infarction

dependent on rate of occlusion, cardiovascular disease, acute decrease of blood pressure (shock), polycythemia, chronic recurrent arrhythmia, CHF
- first crampy, then continuous abdominal pain with acute event
- gross rectal bleeding
- malabsorption with chronic vascular disease + strictures

Signs of mesenteric embolization:
- acute abdominal pain
- cardiac disease predisposing to embolization
- gut emptying (vomiting / diarrhea)
- WBC > 12,000/μl + left shift (80%)

Location: (a) any segment of small bowel
        (b) distal transverse colon, splenic flexure, cecum (most common)

Plain film:
√ gasless abdomen (= fluid-filled loops from exudation) (21%)
√ bowel distension to splenic flexure (perfusion by SMA)(43%)
√ "thumbprinting" (36%) = thickening of bowel wall + valvulae (edema)
√ small bowel pseudoobstruction (most frequently in thrombosis)
√ pneumatosis (= dissection of luminal gas into bowel wall) (28%)
√ mesenteric + portal vein gas (14%)
√ ascites (14%)

Barium:
(a) Acute:
√ "scalloping / thumbprinting" – thickening of wall + valvulae
√ "picket fencing"
√ separation + uncoiling of loops
√ narrowed lumen
√ circumferential ulcer
(b) Subacute:
√ flattening of one border
√ pseudosacculation / pseudodiverticula on antimesenteric border
(c) Chronic:
√ 7 – 10 cm long smooth pliable strictures
√ dilatation of gut between strictures
√ thinned + atrophic valvulae
Cx: obstruction

CT:
(a) Specific findings in 26% only:
√ pneumatosis intestinalis (22 – 57%)
√ portal venous gas (13 – 36%) / mesenteric vein gas (28%)
√ thumbprinting (26%)
(b) Nonspecific findings
√ focal / diffuse bowel dilatation (56 – 71%) with gas (43%) / fluid (29%)
√ thickening of intestinal wall (64%)
√ thrombosis of SMA (7%)
√ pneumoperitoneum (7%)
√ ascites (43%)

Angio:
√ occlusion / vasoconstriction / vascular beading
√ embolus lodges at major branching points distal to first 3 cm of SMA

NUC:
(a) IV / IA Tc-99m sulfur colloid labeled leukocytes, Ga-citrate, Tc-99m pyrophosphate
√ tracer accumulation 5 hours after onset of ischemia (more intense uptake with transmural infarcts)
(b) intraperitoneal injection of Xe-133 in saline is absorbed by intestine
√ decreased washout with abnormal perfusion of strangulated bowel

Prognosis:
(1) Massive infarction of small + large bowel if mesenteric embolization occurs proximal to middle colic artery (= limited collateral flow)
(2) Focal segments of intestinal ischemia if mesenteric embolization occurs distal to middle colic artery (= good collateral flow)

Mortality: 80 – 92% for intestinal infarction

MESOTHELIOMA

= only primary tumor of peritoneum
Age: 55 – 66 years; M >>F
Associated with: asbestos disease
Location: pleura (67%), peritoneum (30%), pericardium (2.5%), processus vaginalis (0.5%)
√ mesenteric, omental, peritoneal, bowel wall thickening
√ nodular masses in anterior parietal peritoneum
√ disproportionately small amount of ascites
CT:
√ nodular irregular thickening of peritoneal surfaces
√ localized masses
√ infiltrating sheets of tissue
√ foci of calcifications
√ ascites near water density
√ stellate configuration of neurovascular bundles
√ pleated thickening of mesenteric leaves
NUC: √ diffuse uptake of Gallium-67

METASTASES TO SMALL BOWEL

Origin: colon > stomach > breast > ovary > uterine cervix > melanoma > lung > pancreas
Spread:
(1) Intraperitoneal seeding: ovary, breast, GI tract
(2) Hematogenous dissemination with submucosal deposits: melanoma, breast, lung, Kaposi sarcoma
(3) Direct extension from adjacent neoplasm: ovary, uterus, prostate, pancreas, colon, kidney
√ fixation + tenting + transverse stretching (= across long axis) of folds secondary to mesenteric + peritoneal infiltration (most common form)
UGI:
√ single mass protruding into lumen resembling annular carcinoma

√ "bull's-eye" lesions = multiple polypoid masses with sizable ulcer craters

√ obstruction from kinking / annular constriction / large intraluminal mass

√ compression by direct extension of primary tumor / involved nodes

CT:

√ soft-tissue density nodules / masses

√ sheets of tissue thickening bowel wall + mesenteric leaves

√ fixation + angulation of bowel loops (tumors with desmoplastic response)

√ ascites

MIDGUT VOLVULUS

= torsion of entire gut around SMA secondary to a short mesenteric attachment of small intestine from incomplete rotation (normally 270° counterclockwise rotation); nonrotation = 90° or less; malrotation = 90 – 270°

Associated with (in 20%):
(1) duodenal atresia
(2) duodenal diaphragm
(3) duodenal stenosis
(4) annular pancreas

• acute symptoms in newborn (medical emergency): bile-stained vomiting (intermittent, postprandial, projectile); abdominal distension; shock

• intermittent obstructive symptoms in older child: recurring attacks of nausea, vomiting and abdominal pain

Plain film:

√ dilated air-filled duodenal bulb + paucity of gas distally

√ "double bubble sign" = air-fluid levels in stomach + duodenum

Barium studies:

√ duodenojejunal junction (ligament of Treitz) located lower than duodenal bulb + to the right of expected position

√ spiral course of midgut loops = "apple peel / corkscrew" appearance

√ duodenal fold-thickening + thumbprinting (mucosal edema + hemorrhage)

√ abnormally high position of cecum

CT:

√ whirllike pattern of small bowel loops + adjacent mesenteric fat converging to the point of torsion (during volvulus)

√ SMV to the left of SMA (NO volvulus)

√ chylous mesenteric cyst (from interference with lymphatic drainage)

Angio:

√ "barber pole sign" = spiraling of SMA

√ tapering / abrupt termination of mesenteric vessels

√ marked vasoconstriction + prolonged contrast transit time

√ absent venous opacification / dilated tortuous superior mesenteric vein

Cx: intestinal ischemia + necrosis in distribution of SMA (bloody diarrhea, ileus, abdominal distension)

MUCOCELE OF APPENDIX

A. MUCOCELE

= distension of appendix with sterile mucus

Etiology:
luminal obstruction by fecalith, foreign body, carcinoid, endometriosis, adhesions, volvulus; mucinous cystadenoma / cystadenocarcinoma of appendix (occasionally)

Incidence: 0.07 – 0.24%

√ globular, smooth-walled, broad-based mass invaginating into cecum

√ peripheral rimlike calcifications frequent

CT:

√ round sharply defined mass with homogeneous low attenuation content

US:

√ ovoid, complex cystic mass with internal echoes

Cx: pseudomyxoma peritonei

B. MYXOGLOBULOSIS

= rare variant of mucocele of the appendix characterized by clusters of pearly white mucous balls intermixed with mucus

• usually asymptomatic

• may appear as acute appendicitis

√ multiple 1 – 10 mm small rounded annular, nonlaminated calcified spherules (PATHOGNOMONIC)

DDx: inverted appendiceal stump, acute appendicitis, carcinoma of the cecum

NECROTIZING ENTEROCOLITIS

= NEC = ischemic bowel disease secondary to hypoxia, perinatal stress, infection (endotoxin), congenital heart disease

Incidence: most common GI emergency in premature infants

Age: develops > 48 – 72 hours after birth; 90% within first 10 days of life

Path: acute inflammation + mucosal ulceration + widespread transmural necrosis

Organism: not yet isolated; often occurs in miniepidemics within nursery

Predisposed:
premature infant (50 – 80%), Hirschsprung disease, bowel obstruction (small bowel atresia, pyloric stenosis, meconium ileus, meconium plug syndrome)

Location: usually in terminal ileum (most commonly involved), cecum, right colon; rarely in stomach, upper bowel

• blood-streaked stools (in 50%); explosive diarrhea

• bile emesis

• mild respiratory distress

• generalized sepsis

√ disarrayed bowel gas pattern (no longer normal array of polygons)

√ distension of small bowel and colon (loops wider than vertebral body L1) ± air-fluid levels, commonly in RLQ (1st sign)
√ tubular loops of bowel
√ bowel wall thickening + "thumbprinting"
√ persisting unchanging loop of bowel for > 24 hours
√ pneumatosis intestinalis (80%) = intramural gas; curvilinear = subserosal; bubbly or cystic = submucosal (gas-forming organisms / dissection of intraluminal gas)
√ "bubbly" appearance (= gas in wall, intraluminal gas, fecal matter); intraluminal contents are composed of blood, sloughed colonic mucosa, intraluminal gas, some fecal material
√ "football" sign = pneumoperitoneum + ascites in 20%
√ gas in portal venous system (frequently transient, does not imply hopeless outcome)
√ ascites
√ pneumoperitoneum (immediate surgery required)
NOTA BENE: Barium enema is contraindicated! May be used judiciously in selected cases with radiologic + clinical doubt!
Cx: inflammatory stricture forming after healing (BE follow-up in survivors)

PELVIC LIPOMATOSIS + FIBROLIPOMATOSIS

= nonmalignant overgrowth of adipose tissue with minimal fibrotic + inflammatory components compressing soft tissue structures within pelvis
Age: 9 – 80 years (peak 25 – 60 years); M:F = 10:1 NO racial predominance of blacks; obesity NOT contributing factor
• often incidental finding
• urinary frequency, flank pain, suprapubic tenderness
• recurrent urinary tract infections
• low back pain, fever
√ elongation + narrowing of rectum
√ elevation of rectosigmoid + sigmoid colon out of pelvis
√ increase in sacrorectal space > 10 mm
√ stretching of sigmoid colon
√ elongation + elevation of urinary bladder with symmetrical inverted pear shape
√ elongation of posterior urethra
√ pelvic lucency; CT confirmatory
√ medial / lateral displacement of ureters
Cx of fibrolipomatosis:
(1) late ureteral obstruction (40% within 5 years)
(2) IVC obstruction

PERITONEAL METASTASES

= intraabdominal spread of tumor
Origin: ovary, stomach, colon, pancreas
√ massive ascites
√ desmoplastic reaction at (a) anterior border of rectum (Blumer shelf) (b) mesenteric side of terminal ileum
CT:
  √ increased density of linear network in mesenteric fat
  √ loculated fluid collections in peritoneal cavity
  √ apparent thickening of mesenteric vessels (= fluid within leaves of mesentery)

√ adnexal mass of cystic / soft-tissue density (= Krukenberg tumor)
√ small nodular densities on peritoneal surface
√ "omental cake" = thickening of greater omentum
√ lobulated mass in pouch of Douglas

PEUTZ-JEGHERS SYNDROME

= autosomal dominant gastrointestinal polyposis
= hamartomatosis; most frequent of polyposis syndromes to involve small intestines
Incidence: 1:7000 live births; in 50% familial, in 50% sporadic
Path: benign polyps as a mixture of mucosa + muscularis mucosae
  (1) hamartomatous polyps in small bowel; NOT premalignant
  (2) adenomatous polyps in stomach + colon
Age: 25 years at presentation (range 10 – 30 years)
Associated with: ovarian cysts / carcinoma, bronchial adenoma, bladder adenoma
• mucocutaneous pigmentation = 1 – 5 mm small melanin spots on mucous membranes (lower lips, gums, palate) + facial skin (lips, nose, cheeks, around eyes) + volar aspects of toes and fingers (100%)
• cramping abdominal pain (small bowel intussusception in 47%)
• rectal bleeding, melena (30%)
• prolapse of polyp through anus
• chronic hypochromic anemia
@ Small bowel (> 95%)
  √ nearly always myriads of 1 – 2 mm nodules = carpet of polyps
@ Colon + rectum (30%)
  √ multiple 1 – 30 mm polyps; NO carpeting
@ Stomach (25%)
@ Esophagus (rare)
@ Respiratory + urinary tract
Cx: (1) transient intussusception (pedunculated polyp)
  (2) carcinoma of stomach, duodenum, colon (in 2%), ovary (in 5%)
Rx: surgery is reserved for obstruction, severe bleeding, malignancy

PNEUMATOSIS CYSTOIDES

= PNEUMATOSIS CYSTOIDES INTESTINALIS
= multiple gas-containing cysts of various sizes located in subserosa (sometimes in submucosa)
Age: adulthood
Location: predominantly in lower colon
Associated with:
  (1) chronic obstructive bronchopulmonary disease
  (2) bowel obstruction (air dissecting distally)
  (3) artificial ventilation
  (4) trauma (sigmoidoscopy, biopsy, BE, postsurgical anastomosis)
  (5) idiopathic
  (6) intestinal ischemia / infarction
  (7) colitis

(8) collagen disease (esp. scleroderma)
(9) steroid therapy
√ best demonstrated on CT
√ segmental mucosal nodularity (DDx: polyposis)
Cx: asymptomatic large pneumoperitoneum (may persist for months / years)

POSTCRICOID DEFECT

= variable defect seen commonly in the fully distended cervical esophagus; no pathologic value
Etiology: redundancy of mucosa over rich postcricoid submucosal venous plexus
Incidence: in 80% of normal adults
Location: anterior aspect of esophagus at level of cricoid cartilage
√ tumor- / weblike lesion with variable configuration during swallowing
DDx: submucosal tumor, esophageal web (persistent configuration)

PRESBYESOPHAGUS

= defect in primary peristalsis + LES relaxation associated with aging
Incidence: 15% in 7th decade; 50% in 8th decade; 85% in 9th decade
Associated with: hiatus hernia, reflux
• usually asymptomatic
√ impaired / no primary peristalsis
√ often repetitive nonperistaltic tertiary contractions in distal esophagus
√ mild / moderate esophageal dilatation
√ poor LES relaxation
DDx: diabetes, diffuse esophageal spasm, scleroderma, esophagitis, achalasia, benign stricture, carcinoma

PROLAPSED ANTRAL MUCOSA

= prolapse of hypertrophic + inflammatory mucosa of gastric antrum into duodenum resulting in pyloric obstruction
√ mushroom- / umbrella- / cauliflower-shaped filling defect at duodenal base
√ filling defect varies in size + shape
√ redundant gastric rugae can be traced from pyloric antrum through pyloric channel
√ gastric hyperperistalsis

PSEUDOMEMBRANOUS COLITIS

Organism: probably overgrowth of Clostridium difficile
Predisposed:
(a) complication of antibiotic therapy with tetracycline, penicillin, ampicillin, clindamycin, lincomycin, amoxacillin, chloramphenicol, cephalosporins
(b) post surgery, intestinal vascular insufficiency, irradiation
(c) uremia
(d) proximal to large bowel obstruction
(e) debilitating diseases: lymphosarcoma, leukemia

Histo: pseudomembranes (exudate composed of leukocytes, fibrin, mucin, sloughed necrotic epithelium) on a partially denuded colonic mucosa (mucosa generally intact)
• profuse diarrhea, abdominal cramps, tenderness
• confluent pseudomembranes seen on endoscopy
Plain film:
√ adynamic ileus pattern = moderate gaseous distension of small bowel + colon
√ edematous, distorted haustral markings
√ transverse bands = marked thickening + distortion of haustra
√ diffusely shaggy + irregular surface (confluent pseudomembranes)
√ "thumbprinting" most prominent in transverse colon
BE (is CONTRAINDICATED):
√ pseudoulcerations = barium filling clefts between pseudomembranes
√ irregular ragged polypoid contour of colonic wall
√ discrete filling defects (DDx: polyposis, nodular form of lymphoma)
CT:
√ irregular colonic wall
√ circumferential wall thickening
√ homogeneous enhancement
Dx: Proctosigmoidoscopy diagnoses confluent pseudomembranes
Cx: Peritonitis
Mortality: 15%
Rx: discontinuation of suspected antibiotic + administration of vancomycin + attention to fluid and electrolyte balance

PSEUDOMYXOMA PERITONEI

= "jelly belly = gelatinous ascites" = slow insidious accumulation of large amounts of intraperitoneal gelatinous material secondary to peritoneal carcinomatosis from mucinous cystadenocarcinoma
Etiology:
ruptured mucinous adenocarcinoma of appendix / ovary; rarely associated with malignancy of colon, stomach, uterus, pancreas, common bile duct, urachal duct, omphalomesenteric duct
• slowly progressive massive abdominal distension
• recurrent abdominal pain
√ thickening of peritoneal + omental surfaces
√ omental cake
√ posterior displacement of bowel loops + mesentery
√ voluminous septated / loculated pseudoascites
√ several thin-walled cystic masses of different size throughout abdominal cavity
√ scalloped contour of liver margins
√ annular / semicircular calcifications (rare but highly suggestive)
DDx: peritoneal metastases, pancreatitis with pseudocysts, pyogenic peritonitis, widespread echinococcal disease
Prognosis: 50% 5-year survival rate

PSEUDOPOLYPOSIS OF COLON
= islands of edematous hyperplastic mucosa surrounded by ulcerated mucosa
Associated with: ulcerative colitis, granulomatous colitis
√ pseudopolyps variable in size, rarely distributed through entire colon
√ pseudopolyps may show "cobblestone" appearance
√ shortened colon diminished in caliber

RADIATION INJURY OF RECTUM
= obliterative endarteritis with irradiation in excess of 4,000 – 6,000 rads
Δ manifestation of radiation colitis can occur up to 15 years
Predisposed: 90% in women (carcinoma of cervix)
• tenesmus, diarrhea, bleeding, constipation
√ ridgelike appearance of mucosa (submucosal fibrosis)
√ irregularly outlined ulcerations (rare)
CT:
  √ narrowed partially distensible rectum
  √ thick homogeneous rectal wall
  √ "target sign" = submucosal circumferential lucency
  √ proliferation of perirectal fat > 10 mm
  √ thickening of perirectal fascia
  √ "halo effect" = increase in fibrosis of pararectal space
Cx: (1) obstruction (2) colovaginal / coloenteric fistula formation

REFLUX ESOPHAGITIS
= esophageal inflammation secondary to reflux of acid-peptic contents of the stomach; reflux occurs if resting pressure of LES < 5 mmHg (may be normal event if followed by rapid clearing)
Reflux preventing features:
  (1) lower esophageal sphincter (2) phrenoesophageal membrane (3) length of subdiaphragmatic esophagus (4) gastroesophageal angle of Hiss (70 – 110°)
May be associated with:
  sliding hiatal hernia, scleroderma, nasogastric intubation
Histo: basal cell hyperplasia with wall thickening + thinning of epithelium, mucosal edema + erosions, inflammatory infiltrate
• heartburn, epigastric discomfort
• choking, globus hystericus
• retrosternal pain
• thoracic / cervical dysphagia
Site: usually lower 1/3
√ interruption of primary peristalsis at inflamed segment
√ nonperistaltic waves in distal esophagus following deglutition (85%)
√ incomplete relaxation of LES (75%), incompetent sphincter (33%)
√ acid test = abnormal motility elicited by acid barium (pH 1.7)
√ segmental esophageal narrowing (edema / spasm / stricture)
√ thickening of esophageal folds ± wall
√ marginal esophagogastric ulcer / erosion

√ prominent mucosal fold ending in polypoid protuberance within hiatal hernia / cardia
REFLUX TESTS
  1. Reflux of barium in RPO position, may be elicited by coughing / deep respiratory movements / swallowing of saliva + water / anteflexion in erect position: only in 50% accurate
  2. Water-siphon test: in 5% false negative; large number of false positives
  3. Tuttle test = measurement of esophageal pH: 96% accurate
Cx of Reflux:
  (a) from acid + pepsin acting on esophageal mucosa:
    (1) motility disturbance (2) stricture (3) Schatzki ring (4) Barrett esophagus (5) iron-deficiency anemia (6) reflux / peptic esophagitis
  (b) from aspiration of gastric contents
    (1) acute aspiration pneumonia (2) Mendelson syndrome (3) pulmonary fibrosis

RETAINED GASTRIC ANTRUM
Cause: retention of endocrinologically active gastric antrum in continuity with pylorus + duodenum
Pathophysiology:
  bathing of antrum in alkaline duodenal juice stimulates secretion of gastrin
Associated with gastric ulcers in 30 – 50%
√ duodenogastric reflux of barium by way of the pylorus (diagnostic)
√ giant marginal ulcer / several marginal ulcers usually on jejunal side of anastomosis (large false-negative + false-positive rate; correct positive rate of 28 – 60%)
√ large amount of secretions
√ edematous mucosa of jejunal anastomotic segment
√ lacy / cobweblike small bowel pattern (hypersecretion)
Cx: gastrojejunocolic fistula

SCHATZKI RING
= LOWER ESOPHAGEAL MUCOSAL RING = constant lower esophageal ring (mucosal thickening) presumed to result from reflux esophagitis = thin annular peptic stricture
Incidence: 6 – 14% of population; old age > young age; M > F
Histo: usually squamous epithelium on upper surface + columnar epithelium on undersurface; may be covered totally by squamous epithelium or columnar epithelium
• asymptomatic (if ring > 20 mm)
• dysphagia (if ring < 13 mm)
Location: near the squamo-columnar junction; above B ring
√ only visible with adequate distension of esophagogastric region and when located above the esophageal hiatus of the diaphragm
√ best demonstrated in prone position during arrested deep inspiration with Valsalva maneuver when barium column passes through esophagogastric region

√ 2 – 4 mm thick shelflike projection into lumen with smooth symmetric margins

√ permanently present transverse ring with constant shape + size (range 3-18 mm)

√ short esophagus + intrahiatal / intrathoracic gastric segment = sliding hiatal hernia if Schatzki ring located 1 – 2 cm above diaphragmatic hiatus

Prognosis: decrease in caliber over 5 years (in 25 – 33%)

Cx: impaction of food bolus (associated with severe chest pain)

Rx: (1) proper mastication of food (2) endoscopic rupture (3) esophageal dilatation (radiographically often lack of caliber change after successful dilatation)

DDx: annular peptic stricture (usually thicker, asymetric, irregular surface, associated with thickened esophageal folds, serration of esophageal margins)

SCLERODERMA

= PROGRESSIVE SYSTEMIC SCLEROSIS = PSS

Age: 30 – 50 years; M:F = 1:3

Histo: vasculitis + submucosal fibrosis extending into muscularis, smooth muscle atrophy

• skin changes, Raynaud phenomenon, arthritis

• abdominal pain, diarrhea, occasional malabsorption

• multiple episodes of pseudoobstruction

Intestinal involvement in 40 – 45% (may precede other manifestations)

@ Esophagus (in 42 – 75%)

  Δ first GI tract location to be involved

  • dysphagia (50%)

  • heartburn (30%)

  √ normal peristalsis above aortic arch (striated muscle in proximal 1/3)

  √ hypotonia / atony + hypokinesia in distal 2/3 of esophagus

  √ deficient emptying in recumbent position

  √ thin / vanished longitudinal folds

  √ mild to moderate dilatation of esophagus

  √ patulous lower esophageal sphincter + gastroesophageal reflux

  √ erosions, superficial ulcers (reflux esophagitis asymptomatic: NO protective esophageal contraction)

  √ fusiform stricture usually 4 – 5 cm above gastroesophageal junction

  √ esophageal shortening + sliding hiatal hernia

@ Stomach (less frequent involvement)

  √ gastric dilatation

  √ decreased motor activity + delayed emptying

@ Small bowel

  • rapidly progressing disease once small intestine is involved

  • malabsorption (delayed intestinal transit time + bacterial overgrowth)

  √ marked dilatation of small bowel (in particular duodenum, jejunum) simulating small bowel obstruction (avoid exploratory surgery)

√ abrupt cutoff at SMA level (atrophy of neural cells with hypoperistalsis)

√ marked delay of transit time with barium retention in duodenum up to 24 hours

√ "hidebound folds" (60%) = sharply defined folds of normal thickness with decreased intervalvular distance (tightly packed folds) within dilated segment

√ pseudodiverticula (10 – 40%) = sacculations = wide-mouthed diverticula

√ pneumatosis cystoides intestinalis + pneumoperitoneum

√ excess fluid with bacterial overgrowth (="pseudo-blind loop syndrome")

√ normal mucosal fold pattern

@ Colon

  • constipation (common), may alternate with diarrhea

  √ pseudosacculations on antimesenteric side (transverse + descending colon)

  √ marked dilatation (may simulate Hirschsprung disease)

  √ stercoral ulceration (from retained fecal material)

  Cx: life-threatening barium impaction

@ Chest

  √ bibasilar interstitial fibrosis

@ Bones

  √ acroosteolysis

  √ soft tissue calcifications

DDx:

  (1) Sprue (increased secretions, segmentation, fragmentation, dilatation most significant in midjejunum, normal motility)

  (2) Obstruction (no esophageal changes, no pseudodiverticula)

  (3) Idiopathic intestinal pseudoobstruction (usually in young people)

SPRUE

= classic disease of malabsorption

A. TROPICAL SPRUE

  Etiology: infectious agent cured with antibiotics; geographic distribution (India, Far East, Puerto Rico)

  Age: any age group

  • glossitis

  • hepatosplenomegaly

  • macrocytic anemia + leukopenia

  Prognosis: spontaneous resolution after months / years

  Rx: responds well to folic acid + broad-spectrum antibiotics

B. NONTROPICAL SPRUE

  = CELIAC DISEASE = GLUTEN-SENSITIVE ENTEROPATHY

  May be hereditary: detected in 15% of 1st degree relatives

  Age: childhood and 30 – 40 years

  Rx: gluten-free diet

Path: villous atrophy (truncation) + elongation of crypts of Lieberkühn + round cell infiltration of lamina propria (plasma cells + lymphocytes)
- diarrhea, steatorrhea
- weakness, weight loss
- anemia (iron / folate / vitamin B_{12} deficiency)
- osteomalacia with bone pain

Location: duodenum + jejunum > remainder of small bowel
√ small bowel dilatation (in 25%) is HALLMARK, best seen in mid + distal jejunum; degree of dilatation related to severity of disease
√ transient nonobstructive intussusception
√ hypersecretion
  √ air-fluid levels in small bowel (rare)
  √ flocculation = coarse granular appearance of barium disintegration due to excess fluid best seen at periphery of intestinal segment; especially with steatorrhea
  √ segmentation = large masses of barium in dilated segments separated by stringlike strands from adjacent clumps due to excessive fluid; best seen on delayed films
  √ fragmentation = scattering = faint irregular stippling of residual barium resembling snowflakes associated with segmentation due to excessive fluid
√ "moulage sign" (50%) = smooth contour with effaced patternless folds resembling tubular wax mold (due to atrophy of the folds of Kerkring) in jejunum CHARACTERISTIC of sprue if seen in duodenum + jejunum
√ long / normal / short transit time
√ nonpropulsive peristalsis (flaccid + poorly contracting loops)
√ normal / thickened / effaced mucosal folds (depending on hypoproteinemia)
√ "jejunization" of ileal loops (= compensatory attempt for decreased jejunal mucosal surface)
√ colonlike haustrations in well-filled jejunum (secondary to spasm + cicatrization from transverse ulcers)

CT:
  √ small bowel dilatation + increased fluid content ± mucosal fold thickening
  √ mild to moderate lymphadenopathy in mesentery / retroperitoneum

Cx:
  (1) multiple duodenojejunal ulcerated strictures (sausagelike appearance) with hemorrhage + perforation
  (2) esophageal carcinoma (in 6%) in 6th – 7th decade
  (3) lymphoma (in 8%): commonly diffuse + nodular
  (4) generalized lymphadenopathy with lymphocytosis (mimicking lymphoma)
  (5) sigmoid volvulus (rare)
Dx: (a) jejunal biopsy
  (b) improvement of small bowel abnormalities after a few months on a gluten-free diet

DDx:
  (1) Esophageal hypoperistalsis: scleroderma, idiopathic pseudoobstruction
  (2) Gastric abnormalities: Zollinger-Ellison syndrome, chronic granulomatous disease, eosinophilic enteritis, amyloidosis, malignancy
  (3) Tiny nodular defects on thickened folds: Whipple disease, intestinal lymphangiectasia, Waldenström macroglobulinemia
  (4) Small 1 – 3 mm nodules: lymphoid hyperplasia associated with giardiasis and immunoglobulin deficiency disease, diffuse lymphoma
  (5) Small nodules of varying sizes: systemic mastocytosis, amyloidosis, eosinophilic enteritis, Cronkhite-Canada syndrome
  (6) Bowel wall narrowing, kinking, scarring, ulceration: regional enteritis, bacterial / parasitic infection, carcinoid, vasculitis, ischemia, irradiation

STRONGYLOIDIASIS
= parasitic infection in tropics + subtropics
Organism: helminthic parasite Strongyloides stercoralis
Cycle: enters body through skin, passes through lung, settles in duodenum + upper jejunum
Path: edema + inflammation of intestinal wall secondary to invasion by larvae; flattening of villi; ova in mucosal crypts
- asymptomatic (in majority)
- pneumonitis
- severe malnutrition (malabsorption, steatorrhea)
- persistent vomiting
- worms, larvae, eggs in stool
√ paralytic ileus (massive invasion)
√ edematous folds, spasm, dilatation of proximal 2/3 of duodenum
√ ulceration
√ stenosis in 3rd + 4th part of duodenum
√ rigid pipestem appearance + irregular narrowing of duodenum (in advanced cases)
Prognosis: high mortality in undernourished patients

SUPERIOR MESENTERIC ARTERY SYNDROME
= vascular compression of 3rd portion of duodenum within aortomesenteric compartment; probably representing a functional reflex dilatation
Etiology:
  A. NORMAL VARIANT:
    asthenic persons, congenitally small vascular angle, prolonged bed rest in supine position (body cast, whole-body burns, surgery)
  B. PRIMARY DUODENAL ATONY
    scleroderma, dermatomyositis, SLE, Chagas disease, aganglionosis, neuropathy, surgical / chemical vagotomy, pancreatitis, cholecystitis, peptic ulcer disease, trauma, altered emotional status
  C. INFLAMMATORY INDURATION OF MESENTERIC ROOT

Crohn disease, tuberculous enteritis, pancreatitis, peptic ulcer disease, strongyloidiasis, metastatic disease
D. OTHERS
exaggerated lumbar lordosis, Abdominal aortic aneurysm, Aorticoduodenal fistula, Chronic idiopathic intestinal pseudo-obstruction
√ megaduodenum = pronounced dilatation of 1st + 2nd portion of duodenum + frequently stomach, best seen in supine position
√ vertical linear pressure defect in transverse portion of duodenum overlying spine
√ relief of compression by postural change into prone knee-elbow position

TERTIARY ESOPHAGEAL CONTRACTIONS
= disordered up-and-down movement of bolus
Causes:
1. Presbyesophagus
2. Diffuse esophageal spasm
3. Hyperactive achalasia
4. Neuromuscular disease
diabetes mellitus, Parkinsonism, amyotrophic lateral sclerosis, multiple sclerosis, thyrotoxic myopathy, myotonic dystrophy
5. Obstruction of cardia
neoplasm, distal esophageal stricture, benign lesion, S/P repair of hiatal hernia
Age: in 5 – 10% of normal adults in 4th – 6th decade
Location: in lower 2/3
√ spontaneous repetitive nonpropulsive contraction
√ "yo-yo" motion of barium
√ "cork screw" apperance = scalloped configuration of barium column
√ "rosary bead" / "shish kebab" configuration = compartmentalization of barium column
√ no lumen-obliterating contractions

TOXIC MEGACOLON
= acute transmural fulminant colitis with neurogenic loss of motor tone + rapid development of extensive colonic dilatation > 5.5. cm in transverse colon (damage to entire colonic wall + neuromuscular degeneration)
Etiology: 1. Ulcerative colitis (most common)
2. Crohn disease
3. Amebiasis, salmonella
4. Pseudomembranous colitis
5. Ischemic colitis
• systemic toxicity
• profuse bloody diarrhea
√ colon ileus, marked dilatation in transverse colon
√ few air-fluid levels
√ increasing caliber of colon on serial radiographs without redundancy
√ pseudopolyposis = mucosal islands in denuded ulcerated colonic wall
√ pneumatosis coli ± pneumoperitoneum
CT:
√ distended colon filled with large amounts of fluid + air

√ distorted haustral pattern
√ irregular nodular contour of thin wall
√ intramural air / small collections
BE: CONTRAINDICATED!
Prognosis: mortality of 20%

TRACHEO-ESOPHAGEAL FISTULA
= incomplete division of primitive foregut into respiratory + digestive tracts occuring at 3rd – 5 th week of intrauterine life
Incidence: 1:2,000 – 4,000 live births; most common sporadic congenital anomaly diagnosed in childhood
Location: between upper 1/3 + lower 1/3 of esophagus just above carina

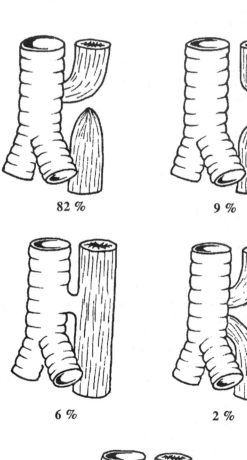

82 %   9 %

6 %   2 %

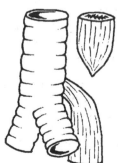

1 %

Types:
- (a) Distal TE fistula (82%)
- (b) Esophageal atresia without fistula (9%)
- (c) H-type fistula without atresia (6%)
- (d) Proximal + distal TE fistula (2%)
- (e) Proximal TE fistula (1%)

Associated anomalies (17 – 70%):
1. Cardiac   (15 – 39%): ASD, VSD
2. Musculoskeletal (24%)   : radial ray, vertebral anomalies
3. Gastrointestinal (20%)   : anorectal anomalies
4. Genitourinary   (12%)   : renal agenesis
5. Chromosomal   (10 – 19%): trisomy 18, 21

mnemonic: "ARTICLES"
Anal atresia
Renal anomaly
TE fistula
Intestinal atresia
Cardiac anomaly (PDA, VSD)
Limb anomaly (radial ray hypoplasia)
Esophageal atresia
Spinal anomalies

mnemonic: "VACTERL"
Vertebral anomalies
Anorectal anomaly
Cardiovascular anomalies
Tracheo-
Esophageal fistula
Renal anomalies
Limb anomalies

- excessive accumulation of pharyngeal secretions
- obligatory regurgitation of ingested fluids
- progressive respiratory distress of variable severity
- √ "coiled tube" = inability to pass feeding tube into stomach
- √ retrotracheal air-filled pouch causing compression / displacement of esophagus
- √ gasless abdomen (esophageal atresia ± proximal TE fistula)
- √ bowel gas present in 90% (esophageal atresia + distal TE fistula / H-type fistula)
- √ non- / hypoperistaltic esophageal segment (6 – 15 cm) in midesophagus
- √ aspiration pneumonia, esp. in dependent upper lobes
- OB-US (anomalies not identified before 24 weeks GA):
  - √ polyhydramnios in 33 – 60% (= obstruction to flow of amniotic fluid)
    - Δ TE-fistula + esophageal atresia is cause of polyhydramnios in only 3%
  - √ absence of fluid-distended stomach (in 10 – 40%; in remaining cases TE-fistula / gastric secretions allow some gastric distention)
  - √ small abdomen (low birth weight in 40%)
  - √ distended proximal pouch of atretic esophagus

Cx after repair:
- (1) Anastomotic leak
- (2) Recurrent TE fistula
- (3) Aspiration pneumonia secondary to
  - (a) esophageal stricture
  - (b) disordered esophageal motility distal to TE fistula
  - (c) gastroesophageal reflux

TUBERCULOSIS
rarely encountered in Western hemisphere, increased incidence in AIDS; usually associated with pulmonary tuberculosis (in 6 – 38%)
Etiology: (a) ingestion of tuberculous sputum
         (b) hematogenous spread from tuberculous focus in lung to submucosal lymph nodes, associated with radiographic evidence of pulmonary TB in < 50%
         (c) primary infection by cow milk (Mycobacterium bovis)
Path: (1) ulcerative form (most frequent): ulcers with their long axis perpendicular to axis of intestine, undermining + pseudopolyps
      (2) hypertrophic form: thickening of bowel wall (transmural granulomatous process)
Organisms: M. tuberculosis, M. bovis, M. avium-intracellulare
Age: 20 – 40 years
- weight loss, abdominal pain (80 – 90%)
- nausea, vomiting
- tuberculin skin test negative in most patients with primary intestinal TB
Location: ileocecal area > ascending colon > jejunum > appendix > duodenum > stomach > sigmoid > rectum

@ Tuberculous peritonitis (in 1/3)
  Δ most common presentation
  Cause: hematogenous spread / rupture of mesenteric node
  1. wet type   = exudative ascites with high protein contents + leukocytes
  2. dry type   = tuberculous adenopathy + adhesions
  3. fibrotic type = abdominal mass with separation + fixation of bowel loops
  CT: √ high-density ascites (30 HU)
       √ predominantly peripancreatic + mesenteric adenopathy with low density centers (caseous necrosis)
       √ irregular soft tissue density of omentum
  Cx: small bowel obstruction (adhesions from serosal tubercles)
@ Ileocecal area (80 – 90%)
  Δ most commonly affected bowel
  Cause: secondary to relative stagnation of intestinal contents + abundance of lymphoid tissue (Peyer patches)

√ Stierlin sign = rapid emptying of narrowed terminal
ileum (persistent irritability)
√ thickened ileocecal valve (mass effect)
√ Fleischner sign = "inverted umbrella" defect = wide
gap between thickened patulous ileocecal valve +
narrowed ulcerated terminal ileum
√ deep fissures + ulcers with sinus tracts /
enterocutaneous fistulas / perforation
DDx: Crohn disease, cecal carcinoma
@ Colon
Site: segmental colonic involvement, esp. on right side
√ rigid contracted cone-shaped cecum
√ spiculations + wall thickening
√ diffuse ulcerating colitis + pseudopolyps
√ shortening + short hourglass strictures
DDx: ulcerative colitis, Crohn disease, amebiasis
(spares terminal ileum), colitis of bacillary
dysentery, ischemic colitis,
pseudomembranous colitis
@ Gastroduodenal
Site: simultaneous involvement of pylorus + duodenum
√ stenotic pylorus with gastric outlet obstruction
√ narrowed antrum (linitis plastica appearance)
√ antral fistula
√ multiple large and deep ulcerations on lesser
curvature
√ thickened duodenal folds with irregular contour /
dilatation
DDx: carcinoma, lymphoma, syphilis
@ Esophagus
least common GI tract manifestation
√ ulceration
√ stricture
√ mass
√ sinus tract formation

TURCOT SYNDROME
= autosomal recessive disease with (1) colonic polyposis
(2) CNS tumors (especially supratentorial glioblastoma)
Age: symptomatic during 2nd decade
Histo: adenomatous polyps
• diarrhea
• seizures
√ multiple 1 – 30 mm polyps in colon + rectum
Cx: malignant transformation of colonic polyps in 100%
Prognosis: death from brain tumor in 2nd + 3rd decade

TYPHLITIS
= necrotizing inflammatory process of cecum in
neutropenic patients; (typhlon = cecum)
Histo: edema + ulceration of entire bowel wall; necrosis
+ perforation possible
Organisms: Pseudomonas, Candida, CMV, Klebsiella,
E. coli, B. fragilis, Enterobacter
Predisposed: aplastic anemia, immunosuppressive
therapy, lymphoma, common in childhood
leukemia
Location: cecum + ascending colon, appendix + distal
ileum may become secondarily involved

• abdominal pain, may be localized to RLQ
• watery diarrhea
• fullness / palpable mass in RLQ
• fever, neutropenia
• hematochezia / occult blood
√ fluid-filled masslike density in RLQ
√ distension of nearby small bowel loops
√ thumb printing of ascending colon
√ circumferential thickening of cecal wall > 4 mm
√ occasionally pneumatosis
CT:
√ circumferential cecal wall thickening (1 – 3 mm)
√ may have intramural pneumatosis
Cx: (1) perforation (BE risky procedure)
(2) abscess formation
DDx: (1) leukemic / lymphomatous deposits (more
eccentric thickening)
(2) appendicitis with periappendicular abscess
(cecal wall thickness normal)
(3) diverticulitis
(4) inflammatory bowel disease

ULCERATIVE COLITIS
= ? hypersensitivity / autoimmune disease primarily limited
to mucosa
Path: predominantly mucosal disease with exudate +
edema + crypt abscesses (HALLMARK) resulting
in shallow ulceration
Age peak: 20 – 40 years + 60 – 70 years; M:F = 1:1
• alternating periods of remission + exacerbation
• bloody diarrhea
• electrolyte depletion, fever, systemic toxicity
• abdominal cramps
Extracolonic manifestations:
• iritis, erythema nodosum, pyoderma gangrenosum
• pericholangitis, chronic active hepatitis, primary
sclerosing cholangitis, fatty liver
• spondylitis, peripheral arthritis, coincidental
rheumatoid arthritis (10 – 20%)
• thrombotic complications
Location: begins in rectum with proximal progression
(rectum spared in 4%)
(1) rectosigmoid in 95% (diagnosed by rectal biopsy);
continuous circumferential involvement often limited
to left side of colon
(2) terminal ileum in 10 – 25% ("backwash ileitis")
Plain film:
√ hyperplastic mucosa, polypoid mucosa, deep ulcers
√ diffuse dilatation with loss of haustral markings
√ toxic megacolon
√ free intraperitoneal gas
√ complete absence of fecal residue (due to
inflammation)
BE:
(a) acute stage
√ narrowing + incomplete filling (spasm + irritability)
√ fine mucosal granularity = stippling of barium coat
(from diffuse mucosal edema + hyperemia +
superficial erosions)

√ spicules + serrated bowel margins (tiny superficial ulcers)

√ "collar button" ulcers (= undermining of ulcers)

√ "double-tracking" = longitudinal submucosal ulceration over several cm

√ hazy / fuzzy quality of bowel contour (excessive secretions)

√ "thumbprinting" = symmetric thickening of colonic folds

√ pseudopolyps = scattered islands of edematous mucosa + reepithelialized granulation tissue within areas of denuded mucosa

√ widening of presacral space

√ obliterated rectal folds = valves of Houston (43%)

(b) subacute stage

√ distorted irregular haustra

√ inflammatory polyps = sessile frondlike / rarely pedunculated lesions (= localized mucosal inflammation resulting in polypoid protuberance)

√ coarse granular mucosa (mucosal replacement by granulation tissue)

(c) chronic stage

√ shortening of colon (= reversible spasm of longitudinal muscles) with depression of flexures

√ "lead-pipe" colon = rigidity + symmetric narrowing of lumen

√ widening of haustral clefts / complete loss of haustrations (DDx: cathartic colon)

√ "burnt-out colon" = fairly distensible colon without haustral markings + without mucosal pattern

√ hazy / fuzzy quality of bowel contour (excessive secretions)

√ postinflammatory polyps (10 – 20%) = small sessile nodules / long wormlike branching + bridging outgrowths (filiform polyposis)

√ "backwash ileitis" (5 – 30%) involving 4 – 25 cm of terminal ileum with patulous ileocecal valve + absent peristalsis + granularity

CT: √ wall thickening < 10 mm

Cx:

(1) Toxic megacolon ± perforation (DDx: granulomatous / ischemic / amebic colitis)

(2) Colonic adenocarcinoma (1 – 16%)
25 x increased risk after 7 – 8 years; higher incidence of multiple carcinomas particularly when total colon involved
Location: distal transverse colon, descending colon, rectum
√ narrowed segment of 2 – 6 cm in length with eccentric lumen + irregular contour + flattened rigid tapered margins = scirrhous carcinoma
√ annular / polypoid carcinoma

(3) Colonic strictures (10%)
smooth contour with fusiform pliable tapering margins, usually short + single; commonly in sigmoid / rectum / transverse colon; usually after minimum of 5 years of disease; rarely cause for obstruction (DDx: colonic carcinoma)

DDx: (1) Familial polyposis (no inflammatory changes)
(2) Cathartic colon (more extensive in right colon)

DDx between CROHN DISEASE versus ULCERATIVE COLITIS
mnemonic: "LUCIFER M"

	Crohn Disease	Ulcerative Colitis
Location	right side	left side
Ulcers	deep	shallow
Contraction	no	yes
Ileocecal valve	thickened	gaping
Fistulae	yes	no
Eccentricity	yes	no
Rate of carcinoma	slight increase	marked increase
Megacolon	unusual	yes

VILLOUS ADENOMA
Villous Adenoma of Colon
Incidence: 7% of all colonic tumors
Age: presentation late in life; M = F
Location: rectum + sigmoid (75%), cecum, ileocecal valve; 2% of all tumors in rectum + colon
Associated with: other GI tumors (25%)

• sensation of incomplete evacuation
• rectal bleeding
• excretion of copious amounts of thick mucus
• fatiguability, weakness
• electrolyte depletion syndrome in 4% (dehydration, hyponatremia, hypokalemia)

√ may completely encircle the colon
√ bulky tumor with spongelike corrugated appearance (barium within interstices)
√ striated "brushlike" surface
√ soft pliable tumor with change in shape
√ innumerable mucosal projections (= fronds) with reticular / granular surface pattern (if villous elements constitute > 75% of tumor, diagnosis can be made on BE)
√ apparent decrease in size on postevacuation films
Cx: malignant transformation / invasion (in 36%) related to size of tumor < 5 cm (9%); > 5 cm (55%); > 10 cm (100%)

Villous Adenoma of Duodenum
More common in colon + rectum; fewer than 50 cases in world literature
√ sessile, soft nonobstructive mass
√ "lace" / "soap bubble" pattern
√ preservation of peristaltic activity + bowel distensibility

WALDENSTRÖM MACROGLOBULINEMIA
= malignant neoplasm of lymphoreticular system with production of abnormal IgM proteins
Histo: hyaline material in lamina propria of small bowel with secondary lymphatic distension
Age: late-life onset
• lymphadenopathy
• hepatosplenomegaly

- dlarrhea, steatorrhea, malabsorption
- anemia, bleeding diathesis
- IgM elevation
- hyperviscosity

Dx: characteristic M-spike in serum electrophoresis

@ Small bowel (rarely involved)
- √   uniform diffuse thickening of valvulae conniventes
- √   granular surface of punctate filling defects (distended villi)

WHIPPLE DISEASE

= INTESTINAL LIPODYSTROPHY

Path: PAS-positive material (periodic acid Schiff) in foamy macrophages in the submucosa of the jejunum (streptococcal material) + fat deposits within intestinal submucosa and lymph nodes causing lymphatic obstruction + dilatation

Organ involvement: small bowel, joints, heart, brain

Age: 40 – 49; M:F = 9:1; Caucasians
- malabsorption, steatorrhea, abdominal pain, weight loss
- recurrent and shifting arthralgias / arthritis
- polyserositis
- generalized lymph adenopathy
- skin pigmentation similar to Addison disease
- √ moderate thickening of jejunal folds with micronodularity (= swollen villi) and wild mucosal pattern
- √ hypersecretion, segmentation, fragmentation (occasionally if accompanied by hyperproteinemia)
- √ NO / minimal dilatation of small bowel
- √ NO rigidity of folds
- √ NO ulcerations
- √ normal transit time (approximately 3 hours)
- √ hepatosplenomegaly

CT:
- √ enlarged low-density lymph nodes in mesenteric root
- √ thickening of intestinal folds
- √ splenomegaly
- √ ascites
- √ pleuropericarditis
- √ sacroiliitis

Dx: jejunal biopsy

Rx: longterm broad-spectrum antibiotics (tetracycline)

DDx: (1) Sprue (marked dilatation, no fold thickening, pronounced segmentation + fragmentation)
         (2) Intestinal lymphangiectasia (thickened folds throughout small bowel)

PSEUDO-WHIPPLE DISEASE IN AIDS

similar clinical picture caused by Mycobacterium avium intracellulare
- √ wall + fold thickening of small bowel loops
- √ mesenteric adenopathy

ZENKER DIVERTICULUM

= posterior hypopharyngeal pouch = pharyngoesophageal diverticulum = pulsion diverticulum with herniation of mucosa + submucosa through oblique + transverse muscle bundles (pseudodiverticulum) of the cricopharyngeal muscle

Etiology: cricopharyngeal dysfunction (cricopharyngeal achalasia / premature closure) results in increased intraluminal pressure

Location: at pharyngoesophageal junction in midline of Killian dehiscence / triangle of Laimer, at level of C5/6
- dysphagia
- regurgitation of food
- √ posterior barium extension in upper half of semilunar depression on the posterior wall of esophagus (cricopharyngeal muscle)
- √ barium-filled sac extending caudally behind + usually to left of esophagus
- √ partial obstruction of esophagus from external pressure of sac contents
- √ partial barium reflux from diverticulum into hypopharynx

ZOLLINGER-ELLISON SYNDROME

Causes:
A. GASTRINOMA = non-beta islet cell tumor with continuous gastrin production
    Location: 87% in pancreas, 13% in medial wall of duodenum
    60% malignant, 40% benign
    Associated with   MEN-Type I (in 10 – 40%)
B. PSEUDO Z-E SYNDROME = antral G-cell hyperplasia (10%)
    (increase in number of G-cells in gastric antrum)
    - lack of gastrin elevation after secretin injection
    - exaggerated gastrin elevation after test meal
- CLINICAL TETRAD:
  (1) Gastric hypersecretion: refractory response to histamine stimulation test concerning HCl concentration; increased basal secretion (> 60% of augmented secretion is diagnostic)
  (2) Diarrhea, steatorrhea (40%): may be sole complaint in 10%, frequently nocturnal; secondary to inactivation of pancreatic enzymes by large volumes of HCl
  (3) Hyperacidity: elevated serum gastrin levels
  (4) Atypical recurrent peptic ulcer disease
- severe intractable pain (90%)
- √ ULCERS (atypical location + course should suggest diagnosis):
  Location: duodenal bulb (60%) + stomach (6%), postbulbar duodenum + jejunum (less common), distal esophagus (exceedingly rare)
  Multiplicity: simultaneous ulcers (in 10%)
  - √ multiple + recurrent / intractable ulcers
  - √ marginal ulcers in postgastrectomy patient
    (a) on gastric side of anastomosis
    (b) on mesenteric border of efferent loop
- √ reflux esophagitis
- √ prominence of area gastricae (hyperplasia of parietal cell mass)
- √ gastric rugal enlargement
- √ sluggish gastric peristalsis (? hypokalemia)

√ "wet stomach" = excess secretions in nondilated nonobstructed stomach

√ dilatation of duodenum + upper small bowel (fluid overload)

√ large folds in duodenum + jejunum (edema)

Cx: (1)   malignant islet cell tumor (in 60%)

      (2)   liver metastases will continue to stimulate gastric secretion (total gastrectomy necessary)

mnemonic: "FUSED"

Folds (thickened, gastric folds)

Ulcers (often multiple, postbulbar)

Secretions increased (refractory to histamine)

Edema (of proximal small bowel)

Diarrhea

DIFFERENTIAL DIAGNOSIS OF UROGENITAL DISORDERS

Absent renal outline on plain film
A. ABSENT KIDNEY
1. Congenital absence
2. S/P nephrectomy
B. SMALL KIDNEY
1. Hypoplasia
2. Renal atrophy
C. RENAL ECTOPIA
1. Pelvic kidney
2. Crossed fused ectopia
3. Intrathoracic kidney
D. OBLITERATION OF PERIRENAL FAT
1. Perirenal abscess
2. Perirenal hematoma
3. Renal tumors

Unilateral large smooth kidney
PRERENAL:
  (a) arterial: Acute arterial infarction
  (b) venous: Acute renal vein thrombosis
INTRARENAL:
  (a) congenital: Duplicated pelvocalyceal system
                      Crossed fused ectopia
                      Multicystic dysplastic kidney
                      Adult polycystic kidney (in 8% unilateral)
  (b) infectious: Acute bacterial nephritis
  (c) adaptation: Compensatory hypertrophy
POSTRENAL:
  (a) collecting system: Obstructive uropathy

mnemonic: "AROMA"
Acute pyelonephritis
Renal vein thrombosis
Obstructive uropathy
Miscellaneous: (compensatory hypertrophy, duplication)
Arterial obstruction (infarction)

Bilateral large kidneys
Average renal length by X-ray: M = 13 cm; F = 12.5 cm
1. PROTEIN DEPOSITION
amyloidosis, multiple myeloma
2. INTERSTITIAL FLUID ACCUMULATION
acute tubular necrosis, acute cortical necrosis, acute arterial infarction, renal vein thrombosis
3. CELLULAR INFILTRATION
  (a) Inflammatory cells: acute interstitial nephritis, acute bacterial nephritis
  (b) Malignant cells : leukemia / lymphoma
4. PROLIFERATIVE / NECROTIZING DISORDERS
  (a) GLOMERULONEPHRITIS:
    acute (poststreptococcal) GN, rapidly progressive GN, idiopathic membranous GN,

membranoproliferative GN, lobular GN, IgA nephropathy, glomerulosclerosis, glomerulosclerosis related to heroin abuse
  (b) MULTISYSTEM DISEASE:
    polyarteritis nodosa, systemic lupus erythematosus, Wegener granulomatosis, allergic angitis, diabetic glomerulosclerosis, Goodpasture syndrome (lung hemorrhage + glomerulonephritis), Schönlein-Henoch syndrome (anaphylactoid purpura), thrombotic thrombocytopenic purpura, focal glomerulonephritis associated with subacute bacterial endocarditis
5. URINE OUTFLOW OBSTRUCTION
bilateral hydronephrosis: congenital / acquired
6. HORMONAL STIMULUS
acromegaly, compensatory hypertrophy, nephromegaly associated with cirrhosis, hyperalimentation, and diabetes mellitus
7. DEVELOPMENTAL
bilateral duplication system, horseshoe kidney, polycystic kidney disease
8. MISCELLANEOUS
acute urate nephropathy, glycogen storage disease, hemophilia, sickle cell disease, Fabry disease, physiologic response to contrast material and diuretics

Unilateral small kidney
A. PRERENAL = VASCULAR
1. Lobar infarction
2. Chronic infarction
3. Renal artery stenosis
4. Radiation nephritis
B. INTRARENAL = PARENCHYMAL
1. Congenital hypoplasia
2. Multicystic dysplastic kidney (in adult)
3. Postinflammatory atrophy
C. POSTRENAL = COLLECTING SYSTEM
1. Reflux nephropathy = Chronic atrophic pyelonephritis
2. Postobstructive atrophy

Bilateral small kidneys
A. PRERENAL = VASCULAR
1. Arterial hypotension (acute)
2. Generalized arteriosclerosis
3. Atheroembolic disease
4. Benign & malignant nephrosclerosis
B. INTRARENAL
1. Hereditary nephropathies: medullary cystic disease, hereditary chronic nephritis (Alport syndrome)
2. Chronic glomerulonephritis
3. Amyloidosis (late)

C. POSTRENAL
   1. Papillary necrosis
D. CAUSES OF UNILATERAL SMALL KIDNEY occurring bilaterally

Depression of renal margins

1. Fetal lobation
   √ notching between normal calices
2. Splenic impression
   √ flattened upper outer margin of left kidney
3. Chronic atrophic pyelonephritis
   √ indentation over clubbed calices
4. Renal infarct
   √ normal calices
5. Chronic renal ischemia
   √ normal calices

Retroperitoneal calcification

A. NEOPLASM
   1. Wilms tumor (in 10 %)
   2. Neuroblastoma (in 50 %): fine, granular / stippled / amorphous
   3. Teratoma: cartilage / bone / teeth, pseudodigits, pseudolimbs
   4. Cavernous hemangioma: phleboliths
B. INFECTION
   1. Tuberculous psoas abscess
   2. Hydatid cyst
C. TRAUMA
   1. Old hematoma

Hyperechoic renal medulla

A. Hyperuricemia
   1. Gout
   2. Lesch-Nyhan syndrome
B. Medullary nephrocalcinosis
   1. Hyperparathyroidism
   2. Milk-alkali syndrome
   3. Hypervitamninosis D
   4. Malignant tumors
   5. Chronic pyelonephritis
   6. Chronic glomerulonephritis
   7. Distal renal tubular acidosis
   8. Sjögren syndrome (distal RTA)
   9. Glycogen storage disease (distal RTA)
   10. Wilson disease (distal RTA)
   11. Primary hypercalcemia
   12. Sarcoidosis
   13. Medullary sponge kidney
C. Hypokalemia
   1. Primary aldosteronism
   2. Pseudo-Bartter syndrome

Enlargement of iliopsoas compartment

A. INFECTION
   (a) from retroperitoneal organs
      1. Renal infection
      2. Complicated pancreatitis
      3. Postoperative aortic graft infection
   (b) from spine
      1. Osteomyelitis / postoperative complication of bone surgery
      2. Discitis / postoperative complication from disc surgery
   (c) from GI tract
      1. Crohn disease
      2. Appendicitis
   (d) others
      1. Pelvic inflammatory disease / postpartum infection
      2. Sepsis
B. HEMORRHAGE
   1. Coagulopathy and anticoagulant therapy
   2. Ruptured aortic aneurysm
   3. Postoperative aneurysm repair / trauma / other surgery
C. NEOPLASTIC DISEASE
   (a) Extrinsic
      1. Lymphoma
      2. Metastatic lymphadenopathy
      3. Bone metastases with soft tissue involvement
      4. Retroperitoneal sarcoma
   (b) Intrinsic
      1. Muscle tumors
      2. Nervous system tumors
      3. Lipoma / liposarcoma
D. MISCELLANEOUS
   1. Pseudoenlargement of psoas muscle compared to de facto atrophy of contralateral side in neuromuscular disease
   2. Fluid collections
      urinoma, lymphocele, pancreatic pseudocyst, enlargement of iliopsoas bursa
   3. Pelvic venous thrombosis
      √ diffuse swelling of all muscles (edema)

RENAL MASS
Unilateral renal masses
SOLID MASSES
   A. TUMORS
      (a) malignant: adenocarcinoma, malignant lymphoma / Hodgkin disease, adult nephroblastoma, metastases, Wilms tumor, sarcoma, oncocytoma, invasive transitional cell carcinoma
      (b) benign: adenoma, hamartoma (angiomyolipoma), mesenchymal tumor (lipoma, fibroma, myoma, hemangioma)
   B. INFLAMMATORY MASSES
      acute focal bacterial nephritis, renal abscess, xanthogranulomatous pyelonephritis, malakoplakia, tuberculoma

FLUID-FILLED MASSES
   A. CYSTS
      (a) Simple renal cyst

(b) Inherited cystic disease:
multicystic dysplastic kidney disease (Potter
Type II), multilocular cystic nephroma
(c) Focal hydronephrosis
B. ARTERIOVENOUS MALFORMATION

Bilateral renal masses
A. TUMORS
1. Malignant lymphoma / Hodgkin disease
2. Metastases
3. Bilateral malignant or benign renal tumors
B. CYSTS
1. Adult polycystic kidney disease
2. Acquired cystic kidney disease

Renal mass in neonate
A. UNILATERAL
1. Multicystic kidney (15 %)
2. Hydronephrosis   (25 %)
(a) UPJ obstruction
(b) upper moiety of duplication
3. Renal vein thrombosis
4. Mesoblastic nephroma
5. Rare: Wilms tumor, Teratoma
B. BILATERAL
1. Hydronephrosis
2. Polycystic kidney disease
3. Multicystic kidney + contralateral hydronephrosis
4. Nephroblastomatosis
5. Bilateral multicystic kidney

Renal mass in older child
A. SINGLE MASS
1. Wilms tumor
2. Multilocular cystic nephroma
3. Focal hydronephrosis
4. Traumatic cyst, abscess
5. Renal cell carcinoma
6. Malignant rhabdoid tumor
7. Teratoma
8. Intrarenal neuroblastoma
B. MULTIPLE MASSES
1. Nephroblastomatosis
2. Multiple Wilms tumors
3. Angiomyolipoma
4. Lymphoma
5. Leukemia
6. Adult polycystic kidney disease
7. Abscesses

Low-density retroperitoneal mass
1. Lipoma
√ sharply marginated, homogeneously fatty mass
2. Lymphangioma
√ similar to lipoma if enough fat content
3. Adrenal myelolipoma
√ density between fat + water
√ usually nonhomogeneous, occasionally with
hemorrhage ± calcifications

4. Renal angiomyolipoma
√ intrarenal component
√ hypervascular with large feeding arteries, multiple
aneurysms, laking without shunting, tortuous
circumferential vessels, whorled parenchymal +
venous phase
5. Xanthogranulomatous pyelonephritis
√ nonfunctioning kidney replaced by low-density
material + central staghorn calculus
6. Metastatic retroperitoneal tumors
7. Renal cell carcinoma
8. Fibrosarcoma, fibrous histiocytoma, mesenchymal
sarcoma, malignant teratoma
√ density close to muscle
9. Liposarcoma

Growth pattern of renal tumors in adults
A. EXPANSILE GROWTH
1. Renal cell carcinoma
2. Oncocytoma
3. Angiomyolipoma
4. Juxtaglomerular tumor
5. Metastatic tumor (e.g. lymphoma)
6. Mesenchymal tumor
B. INFILTRATIVE GROWTH
1. Lymphoma / leukemia
2. Invasive transitional cell carcinoma
3. Metastatic tumor
4. Renal cell carcinoma

Local bulge in renal contour
A. CYST
1. Simple renal cyst
B. TUMOR
1. Adenocarcinoma
2. Angiomyolipoma
3. Pseudotumor
C. INFECTION
1. Subcapsular abscess
2. XGP
D. TRAUMA
1. Subcapsular hematoma
E. DILATED COLLECTING SYSTEM

Multiloculated renal mass
A. NEOPLASTIC DISEASE
1. Multiloculated renal cell carcinoma
2. Multilocular cystic nephroma
3. Cystic Wilms tumor
4. Necrotic tumors
(a) mesoblastic nephroma
(b) clear cell sarcoma
B. RENAL CYSTIC DISEASE
1. Localized renal cystic disease
2. Septated cyst
3. Segmental multicystic kidney
4. Complicated cyst

C. INFLAMMATORY DISEASE
1. Echinococcus
2. Segmental XGP
3. Abscess
4. Malakoplakia
D. VASCULAR LESIONS
1. AV fistula
2. Organizing hematoma

Renal sinus tumor
A. TUMORS
1. Transitional cell carcinoma
2. Lymphoma
3. Metastasis to sinus lymph nodes
4. Mesenchymal tumor
5. Plasmacytoma
B. MISCELLANEOUS
1. Sinus lipomatosis
2. Parapelvic cyst
3. Saccular aneurysm
4. Urinoma
5. Myeloid metaplasia

Hypoechoic renal sinus
1. Fibrolipomatosis
2. Column of Bertin
3. Duplex kidney
4. Multiple parapelvic cysts
5. TCC / RCC
6. Caliectasis
7. Dilated veins

Renal pseudotumor
= anomalies of lobar anatomy which may simulate a tumor
1. **"Dromedary hump"**
secondary to prolonged pressure by spleen during fetal development
Location: in mid portion of lateral border of left kidney
√ triangular contour + elongation of middle calyx
2. **Nodular compensatory hypertrophy**
areas of unaffected tissue in the presence of focal renal scarring from chronic atrophic pyelonephritis (= reflux nephropathy), surgery, trauma, infarction;
√ hypertrophy usually evident within 2 months; less likely to occur > age 50
3. **Lobar dysmorphism**
complete diminutive lobe situated deep within renal substance with its own diminutive calyx in its central portion
4. **Large column of Bertin**
= Large septum of Bertin = cloison of Bertin = large cloison = focal cortical hyperplasia = benign cortical rest = focal renal hypertrophy
= persistence of normal septal cortex / excessive infolding of cortex usually in the presence of partial or complete duplication
Location: between upper and interpolar portion

√ deformation of adjacent calices + infundibula
5. **Hilar lip**
= Supra- / infrahilar bulge = medial part of kidney above and below sinus
6. **Fetal lobation**
= Persistent cortical lobation
14 individual lobes with centrilobar cortex located around calices
Dx: static radionuclide imaging / renal arteriography / CT (ultrasound often not reliable)

ABNORMAL NEPHROGRAM
Abnormal nephrogram due to Impaired Perfusion
1. Systemic hypotensive reaction as reaction to contrast material / cardiac failure / dehydration
Pathophysiology: drop in perfusion pressure after contrast reaches kidney leads to increased salt + water reabsorption and slowed tubular transit
√ prolonged bilateral dense nephrograms = persistent increasing nephrogram
√ decrease in renal size
√ loss of pyelogram after initial opacification
NUC: √ prolonged cortical transit + reduced excretion

2. Impaired Perfusion of Renal Artery
(a) in renal artery stenosis
√ decreased nephrographic opacity + rim nephrogram
√ hyperconcentration in collecting system
√ ureteral notching
NUC: √ decreased perfusion with prolonged excretory phase
(b) in renal artery occlusion (thrombosis, embolism)
√ absent nephrogram

3. Impaired Perfusion of Small Arteries
Trueta shunting = transient rerouting of blood flow from cortex to medulla
Causes:
(a) reflex spasm during arterial angiography secondary to catheter trauma / pressure injection of highly concentrated contrast medium
(b) chronic renal disorders (collagen vascular disease, malignant nephrosclerosis, chronic glomerulonephritis
(c) necrotizing vasculitis (polyarteritis nodosa, scleroderma, hypertensive nephrosclerosis)
CT, Angio:
√ inhomogeneous opacification of cortex
IVP:
√ irregular cortical nephrogram = spotted nephrogram

4. Acute venous outflow obstruction in renal vein thrombosis
√ obstructive nephrogram
√ progressive increase in opacity of entire kidney

Abnormal nephrogram due to <u>Impaired Tubular Transit</u>
Causes:
  A. extrarenal: ureteric obstruction (e.g., stone)
    √ Obstructive nephrogram
    NUC: √ continuous increase in renal activity
        √ dilatation of collecting system
  B. intrarenal:
    (a) segmental: limb of duplication system, calyceal obstruction, interstitial edema
      √ Segmental nephrogram
    (b) protein precipitation: Tamm-Horsfall protein (a normal mucoprotein product of proximal nephrons), Bence-Jones protein (multiple myeloma), uric acid precipitation (acute urate nephropathy), myoglobulinuria, hyperproteinuric state
      √ Striated nephrogram
      NUC:
        √ prolonged cortical transit time + prolonged excretory phase

Abnormal nephrogram due to <u>Abnormal Tubular Function</u>
1. Acute tubular necrosis
  √ immediate persistent nephrogram (common)
  √ progressive increasing opacity (rare)
2. Contrast-induced renal failure

Cortical rim nephrogram
  = rim of cortex continues to receive flow from capsular vessels
  Cause:
    1. Acute total main renal artery occlusion
    2. Renal vein thrombosis
    3. Acute tubular necrosis
    4. Severe chronic urinary obstruction

Increasingly dense nephrogram
  = initially faint nephrogram becoming increasingly dense over hours to days
  Mechanism:
    (a) diminished plasma clearance of contrast material
    (b) leakage of contrast material into renal interstitial spaces
    (c) increase in tubular transit time
  Cause:
    A. VASCULAR = diminished perfusion
      1. Systemic arterial hypotension (bilateral)
      2. Severe main renal artery stenosis (unilateral)
      3. Acute tubular necrosis (in 33 %): due to contrast material nephrotoxicity
      4. Acute renal vein thrombosis
    B. INTRARENAL
      1. Acute glomerular disease
    C. COLLECTING SYSTEM
      1. Intratubular obstruction
        — uric acid crystals (acute urate nephropathy)

        — precipitation of Bence-Jones protein (myeloma nephropathy)
        — Tamm-Horsfall protein (severely dehydrated infants / children)
      2. Acute extrarenal obstruction: ureteral calculus

Striated urographic nephrogram
  = fine linear bands of alternating lucency + density in area of tubules and collecting ducts
  1. Systemic hypotension
  2. Intratubular obstruction (Tamm-Horsfall proteinuria)
  3. Acute bacterial nephritis / pyelonephritis
  4. Renal contusion
  5. Medullary sponge kidney
  6. Medullary cystic disease
  7. Infantile polycystic kidney disease
  8. Renal vein thrombosis
  9. Acute extrarenal obstruction

Striated angiographic nephrogram
  = random patchy densities reflecting redistribution of blood flow from the cortical vasculature to the vasa recta of the medulla
  1. Obliterative diseases of the renal microvasculature polyarteritis nodosa, scleroderma, necrotizing angitis, catheter-induced vasospasm
  2. Acute bacterial nephritis
  3. Renal vein thrombosis

COLLECTING SYSTEM
Caliceal abnormalities
  A. OPACIFICATION OF COLLECTING TUBULES
    1. Pyelorenal backflow
    2. Medullary sponge kidney
  B. PAPILLARY CAVITY
    1. Papillary necrosis
    2. Caliceal diverticulum
    3. Tuberculosis / brucellosis
  C. LOCALIZED CALIECTASIS
    1. Reflux nephropathy = chronic atrophic pyelonephritis
    2. Compound calyx
    3. Hydrocalyx
    4. Congenital megacalyx
    5. Localized postobstructive caliectasis
    6. Localized tuberculosis / papillary necrosis
  D. GENERALIZED CALIECTASIS
    1. Postobstructive atrophy
    2. Congenital megacalices
    3. Obstructive uropathy (hydronephrosis)
    4. Nonobstructive hydronephrosis
    5. Diabetes insipidus

Widened collecting system
  A. Obstructive uropathy
    1. Acute obstruction
    2. Chronic obstruction

B. Nonobstructive widening
  (a) Congenital
    1. Megacalicosis
       underdevelopment of papillae, usually unilateral
    2. Congenital primary megaureter
       widened ureter with normally tapered distal end
    3. Megacystis-megaureter syndrome
    4. Prune-belly syndrome
  (b) Increased urine volume
    1. High-flow states: diabetes insipidus, osmotic diuresis, unilateral kidney
    2. Vesicoureteral reflux
  (c) Atony of collecting system
    1. Infection, i.e., acute pyelonephritis
    2. Pregnancy
       Etiology: ? decreased ureteral tone; obstruction by enlarged ovarian veins / uterus
       Incidence: 3 – 4% of pregnant women
       Time: at end of 1st trimester, maximal in 3rd trimester
       Location: R > L; ureter widened only to pelvic brim
       Prognosis: after delivery resolution within a few weeks to 6 months
  (d) Distended urinary bladder
  (e) Postobstructive atrophy: renal atrophy in spite of relief of obstruction

Nonopaque intraluminal mass in collecting system
A. NONOPAQUE CALCULUS
   uric acid, xanthine, matrix
   √ smooth, rounded, not attached
B. TISSUE SLOUGH
   1. Papillary necrosis
   2. Cholesteatoma
   3. Fungus ball
   4. Inspissated debris ("mucopus")
C. VASCULAR
   1. Blood clot: history of hematuria
      √ change in appearance over time
D. FOREIGN MATERIAL
   1. Air
      from bladder via reverse peristalsis, direct trauma, renoalimentary fistula
   2. Foreign matter

Mucosal mass in collecting system
NEOPLASTIC
A. BENIGN TUMOR
   1. Aberrant papilla = papilla without calix protruding into major infundibulum
   2. Endometriosis
   3. **Fibroepithelial polyp** = fibrous polyp = fibroepithelioma = vascular fibrous polyp = polypoid fibroma = mesodermal tumor with fibrovascular stroma + normal transitional cell epithelium

Age: 20 – 40 years
• Intermittent abdominal / flank pain
• gross hematuria (rare)
√ elongated cylindrical filling defect with smooth margins
√ mobile on thin pedicle
B. MALIGNANT TUMOR
   (a) Uroepithelial tumors
     1. Transitional cell carcinoma (85 – 91%)
     2. Squamous cell carcinoma (10 – 15 %): predisposing factors: calculi (50 – 60%), chronic infection, leukoplakia, phenacetin abuse
        √ infiltrating superficially spreading
     3. Mucinous adenocarcinoma: metaplastic transformation
     4. Sarcoma (extremely rare)
   (b) Metastases: breast (most common), melanoma, stomach, lung, cervix, colon, prostate

INFLAMMATION / INFECTION
   1. Tuberculosis
   2. Candidiasis
   3. Schistosomiasis
   4. Pyeloureteritis cystica
   5. Leukoplakia
   6. Malacoplakia
   7. Xanthogranulomatous pyelonephritis

VASCULAR
   1. Submucosal hemorrhage
      trauma, anticoagulant therapy, acquired circulating anticoagulants, complication of crystalluria / microlithiasis
      √ thumbprinting with progressive improvement
   2. Vascular notching
      ureteropelvic varices, renal vein occlusion, IVC occlusion, vascular malformation, retroaortic left renal vein, "nutcracker" effect on left renal vein between aorta and SMA
   3. Polyarteritis nodosa

PROMINENT MUCOSAL FOLDS
   1. Redundant longitudinal mucosal folds of intermittent hydronephrosis (UPJ obstruction, vesicoureteral reflux) or after relief of obstruction
   2. Chemical / mechanical irritation
   3. Urticaria (Stevens-Johnson syndrome = erythema multiforme bullosa)
   4. Leukoplakia (= squamous metaplasia)
   5. Ureteral diverticulosis
      = rupture of the roofs of cysts in ureteritis cystica

Effaced collecting system
A. EXTRINSIC COMPRESSION
   (1) Unilateral / bilateral global enlargement of renal parenchyma
   (2) Renal sinus masses: hemorrhage; parapelvic cyst; sinus lipomatosis

B. SPASM / INFLAMMATION
  (1) Infection: acute pyelonephritis, acute bacterial
      nephritis, acute tuberculosis
  (2) Hematuria
C. INFILTRATION
  Malignant uroepithelial tumors
D. OLIGURIA
  1. Antidiuretic state
  2. Renal ischemia
  3. Oliguric renal failure

Potter Classification
POTTER SYNDROME
  = any renal condition associated with severe
    oligohydramnios
  • peculiar facies with wide-set eyes, parrot beak nose,
    pliable low-set ears, receding chin
Type I   : infantile PCKD
Type II   : multicystic dysplastic kidney disease,
             multilocular cystic nephroma
      IIa : kidneys of normal / increased size
      IIb : kidneys reduced in size
Type III : adult PCKD, tuberous sclerosis, medullary
             sponge kidney
Type IV   : ureteropelvic junction obstruction with
             development of small cortical cysts / cystic
             dysplasia

Renal cystic disease
A. SIMPLE RENAL CYST
  1. Intrarenal
  2. Parapelvic
D. POLYCYSTIC RENAL DISEASE
  1. Adult PCKD
  2. Infantile PCKD
C. CYSTIC MEDULLARY DISEASE
  1. Uremic medullary cystic disease
  2. Juvenile nephronophtysis
  3. Medullary sponge kidney
D. RENAL DYSPLASIA
  1. Multicystic dysplastic kidney
  2. Segmental / focal renal dysplasia
  3. Familial renal dysplasia
E. NEUROCUTANEOUS DYSPLASIA
  1. Tuberous sclerosis
  2. Von Hippel-Lindau syndrome
F. CYSTIC TUMORS
  1. Multilocular cystic nephroma
  2. Cystic Wilms tumor
  3. Cystic renal cell carcinoma
G. ACQUIRED RENAL CYSTIC DISEASE
  1. Acquired cystic disease of uremia
  2. Infectious cysts (TB, echinococcus, abscess)
  3. Medullary necrosis
  4. Pyelogenic cyst

Syndromes with multiple cortical cysts
1. von Hippel-Lindau syndrome
2. Tuberous sclerosis
3. Meckel-Gruber syndrome
4. Zellweger syndrome = cerebrohepatorenal syndrome
5. Jeune syndrome
6. Conradi syndrome = chondrodysplasia punctata
7. **Oro-facial-digital syndrome**
   X-linked dominant
   √ cleft lip and palate + tongue
   √ clinodactyly, syndactyly, brachydactyly
8. Trisomy 13
9. Turner syndrome

RENAL CALCIFICATION
Calcified renal mass
A calcified renal mass is malignant in about 75% of cases!
A. TUMOR
  1. Renal cell carcinomas calcify in 10%
     √ calcifications generally nonperipheral,
       sometimes along fibrous capsule
  2. Wilms tumor
B. INFECTION
  1. Abscess
     — tuberculous abscess frequently calcifies
     — pyogenic abscess rarely calcifies
  2. Echinococcal cyst
     renal involvement in 3% of hydatid disease; 50% of
     echinococcal cysts calcify
  3. Xanthogranulomatous pyelonephritis
     √ large obstructive calculus in > 70%
C. CYSTS
  calcification related to prior hemorrhage and infection
  1. Simple renal cysts calcify in 1%
  2. Multicystic dysplastic kidney (in adult)
  3. Adult polycystic kidney disease
  4. Milk of calcium (cyst, caliceal diverticulum,
     obstructed hydrocalyx)
  DDx: Residual pantopaque used in cyst puncture
D. VASCULAR
  1. Subcapsular / perirenal hematoma
  2. Renal artery aneurysm
     circular cracked egg-shell appearance
  3. Congenital / posttraumatic arteriovenous fistula

Hypercalcemia
mnemonic: "SHAMPOO DIRT"
  Sarcoidosis
  Hyperparathyroidism
  Alkali-milk syndrome
  Metastases, **M**yeloma
  Paget disease
  Osteogenesis imperfecta
  Osteopetrosis
  D vitamin intoxication
  Immobility
  Renal tubular acidosis
  Thyazides, hyperthyroidism

RENOVASCULAR DISEASE
Renal aneurysm
A. EXTRARENAL ANEURYSM (2/3)
1. Congenital
2. Atherosclerotic
3. Fibromuscular dysplasia
4. Mycotic
   2.5% of all aneurysms
   Cause: bacteremia, SBE, perivascular extension of inflammation
   Organism: streptococcus, staphylococcus, pneumococcus, salmonella
   Locations: thoracic aorta, SMA, peripheral branches of middle cerebral artery, large arteries of extremities, intrarenal (rare), in areas of preexisting vascular disease
5. Neurofibromatosis
6. Trauma + renal artery angioplasty

B. INTRARENAL ANEURYSM (1/3)
in interlobar and more peripheral branches
1. Congenital
   Age at Dx: 30 years; M:F = 1:1
   • hypertension in 25% (from segmental renal ischemia)
   √ aneurysm close to vascular bifurcations, may calcify
2. Atherosclerotic (may calcify)
3. Polyarteritis nodosa
4. SLE
5. Drug abuse vasculitis
   Kidney most commonly affected organ
   Cause:
       (a) immunologic injury from circulating hepatitis antigen-antibody complexes producing a necrotizing angiitis
       (b) bacterial endocarditis
       (c) drug-related
       (d) impurity-related
   Drugs: metamphetamine, heroin, LSD
   √ multiple small aneurysms in interlobar branches near corticomedullary junction
   √ inhomogeneous spotty nephrogram
6. Allergic vasculitis
7. Neoplasm (renal cell carcinoma in 14%; adult Wilms tumor)
8. Hamartoma (angiomyolipoma in 50%)
9. Wegener granulomatosis
10. Metastatic arterial myxoma
11. Transplant rejection
12. Neurofibromatosis
Cx: (1) hypertension (unusual) (2) perinephric / retroperitoneal hemorrhage (3) formation of AV fistula (4) peripheral renal embolization (5) thrombosis

Spontaneous renal hemorrhage
A. COAGULOPATHY

B. RENAL TUMOR
   (a) malignant: RCC, TCC of renal pelvis, Wilms tumor, lipo-, fibro-, angiosarcoma
   (b) benign: lipoma, angiomyolipoma, adenoma, fibromyoma

Subcapsular hematoma
Etiology: trauma, anticoagulation therapy, blood dyscrasia, vasculitis (e.g. polyarteritis nodosa), arteriovenous malformation, ruptured aneurysm, tumor hemorrhage (renal cell carcinoma, angiomyolipoma)
√ subcapsular mass with flattening of renal parenchyma
√ total resorption / formation of pseudocapsule with calcification
Angio: √ avascular mass
Cx: Page kidney (ischemia, release of renin, hypertension)

Renovascular hypertension
1. Atherosclerosis (60%)
2. Fibromuscular dysplasia (35%)
3. Neurofibromatosis
4. Pheochromocytoma
5. Fibrous bands (congenital stenosis)
6. Arteritis (Takayasu disease)
7. Emboli
8. Thrombosis
9. Aneurysm
10. Renal cysts
11. Neoplasm
12. Perirenal hematoma

URETER
Ureteral deviation
A. LUMBAR URETER
   (a) Lateral deviation (common):
       1. Hypertrophy of psoas muscle
       2. Enlargement of paracaval / para-aortic lymph nodes
       3. Aneurysmal dilatation of aorta
       4. Neurogenic tumors
       5. Fluid collections (abscess, urinoma, lymphocele, hematoma)
   (b) Medial deviation:
       1. Retrocaval ureter (on right side only)
       2. Retroperitoneal fibrosis
B. PELVIC URETER
   (a) Medial deviation:
       1. Hypertrophy of iliopsoas muscle
       2. Enlargement of iliac lymph nodes
       3. Aneurysmal dilatation of iliac vessels
       4. Bladder diverticulum at UVJ (Hutch)
       5. Following abdominoperineal surgery + retroperitoneal node dissection
       6. Pelvic lipomatosis
   (b) Lateral deviation with extrinsic compression
       1. Pelvic mass (e.g., fibroids, ovarian tumor)

Ureteral stricture
A. INTRINSIC CAUSE
  (a) MUCOSAL
    1. Primary ureteral tumors
  (b) MURAL
    1. **Endometriosis**
      common disorder in menstruating women (15%)
      ureteral involvement is rare and indicates
      widespread pelvic disease
      √ abrupt smooth stricture of 0.5 – 2.5 cm
        length
      √ BE: rectosigmoid involvement
    2. Tuberculosis, schistosomiasis
    3. Traumatic (ureterolithotomy, endoscopic stone
      extraction, hysterectomy)
    4. Amyloidosis
      √ distal stricture with submucosal calcification
    5. Nonspecific (rare)
B. EXTRINSIC CAUSE
  1. Endometriosis:
    extrinsic form:intrinsic form = 4:1
  2. Abscess: tuboovarian, appendiceal,
    perisigmoidal
  3. Inflammatory bowel disease (e.g., Crohn
    disease, diverticulitis)
  4. Radiation fibrosis
  5. Metastases: cervix, endometrium, ovary,
    rectum, prostate, breast, lymphoma
  6. Iliac artery aneurysm (with perianeurysmal
    fibrosis)

Megaureter
A. VESICOURETERAL REFLUX
  (a) Primary vesicoureteral reflux
    1. Primary reflux megaureter: abnormal ureteral
      tunnel at UVJ
    2. Prune belly syndrome
  (b) Secondary vesicoureteral reflux
    1. Hypertonic neurogenic bladder
    2. Bladder outlet obstruction
    3. Posterior urethral valves
B. OBSTRUCTION
  (a) Primary obstruction
    1. Intrinsic ureteral obstruction (stone, stricture,
      tumor)
    2. Ectopic ureter
    3. Ureterocele
    4. Ureteral duplication: tortuous dilated ureter of
      upper moiety
  (b) Secondary obstruction
    1. Retroperitoneal obstruction: tumor, fibrosis,
      aortic aneurysm
    2. Bladder wall mass
    3. Bladder outlet obstruction: e.g., prostatic
      enlargement
C. NONREFLUX-NONOBSTRUCTED MEGAURETER
  1. Congenital primary megaureter = megaloureter
  2. Polyuria: e.g., diabetes insipidus, acute diuresis

3. Infection
4. Ureter remaining wide after relief of obstruction

Wetting
1. **Enuresis**
  = manifestation of neuromuscular vesicourethral
    immaturity; M:F = 3:2
  • intermittent wetting, usually at night during sleep
  • often positive history of enuresis from one parent
  • normal physical examination
  √ no structural abnormality; urography NOT indicated
2. **Epispadia**
  = some degree of failure of fusion of infravesical portion
    of urinary tract
  • urinary incontinence from incompetent bladder neck /
    urethral sphincter
  √ abnormally wide symphysis pubis (> 1 cm)
3. Sacral agenesis
  = segmental defect (below S_2) with deficiency of
    nerves that innervate bladder, urethra, rectum, feet
    children of diabetic mothers are affected in 17%
4. **Extravesical infrasphincteric ectopic ureter**
  only affects girls as boys do NOT have infrasphincteric
  ureteral orifices
  (a) ureter draining upper pole of duplex system exits
    below urethral sphincter (90%)
  (b) ureter draining single system with ectopic
    extravesical orifice (10%)
5. **Synechia vulvae**
  = adhesive fusion of minor labia directs urine primarily
    into vagina from where it dribbles out post micturition
6. **Vaginal reflux**
  in obese older girls with fat thighs and fat labia
7. Miscellaneous
  posterior urethral valves, urethral stricture, urethral
  diverticula

Polycythemia
= decreased level of erythropoietin in polycythemia rubra
  vera; erythropoietin precursor (produced in kidney +
  converted elsewhere) acts on erythroid stem cells
RENAL
A. INTRARENAL
  1. Vascular impairment
  2. Renal cell carcinoma (5%)
  3. Wilms tumor
  4. Benign fibroma
  5. Simple cyst (14%)
  6. Polycystic kidney disease
B. POSTRENAL
  1. Obstructive uropathy (14%)
EXTRARENAL
A. LIVER DISEASE
  1. Hepatoma
  2. Regenerating hepatic cells
B. ADRENAL DISEASE
  1. Pheochromocytoma
  2. Aldosteronoma
  3. Cushing disease

C. CNS DISEASE
  1. Cerebellar hemangioblastoma
D. Large uterine myomas

NOT found in: renal vein thrombosis
                multicystic dysplastic kidney
                medullary sponge kidney

Diabetes insipidus
1. Hypothalamic diabetes insipidus
   = vasopressin production is reduced to < 10%
   (a) rare autosomal dominant X-linked genetic disorder
   (b) pituitary destruction: craniopharyngioma, surgery, head trauma, complication of meningitis, eosinophilic granuloma
2. Psychogenic water intoxication
   = compulsive intake of large amounts of fluid which leads to inhibition of normal vasopressin production (water deprivation test)
3. Primary nephrogenic diabetes insipidus
   = rare sex-linked recessive genetic disorder with unresponsiveness of tubules + collecting system to vasopressin (in infants + young males)
4. Secondary nephrogenic diabetes insipidus
   drug toxicity, analgesic nephropathy, sickle cell anemia, hypokalemia, hypercalcemia, chronic uremic nephropathy, postobstructive uropathy, reflux nephropathy, amyloidosis, sarcoidosis

ADRENAL GLAND
Adrenal medullary disease
1. Neuroblastoma
2. Ganglioneuroblastoma
3. Ganglioneuroma
4. Pheochromocytoma

Adrenal cortical disease
1. Adrenal hyperplasia
2. Adrenocortical adenoma
3. Adrenocortical carcinoma
4. Cushing syndrome
5. Conn syndrome
6. Adrenogenital syndromes

Small unilateral adrenal tumor
1. Cortical adenoma
2. Metastasis (27% of all tumors): lung (40%), breast (20%), renal cell carcinoma, gastrointestinal tumors, melanoma
3. Pheochromocytoma
4. Asymmetric hyperplasia
5. Granulomatous disease: diffuse enlargement / discrete mass
6. Myelolipoma: rare benign tumor of hematopoietic cells + fat

Large solid adrenal mass
1. Cortical carcinoma

2. Pheochromocytoma
3. Neuroblastoma / ganglioneuroma
4. Myelolipoma
5. Metastasis
6. Hemorrhage
7. Inflammation
8. Abscess

Bilateral large adrenals
1. Hyperplasia
2. Inflammation
3. Hemorrhage
4. Metastases

Cystic adrenal mass
1. Old hemorrhage
2. Cyst: pancreatic pseudocyst, degenerated adenoma, hydatid cyst, endothelial lined vascular cystic space
3. Neuroblastoma (rare)
4. Cystic adenoma

Adrenal calcification
A. TUMOR
  1. Neuroblastoma
  2. Pheochromocytoma
  3. Adrenal adenoma
  4. Adrenal carcinoma
  5. Dermoid
B. VASCULAR
  1. Hemorrhage (neonatal, sepsis)
C. INFECTION
  1. Tuberculosis
  2. Histoplasmosis
  3. Waterhouse-Friderichsen syndrome
D. ENDOCRINE
  1. Addison disease (TB)
E. OTHERS
  1. Wolman disease

URINARY BLADDER
Bilateral narrowing of urinary bladder
A. WITH ELEVATION OF BLADDER FLOOR
  1. Pelvic lipomatosis
  2. Pelvic hematoma
     secondary to trauma, anticoagulant therapy, spontaneous rupture of blood vessels, blood dyscrasia (rare), bleeding neoplasm (rare)
  3. Chronic cystitis
B. WITH SUPERIOR COMPRESSION OF BLADDER
  1. Thrombosis of IVC
     secondary to trauma, hypercoagulability state (oral contraceptives), extension of thrombi from lower extremity, abdominal sepsis, Budd-Chiari syndrome, compression of IVC by neoplasm
     √ collaterals through gonadal veins, ascending lumbar veins, vertebral plexus, retroperitoneal veins, portal vein (via hemorrhoidal veins)
     √ notching of distal ureter by ureteral veins

2. Pelvic lymphadenopathy
   most often secondary to lymphoma
   √ polycystic asymmetric compression of bladder
   √ medial displacement of pelvic segment of
     ureters
   √ lateral displacement of upper ureters
3. Hypertrophy of iliopsoas muscles
4. Bilateral pelvic masses
   — bilateral lymphocysts (following radical pelvic
     surgery)
   — bilateral urinomas
   — bilateral pelvic abscesses

Small bladder capacity
- urinary frequency
√ thickened bladder wall + decreased bladder volume
√ vesicoureteral reflux
1. **Interstitial cystitis**
   Age: postmenopausal female
   - pink pseudoulceration of bladder mucosa
   characteristically at vertex of bladder (= Hummer ulcer)
2. **Hemorrhagic cystitis**
   (a) nonspecific: negative culture
   (b) viral (adenovirus): negative culture, viral exanthem
   (c) cytotoxic: cyclophosphamide (cytoxan), in 15% of
       patients within 1st year of treatment
3. **Tuberculous cystitis**
   √ irritable hypertonic bladder with decreased capacity
   √ usually starts at trigone spreading upwards and
     laterally
   √ calcification of bladder wall (rare)
4. **Schistosomiasis infection of bladder**
   √ calcifications of bladder wall (common)
5. **Cystitis cystica**
   bacterial infection more common in females
   √ cystogram insensitive
6. Radiation cystitis

mnemonic: "SCRITT"
Schistosomiasis
Cytoxan
Radiation
Interstitial cystitis
TB
Transitional cell carcinoma

Bladder wall thickening
Normal bladder wall thickness (regardless of age +
gender):
   < 5 mm in nondistended bladders
   < 3 mm in well distended bladders
A. TUMOR
   1. Neurofibromatosis
B. INFECTION / INFLAMMATION
   1. Cystitis
C. MUSCULAR HYPERTROPHY
   1. Neurogenic bladder
   2. Bladder outlet obstruction (posterior urethral valves)
D. UNDERDISTENDED BLADDER

Bladder wall calcification
A. INFLAMMATION
   1. Schistosomiasis (50 %)
      √ relatively normal distensibility
   2. Tuberculosis
      √ bladder markedly contracted
   3. Postirradiation cystitis
   4. Bacillary UTI (extremely uncommon)
B. NEOPLASM
   TCC, squamous cell carcinoma, leiomyosarcoma,
   hemangioma, neuroblastoma, osteogenic sarcoma

Masses extrinsic to urinary bladder
A. NORMAL / ENLARGED ORGANS
   1. Uterus, leiomyomatous uterus, pregnant uterus
   2. Distended rectosigmoid
   3. Ectopic pelvic kidney
   4. Prostate cancer / BPH
B. OLID PELVIC TUMORS
   1. Lymphadenopathy
   2. Bone tumor from sacrum / coccyx
   3. Rectosigmoid mass
   4. Hip arthroplasty
   5. Neurogenic neoplasm, meningomyelocele
   6. Pelvic lipomatosis
   7. Liposarcoma
C. CYSTIC PELVIC TUMORS
   (a) congenital / developmental
      1. Urachal cyst
      2. Müllerian duct cyst
      3. Gartner duct cyst
      4. Anterior meningocele
      5. Hydrometrocolpos
   (b) related to trauma
      1. Hematoma (e.g., rectus sheath)
      2. Urinoma
      3. Lymphocele
      4. Abscess
      5. Aneurysm
      6. Mesenteric cyst
      7. Rectus sheath hematoma
   (c) cysts in a normal organ
      1. Prostatic cyst
      2. Cyst of seminal vesicle
      3. Cyst of vas deferens
      4. Ovarian cysts
      5. Hydrosalpinx
      6. Vaginal cysts
      7. Bladder diverticula
   (d) GI tract
      1. Peritoneal inclusion cyst
      2. Fluid-filled bowel

Urinary bladder wall masses
A. CONGENITAL
   1. Congenital septum
   2. Simple ureterocele
   3. Ectopic ureterocele

B. BLADDER TUMORS
C. INFLAMMATION / INFECTION
1. Cystitis: hemorrhagic ~, abacterial ~, bullous ~, edematous ~, interstitial ~, eosinophilic ~, granulomatous ~, emphysematous ~, cystitis cystica, cyclophosphamide cystitis, cystitis glandularis (premalignant lesion with villous lesions in bladder dome from proliferation of "intestine-like" glands in submucosa)
2. Tuberculosis
3. Schistosomiasis
4. Malakoplakia
D. HEMATOMA
after instrumentation, surgery, trauma

MALE GENITAL TRACT
Calcifications of male genital tract
A. VAS DEFERENS
1. Diabetes mellitus: in muscular outer layer
2. Degenerative changes
3. TB, syphilis, nonspecific UTI: intraluminal
B. SEMINAL VESICLES
Gonorrhea, TB, schistosomiasis, bilharziosis
C. PROSTATE
Calcified corpora amylacea, TB

Acutely symptomatic scrotum
= acute unilateral scrotal swelling with / without pain
Cause:
epididymitis:torsion = 3:2   < 20 years of age
epididymitis:torsion = 9:1   > 20 years of age
A. Torsion
1. Torsion of testis

2. Torsion of testicular appendages
accounts for 5% of scrotal pathology; both located near upper pole of testes
Frequency:
appendix testis:appendix epididymis = 9:1
3. Scrotal fat necrosis
4. Strangulated hernia
B. Infection / Inflammation
1. Acute epididymitis
2. **Orchitis**
Etiology:
(1) bacterial infection
(2) complication of mumps in 20%: in adolescents + young adults; usually developing 4 – 5 days later; unilateral involvement in > 90%; parotitis precedes orchitis in 84%, simultaneous in 3%, later in 4%, without parotitis in 10%
3. Intrascrotal abscess
C. Hemorrhage
1. Testicular trauma
2. Hemorrhage into testicular tumor

Scrotal mass
1. Inflammation   (48%)
2. Hydrocele   (24%)
3. Torsion   (9%)
4. Varicocele   (7%)
5. Spermatocele   (4%)
6. Cysts   (4%)
7. Malignant tumor   (2%)
8. Benign tumor   (0.7%)

ANATOMY AND FUNCTION OF UROGENITAL TRACT

Urogenital Embryology

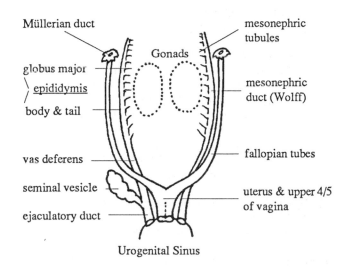

Urogenital Sinus

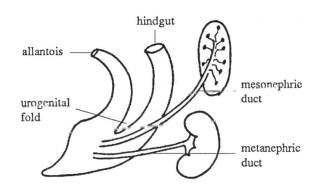

MÜLLERIAN DUCT (grows along mesonephric duct)
   Male: degenerates, remnants are prostatic utricle +
               appendix testis
   Female: uterus, fallopian tubes
PRONEPHROS
   vestigial remnant / completely absent
MESONEPHROS   degenerates
   mesonephric tubules: efferent ductules (M);
                           epinephron (F)
   mesonephric duct: vas deferens, ejaculatory duct,
                        seminal vesicles (M); vanishes (F)
METANEPHROS (kidney)
   (1) metanephric duct buds from mesonephric duct at
        4th week to form ureter, pelvis, calices, collecting
        ducts (10 – 12 generations)
   (2) metanephric vesicles form around terminal
        branches of collecting ducts
        Polycystic kidney disease is believed to be a failure
        of linkage!

Renal Vascular Anatomy

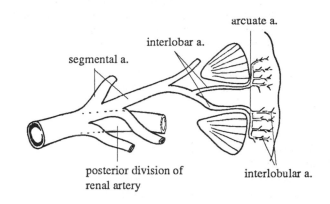

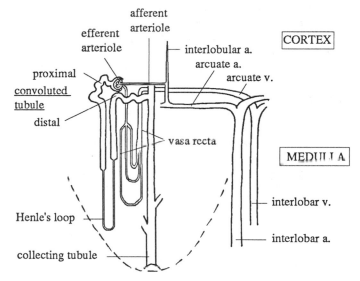

Antidiuretic Hormone (ADH)
Production site: supraoptic nuclei of hypothalamus,
transported to neurohypophysis
Stimulus: fluid loss with increase in osmolality
Effects: (1) 10 x increase in permeability of collecting
              ducts (= concentrated urine)
         (2) decreased blood flow through vasa recta
              leads to increased hypertonicity of
              interstitium (= countercurrent multiplier
              mechanism)

Renal physiology
GLOMERULAR FILTRATION RATE (GFR)
$$[P] \times GFR = [U] \times U_{vol}$$
$$\mathbf{GFR} = \{[U] \times U_{vol}\} / [P] = 125 \text{ ml/min} = 20\% \text{ of RPF}$$
Substrate: inulin; Tc-99m DTPA

TUBULAR SECRETION (Tm)

$[U] \times U_{vol} = [P] \times GFR + Tm$

Tm = { [U] × U$_{vol}$} - {[P] × GFR}

Substrate: p-aminohippurate (PAH); I-131 hippuran

RENAL PLASMA FLOW (RPF)

$[P] \times RPF = [U] \times U_{vol}$

RPF = {[U] × U$_{vol}$} / [P]

Substrate: p-aminohippurate

[P]	= concentration in plasma
GFR	= glomerular filtration rate
[U]	= concentration in urine
U$_{vol}$	= urine volume
Tm	= transport maximum (across tubular cells)
RPF	= renal plasma flow

Renal imaging in newborn infant

Δ low glomerular filtration rate (GFR):
— on first day of life: 21% of adult values
— by 2 weeks of age: 44% of adult values
— at end of 1st year: close to adult values
Δ limited capacity to concentrate urine
IVP: √ occasional failure of renal visualization
NUC: √ improved visualization on radionuclide studies

Contrast excretion

UROGRAPHIC DENSITY depends on

$$[U] = \{[P] \times GFR\} / U_{vol}$$

1. Concentration of contrast material in plasma [P] is a function of
   (a) total iodine dose
   (b) contrast injection rate

(c) volume distribution
Rapid decline of concentration of contrast material in vessels is due to:
   (1) rapid mixing within vascular compartment
   (2) diffusion into extravascular extracellular fluid space (capillary permeation)
   (3) renal excretion
2. Glomerular filtration rate (GFR): 99 % filtered
3. Urine volume (U$_{vol}$) i.e., activity of ADH:
   (a) in dehydrated state with increased ADH activity concentrations of contrast material are higher
        Dehydration is considered a risk-potentiating factor for nephrotoxicity!
   (b) in volume-expanded state with decreased ADH activity concentrations of contrast material are lower
        Patients with CHF require higher doses of contrast material!

MEGLUMINE: no metabolization, excreted by glomerular filtration alone
meglumine effect of osmotic diuresis:
   (a) lower concentration of urinary iodine per ml urine
   (b) greater distension of collecting system
   N.B.: Avoid meglumine in "at risk" patients (higher incidence of contrast reactions than sodium !)
SODIUM: extensive reabsorption by tubules with delayed excretion
sodium effect of reabsorption:
   (a) increased concentration of urinary iodine (improved visualization)
   (b) less distension of collecting system (ureteral compression necessary)

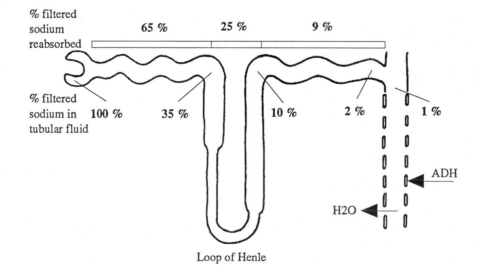

Sodium Reabsorption

hypertonicity is maintained within the medullary interstitium by the countercurrent multiplier system of the loop of Henle and the vasa recta; ADH increases permeability of collecting ducts for water

Abnormal tubular function
A. PROXIMAL TUBULE
   reabsorbs almost all of glucose, amino acids,
   phosphate
   - glycosuria (Toni-Fanconi syndrome)
   - aminoaciduria (cysteinuria)
   - phosphaturia (phosphate diabetes, thiazides)
B. DISTAL TUBULE
   absorbs most of water
   - diabetes insipidus

Renal Tubular Acidosis
= inability of kidney to excrete an acid urine resulting in
  systemic metabolic acidosis
Functional Types:
   A. <u>TYPE I = DISTAL TYPE</u>
      impaired ability to secrete H⁺ in distal tubule
      higher incidence of nephrocalcinosis,
      nephrolithiasis, osteomalacia
      - Acid load test with NH_4Cl
   B. <u>TYPE II = PROXIMAL TYPE</u>
      impaired capacity to absorb HCO_3^- in proximal
         tubule
      most common in renal insufficiency,
      hyperparathyroidism
      - Bicarbonate titration test

Pathophysiology:
   (a) loss of phosphate = osteomalacia / rickets
   (b) loss of calcium   = nephrocalcinosis + renal
                            calculi
   (c) loss of potassium = muscle weakness
   (d) loss of bicarbonate = hyperchloremic acidosis
   - alkaline urine
   - potassium wasting, loss of sodium
   - hypercalciuria (continued mobilization of bone
     calcium)
   - hyperchloremic acidosis (low plasma bicarbonate)

Consequences:
   - chronic renal failure (damage from nephrocalcinosis +
     secondary pyelonephritis)
   - muscle weakness, hyporeflexia, paralysis (due to
     hypokalemia)
   - bone pain (due to osteomalacia)
   √ rickets / osteomalacia
   √ nephrocalcinosis / stone formation (marked reduction
     of urinary citrate)

Categories:
   1. INFANTILE RTA = PRIMARY RTA TYPE II
      = LIGHTWOOD SYNDROME
      late development of enzyme carbonic anhydrase;
      male patients
      spontaneous remission by age 2 in majority of
      patients
      √ nephrocalcinosis in 25%

   2. PRIMARY RTA TYPE I
      autosomal dominant; female patients; presents in
      early adult life
      √ nephrocalcinosis in 75%
      √ osteomalacia in 50%
   3. ACQUIRED RTA
      (a) TYPE I:
          Sjögren syndrome, cryoglobulinemia, light
          chain proteinuria, amphotericin B toxicity,
          toluene toxicity, outdated tetracyclines,
          lithium toxicity, heavy metal intoxication,
          renal transplant, radiation therapy, chronic
          renal disease
      (b) TYPE II
          cystinuria, Wilson disease, primary &
          secondary hyperparathyroidism, Fanconi
          syndrome, glycogen storage disease

Arterial hypotension
= intrarenal hypovolemia, primary vasoconstriction,
  reduced glomerular filtration, depletion of intratubular
  urine volume
May occur as a contrast reaction!
Urogram reverts to normal after reversion of hypotension!
√ bilaterally small smooth kidneys (compared with size on
  preliminary films)
√ increasingly dense nephrogram
√ usually NO opacification of collecting system
√ initially opacification of collecting system if hypotension
  occurs during contrast injection

DEVELOPMENTAL ANOMALIES
A. NUMERARY RENAL ANOMALY
   1. Supernumerary kidney
   2. Complete / partial duplication
   3. Abortive calyx
   4. Unicalyceal (unipapillary) kidney
B. RENAL UNDERDEVELOPMENT
   1. Congenital renal hypoplasia
   2. Renal agenesis
   3. Renal dysgenesis
C. RENAL ECTOPIA
   Normal location of kidneys: 1st – 3rd lumbar vertebra
   1. <u>Longitudinal ectopia</u>
      pelvic, sacral, lower lumbar level, intrathoracic
      (L > R)
      √ must show aberrant arteries
      DDx: displacement through diaphragmatic hernia
             (nonaberrant); hypermobile kidney
   2. <u>Crossed ectopia</u>
      (a) fused (common)
      (b) separate (rare)
      √ invariably aberrant renal arteries
      √ distal ureter inserts into trigone on the side of
        origin
   3. <u>Renal fusion</u>
      = "lump, cake, disc, horseshoe"
      Cx: aberrant arteries may cross and obstruct
            ureter

4. Renal malrotation
   √ collecting structures may be positioned ventrally
   (most common), lateral (rare), dorsal (rarer),
   transverse (along a.p. axis)
   √ "funny looking calices" = developmental usually
   nonobstructive ectasia

ADRENAL ANATOMY

Zona **G**lomerulosa = Mineralocorticoids (aldosterone)
Zona **F**asciculata = Cortisol
Zona **R**eticularis   = Sex hormones (androgen,
                                    estrogen)
Medulla   = norepinephrine, epinephrine

Normal Size   : 3 - 5 x 3 x 1 cm
Normal weight : 3 - 5 g
Visualization by CT : Left side 100 %,   Right side 99 %
            by US : Left side 45 %,   Right side 80 %

ANATOMY OF SCROTAL CONTENTS

Average size of testis   : 3.8 x 3.0 x 2.5 cm (decreasing
                              with age)
Size of globus major   : 11 x 7 x 6 mm (decreasing
                              with age)
Scrotal wall thickness   : 2 – 8 mm (3 – 6 mm in 89%)
Hydrocele   : small to moderate in 14% of
                              normals
Testicular cysts   : in 8% of normals (average size
                              2 – 3 mm), numbers
                              increasing with age
Epididymal cysts   : in 30% of normals (average
                              size 4 mm)
Epididymal calcification : in 3%

DISEASE ENTITIES OF RENAL, ADRENAL, VESICAL, URETERAL, and SCROTAL DISORDERS

ABORTIVE CALYX
= developmental anomaly with short blind-ending outpouching of pyramid without papillary invagination
Location: (a) renal pelvis
          (b) infundibulum (mostly upper pole)

ACQUIRED CYSTIC KIDNEY DISEASE
= ACQUIRED CYSTIC DISEASE OF UREMIA
Cause: patients on long-term hemodialysis (in 43% diffuse bilateral cysts after 5 – 6 years, in 17% < 5 cysts per kidney, in 40% no cysts); successful transplants prevent occurrence of cysts / tumor)
Incidence: in 27 – 47% after approximately 3 years; in 80% after 4 years; approaching 100% after > 5 years
√ small end-stage kidneys (< 280 g)
√ multiple cysts bilaterally (early = small / late = large)
Associated with in 13 – 20%:
  (a) small papillary / tubular / solid clear-cell adenomas 1 cm in diameter
  (b) renal cell carcinoma
Cx: spontaneous hemorrhage

ACUTE CORTICAL NECROSIS
= rare disorder with patchy / universal necrosis of renal cortex + proximal convoluted structures secondary to distension of glomerular capillaries with dehemoglobulinized RBCs, medulla + 1 – 2 mm of peripheral cortex are spared
Etiology:
  (a) Obstetric patient (most often): abruptio placentae = premature separation of placenta with concealed hemorrhage (50%), septic abortion, placenta previa
  (b) Children: severe dehydration + fever, infection, hemolytic uremic syndrome, transfusion reaction
  (c) Adults: sepsis, dehydration, shock, myocardial failure, burns, snakebite, aortic abdominal surgery, hyperacute renal transplant rejection
• protracted + severe oliguria / anuria

EARLY SIGNS
√ diffusely enlarged smooth kidneys
√ absent / faint nephrogram
US: √ hypoechoic cortex
NUC: √ severely impaired renal perfusion
LATE SIGNS
√ small kidney (after a few months)
√ "tramline" / punctate calcifications along margins of viable and necrotic tissue (as early as 24 hours)
US: √ hyperechoic cortex with acoustic shadowing
Prognosis: poor chance of recovery

ACUTE DIFFUSE BACTERIAL NEPHRITIS
= ACUTE SUPPURATIVE PYELONEPHRITIS = more severe and extensive form of acute pyelonephritis which may lead to diffuse necrosis (phlegmon)
Organisms: Proteus, Klebsiella > E. coli
Predisposed: diabetics (60 %)

ACUTE INTERSTITIAL NEPHRITIS
= infiltration of interstitium by lymphocytes, plasma cells, eosinophils, few PMNs + edema
Causes: allergic / idiosyncratic reaction to drug exposure (methicillin, sulfonamides, ampicillin, cephalotin, penicillin, anticoagulants, phenindione, diphenylhydantoin)
• eosinophilia (develops 5 days to 5 weeks after exposure)
√ large smooth kidneys with thick parenchyma
√ normal / diminished contrast density
US: √ normal / increased echogenicity

ACUTE TUBULAR NECROSIS
= temporary reversible marked reduction in tubular flow rate
Etiology:
  (a) DRUGS : bichloride of mercury, ethylene glycol, carbon tetrachloride, bismuth, arsenic, uranium, urographic contrast material (especially when associated with glomerulosclerosis in diabetes mellitus), aminoglycosides (gentamicin, kanamycin)
  (b) ISCHEMIA: cardiogenic shock, crush injury, burns, transfusion reaction, severe dehydration, hemorrhage, renal transplantation, aortic resection
√ smooth large kidneys
√ diminished / absent opacification of collecting system
√ immediate persistent dense nephrogram (75%)
√ increasingly dense persistent nephrogram (25%)
√ diffuse calcifications (rare)
US : √ normal to diminished echogenicity of medulla, normal to increased echogenicity of cortex
Angio: √ normal arterial tree with delayed emptying of intrarenal vessels;
      √ slightly delayed / normal venous opacification
NUC: √ poor concentration of Tc-99m glucoheptonate
      √ well maintained renal perfusion
      √ better renal visualization on immediate postinjection images than on delayed images
      √ progressive parenchymal accumulation of I-131 hippuran
      √ no excretion

ADRENOCORTICAL ADENOMA
A. NONFUNCTIONING
B. HYPERFUNCTIONING
  1. Primary hyperaldosteronism

2. Cushing syndrome (10 %)
3. Virilization
Incidence: 3% at autopsy (nonfunctioning)
√ well-defined sharply marginated 2 – 5 cm large mass
√ adenoma may calcify
√ contralateral atrophic gland (secondary to ACTH -
   suppression with autonomous adenoma)
CT:
    √ HU indicating cystic density (mimicked by high
       cholesterol content)
    √ small adenomas < 1 cm often go undetected
Angio:
    √ tumor blush + neovascularity; occasionally
       hypovascular
    √ pooling of contrast material
    √ enlarged central vein with high flow
    √ arcuate displacement of intraadrenal veins
    √ bilateral adrenal venous sampling in up to 40%
unsuccessful in localizing
MRI: √ isointense to liver on T2

ADRENOCORTICAL CARCINOMA
• 20% nonfunctioning
• 50% functional (often Cushing syndrome)
√ mass usually > 5 cm (median size 12 cm)
√ inhomogeneous enhancement (foci of hemorrhage +
   central necrosis)
√ occasionally calcified
√ enlarged adrenal arteries
√ neovascularity, occasionally with parasitization
√ AV shunting; multiple draining veins
MRI:
    √ hyperintense to liver (SE 2,500 / 80 sequence)
Biopsy: may appear histologically benign in well-
            differentiated adenocarcinoma
Prognosis: 5-year survival rate of 0%

ADRENAL HEMORRHAGE
Cause:
(a) NEWBORN
     Associated with birth trauma (forceps / breech
     delivery), hypoxia (prematurity), infants of diabetic
     mothers, septicemia, hemorrhagic disorders
     Age: 1st week of life
     Site: R > L; bilateral in 10%
(b) ADULT
     Following septicemia (Waterhouse-Friderichsen
     syndrome), trauma, tumor
√ mass displacing renal axis
√ initially echogenic becoming progressively hypoechoic
   (degeneration, lysis)
√ gradual decrease in size
√ peripheral calcification after 1 week

ADRENAL HYPERPLASIA
Responsible for 8% of Cushing syndrome and 10 – 20% of
hyperaldosteronism
Incidence: 4 x increased in patients with malignancy

√ bilateral normal sized / enlarged glands
√ micro- / macronodular configuration (nodules up to
   2.5 cm)
√ normal venogram: may show enlarged gland
√ minimally increased hypervascularity
√ focal accumulation of contrast medium

ADRENOGENITAL SYNDROMES
A. CONGENITAL TYPE
    = impaired cortisol + aldosterone synthesis secondary
       to enzyme defect (21-hydroxylase / 11-beta-
       hydroxylase) with increased ACTH stimulation by
       pituitary gland (negative feedback mechanism)
    M < F
    • virilization of female fetus
    • precocious puberty in male
    • pseudohermaphroditism (clitoral hypertrophy,
       ambiguous external genitalia, urogenital sinus)
B. ACQUIRED TYPE
    M < F
    (a) adrenal hyperplasia / adenoma / carcinoma
    (b) ovarian / testicular tumor
    (c) gonadotropin-producing tumor: pineal,
          hypothalamic, choriocarcinoma
    • virilization
    • Cushing syndrome

AMYLOIDOSIS
= accumulation of extracellular eosinophilic protein
   substances
1. PRIMARY AMYLOIDOSIS
    kidneys involved in 35%
2. SECONDARY AMYLOIDOSIS
    kidneys involved in > 80 %, also affected are breast,
    tongue, alimentary tract, spleen, connective tissue
    Causes: tuberculosis, osteomyelitis, bronchiectasis,
                  ulcerative colitis, rheumatoid arthritis,
                  multiple myeloma, Waldenström
                  macroglobulinemia, familial Mediterranean
                  fever
√ smooth normal to large kidneys (early stage); small
   kidneys (late stage)
√ occasionally attenuated collecting system
√ parenchymal thickness initially increased, renal atrophy
   with time
√ nephrographic density normal to diminished
US: √ normal to increased echogenicity
Cx: renal vein thrombosis

ANALGESIC NEPHROPATHY
= renal damage from ingestion of salicylates in
   combination with phenacetin / acetaminophen in a
   cumulative dose of 1 kg
Incidence: United States (2 – 10%), Australia (20%)
Age: middle-aged; M:F = 1:4
• gross hematuria
• hypertension
• renal colic (passage of renal tissue)

- renal insufficiency (2 – 10% of all endstage renal failures)
- ANALGESIC SYNDROME: history of psychiatric therapy, abuse of alcohol + laxatives, headaches, pain in cervical + lumbar spine, peptic ulcer, anemia, splenomegaly, arteriosclerosis, premature aging
√ papillary necrosis
√ scarring of renal parenchyma ("wavy outlline"); bilateral in 66%, unilateral in 5%
√ renal atrophy
√ papillary urothelial tumors in calices / pelvis (mostly TCC / squamous cell carcinoma), in 5% bilateral

ANGIOMYOLIPOMA
= RENAL HAMARTOMA = benign mesenchymal tumor
Histo: tumor composed of thick-walled blood vessels, smooth muscle, fat
Types:
   (1) Isolated AML (80%) = sporadic AML
      solitary + unilateral, NO stigmata of tuberous sclerosis; M:F = 1:4; commonly in women between 40 – 60 years of age
   (2) AML associated with tuberous sclerosis (in 20%) in 80% of patients with tuberous sclerosis; commonly bilateral + multiple
- flank pain with enlarging mass
- hematuria
√ often large component of extrarenal tumor
√ calcifications (6%)
Plain film: √ fat lucency (in < 10%)
CT: √ fat density (diagnostic)
MRI: √ variable areas of high signal intensity on T1WI (DDx. hemorrhagic cyst, solid tumor)
US: √ intensely echogenic tumor
Angio:
   √ hypervascular mass (95%) with enlarged interlobar + interlobular feeding arteries, tortuous irregular aneurysmally dilated vessels (1/3), venous pooling, "sunburst" / "whorled" / "onion peel" appearance, no AV shunting
Cx: hemorrhagic shock from bleeding into angiomyolipoma or into retroperitoneum
DDx: renal / perirenal lipoma

ARTERIOVENOUS MALFORMATION
   (a) congenital AVM
   (b) acquired AVM: trauma, spontaneous rupture of aneurysm, very vascular malignant neoplasm
Histo:
   (1) cirsoid = multiple coiled vascular channels grouped in cluster; supplied by one / more arteries; draining into one / more veins
   (2) cavernous = single well-defined artery feeding into a single vein (rare)
√ large unifocal mass
√ focally attenuated and displaced collecting system
√ homogeneously enhancing mass
√ curvilinear calcification

US:
√ tubular anechoic structure (DDx: hydronephrosis, hydrocalix)

BLADDER CALCULI
Etiology:
   1. MIGRANT CALCULI
      = renal calculi spontaneously passing into bladder
   2. IDIOPATHIC / PRIMARY / ENDEMIC CALCULI
      in North Africa, India, Indonesia; in young boys of low socioeconomic class (nutritional deficiency?)
   3. STASIS CALCULI
      in bladder outflow obstruction, vesical diverticula, lower urinary tract infection (in particular Proteus), cystocele, neuropathic bladder dysfunction
   4. FOREIGN BODY NIDUS CALCULI
      from self-introduced objects, bladder wall-penetrating bone fragments, prostatic chips, nonabsorbable suture material, fragments of Foley balloon catheter, pubic hair, presence of intestinal mucosa (in bladder augmentation, ileal conduit, repaired bladder exstrophy)
√ single stone in 86%
Rate of recurrence after removal: 41%

BLADDER CONTUSION
= intramural hematoma
√ no extravasation
√ lack of normal distensibility
√ crescent-shaped filling defect in contrast-distended bladder

BLADDER DIVERTICULUM
= cavity formed by herniation of bladder mucosa through muscular wall, joined to the bladder cavity by a constricted neck
Etiology: (a) persistent lower urinary tract obstruction (enlarged prostate, bladder neck stenosis)
         (b) congenital
Average age: 57 years; M:F = 9:1
Sites: areas of congenital weakness of muscular wall at
      (a) ureteral meatus
      (b) posterolateral wall (Hutch diverticulum = paraureteral)
Cx: (1) vesical carcinoma in 0.8 – 7% secondary to chronic inflammation (average age 66 years)
      (2) Ureteral obstruction
      (3) Ureteral reflux

BLADDER RUPTURE
Extraperitoneal Rupture of Bladder (80%)
Cause: pelvic fracture (sharp bony spicule) or avulsion tear at fixation points of puboprostatic ligaments
Location: usually close to base of bladder anterolaterally
Plain film:
   √ "pear-shaped" bladder

√ loss of obturator fat planes
√ paralytic ileus
√ upward displacement of ileal loops
Contrast examination:
    √ flame-shaped contrast extravasation into
      perivesical fat, best seen on postvoid films, may
      extend into thigh / anterior abdominal wall
US:
    √ "bladder within a bladder" = bladder surrounded by
      fluid collection

Intraperitoneal Rupture of Bladder (20%)
Causes:
    (a) usually as a result of invasive procedure
         (cystoscopy), stab wound, surgery
    (b) blunt trauma with sudden rise in intravesical
         pressure (requires distended bladder)
Location: usually at dome of bladder
√ contrast extravasation into paracolic gutters
√ contrast outlining small bowel loops
√ uriniferous ascites

BLADDER TUMORS
3% of all neoplasms; most common tumors of
genitourinary tract
• painless hematuria (60 %)
IVP: 70% accuracy rate

STAGING
T 1	= A	lesions involving mucosa + submucosa
T 2	= B_1	invasion of superficial muscle layer
T 3a	= B_2	invasion of deep muscular wall
T 3b	= C	invasion of perivesical fat
T 4	= D	extension to perivesical organs (seminal vesicles, prostate, rectum)

A. EPITHELIAL TUMORS (95%)
    1. Transitional cell carcinoma (95%):
        multicentric, aniline dyes
    2. Squamous cell carcinoma (4%):
        worst prognosis; secondary to chronic disorders
        (infection, stricture, calculi) in schistosomiasis,
        bladder diverticula
    3. Adenocarcinoma (1%): most common in bladder
        exstrophy, less commonly in cystitis glandularis +
        urachal carcinoma (at dome of bladder in urachal
        remnant)
B. NONEPITHELIAL TUMORS
    (a) PRIMARY BENIGN TUMOR
        1. Leiomyoma (most common):
            • hematuria secondary to ulceration
            Site: submucosal / intramural / subserosal
        2. Rhabdomyoma (rare)
        3. Hemangioma
            compressible, phleboliths, associated with
            cutaneous hemangiomas in 25%
        4. Neurofibroma
            generalized neurofibromatosis in 60%

5. Nephrogenic adenoma
    associated with cystitis cystica / cystitis
    glandularis
6. Endometriosis
    on posterior wall, urinary symptoms in 80%
7. Pheochromocytoma (0.5%)
    from paraganglia of bladder wall; 7% are
    malignant
    • postmicturitional adrenergic attack
(b) PRIMARY MALIGNANT TUMOR
    1. Rhabdomyosarcoma
    2. Leiomyosarcoma
        rarely at trigone; mainly > 40 years of age
    3. Primary lymphoma
        2nd most common nonepithelial tumor of urinary
        bladder
        Age: √ 40 years; M:F = 1:3
        Location: submucosal; at bladder base +
                   trigone
(c) SECONDARY TUMORS
    1. Lymphoma: at autopsy in NHL (15%); Hodgkin
        disease (5%)
    2. Leukemia: at autopsy in 22%; microscopic
        involvement
    3. Metastases: 1.5% of bladder malignancies;
        solitary / multiple nodules
        melanoma > stomach > breast > kidney > lung
    4. Direct extension: (common) from prostate,
        rectum, sigmoid, cervix, ovary

CHOLESTEATOMA
= keratin ball = keratinized squamous epithelium shed into
lumen
• history of UTIs
• repeated episodes of renal colic
Location: renal pelvis > upper ureter
√ mottled / stringy filling defects in collecting system
√ dilatation of pelvicaliceal system (with obstruction)
√ calcification of keratinized material possible
No premalignant condition!

CHRONIC GLOMERULONEPHRITIS
Cause: after acute poststreptococcal
            glomerulonephritis
• late presentation without prior clinically apparent acute
  phase
• hypertension
• renal failure
√ small smooth kidneys with wasted parenchyma
√ normal papillae + calices
√ patchy nephrogram with diminished density of contrast
  material
√ cortical calcification (uncommon)
US:
    √ increased echogenicity
    √ vicarious sinus lipomatosis
Angio:
    √ marked reduction in renal blood flow + reflux of
      contrast material into aorta

√ severely pruned + tortuous interlobar and arcuate arteries
√ nonvisualization of interlobular arteries
√ delayed contrast clearance from interlobar arteries

CONGENITAL RENAL HYPOPLASIA
= miniaturization with reduction in number of renal lobes, number of calices and papillae, amount of nephrons (+ smallness of cells)
VARIANT: **Ask-Upmark kidney** = aglomerular focal hypoplasia
√ unilateral small kidney
√ decreased number of papillae + calices (5 or less)
√ hypertrophied contralateral kidney
√ absent renal artery
√ hypoplastic disorganized renal veins

CONN SYNDROME
= PRIMARY HYPERALDOSTERONISM = excess mineralocorticoid production (sodium resorption, potassium excretion)
M:F = 1:2
• hypertension (secondary to hypernatremia); responsible for 2% of all hypertensions
• depressed renin levels
• hypokalemia + alkalosis
• hyperkaliuria
Path:
   (a) adenoma (89%): solitary aldosteronoma (70%); multiple (13%); microadenomatosis (6 %)
   (b) bilateral hyperplasia (11%): diffuse / nodular
√ small aldosteronoma of 1.7 cm average size (range 0.5 – 3.5 cm); bilateral in 6%
√ usually hypervascular, rarely hypovascular
Adrenal venography   : 76% accuracy
Adrenal venous blood sampling : 91% accuracy, 75% sensitivity
CT   : 70 – 80% sensitivity

CUSHING SYNDROME
Etiology:
   A. ACTH-independent
      1. Exogenous cortisol
      2. Primary adrenal abnormality (20%):
         (a) bilateral adrenal cortical hyperplasia (70 – 80% in adults, 19% in children)
         (b) adrenal adenoma (10% in adults, 15% in children)
         (c) adrenal carcinoma (10% in adults, 66% in children)
   B. ACTH-dependent
      1. Exogenous ACTH
      2. Paraneoplastic ectopic ACTH production (20%): oat cell carcinoma of lung (8%), liver, prostate, ovary, breast, carcinoid, bronchial adenoma, pancreatic islet cell tumor, medullary carcinoma of thyroid, thymoma, pheochromocytoma

      3. CUSHING DISEASE = CNS disease
         (a) Pituitary disease: basophilic/chromophobe adenoma / overactive pituitary
         (b) Hypothalamic abnormality
Incidence: 1:1,000 autopsies; M:F = 1:4
Age: 3rd – 4th decade (highest incidence); more often following pregnancy
• central obesity, buffalo hump, moon face
• striae, acne
• impaired glucose tolerance / diabetes mellitus
• hypertension
• elevated plasma cortisol levels
• excessive excretion of urinary 17-hydroxy-corticosteroids
• dexamethasone suppression test / metyrapone test
√ retarded bone maturation
√ osteoporosis
√ excess callus formation
CT:
   √ normal-sized adrenals in 1/3 of adrenal hyperplasia (micronodular form)

EPIDIDYMITIS
Acute Epididymitis
= ACUTE EPIDIDYMO-ORCHITIS
most common acute pathologic process in postpubertal age secondary to ascending infection
Incidence: < 10 years in 0%; 20 – 30 years in 72%
• fever
• increasing pain over 1 – 2 days
• epididymal swelling + tenderness
• prostatic tenderness (infrequent)
• dysuria + frequency (25%)
• pyuria (95%)
• positive urine culture
• leukocytosis (50%)
Organism: E. coli + St. aureus (85%), Gonococcus (12%), TB (2%)
US:
   √ enlarged epididymis with decreased echogenicity
   √ hydrocele + skin thickening
   √ increase in pulsatile sounds on Doppler US
NUC   (true positive rate of 99%):
   √ symmetrical perfusion of iliac + femoral vessels
   √ markedly increased perfusion through spermatic cord vessels (testicular + deferential arteries)
   √ curvilinear increased activity laterally in hemiscrotum on static images; also centrally if testis involved
   √ increased activity of scrotal contents on static images (hyperemia + increased capillary permeability)
DDx: (1) Testicular abscess (increased perfusion with centrally decreased uptake)
         (2) Hydrocele (normal perfusion, no uptake)
         (3) Testicular tumor (slightly increased perfusion; in-/ decreased uptake)

Cx: (1) focal / diffuse orchitis (20 – 40%)
       (2) epididymal abscess (6%) / testicular
            abscess (6%)
       (3) infarction (3%) from extrinsic compression of
            testicular blood flow
       (4) late testicular atrophy (21%)

Chronic Epididymitis
US: √ enlarged hyperechoic epididymis

GANGLIONEUROBLASTOMA
= transitional phase of cellular maturity from
neuroblastoma to ganglioneuroma

GANGLIONEUROMA
= may represent endstage of maturation of a
neuroblastoma
Age: children + young adults; 60% < 20 years; M < F
Location: adrenal gland (20%); mediastinum (43%)
• rarely hormone-active
√ large-sized mass

HEREDITARY CHRONIC NEPHRITIS
= ALPORT SYNDROME = probably autosomal dominant
trait with presence of fat-filled macrophages ("foam
cells") in the corticomedullary junction and medulla
(a) males: progressive renal insufficiency, death
     usually < age 50
(b) females: nonprogressive
• polyuria
• anemia
• salt wasting
• hyposthenuria
• nerve deafness
• ocular abnormalities (congenital cataracts, nystagmus,
  myopia, spherophakia)
• NO hypertension
√ small smooth kidneys
√ diminished density of contrast material
√ cortical calcifications

HYDROCELE
= collection of fluid between parietal and visceral layers of
tunica vaginalis; most common type of fluid collection in
scrotum
(A) PRIMARY = IDIOPATHIC HYDROCELE
    without predisposing lesion as congenital defect of
    lymphatic drainage
(B) SECONDARY HYDROCELE
    (a) inflammation (epididymitis, epididymo-orchitis)
    (b) testicular tumor (in 10 – 40%)
    (c) trauma / postsurgical
    (d) torsion, infarction
(C) CONGENITAL HYDROCELE
    = ascites in scrotum through communication with
    peritoneal cavity (= open processus vaginalis); may
    be associated with inguinal hernia

(D) INFANTILE HYDROCELE
    = hydrocele with fingerlike extension into funicular
    process but without communication with peritoneal
    cavity
US:
√ anechoic, good back wall, through transmission
√ with low level echoes ± septations: hematocele /
  pyocele / cholesterol crystals

HYDRONEPHROSIS
A. OBSTRUCTIVE UROPATHY = HYDRONEPHROSIS
    = dilatation of collecting structures without functional
    deficit
B. OBSTRUCTIVE NEPHROPATHY = dilatation of
    collecting system with renal functional impairment

Acute Hydronephrosis
Cause:
(1) passage of calculus sites of stone impaction at
     points of ureteral narrowing:
     (a) ureterovesicle junction (70%)
     (b) ureteropelvic junction
     (c) crossing of iliac vessels
(2) passage of blood clot (carcinoma, AV
     malformation, trauma, anticoagulant therapy),
     sloughed necrotic papilla
(3) suture on ureter
(4) ureteral edema following instrumentation
(5) sulfonamide crystallization in nonalkalinized urine
• pain (50%)
• urinary tract infection (36%)
• nausea + vomiting (33%)
√ normal-sized kidney with normal parenchymal
  thickness
√ increasingly dense nephrogram
√ delayed appearance of contrast (decreased
  glomerular filtration)
√ increasingly dense nephrogram over time ("obstructed
  nephrogram")
√ minimally dilated collecting system + ureter
√ widening of forniceal angles
√ may be associated with extravasation from forniceal
  tear (pyelosinus reflux)
√ delayed images demonstrate site of obstruction
√ vicarious contrast excretion through gallbladder
  (uncommon)

Chronic Hydronephrosis
= most frequent cause of abdominal mass in first 6
months of life (25% of all neonatal abdominal
masses)
Causes:
(a) acquired: benign + malignant tumors of the
     ureter; ureteral strictures; retroperitoneal tumor /
     fibrosis; neurogenic bladder; cervical / prostatic
     carcinoma; urethral polyps; urethral neoplasm,
     acquired urethral strictures
(b) congenital: UPJ obstruction (22%), posterior
     urethral valves (18%), ectopic ureterocele

(14%), prune belly syndrome (12%), ureteral +
UVJ obstruction (8%); hypertrophy of
verumontanum, urethral diverticulum, congenital
urethral strictures, anterior urethral valves, meatal
stenosis
- insidious course
√ large kidney with wasted parenchyma
√ diminished nephrographic density (decreased
clearance)
√ early "rim" sign (thin band of radiodensity surrounding
calices)
√ delayed opacification of collecting system
√ moderate to marked widening of collecting system
√ tortuous dilated ureter
NUC:
√ photopenic area during vascular phase
√ accumulation of radionuclide tracer within
hydronephrotic collecting system on delayed
images
Cx: superimposed infection (= pyonephrosis)

US Grading system of hydronephrosis:
Grade 0 = homogeneous central renal sinus complex
without separation
Grade 1 = separation of central sinus echoes of ovoid
configuration; continuous echogenic sinus
periphery; 52% predictive value for
obstruction
Grade 2 = separation of central sinus echoes of
rounded configuration; dilated calices
connecting with renal pelvis; continuity of
echogenic sinus periphery
Grade 3 = replacement of major portions of renal
sinus; discontinuity of echogenic sinus
periphery

Focal Hydronephrosis
= HYDROCALICOSIS = HYDROCALYX = obstructed
drainage of one portion of kidney
Causes: (1) Congenital: partial / complete duplication
(2) Infectious stricture: e.g., TB
(3) Infundibular calculus
(4) Tumor
√ unifocal mass, commonly in upper pole
√ absent polar group of calices (early)
√ dilated polar group (late) with displacement of
adjacent calices
√ delayed opacification in obstructed group
√ focally replaced nephrogram
US: √ anechoic cystic lesion with smooth margins
CT: √ focal area of water density with smooth margin
and thick wall

JUXTAGLOMERULAR TUMOR
= RENINOMA = rare tumor arising from renin-producing
juxtaglomerular cells
Age: young female
- hypertension

√ usually 2 – 3 cm renal mass
√ solid echogenic mass ± areas of necrosis / hemorrhage
√ isodense tumor on NECT, hypodense on CECT
√ angiographically hypovascular tumor
√ renal venous blood sampling (high renin level)

LEUKEMIA
Most common malignant cause of bilateral global renal
enlargement!
(a) Diffuse involvement:
leukemic cells infiltrate the interstitial tissue, tubules
are replaced (more common in lymphocytic than in
granulocytic forms); no relationship to peripheral white
blood cell count
(b) Focal involvement:
rarely cause for unifocal renal mass: chloroma,
myeloblastoma, myeloblastic sarcoma
√ large smooth kidneys bilaterally
√ normal or diminished density on nephrogram
√ occasionally attenuated collecting system with
nonopaque filling defects (clot, uric acid)
√ normal to increased echogenicity
√ retroperitoneal adenopathy
DDx: Hodgkin disease, malignant lymphoma, multiple
myeloma

LEUKOPLAKIA
= KERATINIZING SQUAMOUS METAPLASIA /
DYSPLASIA = DYSKERATOSIS
Cause: associated with chronic infection (80%) / stones
(40%)
Histo: large confluent areas / scattered patches of
squamous metaplasia of transitional cell
epithelium with keratinization + cellular atypia in
deeper layers
Peak age: 4th – 5th decade;
M:F = 1:1 (with involvement of renal pelvis)
M:F = 4:1 (with involvement of bladder)
Location: bladder > renal pelvis > ureter; bilateral in 10%
- hematuria (30%)
- recurrent UTIs
- pathognomonic passage of gritty flakes, soft tissue
stones, white chunks of tissue (desquamated
keratinized epithelial layers) leading to colic, fever, chills
√ corrugated / striated irregularities of pelvocalyceal walls,
localized / generalized
√ plaquelike intraluminal mass with "onion skin" pattern of
contrast material in interstices
√ caliectasis + pyelectasis common (with obstruction)
√ ridging / filling defects of ureter
√ associated with calculi in 25 – 50%
Cx: premalignant condition for epidermoid carcinoma in
12% (controversial!)

LOBAR NEPHRONIA
= ACUTE FOCAL BACTERIAL NEPHRITIS = focal variant
of pyelonephritis with single / multiple areas of
suppuration and necrosis

Organisms: E. coli > Proteus > Klebslella
Predisposed:
  patients with altered host resistance (diabetes [60%], immunosuppression), chronic catheterization, mechanical / functional obstruction, trauma
• fever, flank pain, pyuria
√ focal area of absent nephrogram / distorted pyelogram
√ renal arteries displaced, renal veins compressed
√ hypoechoic mass with ill-defined margins and disruption of corticomedullary border, NO fluid collection
√ low attenuation zone with poorly defined transition to surrounding parenchyma
√ Ga-67 uptake
√ vesicoureteral reflux often present
Cx: (1) scarring (2) abscess

LOCALIZED CYSTIC DISEASE
  = multiple simple cysts involving only one portion of the kidney
• no family history
Histo: dilated ducts and tubules varying in size from mm to several cm
Prognosis: not progressive

LYMPHOMA
  Types:
    (a) NON-HODGKIN LYMPHOMA
        renal involvement detected in 5% of abdominal CT, in 33% of autopsy series
    (b) HODGKIN LYMPHOMA
  Patterns of involvement:
    1. primary renal lymphoma (very rare)
    2. hematogenous dissemination (discrete masses) uni- / bilateral (a) single / multiple foci (b) diffuse infiltration
    3. direct extension from adjacent pararenal lymphomatous disease, usually extranodal
• clinically silent (50%)
• compromise of renal function (urinary tract obstruction, renal vein compression, diffuse infiltration of kidney)
√ unilateral:bilateral = 3:1
√ multiple nodular masses (61%)
√ invasion from perirenal disease (11%)
√ single bulky tumor (7%), small solitary tumor (7%)
√ diffuse infiltration (6%), microscopic infiltration (7%)
√ neovascularity, encasement, vascular displacement (occasionally palisade-like configuration)

MALAKOPLAKIA
  = uncommon chronic inflammatory response to Gram-negative infection
Organism: E. coli (in 94%); diabetes mellitus predisposes
Histo: submucosal histiocytic granulomas containing large foamy mononuclear cells (Hansemann macrophages) with intracytoplasmatic basophilic PAS-positive inclusion bodies (Michaelis-Gutmann bodies) consisting of incompletely

destroyed E. coli bacterium surrounded by lipoprotein membranes
Peak age: 5th – 7th decade; M:F = 1:4
• hematuria
• raised yellow lesion < 3 cm in diameter
Location: bladder > lower 2/3 of ureter > upper ureter > renal pelvis; multifocal in 75%; bilateral in 50%
√ multiple dome-shaped smooth mural filling defects
√ scalloped appearance if lesions confluent
√ generalized pelviureteral dilatation (if obstructive)
√ displacement of pelvocaliceal system + distorted central sinus complex
√ multifocal parenchymal masses may cause diminished / absent nephrogram
DDx: pyeloureteritis cystica

MALPOSITIONED TESTIS
  = MALDESCENDED TESTIS
    testes are normally within scrotum by 28 – 32 weeks MA
Incidence: at birth in 10% (in babies > 2,500 g in 3.4%; in premature babies in 30%); by 3 – 4 months in 0.8%; at puberty in 0.2 – 0.8%
1. **Pseudocryptorchidism**
   = RETRACTILE TESTIS = unusually spastic cremasteric muscle
2. **Cryptorchidism**
   = arrested descent of testis along its normal course bilateral in 10%, anorchia in 3 – 5%
   Location: high scrotal, inguinal canal, abdomen (20%)
3. **Ectopia testis**
   = deviation from the usual pathway
   Location: interstitial (on oblique muscle), pubopenile, perineal, femoral triangle
Cx: (1) Sterility
      (2) Malignancy: most commonly seminoma, 48 x risk, 4 – 11% of all testicular tumors found in cryptorchidism
      (3) Torsion: 10 x risk in cryptorchidism
Test-Sensitivity:
  US   : 20 – 88% (DDx: Lymph node)
  CT   : 95%
  Venography : 50 – 90%

MECKEL-GRUBER SYNDROME
autosomal recessive
Incidence: 1:50,000; more common among Yemenite Jews
Risk of recurrence: 25%
• History of affected siblings
OB-US:
  √ large polycystic kidneys containing 2 – 10 mm cysts
  √ occipital encephalocele
  √ polydactyly
  √ microcephaly
  √ cleft lip and palate
  √ oligohydramnios (onset midtrimester)
  √ inability to visualize urine within fetal bladder

OB-management:
1. Chromosomal analysis to exclude trisomy 13 (if no prior family history)
2. Option of pregnancy termination < 24 weeks GA
3. Nonintervention for fetal distress > 24 weeks GA

Prognosis: invariably fatal at birth due to pulmonary hypoplasia + renal failure

MEDULLARY CYSTIC DISEASE

= variable number of medullary cysts (100 μ to 2 cm) + progressive periglomerular and interstitial fibrosis + tubular atrophy with dilatation of some proximal tubules

Types:
(1) <u>MEDULLARY CYSTIC DISEASE</u> = ADULT ONSET
autosomal dominant, in young adults, rapidly progressive course with uremia + death in 2 years
(2) <u>JUVENILE NEPHRONOPHTHYSIS</u> = JUVENILE ONSET
autosomal recessive, in children, average duration of 10 years before uremia and death occurs

- salt-wasting, polyuria, polydypsia
- failure-to-thrive, growth retardation (in early teens)
- uremia, anemia, normal sediment, hypertension (only in late phase)
√ bilateral normal / small kidneys with smooth contour + thin cortex
√ "medullary nephrogram" = medullary striations persistent for up to 2 hours; occasionally replaced by sharply defined multiple thin-walled lucencies

US / CT:
√ increased parenchymal echogenicity + loss of corticomedullary junction
√ multiple small medullary / corticomedullary cysts

MEDULLARY SPONGE KIDNEY

= dysplastic cystic dilatation of papillary + medullary portions of collecting ducts (first few generations of metanephric duct branchings)

Incidence: 0.5%
Age: young to middle aged adults; sporadic
May be associated with: Ehlers-Danlos syndrome, parathyroid adenoma, Caroli disease

- often asymptomatic
√ medullary nephrocalcinosis (40 – 80%) with one / more calculi up to 5 mm
√ "bunch of flowers" = thick dense streaks of contrast material radiating from pyramids peripherally representing papillary cysts / ectatic ducts (DDx: dense papillary blush in normals)
√ may be unilateral in 25%
√ may involve only one pyramid, involvement of all pyramids (25%)

Cx: urolithiasis, hematuria, infection
DDx:
(1) Normal variant: "papillary blush" w/o distinct streaks / nephrocalcinosis / pyramidal enlargement
(2) Renal tuberculosis: larger more irregular calcifications + cavitations + strictures + ulcerations

(3) Papillary necrosis: sloughed papilla + caliceal ring sign
(4) Medullary nephrocalcinosis: no ectatic ducts / cysts; calcifications beyond pyramids
(5) Juvenile polycystic kidney disease: bilateral renal enlargement + hepatic periportal fibrosis
(6) Caliceal diverticulum: small, solitary, located between pyramid

MEGACALICOSIS

= CONGENITAL MEGACALICES = nonprogressive caliceal dilatation caused by hypoplastic medullary pyramids

Age: any age; M >> F
May be associated with primary megaureter

- normal glomerular filtration rate

Site: entire kidney / part of kidney; unilateral / bilateral
√ kidney usually enlarged with prominent fetal lobation
√ reduced parenchymal thickness (medulla affected, NOT cortex)
√ mosaic-like arrangement of dilated calices (polygonal + faceted appearance, NOT globular as in obstruction)
√ increased number of calices
√ ABSENT caliceal cupping (semilunar instead of pyramidal configuration of papillae)
√ NO dilatation of pelvis / ureters, NORMAL contrast excretion

Cx: (1) hematuria (2) stone formation

MEGACYSTIS-MICROCOLON SYNDROME

= MEGACYSTIS-MICROCOLON-INTESTINAL HYPOPERISTALSIS SYNDROME (MMIH)
= functional obstruction of colon + bladder characterized by
(1) strikingly short small intestine suspended on a primitive dorsal mesentery
(2) small colon
(3) enlarged urinary bladder
(4) markedly enlarged kidneys with little remaining parenchyma

Incidence: 26 cases reported; predominantly in females
May be associated with: diaphragmatic hernia, PDA, natal teeth

- distended abdomen (large bladder + dilated small bowel loops)
- intestinal pseudo-obstruction (NO peristaltic activity)

OB-US:
√ polyhydramnios (in spite of dilated bladder) / normal amount of amniotic fluid
√ megacystis
√ bilateral hydroureteronephrosis
√ female sex

BE:
√ microcolon (transient feature of narrow rectum + sigmoid)
√ malrotation / malfixation or foreshortening of small bowel

VCUG: √ distended unobstructed bladder
Prognosis: lethal in most cases

MEGALOURETER
- = CONGENITAL PRIMARY MEGAURETER = TERMINAL URETERECTASIS = ACHALASIA OF URETER
- = intrinsic congenital dilatation of lower juxtavesical orthotopic ureter

Cause: aperistaltic juxtavesical segment (1.5 cm) secondary to faulty development of muscle layers of ureter (functional, NOT mechanical obstruction)

Incidence: at all ages; M:F = 2:1

Location: L:R = 3:1, bilateral in 20 – 40%
- pain
- asymptomatic (mostly)
- abdominal mass
- hematuria
- infection

Associated disorders (40%):
  (a) contralateral: UPJ obstruction, reflux, ureterocele, ureteral duplication, renal ectopia, renal agenesis
  (b) ipsilateral: caliceal diverticulum, megacalicosis, papillary necrosis

√ prominent localized dilatation of pelvic ureter (up to 5 cm in diameter) usually not progressive, but may involve entire ureter + collecting system
√ vigorous non-propulsive to-and-fro motion in dilated segment
√ functional smoothly tapered narrowing of intravesical ureter
√ NO reflux, NO narrowing

MESOBLASTIC NEPHROMA
- = FETAL RENAL HAMARTOMA = BENIGN CONGENITAL WILMS TUMOR = BENIGN FETAL HAMARTOMA = FETAL MESENCHYMAL TUMOR = LEIOMYOMATOUS HAMARTOMA
- = nonfamilial benign fibromyomatoid mass arising from renal connective tissue

Histo: smooth muscle cells + immature fibroblasts + islands of glomeruli, tubules, vessels + hematopoietic cells + islets of cartilage

Age: most common solid renal mass in neonate; M > F; may occasionally go undetected until adulthood
- hypertension
- large flank mass

√ usually replaces 60 – 90% of renal parenchyma, may produce multiple cystic spaces
√ NO sharp cleavage plane towards normal parenchyma, may extend beyond capsule
√ calcifications (rare)
√ NO venous extension (DDx from Wilms tumor)
OB-US:
  √ polyhydramnios
  √ evenly echogenic tumor resembling uterine fibroids
IVP:
  √ large noncalcified renal mass with distortion of collecting system

√ usually NO herniation into renal pelvis (DDx from MLCN)
Rx: surgery

METASTASES TO KIDNEY
Most common malignant tumor of the kidney (2 x as frequent as primaries)
most common: bronchus, breast, stomach,
less common: chloroma, myeloblastoma, myeloblastic sarcoma, melanoma, osteogenic sarcoma, choriocarcinoma, rhabdomyosarcoma, Hodgkin lymphoma, malignant lymphoma

MULTICYSTIC DYSPLASTIC KIDNEY
- = MULTICYSTIC DYSGENETIC KIDNEY (MCDK)
- = MULTICYSTIC KIDNEY (MCK) = Potter Type II
Second most common cause of an abdominal mass in neonate (after hydronephrosis); most common form of cystic disease in infants

Incidence: 1:10,000 (in bilateral MCDK); M:F = 2:1 (in unilateral MCDK); more common in infants of diabetic mothers

Risk of recurrence: 2 – 3%
Etiology: (sporadic)
  extrarenal obstruction / atresia < 8 – 10 weeks of fetal life leads to aberrant development of collecting ducts and tubules + failure of development of nephrons + cystic expansion of abnormal tubules (after 20 weeks of MA)
Histo: immature glomeruli + tubules reduced in number + whorling mesenchymal tissue, cartilage (33%), cysts
- abdominal mass
- asymptomatic if unilateral (may go undetected until adulthood) or recurrent urinary tract infections, intermittent abdominal pain, nausea + vomiting, hematuria, failure to thrive
- fatal due to pulmonary hypoplasia if bilateral

Associated with   renal anomalies of contralateral side in 30 – 50 %:
  (1) Ureteropelvic junction obstruction (7 – 27%)
  (2) Horseshoe kidney (5 – 9%)
  (3) Ureteral anomalies (5%)
  (4) Renal hypoplasia (4%)
  (5) Vesicoureteral reflux
  (6) Malrotation
Fatal form: bilateral MCDK (4.5 – 21%), contralateral renal agenesis (0 – 11%)

Location:
  1. UNILATERAL multicystic dysplastic kidney secondary to pelvoinfundibular atresia, most common form; L > R
  2. SEGMENTAL / focal renal dysplasia = "multilocular cyst" in upper pole of duplex kidney with high-grade obstruction from an ectopic ureterocele or in a single infundibulum)

3. BILATERAL cystic dysplasia
   in the presence of severe obstruction in utero from
   posterior urethral valves / urethral atresia with
   oligohydramnios + pulmonary hypoplasia
Types:
  (1) MULTICYSTIC KIDNEY (IIA)
      √ large kidney with multiple large cysts + little
        visible renal parenchyma
  (2) HYPOPLASTIC / DIMINUTIVE FORM (IIB):
      √ echogenic small kidney

APPEARANCE RELATED TO SITE OF OBSTRUCTION
  (a) ureteropelvic junction
      √ single / several large / multiple medium-sized
        cysts in large kidney
  (b) distal ureteric / urethral obstruction
      √ small / no cysts in small kidney

APPEARANCE RELATED TO TIME OF INSULT
  (a) early onset between 8th – 11th week
      small / atretic renal pelvis + calices
      √ 10 – 20 cysts + loss of reniform appearance
  (b) late onset = HYDRONEPHROTIC FORM
      √ large central cyst (= dilated pelvis) often
        communicating with cysts
      √ some renal function may be demonstrated

√ large kidney with lobulated contour in infancy / incidental
  finding of small kidney in adults secondary to arrested
  growth
√ ipsilateral atretic ureter
√ contralateral renal hypertrophy
√ calcification: curvilinear / ringlike in wall of cysts in
  30% of adults, rarely in children
IVP + NUC:
  √ no function (rarely faint contrast accumulation)
US:
  √ normal renal architecture replaced
  √ random round anechoic masses separated by septa
    ("cluster of grapes"), predominantly of peripheral
    location, largest cyst not medial, no communication
    between cysts, cysts begin to disappear in infancy
  √ central sinus complex absent
  √ no identification of parenchymal rim or
    corticomedullary differentiation
  √ kidney may be small + atrophic (as little as 1 g) /
    normal / large
  √ oligohydramnios in bilateral MCDK / contralateral
    obstruction
Angio:
  √ absent / hypoplastic renal artery; angiography
    unnecessary since a DDx to long standing
    functionless kidney is not possible
OB-management:
  (1) Routine antenatal care + evaluation by pediatric
      urologist following delivery if unilateral
  (2) Option of pregnancy termination if > 24 weeks GA
  (3) Nonintervention for fetal distress if > 24 weeks GA

MULTILOCULAR CYSTIC NEPHROMA
= MLCN = MULTILOCULAR CYST = CYSTIC
  NEPHROMA = CYSTIC ADENOMA = POLYCYSTIC
  NEPHROBLASTOMA = CYSTIC NEPHROBLASTOMA
  = WELL-DIFFERENTIATED POLYCYSTIC WILMS
  TUMOR = PARTIALLY POLYCYSTIC KIDNEY
= benign neoplasm originating from metanephric blastema
  with malignant potential
Histo: undifferentiated mesenchymal and primitive
         glomerulotubular elements
Age: biphasic age + sex distribution: < 4 years in > 75%
       male; > 4 years in > 90% female; boys 3 months to
       4 years (peak 3 – 24 months) + women 4 – 8th
       decade (peak 50 – 60 years)
√ unilateral unifocal well-circumscribed mass
  (characteristic) usually in lower pole
√ cluster of noncommunicating cysts of various sizes
  separated by thick septa
√ tortuous fine vessels coursing through septa
√ thick fibrous capsule
√ calcifications: peripheral / nonperipheral; linear to
  flocculent (uncommon)
√ echogenicity: mixed anechoic to hyperechoic
√ often herniation into renal pelvis
√ gelatinous fluid
Cx: development into nephroblastoma (in infants) /
      sarcoma (in older patients)

MULTIPLE ENDOCRINE NEOPLASIA
= MEA = MULTIPLE ENDOCRINE NEOPLASIAS (MEN)
= familial autosomal dominant adenomatous hyperplasia

		reminder:
Type I = Wermer syndrome		PPP
Type II = Sipple syndrome (Type IIA)		PMP
Type III = Mucosal neuroma syndrome (Type IIB)		MPM

MEA	Type I	Type II	Type III
Pituitary adenoma	+		
Parathyroid adenoma	+	+	
Medullary thyroid carcinoma		+	+
Pancreatic island cell tumor	+		
Pheochromocytoma		+	+
Mucosal neuroma syndrome			+

Pancreatic islet cell tumors are:
  (a) insulinoma
  (b) gastrinoma = Zollinger-Ellison syndrome
  (c) VIPoma = WDHA-syndrome (watery diarrhea,
      hypokalemia, achlorhydria)

MULTIPLE MYELOMA
Administration of contrast material poses potential
hazards!
It is essential that dehydration is avoided!
• Tamm-Horsfall proteinuria (tubular cell secretion)

Impairment of renal function:
(1) precipitation of abnormal proteins into tubule lumen (30 – 50%)
(2) toxicity of Bence-Jones proteins on tubules
(3) impaired renal blood flow secondary to increased blood viscosity
(4) amyloidosis
(5) nephrocalcinosis from hypercalcemia
√ smooth normal to large kidneys (initially), become small with time
√ occasionally attenuated pelvo-infundibulo-caliceal system
√ normal to diminished contrast material density; increasingly dense in acute oliguric failure
US: √ normal to increased echogenicity

MYCETOMA
= FUNGUS BALL
Organism: typically Candida, Aspergillus, Mucor, Cryptococcus, Phycomycetes, Actinomycetes mostly mycelial (M-form), occasionally yeast cells (Y-form)
Predisposed: diabetics, debilitating illness, prolonged antibiotic therapy, leukemia, lymphoma, thymoma, immunosuppression
• flank pain, passing of tissue, hematuria (extremely rare)
• renal candidiasis associated with candidemia
• candida cystitis preceded by vaginal candidiasis
√ unilateral nonvisualization of kidney (most frequent)
√ large irregular filling defect extending into dilated calices (retrograde study)
√ necrotizing papillitis from candida nephritis (common)
√ lacelike pattern (on antegrade study)

NEPHROBLASTOMATOSIS
= persistent metanephrogenic blastema as a potential precursor of Wilms tumor; primitive renal tissue normally present up to 36 weeks gestational age
Incidence: in 30% of kidneys with single and 100% of kidneys with bilateral Wilms tumor
Age: neonatal period, infancy, childhood
Associated with:
hemihypertrophy, sporadic aniridia, pseudohermaphroditism, Klippel-Trenaunay syndrome, Beckwith-Wiedemann syndrome, splenic agenesis with hepatic malformation
√ kidneys may be enlarged
√ deformity of pelvocaliceal system
US:
√ subtle subcapsular nodules (hypo- / iso- / hyperechoic)
CT:
√ hypodense subcapsular nodules after contrast enhancement

NEPHROCALCINOSIS
Medullary Nephrocalcinosis
= calcifications involving the distal convoluted tubules in the loops of Henle

Incidence: 95% of all nephrocalcinoses
Causes:
A. HYPERCALCURIA
(a) ENDOCRINE
1. Hyperparathyroidism in 5% (primary >> secondary)
2. Paraneoplastic syndrome of lung + kidney primary (ectopic parathormone production)
3. Cushing syndrome
4. Diabetes insipidus
5. Hyperthyroidism
(b) ALIMENTARY
1. Milk-alkali syndrome (excess calcium + alkali = milk + antacids)
2. Hypervitaminosis D
3. Beryllium poisoning
(c) OSSEOUS
1. Osseous metastases and multiple myeloma
2. Prolonged immobilization
3. Progressive senile osteoporosis
(d) RENAL
1. Renal tubular acidosis (in 73% of primary RTA)
2. Medullary sponge kidney
(e) DRUG THERAPY
1. Furosemide
2. Steroids
(f) MISCELLANEOUS
1. Sarcoidosis
2. Idiopathic hypercalcuria
3. Idiopathic hypercalcemia
B. HYPEROXALURIA = OXALOSIS
1. **Primary hyperoxaluria**
= Hereditary hyperoxaluria (more common) rare autosomal recessive inherited enzyme deficiency of carboligase with diffuse oxalate deposition in kidneys, heart, blood vessels, lung, spleen, bone marrow
Age: usually < 5 years
Prognosis: early death in childhood
2. **Secondary hyperoxaluria** = Enteric hyperoxaluria (rare)
secondary to disturbance of bile acid metabolism after jejunoileal bypass, ileal resection, blind loop syndrome, Crohn disease, increased ingestion (green leafy vegetables), pyridoxine deficiency, ethylene glycol poisoning, methoxyflurane anesthesia
C. HYPERURICOSURIA
gouty kidney, Lesch-Nyhan syndrome
D. URINARY STASIS
1. Milk-of-calcium in pyelocaliceal diverticulum
2. Medullary sponge kidney
E. DYSTROPHIC CALCIFICATION
1. Renal papillary necrosis

√ normal sized / occasionally enlarged kidneys (medullary sponge kidney)

√ grouped rounded / linear calcifications
√ small poorly defined / large coarse granular calcifications in renal pyramids
US:
√ absence of hypoechoic papillary structures (earliest sign)
√ hyperechoic rim at corticomedullary junction + around tip and sides of pyramids
√ solitary focus of hyperechogenicity at tip of pyramid near fornix
√ increased echogenicity of renal pyramids ± shadowing
√ no acoustic shadowing with small + light calcifications
DDx of hyperechoic medulla in newborns:
Oliguria with transient tubular blockage by Tamm-Horsfall proteinuria
Cx: often followed by urolithiasis

Cortical Nephrocalcinosis
Incidence: 5% of all nephrocalcinoses
Causes:
1. Acute cortical necrosis
2. Chronic glomerulonephritis
3. Alport syndrome = hereditary nephritis + deafness
4. Congenital oxalosis, Primary hyperoxaluria
5. Chronic paraneoplastic hypercalcemia
6. Rejected renal transplant
US:
√ homogeneously increased echogenicity of renal parenchyma > liver echogenicity

NEUROBLASTOMA
Most common solid abdominal mass of infancy (12.3% of all perinatal neoplasms), 3rd most common malignant tumor in infancy (after leukemia + CNS tumors), 2nd most common tumor in childhood (Wilms tumor more common in older children), 7% of all childhood cancers; 15% of cancer deaths in children
Origin: neural crest
Path: round irregular lobulated mass of 50 – 150 g with areas of hemorrhage + necrosis
Histo: small round cells slightly larger than lymphocytes with scant cytoplasm; Horner-Wright rosettes = one / two layers of neuroblasts surrounding a central zone of tangled neurofibrillary processes
Incidence: 1:7,100 to 1:10,000 live births; 500 cases per year in USA; 20% hereditary
Age: 25% during 1st year; 50% < 2 years; 75% in < 4 years; 90% in < 8 years; occasionally present at birth; M:F = 1:1
May be associated with aganglionosis of bowel, CHD
- pain + fever (30%)
- palpable abdominal mass (45 – 54%)
- bone pain, limp, inability to walk (20%)
- myoclonus of trunk + extremities
- cerebellar ataxia, nystagmus (20%)
- opsoclonus = spontaneous conjugate + chaotic eye movements (sign of cerebellar disease)

- orbital ecchymosis / proptosis (12%)
- intractable diarrhea (9%) due to increase in vasoactive intestinal polypeptides (VIP)
- increased catecholamine production (75 – 90%): in 95% excreted in urine as vanillylmandelic acid (VMA) / homovanillic acid (HVA)
  - hypertension (up to 30%)
  - acute cerebellar encephalopathy
  - paroxysmal episodes of flushing, tachycardia, headaches, sweating
  - rise in body temperature
  - hyperglycemia
Stages
  I   limited to organ of origin
  II   regional spread not crossing midline
  III   extension across midline
  IV   metastatic to distant lymph nodes, liver, bone, brain, lung
  IVs   stages I + II with disease confined to liver, skin, bone marrow WITHOUT radiographic evidence of skeletal metastases
Metastases:
bone (60%), regional lymph nodes (42%), liver (15%), intracranial (14%), lung (10%)
Δ metastases are first manifestation in up to 60%
Hutchinson syndrome
(1) primary adrenal neuroblastoma (2) extensive skeletal metastases, particularly skull (3) proptosis (4) bone pain
Pepper syndrome
(1) primary adrenal neuroblastoma (2) massive hepatomegaly from metastases
Blueberry muffin syndrome
(1) primary adrenal neuroblastoma (2) multiple metastatic skin lesions
Δ bone marrow aspirate positive in 50 – 70% at time of initial diagnosis
Δ 2/3 of patients > 2 years have disseminated disease
@ Skeletal metastases:
√ periosteal reaction
√ osteolytic focus / multicentric lytic lesions
√ lucent horizontal metaphyseal line
√ vertical linear radiolucent streaks in metadiaphysis of long bones
√ pathologic fracture
√ vertebral collapse
√ widened cranial sutures (subjacent dural metastases)
√ sclerotic lesions with healing
DDx: Ewing sarcoma, rhabdomyosarcoma, leukemia, lymphoma
@ Intracranial + maxillofacial metastases:
Site: dura, brain substance
@ Pulmonary metastases:
√ nodular infiltrates
√ rib erosion
√ mediastinal + retrocrural lymphadenopathy (common)

Location: anywhere within sympathetic neural chain
(1) abdomen
    (a) adrenal (36%): almost always unilateral
    (b) bilateral adrenals (7 – 10%)
    (c) extraadrenal in sympathetic chain (18%)
(2) thorax + posterior mediastinum (14%)
(3) neck (5%)
(4) pelvis (5%)
(5) skull / esthesioneuroblastoma of olfactory bulb,
    cerebellum, cerebrum (2%)
(6) other sites (10%): e.g., intrarenal (very rare)
(7) unknown (10%)

√ large suprarenal mass with irregular shape + margins
(82%)
√ heterogeneous with low density areas from hemorrhage
+ necrosis (55%)
√ stippled / coarse calcifications (36 – 70%)
√ "drooping lily" sign = displacement of kidney
inferolaterally without distortion of collecting system
√ hydronephrosis (24%)
√ inseparable from kidney ± invasion of kidney (32%)
√ propensity for extension into spine + erosion of pedicles
(15%)
√ extension across midline (55%) (DDx: Wilms tumor)
√ retroperitoneal adenopathy / contiguous extension
(73%)
√ retrocrural adenopathy (27%)
√ encasement of IVC + aorta, celiac axis, SMA (32%)
√ caval involvement = indicator of unresectability
√ tracer uptake on bone scan (60%)
√ liver metastases (18 – 66%); invasion of liver (5%)
Angio:
    √ hypo- / hypervascular mass
US:
    √ hyper- / hypoechoic mass with acoustic shadows
OB-US:
    • maternal symptoms of catecholamine excess
    √ mixed cystic + solid mass in adrenal region
    √ may exhibit acoustic shadowing (calcifications)

Prognosis versus Age at Presentation (2-year survival):
    60%   if patient's age < 1 year
    20%   if patient's age 1 – 2 years
    10%   if patient's age > 2 years
    Δ may revert to benign ganglioneuroma in 0.2%

Survival rate versus Stage:
    Stage I   80% survival rate
    Stage II   60% survival rate
    Stage III   30% survival rate
    Stage IV   7% survival rate
    Stage IVs 75 – 87% survival rate

DDx: exophytic Wilms tumor, mesoblastic nephroma,
    multicystic kidney, retroperitoneal teratoma,
    adrenal hemorrhage, hepatic hamartoma /
    hemangioma

NEUROGENIC BLADDER
Bladder innervation of detrusor muscle by
parasympathetic nerves S2 – S4
Etiology: Congenital (myelomeningocele); trauma;
    neoplasm (spinal, CNS); infection (herpes,
    polio); inflammation (multiple sclerosis, syrinx);
    systemic disorder (diabetes, pernicious
    anemia)
A.   SPASTIC BLADDER
    "upper motor neuron" lesion above conus
B.   ATONIC BLADDER
    "lower motor neuron lesion" below conus

PAGE KIDNEY
= renin-angiotensin mediated hypertension caused by
    renal compression in a perinephric / subcapsular
    location
Etiology: (1) spontaneous hematoma (most common)
    (2) blunt trauma (3) cyst (4) tumor
√ stretching + splaying of intrarenal vessels
√ slow arterial washout
√ distortion of renal contour + thinning of renal
    parenchyma
√ enlarged + displaced capsular artery

PAPILLARY NECROSIS
= NECROTIZING PAPILLITIS = ischemic necrobiosis of
    medulla (loops of Henle + vasa recta) secondary to
    interstitial nephritis (interstitial edema) or intrinsic
    vascular obstruction
Causes :
    mnemonic: "POSTCARD"
    Pyelonephritis
    Obstruction
    Sickle cell disease
    Tuberculosis
    Cirrhosis = alcoholism
    Analgesic nephropathy
    Renal vein thrombosis
    Diabetes
  also: dehydration, hemophilia, Christmas disease,
    severe infantile diarrhea, transplant rejection,
    postpartum state, high-dose urography,
    intravesical instillation of formalin, thyroid cancer
Types:
  1.   Necrosis in situ = necrotic papilla detaches but
    remains unextruded within its bed
  2.   Medullary type (partial papillary slough) = single
    irregular cavity located concentric / eccentric in
    papilla with long axis paralleling the long axis of the
    papilla + communicating with calyx
  3.   Papillary type (total papillary slough)
Phases:
  (1)   enlargement of papilla (papillary swelling)
  (2)   fine projections of contrast material alongside
    papilla (tract formation)
  (3)   medullary cavitation / complete slough of papilla
• flank pain, dysuria, fever, chills

- ureteral colic, hematuria
- acute oliguric renal failure
- hypertension
- proteinuria, pyuria, hematuria, leukocytosis

Location:
- — localized / diffuse
- — bilateral distribution (systemic cause)
- — unilateral (obstruction, renal vein thrombosis, acute bacterial nephritis)

√ normal or small kidney (analgesic nephropathy) / large kidney (acute fulminant)
√ smooth / wavy renal contour (analgesic nephropathy)
√ diminished density of contrast material in nephrogram; rarely increasingly dense
√ wasted parenchymal thickness
√ widened fornix (necrotic shrinkage) + club-shaped calyx (detached papilla)
√ displaced collecting system (enlarged septal cortex from edema)
√ intraluminal filling defect (sloughed papilla)
√ calcifications: papillary / curvilinear / ringlike (attached papilla)
US: √ multiple round / triangular cystic spaces in medulla
Cx: higher incidence of transitional cell carcinoma in analgesic abusers (8 x); higher incidence of squamous cell carcinoma
DDx: (1) postobstructive renal atrophy
(2) congenital megacalices (normal renal function)

PARATESTICULAR TUMORS
Only 4% of all scrotal tumors
A. BENIGN TUMOR
1. **Adenomatoid tumor** (30%)
= benign slow-growing neoplasm within epididymis (particularly in globus minor), 2nd – 4th decade
√ well-marginated mass with echogenicity equal to / greater than testis
2. Polyorchidism
3. Others: carcinoid, papillary cystadenoma of epididymis, leiomyoma, fibroma, adrenal rest, cholesteatoma, lipoma
B. MALIGNANT TUMOR
1. Sarcomas: rhabdomyo-, leiomyo-, lipo-, fibro-, embryonal sarcoma
2. Metastases

PHEOCHROMOCYTOMA
= rare tumor of chromaffin tissue; responsible for 0.1% of hypertensions
Incidence: 0.13% in autopsy series; sporadic occurrence in 94%
Symptomatology secondary to excess catecholamine production:
- asymptomatic (9%)
- headaches, sweating, flushing, palpitations, anxiety, tremor
- nausea, vomiting, abdominal pain, chest pain

- paroxysmal (47%) / sustained (37%) hypertension
(a) elevated catecholamine
(b) functional renal vasoconstriction
(c) renal artery stenosis (fibrosis, intimal proliferation, tumor encasement)
- hypoglycemia during hypertensive crisis
- elevated urine vanillylmandelic acid (VMA) in 54%; in up to 22% false-negative result because VMA not excreted
Associated with:
(1) Multiple endocrine adenomas (MEA) in 6%:
(a) Sipple syndrome = MEA Type II
= medullary carcinoma of thyroid + parathyroid adenoma + pheochromocytoma
(b) **Mucosal neuroma syndrome** = MEA Type III
= medullary carcinoma of thyroid + intestinal ganglioneuromatosis + pheochromocytoma
- long slender extremities (Marfanoid)
- prominent lips
- nodular deformity of tongue
- corneal limbus thickening
√ thickened colonic folds + abnormal haustral pattern + diverticula
(2) von Hippel-Lindau syndrome
(3) Neurofibromatosis
(4) Familial pheochromocytosis

Location: subdiaphragmatic in 98%
(a) adrenal gland (90%)
(b) extraadrenal (10% in adults, 31% in children) para-aortic sympathetic chain, organ of Zuckerkandl at origin of inferior mesenteric artery (2%), gonads, urinary bladder

MULTIPLICITY (in > 80% solitary; in 5% multiple):
10% in nonfamilial adult cases
32% in nonfamilial childhood cases
65% in familial syndromes

RULE OF TENS:
10% bilateral / multiple   **10%** extraadrenal
10% malignant   **10%** familial

CT: localization accurate in 91% with tumor > 2 cm in size; up to 40% in extraadrenal location are missed by CT
√ solid / cystic / complex mass with low-density areas secondary to hemorrhage / necrosis
√ mean size 5 cm (range 3 – 12 cm)
√ calcifications may be present
NUC: I-131 MIBG (metaiodobenzylguanidine) scan sensitivity of 80 – 90%; specificity of > 90%
MRI:
√ much higher intensity than liver (on SE 2,500 / 80 sequence)
Angio: intraarterial injection CONTRAINDICATED (induces hypertensive crisis)
√ venous blood sampling (at different levels in IVC)

√ localization by aortography in > 91%
√ usually hypervascular lesion with intense tumor blush
√ enlarged feeding arteries + neovascularity ("spoke wheel" pattern)
√ parasitization from intrarenal perforating branches
Cx: malignancy in 14%; metastases (may be hormonally active) to bone, lymph nodes, liver, lung

POLYARTERITIS NODOSA
= PERIARTERITIS NODOSA = systemic vascular disease with focal necrotizing inflammation of vessel walls affecting medium + small arteries; mucoid degeneration + fibrinoid necrosis begins within media; main vessels spared (DDx: necrotizing angiitis, mycotic aneurysm); M > F
• malaise, low-grade fever, weight loss
• renal failure
@ Kidney is most frequently affected organ (85%)
√ multiple small intrarenal aneurysms (interlobar, arcuate, interlobular arteries)
√ aneurysms may disappear (thrombosis) or appear in new locations
√ arterial narrowing + thrombosis (chronic stage / healing stage)
√ multiple small cortical infarcts
Cx: perinephric / subcapsular hemorrhage (rupture of aneurysm)
@ Liver (66%)
@ Mesenteric vessels (50%)
• abdominal pain, ulcer formation, GI bleeding, intestinal infarction
@ Skeletal muscle (39%)
@ Skin (20%)

POLYCYSTIC KIDNEY DISEASE
Autosomal Dominant Polycystic Kidney Disease
= ADULT POLYCYSTIC KIDNEY DISEASE = slowly progressive disease with nearly 100% penetrance and great variation in expressivity
Risk of recurrence: 50%
Incidence: 1:1,000 people carry the mutant gene; 3rd most prevalent cause of chronic renal failure
Histo: abnormal rate of tubule divisions (Potter Type III) with hypoplasia of portions of tubules left behind as the ureteral bud advances; cystic dilatation of Bowman capsule, loop of Henle, proximal convoluted tubule, coexisting with normal tissue
Mean age at diagnosis: 43 years (neonatal / infantile onset has been reported); M:F = 1:1
Δ isolated cases reported in utero / neonatal period (simulating infantile PCKD)
Associated with:
(a) cysts in: liver (30 – 50%), pancreas (9%); rare in lung, spleen, thyroid, ovaries, uterus, testis, seminal vesicles, epididymis

(b) aneurysm: saccular "berry" aneurysm of cerebral arteries (10 – 30%)

• symptomatic at mean age of 35 years (cysts are growing with age)
• hypertension (50 – 70%)
• azotemia
• hematuria, proteinuria
• lumbar / abdominal pain
√ bilaterally large kidneys with multifocal round lesions; unilateral enlargement may be the first manifestation of the disease
√ cysts may calcify
√ elongated + distorted + attenuated collecting system
√ nodular puddling of contrast material on delayed images
√ "swiss cheese" nephrogram = multiple lesions of varying size with smooth margins
√ polycystic kidneys shrink after beginning of renal failure, after renal transplantation, or on chronic hemodialysis
NUC: poor renal function on Tc-99m DTPA scan
√ multiple areas of diminished activity, cortical activity only in areas of functioning cortex
US:
√ multiple anechoic masses (adults)
√ diffusely echogenic when cysts small (children)
OB-US:
√ enlarged kidneys with increased echogenicity / multiple cysts (usually in 3rd trimester), may appear unilateral
√ oligohydramnios / normal amount of amniotic fluid
Cx:
(1) Death from azotemia / cerebral hemorrhage (secondary to hypertension or ruptured aneurysm [10%]) / cardiac complications (mean age 50 years)
(2) Renal calculi
(3) Urinary tract infection
DDx:
(1) multiple simple cysts (less diffuse, no family history)
(2) von Hippel-Lindau disease (cerebellar hemangioblastoma, retinal hemangiomas, occasionally pheochromocytomas)
(3) Acquired uremic cystic disease (kidneys small, no renal function, transplant)
(4) infantile PCKD (usually microscopic cysts)

Autosomal Recessive Polycystic Kidney Disease
= INFANTILE POLYCYSTIC KIDNEY DISEASE
= POLYCYSTIC DISEASE OF CHILDHOOD = Potter Type I
Incidence: 1: 6,000 to 1:50,000 live births; F > M
Path:
(a) kidney: abnormal proliferation + dilatation of renal tubules resulting in multiple 1 – 2 mm cysts

(b) liver: periportal fibrosis often with proliferation + dilatation of bile ducts

(c) pancreas: pancreatic fibrosis

A. ANTENATAL FORM (most common)

90% of tubules show cystic changes
- onset of renal failure in utero
- √ oligohydramnios and dystocia (large abdominal mass)

Prognosis:
death from renal failure / respiratory insufficiency (pulmonary hypoplasia) within 24 hours in 75%, within 1 year in 93%; uniformly fatal

B. NEONATAL FORM

60% of tubules show ectasia + minimal hepatic fibrosis + bile duct proliferation
- onset of renal failure within 1st month of life

Prognosis:
death from renal failure / hypertension / left ventricular failure within 1st year of life

C. INFANTILE FORM

20% of renal tubules involved + mild / moderate periportal fibrosis
- disease appears by 3 – 6 months of age

Prognosis:
death from chronic renal failure / arterial hypertension / portal hypertension

D. JUVENILE FORM

10% of tubules involved + gross hepatic fibrosis + bile duct proliferation
- disease appears at 1 – 5 years of age

Prognosis: death from portal hypertension

The less severe the renal findings the more severe the hepatic findings!

@ Lung
- √ severe pulmonary hypoplasia
- √ pneumothorax / pneumomediastinum

@ Liver
- portal venous hypertension
- √ tubular cystic dilatation of small intrahepatic bile ducts, congenital hepatic fibrosis

@ Kidneys
- √ bilateral gross renal enlargement
- √ on initial images: faint nephrogram + blotchy opacification
- √ increasingly dense nephrogram
- √ poor visualization of collecting system
- √ on delayed images: "sunburst nephrogram"
  = striated nephrogram with persistent radiating opaque streaks (collecting ducts)
- √ prominent fetal lobation

CT:
- √ prolonged corticomedullary phase

US:
- √ hyperechoic enlarged kidneys (cyst size 1 – 2 mm)
- √ occasionally discrete macroscopic cysts
- √ compressed / minimally dilated collecting system

- √ loss of corticomedullary differentiation

OB-US (as early as 17 weeks GA):
- √ renal circumference:abdominal circumference ratio > 0.30
- √ hyperechoic renal parenchyma
- √ nonvisualization of urine in fetal bladder
- √ oligohydramnios

OB-management:
(1) Chromosome studies to determine if other malformations present (e.g., trisomy 13 / 18)
(2) Option of pregnancy termination < 24 weeks
(3) Nonintervention for fetal distress > 24 weeks if severe oligohydramnios present

Risk of recurrence: 25%

POSTERIOR URETHRAL VALVES

= congenital thick folds of mucous membrane located in posterior urethra (prostatic + membranous portion) distal to verumontanum

Type I: (most common) mucosal folds (vestiges of Wolffian duct) extending anteroinferiorly from the caudal aspect of the verumontanum, often fusing anteriorly at a lower level

Type II: (rare) mucosal folds extending anterosuperiorly from the verumontanum toward the bladder neck (nonobstructive normal variant, probably a consequence of bladder outlet obstruction)

Type III: diaphragmlike membrane located below the verumontanum (= abnormal canalization of urogenital membrane)

Time of discovery: prenatal (8%), neonatal (34%), 1st year (32%), 2nd – 16th year (23%), adult (3%)

- urinary tract infection (fever, vomiting) in 36%
- obstructive symptoms in 32% (hesitancy, straining, dribbling [20%], enuresis [20%])
- palpable kidneys / bladder in neonate (21%)
- failure to thrive (13%)
- hematuria (5%)

VCUG:
- √ vesicoureteral reflux, mainly on left side (< 50%)
- √ fusiform distension + elongation of proximal posterior urethra persisting throughout voiding
- √ transverse / curvilinear filling defect in posterior urethra
- √ diminution of urethral caliber distal to severe obstruction
- √ hypertrophy of bladder neck
- √ trabeculation + sacculation of bladder wall
- √ large postvoid bladder residual

OB-US:
- √ male gender
- √ oligohydramnios (related to severity + duration of obstruction)
- √ hypoplastic / multicystic dysplastic kidney (if early occurrence)
- √ overdistended urinary bladder (megacystis) in 30%
- √ thick-walled urinary bladder + trabeculations (best seen after decompression)

√ bilateral hydroureteronephrosis (+ pulmonary hypoplasia)

√ dilated renal pelvic may be absent in renal dysplasia / rupture of bladder / pelviureteric atresia

√ urine leak: urinoma, urine ascites, urothorax

OB-management:
  (1) Induction of labor as soon as fetal lung maturity established if diagnosed during last 10 weeks of pregnancy
  (2) Vesicoamniotic shunting may be contemplated if diagnosed remote from term (68% survivors)

Cx: (1) neonatal urine leak (ascites, urothorax, urinoma) in 13%
  (2) neonatal pneumothorax / pneumomediastinum in 9%
  (3) renal dysplasia (if obstruction occurs early during gestation)
  (4) prune-belly syndrome

Prognosis: depends upon duration of obstruction prior to corrective surgery; nephrectomy for irreversible damage (13%)

DDx: (1) UPJ obstruction (2) UVJ obstruction (3) Primary megaureter (4) Massive vesicoureteral reflux (5) Megacystis-microcolon-intestinal hypoperistalsis syndrome

POSTINFLAMMATORY RENAL ATROPHY

= acute bacterial nephritis with irreversible ischemia as an unusual form of severe gram-negative bacterial infection in patients with altered host resistance in spite of proper antibiotic treatment

Histo: occlusion of interlobar arteries / vasospasm

√ small smooth kidney

√ papillary necrosis in acute phase

POSTOBSTRUCTIVE RENAL ATROPHY

= generalized papillary atrophy usually following successful surgical correction of urinary tract obstruction and progressing in spite of relief of obstruction

√ small smooth kidney, usually unilateral

√ dilated calices with effaced papillae

√ thinned cortex

PRUNE-BELLY SYNDROME

= EAGLE-BARRETT SYNDROME = congenital nonhereditary multisystem disorder; almost exclusively in males

TRIAD: 1. Absent abdominal wall musculature
  2. Urinary tract obstruction
  3. Cryptorchidism

Etiology: massive abdominal distension secondary to urethral obstruction / transient ascites / intestinal duplication cyst / megacystis-microcolon syndrome causes pressure atrophy of abdominal wall muscles; bladder distension interferes with descent of testes

Groups:
  (1) obstruction of urethra (most commonly urethral atresia)
    Associated with: malrotation, intestinal atresia, imperforate anus, skeletal abnormalities, CHD, Hirschsprung disease, congenital cystic adenomatoid malformation
    √ bladder wall hypertrophy
    Prognosis: death shortly after birth
  (2) functional abnormality of bladder emptying (more common)
    no associated abnormalities
    √ large floppy urinary bladder
    √ large urachal remnant
    Prognosis: chronic urinary tract problems

Incidence: 1:35,000 to 1:50,000 live births; almost exclusively in males

• wrinkled flaccid appearance of hypotonic abdominal wall with bulging flanks (agenesis / hypoplasia of muscles in lower + medial parts of abdominal wall)

• bilateral cryptorchidism

√ impaired renal function

√ no / mild hydronephrosis

√ dilated tortuous laterally placed ureters

√ large distended urinary bladder

√ persistence of urachal remnant

√ dilated prostatic urethra (absence of prostate)

VCUG:
  √ ± reflux into ureters
  √ reflux into utriculus / seminal vesicles
  √ diverticula of urethra (megalourethra)

√ urethral obstruction (occasionally posterior urethral valves), renal dysplasia, oligohydramnios, pulmonary hypoplasia (in severe cases)

Cx: respiratory infections (ineffective cough)

PYELOCALICEAL DIVERTICULUM

= PYELOGENIC CYST = PERICALICEAL CYST = CALICEAL DIVERTICULUM

= uroepithelium-lined pouch extending from a peripheral point of the collecting system into adjacent renal parenchyma

TYPE I (calyx):
  more common; connected to caliceal cup, usually at fornix; bulbous shape; narrow connecting infundibulum of varying length; few millimeters in diameter; in polar region especially upper pole

TYPE II (pelvis):
  interpolar region; communicates directly with pelvis; usually larger and rounder; neck short and not easily identified

Cause:
  (1) developmental origin from ureteral bud remnant (obstruction of peripheral aberrant "minicalyx")
  (2) acquired: reflux, infection, rupture of simple cyst / abscess, infundibular achalasia / spasm, hydrocalyx secondary to inflammatory fibrosis of an infundibulum

√ formation of single / multiple stones (50%) or milk of calcium (fluid-calcium level)

√ opacification may be delayed and remain so for prolonged period

√ mass effect on adjacent pelvocaliceal system if large enough

DDx: ruptured simple nephrogenic cyst, evacuated abscess / hematoma, renal papillary necrosis, medullary sponge kidney, hydrocalyx due to infundibular narrowing from TB / crossing vessel / stone / infiltrating carcinoma

PYELONEPHRITIS

Acute Pyelonephritis

= episodic urinary tract infection

Etiology:
infected urine from lower tract during adulthood; in 5% anatomic abnormality (obstruction, stone, stasis); (DDx: chronic atrophic pyelonephritis secondary to vesicoureteral reflux in infancy)

Pathway of infection:
(a) ascending via vesicoureteral reflux + pyelotubular backflow (80 – 90%) with Gram-negative rods
(b) hematogenous spread (12 – 20%) with Gram-positive cocci

Organism: E. coli > Proteus > Klebsiella, Enterobacter, Pseudomonas

Age: 15 – 40 years; M << F

• fever + chills + flank pain
• leukocytosis
• microscopic hematuria
• pyuria

Indication for imaging:
(1) diabetes (2) analgesic abuse (3) neuropathic bladder (4) history of urinary tract stones (5) atypical organism (6) poor response to antibiotics (7) frequent recurrences

√ normal urogram in 75%!

√ smooth normal / enlarged kidney(s), focal >> diffuse involvement of kidney

√ delayed opacification of collecting system

√ compression of collecting system (edema)

√ nonobstructive ureteral dilatation (rare, effect of endotoxins)

√ immediate persistent dense nephrogram, rarely striated

√ diminished nephrographic density (global / wedge-shaped / patchy)

√ nonvisualization of kidney (in severe pyelonephritis, rare)

√ "tree-barking" = mucosal striations (rare)

US: √ swollen kidney with decreased echogenicity
    √ thickened sonolucent corticomedullary bands
    √ loss of corticomedullary junction demarcation
    √ loss of central sinus echoes
    √ wedge-shaped zones of decreased attenuation

CT: √ small foci of low attenuation (= microabscesses 1 – 5 mm) without mass defect

√ delayed / decreased enhancement

Prognosis: quick response to antibiotics leaving no scars

Emphysematous Pyelonephritis

= fulminant infection of kidney + perirenal tissues with gas in and around enlarged nonfunctioning kidney + formation of abscess

Organism: E. coli > Proteus >> Clostridia (rare)

Predisposed: diabetics (in 90% of cases); obstructed kidney (in 40%); F > M

√ gas within collecting system

√ streaks / bubbles of gas in interstitium of renal parenchyma radiating from medulla to cortex

√ subcapsular / perinephric gas

Mortality: 40 – 50%

Rx: prompt surgical drainage

Xanthogranulomatous Pyelonephritis

= chronic suppurative granulomatous infection in chronic obstruction (calculus, stricture, carcinoma) originating in medulla

Incidence: 681,000 surgically proven cases of chronic pyelonephritis

Organisms: Proteus mirabilis, E. coli

Histo: diffuse infiltration by plasma cells + lipid-laden macrophages (xanthoma cells); calices filled with pus and debris

Peak age: 4th – 5th decade; all ages affected, may occur in infants; M:F = 1:3

• pyuria (95%)
• flank pain (80%)
• fever (70%)
• palpable mass (50%)
• weight loss (50%)
• microscopic hematuria (50%)
• reversible hepatic dysfunction with elevated liver function tests (50%)

A. DIFFUSE XGP (83 – 90%)
B. SEGMENTAL / FOCAL XGP (10 – 17%)
= tumefactive form due to obstructed single infundibulum / one moiety of duplex system

√ kidney globally enlarged (smooth contour uncommon) / focal renal mass

√ contracted pelvis with dilated calices

√ totally absent / focally absent nephrogram

√ central obstructing calculus: staghorn calculus in 75%

√ extension of inflammation into perirenal space, psoas muscle, colon, spleen, diaphragm, flank

Retrograde:
√ destroyed collecting system with cavitation

CT:
√ low attenuation masses replacing renal parenchyma

US:
√ hypoechoic calices with echogenic rim

√ parenchymal calcifications are uncommon
Angio:
appearance of (a) hydronephrosis (b) avascular tumor
√ fine neovascularity may be present
√ venous encasement + occlusion

PYELORENAL BACKFLOW
Etiology: increased pressure in collecting system from
retrograde pyelography, IV urogram with large
dose of contrast, ureteral obstruction, external
compression on ureter
1. Pyelotubular backflow
= opacification of terminal portions of collecting ducts
(= papillary ducts = ducts of Bellini) as a physiologic
phenomenon (in 13% with low osmolality + in 0.4%
with high osmolality contrast media), wrongly termed
"backflow"
√ wedge-shaped brushlike lines from calyx towards
periphery
2. Pyelosinus backflow
= contrast extravasation from ruptured fornices along
infundibula, renal pelvis, proximal ureter; most
common form
Cx: urinoma, retroperitoneal fibrosis
3. Pyelointerstitial backflow
= contrast flow from pyramids into subcapsular tubules
4. Pyelolymphatic backflow
= contrast extravasation into periforniceal + peripelvic
lymphatics
√ visualization of small lymphatics draining medially
5. Pyelovenous backflow
= forniceal rupture into interlobar / arcuate veins; very
rare

PYELOURETERITIS CYSTICA
Cause: chronic urinary tract irritant (stone / infection)
Histo: numerous small submucosal epithelial-lined cysts
representing cystic degeneration of epithelial cell
nests within lamina propria (cell nests of von
Brunn) formed by downward proliferation of buds
of surface epithelium that have become detached
from the mucosa
Organisms: E. coli > M. tuberculosis, Enterococcus,
Proteus, Schistosomiasis)
Predisposed: diabetics
Age: 6th decade; more prevalent in women
Location: bladder >> proximal 1/3 of ureter >
ureteropelvic junction; unilateral >> bilateral
√ multiple small round smooth lucent defects of 1 – 3 mm
in size; scattered discrete / clustered
√ persist unchanged for years in spite of antibiotic therapy
DDx: (1) spreading / multifocal TCC
(2) vascular ureteral notching

PYONEPHROSIS
= pyelonephritis in chronic obstruction leading to early
development of microabscesses + necrotizing papillitis

Cx: 1. XGP
2. Renal abscess
3. Perinephric abscess
4. Fistula to duodenum, colon, pleura

RHABDOMYOSARCOMA
= most common soft tissue tumor in childhood
Incidence: 4 – 8% of all malignant tumors in children
< 15 years of age; 10 – 25% of all sarcomas
Age: 75% < 5 years of age; peak age 2 – 6 years
M:F = 2:1
Histo: (1) embryonal (> 50 %)
Subtype: polyploidal form = sarcoma
botryoides = grapelike
(2) alveolar (worst prognosis)
(3) pleomorphic (mostly in adults)
Location: head + neck (28 – 36%), trigone + bladder
neck (18 – 21%), orbit (10%), extremities (18 –
23%), trunk (7 – 8%), retroperitoneum (6 –
7%), perineum + anus (2%), other sites (7%)
Points of origin in genitourinary rhabdomyosarcoma:
trigone, prostate, seminal vesicles, spermatic cord,
vulva, vagina, cervix, uterus (arising from the
mesenchyme of urogenital ridge)
• urinary frequency
• dysuria
• palpable bladder
• hematuria (late manifestation)
• strangury (= painful urge to void without success)
• vaginal discharge / protruding grapelike mass
√ obstruction of bladder neck with large postvoid residual
√ lobulated grapelike tumor mass with elevation of bladder
floor
√ homogeneous echogenicity similar to muscle ±
hypoechoic areas (hemorrhage / necrosis)
√ retroperitoneal lymph node enlargement
Angio: √ diffuse tumor vascularity
Prognosis: (a) 14 – 35% 5-year survival with radical
surgery
(b) 60 – 90% 3-year survival with
chemotherapy

RADIATION NEPHRITIS
Histo: interstitial fibrosis, tubule atrophy, glomerular
sclerosis, sclerosis of arteries of all sizes,
hyalinization of afferent arterioles, thickening of
renal capsule
Threshold dose: 2300 rads over 5 weeks
• clinically resembling chronic glomerulonephritis
√ normal / small smooth kidney consistent with radiation
field
√ parenchymal thickness diminished (globally / focally
— related to radiation field)
√ diminished nephrographic density

REFLUX ATROPHY
Cause: increased hydrostatic pressure of pelvocaliceal
urine with atrophy of nephrons secondary to
long standing vesicoureteral reflux

√ small smooth kidney with loss of parenchymal thickness
√ widened collecting system with effaced papillae
√ longitudinal striations from redundant mucosa when
collecting system is collapsed
NOT to confuse with reflux nephropathy !

REFLUX NEPHROPATHY
= CHRONIC ATROPHIC PYELONEPHRITIS = ascending
bacterial urinary tract infection secondary to reflux of
infected urine from lower tract + tubulointerstitial
inflammation in childhood (hardly ever endangers adult
kidney); most common cause of small scarred kidney
Etiology:
   3 essential elements: (1) infected urine
                         (2) vesicoureteral reflux
                         (3) intrarenal reflux
Age: usually young adults (subclinical diagnosis starting
     in childhood); M < F
• fever, flank pain, frequency, dysuria
• hypertension, renal failure
• may have no history of significant symptoms
Site: predominantly affecting poles of kidneys secondary
     to presence of compound calyces having distorted
     papillary ducts of Bellini (= papillae with gaping
     openings instead of slitlike openings of interpolar
     papillae)
√ normal / small kidney; uni- / bilateral; uni- / multifocal
√ focal parenchymal thinning with contour depression in
upper / lower pole (more compound papillae in upper
pole), scar formation only up to age 4
√ retracted papilla with clubbed calyx subjacent to scar
√ contralateral / focal compensatory hypertrophy
(= pseudotumor)
√ dilated ureters (secondary to reflux) sometimes with
linear striations
(redundant / edematous mucosa)
US:
   √ focally increased echogenicity within cortex (scar)
Angio:
   √ small tortuous intrarenal arteries, pruning of intrarenal
     vessels
   √ vascular stenoses, occlusion, aneurysms
   √ inhomogeneous nephrographic phase
NUC (Tc99m-glucoheptonate / DMSA) most sensitive
method:
   √ focal / multifocal photon deficient areas

RENAL / PERIRENAL ABSCESS
= usually complication of renal inflammation with
liquefaction; 2% of all renal masses
Pathway of infection:
   (a) ascending (80%): associated with obstruction
       (UPJ, ureter, calculus)
   (b) hematogenous (20%): infection from skin, teeth,
       lung, tonsils (St. aureus), endocarditis,
       intravenous drug abuse
Organisms: E. coli, Proteus
• urine culture often negative

Renal Abscess
IVP:
   √ focal mass focally displacing collecting system
CT:
   √ focal renal mass with thick enhancing wall +
     thickened Gerota fascia
   √ centrally diminished attenuation
US:
   √ slightly hypoechoic (early), hypo- to anechoic (late)
     mass with irregular margins + increased through-
     transmission ± septations
NUC (Ga67-citrate / In111-leukocytes):
   √ hot spot
DDx: cystic renal cell carcinoma

Carbuncle
= collection of many small abscesses

Perinephric Abscess
= extension of renal abscess through capsule
Predisposed: diabetics (in 30%), urolithiasis
√ loss of psoas margin / obscuration of renal contour
√ renal displacement
√ focal renal mass
√ scoliosis concave to involved side
√ respiratory immobility of kidney
√ gas in renal fossa
√ unilateral impaired excretion
√ pleural effusion

RENAL ADENOMA
most common cortical lesion, in 1% of individuals (autopsy
statistic)
usually < 3 cm in size; M > F
TYPES:
   (1) Papillary / cystadenoma (38%)
   (2) Tubular adenoma (38%)
   (3) Mixed type adenoma (21%)
   (4) Alveolar adenoma (3%) = precursor of
       hypernephroma

Proximal Tubular Adenoma
= ONCOCYTOMA = BENIGN OXYPHILIC ADENOMA
Path:
   well-encapsulated tan-colored tumor of well-
   differentiated proximal tubular cells (benign adenoma)
   + oncocytes = large eosinophilic / oxophilic cells
   (granular eosinophilic cytoplasm with large number of
   mitochondria); similar tumors seen in thyroid,
   parathyroid, salivary glands, adrenals; pathologic
   diagnosis requires entire tumor because well-
   differentiated renal cell carcinoma may have
   oncocytic features
Age: usually solitary tumor, middle aged subjects;
      M:F = 2:1
√ renal mass of 6 cm average size (1 – 14 cm)
√ tumor of homogeneous low attenuation /
hypoechogenicity (> 50%)

√ well-demarcated with pseudocapsule
√ central stellate scar (in large lesions only) in 30%
Angio:
  √ spokewheel configuration (80%), homogeneous parenchymal phase (71%)
Tc99m-DMSA:
  √ photopenic area (tubular cells do not function normally)

RENAL AGENESIS
Mechanism:
  (a) FORMATION FAILURE
    = failure of ureteral bud to form
    • absence of ipsilateral hemitrigone and ureteral orifice
  (b) INDUCTION FAILURE
    = failure of growing ureteral bud to induce metanephric tissue
    • blind ending ureter

A. UNILATERAL RENAL AGENESIS
  Incidence: 1:600 – 1,000 pregnancies
  Risk of recurrence: 4.5%
  Often coexist with other anomalies:
    genital tract anomalies (40% of females, 12% of males); Turner syndrome, trisomy, Fanconi anemia, Laurence-Moon-Biedl syndrome
  √ absent adrenal gland (11%)
  √ absent renal vessels
  √ colon occupies renal fossa
  √ compensatory contralateral renal hypertrophy (50%)

B. BILATERAL RENAL AGENESIS (= Potter syndrome)
  Incidence: 1:3,000 to 1:10,000 pregnancies;
                  M:F = 2.5:1
  Risk of recurrence: < 1%
  • Potter's facies = low set ears, redundant skin, parrot-beaked nose, receding chin,
  √ oligohydramnios (after 14 weeks MA)
  √ bilateral absence of renal outline (after 12 weeks)
  √ flat discoid adrenals (simulating kidneys with hypoechoic rim + thin central sinus)
  √ inability to visualize urine in fetal bladder (after 13 weeks); negative furosemide test (20 – 60 mg IV) not diagnostic!
  √ bell-shaped thorax (pulmonary hypoplasia)
  √ compression deformities of extremities = clubfoot, flexion contractures, joint dislocations
  Prognosis: stillbirths (24 – 38 %); invariably fatal in the first days of life (pulmonary hypoplasia)
  DDx: functional cause of in utero renal failure

RENAL ARTERY STENOSIS
responsible for 5 – 10% of systemic arterial hypertension
Hemodynamic significance determined by:
  (1) elevated renin levels in renal vein of affected kidney ≥ 1.5:1
  (2) collateral vessels
  (3) greater than 70% stenosis with poststenotic dilatation

  (4) transstenotic intraarterial pressure gradient ≥ 40 mmHg
  (5) decrease in renal size
Causes:
  1. atheromatous lesion (mostly proximal 2 cm)
  2. fibromuscular dysplasia
  3. Uncommon: renal artery aneurysm, arteriovenous malformation / fistula, Takayasu disease, thrombangitis obliterans, syphilitic arteritis, dissecting aortic aneurysm, postradiation artery stenosis, neurofibromatosis, thrombosis, embolus (atrial fibrillation, prosthetic valve thrombi, cardiac myxoma, paradoxical emboli, atheromatous emboli), trauma, aortic dissection
Histo: tubular atrophy and shrinkage of glomeruli
  • abdominal / flank pain
  • hematuria
  • hypertension
  • oliguria, anuria
  • low urine sodium concentration
  √ normal / decreased renal size (R 2 cm < L; L 1.5 cm < R) with smooth contour
  √ delayed appearance of contrast material (decreased glomerular filtration)
  √ increased density of contrast material (increased water reabsorption)
  √ delayed washout of contrast material (prolonged urine transit time)
  √ lack of distension of collecting system
  √ global attenuation of contrast density, urogram may be normal with adequate collateral circulation
  √ notching of proximal ureter (enlargement of collateral vessels)
  √ vascular calcifications (aneurysm / atherosclerosis)
NUC:
  √ reduced / absent perfusion of kidney
  √ poor visualization / nonvisualization on delayed images

Arteriosclerosis of Kidney
  Age: > 50 years; M > F
  Path: lesion primarily involving intima
  Location: main renal artery (93%) + additional stenosis of renal artery branch (7%); bilateral in 31%
  Associated with arteriosclerosis of aorta
  √ eccentric stenosis proximal 2 cm of renal artery, frequently involving orifice

Fibromuscular Dysplasia of Renal Artery
  Incidence: 35% of renal artery stenoses
  Age: most common cause of renovascular hypertension in children + young adults < 40 years; M:F = 1:3
  • hypertension
  • progressive renal insufficiency

Sites: mid- and distal main renal artery (79%), renal
artery branches (4%), combination (17%);
proximal third of main renal artery spared in
98%; bilateral in 2/3; R:L = 4:1
Associated with fibromuscular dysplasia of other aortic
branches in 1 – 2%: celiac, hepatic, splenic,
mesenteric, iliac, internal carotids
Cx: (1) Giant aneurysm
(2) AV fistula between renal artery + vein (in
medial fibroplasia)

1. INTIMAL FIBROPLASIA (1 – 2%)
Path: circumferential / eccentric fibrous tissue
between intima + internal elastic lamina
Age: children + young adults
Site: main renal artery + major segmental
branches; often bilateral
√ narrow annular radiolucent band
√ poststenotic fusiform dilatation
2. MEDIAL FIBROPLASIA (60 – 70%)
Path: multiple fibromuscular ridges + severe mural
thinning with loss of smooth muscle +
internal elastic lamina
Site: mid + distal renal artery + branches
√ "string of beads" = alternating areas of stenoses +
aneurysms
3. MEDIAL HYPERPLASIA (5 – 15%)
Path: smooth muscle hyperplasia within arterial
media
Site: main renal artery and branches
√ long smooth tubular narrowing
4. PERIMEDIAL FIBROPLASIA (20%)
Path: fibroplasia of outer 1/2 of media replacing
external elastic lamina
Site: distal main renal artery
√ long irregular stenosis, beading
NO aneurysm formation (not wider than
unaffected segment)
5. MEDIAL DISSECTION (5 – 10%)
Path: new channel in outer 1/3 of media within
external elastic lamina
Site: main renal artery + branches
√ false channel, aneurysm
6. ADVENTITIAL FIBROPLASIA (< 1%)
Path: adventitial + periarterial proliferation in
fibrofatty tissue
Site: main renal artery, large branches
√ long segmental stenosis

Neurofibromatosis
Hypertension in neurofibromatosis due to:
(1) pheochromocytoma
(2) renal artery stenosis
Renal artery involvement mainly seen in children!
Types:
(a) mesodermal dysplasia of arterial wall with fibrous
transformation (common)
(b) narrowing of main renal artery by neurofibroma
(rare)

√ saccular funnel-shaped aneurysm involving aorta /
main renal artery
√ smooth / nodular stenosis (mural / adventitial
neurofibroma) in proximal renal artery
√ intrarenal aneurysm (rare)
DDx: Fibromuscular dysplasia; congenital renal
artery stenosis

RENAL CELL CARCINOMA
= RCCa = RENAL ADENOCARCINOMA
= HYPERNEPHROMA
= 80% of all renal malignant primaries
Peak age: 55 years (generally > 40 years); may occur
in children; M:F = 2:1
Path:
arises from proximal tubular cells; 30% found
incidentally with imaging
Types:
(a) clear cell carcinoma (95%): hypervascular,
> 50 years
(b) papillary adenocarcinoma (5%): hypovascular,
40 – 50 years, slow growing, well encapsulated,
metastasize late
Predisposed:
(1) tobacco; phenacetin abuse
(2) von Hippel-Lindau syndrome (10 – 25%) often
small intracystic tumors (hemangioblastoma, retinal
angioma, renal cysts)
(3) acquired cystic disease of dialysis (7 x increased
risk)
Multiple RCCa: commonly in von Hippel-Lindau
syndrome, bilateral in 3%
Stage I : tumor confined to renal capsule
√ sharply defined convex interface with
perirenal fat
II : confined to Gerota fascia = perirenal fascia
√ irregular interface between tumor + fat
III: extension into renal vein or IVC ± positive
lymph nodes; extension into perirenal fat
IV: extension into adjacent organs; distant
metastases
Regional extension: into lymph nodes (9 – 20%);
into IVC (4 – 10%)
Metastases to:
lung (55%); lymph nodes (34%); liver (33%); bone
(32%); adrenals (19%); contralateral kidney (11%); brain
(6%); heart (5%); spleen (5%); bowel (4%); skin (3%);
ureter (rare)
• hematuria (56%), flank pain (36%), weight loss (27%),
fever (11%)
• varicocele (2%)
• anemia (40%)
• Stauffer syndrome (15%) = abnormal liver function in
absence of hepatic metastases
• Paraneoplastic syndromes: polycythemia (4%),
hypercalcemia
√ mass, bulge, discontinuity of renal contour
√ calcification (10 – 20%): usually central + amorphous

√ extrinsic compression + displacement of pelvis + calices
√ cysts: (a) cystic necrotic tumor (40%)
       (b) cystadenocarcinoma (2 – 5%)
       (c) renal cell carcinoma in wall of cyst (3 %)
√ diminished function (parenchymal replacement, hydronephrosis)
√ tumor growth into renal vein / IVC (30%)
√ variable echogenicity (DDx: complicated cyst, angiomyolipoma)
MRI (best modality to assess stage III + IV disease):
   √ low to medium signal intensity on T1WI, hyperintense areas are usually hemorrhage
   √ heterogeneous signal intensity on T2WI
Angio:
   √ typically hypervascular (95%) + puddling of contrast + occasional AV shunting
   √ enlarged tortuous poorly tapering feeding vessels
   √ coarse neovascularity + formation of small aneurysms
   √ parasitization of lumbar, adrenal, subcostal, mesenteric artery branches
   √ poorly defined tumor margins
Prognosis: 10 year-survival rate for stage I + II 60 – 70%, Stage III 40%, Stage IV 0%
Recurrence: in 11% after 10 years

RENAL CYST
Simple Cortical Cyst
acquired lesion possibly secondary to tubular obstruction; account for 62% of all renal masses
Incidence: in 1 – 2% of all urograms; in 3 – 5% of all autopsies; increasing frequency with age (in 50% over age 50)
May be associated with: tuberous sclerosis, von Hippel-Lindau disease, Caroli disease, neurofibromatosis
√ large and unifocal when peripheral
√ focally attenuated + displaced collecting system
√ focally replaced nephrogram with smooth margin, thin wall and "beak sign"
√ peripheral + curvilinear calcification (1%) after hemorrhage + infection
US (90 – 100% accuracy of US & CT):
   √ anechoic with sound through transmission and smooth sharply defined wall, may develop delicate septa after hemorrhage (10 – 15%) / infection
CT:
   √ near water density lesion, no enhancement, thin wall, smooth interface with renal parenchyma
Cystography:
   √ smooth wall, clear aspirate with low lactic dehydrogenase, no fat content
Cx: (1) hemorrhage (2) infection (3) tumor within cyst in < 1%

Complicated Cyst
(a) hemorrhagic
(b) infected
US: √ thick-walled with internal echoes

CT: √ increased density secondary to hemorrhage / high protein contents

Parapelvic Cyst
= spherical fluid-filled masses intimately attached to renal pelvis without connection to pelvocaliceal system
Incidence: 4% of all renal cysts
Etiology: probably ectatic lymphatic channels / ? from urine extravasation
• serous fluid
√ soft tissue density in renal sinus
√ focal displacement + smooth effacement of collecting system
√ stretching of collecting system when generalized
√ obstructive caliectasis may occur
√ rarely curvilinear calcification of cyst wall (4%)
US:
   √ anechoic mass with acoustic enhancement, irregular shape

RENAL DUPLICATION
Complete Duplication
in 15% bilateral
(1) Upper pole moiety
    Ectopic ureter inserts below and medial to orthotopic ureter
    Subject to OBSTRUCTION (ectopic insertion, aberrant artery crossing)
(2) Lower pole moiety
    Orthotopic ureter drains lower pole and interpolar portion
    Subject to VESICOURETERAL REFLUX with reflux atrophy / chronic pyelonephritis
√ atrophic system may simulate a renal mass = nubbin sign
√ obstructed upper pole moiety with tortuous dilated ureter
√ faintly visualized diminutive collecting system
√ paucity of cranial calices
√ flattening of lower pole
√ vesicoureteral reflux into atrophied lower pole

Partial Duplication
√ bifid ureter (in early branching)
√ bifid pelvis (in late branching)
√ "yo-yo" peristalsis = urine moves down the cephalad ureter + refluxes up the lower pole ureter
√ upper pole ureter may end blindly (seen on retrograde injection only)

RENAL DYSGENESIS
= undifferentiated tissue of renal anlage
Pathologic NOT radiologic diagnosis
√ renal vessels usually absent; occasionally small vascular channels

RENAL INFARCTION

Causes:
1. TRAUMA: blunt abdominal trauma, traumatic avulsion of renal artery, surgery
2. EMBOLISM:
   (a) Cardiac: rheumatic heart disease with arrhythmia (atrial fibrillation), myocardial infarction, prosthetic valves, myocardial trauma, left atrial / mural thrombus, myocardial tumors, subacute bacterial endocarditis
   (b) Catheters: angiographic catheter manipulation, umbilical artery catheter above level of renal arteries
3. THROMBOSIS: arteriosclerosis, thrombangitis obliterans, polyarteritis nodosa, syphilitic cardiovascular disease, aneurysm (aorta / renal artery), sickle cell disease
4. Sudden complete renal vein thrombosis

Acute Renal Infarction
√ normal / large kidney with smooth contour
√ normal / expanded parenchymal thickness
√ normal / attenuated collecting system, often only opacified by retrograde pyelography
√ absent / diminished nephrogram with cortical rim enhancement, rarely striations
US:
   √ normal / diminished echogenicity

Lobar Renal Infarction
Early signs:
√ focal attenuation of collecting system (tissue swelling)
√ focally absent nephrogram (triangular with base at cortex)
Late signs:
√ normal / small kidney(s)
√ focally wasted parenchyma with NORMAL interpapillary line (portion of lobe / whole lobe / several adjacent lobes)
CT: √ nonperfused area corresponding to vascular division, cortical rim sign
US: √ focally increased echogenicity

Chronic Renal Infarction
Path: all elements of kidney atrophy with replacement by interstitial fibrosis
√ normal / small kidney with smooth contour
√ globally wasted parenchyma
√ diminished / absent contrast material density
US:
   √ increased echogenicity
Angio:
   √ normal intrarenal venous architecture
   √ late visualization of renal arteries on abdominal aortogram

Atheroembolic Renal Disease
= dislodgement of multiple atheromatous emboli from the aorta into renal circulation (below level of arcuate arteries)
√ normal / small kidneys with smooth contour or shallow depressions
√ wasted parenchymal thickness
√ diminished density of contrast material
CT:
   √ patchy nephrographic distribution
Angio:
   √ embolic occlusion

Arteriosclerotic Renal Disease
= disseminated process involving most of the interlobar + arcuate arteries causing uniform shrinkage of kidneys
Age: generally over 60 years
accelerated development in: scleroderma, polyarteritis nodosa, chronic tophaceous gout
• often associated with hypertension (NEPHROSCLEROSIS)
√ normal / small kidneys
√ smooth contour with random shallow contour depressions (infarctions)
√ uniform loss of cortical thickness
√ normal / effaced collecting system (fat proliferation)
√ increased pelvic radiolucency (vicarious sinus fat proliferation)
√ calcification of medium-sized intrarenal arteries
US:
   √ increased echogenicity possible
   √ increased size of renal sinus echoes (fatty replacement)

Nephrosclerosis
Histo: thickening + hyalinization of afferent arterioles, proliferative endarteritis, necrotizing arteriolitis, necrotizing glomerulitis
• arterial hypertension
(a) BENIGN NEPHROSCLEROSIS
(b) MALIGNANT NEPHROSCLEROSIS (rapid deterioration of renal function)
√ radiographic appearance similar to arteriosclerotic kidney

RENAL VEIN THROMBOSIS

Causes:
A. Intrinsic
   (a) children: dehydration from vomiting, diarrhea, glycosuria in infants of diabetic mothers, sepsis, umbilical vein catheterization, enterocolitis
   (b) adults: membranous GN, pyelonephritis, amyloidosis, polyarteritis nodosa, sickle cell anemia, thrombosis of IVC, renal neoplasia (50%), low flow states (CHF, constrictive pericarditis), diabetic nephropathy, lupus nephropathy, sarcoidosis, hypercoagulable states, trauma

B. Extrinsic
    carcinoma of pancreatic tail invading renal vein (in
    75%), lymphoma, metastases to retroperitoneum
    (bronchogenic carcinoma)

Radiographic appearance varies with:
    (1) rapidity of venous occlusion (2) extent of occlusion
    (3) availability of collateral circulation (4) site of
    occlusion in relation to collateral pathways

Acute renal vein thrombosis
    = no time for effective development of collaterals;
      hemorrhage from ruptured venules + capillaries
    • gross hematuria
    • flank mass
    • consumptive thrombocytopenia
    • anuria
    √ smooth enlargement of kidney
    √ diminished radiographic density
    √ little / no pyelocaliceal visualization
    √ focal hemorrhagic infarction + capsular rupture
    US: √ diminished echogenicity
           √ dilated renal vein / IVC with thrombus
    CT: √ exaggerated + prolonged corticomedullary
              differentiation
           √ retroperitoneal hemorrhage
    Angio: √ absent inflow from renal vein into IVC
           √ thrombus extending into IVC
    NUC: √ no characteristic pattern on sequential
              functional study
    Cx: (1) pulmonary emboli (50 %)
           (2) severe renal atrophy (may show complete
                recovery)

Subacute renal vein thrombosis
    = good collateral drainage; impaired function with
      steady state or recanalization
    √ enlarged edematous boggy kidney
    √ slightly diminished / normal nephrographic density
       (may increase over time)
    √ compression of collecting system ("spidery calices")

Chronic renal vein thrombosis
    = indolent stage
    • 80 – 90% asymptomatic
    • nephrotic syndrome (proteinuria,
       hypercholesterolemia, anasarca)
    √ normal excretory urogram in 25% (with good
       collateral circulation especially if left side affected)
    √ notching of proximal ureter
    √ retroperitoneal dilated collaterals
    US: √ increased echogenicity
    CT: √ renal vein + IVC thrombus (24%); perirenal
           collaterals
        √ prolonged corticomedullary differentiation
        √ delayed / absent pyelocaliceal opacification +
           attenuated collecting system
        √ thickening of Gerota fascia

RETROCAVAL URETER
    = CIRCUMCAVAL URETER = abnormality in
      embryogenesis of IVC with abnormal persistence of
      right subcardinal vein ventral to ureter (instead of right
      supracardinal vein which is dorsal to right ureter)
    Incidence: 0.07%;   M:F = 3:1
    • symptoms of right ureteral obstruction
    √ ureteral course swings medially over pedicle of L3/4,
       passing behind IVC, and then exiting anteriorly between
       IVC and aorta returning to its normal position
    √ varying degrees of hydronephrosis + proximal
       hydroureteronephrosis

RETROPERITONEAL FIBROSIS
    = ORMOND DISEASE = CHRONIC PERIAORTITIS
    Path: dense hard fibrous tissue enveloping the
               retroperitoneum with effects on ureter,
               lymphatics, great vessels
    Causes:
    A. PRIMARY RETROPERITONEAL FIBROSIS (2/3)
        Probably autoimmune disease with antibodies to
        ceroid (by-product of aortic plaque which has
        penetrated into media) leading to systemic vasculitis;
        associated with fibrosis outside retroperitoneum in 8
        – 15%
        Age: 31 – 60 years (in 70%); M:F = 2:1
        Rx: responsive to corticoids
    B. SECONDARY RETROPERITONEAL FIBROSIS
        (1/3)
        (1) Drugs (12%):   methysergide, phenacetin,
            hydralazine, ergotamine, methyldopa,
            amphetamines, LSD
        (2) Tumor (8%): lymphoma, carcinoid,
            retroperitoneal metastases, Hodgkin disease
        (4) Retroperitoneal trauma, surgery, infection
        (3) Aneurysm of aorta / iliac arteries (desmoplastic
            response)
        (5) Connective tissue disease: e.g., polyarteritis
            nodosa
    Peak age: 40 – 60 years.; M:F = 2:1
    • renal insufficiency (50 – 60%)
    • dull pain in flank, back, abdomen (90%)
    • hypertension
    • edema, fever, hydrocele (10%)
    Location: around aorta + beyond common iliac
               bifurcation, rarely extends below pelvic rim,
               may extend into mediastinum
    √ medial deviation of ureters in middle third, typically
       bilateral
    √ hydroureteronephrosis
    √ pyeloureterectasis at L4/5 (interference with peristalsis)
    √ gradual tapering of ureter (extrinsic compression)
    US:
       √ hypoechoic homogeneous mass
    CT:
       √ periaortic mass of attenuation similar to muscle
       √ may show contrast enhancement (active
          inflammation)

NUC:
- √ gallium uptake during active inflammation

Rx: (1) withdrawal of possible causative agent
(2) surgical relief of obstruction
(3) corticosteroids

RETROPERITONEAL LIPOSARCOMA

= most common primary retroperitoneal tumor, rarely arising from lipoma, 95% of all fatty retroperitoneal tumors

Histo:
(a) myxoid form (most common): varying degrees of mucinous + fibrous tissue + relatively little lipid
(b) lipogenic form: malignant lipoblasts with large amounts of lipid + scanty myxoid matrix
(c) pleomorphic type: marked cellular pleomorphism, paucity of lipid + mucin

Age: most commonly 40 – 60 years; M > F
Sites: lower extremity 45%, abdominal cavity + retroperitoneum (14%), trunk (14%), upper extremity (7.6%), head & neck (6.5%), miscellaneous (13.5%)

CT:
- √ solid pattern: inhomogeneous poorly marginated infiltrating mass with contrast enhancement
- √ mixed pattern of focal fatty areas (-40 to -20 HU) + areas of higher density (+ 20 HU)
- √ pseudocystic pattern: water-density mass (averaging of fatty + solid connective tissue elements)

Angio:
- √ hypovascular without vessel dilatation / capillary staining / laking

Prognosis: most radiosensitive of soft tissue sarcomas; 32% overall 5-year survival

SCHISTOSOMIASIS

= BILHARZIASIS

Organism: S. haematobium (GU tract) > 95%; S. mansoni (GI tract) < 5%

Lifecycle: female parasite discharges eggs into urine + feces; hatch within fresh water into miracidia; penetrate snail (intermediate host); develop into cercaria; penetrate human skin (usually foot) + pass into lymphatics; settle in portal veins + migrate into pelvic venous plexus; eggs erode bladder mucosa

- frequency, urgency, dysuria
- dull flank pain (from hydronephrosis)
- hematuria
- √ calcifications: linear + continuous bladder wall calcification (in 4 – 56%), vesical calculi (in 39%), distal ureteral calcification (in 34%), honey-combed calcification of seminal vesicles
- √ multiple inflammatory pseudopolyps in bladder + ureter secondary to granulomas (= bilharziomas)
- √ ureteral dilatation (atony secondary to fibrosis / perineuritis)
- √ ureteritis cystica / ureteritis calcinosa (punctate calcifications)

- √ ureteral strictures in distal third (in 8%) (most commonly in intravesical portion with cobrahead configuration = pseudoureterocele); Makar stricture = focal stricture at L3
- √ vesicoureteral reflux
- √ thick-walled fibrotic "flat-topped" bladder with high insertion of ureters
- √ reduced bladder capacity with significant postvoid residual (fibrotic stage)
- √ urethral stricture with perineal fistulas

Cx: (1) Portal hypertension
(2) Squamous cell carcinoma of bladder (discontinuous calcifications, irregular filling defect)

SCLERODERMA

= PROGRESSIVE SYSTEMIC SCLEROSIS (PSS)
Renal disease common within 3 years of onset

Histo: fibrinoid necrosis of afferent arterioles (also in malignant hypertension)
- √ renal cortical necrosis
- √ spotty inhomogeneous nephrogram (constriction & occlusion of arteries)
- √ concomitant arterial ectasia

SCROTAL ABSCESS

Etiology:
(a) complication of epididymo-orchitis (often in diabetics), missed testicular torsion, gangrenous tumor, infected hematoma, primary pyogenic orchitis
(b) systemic infection: mumps, small pox, scarlet fever, influenza, typhoid, syphilis, TB
(c) septic dissemination from: sinusitis, osteomyelitis, cholecystitis, appendicitis

NUC:
- √ marked increase in perfusion, hot hemiscrotum with photondeficient area representing the abscess

US:
- √ hypoechoic / complex fluid collection with low-level echoes, intra- from extratesticular abscess location can be differentiated

Cx: (1) pyocele (2) fistulous tract to skin

SINUS LIPOMATOSIS

= PERIPELVIC LIPOMATOSIS
= PELVIC FIBROLIPOMATOSIS
= PERIPELVIC FAT PROLIFERATION

Etiology:
(1) normal increase with aging and obesity
(2) vicarious proliferation of sinus fat with destruction / atrophy of kidney
(3) extravasation of urine leads to proliferation of fatty granulation tissue

- √ elongated "spiderlike / trumpetlike" pelvocaliceal system
- √ infundibula arranged in "spoke wheel" pattern
- √ parenchymal thickness diminished with underlying disease

√ occasionally focal fat deposit with localized deformity of collecting system

Plain film:	√ diminished sinus density
CT:	√ unequivocal fat values
US:	√ echodense / patchy hypoechoic appearance

STRESS INCONTINENCE
Chain cystography:
√ posterior urethrovesical angle (= angle between posterior urethra + bladder base) increased > 100°
√ upper urethral axis (= angle between upper urethra + vertical) increased > 35°

SUPERNUMERARY KIDNEY
= aberrant division of nephrogenic cord into 2 metanephric tails (rare)
Associated with: horseshoe kidney, vaginal atresia, duplicated female urethra, duplicated penis
Location: most commonly on left side of abdomen caudal to normal kidney
√ supernumerary ureter may insert into ipsilateral kidney / directly into bladder / ectopic site
Cx: hydronephrosis, pyonephrosis, pyelonephritis, cysts, calculi, carcinoma, papillary cystadenoma, Wilms tumor

SYSTEMIC LUPUS ERYTHEMATOSUS
Kidneys involved in 100%, renal disease develops in 50%
Histo: focal membranous glomerulonephritis
Incidence: Blacks:Caucasians = 3:1; M < F; increased risk in relatives
√ nonerosive arthritis of hands (characteristic)
√ aneurysms in interlobular + arcuate arteries (similar to polyarteritis nodosa)
√ normal / decreased renal size
US:
√ increased parenchymal echogenicity
Cx: (1) nephrotic syndrome (common)
(2) renal vein thrombosis (rare)
Prognosis: end stage renal disease is common cause of death

TESTICULAR INFARCT
Etiology: torsion, trauma, leukemia, bacterial endocarditis, polyarteritis nodosa, Henoch-Schönlein purpura
√ diffusely hypoechoic small testis
√ hyperechoic regions (hemorrhage / fibrosis)

TESTICULAR TORSION
most common scrotal disorder in children, 20% of acute scrotal pathology in
Incidence: 1:160, 10 fold risk in undescended testis compared with normal annual incidence of 1:4,000 males
Etiology:
(1) "bell and clapper" deformity = high insertion of tunica vaginalis on spermatic cord

(2) abnormally loose mesorchium between testis + epididymis
in 5% bilateral (anomalous suspension of contralateral testis found in 50 – 80%)
Peak age: newborn period + puberty (13 – 16 years); < 20 years in 74%; > 21 years in 26%; > 30 years in 9%
• sudden severe pain in 100% (frequently at night)
• negative urine analysis (98%)
• history of similar episode in same / contralateral testis (42%)
• nausea + vomiting (50%)
• scrotal swelling + tenderness (42%)
• leukocytosis (32%)
• low-grade fever (20%)
• history of trauma / extreme exertion (13%)

Salvage rate: time interval between onset of pain and surgery

< 6 hours	80 – 100%
6 – 12 hours	76%
12 – 24 hours	20%
> 24 hours	near 0%

Spontaneous detorsion in 7%
Testis viable for only 3 – 6 hours
Cx: testicular atrophy (in 33 – 45%)

Acute Torsion
US (80 – 90% sensitivity):
√ testicular + epididymal enlargement with decreased echogenicity
√ increase in size of spermatic cord
√ scrotal skin thickening
√ hydrocele (occasionally)
√ loss of spermatic cord Doppler signal (sensitivity 44%, specificity 67%)
NUC (accuracy 98%):
Dose: 5 – 15 mCi Tc 99m-pertechnetate
Imaging: at 2 – 5 seconds intervals for 1 minute (vascular phase); at 5 minutes intervals for 20 minutes (tissue phase)
√ decreased perfusion / occasionally normal
√ nubbin sign = bump of activity extending medially from iliac artery denoting reactive increased blood flow in spermatic cord with abrupt termination
√ rounded cold area replacing testis (requires knowledge of testis location)

Missed Torsion
= torsion present for > 24 hours
√ enlarged / normal-sized testis with heterogeneous texture
√ normal NUC angiogram / nubbin sign
√ "doughnut" sign = decreased testicular activity with rim hyperemia of dartos perfusion

TESTICULAR TRAUMA
Testicular rupture is indication for immediate surgical intervention!

Salvageability:
   90% if surgical repair occurs < 72 hours after trauma;
   55% if surgical repair occurs > 72 hours after trauma
√ areas of decreased / increased echogenicity
   (hemorrhage ± necrosis)
√ thickened scrotal wall
√ visualization of fracture plane
√ hematocele, may show thickening + calcification of
   tunica vaginalis if chronic
√ uriniferous hydrocele from perforated bulbous urethra

TESTICULAR TUMOR
most common neoplasm in males between ages 25 – 34
years; 1 – 2% of all cancers in males; 1.5% of all
childhood malignancies; 4th most common cause of death
from malignancy between ages 15 – 34 years (12%)
Incidence per year: 5:100,000
Peak age: 25 – 35 years
Risk factors:
   (a) Caucasian race, Jewish religion
   (b) family history of testicular cancer, previous
         testicular neoplasm
   (c) testicular maldescent / atrophy (10 x) abdominal
         site affected in 5%, inguinal site affected in 1.25%
Prognosis: complete remission under chemotherapy in
               65 – 75%; relapse in 10 – 20% within 18
               months
Tumor activity: monitored by levels of alpha-fetoprotein +
   beta-HCG
Metastases: at presentation in 4 – 14% to lung, liver,
   bones, brain, lymph nodes
STAGING
   Stage I   limited to testis + spermatic cord
   Stage II   metastases to lymph nodes below
               diaphragm
      II A nonpalpable
      II B bulky mass
   Stage III   metastases beyond diaphragm / extranodal
               metastases
Prognosis: > 93% 5-year survival rate for stage I
               85 – 90% 5-year survival rate for stage II

Germinal Cell Tumors (95%)
— one histologic type in 65%
— mixed lesion in 35%
   1. Teratocarcinoma (= teratoma + embryonal cell
       carcinoma)
       2nd most common after seminoma, may
       occasionally undergo spontaneous regression
   2. Embryonal cell carcinoma + seminoma
   3. Seminoma + teratoma

A. **SEMINOMA** (40 – 50%)
   peak age 4th – 5th decade, in 25% metastasized
   on initial presentation, pulmonary mets develop in
   19%, most common tumor in undescended testis,
   sensitive to radiation + chemotherapy, 10-year
   survival rate of 75 – 85%

   • beta-HCG elevation in 10%
   √ usually uniformly hypoechoic + confined within
      tunica albuginea

B. NONSEMINOMA
   1. **Embryonal Cell Carcinoma** (20 – 25%)
      = Endodermal sinus tumor
      equivalent to yolk sac tumor in children, peak age
      2nd – 3rd decade and < 2 years; most aggressive
      testicular tumor, visceral metastases; 5-year
      survival rate of 30 – 35%
      • AFP elevation
      √ hypoechoic mass with areas of increased +
         cystic areas (hemorrhage / necrosis)
      √ may show invasion of tunica albuginea
   2. **Teratoma** (4 – 10%)
      consists of elements from more than one germ
      cell layer; benign in children; may transform into
      malignancy in adulthood with metastases to
      lymph nodes, bone, liver in 30% within 5 years
      √ mixed echotexture with sonolucent + highly
         echogenic components
   3. **Choriocarcinoma** (1 – 3%)
      may rapidly metastasize without evidence of
      choriocarcinoma in primary lesion, pulmonary
      metastases develop in 81%, 5-year survival rate
      of nearly 0%
      √ mixed echotexture (hemorrhage, necrosis,
         calcifications)

Stromal Cell Tumors = Interstitial Cell Tumors
(3%)
   • gynecomastia
   • loss of libido
   • precocious virilism (children)
   • impotence (adults)
   1. **Leydig Cell Tumor**
      generally benign with 10% malignant; may secrete
      androgens / estrogens
      benign:malignant = 9:1
   2. **Sertoli Cell Tumor**
      generally benign with 10% malignant; may secrete
      estrogens
   3. Primitive gonadal stroma tumor (exceedingly rare)

Metastases to testis (0.06%)
   (a) in adults: prostate > lung > kidney > GI tract,
         bladder, thyroid, melanoma
   (b) in children: neuroblastoma
   √ often multiple and bilateral, mostly hypoechoic,
      occasionally echogenic masses

Lymphoma / Leukemia of testis
6.7% of all testicular tumors
occult testicular tumor often found in patients in bone
marrow remission ("gonadal barrier" to chemotherapy)
√ diffuse / focal process of decreased echogenicity

Burned Out Tumor
= AZZOPARDI TUMOR
= spontaneous regression of testicular malignancy
(teratocarcinoma)
√ highly echogenic focal lesion ± shadowing

SECOND TESTICULAR TUMOR
Risk for second tumor in cryptorchidism:
15% for inguinal, 30% for abdominal location
Risk for second contralateral tumor:
500 – 1,000 x ; bilaterality in 1.1 – 4.4%;
Δ development interval between 1st + 2nd tumor:
4 months – 25 years
Δ detected in 47% by 2 years; in 60% by 5 years,
in 75% by 10 years
Δ synchronous contralateral tumor in 8 – 10%
US: a testicular abnormality is only malignant in
50%!

TRANSPLANT
COMPLICATIONS in 10%
problematic period between 4 days and 3 weeks after
surgery
• hypertension in 50% (from rejection / arterial stenosis)
• development of lymphoma in 20%
Prognosis: 85% 2-year survival of transplant from living
related donor

Urologic problems with renal transplant
1. URETERAL OBSTRUCTION (1 – 10%)
   (a) acute: secondary to technical problems
   (b) late: secondary to ischemia or previous
   extravasation
   Causes: stricture (most commonly at
   ureterovesicle junction), ureteral kinking,
   edema at ureteroneocystostomy,
   ureteropelvic fibrosis, crossing vessels,
   blood clot, lymphocele, fungus ball,
   calculus
2. URINARY EXTRAVASATION (3 – 10%)
   Causes:
   (a) distal ureteral necrosis secondary to
   interruption of blood supply (early) / vascular
   insufficiency due to rejection (late)
   (b) leakage from ureteroneocystostomy site
   (c) segmental renal infarction
   (d) leakage from anterior cystostomy closure
   site
   Prognosis: high morbidity + mortality (death from
   transplant infection + septicemia)
3. PARARENAL FLUID COLLECTIONS
   = lymphocele (in 50% multiseptated), urinoma
   (rarely septated), abscess, hematoma
   √ photopenic region with displacement / impression
   on kidney / urinary bladder

Vascular problems with renal transplant
A. Prerenal
1. RENAL ARTERY STENOSIS (1 – 12%)
   (a) short-segment stenosis at anastomosis:
   technical (75 %), clamp, cannula, trauma,
   ischemia of donor vessel
   (b) long-segment stenosis: trauma during
   allograft harvesting, faulty operative
   technique, chronic rejection, atherosclerosis,
   kinking, scar formation
   • recent onset of hypertension
   • renal insufficiency
   √ increased peak frequency shift at stenotic site
   > 7.5 kHz (3 MHz transducer) or > 12 kHz
   (5 MHz transducer) + turbulence
   √ dampened signals distal to stenosis
2. RENAL ARTERY OCCLUSION (1 – 5%)
   Predisposed: allografts with disparate vessel
   size, multiple anastomoses, intramural injury
   due to handling, rejection
   • early sudden onset of anuria
   √ global absence of perfusion, uptake,
   excretion
   √ segmental infarction due to occlusion of polar
   artery
   √ hypo- / hyperechoic area ± cortical thickening
   √ no flow in affected area
3. Pseudoaneurysm
   (a) at anastomotic site: due to suture rupture,
   anastomotic leakage, vessel wall ischemia
   (b) mostly of arcuate arteries within allograft:
   following needle biopsy, mycotic infection
   √ hypoechoic mass
   √ mixed arterial + venous pulsations within
   mass
   Prognosis: mostly spontaneous regression
4. Arteriovenous fistula
   following percutaneous biopsy with vascular
   injury
   • hypertension, hematuria, high-output cardiac
   failure
   √ arterialization of waveform in draining vein
   √ turbulence + high frequency velocity shift
B. Postrenal
1. VENOUS THROMBOSIS (renal / iliac vein)
   √ enlargement of transplant
   √ prolonged arterial transit time without arterial
   occlusions + arterial spasms
   √ diminished cortical perfusion
   √ absent venous opacification (venogram
   essential for diagnosis)

High vascular impedance
= Pulsatility index (A–B/mean) or resistive index
(A–B/B) of Doppler signals greater than 1.8 or 0.9
indicate a reduction in diastolic flow velocity
Causes:
(a) Intrinsic vascular obstruction
   1. Acute vascular rejection

2. Renal vein obstruction
(b) Increased intraparenchymal pressure
1. Severe ATN
2. Severe pyelonephritis:
CMV, herpes, E. coli, C. albicans
3. Extrarenal compression:
large collection, hematoma
4. Drug-related nephrotoxic reaction

Gastrointestinal problems with renal transplant
Incidence: 40%
1. GASTROINTESTINAL HEMORRHAGE
(a) Upper GI tract bleeding
gastric erosions, gastric / duodenal ulcers
Mortality rate: 2 – 3 x of normal
(b) Lower GI tract bleeding
hemorrhoids, pseudomembranous colitis, cecal
ulcers, colonic polyps
2. SPONTANEOUS PERFORATION
Causes: antacid impaction, perinephric abscess,
diverticular disease
Location: colonic > small bowel > gastroduodenal
Mortality rate: approaches 75% (because of
delayed diagnosis)

Aseptic necrosis with renal transplant
Most common long-term disabling complication, bilateral
hip / knee involvement is common
Frequency: 2 – 17%
Time of onset: usually develops 5 – 18 months after
transplantation
Pathophysiology of corticosteroid therapy:
(1) fat embolism (fat globules occlude subchondral
end arteries)
(2) increase in fat cell volume in closed marrow
space (increase in intramedullary pressure leads
to diminished perfusion)
(3) osteopenia (increased bone fragility)
(4) reduced sensibility to pain (loss of protection
against excessive stress)
Histo: fragmentation, compression, resorption of dead
bone, proliferation of granulation tissue,
revascularization, production of new bone
• 40% asymptomatic
• joint pain
• restriction of movement
Sites: femoral head, femoral condyles (lateral > medial
condyle), humeral head
√ subchondral bone resorption
√ patchy osteosclerosis
√ collapse / fragmentation of bone
Bone scan:
√ decreased uptake (early) = interruption of blood
supply
√ increased uptake (late) secondary to
(a) revascularization + bone reparation
(b) degenerative osteoarthritis

Acute tubular necrosis in renal transplant
= primary nonfunctioning with improvement over time
(few days – 1 month)
— ATN more frequent in cadaveric kidney
transplants than living-related donor transplant
— ATN greater in transplants with more than one
renal artery
— ATN related to length of ischemic interval
• no constitutional symptoms
• elevated urine sodium
• oliguria may begin immediately after transplantation /
may be delayed for several days
√ enlargement of transplant
√ normal / slightly decreased transplant perfusion
√ decreased + delayed radiopharmaceutical uptake
√ delayed / decreased / absent excretion of Tc-99m
DTPA scan:
√ reduction in diastolic blood flow (63%) (DDx acute
vascular rejection)
DDx: acute rejection (serial renal studies help to
differentiate)

Rejection of renal transplant
most common cause of parenchymal failure
A. **Hyperacute Rejection**
= humeral rejection with circulating antibodies
present in recipient at time of transplantation
Path: thrombosed arterioles + cortical necrosis
Time of onset: within minutes – 2 days after
transplantation
Rx: requires immediate reoperation
B. **Acute Rejection**
= cellular rejection predominantly dependent on
cellular immunity
Time of onset: after 1st week; peak incidence at
2nd – 5th week
Path:
(a) Acute interstitial rejection
= edema of interstitium with lymphocytic
infiltration of capillaries + lymphatics
(b) Acute vascular rejection
= proliferative endovasculitis + vessel
thrombosis
• low urine sodium, increase in serum creatinine
• hypertension
• oliguria
• fever
• tenderness of transplant
• weight gain
√ mild renal enlargement
√ ill-defined corticomedullary junction
√ poor cortical perfusion (more marked than in
ATN)
√ decreased + delayed tracer uptake
√ prolonged excretory phase
√ poor and inhomogeneous nephrogram
√ decrease in diastolic flow velocity + increase in
resistive index

√ rapid tapering + pruning of interlobar arteries
√ multiple stenoses + occlusions
√ nonvisualization of interlobular arteries
√ prolonged arterial opacification (normally < 2 seconds)

C. **Chronic Rejection**
Path: endothelial proliferation in small arteries + arterioles; glomerular lesions (? recurrence of patient's original glomerulonephritis)
Time of onset: months to years after transplantation
√ small kidney
√ diminished number of intrarenal vessels
√ vascular pruning / stenoses / occlusions

TUBERCULOSIS
Urogenital tract is the second most common site after lung; almost always affects the kidney first as a hematogenous focus from lung / bone / GI tract; evidence of previous TB on CXR in 10 – 15%; < 5% have active pulmonary disease
Age: usually before age 50; M > F
• gross / microscopic hematuria
• "sterile" pyuria
• frequency, urgency, dysuria
• history of previous clinical TB (25%)
@ EXTRARENAL SIGNS ON ABDOMINAL PLAIN FILM
√ osseous / paraspinous changes of TB (discitis + psoas abscess)
√ calcified granulomas in liver, spleen, lymph nodes, adrenals
@ RENAL MANIFESTATIONS
unilateral involvement in 75% with hematogenous spread
√ displacement of collecting system secondary to tuberculoma (initial infection)
√ dystrophic amorphous calcifications in tuberculomas of renal parenchyma (in 25%)
√ kidney enlarged (early) / small (late) / normal
√ "smudged" papillae = irregularities of surface of papillae
√ "moth-eaten" calyx = caliceal erosion (early change)
√ irregular tract formations from calyx into papilla
√ large irregular cavities with extensive destruction = papillary necrosis
√ dilated calices (hydrocalicosis) often with sharply defined circumferential narrowings (infundibular strictures) at one / several sites (most common finding)
√ renal calculi (in 10%)
√ "putty kidney" = tuberculous pyonephrosis from ureteral stricture
√ autonephrectomy = small shrunken scarred nonfunctioning kidney ± dystrophic calcifications
√ infection may extend into peri- / pararenal space + psoas
@ URETERAL MANIFESTATIONS
always with evidence of renal involvement as it spreads from kidney

Location: either end of ureter (most commonly distal 1/3), usually asymmetric, may be unilateral
√ ureteral filling defects (= mucosal granulomas)
√ "saw tooth ureter" = irregular jagged contour secondary to dilatation + multiple small mucosal ulcerations + wall edema (early changes)
√ strictures (late changes):
"beaded ureter"   = alternating areas of strictures + dilatations
"corkscrew ureter" = marked tortuosity with strictures + dilatations
"pipestem ureter"   = rigid aperistaltic short thick and straight ureter
√ vesicoureteral reflux through "fixed" patulous orifice
√ ureteral calcifications uncommon (usually in distal portion)
@ BLADDER MANIFESTATIONS
infection from renal source causing interstitial cystitis
√ thickened bladder wall (= muscle hypertrophy + inflammatory tuberculomas)
√ bladder wall ulcerations
√ "shrunken bladder" = scarred bladder with diminished capacity
√ bladder wall calcifications are rare
Cx: fistula / sinus tract
@ SEMINAL VESICULAR + EPIDIDYMAL MANIFESTATIONS
hematogenous infection (NOT ascending)
√ calcifications in 10% (diabetes more common cause)
DDx: Brucellosis, fungal infections (identical picture)

UNICALICEAL (UNIPAPILLARY) KIDNEY
Path: OLIGOMEGANEPHRONIA = reduced number of nephrons and enlargement of glomeruli
Associated with: absence of contralateral kidney, other anomalies
• hypertension
• proteinuria
• azotemia

URACHAL CARCINOMA
= rare tumor arising from the urachus (vestigial remnant of cloaca + allantois) within space of Retzius
Incidence: 0.2 – 0.34% of all bladder cancers; 20 – 40% of all primary bladder adenocarcinomas
Histo: (a) adenocarcinoma (90%) from malignant transformation of columnar metaplasia, in 75% mucin producing
(b) TCC, sarcoma, squamous cell carcinoma
Age: 41 – 70 years; M:F = 3:1
• suprapubic mass, abdominal pain
• hematuria (71%)
• discharge of blood, pus, mucus from umbilicus
• irritative voiding symptoms
• mucous micturition (25%)

Location: supravesical, midline, anterior (80%), in space of Retzius (bounded by transversalis fascia ventrally + peritoneum dorsally)
√ mass anterosuperior to vesical dome with predominantly muscular / extravesical involvement
√ invasion of bladder dome (88%)
√ low attenuation mass in 60% (mucin)
√ often peripheral psammomatous calcifications (70%)
√ markedly increased signal intensity on T2-weighted images
Prognosis: 16% 5-year survival rate

URETEROCELE
= cystic ectasia of subepithelial segment of intravesical ureter

Simple Ureterocele
= ORTHOTOPIC URETEROCELE = congenital prolapse of dilated distal ureter + orifice into bladder lumen at the usual location of the trigone, typically seen with single ureter
Presentation: incidental finding in adults; M:F = 2:3; bilateral in 33%
√ early filling of bulbous terminal ureter ("cobra head")
√ radiolucent halo (= ureteral wall + adjacent bladder urothelium)
√ round / oval lucent defect near trigone
Cx: (1) pyelocaliceal dilatation
(2) prolapse into bladder neck / urethra causing obstruction (rare)
(3) wall thickening secondary to edema from impacted stone / infection

Ectopic Ureterocele
= ureteral bud arising in an abnormal cephalad position from the mesonephric duct and moving caudally with it resulting in an ureteral orifice distal to trigone within / outside bladder
Incidence: in 10% bilateral
(a) in single non-duplicated system (20%)
M:F = 1:1
• hypoplastic / absent ipsilateral trigone
√ poor / non-visualized kidney
√ small / poorly functioning kidney
(b) in upper moiety ureter of duplex kidney (80%)
M:F = 1:4

Weigert-Meyer rule = upper moiety ureter passes through the bladder wall to insert inferior + medial to lower moiety ureter below the level of trigone
SITE OF ECTOPIC INSERTION:
M: proximal to external sphincter:
low in bladder, bladder neck, prostatic urethra, vas deferens, seminal vesicle (seminal vesical cyst), ejaculatory duct
• NO WETTING in males as insertion is always above external sphincter
• epididymitis in preadolescent male

• urge incontinence (insertion into posterior urethra)
F: infrasphincteric insertion:
distal urethra, vaginal vestibule, vagina, cervix, uterus, fallopian tube, rectum
• WETTING in females only if insertion is below external sphincter
• intermittent / constant dribbling

UPPER MOIETY URETER
= subject to ureteral obstruction from ectopic insertion / aberrant artery crossing
√ hydroureteronephrosis of upper pole of duplex kidney + poor function
√ tortuous dilated lower pole ureter
√ poor / nonvisualization of upper pole collecting system (delayed films)
√ "drooping lily" appearance = displacement of lower pole collecting system
√ lateral displacement of lower pole collecting system + ureter
Cx:
(1) bladder outlet obstruction (if ureterocele prolapses into bladder neck / urethra)
(2) contralateral ureteral obstruction (if ectopic ureter large)
(3) multicystic dysplastic kidney (the further the orifice from normal site of insertion, the more dysplastic the kidney!)

LOWER MOIETY URETER
= subject to vesicoureteral reflux
√ displacement of proximal orifice upward (shortened course results in reflux)
√ voiding cystogram may show reflux (rare)
Cx: lower pole of duplex kidney may atrophy (in 50%) secondary to chronic pyelonephritis
= reflux nephropathy (from reflux ± infection)
√ clubbed calices underneath focal scars

Pseudoureterocele
= obstruction of an otherwise normal intramural ureter mimicking ureterocele
Causes:
(a) Tumor: bladder tumor (most common in adults), invasion by cervical cancer, pheochromocytoma of intravesical ureter
(b) Edema: from impacted ureteral calculus (most common in children), radiation cystitis, following ureteral instrumentation
√ thick, irregular halo in urinary bladder
√ "cobra-head" / "spring-onion" appearance of distal ureter
√ NO protrusion of ureter into bladder lumen (oblique views + cystocopy normal)

URETEROPELVIC JUNCTION OBSTRUCTION
M:F = 5:1
Intrinsic causes: primarily functional with impaired
formation of urine bolus
(1) partial replacement of UPJ muscle by collagen
(2) abnormal arrangement of junction muscles causing
dysmotility (69%) (3) mucosal folds (4) eosinophilic
ureteritis (5) ischemia
Extrinsic causes:
(1) aberrant vessels (2) adventitial bands (3) renal cyst
(4) XGP (5) aortic aneurysm
Associated anomalies (27%):
vesicoureteral reflux, bilateral ureteral duplication,
bilateral obstructed megaureter, contralateral
nonfunctioning kidney, contralateral renal agenesis,
meatal stenosis, hypospadia
Location: unilaterally on left > right side; bilateral (30%)
IVP:
√ sharply defined narrowing at UPJ
√ widening of the pelvocaliceal system
√ anterior rotation of pelvis
√ broad tangential sharply defined extrinsic
compression (in arterial crossing)
√ longitudinal striae of redundant mucosa (in
dehydrated state)
√ late changes: unilateral renal enlargement, diminished
opacification, wasting of kidney substance
OB-US:
√ enlarged renal pelvis + branching infundibula +
calices
√ anteroposterior diameter of renal pelvis ≥ 10 mm
√ large unilocular fluid collection (severely dilated
collecting system)
DDx: Multicystic dysplastic kidney, Perinephric urinoma
ADDITIONAL TESTS:
— Diuresis excretory urography (Whitfield):
accurate in 85%
— Diuresis renography (Iodine-131-iodohippurate
sodium / Tc-99m-DTPA)
— Pressure flow urodynamic study (Whitaker)

URETHRAL TUMORS
BENIGN LESIONS
(a) Polyps
1. **Fibroepithelial polyp**
in child / young adult; transitional cell epithelium
√ solitary, pedunculated fingerlike filling defect
attached near verumontanum
Cx: bladder outlet obstruction
2. **Transitional cell papilloma**
older patient; in prostatic / bulbomembranous
urethra; frequently associated with concomitant
bladder papillomas
3. **Adenomatous polyp**
young men; adjacent to verumontanum
Histo: columnar epithelium from aberrant
prostatic epithelium
• hematuria

4. **Penile squamous papilloma / condyloma
acuminata**
in 5% of patients with cutaneous disease (glans
penis)
√ verrucous lesion in distal urethra, rarely
extension into bladder
5. Others: caruncle, urethral mucosal prolapse,
inflammatory tags (in female)

MALIGNANT NEOPLASMS
Incidence: 6th – 7th decade, M:F = 1:5
(a) female
• urethral bleeding
• obstructive symptoms
• dysuria
• mass at introitus
1. Squamous cell carcinoma (70%):
distal 2/3 of urethra
2. Transitional cell carcinoma (8 – 24%):
posterior 1/3 of urethra
3. Adenocarcinoma (18 – 28%):
from periurethral glands of Skene
(b) males
• palpable urethral mass
• periurethral abscess
• obstructive symptoms
• cutaneous fistula
• bloody discharge
Site: bulbomembranous urethra (60%); penile
urethra (30%); prostatic urethra (10%)
1. Squamous cell carcinoma (70%)
secondary to chronic urethritis from venereal
disease (44%) + urethral strictures (88%)
2. Transitional cell carcinoma (16%)
part of multifocal urothelial neoplasia, in 10%
after cystectomy for bladder tumor
3. Adenocarcinoma (6%)
in bulbous urethra originating in glands of
Cowper / Littre
4. Melanoma, Rhabdomyosarcoma, Fibrosarcoma
(rare)
5. Metastases from bladder / prostatic carcinoma
(rare)

UROEPITHELIAL TUMORS
Incidence: 6 – 10% of all malignant renal tumors
Age: 6th decade; M:F = 2:1
√ intraluminal mass (60 – 70%): single / multiple; papillary
/ broad based
√ nonopacification of kidney (in advanced tumor with loss
of function)
√ hydronephrosis
√ parenchymal mass (invasive TCC)
√ thickening of pelvocaliceal wall (with superficial spread
over large areas)
√ stippled appearance (contrast material trapped in
interstices)
√ coarse punctate calcific deposits (0.7 – 6.7%)

A. PAPILLARY MUCOSAL MASS (80%)
√ "goblet sign" = "Bergman sign" = ureter dilated distal to obstructing mass (probably secondary to to-and-fro peristalsis of mass)
√ "catheter-coiling sign" = coiling of catheter on retrograde catheterization
B. INFILTRATING FORM (20%)
√ stricture which may simulate extrinsic cause
√ arterial encasement + occlusion + neovascularity
√ enlarged pelvic + ureteric arteries
√ occlusion of renal vein / branches (41%)

Transitional Cell Carcinoma
85% of all uroepithelial tumors
√ papillary, bulky, sessile
High-risk group to develop TCC of upper tract:
(1) high-grade high-stage bladder TCC (2) cystectomy for carcinoma in situ (3) analgesic abuser (8 x increase) (4) employee in aniline dye factory (5) patient from Balkan (6) bladder tumor + vesicoureteral reflux (7) exposure to urothelial carcinogens (cyclophosphamide, tobacco smoke)
Ureteral site: lower 1/3 (70%), mid 1/3 (15%), upper 1/3 (15%)
SYNCHRONOUS TCC
(a) with primary ureteral TCC in 39%
(b) with primary renal TCC in 24%
(c) with primary bladder TCC in 2%

METACHRONOUS TCC IN UPPER TRACT
(a) with primary renal + ureteral TCC in 12% after 25 months
(b) with primary bladder TCC in 4% (2/3 within 2 years, up to 20 years)

METACHRONOUS TCC OF BLADDER
(a) after primary renal TCC in 23 – 40% after 15 – 48 months
(b) after primary ureteral TCC in 20 – 50% after 10 – 24 months

URINOMA
= uriniferous perirenal pseudocyst secondary to tear in collecting system with continuing renal function due to lower urinary tract obstruction / trauma
Etiology:
(a) nonobstructive: blunt / penetrating trauma
(b) obstructive:
(1) ureteral obstruction (calculus, surgical ligature, neoplasm)
(2) bladder outlet obstruction (posterior urethral valves)
√ extravasation of contrast material
√ smooth thin-walled cavity (-10 to +30 HU)
√ sickle-shaped collection (SUBCAPSULAR urinoma)
√ cystic mass in perirenal space (LOCALIZED PERIRENAL urinoma)
√ cystic mass filling entire perirenal space (DIFFUSE PERIRENAL urinoma)
√ encapsulated expanding intrarenal cystic mass separating renal tissue fragments (INTRARENAL urinoma)
√ frequently associated with urine ascites

UROLITHIASIS
Anderson-Carr-Randall theory of renal stone formation: in the presence of abnormally high calcium excretion exceeding lymphatic capacity, microaggregates of calcium (present in the normal kidney) occur in medulla, increase in size, migrate toward caliceal epithelium, and rupture into calices to form calculi

Mineral composition	Opacity
A. CALCIUM STONES (90%)	
1. Calcium oxalate monohydrate (= whewellite) + dihydrate (wedellite) (34 %)	+++
√ small, densely opaque, mamillated (stippled appearance)	
2. Calcium oxalate plus apatite (34%)	+++
3. Calcium phosphate (= apatite) (6%)	+++
rarely pure (= laminated), occasionally forms in infected alkaline urine	
4. Calcium hydrogen phosphate (= brushite)	+++
5. Magnesium ammonium phosphate (= struvite)(1%)	++
laminated, result of urea-splitting organisms (usually Proteus), most common constituent of staghorn calculus	
6. Struvite plus calcium phosphate (14%)	++
associated with infection	
B. Cystine (3%): mildly opaque	+
C. Uric acid (7%): radiolucent	-
D. Xanthine (extremely rare): nonopaque	-
E. Matrix (Mucoprotein / Mucopolysaccharide) (rare): nonopaque	-

Incidence: 1:1,000; M > F
Causes:
1. Idiopathic urolithiasis
2. Calcium stones
    (a) with hypercalcemia:
        hyperparathyroidism, milk-alkali syndrome,
        hypervitaminosis D, neoplastic disorders,
        sarcoidosis, Cushing syndrome
    (b) with normocalcemia:
        obstruction, urinary tract infection, vesical
        diverticulum, horseshoe kidney, medullary
        sponge kidney, prolonged immobilization, renal
        tubular acidosis, idiopathic hypercalcuria
3. Hyperoxaluria
4. Uric acid lithiasis (stones form in acid urine)
    (a) with hyperuricemia:
        gout (25%), myeloproliferative diseases,
        antimitotic drugs, chemo- / radiation therapy,
        uricosuric agents, Lesch-Nyhan syndrome
    (b) with normouricemia:
        idiopathic; occurrence in acid concentrated urine
        (hot climate, ileostomy)
5. Cystinuria (stones form in acid urine)
    inherited autosomal recessive disorder of amino acid
    transport in renal tubules
    Age of onset: after 10 years
    Rx: (1) decreased intake of methionine
           (2) alkalinization of urine
6. Xanthinuria
    inherited autosomal recessive deficiency of xanthine
    oxidase (failure of normal oxidation of purines)
7. Urinary tract infection
    may lead to magnesium ammonium phosphate
    = struvite stones
8. Any condition causing nephrocalcinosis
Cx: Xanthogranulomatous pyelonephritis

VARICOCELE
= dilatation + tortuosity of plexus pampiniformis
Components of pampiniform plexus:
    (1) internal spermatic vein (ventral location) draining
        testis
    (2) vein of vas deferens (mediodorsal location) draining
        epididymis
    (3) cremasteric vein (laterodorsal location) draining
        scrotal wall
Etiology:
    (a) retrograde flow into internal spermatic vein
        secondary to incompetent / absent valve at level of
        left renal vein / IVC on right side
    (b) compression of left renal vein by tumor, aberrant
        renal artery, obstructed renal vein
Incidence:
    (a) Clinical varicocele: in 10 – 15% of adult males, in
        21 – 39% of infertile men
    (b) Subclinical varicocele: in 40 – 75% of infertile men

Theoretical causes for infertility:
    (1) increase in local temperature (2) reflux of toxic
    substances from adrenal gland (3) alteration in Leydig
    cell function (4) hypoxia of germinative tissue
    • scrotal pain
    • scrotal swelling
    • abnormal spermatogram (impaired motility, immature
      sperm, oligospermia)
Location: left side (78%), bilateral (16%), right side (6%)
Bidirectional Doppler sonography (erect with quiet
breathing):
    (1) SHUNT TYPE : insufficent distal valves allow
        spontaneous + continuous reflux from internal
        spermatic vein (retrograde flow) into cremasteric
        vein + vein of vas deferens (orthograde flow) via
        collaterals
        • sperm quality diminished
        • clinically plexus type (Grade II + III)
          = medium-sized + large varicoceles
    (2) STOP TYPE / PRESSURE TYPE : intact distal
        valves allow only brief period of reflux from
        spermatic vein into pampiniform plexus under
        Valsalva maneuver
        • sperm quality normal
        • clinically central type (Grade 0 + I)
          = subclinical + small varicocele
US: diameter of dominant vein in upright
        position at inguinal canal

	relaxed	during Valsalva
normal	2.2 mm	2.7 mm
small varicocele	2.5 – 4.0	increase of 1.0 mm
moderate varicocele	4.0 – 5.0	increase of 1.2 – 1.5 mm
large varicocele	> 5.0	increase of > 1.5 mm

VESICOURETERAL REFLUX
Prevalence in school girls: 1.4%
A. CONGENITAL REFLUX = PRIMARY REFLUX
    = incompetence of ureterovesical junction
      unassociated with morphologic abnormalities
    • short submucosal ureteral tunnel (normally has a
      length/width ratio of 4:1)
    • large laterally located ureteral orifice
B. ACQUIRED REFLUX = SECONDARY REFLUX
    1. paraureteric diverticulum = Hutch diverticulum
    2. duplication with ureterocele
    3. cystitis (in 29 – 50%)
    4. urethral obstruction (urethral valves)
    5. neurogenic bladder
    6. absence of abdominal musculature (Prune belly
       syndrome)
Cx: renal scarring with UTI (30 – 60%)

GRADES OF REFLUX (VCUG):
Grade I : √ reflux into distal ureters

Grade II : √ reflux into collecting system (without caliceal dilatation / blunting)

Grade III: √ all of the above + mild dilatation of pelvis and calices

Grade IV: √ all of the above + moderate dilatation (clubbing of calices)

Grade V : √ all of the above + severe tortuosity of ureter

> *Prognosis:* (a) Grade I – III resolve with maturation of the ureterovesical junction
> (b) Grade IV – V require surgery

Radionuclide cystography:

Δ lower radiation dose to gonads than fluoroscopic cystography (5 mrad)

Δ evaluation of bladder volume at reflux, volume of refluxed urine, residual urine volume, ureteral reflux drainage time

  (a) indirect: IV injection of Tc-99m DTPA
  (b) direct: instillation of 1 mCi Tc-99m pertechnetate (more sensitive for reflux during filling phase which occurs in 20%)

VON HIPPEL-LINDAU SYNDROME

= inherited neurocutaneous dysplasia complex, autosomal dominant with variable penetrance and delayed expression

Age at onset: 2nd – 3rd decade

• visual disturbances (hemorrhage, retinal detachment, glaucoma, uveitis)
• neurologic disorders (from hemangioblastomas)
• polycythemia

@ CNS

1. Hemangioblastomas
   most frequent cause of morbidity and mortality
   (a) cerebellar (most common)
       √ large cystic lesion in posterior fossa with enhancing mural nodule
   (b) medullary
   (c) spinal
2. Retinal angiomatosis (in 45%)

@ KIDNEYS

1. Cortical renal cysts (75%)
   multiple + bilateral (may be confused with adult polycystic kidney disease)
2. Renal cell carcinoma (12 – 83%)
   second most frequent cause of mortality
   √ multicentric in 87%, bilateral in 75%, may arise from cyst wall
   50% metastatic at time of discovery
3. Renal adenoma
4. Renal hemangioma

@ ADRENAL

1. Pheochromocytoma (in 17%): confined to certain families

@ PANCREAS

1. Pancreatic cystadenoma / cystadenocarcinoma
2. Pancreatic islet cell tumor

3. Pancreatic hemangioblastoma
4. Pancreatic cysts (in 30%); incidence in autopsies up to 72%
   √ usually multiple and multilocular cysts

@ LIVER

1. Liver hemangioma
2. Adenoma

@ OTHERS

1. Paraganglioma
2. Cysts in virtually any organ: liver, spleen, adrenal, epididymis, omentum, mesentery, lung, bone

WILMS TUMOR

= NEPHROBLASTOMA

Δ most common malignant abdominal neoplasm in childhood (10 %)

Δ 3rd most common malignancy in childhood (after leukemia + brain tumors), (neuroblastoma more common in infancy)

Δ 3rd most common of all renal masses in childhood (after hydronephrosis + multicystic dysplastic kidney)

Incidence: 1:10,000 live births; rare during first year; 50% before 3 years, 75% before 5 years; 90% before 8 years; rare in adults; multifocal in 10 %; bilateral in 5 – 9%

Mean age: 2.5 – 3 years (range of 3 months – 8 years); 90% by 8 years; M:F = 1:1

Histo: arises from undifferentiated metanephrogenic blastema as nephroblastomatosis, recapitulates the developing embryonic kidney
   (1) aggregates of small blastemal cells
   (2) neoplastic nodules
   (3) elongated mesenchymal cells

In 14% associated with:

(1) Beckwith-Wiedemann syndrome (exophthalmos, macrosomia, macroglossia, hepatomegaly, omphalocele, hyperglycemia from islet cell hyperplasia)

(2) Sporadic aniridia

(3) Hemihypertrophy: total / segmental / crossed (2.5%)

(4) Drash syndrome (pseudohermaphroditism, glomerulonephritis, nephrotic syndrome)

(5) Renal anomalies (horseshoe kidney, duplex / solitary / fused kidney)

(6) Genital anomalies (cryptorchidism, hypospadia, ambiguous genitalia)

STAGE:

I tumor limited to kidney

II local extension into perirenal tissue / renal vessels outside kidney / lymph nodes

III not totally resectable (peritoneal implants, other than paraaortic nodes involved, invasion of vital structures)

IV hematogenous metastases (lung, liver, bone [rare], brain)

V bilateral renal involvement (5 – 10%)

• palpable abdominal mass (90%)

- hypertension (50 – 60%)
- abdominal pain (25%)
- fever (15%)
- gross hematuria (7%)
- microscopic hematuria (15 – 20%)
√ large tumor (average size 12 cm) with pseudocapsule
√ partially cystic = focal hemorrhage and necrosis (common)
√ curvilinear / phlebolithic calcifications (15%); (not stippled as in neuroblastoma)
√ distorted "clobbered" calices
√ tumor may invade IVC / right atrium (4 – 10%)
√ tumor may cross midline
√ hypervascular tumor: enlarged tortuous vessels, coarse neovascularity; small arterial aneurysms, vascular lakes
√ parasitization of vascular supply
NUC:
  √ nonfunctioning kidney (10%)
  √ hypo- / iso- / hyperperfusion on radionuclide angiogram
  √ absent tracer accumulation on delayed static images
  √ displacement of kidney + distortion of collecting system

VARIANT: **Cystic Partially Differentiated Nephroblastoma**
= combination of MLCN + Wilms tumor elements
Incidence: M < F
√ multiple noncommunicating locules
√ polypoid masses within locules

WOLMAN DISEASE
= FAMILIAL XANTHOMATOSIS
= rare autosomal recessive lipidosis with accumulation of cholesteryl esters and triglycerides in visceral foam cells + various tissues
Etiology: deficiency of lysosomal acid lipase
- poor development in neonatal period: failure to gain weight
√ hepatosplenomegaly
√ extensive bilateral punctate calcifications throughout enlarged adrenals (retaining normal shape)
√ generalized osteoporosis
Prognosis: death occurs within first few months of life

ZELLWEGER SYNDROME
= CEREBROHEPATORENAL SYNDROME
autosomal recessive,
- muscular hypotonia
- hepatomegaly + jaundice
- craniofacial dysmorphism
- seizures, mental retardation
√ brain dysgenesis (lissencephaly, macrogyria, polymicrogyria)
√ renal cortical cysts
Prognosis: death in early infancy

DIFFERENTIAL DIAGNOSIS OF OBSTETRICAL AND GYNECOLOGICAL DISORDERS

OBSTETRICS
Level I obstetrical ultrasound
Indication: MS-AFP > 2 multiples of mean (MOM) on 2
occasions between 14 and 18 weeks MA
Scope of examination:
1. Fetal number
2. Fetal lie
3. Documentation of fetal life
4. Placental location
5. Amniotic fluid volume
6. Gestational dating
7. Detection + evaluation of maternal pelvic masses
8. Survey of fetal anatomy (2nd + 3rd trimester)

Level II obstetrical ultrasound
Indication: AF-AFP > 3 standard deviations above mean
Scope of examination:
1. Spina bifida
2. Ventral wall defect (gastroschisis, omphalocele)
3. Upper GI obstruction
4. Cystic hygroma
5. Renal anomalies (obstructive uropathy, renal
agenesis)

Elevated alpha-fetoprotein
Origin: formed by yolk sac + fetal liver; levels peak in
early 2nd trimester and decline to low levels at
end of pregnancy (a) detectable in amniotic fluid
secondary to leakage of fetal serum
(transudation, proteinuria) (b) detectable in
maternal circulation secondary to leakage from
placenta / amniotic fluid
• screening at 14 – 18 weeks
(a) Elevation in MATERNAL SERUM (MS-AFP)
   = defined as 2.5 multiples of the median / equivalent
   to the 5th percentile
   Incidence: 5 – 7% of all 2nd trimester pregnancies
(b) Elevation in AMNIOTIC FLUID (AF-AFP)
   Δ elevation of 3 – 5 multiples of the median in
   2 – 3:1,000; 1/4 deliver normal babies
   Δ elevation > 5 multiples of the median in 1 – 2:1,000
Associated with:
   A. FETAL ANOMALIES (61%)
      1. Neural tube defects: anencephaly, meningocele,
         myelomeningocele, encephalocele,
         holoprosencephaly, ventriculomegaly (in 2 – 5%
         missed by US)
         Risk of recurrence: 3% after one affected child;
                              6% after 2 affected children
      2. Ventral wall defects (gastroschisis,
         omphalocele): sensitivity of 50%
      3. Upper GI obstruction (esophageal / duodenal
         atresia)

      4. Cystic hygroma, teratoma
      5. Chorioangioma
      6. Congenital nephrosis
      7. Hepatitis
   B. ERRONEOUS DATES (18%)
   C. MULTIPLE GESTATIONS (14%)
   D. FETAL DEATH IN UTERO (7%) / fetal distress /
      threatened abortion
   E. LOW BIRTH WEIGHT / premature labor

Low alpha-fetoprotein
= MS-AFP ≤ 0.5 / AF-AFP ≤ 0.72 multiples of the
median
Trisomy syndromes (trisomy 21 & 18)

Use of chromosome analysis
Frequency: 11 – 35% of fetuses with sonographically
identified abnormalities have chromosomal
abnormalities
1. CNS anomalies: holoprosencephaly (43 – 59%),
   Dandy-Walker malformation (29 – 50%), cerebellar
   hypoplasia, agenesis of corpus callosum;
   myelomeningocele (33 – 50%)
2. Cystic hygroma
3. Omphalocele (30 – 40%)
4. Cardiac malformations
5. Nonimmune hydrops
6. Duodenal atresia
7. Severe IUGR

Uterus large for dates
1. Multiple gestation pregnancy
2. Inaccurate menstrual history
3. Fibroids
4. Polyhydramnios
5. Hydatidiform mole
6. Fetal macrosomia

First trimester bleeding
Affects 25% of all pregnancies of which 50% terminate in
abortion
A. with intrauterine conceptus identified
   1. blighted ovum / blighted twin
   2. threatened abortion
   3. implantation bleed
   4. gestational trophoblastic disease
B. with normal central stripe
   (a) with beta-hCG level > 1,800 mIU/ml
      1. recent spontaneous abortion
      2. ectopic pregnancy
   (b) with beta-hCG level < 1,800 mIU/ml
      1. very early IUP
      2. ectopic pregnancy

Empty gestational sac
1. Normal early IUP between 5-7 weeks MA
2. Blighted ovum

DDx: Pseudosac of ectopic pregnancy

Polyhydramnios
Incidence: 2%
Etiology:
  A. <u>IDIOPATHIC</u> (60%)
  B. <u>MATERNAL CAUSES</u> (20%)
    1. Diabetes
    2. Rh incompatibility
    3. Placental tumors
  C. <u>FETAL ANOMALIES</u> (20%)
    (a) NEURAL TUBE DEFECTS (9%)
    (b) GASTROINTESTINAL ANOMALIES (6%)
      impairment of fetal swallowing (esophageal atresia in 3 %); high intestinal atresias (1.2 – 1.8%)
    (c) CARDIAC ANOMALIES (7%)
      septal rhabdomyoma, arrhythmia, CHD
    (d) CHEST ANOMALIES
      cystic adenomatoid malformation, primary pulmonary hypoplasia, extralobar sequestration, congenital chylothorax
    (e) GENITOURINARY ANOMALIES
      multicystic dysplastic kidneys, mesoblastic nephroma
    (f) SKELETAL DYSPLASIA
      Dwarfism
    (g) MISCELLANEOUS
      cystic hygroma, teratoma, congenital pancreatic cyst
    mnemonic: "TARDI"
      Twins
      Anomalies, fetal
      Rh incompatibility
      Diabetes
      Idiopathic

Oligohydramnios
Etiology:
  mnemonic: "DRIPP"
    Demise of fetus
    Renal anomalies (inadequate urine production): infantile polycystic kidney disease, posterior urethral valves, prune-belly syndrome
    IUGR
    Premature rupture of membranes
    Post dates
N.B.:   bilateral renal obstruction, if combined with intestinal obstruction, may be associated with polyhydramnios
Cx: pulmonary hypoplasia

Dilated cervix
1. INEVITABLE ABORTION
2. INCOMPETENT CERVIX
  = gaping cervix usually develops during 2nd trimester
  Predisposed: cervical trauma (D & C, cauterization), DES exposure in utero with cervical hypoplasia, estrogen medication
  √ visualization of fetal parts / amniotic fluid within dilated endocervical canal (stress test: patient standing with bladder empty)
  Prognosis: 14th – 18th week best time for Rx prior to significant cervical dilatation
3. PREMATURE LABOR
  = spontaneous onset of palpable, regularly occurring uterine contractions between 20th – 37th weeks

Umbilical cord masses
1. **False Knot**
  = varix of umbilical vessel
  √ irregular protrusions from the cord
2. **True Knot**
  caused by excessive fetal movements
  Incidence: 1% of pregnancies
  Predisposed: long cord, male fetus, multiparity
  √ localized distension of umbilical vein
  √ tortuosity of cord at level of knot
  Cx: vascular occlusion + fetal death in utero
3. **Umbilical Cord Hematoma**
  = rupture of the wall of the umbilical vein secondary to mechanical trauma (torsion, loops, knots, traction) / congenital weakness of vessel wall
  Incidence: 1:5,505 to 1:12,699 deliveries
  Location: near fetal insertion of umbilical cord (most common)
  √ hyper- / hypoechoic mass 1 – 2 cm in size, may be multiple (18%)
  Cx: rupture into amniotic cavity with exsanguination
  Prognosis: overall perinatal fetal mortality is 52%
4. **Allantoin Duct Cyst**
  (a) true cyst = remnant of umbilical vesicle / allantois located close to fetus
  (b) false cyst = liquefaction of Wharton jelly
5. NEOPLASM
  (a) **Angiomyxoma / Hemangioma**
    Histo: multiple channels lined by benign endothelium surrounded by edema + myxomatous degeneration of Wharton jelly
    Location: more frequently toward placental end of umbilical cord
    √ hyperechoic mass within cord
    √ may be associated with pseudocyst (= localized collection of edema)
    Cx: (1) nonimmune hydrops
  (b) Other tumors: myxosarcoma, dermoid, teratoma
6. **Umbilical Hernia**
  = protrudes from anterior abdominal wall with normal insertion of umbilical vessels
  Predisposed: Blacks, low-birth-weight infants, trisomy 21, congenital hypothyroidism, mucopolysaccharidoses, Beckwith-Wiedemann syndrome

Prognosis: spontaneous closure in first 3 years of life
7. **Umbilical vein varix**
   Incidence: < 4% of all umbilical cord abnormalities
   Site: intraamniotic, intraabdominal
   √ fusiform dilatation of umbilical vein
   Cx: (1) thrombosis with subsequent fetal death
   (2) partial thrombosis with IUGR

Abnormal placental size
A. ENLARGEMENT
   = > 5 cm in sections obtained at right angles to long
   axis of placenta
   (a) maternal disease
       1. diabetic mothers (= villous edema)
       2. Intrauterine infections
       3. anemic mothers (= normal histology)
   (b) fetal disease
       1. hemolytic disease of the newborn (= villous
          edema + hyperplasia)
       2. Umbilical vein obstruction
       3. Fetal high-output failure: large chorioangioma,
          sacrococcygeal teratoma, arteriovenous fistula
B. DECREASE IN SIZE
   1. Preeclampsia
      associated with placental infarcts in 33 – 60%

Vascular spaces of the placenta
1. "PLACENTAL CYSTS"
   = large fetal veins located between amnion + chorion
   anastomosing with umbilical vein
   √ sluggish blood flow (detectable by real-time
   observation)
2. BASAL VEINS
   = decidual + uterine veins
   √ lacy appearing network of veins underneath
   placenta
   DDx: placental abruption
3. INTRAPLACENTAL VENOUS LAKES
   √ intraplacental sonolucent spaces
   √ whirlpool motion pattern of flowing blood

Macroscopic lesions of the placenta
1. SUBCHORIONIC FIBRIN DEPOSITION (10 – 15%)
   = laminated collection of fibrin deposition as a result
   of thrombosis of maternal blood in intervillous
   spaces
   √ subchorionic sonolucent area
2. INTERVILLOUS THROMBOSIS (3 – 50%)
   = interplacental areas of hemorrhage
   √ sonolucent intraplacental lesions (mm – cm range)
3. PERIVILLOUS FIBRIN DEPOSITION
   = nonlaminated collection of fibrin deposition as a
   result of thrombosis of intervillous spaces
4. PLACENTAL INFARCT (25%)
   = coagulation necrosis of villi
   • increased frequency in preeclampsia + essential
   hypertension
   √ sonolucent lesion in early phase

√ may undergo organization + calcification
5. CHORIOANGIOMA (1%)
6. HYDATIDIFORM MOLE

Nuchal skin thickening
= skin thickening of posterior neck > 5 mm
Causes:
   A. Normal variant (0.06%)
   B. Chromosomal disorders: Trisomy 21 (in 45 – 80%),
      trisomy 18, XXXX syndrome, XXXXY syndrome,
      18p-syndrome, 13q-syndrome
   C. Nonchromosomal disorders:
      1. Multiple pterygium syndrome = Escobar
         syndrome
      2. Klippel-Feil syndrome (fusion of cervical
         vertebrae, CHD, deafness (30%) cleft palate
      3. Zellweger syndrome = cerebrohepatorenal
         syndrome (large forehead, flat facies, macrogyria,
         hepatomegaly, cystic kidney disease,
         contractures of extremities)

FETAL CNS ANOMALIES
A. HYDROCEPHALUS
   1. Aqueductal stenosis
   2. Communicating hydrocephalus
   3. Dandy-Walker malformation
   4. Choroid plexus papilloma
B. NEURAL TUBE DEFECT
   1. Spina bifida
   2. Anencephaly
   3. Acrania
   4. Encephalocele
   5. Porencephaly
   6. Hydranencephaly
   7. Holoprosencephaly
   8. Iniencephaly
   9. Microcephaly
   10. Agenesis of corpus callosum
   11. Lissencephaly
   12. Arachnoid cyst
   13. Choroid plexus cyst
   14. Vein of Galen aneurysm

FETAL CHEST ANOMALIES
1. Cystic adenomatoid malformation
2. Lung sequestration
3. Bronchogenic cyst
4. Diaphragmatic hernia

Cystic chest mass
1. Bronchogenic cyst
2. Enteric cyst
3. Neurenteric cyst
4. Cystic adenomatoid malformation (Type I)
5. Diaphragmatic abnormalities
6. Pericardial cyst

Complex chest mass
1. Diaphragmatic abnormalities
2. Cystic adenomatoid malformation (Type I, II, III)
3. Pulmonary sequestration
4. Complex enteric cyst

Solid chest mass
1. Diaphragmatic abnormalities
2. Cystic adenomatoid malformation (Type III)
3. Pulmonary sequestration
4. Bronchial atresia
5. Pericardial tumor

FETAL CARDIAC ANOMALIES
Antenatal sonographic diagnosis to prompt cardiac evaluation:
A. Abnormalities of cardiac position
B. CNS
  1. Hydrocephalus
  2. Microcephaly
  3. Agenesis of corpus callosum
  4. Encephalocele (Meckel-Gruber syndrome)
C. Gastrointestinal
  1. Esophageal atresia
  2. Duodenal atresia
  3. Situs abnormalities
  4. Diaphragmatic hernia
D. Ventral wall defect
  1. Omphalocele
  2. Ectopia cordis
E. Renal
  1. Bilateral renal agenesis
  2. Dysplastic kidneys
F. Twins
  1. Conjoined twins

Risk factors for congenital heart disease
Prenatal risk factors for congenital heart disease:
A. FETAL RISK FACTORS
  1. Symmetrical IUGR
  2. Fetal bradycardia
  3. Abnormal karyotype (CHD in Down syndrome in 40%; in Trisomy 18 / 13 in > 90 %; in Turner syndrome in 35%)
  4. Somatic anomalies by US (omphaloceles in 20%, fetal hydrops in 35%)
     60% of CHD have associated extracardiac anomalies!
  5. Oligo- / polyhydramnios
B. MATERNAL RISK FACTORS
  1. Insulin-dependent diabetes mellitus
  2. Collagen vascular disease: SLE
  3. Maternal heart disease
  4. Infection: rubella
  5. Drugs
     (a) phenytoin (in 2% PS, AS, coarctation, PDA)
     (b) trimethadione (in 20% transposition, tetralogy, hypoplastic left heart)
     (c) sex hormones (in 3%)
     (d) lithium (Ebstein anomaly, tricuspid atresia)
     (e) alcohol (VSD, ASD)
C. FAMILIAL RISK FACTORS FOR RECURRENCE OF HEART DISEASE
  — overall incidence : 6 – 8:1,000 live births
  — affected sibling　: 1 – 4% (risk doubled)
  — affected parent　: 2.5 – 4%
POOR PROGNOSTIC FEATURES:
  (1) intrauterine cardiac failure (hydrops)
  (2) extracardiac anomalies
  (3) delivery in center without pediatric cardiology

In utero detection of cardiac anomalies
A. Abnormal 4-chamber view:
  1. Septal rhabdomyoma
  2. Endocardial cushion defect
  3. Ventricular septal defect
  4. Epstein anomaly
  5. Single ventricle
B. Ventricular disproportion:
  1. Hypoplastic right / left ventricle
  2. Hypoplastic aortic arch
  3. Aortic / subaortic stenosis
  4. Coarctation of aorta
  5. Ostium primum defect
C. Increased aortic root dimension:
  1. Tetralogy of Fallot
  2. Truncus arteriosus
  3. Hypoplastic left ventricle with transposition
D. Decreased aortic root dimension
  1. Coarctation of aorta
  2. Hypoplastic left ventricle

Structural cardiac abnormalities + fetal hydrops
1. Atrioventricular septal defect + complete heart block
2. Hypoplastic left heart
3. Critical aortic stenosis
4. Cardiac tumor
5. Ectopia cordis
6. Dilated cardiomyopathy
7. Ebstein anomaly
8. Pulmonary atresia

FETAL GASTROINTESTINAL ANOMALIES
1. Esophageal atresia ± TE fistula
2. Duodenal atresia
3. Meconium peritonitis
4. Hirschsprung disease
5. Choledochal cyst
6. Mesenteric cyst

Nonvisualization of fetal stomach
Incidence:　2% (stomach is visualized in almost all normal fetuses by 14 weeks + in all normal fetuses by 19 weeks)
1. physiologic gastric emptying / intermittent swallowing (repeat scan after 30 minutes)

2. decreased amniotic fluid volume
3. CNS abnormalities
4. GI tract abnormalities: congenital diaphragmatic hernia, TE-fistula with esophageal atresia
5. cleft palate

Double bubble sign
frequently associated with Trisomy 21
1. Duodenal atresia
2. Duodenal stenosis
3. Duodenal web
4. Annular pancreas
5. Preduodenal portal vein
6. Ladd bands
7. Malrotation

Dilated bowel
1. Meconium ileus
   Δ   all newborns with meconium ileus have cystic fibrosis
   Δ   10 – 15% of newborns with cystic fibrosis present with meconium ileus
2. "Apple peel" atresia of small bowel
3. Jejunal atresia
4. Megacystic-microcolon intestinal hypoperistalsis syndrome
5. Colonic aganglionosis = Hirschsprung disease (may be associated with Down syndrome)
6. Anorectal atresia (associated with CNS abnormalities, part of VACTERL complex)

Bowel obstruction
Etiology: Intestinal atresia / stenosis secondary to vascular accident, volvulus, meconium ileus, intussusception after organogenesis
Incidence: imperforate anus 1:3,000; small bowel 1:5,000; colon 1:20,000
Pathologic types:
   I   one / more transverse diaphragms
   II   blind-ending loops connected by fibrous string
   III   complete separation of blind-ending loops
   IV   apple-peel atresia of small bowel (occlusion of SMA branch)
Associated with: GI anomalies in 45% (malrotation, duplication, microcolon, esophageal atresia)
√ multiple distended bowel loops > 7 mm in diameter
√ increased peristalsis
√ polyhydramnios (not seen in distal intestinal obstruction)
Cx: Meconium peritonitis (50%)
DDx: (1)   Other cystic masses: duodenal atresia, hydronephrosis, ovarian cyst, mesenteric cyst
   (2)   Chronic chloride diarrhea

Intraabdominal calcifications
A. Peritoneal
   1. Meconium peritonitis
   2. Plastic peritonitis associated with hydrometrocolpos
B. Tumors
   1. Hemangioma / hemangioendothelioma
   2. Hepatoblastoma
   3. Metastatic neuroblastoma
   4. Teratoma
   5. Ovarian dermoid
C. Congenital infection
   1. Toxoplasmosis
   2. Cytomegalovirus

Cystic mass in fetal abdomen
A. posterior mid abdomen
   1. Cysts of renal origin
   2. Hydroureteronephrosis
   3. Multicystic dysplastic kidney
   4. Paranephric collection
B. right upper quadrant
   1. Liver cyst
   2. Choledochal cyst
C. left upper quadrant
   1. Splenic cyst
D. anterior mid abdomen
   1. Duplication cyst
   2. Mesenteric cyst
   3. Meconium pseudocyst
   4. Dilated bowel
   5. Urachal cyst
E. lower abdomen
   1. Adnexal cyst
   2. Hydrometrocolpos
   3. Meningocele
   4. Sacrococcygeal teratoma

FETAL URINARY TRACT ANOMALIES
1. Bilateral renal agenesis
2. Infantile polycystic kidney disease
3. Adult polycystic kidney disease
4. Multicystic dysplastic kidney
5. Ureteropelvic junction obstruction
6. Megaureter
7. Posterior urethral valves
8. Prune-belly syndrome
9. Megacystis-microcolon-intestinal hypoperistalsis syndrome
10. Mesoblastic nephroma
11. Wilms tumor
12. Neuroblastoma

FETAL SKELETAL DYSPLASIA
= heterogeneous group of bone growth disorders resulting in abnormal shape + size of the skeleton
Birth prevalence: 2.4:10,000 births
Prognosis: 23% stillbirths, 32% death in 1st week of life

	Birth prevalence	Perinatal deaths
Thanatophoric dysplasia	0.69:10,000	1:246
Achondroplasia	0.37:10,000	none
Achondrogenesis	0.23:10,000	1:639
Osteogenesis imperf. type II	0.18:10,000	1:799
Osteogenesis imperf., others	0.18:10,000	none
Asphyxiating thoracic dysplasia	0.14:10,000	1:3196
Chondrodysplasia punctata	0.09:10,000	none
Campomelic dysplasia	0.05:10,000	1:3196
Chondroectodermal dysplasia	0.05:10,000	1:3196

CLASSIFICATION
(1) Osteochondrodysplasias
   = abnormalities of cartilage / bone growth and development
(2) Dysostoses
   = malformation of individual bones singly / in combination
(3) Idiopathic osteolyses
   = disorders associated with multifocal resorption of bone
(4) Chromosomal aberrations
(5) Primary metabolic disorders

TERMINOLOGY
Micromelia = shortening involves entire limb (e.g.,humerus, radius + ulna, hand)
Rhizomelia = shortening involves proximal segment (e.g., humerus)
Mesomelia = shortening involves intermediate segment (e.g., radius + ulna)
Acromelia = shortening involves distal segment (e.g., hand)

Lethal bone dysplasia
in order of frequency
1. Thanatophoric dysplasia
2. Osteogenesis imperfecta type II
3. Achondrogenesis type I + II
4. Jeune syndrome (may be nonlethal)
5. Hypophosphatasia, congenital lethal form
6. Chondroectodermal dysplasia (usually nonlethal)
7. Chondrodysplasia punctata, rhizomelic type
8. Camptomelic dysplasia
9. Short-rib polydactyly syndrome
10. Homozygous achondroplasia

Narrow chest
1. Short-rib polydactyly syndrome
2. Asphyxiating thoracic dysplasia
3. Chondroectodermal dysplasia
4. Campomelic dysplasia
5. Thanatophoric dwarfism
6. Homozygous achondroplasia
7. Achondrogenesis
8. Hypophosphatasia

Spine demineralization
1. Achondrogenesis

Large head
1. Achondroplasia
2. Thanatophoric dysplasia

Bowed long bones
1. Campomelic syndrome
2. Osteogenesis imperfecta
3. Thanatophoric dysplasia
4. Hypophosphatasia

Bone fractures
1. Osteogenesis imperfecta
2. Hypophosphatasia
3. Achondrogenesis

Extreme micromelia
1. Achondrogenesis
2. Thanatophoric dysplasia
3. Fibrochondrogenesis
4. Short rib-polydactyly syndrome
5. Diastrophic dysplasia

GYNECOLOGY
Frequency of pelvic masses
1. Benign adnexal cyst   34%
2. Leiomyoma   14%
3. Cancers   14%
4. Dermoid   13%
5. Endometriosis   10%
6. Pelvic inflammatory disease 8%

Cystic pelvic masses
A. Cystic adnexal masses
B. Extraadnexal cystic masses
   1. Peritoneal inclusion cyst
   2. Mesenteric cyst
   3. Lymphocele
   4. Bladder diverticulum
   5. Ectopic gestation
   6. Fluid-distended bowel
   7. Loculated pelvic abscess
      — appendiceal
      — diverticular
      — postoperative

Uterine masses
A. BENIGN
   1. Uterine fibroids (99%)
   2. Pyometrium
   3. Hemato- / hydrocolpos
   4. Transient uterine contraction (during pregnancy)
   5. Bicornuate uterus
   6. Adenomyosis
   7. Intrauterine pregnancy

B. <u>MALIGNANT</u>
1. Cervical carcinoma
2. Endometrial carcinoma
3. Leiomyosarcoma
4. Invasive trophoblastic disease

Extrauterine pelvic masses
1. Solid adnexal mass
2. Metastatic disease
3. Lymphoma
4. Pelvic kidney
5. Rectosigmoid carcinoma
6. Prostate carcinoma
7. Benign prostatic enlargement
8. Bladder carcinoma
9. Retroperitoneal tumor
10. Intraperitoneal fat
11. Vascular mass / malformation
12. Hematoma
13. Bowel

Adnexal masses
A. CYSTIC
1. Functional cysts
   — Graafian follicle
   — Follicular cyst
   — Corpus luteum cyst
   — Theca lutein cyst
2. Endometrioma
3. Tuboovarian abscess
4. Dermoid cyst
5. Serous cystadenoma
6. Hydrosalpinx
7. Mucinous cystadenome
8. Ectopic pregnancy
9. Paraovarian cyst
10. Hydatid cyst of Morgagni
11. Serous cystadenocarcinoma
12. Mucinous cystadenocarcinoma
13. Hyperstimulation cysts
B. SOLID
1. Ovarian tumor
2. Ovarian torsion
3. Fallopian tube carcinoma
4. Polycystic ovaries
   (DDx: Pedunculated leiomyoma)

Solid ovarian tumor
1. Fibroma
2. Thecoma
3. Granulosa cell tumor
4. Sertoli-Leydig cell tumor
5. Brenner tumor
6. Sarcoma
7. Dysgerminoma
8. Endodermal sinus tumor
9. Teratoma
10. Metastasis
11. Endometrioma

Ovarian tumors
- pressure symptoms: abdominal discomfort, vomiting, flatulence, dyspnea
- pain from adhesions, impaction, torsion
- menstrual irregularity

Cx: (1) torsion (in 10 – 20%)
     (2) rupture (rare)
     (3) infection

CLASSIFICATION
A. <u>Estrogen-producing tumors</u>
1. Granulosa-cell tumor
2. Theca cell tumor = thecoma
B. <u>Tumors of surface epithelium</u>
1. Serous ovarian tumor
2. Mucinous ovarian tumor
3. Endometrioid tumor
4. Cystadenofibroma
5. Clear-cell adenocarcinoma
6. Brenner tumor
C. <u>Germ-cell tumors</u>
40% of germ cell tumors are malignant
(a) benign
   1. Dermoid cyst = mature teratoma (most common)
(b) malignant
   account for 2/3 of ovarian cancers in 1st – 2nd decade of life; < 5% of all ovarian neoplasms
   1. Dysgerminoma
   2. Endodermal sinus tumor
   3. Immature teratoma
   4. Choriocarcinoma
   5 Embryonal carcinoma
D. <u>Sex cord-mesenchyme tumors</u>
1. Granulosa cell tumor
2. Theca cell tumor
3. Luteal cell tumor
4. Arrhenoblastoma
E. <u>Connective tissue tumor</u>
1. Fibroma
2. Fibrosarcoma
F. <u>Secondary ovarian tumors</u>
metastases from: pelvic organs, upper GI tract, breast, bronchus, reticuloendothelial tumors, leukemia
G <u>Androgen-producing tumors</u>
1. Arrhenoblastoma
2. Sertoli-Leydig cell tumor
3. Clear cell tumor

Calcifications of female genital tract
A. <u>Uterus</u>
1. Uterine fibroids
B. <u>Ovaries</u>
1. Dermoid cyst (50%)
2. Papillary cystadenoma (psammomatous bodies)
3. Cystadenocarcinoma
4. Hemangiopericytoma
5. Gonadoblastoma

6. Chronic ovarian torsion
7. Pseudomyxoma peritonei
C. Fallopian tubes
   1. Tuberculous salpingitis
D. Placenta
E. Lithopedion

Free fluid in cul-de-sac

1. Follicular rupture
2. Ovulation
3. Ectopic pregnancy
4. S/P culdocentesis
5. Ovarian neoplasm
6. Pelvic inflammatory disease

Thickened irregular endometrium

Normal endometrial thickness: < 1 cm

1. **Endometrial Polyps**
   Age: mainly 30 – 60 years
   Histo: projections of endometrial glands + stroma into uterine cavity
   Malignant transformation: in 0.4 – 3.7%
2. **Endometrial Hyperplasia**
   secondary to prolonged endogenous / exogenous estrogen stimulation
   (a) glandular-cystic hyperplasia
   (b) adenomatous hyperplasia
   √ endometrial thickening > 6 mm
   Cx: precursor of endometrial cancer
3. Endometritis
4. Primary carcinoma of the endometrium
   Location: predominantly in uterine fundus; 24% in isthmic portion)
5. Metastatic carcinoma (ovary, cervix, fallopian tube, leukemia)
6. Hydatidiform mole
   √ echogenic mass with irregular sonolucent areas
7. Incomplete abortion

ANATOMY AND PHYSIOLOGY OF FEMALE REPRODUCTIVE SYSTEM

Human Chorionic Gonadotropin
= hCG = glycoprotein elaborated by placental trophoblastic cells beginning the 8th day after conception

A. Immunologic Pregnancy Test
= indirect agglutination test for hCG in urine; cross reaction with other hormones / medications possible
Becomes positive at 5 weeks MA

Advantages:	readily available, easily + rapidly performed
Disadvantages:	frequently false-positive + false-negative results

Sensitivity:
(a) slide: 400 – 15,000 mIU/ml (2 min test time)
(b) test tube: 1,000 – 3,000 mIU/ml (2 hours test time)

B. Radioimmunoassay Pregnancy Test
= measures beta subunit of hCG in serum
Becomes positive at 3 weeks MA

Advantages:	specific for hCG, sensitive
Disadvantages:	requires specialized lab + 3 – 24 hours for completion

Sensitivity:
(a) qualitative: 25 – 30 mIU/ml (3 hours test time)
(b) quantitative: 3 – 4 mIU/ml (24 hours test time)
Rise:
> 66% increase of initial beta-hCG level over 48 hours in 86% of normal pregnancies
< 66% increase of initial beta-hCG level seen in 87% of ectopic pregnancies

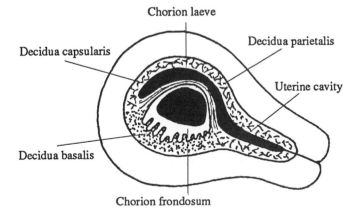

Choriodecidua
Chorion = trophoblast + fetal mesenchyme with villous stems protruding into decidua; provides nutrition for developing embryo

(a) chorion frondosum = part adjacent to decidua basalis, forms primordial placenta
(b) chorion laeve = smooth portion of chorion with atrophied villi
(c) "chorionic plate" = amnionic membrane covering the chorionic plate of the placenta

Decidua
(a) decidua basalis = between chorion frondosum + myometrium
(b) decidua capsularis = portion protruding into uterine cavity
(c) decidua parietalis = decidua vera = portion lining the uterine cavity elsewhere

Gestational Sac
Arises from blastocyst which implants into secretory endometrium; first seen when sac diameter exceeds 5 mm, surrounded by echogenic trophoblast

SAC SIZE: 17 mm by 6th week MA
24 mm by 7th week MA
31 mm by 8th week MA

mean sac diameter grows 1.13 (range 0.71 – 1.75) mm/day; fills chorionic cavity by 11 – 12 weeks MA

VISUALIZATION OF GESTATIONAL SAC
A. in relation to BETA-HCG LEVELS (2nd International Standard):
(serum beta-hCG becomes positive 7 – 10 days following conception)
beta-hCG levels double every 2 – 3 days during first 60 days of pregnancy
(a) on transabdominal scan:
in 100% with beta-hCG levels of > 1,800 IU/l
(b) on transvaginal scan:
in 20% with beta-hCG levels of < 500 IU/l
in 80% with beta-hCG levels of 500 – 1,000 IU/l
in 100% with beta-hCG levels of > 1,000 IU/l
B. in relation to MENSTRUAL AGE
(a) on transabdominal scan:
earliest by 5.5 weeks (diameter of 10 – 12 mm)
(b) on transvaginal scan:
routinely seen by 5 – 5.5 weeks
√ double decidual sac (DDS): visualization correlates with presence of pregnancy in 98 %, may be seen at < 5 weeks on transvaginal scans

Embryo
Developmental stages
PREEMBRYONIC PERIOD: 2nd – 4th menstrual week
TRILAMINAR EMBRYONIC DISC: 5th week
EMBRYONIC PERIOD: 6th – 10th menstrual week
FETAL PERIOD: 11th week – term
Average growth rate:
0.6 mm per day / 1.5 mm every 2 days

VISUALIZATION OF EMBRYO in relation to
GESTATIONAL SAC in 100 %:
  (a) by transabdominal scan:
      with average gestational sac size ≥ 27 mm
  (b) by endovaginal scan:
      with average gestational sac size ≥ 12 mm

VISUALIZATION OF CARDIAC ACTIVITY in 100 %:
  A. in relation to CRL:
     (a) by transabdominal scan : ≥ 9 mm CRL
     (b) by transvaginal scan   : ≥ 5 mm CRL
  B. in relation to MENSTRUAL AGE:
     (a) by transabdominal scan : 7 weeks
     (b) by endovaginal scan   : 5 – 6 weeks
  Δ Cardiac activity predicts a favorable outcome in
    90 – 97% of gestations!
  Δ Nonvisualization of cardiac activity with CRL of
    2 – 12 mm means embryonic demise in 94%!

Yolk sac
  = rounded sonolucent structure (outside amniotic cavity)
  within chorionic sac (= extracoelomic cavity) connected
  to umbilicus via a narrow stalk, formed by proliferation of
  endodermal cells, part of yolk sac is incorporated into
  fetal gut, the rest persists as a sac connected to the
  fetus by the vitelline duct
Function: transfer of nutrients from trophoblast to
             embryo, early blood formation, formation of
             primitive gut, source of primordial germ cells
Earliest visualization: 5 – 7 weeks MA

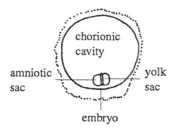

Simple double bleb stage
(earliest detection at 5.5 weeks GA, embryo 2 mm in length

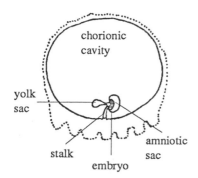

Double bleb + separated yolk sac

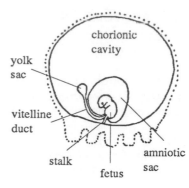

Double bleb + vitelline duct

Size: 3.0 mm by 6th week; 4.5 mm by 7th week; 5.0
         mm by 9th week; greatest size of 7 mm by 10th –
         11th week MA; disappears around 12 weeks MA
Δ Presence / absence of yolk sac does not allow accurate
  prediction of living embryo!

Amnionic membrane
  = curvilinear echogenic line within chorionic sac; fills
  chorionic cavity by 11 – 12 weeks MA; fuses with
  chorionic membrane at approximately 16 weeks MA
  to form the chorionic plate
Incomplete fusion with chorion frequent
(DDx: subchorionic hemorrhage, twin abortion)

Fetal mensuration
US is more reliable than LMP / physical examination

FETAL AGE = GESTATIONAL AGE (GA)
= "MENSTRUAL AGE" (MA)
  = age of pregnancy based on woman's regular last
    menstrual period (LMP) projecting the estimated date
    of confinement (EDC) at 40 weeks
  Accuracy: 1 – 2 weeks

GESTATIONAL SAC
  = average of 3 diameters of anechoic space within sac
    walls
  Δ used for dating between 6 – 12 weeks MA
  Accuracy: ± 1 week
  Identified as early as 5 weeks MA (transabdominal
  scan)

CROWN-RUMP LENGTH (CRL)
  = length of embryo; useful up to 12 weeks MA
  Accuracy: ± 5 to 7 days
  Rule of thumb: MA (in weeks) = CRL (in cm) + 6
  Usually identified by 7 weeks MA (transabdominal scan)

BIPARIETAL DIAMETER (BPD)
  = measured from leading edge to leading edge of
    calvarial table at widest transaxial plane of skull
    = level of thalami + cavum septi pellucidi + Sylvian
    fissures

Δ excellent means of estimating GA in 2nd trimester >
12 weeks MA
Accuracy of BPD measurement (= "between occasion
error"): 2 mm
  (a) in 2nd trimester (< 24 weeks): ± 5 to 7 days
     (± 9 %)
  (b) in 3rd trimester: 2 – 4 weeks
     less reliable for dating in 3rd trimester because of
     increasing biologic variability

CEPHALIC INDEX (CI)
  = BPD / OFD; measurements of BPD and
  occipitofrontal diameter (OFD) are both taken from
  outer to outer edge of calvarium
  Δ confirms appropriate use of BPD if ratio is between
  0.70 - 0.86 (2 SD)

HEAD CIRCUMFERENCE (HC)
  used if ratio of BPD/OFD outside 0.70 – 0.86
  HC = ([BPD + OFD]/2) X Π
  Accuracy: slightly less than for BPD

ABDOMINAL CIRCUMFERENCE (AC)
  = measured at level of vascular junction of umbilical
  vein with left portal vein ("hockey stick" appearance)
  where it is equidistant from the lateral walls in a plane
  perpendicular to long axis of fetus; measured from
  outer edge to outer edge of soft tissues
  Δ allows evaluation of head-to-body disproportion
  Δ better predictor of fetal weight than BPD

FEMUR LENGTH (FL)
  FL > 5 mm below 2 standard deviations suggest skeletal
  dysplasia!
  — distal femoral epiphysis present at 32 – 33 weeks
  — proximal tibial epiphysis present at 36 weeks
  — proximal humeral epiphysis present at 38 weeks

DISCORDANT ESTIMATED DATE OF CONFINEMENT (EDC) AND BPD:
  1. Methodological error in measurement
    (a) wrong axial section
    (b) cranial compression (multiple gestation, breech
      presentation, oligohydramnios, dolichocephaly)
  2. Erroneous LMP
    other measurements (AC, FL) correlate with BPD
  3. Abnormal head growth
    (a) BPD less than AC: microcephaly, fetal
                    macrosomia
    (b) BPD more than AC: intracranial abnormality,
                    asymmetrical IUGR

Placental grading
according to echo appearance of basal zone, chorionic
plate, placental substance

GRADE 0
  √ homogeneous placenta + straight line of chorionic
  plate

Time: < 30 weeks MA
GRADE 1
  √ undulated chorionic plate + scattered bright placental
  echoes
  Time: seen at any time during pregnancy; in 40% at
       term
  Δ in 68% L/S ratio > 2.0
GRADE 2
  √ linear bright echoes parallel to basal plate
  √ confluent stippled echoes within placenta
  ± indentations of chorionic plate
  Time: rarely seen in gestations < 32 weeks MA;
       seen in 40% at term
  Δ in 87% L/S ratio > 2.0
GRADE 3
  √ calcified intercotylidonary septa, often surrounding
  sonolucent center
  Time: rarely seen in gestations < 34 weeks MA;
       in 15 – 20% at term
  Δ in 100% L/S ratio > 2.0 (= strongly correlated with
  lung maturity)

PREMATURE PLACENTAL SENESCENCE
  = grade 3 placenta seen in gestation < 34 weeks MA
  Δ in 50% suggestive of maternal hypertension / IUGR

MULTIPLE GESTATION
Incidence: 1% of all births; in 5 – 50% clinically
           undiagnosed at term
Occurrence:
  twins   in 1:85   pregnancies (= 85^1)
  triplets   in 1:7,600   pregnancies (= 85^2)
  quadruplets in 1:70,000 pregnancies (= 85^3)
At risk for IUGR: monochorionic-monoamniotic >
                monochorionic-diamniotic >
                dichorionic-diamniotic
• uterus large for dates
• may have elevated hCG, hPL (human placental
  lactogen), AFP levels
√ 2 placentas indicate dichorionic diamniotic pregnancy
√ 1 placenta indicates (a) monochorionic pregnancy (b)
  dichorionic pregnancy with fused placenta
√ separating membrane confirms diamniotic pregnancy,
  but does not distinguish between mono- / dichorionic
  pregnancy

Twin Pregnancy
zygote = fertilized egg
√ monozygotic + dizygotic twins sonographically
  indistinguishable
1. MONOZYGOTIC TWINS = "identical twins" (20%)
  = division of a single fertilized ovum; same sex +
  identical genotype
  Occurs after fertilization during earliest stages of
  embryogenesis
  Incidence: 1:250 birth (constant around the world)
  (a) DICHORIONIC DIAMNIOTIC (80%)
    = separation at two cell stage (= blastomere)
    approximately 60 hours after fertilization

√ 2 separate chorionic sacs + 2 separate
amniotic sacs = membrane > 2 mm (92%
accurate for dichorionic diamniotic twins)
√ different fetal gender
√ 2 separate placentas
(b) MONOCHORIONIC DIAMNIOTIC
(most common)
= separation in blastocyst stage between 3rd and
8th day after fertilization (chorion already
developed)
√ 2 separate amniotic sacs within single
chorionic sac
Common monochorionic placenta has vascular
communications in100%
Cx: (1) twin-twin transfusion
(2) DIC in surviving twin from transfer of
thromboplastin; 17% morbidity /
mortality of survivor after fetal death of
twin
(c) MONOCHORIONIC MONOAMNIOTIC
= division of embryonic disc between 8th and
13th day after fertilization (amniotic cavity
already developed)
√ common amniotic + chorionic sac, no
separating membrane
Cx: perinatal mortality up to 50%
(1) entangled umbilical cord (70%)
(2) conjoined twins (umbilical cord with >
3 vessels, shared fetal organs,
continuous fetal skin contour)
Prognosis: 40% survival rate
(d) CONJOINED TWINS
division between 13th and 16th day after
formation of embryonic disc
√ no separating membrane demonstrable
√ fetuses commonly face each other
Cx: perinatal mortality 2.5 times greater than for
dizygotic twins

2. DIZYGOTIC TWINS = "fraternal twins" (70%)
(a) same gender (35%)
(b) different gender (35%)
— arise from two separate ova fertilized by two
separate spermatozoa; determined at ovulation
— superfecundation = two ova fertilized by two
different fathers
Incidence: 1:80 to 1:90 births
Predisposing factors:
(1) advanced maternal age (increased up to age
35)
(2) ovulation-inducing agents (multiple
pregnancies in 5% with clomiphene, in 30%
with pergonal)
(3) maternal history of twinning (3 times as
frequent compared with normal population)
(4) increased parity
(5) maternal obesity
(6) race (more common in blacks)

GROWTH RATES
Twins should be scanned every 3 – 4 weeks> 26 – 28
weeks GA
√ normal individual twins grow at same rate as
singletons up to 30 – 32 weeks GA
√ combined weight gain of both twins equals that of a
singleton pregnancy
√ body length + head size are little affected
√ BDP growth rates similar to singleton fetuses up to
30 – 32 weeks GA

DISCORDANT GROWTH
= weight difference at birth > 25%
Cause: (1) Twin-twin transfusion syndrome
(2) IUGR of one fetus
√ BPD difference > 5 mm (discordant growth in
20 – 30%)
√ discordant HC increases probability of IUGR
√ AC is single most sensitive parameter for IUGR
√ EFW is most sensitive set of combined parameters
for IUGR

"FETUS PAPYRACEUS"
= resorption of fluid resulting in paperlike fetal body +
compression into adjacent membranes
"VANISHING TWIN"
= disappearance of one twin in utero due to
resorption / anembryonic pregnancy
Incidence: 13 – 78% (mean 21%) before 14 weeks
GA
Cx:
(1) DIC in response to release of thromboplastin
from degenerating fetus
(a) into maternal circulation
(b) into monozygotic twin fetus through
shared circulation
(2) Velamentous cord insertion (7 fold increase
compared with singleton pregnancy)

Prognosis:
(1) Perinatal mortality 5 – 10 times that of singleton
pregnancy (91 – 124:1,000 births)
(a) preterm delivery with birthweight < 2500 g
(b) IUGR (2nd most common cause of perinatal
mortality + morbidity)
(c) amniotic fluid infection (60%)
(d) premature rupture of membranes (11%)
(e) twin-twin transfusion syndrome (8%)
(f) large placental infarct (8%)
(g) placenta previa
(h) abruptio placenta
(i) preeclampsia
(j) cord accidents
(k) malpresentations
(2) Fetal death in utero (0.5 – 6.8%; 3 times as often
in monochorionic than in dichorionic gestations)
(3) Increased risk of congenital anomalies (23:1,000
births = twice as frequent as in singletons)

Uteroplacental circulation

By 20th week trophoblast invades maternal vessels which transforms spiral arteries into distended tortuous vessels = uteroplacental arteries.

Histo:

(a) in the decidual portion of spiral arteries: proliferating trophoblast from anchoring villi invade lumen of spiral arteries + partially replace endothelium

(b) in the myometrial portion of spiral arteries: disintegration of smooth muscle elements (loss of elastic lamina) leads to easily distensible low resistance vascular system

Uterine blood volume flow:
— 50 ml/min shortly after conception
— 500 – 900 ml/min by term

Intervillous blood flow: 140 ± 53 ml/min (by Xe-133 washout rate)

Doppler waveform:
√ high velocities in diastole similar to those in systole
√ degree of diastolic flow increases as gestation progresses
√ highly turbulent flow

IUGR-lesions:
= narrowing of vascular lumen through
(1) thrombosis of decidual segments of uteroplacental arteries
(2) failure of development of myometrial segments of uteroplacental arteries

ANATOMY & FUNCTION OF FEMALE GENITAL ORGANS

Uterine Size

NEONATE: pear shaped secondary to maternal hormonal stimulation

PREPUBERTAL: about 1.0 – 3.3 cm (L); 0.5 – 1.0 cm (W); 1.0 cm (D), cervix occupies 2/3 of uterine length

MENSTRUATING: cervix occupies 1/3 of uterine length; mean uterine volume = 90 ccm
— nulliparous: 5 – 9 cm (L); 4.0 – 5.5 cm (W); 3 cm (D)
— multiparous: add 2 cm for multiparous dimensions

POSTMENOPAUSAL: cervix occupies 1/3 of uterine length; 3.5 – 6.5 cm (L); 1.2 - 1.8 cm (W); 2 cm (D)

Uterine Zonal Anatomy (on T2WI)

Thickness of zones depends on menstrual cycle + hormonal medication

A. Endometrium
√ high signal intensity similar to fat

B. Junctional zone= innermost portion of myometrium
√ low signal intensity (lower water content)
√ may not be visible in premenarchal + postmenopausal women

C. Myometrium
√ intermediate signal intensity, increases during secretory phase

CERVICAL ZONES
(a) endocervical canal
√ central zone of high signal intensity on T2WI
(b) myometrium
√ outer zone of low signal intensity similar to junctional zone

Endometrium

1. Menstrual phase: 2 – 3 mm thick
√ thin interrupted central interphase

2. Proliferative phase: 4 – 6 mm thick
√ mildly echogenic interphase surrounded by thin hypoechoic band (= inner layer of myometrium)

3. Periovulatory phase: 6 – 8 mm thick
√ moderately echogenic endometrium
√ "halo sign" = inner hypoechoic layer (= high fluid content of inner functional endometrial layer)
√ 1 – 2 cm of fluid within endometrial lumen

4. Secretory phase: 3 – 6 mm
√ very echogenic endometrial texture (= tortuous glands + mucin)

5. Postmenopausal; < 6 – 8 mm thick

Graafian Follicle

Size of mature Graafian follicle: 18 – 27 mm
√ growth rate 3mm/day until the last preovulatory 24 hours followed by a sudden increase in diameter
√ cumulus = 1 mm mural echogenic focus projecting into antrum of follicle + containing oocyte, followed by ovulation within next 36 hours
√ corpus luteum of menstruation = blurred margin around follicle + internal echoes

SIGNS OF OVULATION:
√ development of solid echoes within Graafian follicle
√ decrease in diameter / sudden collapse of dominant follicle 28 – 35 hours after LH peak
√ "ring" structure within uterine fundus
√ free fluid appearing in pouch of Douglas

SIGNS OF OVULATORY FAILURE:
√ development of internal echoes prior to 18 mm size
√ continuous cystic enlargement up to 30 – 40 mm

DISEASE ENTITIES OF OBSTETRICAL AND GYNECOLOGICAL DISORDERS

ABORTION
Rate of spontaneous abortions
  (a) 31 – 43% of all implantations (estimate)
  (b) 10 – 15% of clinically diagnosed pregnancies
Etiology: usually due to abnormal karyotype: autosomal trisomy (52%), triploidy (20%), monosomy (15%)

Incomplete Spontaneous Abortion
= retained products of conception, i.e. a portion of chorionic villi (placental tissue) / trophoblastic tissue (fetal tissue) remains within uterus
  • prolonged bleeding
  • infection
US: overall accuracy 96%
√ gestational sac / collection (64%): retained products in 100%
√ sac with dead fetus (19%): retained products in 100%
√ endometrial thickness > 5 mm (3%): retained products in 100%
√ endometrial thickness 2-5 mm (7%): retained products in 43%
√ endometrial thickness < 2 mm (7%): retained products in 14%
Cx: endometritis, myometritis, peritonitis, septic shock, diffuse intravascular coagulation (with retention > 1 month)

Inevitable Abortion
= gestational sac with fetus having become detached from implantation site; leading to spontaneous abortion within next few hours
Clinical triad:
  • severe pain
  • uterine contractions
  • dilated cervix
√ sac located low within uterus
√ sac surrounded by anechoic zone of blood
√ dilated cervix

Missed Abortion
= dead conceptus within uterine cavity, occurring between 8 – 14 weeks
√ no fetal heartbeat with CRL > 9 mm (on abdominal scans) / CRL > 5 mm (on transvaginal scans)
√ gestation not in correspondence with menstrual age
√ sac > 25 mm in diameter without an embryo
√ distorted angular sac configuration
√ stringlike debris within gestational sac (in 25%)
√ discontinuous / irregular / thin (2 mm) choriodecidual reaction
√ absent double decidual sac
√ low sac position
√ subchorionic collections

Threatened Abortion
= 1st trimester bleeding with a live fetus
Incidence: 20 – 25% of all pregnancies
Clinical triad:
  • mild bleeding
  • cramping
  • closed cervix
Prognosis: 50% develop normally; 50% abort spontaneously
√ living fetus demonstrated (3 – 10% subsequently abort)
Factors with a poor prognosis:
  √ relative fetal inactivity
  √ disproportion between fetal size and gestational sac size
  √ poor sac outline
√ no cardiac activity visible = missed abortion

ACARDIA
= ACARDIAC MONSTER = TWIN REVERSED ARTERIAL PERFUSION SEQUENCE (TRAP)
Incidence: 1:30,000 – 35,000 births
Spectrum:
  (1) Holoacardia = no heart at all
  (2) Pseudoacardia = rudimentary cardiac tissue
√ fused placentas
√ polyhydramnios
A. PUMP TWIN
    at increased risk for fetal demise + preterm labor
    √ morphologically normal
    √ cardiac overload signs: hydrops, IUGR, hypertrophy of right ventricle, hepatosplenomegaly, ascites
B. PERFUSED TWIN
    monochorial placenta (same gender) with vascular anastomosis sustains life of acardiac monster; wide range of abnormalities
    √ absent / rudimentary heart ("acardius")
    √ unidentifiable head / trunk / extremities
Prognosis: mortality of 100% for perfused twin, 50% for pump twin

ADENOMYOSIS
= benign invasion of endometrium into myometrium ("endometrial islands") undergoing the same cyclic changes ("miniature uterine cavities") + diffuse overgrowth of musculature
Age: multiparous women > 30 years (during menstrual life)
Associated with endometriosis (in 36 – 40%)
  • dysmenorrhea
  • menorrhagia
√ smooth uterine enlargement (DDx: diffuse leiomyomatosis)
√ occasionally "swiss cheese" appearance of myometrium

MRI:
√ low intensity lesions on T2, often isointense to band of junctional zone
√ central high-intensity spots corresponding to hemorrhagic areas
Cx: infertility

AMNIOTIC BAND SYNDROME
= rupture of the amnion exposing the fetus to the injurious environment of fibrous mesodermic bands that emanate from the chorionic side of the amnion
Incidence: 1:1,200 to 1:15,000 live births
√ membrane that flaps with fetal movement
√ abnormal sheet / bands of tissue that attach to the fetus
√ restriction of fetal motion secondary to entrapment of fetal parts by bands
Associated with FETAL DEFORMITIES (77%):
1. Limb defects (multiple + asymmetric)
   √ amputation / constriction rings of limbs / digits
   √ distal syndactyly
   √ clubbed feet
2. Craniofacial defects
   √ anencephaly
   √ asymmetric lateral encephalocele
   √ facial clefting of lip / palate
   √ asymmetric microphthalmia
   √ incomplete / absent cranial calcification
3. Visceral defects
   √ gastroschisis ± exteriorization of liver
   √ omphalocele
   √ gibbus deformity of spine
DDx: (1) Chorioamniotic separation
       (2) Intrauterine synechiae

ARRHENOBLASTOMA
Age peak: 25 – 45 years (range 15 – 66 years)
√ solid mass with cystic components (hemorrhage ± necrosis)
√ unilateral (95%), up to 27 cm in diameter
Cx: malignant transformation in 22%

BECKWITH-WIEDEMANN SYNDROME
= EMG SYNDROME (**E**xomphalos = omphalocele, **M**acroglossia, **G**igantism); autosomal dominant
Incidence: 1:13,700 live births
Constellation:
   (1) macroglossia
   (2) visceromegaly
   (3) omphalocele (10 – 15%)
   (4) natal / postnatal gigantism
   (5) nephromegaly
   (6) facial flame nevus
   (7) hepatomegaly
   (8) ear lobe abnormalities
   (9) hemihypertrophy
   (10) cardiac anomalies
   (11) pancreatic hyperplasia
• neonatal polycythemia

• neonatal hypoglycemia (50%)
Cx: development of malignant tumors (in 10 %): nephroblastoma, hepatoblastoma, adrenal tumor

BLIGHTED OVUM
= ANEMBRYONIC PREGNANCY; may occur as a blighted twin
= gestational sac of > 2.5 ml with no identifiable embryo
√ yolk sac identified without embryo
√ empty gestational sac (> 6 – 8 weeks MA)
√ gestational sac too small for dates
√ distorted shape of gestational sac (DDx: compression by bladder, myoma, contraction)
√ stringlike / granular debris / fluid-fluid level within gestational sac (= intrasac bleeding)
√ subchorionic lucencies (DDx: implantation bleed)
√ thin (< 2 mm) weakly hyperechoic / irregular choriodecidual reaction
√ gestational sac growth ≤ 0.6 mm/day (normal growth rate of 1.1 mm / day determines appropriate time interval for follow-up scan, i.e., when sac is expected to be 27 mm)
(a) by transabdominal scan:
    gestational sac usually visualized not before 5 – 5.5 weeks MA; yolk sac forms at 27 – 28 days menstrual age when gestational sac is 3 mm
    embryo usually visualized by 6 weeks
    √ GS size > 20 mm of mean diameter without yolk sac
    √ GS size > 25 mm of mean diameter without embryo
    √ absence of GS growth documented on repeat scan 7 – 14 days later
(b) by transvaginal scan
    √ GS size > 8 mm of mean diameter without yolk sac
    √ GS size > 16 mm of mean diameter without embryo / cardiac activity
Cx: first trimester bleeding

BRENNER TUMOR
Incidence: 1.5 – 2.5%
Associated with: mucinous cystadenoma in 30%
Peak age: 40 – 70 years
• may have estrogenic activity
√ usually hypoechoic solid tumor with well-defined back wall, up to 30 cm in diameter
√ bilateral in 5 – 7%

CERVICAL CANCER
6th most common cancer in women, approximately 13,000 new cases / year with 7,000 deaths; 2nd most common malignancy in women for ages 15 – 34
Incidence: 12:100,000 women per year
Histo: squamous cell carcinoma (95%), adenocarcinoma (5%), unusual clear cell adenocarcinoma in women exposed to DES in utero

Risk factors: lower socioeconomic class, black race, early marriage, increased parity, young onset of sexual relations, multiple sexual partners, positive herpes virus type II titers

STAGE 0   carcinoma in situ
         Ia   microinvasion of stroma
         Ib   invasion confined to cervix
         IIa   vaginal invasion excluding lower 1/3
         IIb   parametrial involvement excepting pelvic sidewall
         IIIa invasion of lower 1/3 of vagina
         IIIb extension to pelvic sidewall / hydronephrosis
         IVa   mucosal involvement of bladder / rectum / beyond true pelvis
         IVb   spread to distant organs (paraaortic / inguinal nodes, intraperitoneal metastasis)

Significance of tumor size:
   > 4 cm: nodal mets (80%), local recurrence (40%), distant mets (28%)
   < 4 cm: nodal mets (16%), local recurrence (5%), distant mets (0%)

Incidence of nodal metastases:
   for stages   0, I a   0.3%
                  I b   16%
                  II a   33%
                  II b   37%

Peak age: 45 – 55 years
• leukorrhea ± vaginal bleeding (< 30%)
• postcoital bleeding / metrorrhagia
√ bulky enlargement of cervix (DDx: cervical fibroid)
√ fluid-filled uterus (secondary to obstruction)
√ signs of parametrial invasion: > 4 mm soft-tissue strands extending from cervix into parametria, cardinal / sacrouterine ligaments, irregularity of cervical margins, eccentric parametrial enlargement, obliteration of fat planes
MRI (81% staging accuracy):
   √ isointense mass on T1WI
   √ hyperintense focal bulge / mass on T2WI (DDx: postbiopsy changes, inflammation, nabothian cysts)
   √ blurring + widening of junctional zone secondary to obstruction of cervical os (retained secretions in uterine cavity)

CHORIOAMNIONIC SEPARATION
(1) normally seen < 16 weeks
     = incomplete fusion of amniotic membrane with chorionic plate
(2) abnormal > 17 weeks MA
     = secondary to hemorrhage
√ membrane extends over fetal surface + stops at origin of umbilical cord
√ elevated membrane thinner than chorionic membrane
Cx: rupture of amniotic membrane may lead to amniotic band syndrome

CHORIOANGIOMA
= benign vascular malformation of proliferating capillaries (= hamartoma)

Incidence: 1:3,500 to 1:20,000 births
Location: usually near the umbilical cord insertion site
√ well-circumscribed intraplacental mass with complex echo pattern protruding from the fetal surface of the placenta
√ polyhydramnios (in 1/3)
√ arterial signal on Doppler ultrasound in angiomatous chorioangioma
Cx: hemorrhage, fetal hydrops, cardiomegaly, congestive heart failure, IUGR, premature labor, fetal demise (in large lesion)

CHORIOCARCINOMA
5% of gestational trophoblastic diseases
Histo: excessive trophoblastic proliferation without villous structures
• continued bleeding
• elevated hCG after expulsion of molar / normal pregnancy (25%)
√ mixed hyperechoic pattern (hemorrhage, necrosis)
Spread: hemorrhagic metastases to lung + brain
   √ radiodense pulmonary masses with hazy borders due to hemorrhage
   √ hyperechoic hepatic foci

CLEAR-CELL ADENOCARCINOMA OF OVARY
Histo: resembles clear-cell tumor of the kidney

CONJOINED TWINS
= incomplete division of embryonic cell mass in monozygotic twins occurring at 13 – 16 days GA
Incidence: 1:30,000 to 1:100,000 live births; 1:600 twin births; M:F = 1:2
Types:
   1. Thoracoomphalopagus (28%)
   2. Thoracopagus (18%): between thoracic walls + CHD (75%)
   3. Omphalopagus (10%): between umbilicus + xiphoid
   4. Incomplete duplication (10): duplication of only one part of body
   5. Craniopagus (6%): between homologous portions of cranial vault
   6. Pygopagus (20%): between buttocks + lower spine
   7. Ischiopagus: between ischia
   8. Xiphopagus: between xiphoid of sternum
OB-US (diagnosed as early as 12 weeks GA):
   √ interamniotic membrane not identified
   √ umbilical cord with > 3 vessels
   √ single cardiac motion
   √ twins not completely separated
   √ polyhydramnios (in almost 50%)
Prognosis: 39% stillborn; 34% die within first days of life

CORPUS LUTEUM CYST
Types:
1. <u>corpus luteum of menstruation</u>
   formed after rupture of follicle + increasing in size until 22nd day of menstrual cycle

√ usually > 12 – 17 mm in size
2. corpus luteum of pregnancy
caused by hCG stimulation during pregnancy
√ usual size 30 – 40 mm, may grow up to 15 cm in diameter
√ reaches maximum size after 8 – 10 weeks
√ usually resolves before 20 weeks GA (12 – 15 weeks), but occasionally persists past 1st trimester
√ thin-walled usually unilateral cyst
√ echogenic (organized clot) / sonolucent (resorbed blood)
√ low-level internal echoes (= frequent hemorrhage)
Cx: rupture with intraperitoneal hemorrhage

CYSTADENOFIBROMA
= variant of serous cystadenoma, rarely malignant
• may produce estrogen excess
√ small multilocular tumor with papillary processes

CYSTIC HYGROMA
= LYMPHANGIOMA = single / multiloculated fluid-filled cavities on either side of fetal neck + head ± trunk secondary to congenital blockage of lymphatic drainage (= noncommunication of jugular lymphatic sac with jugular vein)
Incidence: 1:6,000 pregnancies
Age: 50% present at birth; up to 90% evident by age 2
Path: macroscopic multilocular mass with cysts of varying size lined with single layer of endothelium containing serous / milky fluid
Associated with:
(1) Turner syndrome (45 XO, mosaic) in 73%
(2) Trisomies 13, 18, 21, 13q, 18p, 22
(3) Noonan syndrome
(4) Fetal alcohol syndrome
(5) Distichiasis-lymphedema syndrome
(6) Familial pterygium colli
Location:
posterior neck (75%), mediastinum (3 – 10%, in 1/2 extension from neck), axilla (20%), chest wall (14%), face (10%), retroperitoneum, abdominal viscera, scrotum, bones
√ thin-walled fluid-filled structure with multiple septa + solid cyst wall components
√ isolated nuchal cysts
√ webbed neck (= pterygium colli) after late communication with jugular veins
√ nonimmune hydrops + progressive peripheral edema
√ fetal ascites
√ oligo- / polyhydramnios / normal amount of fluid
√ bradycardia
Cx: (1)   compression of airways
(2)   slow growth / sudden enlargement (hemorrhage, inflammation)
Prognosis: (1) Intrauterine demise (33%)
(2) Mortality of 100% with hydrops
DDx: cervical meningocele, encephalocele, cystic-teratoma, twin sac of blighted ovum, nuchal edema

DERMOID
= DERMOID CYST = MATURE CYSTIC TERATOMA
= congenital tumor containing mature ectodermal elements
Incidence: 11 – 25% of all ovarian neoplasms; most common ovarian neoplasm
Age: reproductive life (80%)
Site: most often unilateral, bilateral in 12%
may contain: struma ovarii, carcinoid tumor
√ "dermoid plug" = Rokitansky nodule / protuberance
= oval / round solid tissue mass (sebaceous material) of 10 – 65 mm projecting into cyst lumen
Plain film (diagnostic in 40 %):
√ tooth / bone
√ fat density
CT:
√ round mass of fat floating in interface between two water-density components (93%)
√ Rokitansky nodule = dermoid plug (81%), usually single, may be multiple
√ fat-fluid level (12%)
√ globular calcifications (tooth) / rim of calcification (56%)
US (sensitivity 77 – 87%):
√ echogenic focus with acoustic shadowing in a predominantly cystic mass (44%) (DDx: bowel)
√ predominantly solid mass (31%)
√ purely cystic tumor (9%)
Cx: (1)   malignant degeneration in 1 – 2% (usually within dermoid plug)
(2)   torsion (4 – 16%)

DYSGERMINOMA
= homologue of testicular seminoma, highly radiosensitive
Incidence: 1 – 2%
Peak age: 2nd – 3rd decade
• no elevation of AFP / HCG (in 5% syncytiotrophoblastic giant cells present which can elevate HCG levels)
√ hyperechoic solid mass, may have areas of hemorrhage + necrosis
√ bilateral in 15 – 17%
√ speckled pattern of calcifications (rare)

ECTOPIA CORDIS
= fusion defect of anterior thoracic wall / sternum / septum transversum prior to 9th week of gestation
A. Thoracic type (60%) = heart outside thoracic cavity protruding through defect in sternum
B. Abdominal type (30%) = heart protruding into abdomen through gap in diaphragm
C. Thoracoabdominal type (7%) = found with pentalogy of Cantrell
D. Cervical type (3%) = displacement of heart into cervical region
Associated with:
(a) Facial deformities
(b) Skeletal deformities
(c) Ventral wall defects

(d) CNS malformations: meningocele, encephalocele
(e) Intracardiac anomalies: tetralogy of Fallot, TGA
(f) Amniotic band syndrome
Prognosis: stillbirth / death within first hours / days of life
in most cases

ECTOPIC PREGNANCY
= implantation outside the endometrial cavity
Incidence: 1:100 – 400 pregnancies; 73,700 cases in
1986 in United States; 1.4% of all reported
pregnancies; coexistent with intrauterine
pregnancy in 1:6,800 – 30,000 pregnancies
Cause: delayed transit of the fertilized zygote secondary
to abnormal angulation of oviduct or adhesions
from inflammation
Risk factors:
— previous tubal surgery
— previous PID
— ovulation induction
— endometriosis
— previous ectopic pregnancy (25% chance of
recurrence)
CLASSIC TRIAD (< 50%):
• abnormal vaginal bleeding (75%)
• pelvic pain
• palpable adnexal mass (30%)
• secondary amenorrhea
• cervical tenderness
• positive urinary pregnancy test (50%)
• positive beta-hCG does not rise > 66% within 48 hours
(lower levels + lower rise compared with intrauterine
pregnancy)
Location:
(a) tubal (95%): (1) ampullary ectopic
(2) isthmic ectopic (92%)
(3) interstitial ectopic (3%)
(b) other (5%): (4) abdominal ectopic
(5) ovarian ectopic
(6) interligamentary ectopic
(7) cervical ectopic (exceedingly
rare)
Spectrum:
Type 1: unruptured live ectopic + heartbeat
Type 2: early embryonic demise without rupture /
embryonic structures / heartbeat
Type 3: ruptured ectopic with blood in pelvis
Type 4: no sonographic signs of ectopic
√ free abdominal fluid / hyperechoic clot in cul-de-sac
√ hydro-/ hematosalpinx
√ adnexal mass (42%) with small anechoic center
= extrauterine gestational sac ± embryo ± heartbeat
√ live embryo in adnexa (6 – 17%) = only specific
sonographic finding
√ hyperechoic decidual thickening ("decidual cast")
√ "pseudogestational sac" = decidual reaction + anechoic
fluid center from bleeding (up to 20%)
√ absence of intrauterine pregnancy (beyond 6 weeks
MA)

(a) no IUP by transvesical US = ectopic pregnancy in
43 – 46%
(b) no IUP by endovaginal US = ectopic pregnancy in
67%
√ corpus luteum within ovary in > 50% on side of ectopic
Doppler-US:
√ high-velocity low-impedance flow around extrauterine
gestation in 54% (up to 4 kHz shift with 3 MHz
transducer, 0.38 ± 0.2 Pourcelot index)
√ absence of peritrophoblastic flow after 36 days (< 0.8
kHz shift with 3 MHz transducer or < 1.3 kHz shift with
5 MHz transducer)

INTERSTITIAL ECTOPIC
√ eccentrically placed gestational sac + incomplete
myometrial mantle
ABDOMINAL ECTOPIC
√ extrauterine location of fetus + placenta
√ uterus compressed with visible endometrial cavity line
√ absence of uterine wall between gestation + bladder /
abdominal wall

Cx: maternal death in 26%
DDx: (1) hemorrhagic corpus luteum / hematoma
(2) adnexal mass: hydrosalpinx, endometrioma
(3) fluid-containing small bowel loops
(4) eccentrically placed GS in bicornuate /
retroflexed / fibroid uterus

ENDODERMAL SINUS TUMOR OF OVARY
= YOLK SAC TUMOR
= rare but highly malignant tumor
Histo: resembles endodermal sinuses of the rat yolk sac
Age: usually adolescence
May be associated with   teratoma, dermoid cyst,
choriocarcinoma
• frequently abdominal enlargement + pain
• elevated serum AFP (common)
√ predominantly hyperechoic solid tumor
√ cystic areas (epithelial-lined cysts / cysts of coexisting
mature teratoma / hemorrhage / necrosis)

ENDOMETRIAL CANCER
Most common invasive gynecologic malignancy;
4th most frequent female cancer;
34,000 new cases per year with 3,000 deaths
Histo: adenocarcinoma (90 – 95%), sarcoma (1 – 3%)
Peak age: 62 years; 74% > age 50
Risk factors: nulliparity, late menopause, exogenous
hormones, polycystic ovaries, obesity,
hypertension, diabetes mellitus
STAGE 0   in situ
I   confined to corpus (in 75% of cases)
I a   uterine cavity < 8 cm
I b   uterine cavity > 8 cm
II   involvement of corpus + cervix
III   extension outside uterus but within true
pelvis (parametria, adnexa, pelvic sidewall,
pelvic nodes)

IV a   extension beyond true pelvis / mucosal
         involvement of bladder / rectum
IV b   distant metastases (paraaortic nodes,
         peritoneal seeding, lung, brain, bone)
Lymph node metastases: 3% with superficial invasion;
                      40% with deep invasion
- postmenopausal bleeding
√ normal sized / enlarged uterus
MRI: staging accuracy 92%
   √ normal endometrium + endometrial cancer have
      similar high signal intensities
   √ endometrial thickness abnormal if > 3 mm
      (postmenopausal woman) / > 10 mm (under estrogen
      replacement)
      DDx: blood clot, uterine secretions, adenomatous
              hyperplasia
   √ disruption / absence of junctional zone (myometrial
      invasion)
   √ penetration of hyperintense areas into myometrium
      (deep muscle invasion; 75% accuracy)

ENDOMETRIOSIS
= encysted functioning endometrial tissue in ectopic
   locations
Incidence: 5 – 15% of all females
Age: 3rd – 4th decade
- severe dysmenorrhea
- pelvic pain (peritoneal adhesions, bleeding)
- dyspareunia
- sterility (with involvement of tubes + ovaries)
Location:
   (a) internal endometriosis (within uterus)
        = ADENOMYOSIS
   (b) external endometriosis
        typical in: pouch of Douglas, ovary, fallopian tube,
                     broad ligament, rectovaginal septum
        rare in   : umbilicus, laparotomy scar, bladder wall,
                     bowel wall, lungs, pleural space, limbs
√ often NO detectable abnormality (when lesions small +
   scattered)
√ frequently multiple cysts bilaterally
√ typically cystic space = endometrioma = "chocolate cyst"
   up to 20 cm in diameter (usually 2 – 5 cm)
   √ anechoic / hypoechoic cyst (homogeneous low level
      echoes = hemorrhagic debris)
   √ may contain echogenic material (= clot) appearing as
      a solid tumor
   √ may show layering of debris
√ thickened wall + loss of definition of borders with pelvic
   organs
MRI (64 – 71% sensitivity; 60 – 82% specificity):
   √ hyperintense lesions on all pulse sequences in 47 %,
      hypointense on all pulse sequences in 27%
BE:
   √ submucosal implants along anterior rectal wall
CXR:
   √ catamenial pneumothorax = spontaneous
      pneumothorax due to endometriosis of diaphragm

Cx: infertility from adhesions (30% of infertility patients
        show endometriosis)

ENDOMETROID TUMOR
Incidence: 15% of all ovarian cancers
Associated with endometrial cancer in 1/3
Histo: resembles endometrial epithelium
√ solid / complex tumor, bilateral in 1/3

FACIAL CLEFTING
= lack of fusion of facial grooves; second most common
   congenital malformation
Incidence: 1.2 – 1.6:1,000 live births
Associated with 72 abnormalities
1. cleft lip (25 %): F > M
   associated with: most frequently club foot
   √ linear defect extending from one side of lip into nostril
   √ bilateral in 20%
2. cleft palate (25%)
   associated anomalies in 50 %: most frequently club foot
3. cleft lip + palate (50%)
   associated anomalies in 13 %: most frequently
   polydactyly
   √ linear defect extends through alveolar ridge + hard
      palate reaching the floor of the nasal cavity / orbit
   √ L > R side; in 25% bilateral

FETAL CARDIAC DYSRHYTHMIAS
normal heart rate: 120 – 160 bpm

Premature Atrial Contractions
= PAC = most common benign rhythm abnormality
√ transient tachycardia / bradycardia

Supraventricular Tachyarrhythmia
Incidence: 1:25,000; most frequent tachyarrhythmia
              in children
Etiology: viral infection, hypoplasia of sinoatrial tract
Pathogenesis:
   (1) automaticity = irritable ectopic focus discharges
        at high frequency
   (2) reentry   = electric pulse reentering the atria
        inciting new discharges
Types:
   1. Supraventricular tachyarrhythmia (SVT)
      (a) Paroxysmal supraventricular tachycardia
      (b) Paroxysmal atrial tachycardia
      √ atrial rate of 180 – 300 bpm + ventricular
         response of 1:1
   3. Atrial flutter
      √ atrial rate of 300 – 460 bpm + ventricular rate of
         60 – 200 bpm
   4. Atrial fibrillation
      √ atrial rate of 400 – 700 bpm + ventricular rate of
         120 – 200 bpm
Hemodynamics:
   fast ventricular rate results in suboptimal filling of
   heart chambers + decreased cardiac output, overload
   of RA, CHF

Associated with cardiac anomalies (5 – 10 %):
ASD, congenital mitral valve disease, cardiac
tumors, WPW syndrome, cardiomyopathy,
thyrotoxicosis
OB-US:
√ M-mode echocardiography with simultaneous
visualization of atrial + ventricular contractions
allows inference of atrioventricular activation
sequence
Cx: Congestive heart failure + nonimmune hydrops
Rx: Intrauterine pharmacologic cardioversion
(digoxin, propranolol, verapamil, procainamide,
quinidine)

Atrioventricular Block
Incidence: 1:20,000 live births; in 4 – 9% of all infants
with CHD
Etiology: (1) immaturity of conduction system
(2) absent connection to AV node
(3) abnormal anatomic position of AV node
Associated with:
(a) Cardiac structural anomalies (45 – 50%):
corrected transposition, univentricular heart,
cardiac tumor, cardiomyopathy
(b) Maternal connective tissue disease: lupus
erythematosus
Types:
1. First-degree heart block = simple conduction delay
√ normal heart rate + rhythm (not reportedly
diagnosed in utero)
2. Second-degree heart block
(a) Mobitz type I
= progressive prolongation of PR interval
finally leading to the block of one atrial
impulse (Luciani-Wenckebach
phenomenon)
√ a few atrial contractions are not followed by
a ventricular contraction
(b) Mobitz type II
= intermittent conduction with a ventricular
rate as a submultiple of the atrial rate (e.g.,
2:1 / 3:1 block)
√ atrial contraction not followed by ventricular
contraction in a constant relationship
3. Third-degree heart block = complete heart block
= complete dissociation of atria + ventricles
√ slow atrial + ventricular contractions
independent from each other
Cx: decreased cardiac output + CHF

FETAL DEATH IN UTERO
= fetal death during 2nd + 3rd trimesters
Specific signs:
√ absent cardiac / somatic motion
Nonspecific signs seen not before 48 hours after death:
√ same / decreased BPD measurement compared to
prior exam
√ development of dolichocephaly

√ "spalding sign" = overlapping fetal skull bones
√ distorted fetus without recognizable structures
√ skin edema (epidermolysis)
√ increased amount of echoes in amniotic fluid (= fetal
tissue fragments)
√ gas in fetal vascular system

FETAL HYDROPS
Nonimmune Hydrops
= excess of total body water evident as extracellular
accumulation of fluid in tissues + serous cavities
without antibodies against RBC
Incidence: 1:1500 to 1:4000 deliveries
Causes:
1. Cardiac anomalies (40%):
(a) structural heart disease (25 %): AV septal
defect, hypoplastic left heart, rhabdomyoma
(b) tachyarrhythmia (15%)
2. Hematologic causes: thalassemia, hemolysis,
fetal blood loss
3. Idiopathic (25 – 44%)
4. Twin-twin transfusion (20%)
5. Chromosomal abnormalities (6 %): Turner
syndrome
6. Skeletal dysplasias: achondroplasia,
achondrogenesis, osteogenesis imperfecta,
thanatophoric dwarfism, asphyxiating thoracic
dysplasia
7. Renal disease (4 %): congenital nephrotic
syndrome
8. Infections: toxoplasmosis, CMV, syphilis,
coxsackie, parvovirus
9. Cervical tumors: teratoma
10. Chest masses: cystic adenomatoid
malformation, extralobar sequestration,
mediastinal tumor, rhabdomyoma of heart,
diaphragmatic hernia
11. Abdominal masses: neuroblastoma,
hemangioendothelioma of liver
12. Placental tumors: chorioangioma
Prognosis: 46% death in utero; 17% neonatal death

Immune Hydrops
= ERYTHROBLASTOSIS FETALIS
= lysis of fetal RBCs by maternal IgG antibodies
Pathophysiology:
Rh negative women (= no D antigen) may become
isoimmunized if exposed to Rh positive blood (= D
allotype present); maternal IgM antibodies develop
initially, later IgG antibodies with ability to cross
placenta (= transplacental passage)
Cause of isoimmunization:
feto-maternal hemorrhage during pregnancy /
delivery / spontaneous or elective abortion
At risk:
Caucasians (15%), Blacks (6%), Orientals (1%);
absence of D antigen originates in Basques

Determination of extent of disease by:
  (1) Optical density shift at 450 nm (= delta OD 450) reflects amount of bilirubin in amniotic fluid
  (2) Percutaneous umbilical cord sampling (PUBS)
√ anasarca (= skin edema)
√ fetal ascites
√ pleural effusion
√ increased diameter of umbilical vein
√ subcutaneous edema (skin thickness > 5 mm)
√ polyhydramnios (75%)
√ placentomegaly > 6 cm
√ pericardial effusion
√ hepatosplenomegaly
Prophylaxis:
  Rh immune globulin (RhoGAM® = antibody against D antigen) blocks antigen sites on Rh positive cells in maternal circulation to prevent initiation of maternal antibody production; RhIg given at 28 weeks to all Rh negative women

FOLLICULAR CYST
= unruptured follicle / ruptured follicle that sealed immediately (after continued stimulation); sign of anovulatory cycle
Predisposed: patients during puberty + menopause; S/P salpingectomy
Prognosis: usually disappears after 1 – 2 menstrual cycles
√ thin-walled, unilocular cyst
√ size usually > 2.5 cm / occasionally up to 10 cm in size
√ usually multiple / may be single

GASTROSCHISIS
= paraumbilical fusion defect usually on right side secondary to premature interruption of right omphalomesenteric artery (normally persists proximally as superior mesenteric artery) / abnormal involution of right umbilical vein at 5 weeks gestational age; may involve thorax; bowel is nonrotated + lacks secondary fixation to dorsal abdominal wall
Incidence: 1:10,000 to 1:20,000 live births, sporadic
Age of occurrence: 37 days of embryonic life
  low incidence of associated anomalies (5%): intestinal atresia / stenosis (25%), IUGR (up to 77%), ectopia cordis
• elevated maternal serum AFP in 75%
√ normal insertion of umbilical cord
√ thickened freely floating bowel loops outside fetal abdomen (lack of peritoneal covering)
√ < 3 – 5 cm defect usually on right side of cord insertion
√ no fetal ascites
√ polyhydramnios may be present
Cx: (1) bowel obstruction / perforation
       (2) immaturity (65%)
Mortality rate: 7.6 – 28%

GESTATIONAL TROPHOBLASTIC DISEASE
= group of disorders as a result of a combination of male + female gametes arising from trophoblastic elements of the developing blastocyst with invasive tendency + hCG-synthesis
1. Benign hydatidiform mole (90%)
2. Invasive mole (5 – 8%)
3. Choriocarcinoma (1 – 2%)

GRANULOSA CELL TUMOR
Most common hormone-active estrogenic tumor of ovary
Incidence: 1 – 3% of all ovarian neoplasms
Age: puberty (5%), reproductive age (45%), postmenopausal (50%)
• precocious puberty
• vaginal bleeding + full breasts
√ multilocular cyst containing fluid / blood (most frequently)
√ size up to 40 cm in diameter, mostly unilateral
√ predominantly hypoechoic mass simulating fibroid
√ endometrial glandular hyperplasia
Cx: malignant transformation is rare

HYDATIDIFORM MOLE
= MOLAR PREGNANCY
Histo: marked edema + enlargement of chorionic villi; disappearance of villous blood vessels + proliferation of trophoblasts
Types:
  1. COMPLETE / CLASSICAL MOLE
     = fertilization of an "empty egg" (= ovum with no active chromosomal material)
     Histo: hydatiform swelling of all villi + trophoblastic proliferation
     • diploid karyotype almost always paternal XX chromosomes
     √ no fetal parts / no chorionic membrane
     Prognosis: in 80% benign, in 20% malignant
  2. COMPLETE MOLE + COEXISTENT FETUS (2%)
     = molar degeneration of one conceptus of an identical twin pregnancy with same risk of malignant degeneration as in classical mole
  3. PARTIAL MOLE
     = areas of molar change alternating with normal villi + fetus with significant congenital anomalies
     Histo: areas of molar change alternating with normal villi
     • triploid karyotype (66% XXY; 33% XXX)
     • early onset of preeclampsia
     √ fetal structures present (e.g., placenta)
     Prognosis: not associated with malignant transformation

• severe eclampsia prior to 24 weeks
• uterus too large for dates
• 1st trimester bleeding
• abnormal elevation of beta-hCG
• passing of grapelike vesicles per vagina

√ uterus larger than dates (in 50%)
√ hyperechoic intrauterine tissue interspersed with
   numerous punctate hypoechoic areas = hydropic villi
√ in 25% atypical appearance: large hyperechoic areas
   (blood clot) + areas of cystic degeneration resembling
   incomplete abortion
√ thick hyperechoic rim around central anechoic zone
√ bilateral theca lutein cysts (18 – 37%) which may take 4
   months to regress after evacuation of a molar
   pregnancy
DDx:
   (1) Hydropic degeneration of the placenta (associated
       with incomplete / missed abortions)
   (2) Degenerated uterine leiomyoma
   (3) Incomplete abortion = retained products with
       hemorrhage
   (4) Choriocarcinoma

HYDRO- / HEMATOMETROCOLPOS
= accumulation of sterile fluid (hydro~) / blood (hemato~) /
  pus (pyo~) within uterus (metria) + vagina (colpos)
Incidence: 1:16,000 female births
Etiology:
   (a) congenital obstruction: persistent urogenital sinus,
       imperforate hymen, transverse vaginal septum,
       vaginal atresia, blind horn of bicornuate uterus
       may be associated with:
          imperforate anus, unilateral renal agenesis /
          hypoplasia, polycystic kidneys, duplication of
          vagina + uterus, sacral hypoplasia, esophageal
          atresia
   (b) acquired obstruction: neoplastic obstruction of
       endocervical canal / vagina, postpartum infection,
       attempted abortion, cervical stenosis after
       radiotherapy, postsurgical scarring, senile
       contraction
Age: most often in adolescence
• "delayed menarche"
• pain during defecation / urination
• asymptomatic / vague pelvic discomfort
√ pear-shaped distended uterus ± vagina
√ anechoic / echogenic uterine ± vaginal contents
OB-US:
   √ cystic / midlevel echogenic retrovesical mass
     (mucous secretions secondary to steroidal stimulation
     during fetal life)
DDx: ovarian cyst, mesenteric cyst, anterior meningocele,
     cystic tumor
Cx: endometritis, myometritis, parametritis (= pelvic
     lymphangitis), pelvic abscess, septic pelvic
     thrombophlebitis, urinary tract infection

IMMATURE TERATOMA OF OVARY
= EMBRYONAL TERATOMA = MALIGNANT TERATOMA
= SOLID TERATOMA
Histo: immature tissue resembling those of the embryo;
        grade 0 – 3 reflect amount of immature
        neuroectodermal tissue

May be associated with gliomatosis peritonei = multiple
   peritoneal implants of mature glial tissue
• elevated AFP levels (50%)
• no elevation of serum hCG levels
√ predominantly solid tumor with numerous cysts of
   varying size
√ scattered calcifications (due to invariable association
   with mature teratoma)

INTRAUTERINE CONTRACEPTIVE DEVICE
√ double echogenic line with plastic IUD
√ reverberation echoes with metal IUD

Types of IUD:
   1. Lippes loop
      √ 4 – 5 echogenic dots on SAG view
      √ horizontal line / dot on TRV view
   2. Saf-T-coil
      √ echogenic solid line on SAG view
      √ series of echoes / dot on TRV view
   3. Copper 7 / Copper T / Progestasert
      √ dot in fundus + solid line in corpus on SAG view
      √ solid line in fundus + dot in corpus on TRV view
   4. Dalkon shield (no longer produced)

"LOST IUD":
= locater device not palpated
1. expulsion of IUD
3. migration of thread
2. detachment of thread
4. uterine perforation of IUD
Abdominal plain film indicated if IUD not identified by
US!
Cx: pelvic inflammatory disease (risk 2 – 3 x that of
      non-IUD users)

IUD + PREGNANCY
√ IUD may not be visualized after 1st trimester (as
   uterus grows IUD is drawn into cavity)
Prognosis: high risk of septic abortion
Rx: early removal of IUD if string remained in vagina

INTRAUTERINE GROWTH RETARDATION
= process resulting in birth of a neonate with weight below
  10th percentile for gestational age; usually not
  detectable before 32 – 34 weeks GA (time of maximal
  fetal growth)
Incidence: 3 – 7% of all deliveries; in 12 – 47% of all
             twin pregnancies
Etiology:
   A. UTEROPLACENTAL INSUFFICIENCY (80%)
      1. MATERNAL CAUSES
          √ asymmetric IUGR / symmetric IUGR (in
             severe cases)
          (a) Deficient supply of nutrients:
              smoking, maternal malnutrition, multiple
              gestations, anemia, life in high altitudes

(b) Maternal vascular disease (more common):
severe diabetes, chronic hypertension,
chronic renal disease, collagen disease
(e.g., SLE) (inadequate placental perfusion)
2. PRIMARY PLACENTAL CAUSES
Extensive placental infarctions, chronic partial
separation, placenta previa
B. PRIMARY FETAL CAUSES (20%)
= decreased intrinsic growth
√ symmetric IUGR
Congenital heart disease, genitourinary anomalies,
CNS anomalies, chromosomal abnormalities
(trisomy 13, 18, 21), viral infection (rubella, CMV)

PHENOTYPES
1. Pure symmetrical IUGR = low profile IUGR
= proportionate reduction of all fetal
measurements due to
(a) intrinsic alteration in growth potential
(b) severe nutritional deprivation overwhelming
protective brain-sparing mechanism occurring
prior to 26 weeks MA + persisting until delivery
2. Asymmetrical IUGR = late flattening IUGR (75%)
= disproportionate reduction of fetal measurements
due to uteroplacental insufficiency with
preferential shunting of blood to fetal brain
occurring after 26 weeks GA
√ small body (AC)
√ high HC/AC and FL/AC ratios (head size + femur
length less affected)

MORPHOLOGIC GROWTH PARAMETERS
AC + EFW have highest sensitivity
√ BPD growth rate < 5th percentile (82% chance of
IUGR; 18% false positive; 17% false negative)
√ HC:AC ratio > 95th percentile (71% chance of
asymmetrical IUGR)
√ reduced amniotic fluid volume < 1 cm in its broadest
dimension anywhere (90% chance of IUGR)
√ abdominal circumference (AC) < 10th percentile
(84% chance for IUGR)
√ grade III placenta

BIOPHYSICAL PROFILE (Platt and Manning)
33% sensitivity, 17% positive predictive value
Parameters   (30 minutes observation period):
1. NST: reactive
2. Fetal breathing movement (FBM):
breathing period at least 60 seconds
3. Fetal body movement:
> 3 discrete movements of limbs / trunk
4. Fetal tone
upper + lower limbs usually fully flexed with head
on chest;
> 1 episode of extension with return to flexion
5. Amniotic fluid volume
largest pocket > 1 cm in vertical diameter without
containing loops of cord

Score: 2 points if normal; 0 points if abnormal
Results:
8 – 10   maximal score
6   equivocal
0 – 4   severe fetal compromise, delivery indicated

AMNIOTIC FLUID INDEX
= sum of the largest amniotic fluid pockets in each
quadrant of uterus expressed in cm

DOPPLER STUDY
1. NON-STRESS TEST (NST)
External monitoring over 20 minutes;
√ at least 4 fetal heart accelerations (> 15 bpm over
baseline lasting > 15 seconds) following fetal
movement > 34 weeks GA
√ no heart accelerations in immaturity, during sleep
cycle, with maternal sedative use
Poor specificity = most abnormal test results occur in
normal fetuses
2. CONTRACTION STRESS TEST (CST)
External monitoring after injection of oxytocin /
maternal breast stimulation to elicit > 3 uterine
contractions in 10-minute period
50% specificity
3. UTERINE + UMBILICAL ARTERY WAVEFORM
√ elevated systolic:diastolic ratio (indicating
increased vascular resistance)
4. FETAL AORTIC FLOW VOLUME
√ decrease in blood flow < 185 – 246 ml/kg/min
Cx: increased risk for perinatal asphyxia, meconium
aspiration, electrolyte imbalance from metabolic
acidosis, polycythemia
Prognosis: 6 – 8 fold increase in risk for intrapartum +
neonatal death
DDx of SGA (fetus small for gestational age):
(1) constitutionally small fetus
(2) primary growth failure associated with congenital
anomalies
(3) IUGR

INVASIVE MOLE
= CHORIOADENOMA DESTRUENS
Histo: excessive trophoblastic proliferation with
presence of villous structure + invasion of
myometrium
• history of previous molar gestation / missed abortion
(75%)
• continued uterine bleeding
• persistently elevated beta-hCG levels
√ hyperechoic tissue with punctate lucencies
√ irregular focal hyperechoic region within myometrium
√ bilateral theca lutein cysts, 4 – 8 cm in size

KRUKENBERG TUMOR
= ovarian tumors from gastric cancer (now including
pancreatic + biliary primaries); 2% of females with
gastric cancer develop Krukenberg tumor

Age: any age, most common in 5th – 6th decade
√ in 80% bilateral hypo- / hyperechoic mass ± cystic
  degeneration

MACROSOMIA
= FETAL GROWTH ACCELERATION
= fetus large for gestational age (LGA) with EFW > 90th
  percentile for age / > 4,000 g at term
√ AC > 3 SD above the mean for age (most reliable
  measurement)
√ estimated fetal weight (EFW) including fetal head,
  abdomen, femur length > 90th percentile (± 15%
  accuracy)
√ low FL:AC ratio
√ low HC:AC ratio
√ enlarged thigh circumference
√ low FL:thigh circumference ratio

MALIGNANT GERM CELL TUMOR OF OVARY
Age: 14 years on average
• pelvic / abdominal pain
• pelvic / abdominal mass
• elevated alpha-fetoprotein (60% in immature teratoma;
  100% in endodermal sinus tumor)
• elevated beta-hCG (30% of endodermal sinus tumors)
√ average diameter of 15 cm
√ unilateral, rarely bilateral
√ calcifications (40%)
√ homogeneously solid (3%), predominantly solid (85%),
  predominantly cystic (12%)

MUCINOUS OVARIAN TUMOR
Incidence: 20% of all ovarian tumors;
             benign:malignant = 7:1
Histo: nonciliated tall columnar epithelium, cysts lined
         by mucus-secreting cells (similar to endocervix)
Age: middle adult life, rare before puberty + after
        menopause
Cx: rupture may lead to pseudomyxoma peritonei
A. MUCINOUS CYSTADENOMA
   Age: reproductive years + postmenopause
   √ multilocular cyst with thin septa
   √ complex cysts with solid elements
   √ usually unilateral, bilateral in 5%
   Cx: malignant transformation in 1 of 8 cases
B. MUCINOUS CYSTADENOCARCINOMA
   difficult to differentiate from benign variety
   √ solid tissue areas within cystic septated adnexal
     mass
   √ usually unilateral, bilateral in 20%
   √ capsular infiltration with loss of definition + fixation

OMPHALOCELE
= persistence of body stalk = midline defect of anterior
  abdominal wall secondary to failure of lateral body folds
  to fuse during 3rd to 4th week of gestation + herniation
  of intraabdominal contents into base of umbilical cord
Incidence: 1:4,000 to 1:5,500 pregnancies

Age: earliest detection at 12 weeks menstrual age
High incidence of ASSOCIATED ANOMALIES (45 - 72%):
  1. Chromosomal (35 – 58%): trisomy 13, 18, 21,
     Turner syndrome (13% with liver in omphalocele,
     77% with bowel in omphalocele)
  2. Genitourinary (40%)
  3. Cardiac (16 – 47%): VSD, ASD, tetralogy of Fallot,
     ectopia cordis in pentalogy of Cantrell, DORV
  4. Neural tube defects (4 – 39%): holoprosencephaly,
     encephalocele, cerebellar hypoplasia
  5. IUGR (20%)
  6. Beckwith-Wiedemann syndrome (10%)
  7. GI tract
     intestinal atresia (vascular compromise); malrotation;
     abnormal fixation of liver, esophageal atresia, facial
     cleft
  8. Limb-body wall deficiency; cystic hygroma
  9. Abnormal amniotic fluid volume
• elevated maternal serum AFP in 40%
√ midline defect
  √ defect over entire ventral abdominal wall (mean size
    2.5 – 5 cm)
  √ widened cord where it joins the skin of the abdomen
√ cord inserting at apex of defect
√ herniation of abdominal viscera at base of umbilical
  cord: liver (27%) ± stomach ± bowel
√ hypoechoic Wharton jelly within herniated sac
√ covering peritoneal-amniotic membrane (may rupture in
  exceedingly rare cases)
√ polyhydramnios (occasionally oligohydramnios)
Cx: (1) infection, inanition
       (2) immaturity (23%)
Mortality rate: 29 – 55% due to frequency of concurrent
                 malformations + chromosomic
                 abnormalities; 10% mortality if isolated
                 abnormality

PSEUDOOMPHALOCELE
= deformation of fetal abdomen by transducer pressure
  coupled with an oblique scan orientation may give the
  appearance of an omphalocele

OMPHALOMESENTERIC CYST
Etiology: persistence + dilatation of a segment of the
           omphalomesenteric duct joining the embryonic
           gut and the yolk sac which is formed during the
           3rd week and closed by the 16th week of
           gestation
Histo: cyst lined by gastrointestinal epithelium
M:F = 3:5
Location: usually in close proximity to fetus
√ umbilical cord cyst up to 6 cm in diameter
Cx: (1) Compression of umbilical vessels by expanding
          cyst
       (2) Erosion of umbilical vein from acid-producing
          gastric mucosal lining
DDx: Allantoic cyst, umbilical cord hematoma

OVARIAN CANCER

3rd most common gynecologic malignancy = 25% of all gynecologic malignancies; highest mortality rate of all female cancers, 4th leading cause of cancer deaths in women, acounts for 50% of cancer deaths of female genital tract
Incidence: 33 cases per year per 100,000 women > age 50 ; 19,000 new cases per year with 12,000 deaths
Peak age: 55 – 59 years
Histo: epithelial (70%), germ cell (15%), metastases (10%), stromal (5%)
    (a) serous tumor resembling ciliated columnar cells of the fallopian tubes (50%)
    (b) endometrioid tumor similar to endometrial adenocarcinoma (15 – 30%)
    (c) mucinous tumor similar to endocervical canal epithelium (15%)
    (d) mesonephroid tumor similar to clear cell carcinoma of kidney (5%)
    (e) undifferentiated tumor (15%)
Increased risk:
    nulliparity, Caucasian race, higher socioeconomic group, Hx of breast cancer (risk factor of 2)
STAGE I a   limited to one ovary
    I b   limited to both ovaries
    I c   + positive peritoneal lavage / ascites
    II a   involvement of uterus / fallopian tubes
    II b   extension to other pelvic tissues
    II c   + positive peritoneal lavage / ascites
    III   intraabdominal extension outside pelvis / retroperitoneal nodes / extension to small bowel / omentum
    IV   distant metastases
At time of diagnosis: 75% of patients have stage III / IV disease, metastases in 2/3 of patients
- occasional pelvo-abdominal pain
- constipation, urinary frequency
- early satiety
- ascites
- paraneoplastic hypercalcemia
US:
    Screening finds adnexal masses in 1 – 10% of postmenopausal women; masses < 5 cm are only in 3% malignant
    √ ovarian size > 1.5 cm, ovarian volume > 2 ml (ovaries may be larger with multiparity, obesity, hormonal replacement); 80% of normal ovaries not visualized
    √ omental / peritoneal masses
    √ pseudomyxoma peritonei
    √ liver metastases
    √ ascites
Prognosis: 20 – 30% overall 5-year survival rate

OVARIAN FIBROMA

Incidence: 3 – 4%
Age: usually menopausal / postmenopausal
- usually asymptomatic
√ hypoechoic mass with sound attenuation

OVARIAN HYPERSTIMULATION SYNDROME

Incidence: severe OHSS in 1.5 – 6% under Perganol therapy
Etiology:
    (a) induced by hCG therapy with human menopausal gonadotropin (Perganol), occasionally with clomiphene (Clomid)
    (b) hydatidiform mole
    (c) chorioepithelioma
    (d) multiple pregnancies
Path: enlarged ovaries with multiple follicular cysts, corpora lutea, edematous stroma (fluid shift secondary to increased capillary permeability)
- abdominal pain (100%)
- abdominal distension (100%)
- nausea (100%)
- vomiting (36%)
- acute abdomen (17%)
- dyspnea (16%)
- thrombophlebitis (11%)
- marked hemoconcentration
- fainting (11%)
- blurred vision (5%)
- anasarca (5%)
- hydrothorax
- enhanced fertility
√ ovary > 5 cm in longest dimension containing large geometrically packed follicles
√ ovarian cyst > 10 cm (100 %): usually disappear after 20 – 40 days
√ ascites (33%)
√ pleural effusion (5%)
√ hydroureter (11%)
Cx: (related to volume depletion):
    (1) hypovolemia + hemoconcentration
    (2) oliguria, electrolyte imbalance, azotemia
    (3) death from intraabdominal hemorrhage / thromboembolic event

PARAOVARIAN CYST

= vestigial remnant of Wolffian body = mesonephric tubules off the mesonephric (= Gartner) duct, paralleling vagina and fallopian tube, usually degenerate into vestigial structures
Location: within the two peritoneal layers of broad ligament, between the tube and hilum of the ovary
Types: (a) mesonephric (Wolffian duct)
    (b) paramesonephric (Müllerian duct)
    (c) mesothelial
1. GARTNER DUCT CYST: inclusion cyst; lateral to vaginal + uterine wall
2. PAROÖPHORON: medial location between tube + hilum of ovary
3. EPOÖPHORON: lateral location between tube + hilum of ovary
4. HYDATID OF MORGAGNI: most lateral + outer end of Gartner duct

√ thin-walled unilocular cyst, up to 18 cm in diameter
√ may arise out of pelvis (if pedunculated + mobile)

PELVIC INFLAMMATORY DISEASE
Incidence: in 1% of women between age 15 – 24 years
Predisposed: Intrauterine contraceptive device
(increased risk 1.5 – 4 x)
Etiology: (a)   bilateral: venereal disease (gonorrhea),
IUD, S/P abortion
(b)   unilateral = nongynecologic: rupture of
appendix, diverticulum, S/P pelvic surgery
Organisms:
(1)   Gonorrhea (most common) with spread from cervix
to tubes producing fibrosis + adhesions
(2)   Staphylococcus / Streptococcus via lymphatics +
veins
(3)   Tuberculosis (hematogenous)
(4)   Actinomycosis in IUD users
May be associated with Fitz-Hugh-Curtis syndrome
(= gonorrheic perihepatitis)
A. **Endometritis**
√   endometrial prominence
√   small amount of fluid within uterine lumen
√   gas reflection within uterine cavity (most specific)
√   pain over uterus
B. **Salpingitis**
not depicted by imaging techniques
C. **Hydro- / pyosalpinx**
=   continued secretion of tubal epithelium into lumen
of a fallopian tube obstructed at two sites
√   funnel-shaped kinked thick-walled cystic structure
filled with sterile fluid / pus
√   free fluid / pus in cul-de-sac
√   loss of definition of uterine borders
Cx: tubal torsion
D. **Tuboovarian Abscess**
√   multilocular complex mass usually in posterior
cul-de-sac extending bilaterally
√   may contain fluid-fluid levels or gas

PENTALOGY OF CANTRELL
= sporadic very rare abnormality
1. midline supraumbilical abdominal defect
2. defect of lower sternum
3. deficiency of diaphragmatic pericardium
4. deficiency of anterior diaphragm: herniation of
intraabdominal organs into thoracic cavity is rare
5. intracardiac abnormality: atrioventricular septal defect
(50%), VSD (18%), tetralogy of Fallot (11%)
√ ectopia cordis

PERITONEAL INCLUSION CYST
Histo: cyst lined by hyperplastic mesothelial cells +
fibroglandular tissue with chronic inflammation
Predisposed: patients with active ovaries + extensive
pelvic adhesions from previous abdominal
surgery / pelvic inflammatory disease /
endometriosis

Pathogenesis: impaired peritoneal clearing of fluid
normally produced by ovaries
√ single / multiloculated cyst contiguous with ovary
Cx: infertility
DDx: paraovarian cyst, ovarian neoplasm, lymphangioma

PLACENTA ACCRETA
= underdeveloped decidualization with chorionic villi
growing into uterine wall
Incidence: 1:2,500 – 7,000 deliveries
Predisposed: areas of uterine scarring
(1)   prior cesarean section (1/4)
(2)   associated with placenta previa (2/3)
Associated with placenta previa
Types:
1.   PLACENTA ACCRETA = chorionic villi in direct
contact with myometrium
2.   PLACENTA INCRETA = villi invade myometrium
3.   PLACENTA PERCRETA = villi penetrate through
uterine serosa
√ absence of subplacental sonolucent space (= venous
complex)
√ placental vessels extending into urinary bladder wall
Cx: retention of placental tissue with persistent
postpartum bleeding

PLACENTA EXTRACHORIALIS
= attachment of placental membranes to the fetal surface
of the placenta rather than to the placental margin
= chorionic plate smaller than basal plate, i.e., the
transition of membranous to villous chorion occurs at a
distance from the placental edge that is smaller than the
basal plate radius

1.   CIRCUMMARGINATE PLACENTA
Incidence: up to 20% of placentas
•   No clinical significance
√   placental margin not deformed
2.   CIRCUMVALLATE PLACENTA
=   attachment of fetal membranes form a folded
thickened ring with underlying fibrin + often
hemorrhage
Incidence: 1 – 2% of pregnancies
Cx: premature labor, threatened abortion,
increased perinatal mortality, marginal
hemorrhage

PLACENTAL ABRUPTION
= ABRUPTIO PLACENTAE = premature separation of
placenta from the myometrium secondary to maternal
hemorrhage into decidua basalis between 20th week
and birth
Incidence: 0.5 – 1.3% of gestations
Risk factors:
previous history of abruption / perinatal death /
premature delivery; hypertension; vascular disease;
smoking; drugs (cocaine); fibroids; trauma; fetal
malformations

Associated with   intraplacental infarction / hematoma
- vaginal bleeding (80%)
- abdominal pain (50%)
- consumptive coagulopathy = DIC (30%)
- uterine rigidity (15%)

Site: marginal (most common site); retroplacental
√ hyperechoic / isoechoic hematoma (initially difficult to distinguish from placenta)
√ hypoechoic / complex collection between uterine wall + placenta in 50% within 1 week (hematoma / placental infraction)
√ anechoic collection within 2 weeks
√ separation / rounding of placental margin
√ abnormally thick + heterogenous placenta with isoechoic blood
√ elevation of chorioamnionic membrane (DDx: incomplete chorioamnionic fusion during 2nd trimester, blighted twin)

Prognosis:
(1) only large hematomas (occupying > 30 – 40% of the maternal surface) result in fetal hypoxia
(2) abruptions with contained hematoma have worse prognosis
(3) responsible for up to 15 – 25% of all perinatal deaths
(4) normal term deliveries in 27% of hematomas seen > 20 weeks GA
(5) normal delivery in 80% of intrauterine hematomas < 20 weeks GA

Cx: (1) perinatal death (5-fold increase)
(2) fetal distress / demise (15 – 27%)
(3) premature labor + premature delivery (23 – 52%) (3-fold increase)
(4) threatened abortion during first 20 weeks
(5) infant small-for-gestational age (6 – 7%)

DDx: (1) Normal draining basal veins
(2) Normal uterine tissue
(3) Retroplacental myoma
(4) Focal contraction
(5) Chorioangioma
(6) Coexistent mole

PLACENTA MEMBRANACEA
= presence of well-vascularized placental villi in the peripheral membranes

Cause: ? endometritis, endometrial hyperplasia, extensive vascularization of decidua capsularis, previous endometrial damage by curettage
- repeated vaginal bleeding extending into 2nd trimester + abortion at 20 – 30 weeks
- postpartum hemorrhage
√ thickened outline over whole gestational sac (0.2 – 3.0 cm)
√ may show additional distinct disc of placenta

PLACENTA PREVIA
= abnormally low implantation of ovum with the placenta covering all / part of internal cervical os

Incidence: 0.5% of all deliveries; in 7 – 11% of women with 2nd + 3rd trimester vaginal bleeding
Predisposed:
defective decidual vascularization in areas of endometrial scarring causing compensatory placental thinning; placenta occupies a greater surface of the uterus with increased probability for encroachment upon internal os
(1) previous uterine incision (cesarian section, myomectomy)
(2) older women
(3) multiparous women

Types:
1. Central / total previa (1/3) = complete covering of internal os
2. Partial previa = internal os partially covered by placenta
3. Low-lying placenta = low placental edge without extension over internal os; palpable by examining finger
- painless vaginal bleeding in 93% (usually 3rd trimester / as early as 20 weeks)

US - FALSE POSITIVES (5 – 7%):
1. Placental "migration" / rotation
= differential growth rates between lower uterine segment + placenta
Δ 63 – 93% will have normal implantation at term
— conversion to normal position: anterior wall > posterior wall of uterus
— NO conversion if placenta attaches to both posterior + anterior walls
2. Overfilled urinary bladder
bladder-induced compression leads to apposition of the lower anterior + posterior uterine walls (cervical length > 3.5 – 4 cm) simulating a placenta previa
3. Focal myometrial contraction (myometrial thickness > 1.5 cm) in the region of the lower uterine segment

US - FALSE NEGATIVES (2%)
1. Obscuring fetal head
remedied by Trendelenburg position / gentle upward traction on fetal head
2. Lateral position of placenta previa; remedied by obtaining oblique scans
3. Blood in region of internal os mistaken for amniotic fluid

Cx: (secondary to premature detachment of placenta from lower uterine segment)
(1) maternal hemorrhage (blood from intervillous space)
(2) premature delivery
(3) IUGR
(4) perinatal death (5%)

POSTMATURITY SYNDROME
= inability of aging placenta to support demands of fetus
Incidence: in 15% of all postterm gravidas
(= undelivered by 42nd week MA which occurs in 7% of all pregnancies)

- meconium-stained amniotic fluid
- √ grade 3 placenta (in 85%), grade 2 (in 15%), grade 1 (in 0%)
- √ decreased subcutaneous fat + wrinkling of skin
- √ long finger nails
- √ decreased vernix
- *Cx:*   meconium aspiration, perinatal asphyxia, thermal instability

PREMATURE RUPTURE OF MEMBRANES
= spontaneous rupture of chorioamniotic membranes before the onset of labor
Types:
   (a) Preterm premature rupture of membranes (PPROM) < 37 weeks GA
   (b) Term premature rupture of membranes (TPROM) > 37 weeks GA
Incidence: overall 2.1 – 17.1%; PPROM 0.9 – 4.4%; in 29% of all preterm deliveries; in 18% of all term deliveries
Cause: ? infection of membranes
Cx
   (a) TPROM:
      — > 24 hours may result in intrapartum fever
      — > 72 hours may result in chorioamnionitis + still-birth
   (b) PPROM: respiratory distress syndrome (9 – 43%), neonatal sepsis (2 – 19%)
Prognosis: 21% of women with PPROM have a similar outcome in following pregnancy

PREPLACENTAL HEMORRHAGE
= BREUS MOLE = SUBCHORIAL HEMORRHAGE
Incidence: in 4% of all placental abruptions
Risk for fetal demise: 67% overall; 100% for hematomas > 60 ml

PRIMARY OVARIAN CHORIOCARCINOMA
= NONGESTATIONAL CHORIOCARCINOMA
Incidence: extremely rare; 50 cases in world literature
Age: < 20 years
- elevated serum hCG
- √ predominantly solid tumor with areas of hemorrhage + necrosis
DDx: metastasis to ovary from gestational choriocarcinoma (reproductive age)

RETROPLACENTAL HEMATOMA
= accumulation of blood behind placenta which may dissect into placenta / myometrium secondary to rupture of spiral arteries
Incidence: 4.5%; 16% of all placental abruptions
- external bleeding
- √ thickened heterogeneous appearing placenta (hematoma of similar echogenicity as placenta)
- √ rounded placental margins + intraplacental sonolucencies

Cx: (1) precipitous delivery
       (2) coagulopathy
       (3) fetal demise (accounts for 15 – 25% of all perinatal deaths);
           risk for fetal demise with hematomas > 60 ml :
           6% before 20 weeks GA; 29% after 20 weeks GA

SEROUS OVARIAN TUMOR
Incidence: 30% of ovarian tumors;
               benign:malignant = 1:9
Histo: lined by tall columnar epithelial cells (like Fallopian tubes), filled with serous fluid
Age: 20 – 50 years (malignant forms later)
A. SEROUS CYSTADENOMA
   second most common benign tumor of the ovary (20%)
   - √ uni- / multilocular thin-walled cyst with an occasional septum
   - √ up to 20 cm in diameter
   - √ mostly unilateral, bilateral cysts in 20 – 30%
   Cx: malignant transformation in 1 of 10 cases
B. SEROUS CYSTADENOCARCINOMA
   = 60% of all ovarian carcinomas
   - √ solid papillomatous areas within cystic mass
   - √ loss of capsular definition + tumor fixation
   - √ mostly bilateral (70%)
   - √ ascites secondary to peritoneal surface implantation
   - √ lymph node enlargement (periaortic, mediastinal, supraclavicular)

SERTOLI-LEYDIG CELL TUMOR OF OVARY
Origin: from hilar cells of ovary
Incidence: < 0.5%
Age: any age; most common in 2nd – 3rd decade
- androgenic
- √ hypoechoic mass simulating fibroid
- √ may have cystic / hemorrhagic degeneration

SINGLE UMBILICAL ARTERY
Etiology: (1) aplasia / atrophy of one umbilical artery
             (2) persistence of normal transient phase of single umbilical artery in body stalk
Incidence:
   1% of singleton births; 5% in dizygotic twins; 2.5% in abortuses; increased incidence in trisomy D / E, diabetic mothers, black patients, spontaneous abortions
Associated with:
   (a) Congenital anomalies (21 %):
      1. CHD (most frequent): VSD, conotruncal anomalies
      2. Abdomen: ventral wall defect, diaphragmatic hernia
      3. CNS: hydrocephalus, holoprosencephaly, spina bifida
      4. GU: hydronephrosis, dysplastic kidney
      5. Esophageal atresia, cystic hygroma, cleft lip
      6. Polydactyly, syndactyly

(b) IUGR
(c) Prematurity
(d) Perinatal mortality (20%): stillbirth (66%)
(e) Marginal (18%) / velamentous (9%) insertion of umbilical cord
(f) Chromosomal anomalies (67%)

Site: L > R
√ axial view of cord shows 2 vessels
√ incurvation of distal aorta toward common iliac artery on the side of patent umbilical artery
√ ipsilateral hypoplastic common iliac artery
√ absence of abdominal portion of umbilical artery on ipsilateral side of missing umbilical artery
Prognosis: 4 fold increase in perinatal mortality (14%)

STEIN-LEVENTHAL SYNDROME
Incidence: 2.5% of all women
Etiology:
deficient aromatase activity (catalyst for conversion of androgen into estrogen) resulting in androgen excess; exaggerated pulsatile release of LH stimulates continued ovarian androgen secretion at the expense of estradiol; reduction of local estrogen impairs FSH activity; this results in accumulation of small- + medium sized-atretic follicles without final maturation into graafian follicles
Path:
pearly white ovaries with multiple cysts below the capsule which are lined by a hyperplastic theca interna layer showing pronounced luteinization; granulosa cells are absent / degenerating; corpora lutea are absent
Age: late 2nd decade
Associated with: Cushing syndrome, basophilic pituitary adenoma, post-pill amenorrhea, virilizing ovarian / adrenal tumor
• secondary amenorrhea / oligomenorrhea
• reduced infertility / sterility
• periodic abdominal discomfort
• obesity
• mild facial / severe generalized hirsutism
• cystic acne
• cephalic hair loss
• elevated LH levels
• normal / decreased FSH
• increased androstenedione / testosterone
• elevated estrone / estradiol
√ normal ovarian size (in 30%)
√ bilaterally enlarged ovaries (70%), volume of 6 – 30 ccm
√ excessive number of developing follicles
(a) multiple (over 5) small cysts 5 – 8 mm in subcapsular location (40%)
(b) hypoechoic ovaries (25%)
(c) isoechoic ovaries (5%)
Cx: endometrial cancer < 40 years of age (due to unopposed chronic estrogen stimulation)
DDx: Ovaries in congenital adrenal hyperplasia
Rx: (1) Ovulation induction with clomiphene (Clomid) / menotropins (Perganol)
(2) wedge resection (transient effect only)

STUCK TWIN
= one twin with IUGR residing within an oligo- / anhydramniotic sac of a diamniotic twin pregnancy
√ amnion invisible secondary to close contact with fetal parts
√ fetus fixed relative to the uterine wall during shift in maternal position
√ diminished / absent active fetal motion
√ absence of intermingling of fetal parts between twins
Prognosis: fetal death in utero

SUCCENTURIATE LOBE
= ACCESSORY LOBE = separate mass of chorionic villi connected to main placenta by vessels within membrane
Incidence: 0.14 – 3%
Cx: (1) retained in utero with postpartum hemorrhage
(2) placenta previa with intrapartum hemorrhage
(3) VASA PREVIA = succenturiate vessels traversing internal os which may rupture resulting in fetal blood loss

SUBCHORIONIC HEMORRHAGE
= separation of chorionic membrane from decidua with accumulation of blood in subchorionic space (placental membranes are more easily stripped from myometrium than from placenta)
Incidence: 81% of all placental abruptions; in 91% before 20 weeks
• may lead to vaginal hemorrhage after dissection through decidua
√ detached placental margin from adjacent myometrium (60%)
√ hematoma contiguous with placental margin (100%)
√ predominant hemorrhage often separate from placenta, even on opposite side of placenta
Prognosis: probably no risk for fetal demise

TERATOMA OF NECK
= germ cell tumor of neck
√ polyhydramnios in 30% (from esophageal obstruction)
√ complex mass in cervical region
Cx: airway obstruction
DDx: Cystic hygroma, goiter, branchial cleft cyst, cervical meningocele, neuroblastoma of neck, hemangioma of neck

TERATOMA OF OVARY
= immature derivatives of all 3 germ cell layers
Incidence: rare
Age: childhood / adolescence
√ cystic / complex mass (most frequently)
√ usually large solid mass with internal echoes

THECA CELL TUMOR OF OVARY
= THECOMA
Incidence: 1 – 2% of all ovarian neoplasms
Age: > 30 years (30%), postmenopausal (70%)

- estrogenic
- √ hypoechoic mass with sound attenuation
- √ unilateral

THECA LUTEIN CYST
- associated with abnormally high levels of hCG secondary to
  - (1) multiple gestations
  - (2) trophoblastic disease (hydatidiform mole, choriocarcinoma)
  - (3) normal pregnancy (uncommon)
- √ multiple bilateral large septated cysts
- √ several cm in size
- √ involution after source of gonadotropin removed

TWIN-TWIN TRANSFUSION SYNDROME
= MONOVULAR TWIN TRANSFUSION
= INTRAUTERINE PARABIOTIC SYNDROME
= complication of monozygotic twinning with one placenta / one fused placenta secondary to unbalanced intrauterine shunting of blood

Incidence: 5 – 18% of twin pregnancies; 15 – 20% of monozygotic twins
Time of onset: 2nd trimester
Path: large subchorionic communications between arterial circulation of one twin and venous circulation of the other twin through arteriovenous shunts (= common villous district)
- √ discrepant amniotic fluid volume (75%)
- √ discordant BPD by > 5 mm (57%)
- √ discordant estimated fetal weight > 25% (67 – 100%)
- A. <u>DONOR TWIN</u>
  - = twin which transfuses the recipient twin
  - • anemic + hypovolemic
  - • high output failure + hydrops (rare)
  - √ oligohydramnios (75 – 80%) / "stuck twin" = severe oligohydramnios (60%)
  - √ growth retardation (common)
  - √ morphologically normal
- B. <u>RECIPIENT TWIN</u>
  - • polycythemia + plethora (volume overload)
  - √ polyhydramnios (70 – 75%)
  - √ fetal hydrops (10 – 50%)
  - √ fetus papyraceus = macerated dead fetus
Cx: Premature labor with 40 – 70% perinatal mortality
DDx: IUGR of one twin (two separate placentas, two different sexes)

UTERINE ANOMALIES
= anomalies of fusion of paramesonephric duct (= Müllerian duct) completed by 18th week of fetal life
Incidence: 0.1 – 3%
Associated with:
    urinary tract anomalies in 20 – 50 %; possibly increased familial occurrence of limb reduction
CLASSIFICATION:
- A. <u>Arrested Müllerian duct development</u>
  - 1. bilateral: **Uterine aplasia**

- 2. unilateral: **Unicornuate uterus** = Uterus unicornis unicollis
  Incidence: 3 – 6% of uterine anomalies
  May be associated with ipsilateral renal agenesis
  - • infertility in 5 – 20%
  - √ solitary fusiform uterine cavity with lateral deviation within pelvis terminating in a single fallopian tube

- B. <u>Total / partial failure of Müllerian duct fusion</u> (75% of uterine anomalies)
  - 1. **Uterus didelphys**
    - = complete duplication with 2 vaginas + 2 cervices + 2 uteri
    - √ two widely spaced uterine corpora, each with a single fallopian tube
    - *Cx:*   unilateral hematometrocolpos

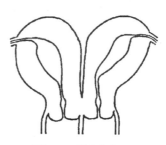

Uterus didelphys

  - 2. **Bicornuate uterus** = uterus bicornis
    - (a) bicollis = 2 uterine horns, 2 cervices, 1 vagina
    - (b) unicollis = 2 uterine horns, 1 cervix, 1 vagina
    - √ separation of uterine horns with wide intercornual angle
    - √ fusiform shape of each uterine horn with lateral convex margins
    - √ discrepancy in size of the 2 uterine horns
    - √ elongation + widening of cervical canal + isthmus
    - √ external morphology as the ONLY reliable sign: bilobed fundal configuration
    - *Cx:*   repeated spontaneous abortions (frequently in 2nd – 3rd trimester), premature rupture of membranes, premature labor, persistent malpresentations (transverse lie)

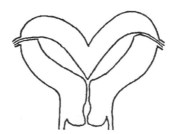
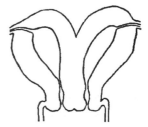

Uterus bicornis unicollis   **Uterus bicornis bicollis**

C. Nonresorption of sagittal uterine septum
   (a) total: **Uterus septus**
      √ very acute angle between uterine cavities
   (b) partial: **Uterus subseptus**

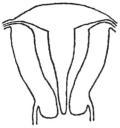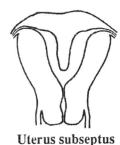

Uterus septus   **Uterus subseptus**

   (c) **Uterus arcuatus**
      most common anomaly, not associated with
      reproductive failure
      √ NOT depicted on US
      √ "saddle-shaped" uterine fundus
      √ increased transverse diameter of uterine cavity
      √ normal external morphology

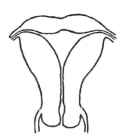

Arcuate uterus

D. inadequate hormonal stimulation during fetal
   development
   1. **Infantile uterus**
   2. **Uterine hypoplasia**
      associated with diethylstilbestrol (DES) exposure in
      utero
      √ mean uterine volume = 50 ccm
   3. **T-shaped uterus**
      encountered in 15% of women exposed to DES
      (diethylstilbestrol) in utero
      √ low uterine volume
      √ uterine fundus thinner than cervix
      √ greater width than depth of corpus + fundus over
      cervix
      √ T-shaped lumen on hysterosalpingogram

UTERINE FIBROID
   = LEIOMYOMA = benign overgrowth of smooth muscle +
   connective tissue; commonest cause for uterine
   enlargement after pregnancy

Hormonal dependency:
   grows secondary to increase in estrogen production in
   10 – 20 %; shrinks after menopause
Incidence: in 20% > age 35; more prevalent in black
               women
• palpable mass
• pelvic pain (torsion, infarction, necrosis)
• heavy prolonged periods
• infertility
Location: mostly in fundus + corpus; in 3% in cervix
   1. intramural (within confines of uterine outline) in 95%
   2. subserosal = exophytic
      (a) parasitic fibroid = subserosal fibroid which has
          become detached secondary to circulatory
          occlusion of vessels in pedicle, revitalised
          through omental / mesenteric blood supply
      (b) intraligamentous fibroid
   3. submucosal
      (a) fibroid polyp = partial / complete extrusion of
          pedunculated submucosal fibroid through
          cervical canal
   √ uterine enlargement
   √ lobulated / nodular distortion of uterine outline +
   indentation of urinary bladder
   √ speckled / ringlike / popcorn calcification
   √ intramural soft tissue mass, usually multiple, solitary in
   2%
   √ distortion / obliteration of the contour of the uterine
   cavity
   US (sensitivity 60 %, specificity 99 %, accuracy 87%):
      √ nodular distortion of uterine outline
      √ hypoechoic solid concentric mass (< 30 %) (= muscle
      component prevails)
      √ echogenic mass (= fibrous component prevails)
      √ anechoic features (secondary to internal
      degeneration: atrophic, hyaline, cystic, myxomatous,
      lipomatous, calcareous, carneous, necrobiotic,
      hemorrhagic, proteolytic degeneration)
   CT:
      √ hypo- / iso- / hyperdense mass containing mixed
      hyperechoic areas
   MRI (86 – 92 % sensitivity, 100 % specificity, 97%
      accuracy):
      √ well-circumscribed low signal intensity mass on T2WI
      with high signal intensity areas (from hemorrhage /
      hyaline degeneration)
   Hysterosalpingography (9 % sensitivity, 97 % specificity,
      76% accuracy)
   Cx:
      (1) Infertility in 35% (a) if isthmic portion of tube
          involved (b) from impingement on endometrium
          interfering with implantation
      (2) Increased frequency of spontaneous abortions
      (3) Increased frequency of IUGR
      (4) Preterm labor in 7% + premature rupture of
          membranes
      (5) Uterine dyskinesia, uterine inertia during labor
      (6) Dystocia, obstruction of birth canal during vaginal
          delivery

(7) Postpartum hemorrhage
(8) Hydroureteronephrosis
(9) Malignant transformation (in 0.2%)

DDx of necrotic leiomyoma:
  (1) Ovarian mass (ovarian cyst, hemorrhagic cyst,
       endometrioma, cystic dermoid, cystadenoma,
       malignancy)
  (2) Ectopic interstitial pregnancy
  (3) Intrauterine gestational sac
  (4) Intrauterine fluid collection
  (5) Hydatidiform mole
  (6) Myometrial contraction (last for 15 – 30 minutes)
  (7) Cervical tumor
  (8) Hematoma of broad ligament

VAGINAL AGENESIS
2nd most common cause of primary amenorrhea
Incidence: 1:5,000
• cyclic abdominal pain
May be associated with:
  (a) uterine + partial tubal agenesis (90%)
  (b) unilateral renal agenesis / ectopia (34%)
  (c) skeletal malformations (12%)
  (d) McKusick-Kaufman syndrome (hydrometrocolpos +
       polydactyly + heart defects)
  (e) Ellis-van Creveld syndrome

VELAMENTOUS INSERTION
= attachment of cord to chorion laeve
Incidence: 0.09 to 1.8%
Associated with congenital anomalies (in 5.9 – 8.5%):
    esophageal atresia, obstructive uropathy, asymmetrical
    head shape, spina bifida, VSD, cleft palate
Cx: (1) IUGR
         (2) Preterm labor

NUCLEAR MEDICINE

TABLE OF DOSE, ENERGY, HALF-LIFE, AND RADIATION DOSE

Organ	Pharmaceutical	Dose	keV	T1/2 phys	(bio)
Brain	Tc-99m pertechnetate	10 - 30 mCi	140	6 h	
	Tc-99m DTPA	10 mCi	140	6 h	
	Tc-99m glucoheptonate	10 mCi	140	6 h	
CSF	In-111 DTPA	500 µCi	173, 247	2.8 d	
Cardiac	Tl-201	1 - 2 mCi	71, 135, 167	73 h	
	Tc-99m pyrophosphate	15 mCi	140	6 h	
	Tc-99m pertechnetate	15 - 25 mCi	140	6 h	
	Tc-99m labeled RBC	10 - 20 mCi	140	6 h	
Liver	Tc-99m sulfur colloid	3 - 5 mCi	140	6 h	
	Tc-99m HIDA	4 - 5 mCi	140	6 h	
Lung	Xe-127	5 - 10 mCi	172, 203	36.4 d	(13 s)
	Xe-133	10 - 20 mCi	80	5.3 d	(20 s)
	Kr-81m	20 mCi	176, 188, 190	13 s	
	Tc-99m MAA	3 mCi	140	6 h	(8 h)
Kidney	Tc-99m DTPA	15 - 20 mCi	140	6 h	
	Tc-99m DMSA	2 - 5 mCi	140	6 h	
	Tc-99m glucoheptonate	15 - 20 mCi	140	6 h	
	I-131 hippuran	250 µCi	364	8 d	(18 min)
Thyroid	Tc-99m pertechnetate	5 - 10 mCi	140	6 h	
	I-123	50 - 200 µCi	159	13.6 h	
	I-125	30 - 100 µCi	27, 35	60 d	
	I-131	30 - 100 µCi	364	8 d	
Testes	Tc-99m pertechnetate	10 mCi	140	6 h	
Mucosa	Tc-99m pertechnetate	50 µCi / kg	140	6 h	
Gallium	Ga-67 citrate	3 - 5 mCi	92, 184, 296, 388	78 h	

RADIATION DOSE

	Critical organ	rad/mCi
I-131	Thyroid	1,000
I-125	Thyroid	900
I-123	Thyroid	15
In-111 DTPA	Spinal cord	12.0
In-111 oxine WBC	Spleen	
Tl-201	Kidney	1.5
Ga-67 citrate	Colon	1.0
Tc-99m MAA	Lung	0.4
Tc-99m albumin microspheres	Lung	0.4
Tc-99m DISIDA	Large bowel	0.39
Tc-99m sulfur colloid	Liver	0.33
Tc-99m glucoheptonate	Kidney	0.2
Tc-99m pertechnetate (+ perchlorate)	Colon	0.2
Tc-99m pertechnetate	Intestine	
	Thyroid	0.15
Tc-99m DTPA	Bladder	
Tc-99m pyrophosphate	Bladder	0.13
Tc-99m phosphate	Bladder	0.13
Tc-99m tagged RBCs	Spleen	
Tc-99m albumin	Blood	0.015
Xe-133	Trachea	

STATISTICS

Incidence = number of diseased people per 100,000 population per year

Prevalence = number of existing cases per 100,000 population at a target date

Mortality = number of deaths per 100,000 population per year

Fatality = number of deaths per number of diseased

Decision Matrix:

TP	FP	T+
FN	TN	T-
D+	D-	total

TP = test positive in diseased subject
FP = test positive in nondiseased subject
FN = test negative in diseased subject
TN = test negative in nondiseased subject
T+ = abnormal test result
T- = normal test result
D+ = diseased subjects
D- = nondiseased subjects

Sensitivity
= ability to detect disease
= probability of having an abnormal test given disease
= number of correct positive tests / number with disease
= True positive ratio = TP / TP + FN = TP / D+
• D+ column in decision matrix

Specificity
= ability to identify absence of disease
= probability of having a negative test given no disease
= number of correct negative tests / number without disease
= True negative ratio = TN / TN + FP = TN / D-
• D- column in decision matrix

Accuracy
= number of correct results in all tests
Δ depends much on the proportion of diseased + nondiseased subjects in studied population
= number of correct tests / total number of tests
= [TP + TN] / total

Positive predictive value
= positive test accuracy
= relationship between a positive test result and the presence of disease
= number of correct positive tests / number of positive tests
= TP / TP + FP = TP / T+
• T+ row in decision matrix

Negative predictive value
= negative test accuracy
= relationship between a negative test result and the absence of disease
= number of correct negative tests / number of negative tests
= TN / TN + FN = TN / T-
• T- row in decision matrix

False-positive ratio
= proportion of nondiseased patients with an abnormal test result
• D- column in decision matrix
= FP / D-

False-negative ratio
= proportion of diseased patients with a normal test result
• D+ column in decision matrix
= FN / D+

Disease prevalence
= proportion of diseased subjects to total population
= D+ / total
Δ affects predictive values + accuracy of a test result
Δ sensitivity + specificity are independent of prevalence

Receiver operating characteristics (ROC)
= curve generated by calculating TP ratio (X-axis) and FP ratio (Y-axis) for a number of different test values (as "cutoff point")
Interpretation:
Δ the most sensitive point is the point with the highest TP ratio
Δ the most specific point is the highest point with the highest TN ratio / lowest FP ratio
Δ the ROC curve closest to the Y-axis represents the best diagnostic test
Δ does not consider disease prevalence in the population

QUALITY CONTROL

Quality control logs should be kept for 3 years.

Radiopharmaceuticals
1. RADIONUCLIDE IMPURITY
   = amount (µCi) of radiocontaminant per amount (µCi / mCi) of desired radionuclide
   Tc-99m:
   allowable contamination of 1:1,000 (= 0.15 µCi Mo-99 per 1 mCi of Tc-99m), and < 5 µCi Mo-99 per administered dose; measured after lead shielding of vial (filters 140 keV but permits 452 keV of Mo-99 to pass through)
2. RADIOCHEMICAL IMPURITY
   Precise registration of different compounds of Tc-99m with other substances or free pertechnetate can be monitored by paper chromatography
3. CHEMICAL IMPURITY
   Chemicals from elution process are restricted in their amount;
   Tc-99m: < 10 µg Al per 1 ml eluate if radionuclide from fission generator;
   < 20 µg Al per 1 ml eluate if radionuclide from neutron bombardment

Calibrators
quality control required 4 x per year
1. LINEARITY
   = accurate measurement over large range of activity levels
   Method: 1 mCi source activity is measured every 4 hours for 10 / more measurements
   Evaluation: measurements must fall within ± 5% of the calculated physical decay curve

2. PRECISION (quality control required every day)
   = reproducibility over time
   Method: daily measurement of a Co-57 standard
   Evaluation: measurement must fall within ± 5% of the calculated activity

3. ACCURACY
   Method: measurements of three different activity standards whose amount is certified by the National Bureau of Standards (NBS)
   Co-57: 123 keV, half-life of 270 days
   Ba-133: 354 keV, half-life of 7.2 years
   Cs-137: 662 keV, half-life of 30 years
   Evaluation: measurements must fall within expected range

4. GEOMETRY
   = to assure that measurement is not dependent upon location of tracer within ionization chamber, usually done by manufacturer

Scintillation camera
Field uniformity
= ability of camera to reproduce a uniform radioactive distribution = variability of observed count density with a homogeneous flux
(a) Integral uniformity = maximum deviation
(b) Differential uniformity = maximum rate of change over a specified distance (5 pixels)
Causes for nonuniformity:
(1) high kilovoltage drift of photomultiplier (PM) tubes
(2) physical damage to collimator
(3) improper photopeak setting
(4) contamination
Frequency of quality control: every day

A. INTRINSIC FIELD UNIFORMITY TEST
   (without collimator)
   1. Remove collimator + replace with lead ring (to eliminate edge packing)
   2. Place a point source at a distance of at least 5 crystal diameters from detector (4 – 5 feet for small, 7 – 9 feet for large crystals)
   3. Point source contains 200 – 400 µCi of Tc-99m for minimal personnel exposure (avoid contamination of crystal)
   4. Set count rate below limit of instrument (< 30,000 counts)
   5. Adjust the pulse height selector to normal window settings by centering at 140 keV with a window of 20% (for Tc-99m studies only)
   6. Use the same photographic device
   7. Acquire 1.25 million counts for a 10" field of view, 2.5 million counts for a 15" field of view
   8. Register counts, time, CRT intensity, analyzer settings, initials of controller

B. EXTRINSIC FIELD UNIFORMITY TEST
   (with collimator)
   1. Collimator is kept in place
   2. Sheet source / flood of 2 – 10 mCi activity is placed on collimator
      (a) fillable floods: mix thoroughly, avoid air bubbles, check for flat surface
      (b) nonfillable: commercially available Co-57 source
   3. Other steps as described above
   Evaluation:
   (1) Compare uncorrected with corrected images. Note acquisition time!
   (2) Store correction flood
   (3) Rerecord image with corrected flood + check for uniformity

Spatial resolution / linearity

A. <u>Spatial resolution</u> = parameter of scintillation camera which characterizes its ability to accurately determine the original location of a gamma ray on a X,Y plane; measured in both X and Y directions; expressed as full width at half maximum (FWHM) of the line spread function in millimeters
   - (a) Intrinsic spatial resolution
   - (b) System spatial resolution

B. <u>Intrinsic spatial linearity</u> = parameter of a scintillation camera which characterizes the amount of positional distortion caused by the camera with respect to incident gamma events entering the detector
   - (a) Differential linearity = standard deviation of line spread function peak separation (in mm)
   - (b) Absolute linearity = maximum amount of spatial displacement (in mm)

Frequency of quality control: every week
1. Mask detector to collimated field of view (lead ring)
2. Lead phantom is attached to front of crystal
   - (a) Four-quadrant bar pattern (3 pictures each after 90° rotation to test entire crystal)
   - (b) Parallel line equal spacing (PLES) bar pattern (2 pictures)
   - (c) Smith orthogonal hole test pattern (OHP) (1 picture only)
   - (d) Hine-Duley phantom (2 pictures)
3. Set symmetrical analyzer window to width normally used
4. Place a point source (1 – 3 mCi) at a fixed distance of at least 5 crystal diameters from detector on central axis (remove all sources from immediate area so that background count rate is low)
5. Acquire 1.25 million counts for a small field, 2.5 million counts for a large field on the same media used for clinical studies
6. Record counts, time, CRT intensity, analyzer setting, initials of controller
(All new cameras are equipped with a spatial distortion correction circuit)
Evaluation:
   Visual assessment of (1) spatial resolution over entire field (2) linearity

Intrinsic energy resolution

– ability to distinguish between primary gamma events and scattered events; performed without collimator; expressed as ratio of photopeak FWHM to photopeak energy (in %)

CRT-output / photographic device

(1) Check for dirt, scratches, burnt spots on CRT face plates
(2) Adjust grey scale + contrast settings to suit film

Sources of artifacts

A. <u>Attenuator between source and detector</u>
   materials: cable, lead marker, solder dropped into collimator during repair, belt buckle / watch / key on patient, defective collimator
   - (a) at time of correction flood procedure:
      √ hot spot
   - (b) after correction flood procedure:
      √ cold spot

B. <u>Cracked crystal</u>
   √ white band with hot edges

C. <u>PMT failure + loss of optical coupling between PMT and crystal</u>
   √ cold defect

D. <u>Problems during film exposure + processing</u>
   1. Double exposed film
   2. Light leak in multiformat camera
   3. Water lines from film processing
   4. Frozen shutter: √ part of film cut off
   5. Variations in film processing

E. <u>Improper window setting</u>
   1. Photopeak window set too high: √ hot tubes
   2. Photopeak window set too low: √ cold tubes

F. <u>Administration of wrong isotope</u>
   √ atypically imaged organs

G. <u>Excessive amounts of free Tc-99m pertechnetate</u>
   √ too much uptake in choroid plexus, salivary glands, thyroid, stomach

H. <u>Faulty injection technique</u>
   e.g., inadvertently labeled blood clot in syringe leading to iatrogenic pulmonary emboli

I. <u>Contamination with radiotracer</u>
   on patient's skin, stretcher, collimator, crystal

J. <u>CRT problems</u>
   1. Burnt spot on CRT phosphor
   2. Dirty / scratched CRT face plates

POSITRON EMISSION TOMOGRAPHY

= PET = technique that permits non-invasive in vivo examination of metabolism, blood flow, electrical activity, neurochemistry

Physics:
positron matter-antimatter annihilation reaction with an electron results in formation of annihilation photons which are emitted in exactly opposite directions (511 keV each); detected by coincidence circuitry through simultaneous arrival at detectors (bismuth germanate) on opposite sides of the patient; collimation not necessary; spatial reconstruction similar to transmission CT

Agents: positron-emitting radionuclides of C-11 (20 min. half-life), F-18 (110 min half-life, commonly used within 500 mile radius of cyclotron facility as fluorodeoxyglucose), N-13 (as NH_3; 10 min half-life), O-15 (as O_2, H_2O, CO_2, CO; 2 min half-life), Ga-68, Rb-Isotopes

Applications:
1. Focal epilepsy prior to seizure surgery
   √ measurement of regional glucose metabolism (70% sensitivity)
   √ measurement of opiate receptor density
2. Brain tumor grading / recurrence
   √ hypermetabolic glucose metabolic grade
3. Coronary artery disease
   sensitivity of > 95%
4. Stroke
   √ disassociated oxygen metabolism + brain blood flow
5. Schizophrenia
   √ abnormally reduced glucose activity in frontal lobes
   √ dopamine receptors in caudate / putamen elevated to 3 x of normal levels
6. Alzheimer disease
   √ characteristic pattern of distribution of regional blood flow, glucose metabolism, oxygen metabolism involving the parietal lobes in a relatively symmetric fashion

A. REGIONAL CEREBRAL BLOOD FLOW
   (a) breathing of carbon monoxide (C-11 and O-15) which concentrates in RBCs
   (b) Xe-133 inhalation / injection into ICA / IV injection after dissolution in saline: volume distribution is in the water space of the brain; no correction for recirculation necessary because all Xe is exhaled during lung passage, but correction for scalp + calvarial activity is required (for inhalation method)
       √ washout rate of grey matter:white matter = 4 – 5:1

B. GLUCOSE METABOLISM
   for measurements of metabolic rate + mapping of functional activity
   (a) C-11 glucose: rapid uptake, metabolization, and excretion by brain
   (b) F-18 fluorodeoxyglucose: metabolically trapped by brain cells

GALLIUM SCINTIGRAPHY

Gallium-67 citrate

Ga-67 acts as an analogue of ferric ion; used as gallium citrate (water-soluble form)

Production: bombardment of zinc targets (Zn-67, Zn-68) with protons (cyclotron); virtually carrier-free after separation process

Decay: by electron capture to ground state of Zn-67

Energy levels:
   (a) used: 92 keV (40%), 184 keV (23%), 296 keV (21%)
   (b) unused: 91 keV (2%), 206 keV (2%), 388 keV (8%)

Physical half-life: 3.3 d (=78 hours)

Biologic half-life: 2 – 3 weeks

Adult dose: 3 – 6 mCi or 50 µCi/kg

Radiation dose:
   0.3 rads/mCi for whole body; 0.9 rads/mCi for distal colon (= critical organ); 0.58 rads/mCi for red marrow; 0.56 rads/mCi for proximal colon; 0.46 rads/mCi for liver; 0.41 rads/mCi for kidney; 0.24 rads/mCi for gonads

Physiology:

Ga-67 is bound to iron-binding sites of various proteins (strongest bond with transferrin in plasma, lactoferrin in tissue); multiexponential + slow plasma disappearance; competitive iron administration (Fe-citrate) enhances target-to-background ratio by increasing Ga-67 excretion

BINDING SITES:
   (a) Fluid spaces
      1. transferrin, haptoglobin, albumin, globulins in blood serum
      2. interstitial fluid space (increased capillary permeability and hyperemia in inflammation + tumor)
      3. lactoferrin in tissue
   (b) Cellular binding
      1. viable PMNs (incorporate 10% of Ga-67 bound to lactoferrin in intracytoplasmic granules)
      2. nonviable PMNs + their protein exudate (deposition of iron-binding proteins extracellularly at sites of inflammation sequesters needed iron from bacteria)
      3. lymphocytes have lactoferrin-binding surface receptors
      4. phagocytic macrophages engulf protein-iron complexes
      5. bacteria + fungi (siderophores = lysosomes have iron-transporting protein mechanism)
      6. tumor cell-associated transferrin receptor + transportation into cell ((lymphocytes bind Ga-67 less avidly than PMNs, RBC do not bind Ga-67)

UPTAKE:
   at 24 hours: most intense in RES, liver, spleen (4%), bone marrow (lumbar spine, sacroiliac joints), bowel wall (chiefly colonic activity on delayed images), renal

cortex, nasal mucosa, lacrimal + salivary glands, blood pool (20%), lung (< 3% = equivalent to background activity), breasts
   at 72 hours: activity in liver, skeleton, colon, nasal mucosa, occiput; kidney activity no longer detectable; lacrimal + salivary glands may still be prominent

EXCRETION:
   (a) via GI tract (10 – 20%)
      hepatobiliary pathway + colonic mucosal excretion: enemas + laxatives promote clearing of bowel activity
   (b) via urinary tract (10 – 20% within 24 hours)
      no activity in kidneys + urinary bladder after 24 hours
   (c) via various body fluids
      e.g., human milk (mandates to stop nursing for 2 weeks)

TIME OF IMAGING: usually 24, 48, 72 hours
   Δ generally best target-to-background ratio at 72 hours
   Δ optimal target-to-background ratio at 6 – 24 hours for abscess
   Δ optimal target-to-background ratio at 24 – 48 hours for tumor

DEGRADING FACTORS OF IMAGING
   √ lesions < 2 cm are not detectable
   √ photon scatter within overlying tissues
   √ physiologic high activity of liver, spleen, bones, kidney, GI tract may obscure lesion

NORMAL VARIANTS OF Ga-67 UPTAKE
   1. breasts: increased uptake under stimulus of menarche, estrogens, pregnancy, lactation, phenothiazine medication
   2. liver: suppressed uptake by chemotherapeutic agents / high levels of circulating iron / irradiation / severe acute liver disease
   3. lung: prominent uptake after lymphangiography
   4. spleen: increased uptake in splenomegaly
   5. thymus: uptake in children
   6. salivary glands: uptake within first 6 months after radiation therapy to neck (may persist for years)
   7. epiphyseal plates in children

INDICATIONS:
   A. Infection:
      1. Occult infection
      2. Osteomyelitis
   B. Tumor:
      1. Staging of Hodgkin disease + non-Hodgkin lymphoma
      2. Staging of lung cancer
      3. Detection of tumor recurrence
      4. DDx of focal cold liver lesions on Tc-99m sulfur colloid scan

NO UPTAKE: most benign neoplasms; hemangioma; cirrhosis; cystic disease of the breast, liver, thyroid; reactive lymphadenopathy; inactive granulomatous disease

Gallium imaging in inflammation

Pathophysiology:
leakage of protein-bound Ga-67 into extracellular space secondary to increased capillary permeability; Ga-67 is preferentially bound to nonviable PMNs + macrophages
1. Leukocyte incorporation (rich in lactoferrin)
2. Bacterial uptake (siderophores)
3. Inflammatory tissue stimulates lactoferrin production

CHRONIC ABDOMINAL INFLAMMATION
67% sensitivity, 64% specificity, 13% false-negative rate, 5% false-positive rate
Dose: 5 mCi
Imaging: at 24, 48, 72 hours
√ diffuse uptake in peritonitis
√ localized uptake in acute pyogenic abscess, phlegmon, acute cholecystitis, acute pancreatitis, acute gastritis, diverticulitis, inflammatory bowel disease, surgical wound, pyelonephritis, perinephric abscess

Gallium in bone Imaging

Increased activity in:
1. Active osteomyelitis (90 % sensitivity is higher than for Tc-99m MDP)
2. Sarcoma
3. Cellulitis
4. Septic arthritis, rheumatoid arthritis
5. Paget disease
6. Metastases (65% sensitivity, less than for bone agents)

Gallium in tumor imaging

Particularly useful in evaluating extent of known tumor disease + in detection of tumor recurrence
A. USEFUL CATEGORY
1. Hodgkin disease + histiocytic form of NHL 95% specificity; 95% sensitivity for mediastinal disease, 80% sensitivity for cervical + superficial lesions; poor sensitivity below diaphragm
2. Burkitt lymphoma: almost 100% sensitivity
3. Hepatoma: 90% sensitivity
4. Melanoma: 90% sensitivity
5. Leukemia
B. POSSIBLY USEFUL
1. NHL: good for large + mediastinal lesions
2. Nodal metastases from seminoma + embryonal cell carcinoma: 87% sensitivity
3. Nonsmall cell lung cancer: 85% sensitivity for primary of any histologic type, 90% probability for uptake in mediastinal nodes, 67% probability for uptake in normal mediastinal nodes, 90% probability for uptake in extrathoracic metastases
C. NOT USEFUL
Head & neck tumors, GI tumors (especially adenocarcinomas), breast tumors, gynecologic tumors, pediatric tumors

Gallium in lung imaging

Scans at 48 hours because 50% of normals show activity at 24 hours
A. FOCAL UPTAKE
1. Primary pulmonary malignancy (> 90% sensitivity)
2. Benign disorders: granuloma, abscess, pneumonia, silicosis
B. MULTIFOCAL / DIFFUSE UPTAKE
(a) Infection
1. Tuberculosis
√ intense uptake in active lesions (97%) = parameter of activity
√ diffuse uptake in miliary TB + rapidly progressive TB pneumonia
2. Pneumocystis carinii
√ increased uptake at time when physical signs, symptoms, and roentgenographic changes are unimpressive
3. Cytomegalovirus
(b) Inflammation
1. Sarcoidosis
70% sensitivity for active parenchymal disease, 94% sensitivity for hilar adenopathy, indicator of therapeutic response to steroids
2. Interstitial lung disease
pneumoconiosis, idiopathic pulmonary fibrosis, lymphangitic carcinomatosis
3. Exudative stage of radiation pneumonitis
(c) Drugs
1. Bleomycin toxicity
2. Amiodarone
(d) Contrast lymphangiography (in 50%)

GALLIUM UPTAKE + NORMAL CHEST FILM
1. Pulmonary drug toxicity
2. Tumor infiltration
3. Sarcoidosis
4. Pneumocystis carinii

Gallium in renal imaging

abnormal uptake on delayed images at 48 – 72 hours
(a) Renal tumor
1. Primary renal tumor (variable uptake)
2. Lymphoma / leukemia
3. Metastases (e.g., melanoma)
(b) Renal inflammation
1. Acute pyelonephritis (88% sensitivity): √ diffuse / focal uptake
2. Lobar nephronia
3. Renal abscess
(c) Others
1. Collagen-vascular disease, vasculitis, Wegener granulomatosis
2. Amyloidosis, hemochromatosis
3. Hepatic failure
4. Administration of antineoplastic drugs

(d) Transplant
  1. Acute / chronic rejection
  2. Acute tubular necrosis
(e) Urinary bladder: cystitis, tumor

Gallium imaging in lymphoma
  1. Hodgkin Disease
     50 – 70% average sensitivity dependent on size, location, technique
  2. Non-Hodgkin Lymphoma
     30% sensitivity for lymphocytic subtype, 70% sensitivity for histiocytic subtype
     Sensitivity: 90% for mediastinal nodes
                       80% for neck nodes
                       48% for periaortic nodes
                       47% for iliac nodes
                       36% for axillary nodes

Gallium imaging in malignant melanoma
  TYPES:
  1. Lentigo maligna: low invasiveness, low metastatic potential
  2. Superficial spreading melanoma: intermediate prognosis
  3. Nodular melanoma: most lethal
  PROGNOSIS (level of invasion versus 5-year survival):
  Level I   (in situ)   100%
  Level II   (within papillary dermis)   100%
  Level III   (extending to reticular dermis)   88%
  Level IV   (invading reticular dermis)   66%
  Level V   (subcutaneous infiltration)   15%
  Ga-67:
     > 50% sensitivity for primary + metastatic sites; detectability versus tumor size: 73% sensitivity > 2 cm; 17% sensitivity < 2 cm
  Bone, brain, liver scintigraphy :
     show very low yield in detecting metastases at time of preoperative assessment and are not indicated

Agents for Inflammation
  1. Ga-67 citrate
     overall 58 – 100% sensitivity; 75 – 100% specificity (lower for abdominal inflammation); most helpful in chronic low-grade infections

  2. In-111 oxine labeled autologous leukocytes
     80% sensitivity; 97% specificity, 91% accuracy (superior to Ga-67 citrate); most helpful in acute infections; no activity in intestinal contents / urine
     Technique:
        harvesting of cells (inadequate in children + neutropenia) followed by washing off plasma; chelating agents (oxine = 8-hydroxyquinoline / tropolone) used for labeling; lipophilic oxine-indium complex penetrates cell membrane of white cells; intracellular proteins scavenge the indium from oxine; oxine diffuses out from cell; requires 2 hours of preparation time
        Recovery rate: 30% at 1 – 4 hours after injection
     Dose: 0.5 – 1 mCi
     Half-life: 67 hours
     Useful photopeaks: 173 keV, 247 keV
     Radiation dose:
        18 rad/mCi for spleen; 3.8 rad/mCi for liver; 0.65 rad/mCi for red marrow; 0.45 rad/mCi for whole body; 0.29 rad/mCi for testes; 0.14 rad/mCi for ovaries (compared with Ga-67 higher to spleen, but lower to all other organs)
     Imaging: best at 18 – 24 hours following injection of cell preparation; 4-hour views may be helpful (e.g., in inflammatory bowel disease)
     √ focal activity greater than in spleen is typical for abscess (comparison based on liver, spleen, bone marrow activity)
     √ activity equal to liver (significant inflammatory response)

     False-positives:
     @ Chest: CHF, RDS, embolized cells, cystic fibrosis
     @ Abdomen: accessory spleen, colonic accumulation, renal transplant rejection, GI hemorrhage, vasculitis, ischemic bowel disease, following CPR, uremia, postradiation therapy, Wegener granulomatosis, ALL
     @ Miscellaneous: IM injection, histiocytic lymphoma, cerebral infarction, arthritis, skeletal metastases, thrombophlebitis, hematoma, hip prosthesis, cecal carcinoma, postsurgical pseudoaneurysm, necrotic tumors which harvest WBCs
     False-negatives:
     Chronic infection, aorto-femoral graft, LUQ abscess, infected pelvic hematoma, splenic abscess, hepatic abscess (occasionally)

BONE SCINTIGRAPHY

Bone agents
A. POLYPHOSPHATES = LINEAR PHOSPHATES
= CONDENSED PHOSPHATES
First agents described; contain up to 46 phosphate residues; simplest form contains 2 phosphates = PYROPHOSPHATE (PYP)
B. DIPHOSPHONATES
Organic analogs of pyrophosphate characterized by P-C-P bond; chemically more stable; not susceptible to hydrolysis in vivo; most widely used agents:
1. ethylene hydroxydiphosphonate (EHDP)
= ethane-1-hydroxy-1,1 diphosphonate
2. methylene diphosphonate (MDP)
C. IMIDODIPHOSPHONATES (IDP)
Characterized by P-N-P bond
Indications:
1. Imaging of bone, myocardial / cerebral infarct, ectopic calcifications, some tumors (neuroblastoma)
2. Rx for Paget disease, myositis ossificans progressiva, calcinosis universalis (inhibits formation + dissolution of hydroxyapatite crystals)
Usual dose: 20 mCi
Radiation dose: 0.13 rad/mCi for bladder (critical organ),
0.04 rad/mCi for bone,
0.01 rad/mCi for whole body
Imaging:
@ bone: 2 – 3 hours post injection (fractures may not show positive uptake until 3 – 10 days depending on age of patient)
@ myocardium: 90 – 120 minutes post injection (ideal imaging time 1 – 3 days post infarction)
Labeling: Tc (VII) is eluted as a pertechnetate ion; chemical reduction with Sn (II) chloride; chelated into a complex of Tc-99m (IV)-tin-phosphate
Quality Control:
(1) < 10% Tc-99m tin colloid / free Tc-99m pertechnetate (a good preparation is 95% bound)
(2) agent should not be used prior to 30 minutes after preparation
(3) avoid injection of air in preparation of multidose vials (oxidation results in poor Tc bond)
Uptake:
(a) rapid distribution in ECF; blood clearance rate determines ECF (= background) activity (at 4 hours 1% for diphosphonates, 5% for pyrophosphate / polyphosphate secondary to greater degree of protein binding)
(b) chemisorbs on hydroxyapatite crystals in bone + in calcium crystals in mitochondria; 50 – 60% (58% for MDP, 48% for EHDP, 47% for PYP) are localized in bone by approx. 3 hours depending on blood flow + osteoblastic activity; myocardial uptake depends on at least some revascularization of infarcted muscle

Excretion: via urinary tract (forcing fluids + frequent voiding reduces radiation dose to bladder) by 6 hours 68% of MDP/EHDP, 50% of PYP, 46% of polyphosphates

Technetium-99m pertechnetate
Physical decay: 10 mCi Tc-99m decays to 2.7×10^{-7} mCi Tc-99
Physical half-life: 2×10^5 years
Biologic half-life: 6 hours
Administration: oral / IV
Pharmacokinetics:
Uptake: in thyroid, salivary glands, gastric mucosa, choroid plexus
Excretion: mostly in feces, some in urine
QUALITY CONTROL
(1) < 0.1% Mo-99 (= 1μCi/mCi), maximum of Mo-99 at 5 μCi
(2) < 0.5 mg aluminum / 10 mCi Tc-99m
(3) < 0.01% radionuclide impurities

Bone marrow agents
for assessment of hematopoiesis/ phagocytosis by RES; shows
(1) expansion of hematopoietically active bone marrow
(2) local defect due to displacement by infiltrating disease
1. Tc-99m sulfur colloid
2. In-111 chloride
3. Tc-99m MMAA (mini-microaggregated albumin colloid = not FDA approved) for liver, spleen, hematopoietic marrow
Particle size: 30 - 100 microns
Dose: 10 mCi
Marrow dose: 0.55 rad
Marrow accumulation at 1 hour :
6 x higher than sulfur colloid
3 x higher than antimony-sulfur colloid

Superscan
Causes:
A. Metabolic
1. Renal osteodystrophy
2. Osteomalacia
√ randomly distributed focal sites of intense activity = Looser zones = pseudofractures = Milkman fractures (most characteristic)
3. Hyperparathyroidism
√ focal intense uptake corresponds to site of brown tumors
4. Hyperthyroidism
rate of bone resorption more increased than rate of formation (= decrease in bone mass)
• hypercalcemia (occasionally)
• elevated alkaline phosphatase
√ NOT visible on radiographs
√ susceptible to fractures

B. Widespread bone lesions
1. Diffuse skeletal metastases (most frequent) from breast, lung, prostate, bladder, lymphoma
2. Myelofibrosis / myelosclerosis
3. Systemic mastocytosis
4. Paget disease

√ diffusely increased activity in bones: particularly prominent in axial skeleton, calvarium, mandible, costochondral junctions (= "rosary beading"), sternum (= "tie sternum"), long bones
√ increased metaphyseal + periarticular activity
√ increased bone-to-soft-tissue ratio
√ "absent kidney sign" = little / no activity in kidneys
√ femoral cortices become visible

Soft tissue uptake
A. Radiochemical impurity (free pertechnetate)
   √   activity in mouth (saliva), thyroid, stomach (mucus-producing cells), GI tract (direct secretion + intestinal transport from gastric juices)
B. Tumor
   1. Primary tumors
      (a) Osteosarcoma: bone foming
      (b) Neuroblastoma (50%): calcifying tumor
      (c) Breast carcinoma
   2. Metastases
      (a) in liver: mucinous carcinoma of colon, breast carcinoma
      (b) in lung: osteosarcoma
C. Inflammation
   1. Inflammatory process (abscess, pyogenic / fungal infection):
      (a) adsorption onto calcium deposits (b) binding to denatured proteins, iron deposits, immature collagen (c) hyperemia
   2. Myositis ossificans / polymyositis
   3. Dermatomyositis
D. Trauma
   1. Healing soft tissue wounds
   2. Intramuscular injection sites:
      especially Imferon (= iron dextran) injections with resultant chemisorption
   3. Bowel infarction (late uptake)
E. Metabolic
   1. Hypercalcemia: uptake in stomach, lung, kidneys, myocardium
   2. Diffuse interstitial pulmonary calcifications: hyperparathyroidism, mitral stenosis
   3. Amyloid deposits
F. Dystrophic soft- tissue calcifications
   Necrotic tumor with dystrophic calcification
   @ Spleen: infarct (sickle cell anemia in 50%), microcalcification secondary to lymphoma, thalassemia major, hemosiderosis, glucose-6-phosphate-dehydrogenase deficiency
   @ Liver: massive hepatic necrosis
   @ Heart: acute myocardial infarction, valvular calcification, amyloid deposition
   @ Muscle: traumatic / ischemic skeletal muscle injury
   @ Brain: cerebral infarction

Photon-deficient bone lesion
= decreased radiotracer uptake
Causes:
   A. Interruption in local bone blood flow
      = vessel trauma or vascular obstruction by thrombus / tumor
      1. Early osteomyelitis
      2. Radiation therapy
      3. Posttraumatic aseptic necrosis
      4. Sickle cell crisis
   B. Replacement of bone by destructive process
      1. Metastases: central axis skeleton > extremity, most commonly in carcinoma of kidney + lung + breast + multiple myeloma
      2. Primary bone tumor (exceptional)

Long segmental diaphyseal uptake
A. BILATERALLY SYMMETRIC
   1. Hypertrophic pulmonary osteoarthropathy
   2. "Shin splints"
   3. Ribbing disease
   4. Engelmann disease = progressive diaphyseal dysplasia
B. UNILATERAL
   1. Inadvertent arterial injection
   2. Melorheostosis
   3. Chronic venous stasis
   4. Osteogenesis imperfecta
   5. Vitamin A toxicity
   6. Osteomyelitis
   7. Paget disease
   8. Fibrous dysplasia

Pediatric indications for bone scan
A. Back pain
   1. Discitis
   2. Pars interarticularis defect
   3. Osteoid osteoma
   4. Sacroiliac infection
B. Nonaccidental trauma

Benign bone lesions
A. NO TRACER UPTAKE
   1. Bone island
   2. Osteopoikilosis
   3. Osteopathia striata
   4. Fibrous cortical defect
   5. Nonossifying fibroma
B. INCREASED TRACER UPTAKE
   1. Fibrous dysplasia
   2. Eosinophilic granuloma
   3. Melorheostosis
   4. Osteoid osteoma

Fractures

TYPICAL TIME COURSE
1. Acute phase (3 – 4 weeks)
   abnormal in 80% < 24 hours, in 95% < 72 hours
   elderly patients show delayed appearance of positive scan
   √ broad area of increased tracer uptake (wider than fracture line)
2. Subacute phase (2 – 3 months)
   time of most intense tracer accumulation
   √ focally increased tracer uptake corresponding to fracture line
3. Chronic phase (1 – 2 years)
   √ slow decline in tracer accumulation
   √ in 65% normal after 1 year; in > 95% normal after 3 years

RETURN TO NORMAL
rib fractures return to normal most rapidly; delayed in weight-bearing extremities; complicated fractures with orthopedic fixation devices take longest to return to normal
1. Simple fractures: 90% normal by 2 years
2. Open reduction / fixation: < 50% normal by 3 years
3. Delayed union: slower than normal for type of fracture
4. Nonunion: persistent intense uptake in 80%
5. Complicated union (true pseudarthrosis, soft tissue interposition, impaired blood supply, presence of infection)
   √ intense uptake at fracture ends
   √ decreased uptake at fracture site

VERTEBRAL COMPRESSION FRACTURES
return to normal   in 60% by 1 year
in 90% by 2 years
in 97% by 3 years

BRAIN SCINTIGRAPHY

Radionuclide angiography

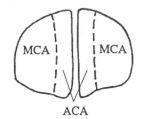

anterior view

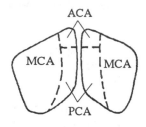

posterior view

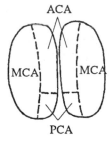

high axial view

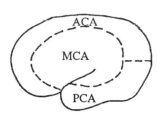

left lateral view

Mechanism of accumulation:
disruption of blood-brain barrier
Agents:
A. Tc-99m glucoheptonate
15 – 20 mCi bolus injection in < 2 ml saline; 30 flow images of 2 seconds duration; static image of 1 million counts after 4 hours; delayed image after 24 hours (higher target-to-background ratio than DTPA)
B. Tc-99m DTPA
C. Thallium-201: best predictor for tumor burden
√ increased perfusion in
1. primary / metastatic brain tumor
2. AVM, large aneurysm, tumor shunting
3. luxury perfusion after infarction
4. infections (e.g., herpes simplex encephalitis)
5. extracranial lesions: bone metastasis, fibrous dysplasia, Paget disease, eosinophilic granuloma, fractures, burr holes, craniotomy defects
√ asymmetrical decreased perfusion in acute / chronic cerebrovascular disease + mass lesions (tumor, hemorrhage, subdural hematoma)
√ "flip-flop" phenomenon (= decreased perfusion in arterial phase, equalization of activity in capillary phase, increased activity in venous phase) in CVA secondary to late arrival of blood via collaterals + slow washout
√ bilateral absent flow in brain death

Seizures
Abnormal cerebral radionuclide angiography within 1 week of seizure activity even without underlying organic lesion
Etiology:
(1) 35% cerebral tumors (meningioma in 34%, metastases in 17%)
(2) Cerebral vascular disease (more common in age > 50 years)
(3) Trauma, inflammation, CNS effects of systemic disease
√ transient hyperperfusion of involved hemisphere

Brain tumor
Good correlation between hyperperfusion and enlarged supplying vessels
Etiology:
meningioma (increased activity in 60 – 80%);
metastases (increased activity in 11 – 23%);
vascular metastases: thyroid, renal cell, melanoma, anaplastic tumors from lung / breast

Cerebral death
Increased intracranial pressure results in markedly decreased cerebral perfusion, thrombosis, total cerebral infarction
Path: severe brain edema, diffuse liquefactive necrosis
√ carotid arteries visualized (= confirmation of good bolus)
√ activity stops abruptly at the skull base
√ sagittal sinus not visualized
√ activity in arteries of face + scalp with "hot nose" sign
DDx by EEG:
severe barbiturate intoxication may produce a flat EEG response in the absence of brain death

Arterial stenosis
Radionuclide angiography of limited value!
(1) complete occlusion / > 80% stenosis of ICA: 53 – 80% sensitivity
(2) 50 – 80% stenosis of ICA: 50% sensitivity
(3) < 50% stenosis of ICA: 10% sensitivity
Problematic lesions:
(1) Bilaterally similar degree of stenosis
(2) Occlusion of MCA + unilateral ACA
(3) Vertebrobasilar occlusive disease (20% sensitivity)

Radionuclide cisternography
Indications: 1. suspected normal pressure hydrocephalus
2. occult CSF rhinorrhea / otorrhea
3. ventricular shunt
4. porencephalic cyst, leptomeningeal cyst, posterior fossa cyst

Technique:
1. Measurement of spinal subarachnoid pressure
2. Sample of CSF for analysis
3. Subarachnoid injection of radiotracer

Normal study: (completed within 48 hours) symmetrical activity sequentially from basal cisterns, up the Sylvian fissures + anterior commissure, eventual ascent over cortices with parasagittal concentration
√ activity in basal cistern by 2 – 4 hours
√ activity at vertex by 24 – 48 hours
√ no / minimal lateral ventricular activity (may be transient in older patients)

Agents:
1. <u>Indium-111 DTPA</u>
   Physical half-life: 2.8 days
   Gamma photons: 173 keV (90%), 247 keV (94%) detected with dual pulse height analyzer
   Dose: 250 – 500 µCi
   Radiation dose: 9 rads / 500 µCi for brain + spinal cord (in normal patients)

Imaging: at 10 minute intervals / 500,000 counts up to 4 – 6 hours; repeat scans at 24, 48, 72 hours
2. <u>Technetium-99m DTPA</u>
   not entirely suitable for imaging up to 48 – 72 hours; DTPA tends to have faster flow rate than CSF; used for shunt evaluation
   Dose: 4 – 10 mCi
   Radiation dose: 4 rads for brain + spinal cord
3. <u>Iodine-131 serum albumin</u> (RISA)
   prototype agent; beta emitter
   Physical half-life:
      8 days; high radiation dose of 7.1 rads / 100 µCi no longer used secondary to pyrogenic reactions
D. <u>Ytterbium-169 DTPA</u>
   Physical half-life: 32 days
   Gamma decay: 63 keV; 177 keV (17%); 198 keV (25%); 308 keV
      dual pulse height analyzer set for 177 + 198 keV
   Dose: 500 µCi
   Radiation dose: 9 rads / 500 mCi for brain + spinal cord (in normal patients)

LUNG SCINTIGRAPHY

Perfusion agents

Tc-99m macroaggregated albumin

Preparation:
  human serum albumin (HSA) is heat-denatured + pH adjusted; added stannous chloride precipitates albumin into tin-containing macroaggregates; lyophilization prolongs stability; added Tc-99m pertechnetate is reduced by $SnCl_2$ and tagged onto the MAA particles

Quality Control (USP guidelines):
  (1) 90% of particles should have a diameter between 10 – 90 μ
  (2) No particle should exceed 150 μ
  (3) Should be at least 90% pure (by ascending chromatography)
  (4) A batch of Tc-99 m MAA should not be used > 8 hours after preparation
  (5) Preparation should not be backflushed into syringe

Physical half-life: 6 hours
Biological half-life: 6 hours
Usual dose: approximately 4 mCi + > 60,000 particles (recommended number of 200,000 – 500,000 particles for adequate spatial distribution + good image quality)
  CAVE: critically ill patients with pulmonary hypertension, infants, children up to age 3 need dose reduction!
Radiation dose (rads/mCi):   0.013 for whole body, 0.25 for lung (critical organ), 0.01 for gonads

PHYSIOLOGY
90% of MAA particles will be trapped in lung capillaries on first pass; 0.22% (= 2 of 1000) capillaries become occluded; protein is lysed within 6 – 8 hours and taken up by RES; particles < 1μ are trapped by RES in liver + spleen

IMAGING
large field view scintillation camera + parallel hole low-energy collimator
Views: anterior, posterior, lateral, posterior oblique (additional information in 50%), anterior oblique (additional information in 15%); oblique views reduce equivocal findings from 30% to 15%; recording times should be identical for corresponding views

Tc-99m human albumin microspheres
Particle size: 20 – 30 μ
Biological half-life: 8 hours

Ventilation agents

Xenon-133
Fission product of U-235
Decay: to stable Cs-133 under emission of beta particle (374 keV), gamma ray (81 keV), X-ray (31 keV); beta-component responsible for high radiation dose of 1 rad to lung)
Physical half-life: 5.2 days
Biological half-life: 2 – 3 minutes
Physical properties: highly soluble in oil + grease, absorbed by plastic syringe
Administration: via mouth piece with a disposable breathing unit
Dose: 15 mCi

TECHNIQUE
Ventilation study preferably done before perfusion scan to avoid interference with higher-energetic Tc-99m (Compton scatter from Tc-99m into lower Xe-133 photopeak); feasible however if dose of Tc-99m MAA is kept below 2 mCi + concentration of Xe-133 is above 10 mCi/l of air and if Xe-133 acquisition times for wash-in, equilibrium, wash-out images are kept to about 30 seconds
1. Phase
  = Single breath phase = inhalation of 10 – 20 mCi Xe-133 to vital capacity in supine position over 10 – 20 seconds (65% sensitivity for abnormalities)
2. Phase
  = Tidal breathing = closed loop rebreathing of Xe-133 + oxygen for 3 – 5 minutes = equilibrium phase for tracer to enter poorly ventilated areas; also functions as internal control for air leaks
3. Phase
  = Washout / clearance phase; tracer retention at 3 minutes reveals areas of air-trapping; exhaled Xe-133 is stored in charcoal trap

√ poor image quality secondary to significant scatter
√ abnormal scan:
  (a) delayed wash-in (initial 30 seconds of tidal breathing)
  (b) tracer accumulation on equilibrium views (partial obstruction with collateral air drift + diffusion into affected area via blood stream)
  (c) delayed wash-out = retention > 3 minutes
  (d) tracer retention in regions not seen on initial single breath view

Xenon-127
cyclotron-produced with high cost
Physical half-life: 36.4 days
Photon energies: 172 keV (22%), 203 keV (65%)

Advantages:
  (1) high photon energy allows ventilation study following perfusion study
  (2) Decreased radiation dose (0.3 rad)
  (3) Storage capability because of long physical half-life

Krypton-81 m
eluted from Rb-81 generator (half-life of 4.7 hours)
Physical half-life: 13 seconds
Biological half-life: < 1 minute
Principal photon energy: 190 keV (65% abundance)
Advantages:
  (1) higher photon energy than Tc-99m so that ventilation scan can be performed following perfusion study
  (2) each ventilation scan can be matched to perfusion scan without moving patient
  (3) can be used in patients on respirator (no contamination due to short half-life)
  (4) low radiation dose (during continuous inhalation for 6 – 8 views 100 mrad are delivered)
  √ lack of activity = abnormal area (tracer activity is proportional to regional distribution of tidal volume because of short biological half-life, washout phase not available)

Tc-99m DTPA aerosol
Delivery through a nebulizer during inspiration; less physiological indicator of ventilation + subject to nebulization technique

Carbon dioxide tracer
O-15 labeled carbon dioxide
Physical half-life: 2 minutes (requires on-site cyclotron)
PHYSIOLOGY:
  inhalation of carbon dioxide; rapid diffusion across alveolar-capillary membrane; clearance from lung within seconds
  √ cold spot due to failure of tracer entry into airway = airway disease
  √ hot spot due to delayed / absent tracer clearance = perfusion defect
  87% sensitivity, 92% specificity
INDICATIONS:
  1. emboli can be detected in preexisting cardiopulmonary disease
  2. in equivocal / indeterminate V/Q studies

Unilateral lung perfusion
Incidence: 2%
A. PULMONARY EMBOLISM (23%)
B. AIRWAY DISEASE
  (a) Unilateral pleural / parenchymal disease (23%)
  (b) Bronchial obstruction
    1. Bronchogenic carcinoma (23%)
    2. Bronchial adenoma
    3. Aspirated endobronchial foreign body
C. CONGENITAL HEART DISEASE (15%)
D. ARTERIAL DISEASE
  1. Swyer-James syndrome (8%)
  2. Congenital pulmonary artery hypoplasia / stenosis
  3. Shunt procedure to pulmonary artery (e.g., Blalock-Taussig)
E. ABSENT LUNG
  1. Pneumonectomy (8%)
  2. Unilateral pulmonary agenesis

Perfusion defects
A. VASCULAR DISEASE
  (a) Acute / previous pulmonary embolus
    1. Pulmonary thromboembolic disease
    2. Fat embolism
      √ nonsegmental perfusion defect
    3. Air embolism
      √ characteristic decortication appearance in uppermost portion on perfusion scintigraphy
    4. Embolus of tumor / cotton wool / balloon for occlusion of AVM / obstruction by Swan-Ganz catheter, other foreign body
    5. Dirofilaria (dog heart worm): clumps of heart worms break off cardiac wall + embolize pulmonary arterial tree
  (b) Vasculitis
    1. Collagen vascular disease
    2. IV drug abuse
    3. Previous radiation therapy:
      √ defect localized to radiation port
    4. Tuberculosis
  (c) Vascular compression
    1. Bronchogenic carcinoma:
      √ perfusion defect depending on tumor size + location
    2. Lymphoma / lymph node enlargement
    3. Fibrosing mediastinitis
    4. Idiopathic pulmonary fibrosis:
      √ small subsegmental defects in both lungs
    5. Aortic aneurysm
  (d) Altered pulmonary circulation
    1. Absence / hypoplasia of pulmonary artery
    2. Peripheral pulmonary stenosis
    3. Bronchopulmonary sequestration
    4. Primary pulmonary hypertension
      √ upward redistribution + large hilar defects
      √ multiple small peripheral perfusion defects
    5. Pulmonary venoocclusive disease
    6. Mitral valve disease
      √ predilection for right middle lobe + superior segments of lower lobes
    7. Congestive heart failure
      √ diffuse nonsegmental VQ mismatch
      √ enlargement of cardiac silhouette + perihilar regions
      √ reversed distribution: more activity anteriorly than posteriorly
      √ accentuation of fissures

√ flattening of posterior margins of lung (lateral view)
√ pleural effusion

B. AIRWAY DISEASE
1. Asthma, chronic bronchitis, bronchospasm, mucous plugging
2. Bronchiectasis (bronchiolar destruction)
3. Emphysema (bulla / cyst)
4. Pneumonia / lung abscess
5. Lymphangitic carcinomatosis
√ perfusion defects in area of hypoxia (reflex vasoconstriction)
√ abnormal ventilation to a similar / more severe degree
√ mostly nonanatomic multiple defects (in 20%)

PULMONARY EMBOLIC DISEASE

Segmental defect = involves > 75% of a known bronchopulmonary segment
Subsegmental defect = involves 25 – 75% of a known bronchopulmonary segment

Perfusion images will detect:
(a) 90% of emboli which completely occlude a vessel > 1 mm in diameter
(b) 90% of surface perfusion defects that are larger than 2 x 2 cm

Therapeutic implications:
(a) high probability scan : treat for PE
(b) indeterminate scan : pulmonary angiogram
(c) low probability scan : consider other diagnosis, unless clinical suspicion very high

Indications for pulmonary angiography:
1. Embolectomy considered
2. Indeterminate V/Q scan with high clinical suspicion + risky anticoagulation therapy
3. Specific diagnosis necessary for proper management (vasculitis, drug induced, lung cancer with predominant vascular involvement)

Overall accuracy:
perfusion scan only (68%), ventilation-perfusion scan (84%)
False-positive scans: nonthrombotic emboli, IV drug abuser, vasculitis, redistribution of flow
False-negative scans: saddle embolus
√ associated with normal ventilation scan in > 90%
√ "stripe sign" = peripheral rim of activity indicates nonembolic cause

Perfusion	Ventilation	CXR	Interpretation	on Angio
Normal	normal	normal	normal	0%
< 2 segmental defects	normal	normal	low p	14%
Single defect < than CXR abnormality	matched defect	infiltrate	low p	7%
Single defect = to CXR abnormality	matched defect	infiltrate	low p	26%
Multiple nonanatomic defects	multiple areas of retention	normal / COPD	moderate p	34%
Single defect > than CXR abnormality	matched defect	infiltrate	indeterminate	89%
≥ 2 segmental defects	normal	normal	high p	93%

HEART SCINTIGRAPHY

Imaging choices:
1. PLANAR imaging
2. SPECT imaging
   improves object contrast by removing overlying tissues
3. QUANTITATIVE analysis
   = circumferential profiles = plotting of average counts along equally spaced radii emanating from center of LV makes interpretation more objective + reproducible

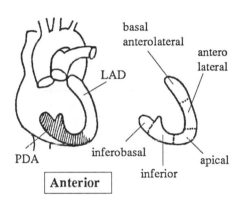

Anterior

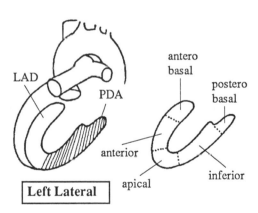

Left Lateral

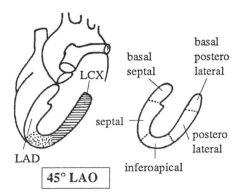

45° LAO

LAD supplies: upper 2/3 of interventricular septum
                  anterior wall
                  part of lateral wall
                  apex of left ventricle (in most patients)
LCX supplies: posterior portion of left ventricle
                  lateral portion of left ventricle
RCA supplies: lower 1/3 of interventricular septum
                  inferior wall of right + left ventricle

Left ventricular anatomy and projections

A. AP
   displays anterolateral wall, apex, inferior wall
   √ decreased activity at apex of LV due to thinning in 50%
B. LEFT LATERAL
   displays inferior wall, anterior wall
C. LAO 40° / LAO 70°
   Δ most often used projection; for all exercise studies displays interventricular septum, posterior wall, inferior wall
   √ best projection to separate right + left ventricles
   √ best projection to evaluate septal + posterior LV wall motion
D. RAO 45°
   displays anterior + inferior ventricular wall
   √ useful during 1st-pass studies with temporal separation of ventricles
E. LPO 45° (rarely used)
   10° caudal tilt minimizes LA contamination of LV region
   displays anterior + inferior ventricular wall
   √ preferred over RAO 45° because LV is closer to camera

Ejection fraction

Ejection fraction (EF) = stroke volume (SV) divided by end-diastolic volume (EDV)
   stroke volume = end-diastolic volume (EDV) minus end-systolic volume (ESV)

$$\mathbf{EF = [EDV - ESV] / [EDV]}$$
$$= [ED_{counts} - ES_{counts}] / [ED_{counts} - BKG_{counts}]$$

sensitive indicator of left ventricular function
Accuracy in detection of coronary artery disease:
   (a) Exercise EF: 87% sensitivity; 92% specificity
   (b) Exercise ECG: 60% sensitivity; 81% specificity
Interpretation:
   @ Left ventricle
      Mean normal value = 67 ± 8%
         (increase under stress normally > 5 – 7%)
      Probably abnormal ≤ 55%
      Definitely abnormal < 50%

@   Right ventricle
    mean normal value > 45%
        (RV ejection fraction is smaller than for LV
        because RV has greater EDV than LV but the
        same stroke volume)
    False-positive with   (a) inadequate exercise
                          (b) recent ingestion of meal
√ EF unchanged / decreased in coronary artery disease
√ new regional wall motion abnormality under exercise in
  coronary artery disease
√ correlates well with clinical severity of myocardial
  infarction

Intravascular agents
Tc-99m labeled RBCs
= agent of choice because of good heart-to-lung ratio
Technique:
    (1) IN VITRO-LABELING
         } 50 ml drawn blood incubated with Tc-99m
            reduced by stannous ion; RBCs washed and
            reinjected
         Δ expensive + time-consuming method
    (2) IN VIVO-LABELING
         } IV injection of stannous pyrophosphate (1 vial
            PYP diluted with 2 cc sterile saline = 15 mg
            sodium pyrophosphate containing 3.4 mg
            anhydrous stannous chloride)
         } 15 – 30 minutes later injection of Tc-99m
            pertechnetate (+7) which binds to "pretinned"
            RBCs (reduction to Tc-99m [+4])
         Δ least time-consuming + easiest method
         Δ worst labeling efficiency (30% not tagged to
            RBCs + excreted in urine)
    (3) IN VIVTRO-LABELING
         = MODIFIED IN VIVO-METHOD
         } 10 minutes after IV injection of 1 mg stannous
            pyrophosphate 10 ml of blood are drawn +
            incubated with Tc-99m pertechnetate for 10 –
            20 minutes with small amount of heparin added
            + reinjected (3-way stop-cock technique)
         Δ preferred method because of high labeling
            efficiency with little free pertechnetate
N.B.: poor tagging in (1) heparinized patient
                       (2) injection through IV line (adherence to wall)
                       (3) syringe flushed with dextrose instead of saline
Dose: 15 – 30 mCi
         Δ larger dose required for stress MUGA + obese
            patients
         Δ for children: 200 μCi / kg (minimum dose of
            2 – 3 mCi)
Radiation dose: 1.5 rad for heart, 1.0 rad for blood,
                    0.4 rad for whole body

Tc-99m HSA
HSA = human serum albumin
Indication: drug interference with RBC labeling (e.g.,
                heparinized patient)
Physiology: (1) albumin slowly equilibrates throughout
                     extracellular space

(2) poorer heart-to-lung ratio than with
     labeled RBCs

Thallium-201 chloride
= cation produced in cyclotron from Tl-203
Decay: by electron capture to Hg-201
Energy spectrum: 71 keV of Hg-K x-rays (98%
                     abundance); 135 keV (3%) +
                     167 keV (10%) gamma-rays
Physical half-life: 73 hours
Biological half-life: 10 ± 2.5 days
Dose: 1.5 – 3 mCi
Radiation dose:
    3 rad for kidneys (critical organ) (1.2 rad/mCi); 1.2 rad
    for gonads (0.6 rad/mCi); 0.7 rad for heart + marrow
    (0.34 rad/mCi); 0.5 rad for whole body (0.24 rad/mCi)
Quality control: should contain < 0.25% Pb-203,
                     < 0.5% Tl-202 (439 keV)

Indications:
    1. ACUTE MYOCARDIAL INFARCTION
    2. CORONARY ARTERY DISEASE
       particularly useful over ECG in:
       (a) conduction disturbances (e.g., bundle branch
           block, preexitation syndrome)
       (b) previous infarction
       (c) under drug influence (e.g., digitalis)
       (d) left ventricular hypertrophy
       (e) hyperventilation
       (f) ST-depression without symptoms
       (g) if stress ECG impossible to obtain
Sensitivity: overall 82 – 84% for stress Tl-201
                 (60 – 62% for exercise ECG)
    (a) increased with: (1) severity of stenosis (> 50%)
        (2) greater number of involved arteries
        (3) stenosis of left main > LAD > RCA > LXC
    (b) decreased with: (1) presence of collateral
        (2) beta blockers (3) time delay for poststress
        images
Specificity: overall 91 – 94% for stress Tl-201
                 (81 – 83% for exercise ECG)

IMAGING
    1. FIRST-PASS EXTRACTION = exercise image
       = Stress thallium image = map of regional perfusion
       obtained within minutes after injection to assess
       initial distribution dependent on perfusion; 300,000 –
       400,000 counts / view (approximately 10 minutes
       sampling time)
    2. REDISTRIBUTION IMAGE = delayed image
       = equilibrium between tracer uptake and efflux
       dependent on blood flow + mass of viable tissue +
       concentration gradients
       = map of viable cell mass obtained at rest after 2 – 6
       hours; washout half-life from myocardium is 54
       minutes

INTERPRETATION OF STRESS THALLIUM IMAGES

Immediate Image	Delayed Image	Diagnosis
normal	normal	normal
defect	fill-in	transient ischemia
defect	unchanged	myocardial scar
defect	partial fill-in	scar + ischemia / persistent ischemia

1. Initial phase = first-pass extraction
   - √ temporary defect accentuated by exercise
   - √ defect > 15% of ventricular surface suggests > 50% stenosis of coronary artery
2. Redistribution phase (on 2 – 4 hours-images)
   - √ wash out in normal areas + increased uptake in viable ischemic zones
   - √ permanent defect = myocardial infarction / fibrosis
   - √ increased lung activity (= > 50% of myocardial count) indicative of
     - (a) left ventricular failure due to severe LCA disease / myocardial infarction
     - (b) pulmonary venous hypertension due to cardiomyopathy / mitral valve disease
   - √ activity in right ventricle due to
     - (a) increase in ventricular systolic pressure
     - (b) increase in mean pulmonary artery pressure
     - (c) increase in total pulmonary vascular resistance

FALSE-POSITIVE THALLIUM TEST
   - A. Infiltrating myocardial disease:
     1. Sarcoidosis
     2. Amyloidosis
   - B. Cardiac dysfunction:
     1. Cardiomyopathy
     2. IHSS
     3. Valvular aortic stenosis
     4. Mitral valve prolapse (rare)
   - C. Decreased cardiac perfusion other than myocardial infarction:
     1. Cardiac contusion
     2. Myocardial fibrosis
     3. Coronary artery spasm (sever unstable angina may cause defect after stress + on redistribution images, but will be normal at rest!)
   - D. Normal variant:
     1. Apical myocardial thinning
     2. Attenuation due to diaphragm, breast, implant, pacemaker

FALSE-NEGATIVE THALLIUM TEST
   1. Under influence of beta-blocker (e.g., propranolol)
   2. "Balanced ischemia" = symmetric 3-vessel disease
   3. Insignificant obstruction
   4. Inadequate stress
   5. Failure to perform delayed imaging
   6. Poor technique

Thallium uptake & distribution
Intracellular uptake via Na/K-ATPase analogue to ionic potassium, but less readily released from cells than potassium; distribution is proportional to regional blood flow; uptake depends on quality of regional perfusion + integrity of sodium-potassium pump
- @ Blood pool
  - } < 5% remain in blood pool 15 minutes post injection
- @ Myocardium:
  - } uptake depends on (a) myocardial perfusion (b) myocardial mass (c) myocardial cellular integrity
  - } first-pass extraction efficiency is 88%
  - } 4% of total dose localizes in myocardium (myocardial blood flow = 4% of cardiac output)
  - } peak myocardial activity at 5 – 15 minutes after injection
  - } uptake can be increased by 1 – 2% through exercise / myocardial hypertrophy
  - } right heart faintly visualized during rest (15% of perfusion to right side); well seen during stress test, tachycardia, volume/pressure overload
- @ Skeletal muscle + Splanchnicus:
  - } first-pass extraction efficiency is 65%
  - } accumulate 40% of injected dose
  - } 4 – 6 hours fast + exercise decrease flow to splanchnicus and increase cardiac uptake
- @ Lung:
  - } 10% of total dose localizes in lung
  - } < 5% activity over lung is normal
  - } augmented pulmonary extraction with left ventricular dysfunction, bronchogenic carcinoma, lymphoma of lung
- @ Kidney:
  - } accumulates 4% of injected dose
  - } excretion of 4 – 8% within 24 hours
- @ Thyroid:
  - } increased uptake > 1% in Graves disease + thyroid carcinoma
- @ Brain:
  - } uptake only after disruption of blood-brain barrier

Stress test
Rationale:
   increased heart rate will unveil insufficient regional perfusion secondary to coronary artery disease
Technique:
   } exercise in erect position (peak heart rate lower if supine) on treadmill or bicycle; isometric handgrip exercise raises blood pressure less (but adequate for evaluation)

} starting point of workload selected according to preliminary exercise results (at an average of 200 kilowatt pounds)
} workload increments by 200 kilowatt pounds up to 85% of predicted maximum heart rate (= 220 - age) / exercise limited by symptoms of chest pain, dyspnea, fatigue, arrhythmia, ischemic ECG (cardiologist with crash cart should be available)
} Pharmacologic stress test = stress test substitute (in patients who cannot exercise): IV infusion of 0.14 mg/kg/min dipyridamole (vasodilator) for 4 minutes (effect reversible by administration of aminophylline)

End-points for discontinuing exercise:
a. Symptoms: chest pain, dyspnea, fatigue, leg cramps, dizziness
b. Signs: fall in BP > 10 mmHg below previous stage, ventricular tachycardia, run of 3 successive ventricular premature beats

Problems of exercise imaging:
(1) Sensitivity to detect ischemic lesions decreases with suboptimal exercise (in particular for older population)
(2) Higher false-positive tests in women (artifacts from overlying breast tissue)
(3) Propranolol (beta blocker) interferes with stress test

Applied to:
1. Thallium imaging (redistribution images after stress test):
   injection of 1.5 – 2 mCi of Tl-201 during peak exercise, continuation of exercise for additional 60 seconds before imaging commences
   Clues for stress images:
   √ RV myocardium well visualized
   √ little pulmonary background activity
   √ little activity in liver, stomach, spleen
   √ distribution more uniform after stress than during rest
   Degree of liver uptake useful as direct measure of level of exercise!
2. Gated blood pool imaging (response of EF)
   √ increase in ejection fraction from 63 – 93% in normals
   √ increase in ventricular wall motion (anterolateral > posterolateral > septal)

Ventricular function
First-pass method
= FIRST TRANSIT = recording of initial transit time of an intravenously administered Tc-99m bolus through heart + lungs; limited number of cardiac cycles available for interpretation; additional projections / serial studies require additional bolus injection
Accuracy: good correlation with contrast ventriculography

Agents: pertechnetate, pyrophosphate, albumin, DTPA, sulfur colloid (almost any Tc-99m labeled compound except lung scanning particles)
Indication:
(1) only 15 seconds of patient cooperation required
(2) calculation of cardiac output + ejection fraction (RBCs)
(3) subsequent first-pass studies within 15 – 20 minutes of initial study possible (DTPA)
(4) separate assessment of individual cardiac chambers in RAO projection (temporal separation without overlying atria, pulmonary artery, aortic outflow tract) e.g., for right ventricular EF
Gating:
improved images obtained by selection of time interval corresponding only to RV passage of bolus averaged over several (3 – 5) individual beats; gating may be done intrinsically or with ECG guidance
Imaging:
region of interest (ROI) over RV silhouette in RAO projection; background activity taken over horseshoe-shaped ventricular wall; counts in ROI displayed as function of time; 25 frames / second for 20 – 30 seconds
Evaluation:
1. Evidence of obstruction in SVC region
2. Evidence of reflux from RA in IVC region
3. Evidence of stenosis in pulmonary outflow tract
4. Evidence of R-L shunt
5. Contractility of RV
6. Sequential beating of RA and RV

Equilibrium images
= "blood pool" radionuclide angiography = imaging after thorough mixing of Tc-99m labeled radiopharmaceutical (HSA / RBCs) throughout vascular space
} acquisition of images during selected portions of cardiac cycle gated by R-wave; each image is composed of > 200,000 counts (2 – 10 minutes) obtained over several hundred cycles after equilibrium has been reached; high quality images can be obtained in different projections
} gated acquisition from 16 – 24 equal subdivisions of the R-R cycle allows display of synchronized cinematic images (assembled to composite single-image sequence) of entire cardiac cycle
√ may be displayed as time activity curves reflecting changes in ventricular counts throughout R-R interval
— measured functional indices: preejection period (PEP), left ventricular ejection time (LVET), left ventricular fast filling time ($LVFT_1$), left ventricular slow filling time ($LVFT_2$), PEP/LVET ratio, rate of ejection + filling of LV
} at rest: count density 200 – 250 counts / pixel requires generally 7 – 10 minutes acquisition time for 200,000 – 250,000 counts / frame

} during exercise: 100,000 – 150,000 counts / frame requires an acquisition time of 2 minutes

Evaluation of:
1. LV ejection fraction
2. regional wall motion
3. valvular regurgitation

Interpretation:
1. Heart failure: decreased EF, prolongation of PEP, shortening of LVET, decreased rate of ejection
2. Hypertensive heart: normal systolic indices, normal EF, prolonged LVT_1
3. Hypothyroidism: prolonged PEP, normal EF
4. Aortic stenosis: mild reduction of EF, prolonged LV emptying time, decreased rate of ejection, normal rate of filling

√ area of decreased periventricular uptake secondary to (a) pleural effusion > 100 ml (b) ventricular hypertrophy

Gated blood pool imaging
= MULTIPLE GATED ACQUISITION (MUGA)

Recording of:
(1) ejection fraction (EF) of left ventricle before + after exercise
(2) regional wall motion of ventricular chambers
   (a) at rest: myocardial infarction, aneurysm, contusion
   (b) during exercise: ischemic dyskinesia (detectable in 63%)

PROs: (1) higher information density than 1st-pass method
     (2) assessment of pharmacologic effect possible
     (3) "bad beat" rejection possible

CONs: (1) significant background activity
     (2) inability to monitor individual chambers in other than LAO 45° projection
     (3) plane of AV valve difficult to identify

Radiation dose: 1.5 rad for heart; 1.0 rad for blood; 0.4 rad for whole body

Imaging:
physiologic trigger provided by ECG ("bad beat" rejection program desirable)
(a) gated images obtained for 5 minutes
(b) for each stage of exercise 2 minutes image acquisition time

MYOCARDIAL INFARCT
Hot Spot Imaging
= INFARCT-AVID IMAGING

Agent: Tc-99m pyrophosphate, Hg-203 chlormerodrin, Tc-99m tetracycline, Tc-99m glucoheptonate, F-18 sodium fluoride

Pathophysiology in MYOCARDIAL INFARCTION: pyrophosphate uptake into myocardial necrosis through complexation with calcium deposits > 10 – 12 hours post infarction, requires presence of residual collateral blood flow; maximum accumulation in hypoxic cells under conditions of diminished blood flow by 30 – 40%

Uptake post infarction:
Earliest uptake by 12 – 24 hours;
Maximal uptake by 48 – 72 hours;
Persistent uptake seen up to 7 days with return to normal by 10 -14 days

Sensitivity:
90% for transmural infarction, 40 – 50% for subendocardial (nontransmural) infarction

Dose: 15 – 20 mCi IV (minimal count requirement of 500,000/view)

Imaging: at 3 – 6 hours (60% absorbed by skeleton within 3 hours)

Indications:
1. Lost enzyme pattern = patient admitted 24 – 48 hours after infarction
2. Equivocal ECG + atypical angina:
   (a) left ventricular bundle branch block
   (b) left ventricular hypertrophy
   (c) impossibility to perform stress test
   (d) patient on digitalis
3. ST-depression without symptoms
4. Equivocal enzyme pattern + equivocal symptoms
5. S/P cardiac surgery (perioperative infarction in 10 %, enzymes routinely elevated, ECG always abnormal), requires preoperative baseline study as 40% are preoperatively abnormal
6. for detection of right ventricular infarction

NOT HELPFUL:
1. in differentiating multiple- from single-vessel disease
2. typical angina
3. normal ECG stress test + NO symptoms

SCAN INTERPRETATION
Grade 2+ and above are positive
Grade 0   no activity
Grade 1+ faint uptake
Grade 2+ slightly less than sternum, equal to ribs
Grade 3+ equal to sternum
Grade 4+ greater than sternum

√ "doughnut" pattern = central cold defect (necrosis in large infarct) usually in cases of large anterior + anterolateral wall infarctions

√ uptake in inferior wall extending behind sternum (anterior projection) suggests RV infarction

FALSE-POSITIVES (10%)
A. Cardiac causes
1. Recent injury: myocardial contusion, resuscitation, cardioversion, radiation injury, adriamycin cardiotoxicity, myocarditis, acute pericarditis
2. Previous injury: left ventricular aneurysm, mural thrombus, unstable angina, previous infarction with persistent uptake
3. Calcified heart valves / coronaries (rare) / chronic pericarditis

4. Amyloidosis
B. Extracardiac causes:
   1. Soft tissue uptake: breast tumor / inflammation, chest wall injury, paddle burns from cardioversion, surgical drain, lung tumor
   2. Osseous: calcified costal cartilage (most common), lesions in rib / sternum
   3. Increased blood pool activity secondary to renal dysfunction / poor labeling technique (improvement on delayed images)

FALSE-NEGATIVES (5%)
Myocardial metastasis

PERSISTENTLY POSITIVE SCAN (> 2 weeks)
= ongoing myocardial necrosis indicating poor prognosis, may continue on to cardiac aneurysm, repeat infarction, cardiac death
Δ in 77% of persistent / unstable angina pectoris
Δ in 41% of compensated congestive heart failure
Δ in 51% of ECG evidence of ventricular dyssynergy
Prognosis: the larger the area the worse the mortality + morbidity

Cold spot imaging
= NONAVID IMAGING = myocardial perfusion study for acute myocardial infarction
Agent: Tl-201 (at rest)
Sensitivity   after onset of symptoms:
96% within 6-12 hours, 79% after 48 hours, 59% in remote infarction; sensitivity for SPECT (seven pinhole tomography) 94% > planar scintigraphy 75%
√ fixed permanent defect in acute infarction
√ fixed permanent defect at rest + on stress thallium + redistribution images in old infarction
√ "cold defect" at rest may represent transient ischemia in unstable angina
N.B.:   Tl-201 cannot distinguish between recent + remote infarction!

MYOCARDIAL ISCHEMIA
can be assessed (1) directly with stress Tl-201 imaging (2) indirectly with gated blood pool imaging (wall motion, ejection fraction)
LOCATION OF PERFUSION DEFECTS
(a) Right coronary artery (RCA)
     best seen on left LAT / AP projections
     √ inferior + posteroseptal segments
(b) Circumflex branch of left coronary artery (LCX)
     best seen on LAO projection
     √ posterolateral segment
(c) Anterior descending branch of left coronary artery (LAD)
     √ anteroseptal, anterior, anterolateral segments
N.B.: decreased activity in apical + posterior segments is not reliably correlated with disease of any vessel!

Intracardiac shunts
Agents administered by peripheral IV injection:
Tc-99m macroaggregated albumin, Tc-99m pertechnetate, DTPA, sulfur colloid, labeled RBCs
Method:
C2/C1-method = measures hemodynamic significance of a shunt; raw data obtained from pulmonary activity curve (gamma variate method, two area ratio method, count method); accuracy depends on the shape of the input bolus (single peak of < 2 seconds duration); measuring C1, C2, T1, T2
A. NORMAL
    C2/C1 is < 32%
B. L-R SHUNT
    Indication: ASD, VSD, AV canal, aortopulmonic window, rupture of sinus of Valsalva aneurysm
    √ C2/C1 > 35% (area A = primary pulmonary circulation; area B = L-R shunt; area (A-B) = systemic circulation; Qp / Qs = area A / area (A-B) = 0.91)
C. R-L SHUNT
    Indication: Tetralogy of Fallot, transposition, truncus, Ebstein anomaly
    √ early arrival of tracer in left side of heart + aorta (first-pass method) prior to arrival of activity from lungs to LV
    √ quantification possible only by registration of sum of activity of trapped macroaggregate / microspheres in brain + kidneys
Causes of abnormal non-shunt-related activity:
(1) Radiopharmaceutical breakdown
     √ free pertechnetate activity in salivary glands, gastric mucosa, thyroid, kidney
(2) Hepatic cirrhosis
     abnormal pulmonary vascular channels bypassing the lung (in 10 – 70%)
(3) Pulmonary AVM

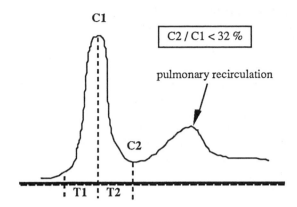

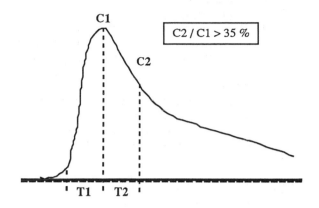

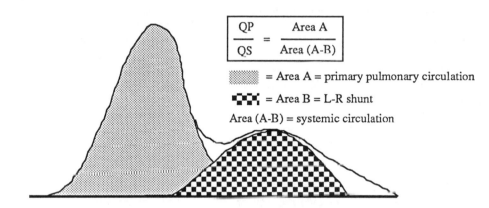

LIVER AND GASTROINTESTINAL TRACT SCINTIGRAPHY

Tc-99m IDA analogs

= Tc-99m acetanilide iminodiacetic acid analogs
= dependent on the substance's lipophility, there is a
  trade-off between renal excretion + hepatic uptake
  (BIDA is the most lipophilic, HIDA the least lipophilic)
1. HIDA (2,6-dimethyl derivative): [H= Hepatic] bilirubin
   threshold of < 18 mg/dl; 15% renal excretion
2. BIDA (parabutyl derivative): bilirubin threshold of < 20
   mg/dl
3. PIPIDA (paraisopropyl derivative): 2% renal excretion
4. DIDA (diethyl derivative)
5. DISIDA (diisopropyl derivative): bilirubin threshold of <
   30 mg/dl
Quality control: the final compound should contain
   —   90 – 100% Tc-99m IDA
   —   < 10% Tc-99m tin colloid
   —   < 10% Tc-99m sodium pertechnetate
Pharmacokinetics:
   peak liver activity 5 – 10 minutes post injection = hepatic
   phase; 85% extracted by hepatocytes; secretion by
   hepatocytes without conjugation; CBD + cystic duct
   visualized within 15 minutes (not always visualized in
   normals); GB visualized by 20 minutes; excretion into
   duodenum by 30 minutes; bowel visualized within 1
   hour; renal excretion seen in most normals; no
   enterohepatic recirculation
Preparation: fasting for 2 – 4 hours
Dose: 5 – 7 mCi
Radiation dose: 2 rad for upper large bowel; 0.55 rad for
   gallbladder; 3 rad/mCi for small bowel; 0.01 rad/mCi for
   whole body
Imaging: at 5 – 10 minutes intervals for 30 minutes; at
   45, 60 minutes; if gallbladder not visualized at
   least up to 4 hours

Technetium-99m sulfur colloid

Indications: liver, spleen, bone marrow, acute rejection in
   renal transplant, lower GI bleeding, gastric
   emptying
Preparation:
   Tc-99m pertechnetate and sodium trisulphate are
   heated in a waterbath (95 ± 5°C) for 10 ± 2 minutes;
   sulfur atoms aggregate to form a "colloid" (average
   particle size 0.1 – 1 µ with a range of 0.001 – 1 µ; true
   colloid has a particle size of 0.001 – 0.5 µ); gelatin is
   added to prevent further growth of particles
Quality control:
   (a)   > 92% remain at origin of ascending
          chromatography
   (b)   upper limit for particle size is 1 µ
   Δ usual cause for poor preparation are excessive /
      prolonged heating or a pH > 7
   Δ preparation should not be used > 6 hours
      (agglomeration of particles with aging)
Dose: usually 3 – 6 mCi

Imaging: 15 – 30 minutes post IV injection
Radiation dose: 0.3 rad/mCi for liver (critical organ);
                     0.02 rad/mCi for whole body;
                     0.025 rad/mCi for bone marrow
Pharmacokinetics:
   accumulation in liver (85%), spleen (10%), bone
   marrow (5%); lung localization is rare (presumably
   secondary to circulating endotoxins + macrophage
   infiltration)
A.   RETICULOENDOTHELIAL LOCALIZATION
      √ colloid shift away from liver in diffuse hepatic
        dysfunction / decreased hepatic perfusion
      √ increased bone marrow activity in hemolytic anemia
      √ increased splenic activity in hypersplenism of
        splenomegaly / cancer / systemic illness
B.   BONE MARROW LOCALIZATION
      hematopoietic system extends into long bones in
      children; recedes to axial skeleton, femora, and
      humeri with age
      Δ bone marrow distribution cannot be used to
        determine sites of erythropoiesis
C.   ABSCESS LOCALIZATION
      sulfur colloid phagocytized by PMNs + monocytes
      Labeling:
      (a)   in vivo: small labeling yield
      (b)   in vitro: 40% labeling efficiency, but difficult +
             time-consuming preparation

Colloid shift

A.   Hepatic dysfunction
      1.   Cirrhosis
      2.   Hepatitis
      3.   Chronic passive congestion
B.   Augmented perfusion of spleen + bone marrow
      1.   Hematopoietic disorders
      2.   Long-term corticosteroid therapy

Focal hot liver lesion

1.   IVC / SVC obstruction
      √   increased perfusion of quadrate lobe (collateral
           pathway via umbilical vein)
2.   Budd-Chiari syndrome
      √   "increased" perfusion of caudate lobe (actually
           decrease of activity elsewhere in liver)
3.   FNH
4.   Regenerating nodules of cirrhosis

Defects in porta hepatis

1.   Normal variant (thinning of hepatic tissue overlying
      portal veins + gallbladder)
2.   Biliary causes: dilatation of bile ducts, gallbladder
      hydrops
3.   Enlarged portal lymph nodes
4.   Metastases
5.   Hepatic cyst

6. Hepatic parenchymal disease (pseudotumor)
7. Hepatic compression by adjacent extrinsic mass
8. Postsurgical changes following cholecystectomy

Focal liver defects
A. Neoplastic
  (a) Primary liver tumor: hepatoma, hemangioma, hepatic adenoma, FNH
  (b) Metastases: 85% sensitivity, 75 – 80% specificity (for lesion > 1 - 2 cm)
B. Infectious disease / abscess
C. Benign cyst
D. Trauma
E. Pseudotumor = normal variant

Mottled hepatic uptake
1. Cirrhosis
2. Acute hepatitis
3. Lymphoma
4. Amyloidosis
5. Granulomatous disease (sarcoid, fungal, viral, parasitic)
6. Chemo- / radiation therapy

Splenic scintigraphy
1. Tc-99m sulfur colloid: 3 – 5 mCi
2. Tc-99m heat denatured erythrocytes
  Indication:
    (1) Splenic trauma (2) Accessory + ectopic spleen
  Technique:
    20 – 30 minutes after injection of pyrophosphate IV 15 – 20 ml of blood are drawn + incubated with 2 mCi of pertechnetate; blood is heated to 49.5°C for 35 minutes and reinjected
    N.B.: fragmentation of RBCs from overheating increases hepatic uptake
  Imaging: 20 minutes post injection

Radionuclide esophogram
Preparation: 4 – 12 hours fasting; imaging in supine / erect position
Dose: 250 – 500 µCi Tc-99m sulfur colloid in 10 ml of water taken through straw
Imaging: when swallowing begins
√ normal transit time: 15 seconds with 3 distinct sequential peaks progressing aborally
√ prolonged transit time: achalasia, progressive systemic sclerosis, diffuse esophageal spasm, nonspecific motor disorders, "nutcracker" esophagus, Zenker diverticulum, esophageal stricture + obstruction
Difficult interpretation in: hiatal hernia, GE reflux, Nissen fundoplication

GASTROESOPHAGEAL REFLUX
89% correlation with acid reflux test
Preparation: 4 hours / overnight fasting; abdominal sphygmomanometer

Dose: 0.5 – 1.0 mCi Tc-99m sulfur colloid in 300 ml of acidified orange juice (150 ml juice + 150 ml 0.1 N hydrochloric acid) followed by "cold" acidified orange juice
Imaging: at 30 – 60 seconds intervals for 30 – 60 minutes, images taken in supine position from anterior; sphygmomanometer inflated at 20, 40, 60, 80, 100 mmHg
Interpretation: Reflux (in %) = ([esophageal counts - background] / gastric counts) x 100
√ up to 3% reflux is normal
√ evidence of pulmonary aspiration (valuable in pediatric age group)

GASTRIC EMPTYING
Dose: 1 – 2 mCi
  (a) Tc-99m sulfur colloid cooked with egg white as solid food
  (b) In-111 DTPA for simultaneous measurement of liquid phase
Imaging: one-minute anterior abdominal images obtained at 0, 10, 30, 60, 90 minutes in erect position
Pharmakokinetics:
  Tracer activity in stomach for solid phase of 79% at 10 minutes; 65% at 30 minutes; 33% at 60 minutes; 10% at 90 minutes; 50% of activity in stomach at time zero should empty by 60 ± 30 minutes
√ acutely delayed emptying in stress (pain, cold), drugs (morphine, anticholinergics, levo-dopa, nicotine, beta adrenergic antagonists), postoperative ileus, acute viral gastroenteritis, hyperglycemia, hypokalemia
√ chronically delayed gastric emptying in gastric outlet obstruction, postvagotomy, gastric ulcer, chronic idiopathic intestinal pseudoobstruction, GE reflux, progressive systemic sclerosis, dermatomyositis, spinal cord injury, myotonia dystrophica, familial dysautonomia, anorexia nervosa, hypothyroidism, diabetes mellitus, amyloidosis, uremia
√ abnormally rapid gastric emptying in gastric surgery, ZE syndrome, duodenal ulcer disease, malabsorption (pancreatic exocrine insufficiency / celiac sprue)

GASTROINTESTINAL BLEEDING
Detection depends on:
  (1) rate of hemorrhage (≥ 0.05 ml/minute); NUC more sensitive than angiogram
  (2) continuous versus intermittent bleeding
  (3) site of hemorrhage
  (4) characteristics of radionuclide agent
Angiography requires a bleeding rate of approximately 0.5 ml/min

1. Tc-99m sulfur colloid
  Indications: Bleeding must be active at time of tracer administration
  Δ disappearance half-life of 3 – 8 minutes (rapidly cleared from blood by RES + low background activity)

Δ active bleeding sites detected with rates as low as 0.05 – 0.1 ml/min

Δ not useful for upper GI-bleeding (interference from high activity in liver + spleen) or bleeding near hepatic / splenic flexure

Dose: 10 mCi

Imaging: (a) every 5 seconds for 1 minute (b) 60 seconds images at 2,5,10, 15, 20, 30, 40, 60 minutes (c) images at 2, 4, 6, 12 hours; (study terminated if no abnormality up to 30 minutes)

√ activity below pubic symphysis in males may be normal (e.g., spongiosa)

√ transplanted kidneys may take up colloid

2. Tc-99m labeled RBCs (in vitro labeling)

Indications: intermittent bleeding (0.35 ml/minute)

Δ remains in vascular system for prolonged period

Δ liver + spleen activity are low allowing detection of upper GI tract hemorrhage

Δ low target-to-background ratio (high activity in great vessels, liver, spleen, kidneys, stomach, colon probably related to free pertechnetate fraction)

Dose: 10 – 20 mCi

Imaging: (a) every 2 seconds for 64 seconds (b) static images for 500,000 counts at 2, 5 and every consecutive 5 minutes up to 1 hour (c) delayed images at 2, 4, 6, 12 hours up to 36 hours; localization of bleeding site may be difficult secondary to rapid transit time or too widely spaced time intervals

√ increase in tracer accumulation over time in abnormal location

√ bleeding site conforms to bowel anatomy

√ change in appearance with time consistent with bowel peristalsis

Sensitivity: in 83 – 91% correctly identified bleeding site (50% within 1st hour, may become positive in 33% only after 12 – 24 hours); superior to sulfur colloid

RENAL AND ADRENAL SCINTIGRAPHY

Renal agents

A. Agents for renal function: Tc-99m DTPA,
                                       I-131 hippuran
B. Renal cortical agents: Tc-99m DMSA
C. Renal combination agent: Tc-99m glucoheptonate

Tc-99m DTPA

= Tc-99m diethylenetriamine penta-acetic acid
= agent of choice for assessment of (1) perfusion (2) glomerular filtration = relative GFR (3) obstructive uropathy (4) vesicoureteral reflux

Pharmacokinetics:
    chelating agent; 5 – 10% bound to plasma protein; extracted with 20% efficiency on each pass through kidney (= filtration fraction); excreted exclusively by glomerular filtration (similar to inulin) without reabsorption / tubular excretion / metabolism

Time-activity behavior:
— abdominal aorta (15 – 20 seconds)
— kidneys + spleen (17 – 24 seconds); liver appears later because of portal venous supply
— renal cortical activity (2 – 4 minutes): mean transit time of 3.0 ± 0.5 minutes; static images of cortex taken at 3 – 5 minutes
— renal pelvic activity (3 – 5 minutes): peak at 10 minutes; asymmetric clearance of renal pelvis in 50%; accelerated by furosemide

Biologic half-life: 20 minutes
Dose: 10 – 20 mCi
Radiation dose: 0.85 rads/mCi for renal cortex; 0.6 rads/mCi for kidney; 0.5 rads/mCi for bladder; 0.15 rads/mCi for gonads; 0.15 rads/mCi for whole body

Tc-99m glucoheptonate

= good all-purpose agent suitable for functional + anatomic studies

Pharmacophysiology:
    rapid plasma clearance + urinary excretion with excellent definition of pelvocalyceal system during 1st hour; extracted by (a) glomerular filtration and (b) tubular excretion (30 – 45% within 1st hour); 5 – 15% of dose accumulate in tubular cells by 1 hour.; cortical accumulation remains for 24 hours

Imaging:
(a) collecting system within first 30 minutes
(b) renal parenchyma after 1 – 2 hours (interference of activity in collecting system)

Biologic half-life: 2 hours
Dose: 15 (range 10 – 20) mCi
Radiation dose: 0.17 rads/mCi for kidney; 0.008 rads/mCi for whole body; 0.015 rads/mCi for gonads

Tc-99m DMSA

= Tc-99m dimercaptosuccinic acid
= suitable for imaging of functioning cortical mass: pseudotumor versus lesion

Pharmacokinetics:
    high protein-binding + slow plasma clearance; 4% extracted per renal passage; 4 – 8% glomerular filtration within 1 hour and 30% by 14 hours; 50% of dose accumulate in proximal + distal renal tubular cells by 1 hour (= cortical agent)

Imaging: after 1 – 24 hours (optimal at 34 hours)
Biologic half-life: > 30 hours
Dose: 5 – 10 mCi
Radiation dose: 0.014 rads/mCi for gonads; 0.015 rads/mCi for whole body

I-131 OIH

= I-131 orthoiodohippurate (Hippuran®)
= good for evaluation of renal tubular function / effective renal plasma flow; agent with highest extraction ratio without binding to renal parenchyma; visualizes kidney even in severe renal failure

Pharmacokinetics:
    80% secreted by proximal tubules; 20% filtered by glomeruli; maximal renal concentration within 5 minutes; normal transit time of 2 – 3 minutes; approximately 2% free iodine (Lugol's solution administered to protect thyroid)

Imaging:
    in 15 – 60 seconds intervals for 20 minutes; renal uptake determined from images obtained by 1 – 2 minutes (patient in supine position for equidistance of kidneys to camera)

Biologic half-life: 10 minutes (with normal renal function)
Dose: 200 (range 150 – 300) µCi
Radiation dose: 0.06 rads/200 µCi for bladder; 0.02 rads/200 µCi for kidney; 0.02 rads/200 µCi for whole body; 0.02 rads/200 µCi for gonads

Differential renal function

Agents:
(1) <u>Tc-99m DTPA</u>:
    measurements prior to excretion within first 1 – 3 minutes; images taken at 1.5 seconds intervals for 30 seconds followed by serial images for next 30 minutes
(2) <u>I-131 hippuran</u>:
    measurements prior to excretion within first 1 – 2 minutes

Evaluation: generation of time-activity curves
√ increased hepatic + soft tissue uptake with impaired renal function

√ measurements usually not significantly affected with differences in renal depth

√ measurements are accurate in renal obstruction if obtained within 1 – 3 minutes

√ prediction about functional recovery not possible following surgical relief of obstruction

I-131 meta-iodobenzylguanidine (MIBG)

Indications:

(1) Pheochromocytoma (80 – 90% sensitivity, > 90% specificity); tumors as small as 0.2 g have been detected

(2) Neuroblastoma, carcinoid, medullary thyroid carcinoma, nonfunctioning retroperitoneal neuroendocrine tumor, middle mediastinal paraganglioma, adrenal metastasis of choriocarcinoma

Pharmakokinetics:

localizes in storage granules of adrenergic tissue; normal activity is seen in liver, spleen, bladder, salivary glands, myocardium, lungs

Method:

Lugol solution administered orally once a day for 4 days (to block thyroid uptake of free iodine)

Dose: 0.5 mCi / 1.73 square meters of body surface MIBG (maximum of 0.5 mCi)

Imaging: 1, 2, 3 days after injection

Radiation dose: 18 rad for adrenal medulla, 0.5 rad for ovaries, 0.2 rad for liver, 0.11 rad for whole body

False-negative scan:

uptake blocked by reserpine, imipramine, other tricyclic depressants, amphetamine-like drugs

THYROID AND PARATHYROID SCINTIGRAPHY

SUPPRESSION SCAN
= to define autonomy of a nodule
√ suppression of a hot nodule following T3/T4
administration is proof that autonomy does not exist
STIMULATION SCAN
= to demonstrate thyroid tissue suppressed by
hyperfunctioning nodule
√ administration of TSH documents functioning thyroid
tissue (rarely done)
PERCHLORATE WASHOUT TEST
= to demonstrate organification defect
√ repeat measurement of radioiodine uptake following
oral potassium perchlorate shows lower values if
organification defect present

Tc-99m pertechnetate
Physical half-life: 6 hours
Decay: by photon emission of 140 keV
Dose: 10 mCi administered IV 20 minutes prior to
imaging (100 – 300 mrad/mCi)
Uptake:
0.5 – 3.7% at 20 minutes (time of maximum uptake)
assessment of trapping function only; NO organification;
may be almost completely discharged by perchlorate
Comparison to iodine:
(a) target-to-background ratio less favorable than with
iodine
(b) greater photon flux than iodine = detectability of
small thyroid lesions (> 8 mm) is improved
(c) lesion with increased uptake without suppression of
remainder of gland require additional iodine study
to exclude Tc-99m avid cancer
IMAGING
(a) Collimator: usually with pinhole collimator for image
magnification (5 mm hole)
(b) Distance: selected so that organ makes up 2/3 of
field of view, significant distortion of organ periphery
occurs if detector too close
(c) Counts: 200,000 – 300,000 counts are usually
acquired within 5 min. after a dose of 5 – 10 mCi of
Tc-99m pertechnetate
(d) Image must include markers for scale + anatomic
landmarks + palpatory findings

Iodine-123
agent of choice for thyroid imaging
Production:
in accelerator; contamination with I-124 dependent on
source (Te-122 in ~ 5%, Xe-123 in ~ 0.5%);
contamination with I-125 increases with time elapsed
after production
Physical half-life: 13.3 hours
Decay: by electron capture with photon emission at 159
keV (83% abundance) + X-ray of 28 keV (87%
abundance)

Dose: 200 – 400 µCi orally 24 hours prior to imaging
(radiation dose of 7.5 mrads/µCi)
Uptake: iodine readily absorbed from GI-tract (10 – 30%
by 24 hours), distributed primarily in extracellular
fluid spaces; trapped + organified by thyroid
gland; trapped by stomach + salivary glands
Excretion: via kidneys in 35 – 75% during first 24 hours
+ GI tract

Iodine-131
Indication: thyroid uptake study, thyroid imaging,
treatment of hyperthyroidism, treatment of functioning
thyroid cancer, imaging of functioning metastases
Production: by fission decay
Physical half-life: 8.05 days (allows storing for long
periods)
Decay: principal gamma energy of 364 keV (82%
abundance) + significant beta decay fraction of a mean
energy of 192 keV (92% abundance)
Dose: 30 – 50 µCi (1.2 rad/µCi = 50 rad for thyroid)
Radiation dose:
(90% from beta decay, 10% from gamma radiation)
0.6 mrad/mCi for whole body; 1.2 mrad/µCi for thyroid
(critical organ)
Kinetics: identical to I-123
Disadvantages:
(a) too energetic for gamma camera, well suited for
rectilinear scanner with limited resolution
(b) high radiation dose prohibits use for diagnostic
purposes
(c) ectopic thyroid tissue just as well detectable with
I-123

Iodine fluorescence imaging
Technique:
collimated beam of 60 keV gamma photons from an
Am-241 source is directed at thyroid, which results in
production of K-characteristic x-rays of 28.5 keV;
x-rays are detected by semiconductor detector
Advantages:
(a) no interference with flooded iodine pool / thyroid
medication
(b) measures total iodine content
(c) low radiation exposure (15 mrad) acceptable for
children + pregnant women
Disadvantage: dedicated equipment necessary

Parathyroid scintigraphy
Technetium-Thallium subtraction imaging
Sensitivity: 72 – 92% (depending on size, smallest
adenoma was 60 mg)
Specificity: 43% (benign thyroid adenomas,
carcinomas, lymph nodes also concentrate
thallium)

Method:

(1) IV injection of 2 – 3 mCi Tl-201 chloride; images recorded for 15 minutes with 2-mm pinhole collimator
   √ concentrates in normal thyroid + enlarged - parathyroid glands

(2) IV injection of 5 – 10 mCi Tc-99m pertechnetate; images recorded at 1 minute intervals for 20 minutes
   √ pertechnetate concentrates only in thyroid

(3) Computerized subtraction

INDEX

T